THE OXFORD HANDBOOK OF

NEUROETHICS

THE OXFORD HANDBOOK OF

NEUROETHICS

Edited by

JUDY ILLES

and

BARBARA J. SAHAKIAN

Assistant Editors

CAROLE A. FEDERICO

and

SHARON MOREIN-ZAMIR

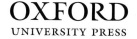

OXFORD

UNIVERSITY PRESS

OXFORD

UNIVERSITY PRESS

Great Clarendon Street, Oxford OX2 6DP

Oxford University Press is a department of the University of Oxford.
It furthers the University's objective of excellence in research, scholarship,
and education by publishing worldwide in

Oxford New York

Auckland Cape Town Dar es Salaam Hong Kong Karachi
Kuala Lumpur Madrid Melbourne Mexico City Nairobi
New Delhi Shanghai Taipei Toronto

With offices in

Argentina Austria Brazil Chile Czech Republic France Greece
Guatemala Hungary Italy Japan Poland Portugal Singapore
South Korea Switzerland Thailand Turkey Ukraine Vietnam

Oxford is a registered trade mark of Oxford University Press
in the UK and in certain other countries

Published in the United States
by Oxford University Press Inc., New York

British Library Cataloguing in Publication Data
Data available

Library of Congress Cataloguing in Publication Data
Library of Congress Control Number: 2011922176

Typeset by Glyph International Bangalore, India
Printed in Great Britain
on acid-free paper by
CPI Antony Rowe, Chippenham, Wiltshire

ISBN 978-0-19-957070-6

1 3 5 7 9 10 8 6 4 2

Whilst every effort has been made to ensure that the contents of this book are as complete,
accurate and up-to-date as possible at the date of writing, Oxford University Press is not
able to give any guarantee or assurance that such is the case. Readers are urged to take
appropriately qualified medical advice in all cases. The information in this book is
intended to be useful to the general reader, but should not be used as a means of
self-diagnosis or for the prescription of medication.

Foreword

Bridging neuroscience and society: research, education, and broad public engagement

Alan I. Leshner

Introduction

Advances in neuroscience are reported widely in the public media, reflecting both the great pace of neuroscientific progress and the extensive interest people have in their own brains, particularly in their minds, and how well they are functioning. This should not be interpreted to imply that there is a deep public understanding of the details of brain or mental functioning, but it does reflect widespread recognition and excitement that scientists are learning more and more as the decades pass about the brain and mind. That high level of public interest in our science is, of course, generally a very good thing.

However, as the public increasingly grasps what science is revealing about the nature of the brain and mental function, some individuals will become less sanguine about what science is revealing. Moreover, the potential use and misuse of various neurotechnologies will likely raise concerns among members of the public. Much of this book is about the current and emerging issues in neuroscience that now or in the future will need attention.

A broad societal context

Since neuroscience is part of the broad science and technology enterprise, some initial comments about the overall science–society relationship are relevant as context for understanding what could happen with neuroscience and its rapport with the broader public. Science and technology are embedded in every aspect of modern life, whether at work, at home, at play, or elsewhere in people's lives. An obvious consequence is that in order to thrive in the modern world, people need a fundamental understanding and comfort with science and technology. That does not mean that all people need to understand the details of most scientific discoveries and issues, but they do need to understand the nature of science, its power and limits, and they need to be able to discriminate science from pseudo-science.

Moreover, every major problem or issue that modern society faces has a science and technology component—either as a cause or a cure. Obvious examples include balancing energy needs with a sustainable environment, the equitable distribution of such resources as water and fertile land, controlling the spread of infectious diseases and ensuring adequate health, and sustaining a viable economy in the world of the future. To deal with those kinds of problems on either a global or a national scale requires that modern countries have at least some significant science and technology capacity, which in turn requires broad public recognition, understanding, and support. These intersecting forces require that the relationship between science and the rest of society be mutually beneficial and strong.

In contrast, the last few decades have been rather Dickensian for science and its relationship with the rest of society—the best of times and the worst of times. On the positive side, scientific advances continue at a very rapid pace. The case of neuroscience is particularly striking; examples can be found throughout this book. For nearly 40 years scientists have been able to credibly maintain that we have learned more about the brain in the past decade than in all of recorded history. Some of these advances have been incremental in character, building systematically on past knowledge, whereas others have appeared more transformative. Many of the most transformative advances have been fueled by the availability of new technologies, like molecular genetics, information and communication technologies, and neuroimaging. The advent of these new technologies has enabled us to ask wholly new questions that could not have been approached before.

We also are seeing great progress in the diagnosis, prevention, and treatment of nervous system disorders, as basic, translational, and clinical neuroscience increasingly inform each other. And neuroscience advances have had significant public and policy implications, as we revise our conceptualization of such illnesses as mental and substance abuse disorders, recognizing their biological origins in brain dysfunction. For example, the policy implications of the recognition that addiction is fundamentally a health issue, a brain disease, are far-reaching.

That is the good news. In contrast, although the last decades have been among the scientifically most productive, they also have been among the rockiest in modern times for the overall science–society relationship. Although it is true that every attitude survey continues to show that, overall, the public has great respect for science and scientists, and that most people believe the benefits of science have outweighed its risks or harms, many people find particular scientific advances disquieting or even dangerous. This is discussed later in this Foreword.

One more set of contextual comments seem relevant. On the one hand, the purpose of science is to tell us about the nature of the natural world, whether we like the answer or not. On the other hand, only scientists are obliged to accept scientific explanations, again whether they like them or not. The rest of the public is free to disregard or, worse, to distort scientific findings at will, and with rather limited immediate consequences. Scientific understanding is only binding on scientists.

SOURCES OF SCIENCE–SOCIETY TENSION

The recent high levels of science–society disharmony come from two types of conflicts. One obvious issue is that some scientific discoveries are simply politically or economically inconvenient. The most obvious recent example has been global climate change and what to do about balancing energy and environmental needs and concerns. The highly expert Intergovernmental Panel on Climate Change (IPCC) has made quite clear that the earth is warming, and that the warming is heavily anthropogenic in origin and related to energy use (Intergovernmental Panel on Climate Change 2007). However, it is both expensive and politically contentious to impose energy use controls on individuals and industries. Therefore, some governments have decided to either ignore or distort the findings, and thus avoid dealing with the contentious issues in productive ways. Importantly, there are no rules that say governments are obliged either to acknowledge or act on scientific evidence and opinion.

But as implied earlier, there is another category of science–society tension that is at least as far-reaching as political or economic issues. Many scientific advances seem to be encroaching upon or abutting against issues of core human values or religious beliefs, and when that happens, values frequently trump science. As a matter of fact, 56% of Americans agree that "scientific research these days doesn't pay enough attention to the moral values of society" (National Science Board 2008).

One example is embryonic stem cell research. The issue here is not whether people understand it in a general way, or even whether they believe this line of research likely will lead to improved diagnosis and treatment of major diseases. They do (Research!America 2009). The problem relates to when one believes life begins, and that, of course, is not a scientific question. Science cannot tell us when life begins; it is a matter of belief. And if one's religion says that life begins at the moment of fertilization, destroying early-stage embryos for research purposes is unacceptable. If, on the other hand, one believes life begins later in gestation, embryonic stem cell research is not a problem.

The teaching of evolution in public schools is another example. Modern understanding of how humans came to be conflicts directly with a literal interpretation of the biblical account of creation. As a result, many Americans do not want their children taught evolution in schools; it conflicts with their religious beliefs. The fact that there have been tens of thousands of scientific studies, from many converging disciplines, that all lead to acceptance of evolution as a core scientific organizing principle is not relevant. For many people, religious beliefs trump science.

One more tension point seems to be emerging: the field of synthetic biology. The fact that scientists may be able to create or recreate aspects of life in the laboratory is beginning to cause some science-society disquiet which is likely to escalate in the future.

NEUROSCIENCE–SOCIETY TENSION POINTS

Many major examples of potential pressure points for neuroscience–society tension are covered in this book. In the aggregate there are many issues leading to the conclusion that this problem merits significant attention. Some pressure points relate to new or emerging neurotechnologies, like pharmacological enhancement of cognitive abilities or lie detection using neuroimaging (Greely *et al.* 2008). The possibility of using neurotechnologies for defense purposes is another (Moreno 2007). Ambivalence surrounding dual-use research is not unique to neuroscience, but the possibility of manipulating minds for potentially nefarious ends seems a particularly likely point of contention.

The use of biomarkers to predict human behavior or mental disorders raises another set of issues where science and human values have clashed (Singh and Rose 2009). All types of concerns, including those related to personal identity, labeling, discrimination, and privacy likely will surround progress in biomarker research.

Another class of issues surrounds the implication of neuroscience advances for how people view their own humanity. Churchland has written eloquently about the implications of neuroscience findings for concepts of free will and personal responsibility (Churchland 2008). If the mind is conceptualized as simply the product of biological events occurring in the brain, what does that say about free will, a core concept of many religions? Moreover, where is one's "soul"? Does the concept lose power if mental activity is reducible to biological events in the brain? Of course, there is no a priori reason one cannot have an integrated mind and brain and still have free will or even a soul; it just means they are contained within the brain. We have not made nearly enough progress in understanding how mental activity emerges from brain structure and function to be able to inform these kinds of questions in a meaningful way.

THE DISORDERED MIND: MENTAL ILLNESS AND ADDICTION

We now get to issues surrounding mental and addictive disorders, and concepts such as personal or even legal responsibility. It is now widely accepted in both the basic and clinical scientific communities that mental disorders like schizophrenia, bipolar disorder, and depression are brain diseases—they come about because of brain dysfunction. Terms like "schizophrenogenic mothers" or "refrigerator parents" are almost never heard anymore. Moreover, the fact that mental disorders are brain diseases is slowly entering public consciousness and will, hopefully, lead both to reduced stigma and an increase in the number of people receiving effective treatment.

But recognizing mental illnesses as brain diseases also raises some difficult questions. For example, if a person commits a crime because their brain is disordered, what does that say about personal responsibility? Do we punish a brain-disordered individual who commits a crime in the same way we might deal with a so-called normal person? Is the person really responsible for the behavior? If not, how should society weigh that fact as an element in criminal justice decisions and policies? These issues are discussed in this book and represent special cases where advances in clinical neurobiology are presenting difficult problems for society.

The fact that addiction is a brain disease is even more complicated. Drug use does begin as a voluntary behavior, for which an individual is wholly responsible, but then that voluntary drug use is converted into addiction (compulsive and often uncontrollable drug craving, seeking, and use) as a result of the effects of prolonged drug exposure on the brain (Leshner 1997). So what level of responsibility do people with addictions have for the antisocial and criminal behaviors that often accompany being addicted? This is a question of significant complexity for society.

Anticipating neuroscience–society tension

How should the scientific community prepare for the likelihood that neuroscience advances will result in increasing tension with the rest of society? This is not as simple a question as it may appear. First, there is the issue of whether the community should become active at all. By and large we do not have a problem now. Would raising these issues in the public's consciousness precipitate problems? Or are they coming anyway, and, therefore, we should try to get ahead of them to help set the stage in as positive a way as possible?

We certainly do not want to cause problems, but there is some evidence that problems are on their way. For example, in 2008 the Discovery Institute—the group at the forefront of the Intelligent Design, anti-evolution movement—posted a blog article condemning "mental materialism" as antithetical to religious belief (Egnor 2008).

In addition, when other fields have acted preemptively to diffuse potential science-society tension, it has been quite successful. The best example is the preparatory work done by the genetics community in anticipation of the Human Genome Project (HGP). The HGP could have been quite threatening to the public with the specter of knowing all of a person's genetic secrets. The National Institutes of Health's Ethical, Legal and Social Implications (ELSI) Research Program has also done much to diffuse potential problems.

I have argued elsewhere (Leshner 2005) and reiterate here that it is time to "go public" with neuroscience and neuroethics issues. It would be better to anticipate the issues rather than only react defensively once they arise. However, this would need to be done in a strategic and measured way.

Approaching the public in a proactive way should only be done with very clear goals. What is the desired outcome, the purpose of "going public"? The straightforward answer is that the goal would be to diffuse potential tension as much as possible, without precipitating more. It is the only way the public can reap the full benefits of the products of neuroscience advances. Moreover, it would be important to ensure that the neuroscience community will not lose public support as a result of the discomfort the work could produce. The most productive goal is to find common ground between the scientific community and the rest of society so that potential conflicts can be pre-empted, recognizing that some issues just cannot be resolved. With these goals in mind, then, what strategy should be taken?

The public engagement approach

The traditional response by the scientific community to tension with the rest of society has been to work on increasing public understanding based on the belief that most problems result simply from a lack of understanding on the part of the populace. "If only they understood us, they'd accept all we have to offer."

However, over the last decade, it has become clear that this approach is not enough. In many cases, the general public does understand enough about the science to know whether it will like it and will accept it or not. The cases of embryonic stem cell research and teaching evolution in the schools discussed earlier are excellent examples of this point.

Oftentimes individuals generally understand the issues but do not like the implications of the science.

An expanded or alternative approach, widely advocated in Europe and by many in the US, has been termed "public engagement with science" and includes but extends attempts to educate the public about scientific issues (Yankelovich 2003). The public engagement approach may begin with public education, but then, using discussion formats and with each community listening and learning from the other, it strives to find common ground and work through contention, as much as possible. Through this approach, the public comes to understand the science better, scientists come to understand the public, and then both groups can work toward common goals.

Different public engagement formats have been used, with varying success. The most popular in the US seems to be a town meeting-type format, where a single expert or panel of experts first presents the science and then offers open microphones for members of the public to respond. But these kinds of events, although often feeling successful, rarely stimulate genuine discussion and mutual learning. It is not uncommon that the microphone becomes usurped by extremists on either side of an issue.

Smaller group discussions seem most productive, particularly if there is a concrete problem to work through. This approach has been used widely and successfully by groups specializing in civic or public engagement, like Public Agenda, often working in partnership with scientific organizations (Wooden 2006).

Principles of public engagement

Although scientists, particularly those who are academics, are quite experienced at educating people about science, public engagement involves a different set of skills, and they are learned, not innate. One needs to be trained explicitly in public engagement with science (Illes *et al.* 2009; Morein-Zamir and Sahakian, 2010). Many scientific organizations, like Research!America, the Aldo Leopold Fellowships program, and the American Association for the Advancement of Science's (AAAS) Communicating Science project (http://www.aaas.org/communicatingscience), have developed training programs for communicating with the public. In addition, many individuals and groups have thought about what works in public engagement and what does not. These include Public Agenda, AAAS, the Royal Society (London), and the European Commission. A recent social issues roundtable on neuroscience and society at the October 2009 Society for Neuroscience annual meeting also discussed many principles of effective public engagement with neuroscience. Henry Greely articulated a list of such principles there. The following is an aggregated and distilled list of some fundamentals from these discussions and groups' writings, which include:

- **Listen carefully to what members of the public are saying**. Tone must attend to people's concerns, and that requires understanding them. Scientists' understanding the public is as important as the public understanding science.
- **Work to improve the understanding of the nature and process of science**. Use the opportunity to clarify the enterprise, its potential, and its limits.

- **Make the issue personally or locally meaningful for members of the public.** People only care about things that affect them directly or closely.

- **Only scientists care about the integrity of science or are bound by it.** If people do not like what science is showing, they are free to disregard or distort it.

- **Never debate an ideologue.** Scientists are bound by the data; others are not. People can and will say anything they want to make a point.

- **Do not be intentionally or overly provocative.** The issues are provocative enough, and one should not try to force one's point of view on others.

- **Pay attention to the subtleties surrounding issues.** Most issues are not as blunt a conflict as that between evolution and creationism.

- **Be humble.** Humility is a powerful tool for scientists to use in public engagement. Members of the public often think scientists are arrogant and condescending, and therefore they need to be convinced we mean to engage with the public. It is important to be sincere in this effort.

Concluding comments

Neuroscience has provided great insights into the nature of the brain and mind, and many of those insights have been translated into improved diagnosis, prevention, and treatment of nervous system disorders. Some of those insights, on the other hand, are likely to threaten core values and beliefs that have long been held by many people in the broader society. Not all points of conflict will be resolvable. However, genuine dialogue and engagement between neuroscientists and the broader public can go a long way toward discovering common ground and will yield much greater likelihood that our work will be broadly put to use for the benefit of humanity. And that, of course, is the ultimate goal of all of science.

References

Churchland, P.S. (2008). The impact of neuroscience on philosophy. *Neuron*, **60**, 409–11.

Egnor, M. (2008). Materialist neuroscience and the 'hard problem' of consciousness. *Discovery Institute Evolution News and Views Blog*. Available at: http://www.evolutionnews.org/

Greely, H., Sahakian, B., Harris, J., *et al.* (2008). Towards responsible use of cognitive-enhancing drugs by the healthy. *Nature*, **456**, 702–5.

Illes, J., Moser, M.A., McCormick, J.B., *et al.* (2009). Neurotalk: improving the communication of neuroscience research. *Nature Reviews Neuroscience*, **11**, 61–9.

Intergovernmental Panel on Climate Change (IPCC) (2007). Fourth Assessment Report. IPCC.

Leshner, A.I. (1997). Addiction is a brain disease and it matters. *Science*, **278**, 45–7.

Leshner, A.I. (2005). It's time to go public with neuroethics. *American Journal of Bioethics*, **5**, 1–2.

Morein-Zamir, S. and Sahakian, B.J. (2010). Neuroethics and public engagement training needed for neuroscientists. *Trends in Cognitive Science*, **14**, 49–51.

Moreno, J. (2007). *Mind Wars: Brain Research and National Defense*. New York: Dana Press.

National Science Board (2008). *Science and Engineering Indicators 2008*. Chapter 7: Science and Technology: Public Attitudes and Understanding. Arlington, VA: National Science Board.

Research!America (2009). Your Congress – Your Health Survey [online]. http://yourcongressyourhealth.org/

Singh, I. and Rose, N. (2009). Biomarkers in psychiatry. *Nature,* **460**, 202–7.

Yankelovich, D. (2003). Winning greater influence for science. *Issues in Science & Technology,* **19** [online].

Wooden, R. (2006). The principles of public engagement: At the nexus of science, public policy influence and citizen education. *Social Research,* **73**, 1057–63.

PREFACE

IT is with great excitement that we present the *Oxford Handbook of Neuroethics*, a compendium of chapters presenting key issues, complementary discussion, and critical debate at the intersection of brain and ethics.

The contributors to the volume join us from around the world and a broad range of sectors of academia and clinical practice spanning the neurosciences, medical sciences, the social sciences and humanities, and law. We are privileged to have engaged authors who wrote for one of the first books on neuroethics (*Neuroethics: Defining the Issues in Theory, Practice and Policy*, edited by J. Illes, 2006) and are well established in the field, in addition to many new contributors. Some are seasoned thinkers in neuroethics; others are newcomers to the field exploring, for the first time, the uncharted terrain and discovering its riches.

We have clinicians who think about ethics daily in their Western practices. Some of them, and others, are taking that thinking outside familiar urban borders, testing and endeavoring to make the world a better place by reducing the burden of suffering from neurologic and psychiatric disease in rural and developing regions of the world, and placing authenticity, consciousness, accountability, sustainability in the forefront of research, care and education. We may call this a movement toward global health neuroethics, drawing upon "... human rights as a key value, [and] global health ethics... [a] moral guidance for world health systems and governance." (Velji and Bryant, *Understanding Global Health*, 2007 International Health).

Certain authors use functional magnetic resonance imaging hands-on to understand how the human mind works, and others use meta-analyses of those data to expound on the implications of such neurotechnology. We have contributors who believe that enhancing cognition pharmacologically with brain devices is an important goal to improve cognition, functional outcome and well-being for children and adults with neuropsychiatric disorders and brain injury. Other contributors believe this goal should not be limited to those suffering from neuropsychiatric disorders or brain injury, but should be considered a natural phenomenon arising from human curiosity and the pursuit of personal betterment. Yet other authors argue fiercely against this position, concerned that the very nature of the human condition, defined by naturalness and authenticity, is at stake.

One author considers gender in the full range of concerns for brain research, healthcare, law, and education. Others look to the future of neurotechnology, genetics, and stem cells. Many tackle the challenges of the aging brain, predictive testing, and still limited therapeutic remedies to the relentless decline associated with dementia. Some promote imaging as a means of understanding of states of consciousness in the brain injured; others share or are even more cautious about what this wave of new research will bring and critical ethical challenges whether it proves to be viable or not. Needless to say, the importance of communication and outreach is a common theme throughout.

Quoting George Khushf in this volume, the importance of the unfettered activity in neuroethics is: "[t]o move ethics upstream... to be located at the place where the research first arises, and it needs to uncover the possibilities inherent within that research... to cultivate responsible research practices that are proactively responsive to broader ramifications of the practices." More than 90 international authors and co-authors have joined together with us and our assistant editors Carole Federico and Dr. Sharon Morein-Zamir, to promote this goal.

No doubt, we have not covered all topics or involved all possible contributors in this volume. Neuroethics is growing so rapidly that it would be impossible to do so. In fact, by way of this *Oxford Handbook of Neuroethics*, we hope to promote this growth and pave the way for other major texts for the field like this one. As Editors, we also do not necessarily agree with all views expressed by contributors. All, however, provide material for stimulating discussion and debate.

With this volume, we hope to reach young neuroscientists as we urge them to consider the research they do within an ethical context. We hope that students reading the Handbook will be inspired to take on leading roles in the rapidly developing field of neuroethics. We also hope to engage the public in active discussion about research findings and the impact discoveries about the brain may have on the lives of individuals and the fabric of society.

Overall, we trust that this Handbook will expand the knowledge base of its readers, as it has for us as Editors, and successfully share our commitment to ethics and neuroscience that is unwavering and profound.

Judy Illes and Barbara J. Sahakian

Acknowledgments

THE editors wish to thank all the authors for their contributions and acknowledge the support they have received from their funders. Judy Illes and Carole Federico extend their deepest gratitude for research funding to the CIHR, NIH/NIMH, the Canadian Foundation for Innovation (CFI), British Columbia Knowledge Development Fund (BCKDF), Foundation for Ethics and Technology, North Growth Foundation, Stem Cell Network, Vancouver Coastal Health Research Institute (VCHRI), Peter Wall Institute for Advanced Studies (PWIAS), the Dana Foundation, the Greenwall Foundation, the Michael Smith Foundation for Health Research (MSFHR), the John D. and Catherine T. MacArthur Foundation Law & Neuroscience Project, and the Canada Research Chairs Program.

Barbara J. Sahakian and Sharon Morein-Zamir thank the Wellcome Trust for a Programme Grant (no. 089589/Z/09/Z) awarded by the Trust to T.W. Robbins, B.J. Sahakian, B.J. Everitt and A.C. Roberts, and to the Medical Research Council and Wellcome Trust for the funding of the Behavioural and Clinical Neuroscience Institute (BCNI) (G0001354).

B.J. Sahakian dedicates her work on this volume to Jacqueline and Miranda Robbins whose keen interest in neuroscience, psychopharmacology, neuroethics, and public engagement in science has provided a great source of support for her activities in these areas and many lively debates.

CONTENTS

PART II RESPONSIBILITY AND DETERMINISM

PART III MIND AND BODY

PART IV NEUROTECHNOLOGY

PART V AGING AND DEMENTIA

PART VI LAW AND PUBLIC POLICY

PART VII SCIENCE, SOCIETY, AND INTERNATIONAL PERSPECTIVES

EPILOGUE

Notes on the Contributors

Marilyn S. Albert is a Professor of Neurology at the Johns Hopkins School of Medicine. She is Director of the Division of Cognitive Neuroscience and Director of the Johns Hopkins Alzheimer's Disease Research Center. Her major area of interest is the early diagnosis of Alzheimer's disease.

Ana Inés Ansaldo is a Professor in the Speech-Language Pathology Department at L' Université de Montréal and also holds a Young Investigator Award position from Fonds de recherche en santé du Québec. She has a Ph.D in Communication Sciences and Disorders with post-doctoral training in neuroimaging. Her research interests are at the crossroads of cognitive neuropsychology, speech-language pathology, and functional neuroimaging, in particular brain plasticity for language processing in healthy and brain damaged populations.

Silke Appel-Cresswell is a movement disorder neurologist and Assistant Professor at the Pacific Parkinson's Research Centre, University of British Columbia, Vancouver, Canada. She trained in neurology, movement disorders, and psychiatry in Germany and the United Kingdom. Her research interests are the clinical and imaging aspects of cognitive and neuropsychiatric symptoms in Parkinson's disease, including impulse control disorders.

Bernard Baertschi graduated from the University of Fribourg and obtained his doctoral degree in Philosophy at the University of Geneva in 1979. He is presently Maître d'Enseignement et de Recherche at the Institute of Biomedical Ethics at the University of Geneva. He is currently working on the ethics of biotechnologies and on neuroethics.

Roger A. Barker is the University Reader in Clinical Neuroscience and Honorary Consultant in Neurology at the University of Cambridge and Addenbrooke's Hospital. His clinical research centers on neurodegenerative disorders and in particular the translation of novel disease-modifying therapies, including cell based treatments.

Mario Beauregard is an Associate Research Professor at the Université de Montréal (Departments of Psychology and Radiology, Neuroscience Research Center). He is the author of more than 100 publications in neuroscience, psychology, and psychiatry. His groundbreaking work on the neurobiology of emotion regulation has received international media coverage.

Mark Bernstein is a neurosurgeon at Toronto Western Hospital and a Professor of Surgery at the University of Toronto. His main clinical interests are caring for patients with brain tumors, and teaching neurosurgery in the developing world. His interests in bioethics include novel resource utilization, patient safety, and neuroethics.

Kent C. Berridge is a James Olds Collegiate Professor of Psychology and Neuroscience at the University of Michigan, Ann Arbor. He aims to improve understanding of the neural mechanisms of emotion, motivation, learning, and reward with implications for motivational disorders such as drug addiction and eating disorders.

Teneille R. Brown is an Associate Professor of Law at the S.J. Quinney College of Law and a member of the Division of Medical Ethics at the University of Utah. Her research is highly interdisciplinary, and analyzes legal and ethical responses to advances in biotechnology and health.

Timothy Caulfield is the Research Director of the Health Law Institute at the University of Alberta, Canada Research Chair in Health Law and Policy, a Professor in the Faculty of Law and the School of Public Health, and a Senior Health Scholar with the Alberta Heritage Foundation for Medical Research.

Camille Chatelle works as a neuropsychologist at the Coma Science Group at the Cyclotron Research Center, Sart Tilman, Liège. She graduated as a neuropsychologist from the University of Brussels (ULB, 2009). She is currently a Ph.D student at the Belgian National Fund of Scientific Research (FNRS).

Daofen Chen is the Program Director in Systems and Cognitive Neuroscience at the National Institute of Neurological Disorders and Stroke. He is responsible for identifying research issues and administering a grant portfolio related to sensorimotor functions and integration, focusing especially on basic and clinical sciences of sensorimotor control, neurorehabilitation, and related neurotechnologies.

Hervé Chneiweiss is a neurologist and neuroscientist, studying molecular mechanisms involved in glial cell fate dynamics that may be involve in brain tumor development. He is currently head of the Glial Plasticity laboratory INSERM/Paris Descartes University, and Research Director at CNRS. He was also the adviser for life sciences and bioethics to the French minister for research from 2000–2002.

Patricia Churchland is a Professor of Philosophy at the University of California, San Diego, and an adjunct Professor at the Salk Institute. Her research focuses on the interface between neuroscience and philosophy. She explores the impact of scientific developments on the understanding of consciousness, the self, free will, decision making, ethics, learning, and religion.

Jonathan Cohen is the Eugene Higgins Professor of Psychology at Princeton University, Co-Director of the Princeton Neuroscience Institute, and Professor of Psychiatry at the Western Psychiatric Institute and Clinic at the University of Pittsburgh. Research in his laboratory focuses on the neurobiological mechanisms underlying cognitive control.

Alasdair Coles is a Senior Lecturer in neuroimmunology at the University of Cambridge. He researches experimental treatments of multiple sclerosis, especially a drug called alemtuzumab. He is also a minister in the Church of England.

Bruno della Chiesa is a Senior Analyst at OECD and Visiting Lecturer on Education at Harvard. He pioneered an international movement to connect brain research results with education policy. Bridging didactics of languages, cultural diversity awareness, neuroscientific insights, and ethics in a globalizing world, he recently developed new theoretical schemes, including the politically controversial "cultural tesseract."

Jessica Evert is Medical Director of Child Family Health International and recipient of Global Health Education Consortium's 2010 Christopher Krogh Award. Dr. Evert is a long-time advocate for global health medical education quality and ethical standards and has completed international work in Kenya, Guatemala, Australia, and Cuba.

Martha J. Farah is the Walter H. Annenberg Professor in the Natural Sciences at the University of Pennsylvania, where she directs the Center for Neuroscience & Society and the Center for Cognitive Neuroscience. She was educated at MIT and Harvard, and has worked most recently on the effects of poverty on brain development and neuroethics.

Carole A. Federico is a Research Coordinator at the National Core for Neuroethics at the University of British Columbia. She completed her undergraduate studies at the University of British Columbia in Biopsychology with an interest in Philosophy. At the Core she examines the need and priorities of neuroimagers and neurodegenerative disease researchers for incorporating neuroethics into their research.

Joseph J. Fins is Chief of the Division of Medical Ethics at Weill Cornell Medical College where he serves as a Professor of Medicine, Professor of Public Health, and Professor of Medicine in Psychiatry. Dr. Fins is also Director of Medical Ethics at New York-Presbyterian Weill Cornell Medical Center and an adjunct faculty member at The Rockefeller University.

Ruth Fischbach is Professor of Bioethics and Director and Co-founder of the Center for Bioethics at Columbia University. Her research interests and scholarly publications have focused on decisions around the end of life, autonomy of the elderly, communication between patients and healthcare professionals, pain assessment, and the management and experiences of research participants, particularly as they relate to privacy and informed consent. Her current work focuses on research ethics and contemporary issues in bioethics including neuroethics, stem cell research, and advances in assisted reproductive technology.

Kurt W. Fischer is the Charles Bigelow Professor of Education and Director of the Mind, Brain and Education Program at Harvard University. He studies cognitive and emotional development and learning from birth through adulthood, combining analysis of the commonalities across people with the diversity of pathways of learning and development. He is founding president of the International Mind, Brain and Education Society and founding editor of the new journal *Mind, Brain, and Education*.

Lachlan Forrow is Associate Professor of Medicine at Harvard Medical School, Director of Ethics and Palliative Care Programs at Beth Israel Deaconess Medical Center, and a member of the Dana Farber/Harvard Cancer Center Institutional Review Board.

Erica Frank is a Professor and Canada Research Chair at the University of British Columbia, Founder of Healthy Doc = Healthy Patient and of Health Sciences Online (a global virtual health sciences training center) and 2008 President of Physicians for Social Responsibility.

Felipe Fregni is an Assistant Professor of Neurology at Harvard Medical School. He is Director of the Laboratory of Neuromodulation at Spaulding Rehabilitation Hospital and

Director of the Collaborative Learning in Clinical Research Program – Principles and Practice of Clinical Research from the Department of Continuing Education, Harvard Medical School.

Giorgio Ganis has a Ph.D in Cognitive Science from the University of California at San Diego and he is an Assistant Professor in Radiology at the Harvard Medical School. He is an established cognitive neuroscientist in the fields of visual and social cognition.

Henry T. Greely is the Deane F. and Kate Edelman Johnson Professor of Law, and Professor, by courtesy, of Genetics at Stanford University. He directs Stanford's Center for Law and the Biosciences and the Stanford Interdisciplinary Group on Neuroscience and Society. He is a co-founder of the Neuroethics Society and member of its Executive Committee.

Benjamin D. Greenberg is Chief of Adult OCD research at the National Institute of Mental Health (NIMH). He studied psychology at Amherst College, and received a Ph.D in neuroscience from UC San Diego, and an MD from the University of Miami. He was a neurology resident at Columbia University, and completed psychiatry residency at Johns Hopkins Hospital and a fellowship at the NIMH. His primary research for more than a decade has been in psychiatric neurosurgery.

Joshua Greene is an Assistant Professor of Psychology at Harvard University and the Director of the Moral Cognition Lab. He studies moral judgment and decision making using neuroscientific and behavioral methods. Professor Greene has a Ph.D. in philosophy, and much of his scientific research is motivated by traditionally philosophical questions.

Michael R. Hadskis is an Assistant Professor in the Schulich School of Law, Dalhousie University, Halifax, Nova Scotia. His research interests include the regulation of human biomedical research and neuroimaging ethics. Professor Hadskis has served on a number of research ethics boards. In 2007, he received a Distinguished Service Award in connection with his service on Dalhousie University's Health Sciences Research Ethics Board.

Patrick Haggard trained in philosophy, experimental psychology and neurophysiology at the Universities of Cambridge and Oxford. He has been at University College London since 1995, where he leads a research group investigating voluntary action.

John Harris is Director of The Institute for Science, Ethics and Innovation and of the Wellcome Strategic Programme in the Human Body, its Scope, Limits and Future, School of Law, University of Manchester, where he is Lord Alliance Professor of Bioethics. He is joint Editor-in-Chief of *The Journal of Medical Ethics* and has been a member of The United Kingdom *Human Genetics Commission* since its foundation in 1999.

John-Dylan Haynes is a Professor for Neuroimaging at the Bernstein Center for Computational Neuroscience in Berlin. He worked in Bremen, Plymouth, and London before starting his own Max Planck research group in Leipzig. His research focuses on the role of awareness in vision and action, neurotechnology, and brain reading.

Gary Heit received his Ph.D in neuroscience from UCLA and his MD from Stanford. After serving as an Assistant Professor of Neurosurgery and Director of Functional Neurosurgery at Stanford, he joined the neurosurgery staff of the Permanente Medical Group of Northern California. Dr. Heit is Co-Founder of Americare Neurosurgery International, dedicated to promoting locally sustainable, modern neurosurgical care in developing countries.

Elisabeth Hildt is a lecturer in the Department of Philosophy at the Johannes Gutenberg University in Mainz, Germany, where she is heading a neuroethics research group. The focus of her research is on theory and ethics in the life sciences, with particular interests in neuro-philosophy, neuroethics and human genetics.

Christina Hinton is a doctoral student at Harvard in neuroscience and education. She works to inform education policy and practice with neuroscience findings, in collaboration with OECD, UNICEF, and the Ross Schools. She lectures internationally on the brain and learning, research schools, and education for global consciousness.

Ging-Yuek Robin Hsiung is an Assistant Professor in the Division of Neurology, Department of Medicine, University of British Columbia, and Director of Clinical Trials Program at the University of British Columbia Hospital Clinic for Alzheimer and Related Disorders. His research interests include clinical and genetic epidemiology of Alzheimer disease and related neurodegenerative disorders, neuropsychological characteristics of cognitive disorders, as well as translational research on neurological health and aging.

Julian C. Hughes is a consultant in old age psychiatry based at North Tyneside General Hospital. He is honorary Professor of Philosophy of Ageing at the Institute for Ageing and Health, Newcastle University. His most recent, co-edited, book is *Supportive Care for the Person with Dementia* (Oxford University Press, 2010).

Robert Huish is Assistant Professor in International Development Studies at Dalhouse University. He is the 2004 Trudeau Scholar and holds a Ph.D in geography from Simon Fraser University in Vancouver, BC and a SSHRC Postdoctoral Fellow at L'Université de Montréal. His research rests between the pursuit of global health equity and the understanding of public health ethics.

Samia Hurst is an Assistant Professor of Bioethics at Geneva University's medical school in Switzerland, ethics consultant to the Geneva University Hospitals' clinical ethics committee, and editor of the Swiss bioethics journal *Bioethica Forum*. Her research focuses on fairness in clinical practice and the protection of vulnerable persons.

Steven E. Hyman is Provost of Harvard University and Professor of Neurobiology at Harvard Medical School. From 1996–2001, he served as Director of the US National Institute of Mental Health (NIMH). Before that he was Director of Harvard University's interdisciplinary Mind, Brain, and Behavior Initiative.

Judy Illes is the Canada Research Chair in Neuroethics and Professor of Neurology at the University of British Columbia, Canada. She also holds academic appointments as Adjunct Professor in the School of Population and Public Health, School of Journalism, and the Department of Computer Science and Engineering at the University of Washington, Seattle, USA. She is a co-founder and Executive Committee Member of the Neuroethics Society, a member of the Dana Alliance for Brain Initiatives, and is past Chair of the Committee on Women in World Neuroscience of the International Brain Research Organization (IBRO).

Adrian J. Ivinson is Director of the Harvard NeuroDiscovery Center since its founding in 2001. Trained as a geneticist, his career has focused on the genetics of single gene disorders and the translation of research into effective medical interventions.

Yves Joanette is a Professor in the Faculty of Medicine at the Université de Montréal, and Laboratory Director at the Centre de recherche of the Institut universitaire de gériatrie de Montréal. He is currently President and CEO of the Fonds de la recherche en santé du Québec.

Evaleen Jones founded the Child Family Health International (CFHI) and holds a position on the Clinical Faculty at Stanford University School of Medicine. Her commitment to underserved people stems from growing up in rural New Jersey and spending her college years in the Appalachian region of Virginia where poverty prevails. CFHI has over 250 global partners, sending more than 700 medical students abroad each year.

Karima Kahlaoui is a Postdoctoral Fellow at the Université de Montréal. Her research includes studies of the semantic processing of words across the hemispheres, semantic memory, and aging. In order to investigate these topics, she has made use of behavioral methods, event-related potentials (ERPs), and near infrared spectroscopy (NIRS). She is also a clinical neuropsychologist with a Ph.D in Psychology from Nice University (France).

George Khushf is Director of the Center for Bioethics and Professor in the Department of Philosophy at the University of South Carolina. He conducts research on the philosophical and ethical aspects of emerging research in engineering and medicine, with a special interest in areas of convergence between nanoscience, biomedicine, information technology, and cognitive science.

Morten L. Kringelbach is Director of the TrygFonden Research Group. He is a Senior Research Fellow in the Department of Psychiatry, University of Oxford and a Professor at Aarhus University, Denmark, as well as Extraordinary Junior Research Fellow and College Lecturer in Neuroscience at The Queen's College, University of Oxford.

Kimberley Lakes is an Assistant Professor in the Department of Pediatrics at the University of California, Irvine. She received her Ph.D from the University of Wisconsin, Madison and completed a postdoctoral fellowship at the Children's Hospital of Orange County and UC Irvine. Dr. Lakes is an elected member of the Society of Pediatric Research.

Steven Laureys leads the Coma Science Group at the Cyclotron Research Center and Department of Neurology, Sart Tilman, in Liège. He graduated as a Medical Doctor from the Vrije Universiteit (Brussels, Belgium) in 1993. He is Clinical Professor and Senior Research Associate (tenure) at the Belgian National Fund of Scientific Research (FNRS).

Alan I. Leshner is the Chief Executive Officer of the American Association for the Advancement of Science (AAAS) and Executive Publisher of the journal Science. Before coming to AAAS, Dr. Leshner was Director of the National Institute on Drug Abuse (NIDA), Deputy Director and Acting Director of the National Institute of Mental Health (NIMH). At the National Science Foundation (NSF) Dr. Leshner focused on basic research in the biological, behavioral and social sciences, science policy, and science education.

Neil Levy is Director of Research at the Oxford Centre for Neuroethics, and Head of Neuroethics at the Florey Neuroscience Institutes. He is the author of five books, including *Neuroethics: Challenges for the 21st Century* (Cambridge University Press, 2007), and Editor-in-Chief of the journal *Neuroethics* (Springer).

Nir Lipsman is a neurosurgery resident at the University of Toronto, having completed his medical education at Queen's University in Kingston, Ontario. His clinical and research interests are in functional neurosurgery, and specifically, the application of novel surgical techniques to the treatment of refractory psychiatric disease.

Scott Loeliger is a family physician, Director of the Mark Stinson Fellowship in Global Health and Underserved Medicine at the Contra Costa Regional Medical Center in California, and Program Director for Global Health Through Education and Training (GHETS) where he works to develop family medicine and primary healthcare in international settings.

Sofia Lombera is a Master of Science student in the Biomedicine, Bioscience and Society (BIOS) program at the London School of Economics and Political Science, UK. Prior to enrolling in the program she was the Research Manager for the National Core for Neuroethics at the University of British Columbia.

Monica Luciana is Professor of Psychology and Child Development at the University of Minnesota and a founding member of the University of Minnesota's Center for Neurobehavioral Development. She has a longstanding interest in the development and neural bases of executive functions in middle childhood and adolescence.

Debra J.H. Mathews is the Assistant Director for Science Programs at the Johns Hopkins Berman Institute of Bioethics, with a secondary appointment in the Institute of Genetic Medicine, and an Assistant Professor of Pediatrics in the School of Medicine. She has a Ph.D in genetics and a MA in bioethics from Case Western Reserve University.

Alexandre Mauron was initially trained as a molecular biologist at the University of Lausanne (Ph.D, 1978) and was a postdoctoral fellow in developmental biology at Stanford. He then moved to the field of bioethics during the late 1980s. He is presently a Professor at the Institute of Biomedical Ethics at the University of Geneva. Professor Mauron is currently working on various bioethical issues, including stem cell research, neuroethics, and enhancement.

Jennifer B. McCormick is an Assistant Professor of Biomedical Ethics and an Associate Consultant, Departments of Medicine and Health Sciences Research Mayo Clinic and College of Medicine. Her research interests include science policy and biomedical ethics, how scientists engage in public and science policy discussions, and the dialogue around social responsibility in science.

Guy M. McKhann is a Professor of Neurology at the Johns Hopkins School of Medicine. He was the founding Chair of the Department of Neurology and subsequently the founding Chair of the Mind Brain Institute. His major areas of interest include Guillian–Barré syndrome, vascular cognitive decline, and Alzheimer's disease.

Thomas Metzinger directs the Theoretical Philosophy Group and coordinates a neuroethics research group at the Johannes Gutenberg University in Mainz, Germany. He is an Adjunct Fellow at the Frankfurt Institute for Advanced Study, and was a Fellow at the Institute for Advanced Study in Berlin. Metzinger is a former president of the German Cognitive Science Society and of the Association for the Scientific Study of Consciousness.

Janet Mindes is a Consultant with the Center for Bioethics, Columbia University, working on a series of projects in bioethics. Her primary interest is in neuroethics. Dr. Mindes' diverse background includes experimental psychology (memory and cognition), and complementary and alternative medicine, and art history. Her primary neuroscience interests are mind/brain/body and affective processes.

Jonathan D. Moreno is the David and Lyn Silfen University Professor of Ethics and Professor of Medical Ethics and of History and Sociology of Science at the University of Pennsylvania. His books include *Mind Wars: Brain Research and National Defense* (2006), and *Undue Risk: Secret State Experiments on Humans* (1999).

Sharon Morein-Zamir is a Research Associate in the Department of Psychiatry at the University of Cambridge, UK. She has a Ph.D in Psychology from the University of British Columbia, Canada. Her research interests include response inhibition, action control, and compulsivity.

Emily R. Murphy is a JD candidate at Stanford Law School. She has a Ph.D. in behavioral neuroscience from the University of Cambridge, completed in 2007, and an undergraduate degree from Harvard in Psychology/Mind, Brain, Behavior. Prior to undertaking law studies she was a postdoctoral fellow in the Program in Neuroethics at the Stanford Center for Biomedical Ethics, then a postdoctoral fellow concurrently at the Center for Law and the Biosciences at Stanford Law School and on the MacArthur Foundation Law and Neuroscience Project.

Adrian M. Owen received his Ph.D from the Institute of Psychiatry, London in 1992. He trained post-doctorally at the Montreal Neurological Institute, Canada and since 1997 has been at the MRC Cognition and Brain Sciences Unit, Cambridge, where he is currently Assistant Director. Since 1990, he has published over 190 scientific articles and chapters. His work on the vegetative state has been widely reported by the world's media and has been the subject of several TV and radio documentaries.

Alvaro Pascual-Leone is Professor of Neurology at Harvard Medical School, Director of the Berenson-Allen Center for Noninvasive Brain Stimulation, and Program Director of the Harvard-Thorndike Clinical Research Center at Beth Israel Deaconess Medical Center in Boston, MA.

Martin P. Paulus studied Medicine at the Johannes Gutenberg University in Mainz. He is Professor in Residence at the University of California San Diego as well as a staff psychiatrist at the San Diego Veterans Affairs Health Care System. Currently, Dr. Paulus is interested in developing functional magnetic resonance imaging as a tool in psychiatry for making clinically important predictions, developing new medications, and examining the degree of dysfunctions in patients.

Remi Quirion is the Executive Director for the CIHR International Collaborative Research Strategy for Alzheimer's disease, a McGill University Full Professor in Psychiatry, and the Scientific Director at the Douglas Mental Health University Institute. Dr. Quirion was the inaugural leader of the Institute of Neurosciences, Mental Health and Addiction.

Peter V. Rabins is Professor of Psychiatry and Behavioral Sciences in the Johns Hopkins Hospital and the Richman Family Professor for Alzheimer's and Related Diseases. His interests include the effectiveness of current treatment for Alzheimer disease, the development of measures of quality of life in persons with Alzheimer disease and the care of patients with late stage dementia.

Eric Racine is the Director of the Neuroethics Research Unit at the Institut de recherches cliniques de Montréal and holds appointments at the University of Montreal and McGill University. He is a principal investigator on several projects examining neuroscience communication and is an associate editor of the journal *Neuroethics*.

Peter B. Reiner is a Professor at the National Core for Neuroethics and the Brain Research Centre at the University of British Columbia. Dr. Reiner has a distinguished track record as a research scientist studying the neurobiology of behavioral states and the molecular underpinnings of neurodegenerative disease, and was President & CEO of Active Pass Pharmaceuticals, a drug discovery company that he founded in 1998 to tackle Alzheimer's disease. Together with Professor Judy Illes, he co-founded the National Core for Neuroethics in 2007 where his scholarly work focuses on issues of neuroessentialism and cognitive enhancement.

Martina Reske received her Ph.D in Psychology from the University of Düsseldorf, Germany. Her research focuses on studying the neural substrates underlying executive dysfunctions in individuals with psychiatric disorders using fMRI. She collaborates with Martin Paulus on stimulant use and now holds an appointment at the Forschungszentrum Jülich, Germany, to apply new MR techniques, among others, to substance use disorders.

J. **Peter Rosenfeld** has a Ph.D in Biopsychology from the University of Iowa and is a Professor of Psychology and Neuroscience at Northwestern University. He is among the pioneers and leaders in the field who use event-related EEG potentials in the study of deception.

Barbara J. Sahakian is Professor of Clinical Neuropsychology at the University of Cambridge, Department of Psychiatry, and the Medical Research Council/Wellcome Trust Behavioural and Clinical Neuroscience Institute. She is co-inventor of the CANTAB neuropsychological tests, which are in use world-wide. She is also a Fellow of the Academy of Medical Sciences, a practicing clinical psychologist, president-elect of the British Association for Psychopharmacology, a member of the CINP council, and a founder and Executive Board member of the Neuroethics Society.

Jerry Samet is a member of the Philosophy Department at Brandeis University. His areas of specialization include the Philosophy of Mind and Cognitive Science and the History of Modern Philosophy.

Anders Sandberg has a background in computational neuroscience from Stockholm University, where he studied the neuroscience of memory. He is currently at the Future of Humanity Institute of Oxford University researching the ethics and social impact of human enhancement, emerging technologies and large-scale risks.

Julian Savulescu is the Uehiro Chair in Practical Ethics at the University of Oxford. He is Director of the Oxford Uehiro Centre for Practical Ethics within the Faculty of Philosophy, and is Director of the Wellcome Centre for Neuroethics, and the James Martin 21st Century School Program on the Ethics of the New Biosciences.

Steve Schmidbauer is Executive Director of Child Family Health International (CFHI), a leading non-governmental organization (NGO) placing health science students on global health education programs in ways that are socially responsible and financially just.

Matthias H. Schmidt is a pediatric radiologist, as well as a diagnostic and interventional neuroradiologist. He is an Associate Professor of Radiology, Psychiatry and Anatomy & Neurobiology at Dalhousie University, a member of the Brain Repair Centre and of the CIHR New Emerging Team in Neuroethics. His research interests encompass the development of innovative imaging techniques for clinical neuroscience, the application of neuroimaging tools to basic human neuroscience, and the safety of child participants in neuroimaging research.

Walter Sinnott-Armstrong is Chauncey Stillman Professor in the Department of Philosophy and Kenan Institute for Ethics at Duke University. He is Co-Director of the MacArthur Law and Neuroscience Project and co-investigator at Oxford's Wellcome Centre for Neuroethics. His current research focuses on moral psychology and neuroscience.

Bernadette Ska obtained a Ph.D in Psychology of the Université Catholique de Louvain (Belgium). She was a fellow in neuropsychology at the Institut universitaire de gériatrie de Montréal. She is currently a Full Professor at the École d'orthophonie et audiologie, Faculté de médecine, Unversité de Montréal and researcher at the centre de recherche of the Institute universitaire de gériatrie de Montréal.

Zachary Stein is currently a student of philosophy and cognitive development pursing a doctorate at the Harvard Graduate School of Education. He is also Deputy Director and Senior Analyst for the Developmental Testing Service, a non-profit dedicated to educational research and development.

Yaakov Stern is a Professor of Clinical Neuropsychology at Columbia University College of Physicians and Surgeons. His research focuses on cognition in normal aging and in diseases of aging, particularly Alzheimer's disease. His approach includes classic neuropsychological and cognitive experimental techniques, with a strong focus on functional imaging.

Megan S. Steven-Wheeler is a Visiting Assistant Professor of Neuroscience at the Center for Cognitive Neuroscience at Dartmouth College where she also serves as the Assistant Dean of Faculty for Administration.

A. Jon Stoessl is a Professor and Acting Head of Neurology at the University of British Columbia, where he holds a Tier 1 Canada Research Chair and directs the Pacific Parkinson's Research Centre and National Parkinson Foundation Centre of Excellence. His research program is focused on the use of functional imaging to study Parkinson's disease, with an interest in compensatory mechanisms, disease progression, complications of disease and therapy, and mechanisms underlying the placebo effect.

Christopher Suhler is a doctoral student in the Department of Philosophy and Interdisciplinary Program in Cognitive Science at the University of California, San Diego. His research is in the philosophy of cognitive science, moral psychology, and philosophy of psychology.

James M. Swanson served as the initial Principal Investigator at UC Irvine for two multisite treatment studies of ADHD (the MTA and PATS), for several clinical trials for the development of new medications for ADHD, and currently for the Orange County CA Vanguard Center of the National Children's Study.

Kate Tairyan is the content director of Health Sciences Online and the Director of the Online School of Public Health at Global University (www.globaluni.info). She is also a global health Lecturer at Simon Fraser University and a research consultant at the National Core for Neuroethics, University of British Columbia.

Stacey A. Tovino is Director of the Health Law and Policy Center and Associate Professor of Law at Drake University Law School in Des Moines, Iowa, where she teaches and conducts research in the areas of health law, bioethics, and the medical humanities.

Craig Van Dyke is a Professor and Director of Global Mental Health for the Department of Psychiatry at the University of California San Francisco. He served as Department Chair from 1994 until 2008. During 2008–2009 he was Special Advisor to the Director of the National Institute of Mental Health (NIMH).

Nora D. Volkow became Director of the National Institute on Drug Abuse (NIDA) in May 2003. Her pioneering use of brain imaging to investigate the toxic effects and addictive properties of drugs was instrumental in demonstrating that drug addiction is a disease of the brain.

Bruce E. Wexler is a Yale Professor with over 100 scientific papers. Dr. Wexler's book *Brain and Culture; Neurobiology, Ideology and Social Change* presents new research and ideas on how cultural environments affect development of our minds and brains, and how these processes change across the lifespan due to changes in neuroplasticity.

Timothy Wigal is an Adjunct Professor of Pediatrics and Director of the University of California Irvine, Child Development Center and is the principal investigator of the Multimodal Treatment study of Children with Attention Deficit Hyperactivity Disorder (ADHD). He is a licensed psychologist with expertise in diagnosis and treatment of ADHD in children and adults.

Maximiliano Wilson has a Ph.D in Neuropsychology of Language from the University of Buenos Aires, Argentina. He held an experienced Researcher fellowship of the European Marie-Curie Research and Training Network "Language and Brain," based in Rome, Italy. He is currently a postdoctoral research fellow at the Centre de Recherche de l'Institut universitaire de gériatrie de Montréal.

Susan M. Wolf is the McKnight Presidential Professor of Law, Medicine & Public Policy at the University of Minnesota, as well as Faegre & Benson Professor of Law, Professor of Medicine, and Faculty Member in the Center for Bioethics. She is an elected Member of the National Academy of Sciences' Institute of Medicine and an elected Fellow of the American Association for the Advancement of Science. Her research is supported by grants from the National Institutes of Health, National Science Foundation, and private foundations including the MacArthur Foundation's Project on Law & Neuroscience.

Amy Zarzeczny is a Research Associate at the Health Law Institute, University of Alberta. Her work is focused on the ethical, legal, social and policy implications of emerging biotechnologies. Prior to this appointment, she completed graduate studies at the London School of Economics and Political Science and practiced law in Edmonton.

LIST OF ABBREVIATIONS

ACC	anterior cingulate cortex
AD	Alzheimer's disease
ADA	Americans with Disabilities Act
ADAAA	Americans with Disabilities Act Amendments Act
ADD	attention deficit disorder
ADHD	attention deficit hyperactivity disorder
AMCANI	Americare Neurosurgery International
AMP	amphetamine
APA	American Psychological Association
APFC	anterior prefrontal cortex
BA	Brodmann area
BCI	brain–computer interface
Beh	behavior modification
BEOS	brain electrical oscillations signature
BIS	bispectral index
BMI	brain–machine interface
BOLD	blood oxygen level-dependent
CAI	computer-assisted instruction
CANTAB	Cambridge Neuropsychological Test Automated Battery
CBCL	Child Behavior Checklist
CDC	Centers for Disease Control and Prevention
CdSe	cadmium selenide
CE	cognitive enhancement
CFHI	Child Family Health International
CHADD	Children and Adults with ADD
CIOMS	Council for International Organizations of Medical Sciences
CIT	Concealed Information Test
CME	continuing medical education
CNS	central nervous system
CQT	Control Question Test

CR	controlled-release
CR	cognitive reserve
CRF	corticotropin releasing factor
CRO	contract research organization
CRS-R	Coma Recovery Scale-Revised
CRUNCH	compensation-related utilization of neural circuits hypothesis
CT	computed tomography
DA	dopamine
DAC	Data Access Committee
DAT	dopamine transporter
DBS	deep brain stimulation
DD	Differentiation of Deception
DLB	dementia with Lewy bodies
DLPFC	dorsolateral prefrontal cortex
DMD	Duchenne muscular dystrophy
DNA	deoxyribonucleic acid
DSM	Diagnostic and Statistical Manual of Mental Disorders
DTI	diffusion tensor imaging
ECT	electroconvulsive therapy
EEG	electroencephalography
EHA	Education of the Handicapped Act
ELSI	ethical, legal, and social issues
ERC	ethics review committee
ERN	error-related negativity
ERP	event-related potential
FDA	Food and Drug Administration
FDG	fludeoxyglucose
FES	functional electrical stimulation
FISH	fluorescent *in situ* hybridization
FMLA	Family and Medical Leave Act
fMRI	functional magnetic resonance imaging
GCS	Glasgow Coma Scale
GID	graft induced dyskinesia
GPi	globus pallidus internus
HAROLD	hemispheric asymmetry reduction in older adults
HD	Huntington's disease
HDE	Humanitarian Device Exemption

HIC	high-income country
HIPAA	Health Insurance Portability and Accountability Act
HKD	hyperkinetic disorder
HSO	Health Sciences Online
IAPS	International Affective Picture System
IBC	International Bioethics Committee
IBID	implantable brain-interfacing device
ICD	International Classification of Diseases
ICD	impulse control disorder
IDEA	Individuals with Disabilities Education Act (US)
IF	incidental finding
IMBES	International Mind, Brain, and Education Society
iPS	induced pluripotent stem
IQ	intelligence quotient
IR	immediate-release
IT	information technology
LMICs	low- and middle-income countries
LIS	Locked in syndrome
LPFC	lateral prefrontal cortex
LSD	lysergic acid diethylamide
LTD	long-term depression
LTP	long-term potentiation
MBT	mood, behavior, and thought
MCI	mild cognitive impairment
MCS	minimally conscious state
MedMgt	medication management
MEG	magnetoencephalography
MFN	medial frontal negativity
MMN	mismatch negativity
MOFC	medial orbitofrontal cortex
MPFC	medial prefrontal cortex
MPH	methylphenidate
MPH	methylphenidate
MRI	magnetic resonance imaging
MTA	Multimodal Treatment study of ADHD
NAc	nucleus accumbens
NIBC	nanoscience, biomedicine, information technology, and cognitive science

NICE	National Institute for Health and Clinical Excellence
NIH	National Institutes of Health
NIMH	National Institute of Mental Health
NMDA	N-methyl-D-aspartic acid
NMR	nuclear magnetic resonance
NNI	National Nanotechnology Initiative
OCD	obsessive–compulsive disorder
OECD	Organization for Economic Cooperation and Development
OFC	orbitofrontal cortex
PAG	periaqueductal gray
PCE	pharmaceutical cognitive enhancer
PCL-R	Psychopathy Checklist-Revised
PD	Parkinson's disease
PET	positron emission tomography
PFC	prefrontal cortex
PKU	phenylketonuria
PTSD	post-traumatic stress disorder
PVS	persistent vegetative state
QD	quantum dot
R&D	research and development
rCBF	regional cerebral blood flow
RCT	randomized control trial
REC	Research Ethics Committee
RNA	ribonucleic acid
RT	reaction time
rTMS	repetitive transcranial magnetic stimulation
SCG	subcallosal cingulate gyrus
SCR	skin conductance response
SDQ	Strengths and Difficulties Questionnaire
SfN	Society for Neuroscience
SMA	supplementary motor area
SMART	Sensory Modality Assessment and Rehabilitation Technique
SNAP	Swanson, Nolan, and Pelham (scale)
SNRI	selective noradrenaline reuptake inhibitor
SPECT	single photon emission computed tomography
SSRI	selective serotonin reuptake inhibitor
STAC	scaffolding theory of aging and cognition

STN	subthalamic nucleus
SUD	substance use disorder
TAT	Thematic Apperception Test
tDCS	transcranial direct current stimulation
TID	three times a day
TMS	transcranial magnetic stimulation
TRD	treatment-resistant depression
UBO	unidentified bright object
UK	United Kingdom
US	United States
VIM	ventral intermediate nucleus
vlPAG	ventrolateral region of the periaqueductal gray
VLPFC	ventrolateral prefrontal cortex
VMPFC	ventromedial prefrontal cortex
VMPFC	ventral mesencephalon
VS	vegetative state
VTA	ventral tegmental area
WMH	white matter hyperintensities
WHIM	Wessex Head Injury Matrix
WSSFN	World Society of Stereotactic and Functional Neurosurgery
ZnS	zinc sulfide

PART I

CONSCIOUSNESS AND INTENTION: DECODING MENTAL STATES AND DECISION MAKING

CHAPTER 1

....

BRAIN READING: DECODING MENTAL STATES FROM BRAIN ACTIVITY IN HUMANS

....

JOHN-DYLAN HAYNES

INTRODUCTION

....

THE ability to read another person's thoughts has always exerted an enormous fascination. Recently, new brain imaging technology has emerged that might make it possible to one day read a person's thoughts directly from their brain activity. This novel approach is referred to as "brain reading" or the "decoding of mental states." This article will first provide a general outline of the field, and will then proceed to discuss its limitations, its potential applications, and also certain ethical issues that brain reading raises.

The measurement of brain activity and brain structure has made considerable progress in recent decades. Computed tomography (CT) and magnetic resonance imaging (MRI) have vastly improved the ability to measure an individual's brain structural composition with high detail and non-invasively. This provides a three-dimensional image of the human brain showing the distribution of gray and white matter, bone, and cerebrospinal fluid. Although these structural neuroimaging techniques are routinely used in neuroradiology to assess injuries of the central nervous system and to diagnose neurological diseases, they provide no information about a person's *current* mental states (such as their current ideas, thoughts, intentions, and feelings). This is because they measure the *structure* of the brain rather than the brain *activity* that changes from moment to moment. In order to read out the current mental state of a person a measurement of their current brain activity is required.

Brain activity can be measured using a number of techniques: electromagnetic brain activity signals can be measured using electroencephalography (EEG) and magnetoencephalography (MEG). These techniques map brain activity with high temporal resolution (in the millisecond range), but their spatial resolution is very low (several centimeters). Already in the 1960s researchers used EEG for brain-based spelling devices. Subjects learned to control the alpha oscillations of their EEG and were then able to transmit Morse code by sending short versus long bursts of alpha activity (Dewan 1967). Such techniques could potentially be useful in helping paralyzed people communicate their thoughts and wishes by deliberately changing their brain activity. The goal in this field of so-called non-invasive brain–computer interfaces (BCIs) is to develop techniques that allow users to control technical devices "with the power of thought." Already today it is possible to control a prosthesis, spell a letter, or steer a wheelchair using EEG-based BCIs. Unfortunately the low spatial resolution of EEG means that it is limited to reading out simple commands, such as spelling texts or moving a computer cursor on a screen. It is difficult to read out more complex ideas (such as an intention or a memory) due to the lack of spatial resolution. The key problem is that the brain represents information in fine-grained columnar maps with a resolution of approximately 0.5mm (Tanaka 1997). These activation patterns are far too small to be resolved with EEG.

Complementary to EEG/MEG, functional magnetic resonance imaging (fMRI) allows measurement of brain activity with high spatial resolution (a few millimeters), but lower temporal resolution (a few seconds). Unlike EEG, fMRI signals are only an indirect marker of the activity of nerve cell clusters, because brain activity is estimated via its effects on the oxygen content of blood. However, fMRI is currently the only available non-invasive procedure that allows for a measurement of brain activity with high spatial resolution without having direct access to the brain through invasive surgical techniques. The resolution achievable with fMRI is just enough to extract some information from fine-grained activity patterns. For this reason, fMRI-based brain reading techniques allow reading out a person's thoughts in much more detail than with EEG. In particular, the combination of fMRI with specialized statistical pattern recognition techniques has provided a new impetus to the field of brain reading.

Brain reading requires that every mental state ("thought") is associated with a characteristic pattern of brain activity. Similar to a fingerprint, a brain activity pattern as a unique and unmistakable brain signal indicates a specific thought. By learning to identify such brain activity patterns it is thus possible to infer what a person is thinking. A typical brain reading procedure starts by measuring the brain activity patterns that occur when a person has a specific thought. Then a computer is trained to recognize the specific patterns of brain activity that are associated with the different thoughts (Figure 1.1). This is done using so-called pattern-recognition algorithms that can classify brain activation patterns in a statistically optimal fashion. Similar algorithms are also used to detect fingerprints or identify faces from surveillance videos. Unlike traditional methods for analyzing brain imaging data, pattern recognition combines information from multiple brain locations and thus maximizes the information that can be read out. By combining fMRI with pattern recognition, the field of "brain reading" has made huge progress in the last few years. It has been possible to read out very detailed contents of a person's thoughts, including detailed visual percepts and ideas, memories, and even intentions and emotions. It is possible to read out implicit and even unconscious mental states, such as unconscious percepts and decisions (for an overview see Haynes and Rees 2006; Norman *et al.* 2006).

Take, for example, the read-out of subjects' intentions from brain signals (Haynes *et al.* 2007). In this experiment we let subjects decide freely between two possible choices, i.e. adding or subtracting numbers. Importantly, participants made their choice covertly and so we initially did not know which choice they had made. Then, after a delay, we showed them the numbers and asked them to do the corresponding calculation. We were able to decode

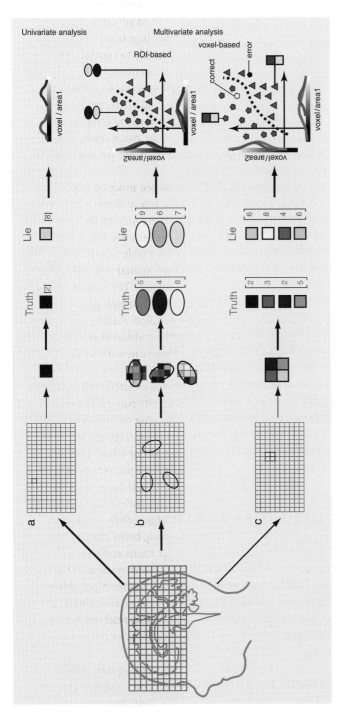

FIG. 1.1 (Also see Plate 1). Decoding mental states from brain activity using statistical pattern recognition techniques. Left: Functional magnetic resonance imaging (fMRI) uses a measurement grid of small volumes ("voxels") with a resolution of typically between 1–3mm. Each of these voxels measures changes of the oxygen content of small blood vessels that are an indicator of neural activity. In order to extract a maximum of information out of the fMRI signals, statistical pattern recognition algorithms or "decoders" are used. These decoders are given the brain activity patterns and the corresponding mental states and learn the mapping between the two. Then they are tested to see if they can correctly classify unknown mental states from their corresponding activity patterns. (a) This shows a hypothetical voxel that responds strongly when a person is lying and weakly when they are telling the truth. In this case, the decision whether the person is lying or not could be made based on the activity in this single voxel because the distributions are widely separated (far right). However, in real neuroimaging data, the responses in individual voxels are only slightly separated and thus individual voxels are not sufficient to tell truth from lie. (b) If the neurocognitive

continued

FIG. 1.1 (*continued*) correlates of deception are specific, global patterns of brain activity, then pattern recognition can be used to recognize deception by training a classifier to identify the occurrence of this pattern of brain activity. The right-hand figure shows the principle of pattern recognition using the average activity in two different brain regions as an example. The average activation values of the two individual regions can be plotted on the x-axis and y-axis yielding a number of measurement points, one for each brain pattern. Red points correspond to global patterns acquired during truthful responding and blue points correspond to global patterns acquired during deception. The decision cannot be made based on individual regions but can easily be made when taking into account the combined activation in both regions. Here the decision is made using a linear decision boundary (dashed line). A key question is, however, whether such unique signature patterns exist that are valid for different people, different situations, and different types of lies. (c) This shows a local decoding approach that can be used to reveal information stored in micro-patterns of local cortical maps (Haynes and Rees, 2006). The right hand figure shows a case where the decision boundary is non-linear. New measurements of brain activity are classified as lie or truth depending on which side of the boundary they fall (black and white symbols). Reproduced from Detecting concealed information using brain-imaging technology, Bles and Haynes, *Neurocase*. Reprinted with permission of the publisher (Taylor and Francis Group http://www/informaworld.com).

their intentions with 70% accuracy based only on their patterns of brain activity—even before they had seen the numbers and began to calculate. Because of a delay between the choice and the presentation of the numbers we were able to exclude that other neural activity, such as the actual carrying out of calculation or the preparation of the buttons to indicate the solution, was used for the prediction. In one area of the brain called the medial prefrontal cortex, we were able to read from fine-grained patterns of brain activity which intention a subject had chosen. In another experiment, we showed that such intentions could be partially predicted from brain activity even several seconds *before* a subject had consciously made up their mind (Soon *et al.* 2008).

Methodological limitations

These recent advances should not obscure the fact that scientific "mind reading" is still in its infancy. But is it only a matter of time until we can build a "universal mind reading machine"? Such a machine should be able to decode arbitrary thoughts of any person virtually in real time. Such a machine will presumably remain a pure fiction for the foreseeable future due to fundamental methodological challenges.

Limitations of measurement technology

The brain imaging technology available today does not have a sufficient resolution to allow differentiating between subtly different brain activity patterns, or their corresponding mental states. This would require increasing the spatial resolution down to around 0.5mm which is the approximate size of cortical columns (see e.g. Tanaka 1997). A cortical column is the smallest topographic unit in the neocortex and contains cells coding for similar contents. Also there are severe limitations to real-time brain reading, such as the low temporal resolution of fMRI or the large computational power required for online decoding. Furthermore, fMRI and EEG signals are contaminated by strong noise originating from limitations of the measurement technology and from physiological background signals (such as heart beat and breathing rhythms). Taken together this severely limits the currently attainable accuracy of brain reading.

Differences between subjects

Coding of the details of mental states in the brain is substantially different from person to person. This is presumably due to the fact that the development of fine-grained cortical topographies is idiosyncratic and follows principles of self-organization. Individual experiences also play an important role in shaping each person's brain topography, for example, the individual associations and connotations that are a vital component of most thoughts. For this reason it is currently very difficult to learn to read the fine-grained details of one person's thoughts by training an algorithm on data from another subject.

Reading arbitrary thoughts

In order to decode a person's thoughts it would be necessary to know how they are encoded in that individual person's brain. Currently, it is not possible to directly "read" the "language" of the brain, that is, to identify mental states based on a systematic *interpretation* of the corresponding brain states. For this reason the mapping from brain activity patterns to thoughts is learned for each specific subject using brute force statistical pattern recognition techniques. This can be thought of like a dictionary that translates brain activity patterns into the corresponding thoughts (Figure 1.2, a). In order to read out a specific thought there has to be an entry in the dictionary, and each entry has to be painstakingly learned by getting a person to think the thought, after which the concurrent brain activity is measured. Obviously this is only possible for a very limited number of mental states. There are first approaches that show how a few simple calibration measurements can be used to read out a large number of simple percepts and even concepts (Kay *et al.* 2008; Mitchell *et al.* 2008). If the brain activity patterns for several mental states are known, it is possible to partially recover other mental states as well, based on interpolation. For example, it might be possible to infer the pattern for "motorbike" by averaging the patterns for "car" and "bicycle" (Figure 1.2, b). Such interpolation can provide a surprisingly powerful approximation; however, it will break down where the relevant mental state violates principles of linearity and compositionality.

Learning and plasticity

Currently, decoding approaches assume a static relationship between thoughts and brain activation patterns. So it remains unclear how to account for the continuous learning and

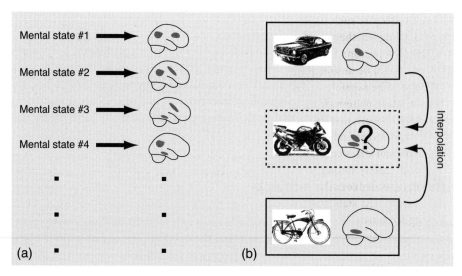

FIG. 1.2 (Also see Plate 2). A major challenge in brain reading is to learn how to decode a possibly infinite number of arbitrary mental states despite only being able to measure the brain activity patterns corresponding to a few thoughts. a) The simplest approach is a look-up table where the brain activity pattern is listed for a number of mental states that have been measured. The problem is that it is virtually impossible to measure the patterns corresponding to all potential thoughts a person might have. b) The way out is to learn to exploit the systematic relationships between different thoughts. If the brain activity patterns for "cars" and "bicycles" are known, then decoding of a "motorcycle" might be possible based on the notion that it is a concept that is "half way" between a car and a bicycle and thus it might have a brain activity pattern that is the average between that of a car and a bicycle. It has been shown that similar basic principles can be extended to many mental states (Kay *et al.* 2008; Mitchell *et al.* 2008).

the change of connotations that are likely to occur throughout the lifespan. For example, the associations that a child and an adult might have with the term "favorite movie" are likely to be quite different. Despite the large body of research on learning and plasticity, currently only little is known about how this affects the decodability of mental states.

APPLICATIONS

For the above mentioned reasons, it is not likely that we can expect a "universal thought reading machine" in the near future, that is, a machine that reads out the mental states of an arbitrary person with high accuracy, online, and without requiring long calibration. However, it is important to note that very powerful commercial applications do not necessarily require such universal thought reading. For example, the identification of a lie requires telling whether a person is lying or not, which is a binary decision. A detailed reconstruction of a person's thoughts (i.e. why they are lying, what they are thinking while they are lying) might be desirable, but is not essential for detection of deception. Importantly, it also seems to be possible to detect deception in one person by using a decoder trained on brain activation patterns from a group of other people. So it should be possible to develop a lie detector that can then be used on a large number of suspects without requiring calibration on each individual. For many similar applications it would be sufficient to classify a person's mental states coarsely. The brain activity patterns for such coarse classification are also approximately similar from person to person. So it is likely that brain reading applications will be available earlier than the advent of a universal thought reading machine in the distant future. The state of the art of two applications of brain reading are outlined in the following sections.

Lie detection

The classical approach to lie detection uses polygraphy, a technique that measures a number of physiological indicators of *peripheral arousal* in parallel, such as skin conductance, heart rate, and respiration rate. The idea is that a person who is lying is highly aroused and thus the peripheral indicators of this arousal will reveal on which question they are lying. Interestingly, polygraphy is indeed reliable when applied to naïve subjects. The problem of classical polygraphy is that it uses arousal as a physiological marker of deception, but arousal can be affected by other mental factors (such as general anxiety) or by deliberate manipulation. For example, it has been repeatedly shown that subjects can deliberately and selectively control their level of arousal in polygraph tests. Instructions on how to do this are freely available on the Internet. Therefore, manipulation of polygraphy results by trained subjects cannot be excluded and the validity of the tests remains doubtful.

An alternative to the measurement of peripheral arousal lies in *brain-based* lie detection (reviewed in Bles and Haynes 2008). The idea is to directly reveal the cognitive processes involved in the generation of a lie. FMRI (and possibly EEG) signals are measured while a test subject is lying in a scanner answering questions related to the crime. A similar approach is to use fMRI and EEG signals to reveal that a subject covertly recognizes crime-related material. Current research shows that EEG and fMRI can be used to detect deception accurately in artificial laboratory settings, where, for example, subjects are asked to lie about whether they have previously been exposed to specific playing cards. However, these laboratory experiments are still far from what would be required in real-world lie detection. Detection of artificial laboratory lies gives no clear indication as to whether a lie could be detected during a criminal investigation. The laboratory situations differ from the real world in a number of important parameters, such as the motivation of the subjects, the personality characteristics of the study sample, and the reward/punishment value of the anticipated consequences. So, although fMRI-based lie detection certainly represents a technical improvement and has considerable development potential, it still awaits clear validation in real-world settings under field conditions.

An important question is the degree to which polygraphy and brain-based lie detection can be *manipulated* by trained subjects. The brain-based approach is presumably more difficult to manipulate due to the difficulty of deliberately obtaining a specific brain activation pattern, whereas it is easier to achieving a specific level of arousal. This would suggest that brain-based lie detection is more reliable. On the other hand, brain-based lie detection requires cooperation by the subject because even the smallest movements inside the scanner make fMRI signals unusable. Thus, fMRI-based lie detection is promising, but still in development. It seems imperative to formulate clear standards of practice before commencement of commercial lie detection applications for which hard scientific evidence from real-world applications is currently not available.

Neuromarketing

Another future application of brain reading technology is so-called "neuromarketing," such as the prediction of consumer behavior from brain activity for optimization of products and advertising. In recent years this area has received tremendous interest and there were repeated attempts to optimize marketing campaigns by adding brain-based sources of information. For neuromarketing applications it is also not necessary to await the development of a universal thought reading machine. Similar to lie detection, many powerful applications would be possible even with a simple binary decoding scheme, such as predicting whether a person is likely to purchase a product or not, or whether a product is experienced pleasant or unpleasant.

Neuromarketing focuses mainly on reward-related brain regions, such as the nucleus accumbens or the orbitofrontal cortex, that are believed to play a key role in governing consumer choices. For example, if one product evokes a higher response in nucleus accumbens this would be seen as an indicator of a desire ("craving") for the product. Importantly, reward-related brain regions are anatomically easy to identify and thus are in predictable positions. This allows development of a technique on one group of subjects which can then be applied to another group of subjects. But although the link from activity in reward-related brain regions to preference is very plausible, further research is still needed to exclude other potential causes of increased brain responses. For example, responses in the nucleus accumbens are also increased by the prominence or "salience" of objects. This means that the activity in this region does not uniquely signify the valence of products. This highlights the pitfall of invalid "reverse inference" (Poldrack 2006). Just because a brain region B is always active during a specific mental state M, this doesn't mean that the presence of activity in B implies the presence of M, simply because B could be active also during other mental processes (Figure 1.3).

Usability

In addition to the feasibility of brain reading applications, their usability is an important factor that will decide on the degree to which neuroscientific technologies enter everyday life. Usability refers to how easy (or complicated) a technique is to use and how much joy (or frustration) arises when using it. Brain reading techniques still need considerable development before they are likely to enter any mass markets. One important usability factor is mobility. Only EEG and near-infrared spectroscopy are partially suitable for mobile applications.

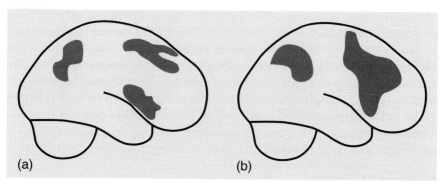

(a)   (b)

FIG. 1.3 Similarity between brain patterns characteristic for deception (a) and response inhibition (b). There are several individual brain regions in prefrontal and parietal cortex that are active in both cases. Thus, one has to be careful to avoid invalid "reverse inference" (Poldrack 2006) when inferring mental states from brain activity. Just because a brain region B is always active during a specific mental state M, this doesn't mean that the presence of B implies the presence of M, simply because B could be active also during other mental processes. However, when considering the whole brain activation pattern using pattern recognition techniques the danger of a false inference is much lower. Schematically redrawn from Spence, S. A., Farrow, T. F., Herford, A. E., *et al.* (2001). *Neuroreport*, **12**, 2849–53, Figure 1 and Blasi, G., Goldberg, T. E., Weickert, T., *et al.* (2006). *European Journal of Neuroscience*, **23**, 1658–64, Figure 1b.

In contrast, in the foreseeable future fMRI will remain a stationary technology due to the high weight of scanners and the tight security restrictions (that are in turn due to the use of strong magnetic fields). Nevertheless, certain applications do not require mobility. For example, it is not necessary to perform lie detection in real-world situations; instead a test subject can be taken to a scanner. A different constraint to usability is that the present use of EEG and fMRI is still very cumbersome. For EEG, recording electrodes must be placed in contact with the scalp and attached with a special electrode paste. This requires a substantial set-up time of up to an hour (depending on the number of electrodes). For certain applications such as neuromarketing or lie detection such difficulties might be acceptable, but for everyday applications (such as the remote control of a TV or computer using EEG) they are certainly not. In contrast, MRI is contact-free but preparation here is tedious in other ways. It involves a number of safety procedures and several exclusion criteria need to be considered due to the use of strong magnetic fields. Subjects who suffer from claustrophobia or subjects with pacemakers, brain stimulators, or certain metals in their body (e.g. surgical screws) have to be excluded. Furthermore, the procedures are not very comfortable and involve high noise levels and require the subject not to move during the measurement period of up to 1 hour.

ETHICAL ASPECTS

As outlined earlier, brain reading is an emerging technology that has strong limitations but which might allow for certain simple commercial applications within the coming years.

But should we allow commercial technologies that read a person's thoughts? As in many areas of biomedical research one is faced with a dilemma. On the one hand, new findings raise hope for improvement of clinical and technical applications. For example, BCIs can help identify residual mental processes in waking coma patients (Owen *et al.* 2006; Coleman *et al.* 2009), or can help paralyzed patients communicate with their environment or control artificial prostheses (Blankertz *et al.* 2008). Such clinical applications are likely to be uncontroversial. Other applications might, on the other hand, be viewed critically. This includes commercial applications, such as reading a product preference for marketing purposes, or measuring the attitude of job candidates towards a future employer. Several important ethical aspects are raised by brain reading, both in research and in applications.

Mental privacy It is fundamental to our self-model that our thoughts are private and cannot be read from the outside. Typically, the belief that someone could read or control my thoughts could be considered an indicator of a psychiatric condition. This means that any technical applications that can read a person's mental states must be handled with particular sensitivity because they can be used to invade a person's "mental privacy" (Farah 2005). It is important to discuss any potential consequences that would follow if a person were found to be engaged in deliberating criminal actions. We normally tend to consider it fully legal if a person thinks about committing a criminal act as long as they don't put it into action. However, what if it were possible to decode that a person was truly committed to performing a criminal offense? Should the person be stopped before they a crime? Current research shows that it should be possible tell whether a person is thinking about a specific intention, but it is not clear whether it is possible to tell whether they are truly committed to it.

Data security Most current neuroimaging research takes place in academic institutions that have strict data protection policies. With the progressive use of such technologies for commercial applications, it is foreseeable that large amounts of sensitive personal information will end up in the hands of private companies that could potentially extract critical personal information, even beyond the information for which a test was originally planned. For example, say a subject has consented to a neuromarketing study with a private company. With the advent of techniques that allow for the prediction of diseases from brain imaging recordings, the data obtained during the neuromarketing session could potentially be used to read out certain aspects of a person's medical condition. The possibility to decode such "collateral information" might not be apparent to date, but might become available with further progress of techniques for decoding of medical states from neuroimaging data (Kloppel *et al.* 2008).

Quality There are currently no guidelines that define quality standards for successful decoding of mental states. This is problematic because commercial companies are already marketing brain reading applications without a widely acknowledged scientific assessment of the validity of such techniques. There are published studies on the reliability of MRI lie detectors, but these relate to artificial laboratory situations, which do not allow to tell how well they perform in real-world scenarios. Thus, scientists need to begin defining guidelines and quality standards in this emerging field.

To summarize, modern neuroimaging techniques have made substantial progress over the last few years and now have shown that it is possible to decode a person's mental states from their brain activity. There are still many technical and methodological challenges in this field that render it highly unlikely that a universal thought reading technology will be available in the near future. But nonetheless, the first applications are beginning to emerge thus making it necessary to monitor and discuss their ethical implications.

References

Blankertz, B., Losch, F., Krauledat, M., Dornhege, G., Curio, G., and Müller, K.R. (2008). The Berlin Brain–Computer Interface: accurate performance from first-session in BCI-naïve subjects. *IEEE Transactions on Biomedical Engineering*, **55**, 2452–62.

Bles, M. and Haynes, J.D. (2008). Detecting concealed information using brain-imaging technology. *Neurocase*, **14**, 82–92.

Coleman, M.R., Davis, M.H., Rodd, J.M., *et al.* (2009). Towards the routine use of brain imaging to aid the clinical diagnosis of disorders of consciousness. *Brain*, **132**, 2541–52.

Dewan, E.M. (1967). Occipital alpha rhythm, eye position and lens accommodation. *Nature*, **214**, 975–7.

Edelman, S., Grill-Spector, K., Kushnir, T., and Malach, R. (1998). Toward direct visualization of the internal shape representation space by fMRI. *Psychobiology*, **26**, 309–21.

Farah, M.J. (2005). Neuroethics: the practical and the philosophical. *Trends in Cognitive Sciences*, **9**, 34–40.

Haynes, J.-D. (2008). Decoding the contents of visual consciousness from human brain signals. *Trends in Cognitive Sciences*, **13**, 194–202.

Haynes, J.-D. and Rees, G. (2006). Decoding mental states from brain activity in humans. *Nature Reviews Neuroscience*, **7**, 523–34.

Haynes, J.-D., Sakai, K., Rees, G., Gilbert, S., Frith, C., and Passingham, R.E. (2007). Reading hidden intentions in the human brain. *Current Biology*, **17**, 323–8.

Kay, K.N., Naselaris, T., Prenger, R.J., and Gallant, J.L. (2008). Identifying natural images from human brain activity. *Nature*, **452**, 352–5.

Kloppel, S., Stonnington, C.M., Chu, C., *et al.* (2008). Automatic classification of MR scans in Alzheimer's disease. *Brain*, **131**, 681–9.

Mitchell, T.M., Shinkareva, S.V., Carlson, A., *et al.* (2008). Predicting human brain activity associated with the meanings of nouns. *Science*, **320**, 1191–5.

Norman, K.A., Polyn, S.M., Detre, G.J., and Haxby, J.V. (2006). Beyond mind-reading: multi-voxel pattern analysis of fMRI data. *Trends in Cognitive Sciences*, **10**, 424–30.

Owen, A.M., Coleman, M.R., Boly, M., Davis, M.H., Laureys, S., and Pickard, J.D. (2006). Detecting awareness in the vegetative state. *Science*, **313**, 1402.

Poldrack, R.A. (2006). Can cognitive processes be inferred from neuroimaging data? *Trends in Cognitive Sciences*, **10**, 59–63.

Soon, C.S., Brass, M., Heinze, H.J. and Haynes, J.-D. (2008). Unconscious determinants of free decisions in the human brain. *Nature Neuroscience*, **11**, 543–5.

Tanaka, K. (1997). Mechanisms of visual object recognition: monkey and human studies. *Current Opinion in Neurobiology*, **7**, 523–9.

CHAPTER 2

....

THE NEUROBIOLOGY
OF PLEASURE AND
HAPPINESS

....

MORTEN L. KRINGELBACH AND KENT C. BERRIDGE

INTRODUCTION

HAPPINESS is an elusive state, difficult to define, and therefore challenging to measure—partly due to its clearly subjective, and perhaps uniquely human, nature. But how can one get a scientific handle on such a slippery concept?

Since Aristotle, happiness has been thought of as consisting of at least two aspects: hedonia (pleasure) and eudaimonia (a life well-lived) (Waterman 1993). In contemporary psychology these aspects are usually referred to as pleasure and meaning, and scientists have recently proposed to add a third distinct component of engagement related to feelings of commitment and participation in life (Seligman *et al.* 2005).

Using these definitions scientists have made substantial progress in defining and measuring happiness in the form of self-reports of subjective well-being (Kahneman 1999; Ryan and Deci 2001; Diener *et al.* 2003; Seligman *et al.* 2005). This research shows that while there is clearly a sharp conceptual distinction between pleasure versus engagement-meaning components, hedonic and eudaimonic aspects empirically cohere together in happy people.

For example, in happiness surveys over 80% of people rate their overall eudaimonic life satisfaction as "pretty to very happy", and comparably, 80% also rate their current hedonic mood as positive (e.g. positive 6–7 on a 10-point valence scale where 5 is hedonically neutral) (Kesebir and Diener 2008). A lucky few may even live consistently around a hedonic point of 8—although excessively higher hedonic scores may actually impede attainment of life success, as measured by riches, education, or political participation (Oishi *et al.* 2007).

While these surveys are interesting indications of mental well-being, they offer little evidence of the underlying neurobiology of happiness. In this review we will therefore focus on the substantial progress in understanding the psychology and neurobiology of sensory pleasure that has been made over the last decade (Berridge and Kringelbach 2008; Kringelbach and Berridge 2010).

These advances make the hedonic side of happiness most tractable to a scientific approach to the neural underpinnings of happiness. Supporting a hedonic approach, it has been suggested that the best measure of subjective well-being may be simply to ask people how they hedonically feel right now—again and again—so as to track their hedonic accumulation across daily life (Kahneman 2000; Diener *et al.* 2003; Gilbert and Wilson 2007). These repeated self-reports of hedonic *states* could also be used to identify more stable neurobiological hedonic brain *traits* that dispose particular individuals toward happiness. Further, a hedonic approach might even offer a toehold into identifying eudaimonic brain signatures of happiness, due to the empirical convergence between the two categories, even if pleasant mood is only half the happiness story (Kringelbach and Berridge 2009).

It is important to note that our focus on the hedonia component of happiness should not be confused with hedonism, which is the pursuit of pleasure for pleasure's own sake, and more akin to the addiction features we describe later. Also, to focus on hedonics does not deny that some ascetics may have found bliss through painful self-sacrifice, but simply reflects that positive hedonic tone is indispensable to most people seeking happiness.

A SCIENCE OF PLEASURE

The link between pleasure and happiness has a long history in psychology. It was stressed in the early writings of Sigmund Freud (Freud and Riviere 1930), when he posited that people "strive after happiness; they want to become happy and to remain so. This endeavor has two sides, a positive and a negative aim. It aims, on the one hand, at an absence of pain and displeasure, and, on the other, at the experiencing of strong feelings of pleasure" (Freud and Riviere 1930, p. 76). Emphasizing a positive balance of affect to be happy implies that studies of hedonic brain circuits can advance the neuroscience of both pleasure and happiness.

A related but slightly different view is that happiness depends most chiefly on eliminating negative "pain and displeasure" to free an individual to pursue engagement and meaning. Positive pleasure by this view is somewhat superfluous. This view may characterize the 20th century medical and clinical emphasis on alleviating negative psychopathology and strongly distressing emotions. It fits also with William James's early quip that "Happiness, I have lately discovered, is no positive feeling, but a negative condition of freedom from a number of restrictive sensations of which our organism usually seems the seat. When they are wiped out, the clearness and cleanness of the contrast is happiness. This is why anaesthetics make us so happy. But don't you take to drink on that account." (James 1920, vol 2, p. 158).

Focusing on eliminating negative distress seems to leave positive pleasure outside the boundary of happiness, perhaps as an extra bonus or even an irrelevancy for ordinary pursuit. In practice, many mixtures of positive affect and negative affect may occur in individuals (Ryff *et al.* 2006) and cultures may vary in the importance of positive versus negative affect for happiness. For example, positive emotions are linked most strongly to ratings of life satisfaction overall in nations that stress self-expression, but alleviation of negative emotions may become relatively more important in nations that value individualism (Kuppens *et al.* 2008).

By either view, psychology seems to be moving away from the stoic notion that affect states such as pleasure are simply irrelevant to happiness. The growing evidence for the importance of affect in psychology and neuroscience shows that a scientific account will have to involve hedonic pleasures and/or displeasures. To move towards a neuroscience of happiness, a neurobiological understanding is required of how positive and negative affect are balanced in the brain.

Given the potential contributions of hedonics to happiness, we now survey developments in understanding brain mechanisms of pleasure (Berridge and Kringelbach 2008; Leknes and Tracey 2008). The scientific study of pleasure and affect was foreshadowed by the pioneering ideas of Charles Darwin, who examined the evolution of emotions and affective expressions, and suggested that these are adaptive responses to environmental situations. In that vein, pleasure "liking" and displeasure reactions are prominent affective reactions in the behavior and brains of all mammals (Steiner *et al.* 2001), and likely had important evolutionary functions (Kringelbach 2009). Neural mechanisms for generating affective reactions are present and similar in most mammalian brains, and thus appear to have been selected for and conserved across species (Kringelbach 2010). Indeed, both positive affect and negative affect are recognized today as having adaptive functions (Nesse 2004), and positive affect in particular has consequences in daily life for planning and building cognitive and emotional resources (Fredrickson *et al.* 2008; Dickinson and Balleine 2010).

Such functional perspectives suggest that affective reactions may have objective features beyond subjective ones (Kringelbach 2004a). Progress in affective neuroscience has been made recently by identifying objective aspects of pleasure reactions and triangulating toward underlying brain substrates. This scientific strategy divides the concept of affect into two parts: the *affective state*, which has objective aspects in behavioral, physiological, and neural reactions; and *conscious affective feelings*, seen as the subjective experience of emotion (Kringelbach 2004a). Note that such a definition allows conscious feelings to play a central role in hedonic experiences, but holds that the affective essence of a pleasure reaction is more than a conscious feeling.

Evidence so far available suggests that brain mechanisms involved in *fundamental* pleasures (food and sexual pleasures) overlap with those for *higher-order pleasures* (for example, monetary, artistic, musical, altruistic, and transcendent pleasures) (Small *et al.* 2001; Kahneman *et al.* 2004; Kringelbach 2005; Peciña *et al.* 2006; Gottfried 2010; Kringelbach 2010; Kringelbach *et al.* 2010; Veldhuizen *et al.* 2010).

From sensory pleasures and drugs of abuse (Robinson and Berridge 2003) to monetary, aesthetic, and musical delights, all pleasures seem to involve the same hedonic brain systems, even when linked to anticipation and memory (Skov 2010; Vuust and Kringelbach 2010). Pleasures important to happiness, such as socializing with friends (Kahneman 1999; Ryan and Deci 2001; Diener *et al.* 2003; Kahneman *et al.* 2004; Seligman *et al.* 2005), and related traits of positive hedonic mood are thus all likely to draw upon the same neurobiological roots that evolved for sensory pleasures. The neural overlap may offer a way to generalize from fundamental pleasures that are best understood and so infer larger hedonic brain principles likely to contribute to happiness.

We note the rewarding properties for all pleasures are likely to be generated by hedonic brain circuits that are distinct from the mediation of other features of the same events (e.g. sensory, cognitive) (Kringelbach 2005). Thus pleasure is never merely a sensation or a thought (Frijda 2010), but is instead an additional hedonic gloss generated by the brain via dedicated systems.

The neuroanatomy of pleasure

How does positive affect arise? Affective neuroscience research on sensory pleasure has revealed many networks of brain regions and neurotransmitters activated by pleasant events and states (Figures 2.1 and 2.2). Identification of hedonic substrates has been advanced by recognizing that pleasure or "liking" is but one component in the larger composite psychological process of reward, which also involves "wanting" and "learning" components (Smith *et al.* 2010). Each component also has conscious and non-conscious elements that can be studied in humans—and at least the latter can also be probed in other animals.

Hedonic hotspots

Despite having an extensive distribution of reward-related circuitry, the brain appears rather frugal in "liking" mechanisms that cause pleasure reactions. As shown in later paragraphs, some hedonic mechanisms are found deep in the brain (nucleus accumbens, ventral pallidum, brainstem) and other candidates are in the cortex (orbitofrontal, cingulate, medial prefrontal, and insular cortices) (Berridge 1996; Cardinal *et al.* 2002; Kringelbach *et al.* 2003; Kringelbach and Rolls 2004; Everitt and Robbins 2005; Amodio and Frith 2006; Kringelbach 2010; Watson *et al.* 2010). Pleasure-activated brain networks are widespread, but compelling evidence for pleasure causation (detected as increases in "liking" reactions consequent to brain manipulation) has so far been found for only a few hedonic hotspots in the subcortical structures. Each hotspot is merely a cubic millimeter or so in volume in the rodent brain (and should be a cubic centimeter or so in humans, if proportional to whole brain volume). Hotspots are capable of generating enhancements of "liking" reactions to a sensory pleasure such as sweetness, when stimulated with opioid, endocannabinoid, or other neurochemical modulators (Smith *et al.* 2010).

Hotspots exist in nucleus accumbens shell and ventral pallidum, and possibly other forebrain and limbic cortical regions, and also in deep brainstem regions including the parabrachial nucleus in the pons (Figure 2.2d) (Peciña *et al.* 2006). The pleasure-generating capacity of these hotspots has been revealed in part by studies in which microinjections of drugs stimulated neurochemical receptors on neurons within a hotspot, and caused a doubling or tripling of the number of hedonic "liking" reactions normally elicited by a pleasant sucrose taste (Smith *et al.* 2010). Analogous to scattered islands that form a single archipelago, hedonic hotspots are anatomically distributed but interact to form a functional integrated circuit. The circuit obeys control rules that are largely hierarchical and organized into brain levels. Top levels function together as a cooperative heterarchy, so that, for example, multiple unanimous "votes" in favor from simultaneously-participating hotspots in the nucleus accumbens and ventral pallidum are required for opioid stimulation in either forebrain site to enhance "liking" above normal (Smith and Berridge 2007).

In addition, as mentioned earlier, pleasure is translated into motivational processes in part by activating a second component of reward termed "wanting" or incentive salience, which makes stimuli attractive when attributed to them by mesolimbic brain systems (Berridge and Robinson 2003). Incentive salience depends in particular on mesolimbic

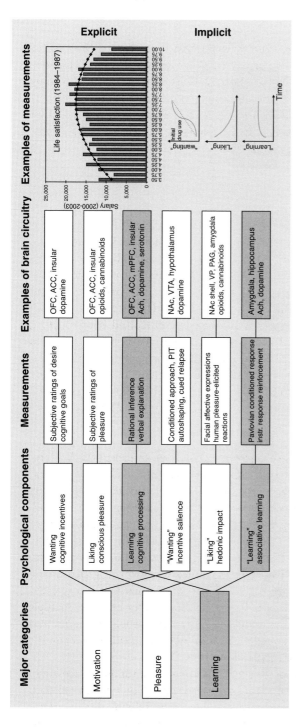

FIG. 2.1 Measuring reward and hedonia. Reward and pleasure are multifaceted psychological concepts. Major processes within reward (first column) consist of motivation or wanting (white), learning (gray), and—most relevant to happiness—pleasure liking or affect (light gray). Each of these contains explicit (top three rows) and implicit (bottom three rows) psychological components (second column) that constantly interact and require careful scientific experimentation to tease apart. Explicit processes are consciously experienced (e.g. explicit pleasure and happiness, desire, or expectation), whereas implicit psychological processes are potentially unconscious in the sense that they can operate at a level not always directly accessible to conscious experience (implicit incentive salience, habits and "liking" reactions), and must be further translated by other mechanisms into subjective feelings. Measurements or behavioral procedures that are especially sensitive markers of the each of the processes are listed (third column). Examples of some of the brain regions and neurotransmitters are listed (fourth column), as well as specific examples of measurements (fifth column), such as an example of how highest subjective life satisfaction does not lead to the highest salaries (top) (Haisken-De New and Frick 2005). Another example shows the incentive-sensitization model of addiction and how "wanting" to take drugs may grow over time independently of "liking" and "learning" drug pleasure as an individual becomes an addict (bottom) (Robinson and Berridge 1993). ACC, anterior cingulate cortex; Ach, acetylcholine; OFC, orbitofrontal cortex; mPFC, medial *prefrontal* cortex; NAc, nucleus accumbens; PAG, periaqueductal gray; VP, ventral pallidum; VTA, ventral tegmental area.

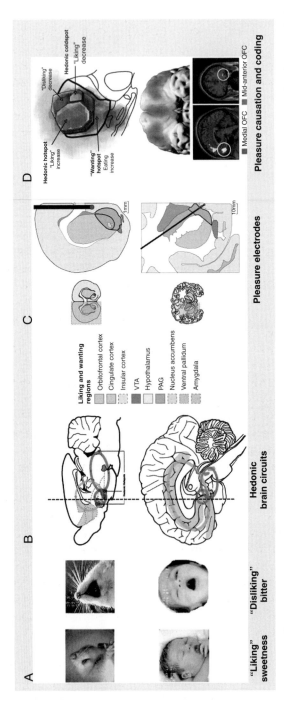

FIG.2.2 (Also see Plate 2). Hedonic brain circuitry. The schematic figure shows the brain regions for causing and coding fundamental pleasure in rodents and humans. (a) Facial "liking" and "disliking" expressions elicited by sweet and bitter taste are similar in rodents and human infants. (b, d) Pleasure causation has been identified in rodents as arising from interlinked subcortical hedonic hotspots, such as in nucleus accumbens and ventral pallidum, where neural activation may increase "liking" expressions to sweetness. Similar pleasure coding and incentive salience networks have also been identified in humans. (c) The so-called "pleasure" electrodes in rodents and humans are unlikely to have elicited true pleasure but perhaps only incentive salience or "wanting." (d) The cortical localization of pleasure coding may reach an apex in various regions of the orbitofrontal cortex, which differentiate subjective pleasantness from valence processing of aspects of the same stimulus, such as a pleasant food. PAG, periaqueductal gray; VTA, ventral tegmental area.

dopamine neurotransmission (though other neurotransmitters and structures also are involved).

Importantly, incentive salience is not hedonic impact or pleasure "liking" (Berridge 2007). This is why an individual can "want" a reward without necessarily "liking" the same reward. Irrational "wanting" without liking can occur especially in addiction via incentive-sensitization of the mesolimbic dopamine system and connected structures (Robinson and Berridge 2003). At extreme, the addict may come to "want" what is neither "liked" nor expected to be liked, a dissociation possible because "wanting" mechanisms are largely subcortical and separable from cortically-mediated declarative expectation and conscious planning. This is a reason why addicts may compulsively "want" to take drugs even if, at a more cognitive and conscious level, they do not want to do so. That is surely a recipe for great unhappiness (Figure 2.2, bottom right).

Cortical pleasure

In cortex, hedonic evaluation of pleasure valence is anatomically distinguishable from precursor operations such as sensory computations, suggesting the existence of a hedonic cortex proper (Figure 2.2) (Kringelbach 2004b). Hedonic cortex involves regions such as the orbitofrontal (Kringelbach 2005), insula (Craig 2002), medial prefrontal (Amodio and Frith 2006), and cingulate cortices (Beckmann *et al.* 2009), which a wealth of human neuroimaging studies have shown to code for hedonic evaluations (including anticipation, appraisal, experience, and memory of pleasurable stimuli) and have close anatomical links to subcortical hedonic hotspots. It is important, however, to again make a distinction between brain activity *coding* and *causing* pleasure. Neural *coding* is inferred in practice by measuring brain *activity correlated to a pleasant stimulus*, using human neuroimaging techniques (Gottfried 2010), or electrophysiological or neurochemical activation measures in animals (Aldridge and Berridge 2010). Causation is generally inferred on the basis of a *change* in pleasure as a *consequence of a brain manipulation* such as a lesion or stimulation (Green *et al.* 2010; Smith *et al.* 2010). Coding and causation often go together for the same substrate, but they may diverge so that coding occurs alone.

Pleasure encoding may reach an apex of cortical localization in a mid-anterior subregion within the orbitofrontal cortex, where neuroimaging activity correlates strongly to subjective pleasantness ratings of food varieties (Kringelbach *et al.* 2003)—and to other pleasures such as sexual orgasms (Georgiadis *et al.* 2006), drugs (Völlm *et al.* 2004), chocolate (Small *et al.* 2001), and music (Blood and Zatorre 2001). Most importantly, mid-anterior orbitofrontal activity tracks changes in subjective pleasure, such as a decline in palatability when the reward value of one food was reduced by eating it to satiety (while remaining high to another food) (Kringelbach 2005)ʼ (Kringelbach *et al.* 2003). The mid-anterior subregion of orbitofrontal cortex is thus a prime candidate for the coding of subjective experience of pleasure (Kringelbach 2005).

Another coding site for positive hedonics in orbitofrontal cortex is along its medial edge that has activity related to the positive and negative valence of affective events (Kringelbach and Rolls 2004), contrasted to lateral portions that have been suggested to code unpleasant events (O'Doherty *et al.* 2001) (although lateral activity may reflect a signal to escape the situation, rather than displeasure per se (Iversen and Mishkin 1970; Kringelbach and

Rolls 2003; Hornak *et al.* 2004; Kringelbach and Rolls 2004)). This medial–lateral hedonic gradient interacts with an abstraction–concreteness gradient in the posterior–anterior dimension, so that more complex or abstract reinforcers (such as monetary gain and loss) (O'Doherty *et al.* 2001) are represented more anteriorly in the orbitofrontal cortex than less complex sensory rewards (such as taste) (Small *et al.* 2001). The medial region that codes pleasant sensations does not, however, appear to change its activity with reinforcer devaluation, and so may not reflect the full dynamics of pleasure.

Other cortical regions implicated in coding for pleasant stimuli include parts of the mid-insular (Craig 2009) and anterior cingulate cortices (Beckmann *et al.* 2009). As yet, however, it is not as clear as for the orbitofrontal cortex whether those regions specifically code pleasure or only emotion more generally (Feldman Barrett and Wager 2006). A related suggestion has emerged that the frontal left hemisphere plays a special lateralized role in positive affect more than the right hemisphere (Davidson and Irwin 1999), though how to reconcile left-positive findings with many other findings of bilateral activations of orbitofrontal and related cortical regions during hedonic processing remains an ongoing puzzle (Kringelbach 2005).

It remains still unknown, however, if mid-anterior orbitofrontal cortex or medial orbitofrontal cortex or any other cortical region actually causes a positive pleasure state. Clearly, damage to orbitofrontal cortex does impair pleasure-related decisions, including choices and context-related cognitions in humans, monkeys, and rats (Butter *et al.* 1963; Nauta 1971; Baylis and Gaffan 1991; Anderson *et al.* 1999; Baxter *et al.* 2000; Beer *et al.* 2003; Hornak *et al.* 2003; Pickens *et al.* 2003, 2005). But some caution regarding whether cortex generates positive affect states per se is indicated by the consideration that patients with lesions to the orbitofrontal cortex do still react normally to many pleasures, although sometimes showing inappropriate emotions (Damasio 1996; Anderson *et al.* 1999; Beer *et al.* 2003; Hornak *et al.* 2003). Hedonic capacity after prefrontal damage has not, however, yet been studied in careful enough detail (e.g. using selective satiation paradigms (Kringelbach *et al.* 2003)), and it would be useful to have more information on the role of orbitofrontal cortex, insular cortex, and cingulate cortex in generating and modulating hedonic states.

Pleasure causation has been so far rather difficult to assess in humans given the limits of information from lesion studies, and the correlative nature of neuroimaging studies. A promising tool, however, is deep brain stimulation (DBS) which is a versatile and reversible technique that directly alters brain activity in a brain target and where the ensuing whole-brain activity can be measured with magnetoencephalography (MEG) (Kringelbach *et al.* 2007b). Pertinent to a view of happiness as freedom from distress, at least pain relief can be obtained from DBS of periaqueductal gray in the brainstem in humans (Gildenberg 2005), where specific neural signatures of pain have been found (Green *et al.* 2009), and where the pain relief is associated with activity in the mid-anterior orbitofrontal cortex, perhaps involving endogenous opioid release (Kringelbach *et al.* 2007a). Similarly, DBS may alleviate some unpleasant symptoms of depression, though without actually producing positive affect.

Famously, also, pleasure electrodes were reported to exist decades ago in animals and humans when implanted in subcortical structures including the nucleus accumbens, septum, and medial forebrain bundle (Olds and Milner 1954; Heath 1972) (Figure 2.2c). However, recently we and others have questioned whether most such electrodes truly caused pleasure, or instead, only a psychological process more akin to "wanting" without "liking"

(Berridge and Kringelbach 2008). In our view, it still remains unknown whether DBS causes true pleasure, or if so, where in the brain electrodes produce it.

Loss of pleasure

The lack of pleasure, anhedonia, is one of the most important symptoms of many mental illnesses including depression. It is difficult to conceive of anyone reporting happiness or well-being while so deprived of pleasure. Thus anhedonia is another potential avenue of evidence for the link between pleasure and happiness (Gorwood 2008).

The brain regions necessary for pleasure—but disrupted in anhedonia—are not yet clear. Core "liking" reactions to sensory pleasures appear relatively difficult to abolish absolutely in animals by a single brain lesion or drug, which may be very good in evolutionary terms. Only the ventral pallidum has emerged among brain hedonic hotspots as a site where damage fully abolishes the capacity for positive hedonic reaction in rodent studies, replacing even "liking" for sweetness with "disliking" gapes normally reserved for bitter or similarly noxious tastes (Cromwell and Berridge 1993; Aldridge and Berridge 2010). Interestingly, there are extensive connections from the ventral pallidum to the medial orbitofrontal cortex (Öngür and Price 2000).

On the basis of this evidence, the ventral pallidum might also be linked to human anhedonia. This brain region has not yet been directly surgically targeted by clinicians but there is anecdotal evidence that some patients with pallidotomies (of nearby globus pallidus, just above and behind the ventral pallidum) for Parkinson's patients show flattened affect (Parkin *et al.* 2002) (T. Z. Aziz, personal communication), and stimulation of globus pallidus internus may help with depression (Kosel *et al.* 2007). A case study has also reported anhedonia following bilateral lesion to the ventral pallidum (Miller *et al.* 2006).

Alternatively, core "liking" for fundamental pleasures might persist intact but unacknowledged in anhedonia, while instead only more cognitive construals, including retrospective or anticipatory savoring, becomes impaired. That is, fundamental pleasure may not be abolished in depression after all. Instead, what is called anhedonia might be secondary to motivational deficits and cognitive misappraisals of rewards, or to an overlay of negative affective states. This may still disrupt life enjoyment, and perhaps render higher pleasures impossible.

Other potential regions targeted by DBS to help with depression and anhedonia include the nucleus accumbens (Schlaepfer *et al.* 2008) and the subgenual cingulate cortex (Mayberg *et al.* 2005). In addition, lesions of the posterior part of the anterior cingulate cortex have been used for the treatment of depression with some success (Steele *et al.* 2008).

Bridging pleasure to meaning

It is potentially interesting to note that all these structures either have close links with frontal cortical structures in the hedonic network (e.g. nucleus accumbens and ventral pallidum) or belong to what has been termed the brain's default network which changes over early development (Fransson *et al.* 2007; Fair *et al.* 2008) (Figure 2.3).

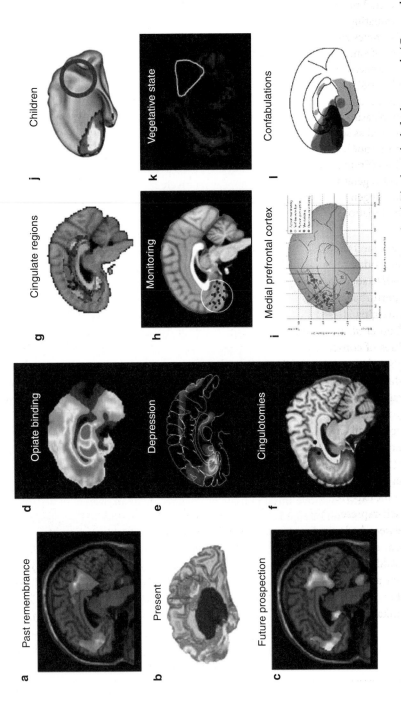

FIG. 2.3 (Also see Plate 3). The brain's default network and eudaimonic–hedonic interaction. (a–c) The brain's default network (Gusnard and Raichle 2001; Addis *et al.* 2007) has been linked to self-awareness, remembering the past and prospecting the future (Addis *et al.* 2007). Some components overlap with pleasure networks, including midline structures such as the orbitofrontal, medial prefrontal, and cingulate cortices.

FIG. 2.3 (*continued*) We wonder whether happiness might include a role for the default network, or for related neural circuits that contribute to computing relations between self and others, in evaluating eudaimonic meaning and interacting with hedonic circuits of positive affect. Examples show (d) key regions of the default network such as the anterior cingulate and orbitofrontal cortices that have a high density of opiate receptors (Willoch *et al.* 2004), (e) have been linked to depression (Drevets *et al.* 1997), and (f) its surgical treatment (Steele *et al.* 2008). (g) Subregional localization of function may be indicated by connectivity analyses of cingulate cortex (Beckmann *et al.* 2009) and related structures, (h) important in pleasure-related monitoring, learning, and memory (Kringelbach and Rolls 2004), (i) as well as self-knowledge, person perception, and other cognitive functions (Amodio and Frith 2006). (j) The default network may change over early life in children and pre-term babies (Fransson *et al.* 2007; Fair *et al.* 2008), (k) in pathological states including depression and vegetative states (Laureys *et al.* 2004), (l) and after lesions to its medial orbitofrontal and subgenual cingulate cortices that disrupt reality monitoring and create spontaneous confabulations (Schnider 2003).

Mention of the default network brings us back to the topic of eudaimonic happiness, and to potential interactions of hedonic brain circuits with circuits that assess meaningful relationships of self to social others. The default network is a steady-state circuit of the brain which becomes perturbed during cognitive tasks (Gusnard and Raichle 2001). Most pertinent here is an emerging literature that has proposed the default network to carry representations of self (Lou *et al.* 1999), internal modes of cognition (Buckner *et al.* 2008), and perhaps even states of consciousness (Laureys *et al.* 2004). Such functions might well be important to higher pleasures as well as meaningful aspects of happiness.

Although highly speculative, we wonder whether the default network might deserve further consideration for a role in connecting eudaimonic and hedonic happiness. At least, key regions of the frontal default network overlap with the hedonic network discussed earlier, such as the anterior cingulate and orbitofrontal cortices (Kringelbach and Rolls 2004; Amodio and Frith 2006; Steele *et al.* 2008; Beckmann *et al.* 2009), and have a relatively high density of opiate receptors (Willoch *et al.* 2004). And activity changes in the frontal default network, such as in the subgenual cingulate and orbitofrontal cortices, correlate to pathological changes in subjective hedonic experience, such as in depressed patients (Drevets *et al.* 1997).

Pathological self-representations by the frontal default network could also provide a potential link between hedonic distortions of happiness that are accompanied by eudaimonic dissatisfaction, such as in cognitive rumination of depression (Williams *et al.* 1996; Schnider 2003; Addis *et al.* 2007). Conversely, mindfulness-based cognitive therapy for depression, which aims to disengage from dysphoria-activated depressogenic thinking, might conceivably recruit default network circuitry to help mediate improvement in happiness via a linkage to hedonic circuitry (Teasdale *et al.* 2000).

CONCLUDING REMARKS

The most difficult questions facing pleasure and happiness research remain the nature of its subjective experience and the relation of hedonic components (pleasure or positive affect) to eudaimonic components (cognitive appraisals of meaning and life satisfaction). While some progress has been made in understanding brain hedonics, it is important not to over-interpret. In particular we have still not made substantial progress towards understanding the functional neuroanatomy of happiness.

In this review we have, however, identified a number of brain regions that are important in the brain's hedonic networks, and speculated on potential interaction with eudaimonic networks. While it remains unclear how pleasure and happiness are exactly linked, it may be safe to say at least that the pathological lack of pleasure, in anhedonia or dysphoria, amounts to a formidable obstacle to happiness.

In social animals like humans, social interactions with conspecifics are fundamental and central to enhancing the other pleasures. Humans are intensely social, and data indicate that one of the most important factors for happiness is social relationships with other people. Social pleasures may still include vital sensory features such as visual faces, touch features of grooming and caress, as well as in humans more abstract and cognitive features of social reward and relationship evaluation (Adolphs 2003).

In particular, adult pair bonds and attachment bonds between parents and infants are likely to be extremely important for the survival of the species (Kringelbach *et al.* 2008). The breakdown of these bonds is all too common and can lead to great unhappiness. And even bond formation can potentially disrupt happiness, such as in transient parental depression after birth of an infant (in over 10% of mothers and approximately 3% of fathers (Cooper and Murray 1998)). Progress in understanding the hedonics of social bonds could be useful in understanding happiness.

Social neuroscience is beginning to unravel some of the complex dynamics of human social interactions. One of its major challenges is to map the developmental changes in reward processing over a lifespan. Another challenge is to understand how brain networks underlying fundamental pleasure relate to higher pleasures such as music, dance, play and flow, and to happiness.

Further, so far as positive affect contributes to happiness, then considerable progress has been made in understanding the neurobiology of pleasure in ways that might be relevant. For example, we can imagine several possibilities to relate happiness to particular hedonic psychological processes discussed previously. Thus, one way to conceive of hedonic happiness is as "liking" without "wanting." That is, a state of pleasure without disruptive desires, a state of contentment (Kringelbach 2009). Another possibility is that moderate "wanting" matched to positive "liking" facilitates engagement with the world. A little incentive salience may add zest to the perception of life and perhaps even promote the construction of meaning, just as in some patients DBS may help lift the veil of depression by making life events more appealing. However, too much "wanting" can readily spiral into maladaptive patterns such as addiction, and is a direct route to great unhappiness. Finally, happiness might spring from higher pleasures, positive appraisals of life meaning, and social connectedness, all combined and merged by interaction between the brain's default networks and pleasure networks. Achieving the right hedonic balance in such ways may be crucial to keep one not just ticking over but perhaps even happy.

Future scientific advances may provide a better sorting of psychological features of happiness and its underlying brain networks. If so, it remains a distinct possibility that more among us may be one day shifted into a better situation to enjoy daily events, to find life meaningful and worth living—and perhaps even to achieve a degree of bliss.

ACKNOWLEDGMENTS

We thank Christopher Peterson, Eric Jackson, Kristine Rømer Thomsen, Christine Parsons, and Katie Young for helpful comments on an earlier version of this manuscript. Our research has been supported by grants from the TrygFonden Charitable Foundation to MLK and from the NIMH and NIDA to KCB. This chapter is based on a previously published article.

REFERENCES

Addis, D.R., Wong, A.T., and Schacter, D.L. (2007). Remembering the past and imagining the future: common and distinct neural substrates during event construction and elaboration. *Neuropsychologia, 45,* 1363–77.

Adolphs, R. (2003). Cognitive neuroscience of human social behaviour. *Nature Reviews Neuroscience, 4,* 165–78.

Aldridge, J.W. and Berridge, K.C. (2010). Neural coding of pleasure: "rose-tinted glasses" of the ventral pallidum. In M.L. Kringelbach, and K.C. Berridge (eds.) *Pleasures of the Brain,* pp. 62–73. New York: Oxford University Press.

Amodio, D.M. and Frith, C.D. (2006). Meeting of minds: the medial frontal cortex and social cognition. *Nature Reviews Neuroscience, 7,* 268–77.

Anderson, S.W., Bechara, A., Damasio, H., Tranel, D., and Damasio, A.R. (1999). Impairment of social and moral behavior related to early damage in human prefrontal cortex. *Nature Neuroscience, 2,* 1032–7.

Baxter, M.G., Parker, A., Lindner, C.C., Izquierdo, A.D., and Murray, E.A. (2000). Control of response selection by reinforcer value requires interaction of amygdala and orbital prefrontal cortex. *Journal of Neuroscience, 20,* 4311–19.

Baylis, L.L. and Gaffan, D. (1991). Amygdalectomy and ventromedial prefrontal ablation produce similar deficits in food choice and in simple object discrimination learning for an unseen reward. *Experimental Brain Research, 86,* 617–22.

Beckmann, M., Johansen-Berg, H., and Rushworth, M.F. (2009). Connectivity-based parcellation of human cingulate cortex and its relation to functional specialization. *Journal of Neuroscience, 29,* 1175–90.

Beer, J.S., Heerey, E.A., Keltner, D., Scabini, D., and Knight, R.T. (2003). The regulatory function of self-conscious emotion: insights from patients with orbitofrontal damage. *Journal of Personality and Social Psychology, 85,* 594–604.

Berridge, K. (2007). The debate over dopamine's role in reward: the case for incentive salience. *Psychopharmacology, 191,* 391–431.

Berridge, K.C. (1996). Food reward: brain substrates of wanting and liking. *Neuroscience and Biobehavioral Reviews, 20,* 1–25.

Berridge, K.C. and Kringelbach, M.L. (2008). Affective neuroscience of pleasure: Reward in humans and animals. *Psychopharmacology, 199,* 457–80.

Berridge, K.C. and Robinson, T.E. (2003). Parsing reward. *Trends in Neurosciences, 26,* 507–13.

Blood, A.J. and Zatorre, R.J. (2001). Intensely pleasurable responses to music correlate with activity in brain regions implicated in reward and emotion. *Proceedings of the National Academy of Sciences of the United States of America, 98,* 11818–23.

Buckner, R.L., Andrews-Hanna, J.R., and Schacter, D.L. (2008). The brain's default network: anatomy, function, and relevance to disease. *Annals of the New York Academy of Sciences*, **1124**, 1–38.

Butter, C.M., Mishkin, M., and Rosvold, H.E. (1963). Conditioning and extinction of a food-rewarded response after selective ablations of frontal cortex in rhesus monkeys. *Experimental Neurology*, **7**, 65–75.

Cardinal, R.N., Parkinson, J.A., Hall, J., and Everitt, B.J. (2002). Emotion and motivation: the role of the amygdala, ventral striatum, and prefrontal cortex. *Neuroscience and Biobehavioral Reviews*, **26**, 321–52.

Cooper, P.J. and Murray, L. (1998). Postnatal depression. *British Medical Journal*, **316**, 1884–6.

Craig, A.D. (2002). Opinion: How do you feel? Interoception: the sense of the physiological condition of the body. *Nature Reviews Neuroscience*, **3**, 655–66.

Craig, A.D. (2009). How do you feel—now? The anterior insula and human awareness. *Nature Reviews Neuroscience*, **10**, 59–70.

Cromwell, H.C. and Berridge, K.C. (1993). Where does damage lead to enhanced food aversion: the ventral pallidum/substantia innominata or lateral hypothalamus? *Brain Research*, **624**, 1–10.

Damasio, A.R. (1996). The somatic marker hypothesis and the possible functions of the prefrontal cortex. *Philosophical Transactions of the Royal Society B: Biological Sciences*, **351**, 1413–20.

Davidson, R.J. and Irwin, W. (1999). The functional neuroanatomy of emotion and affective style. *Trends in Cognitive Science*, **3**, 11–21.

Dickinson, A. and Balleine, B. (2010). Hedonics: the cognitive–motivational interface. In M.L. Kringelbach and K.C. Berridge (eds.) *Pleasures of the Brain*, pp. 74–84. New York: Oxford University Press.

Diener, E., Oishi, S., and Lucas, R.E. (2003). Personality, culture, and subjective well-being: emotional and cognitive evaluations of life. *Annual Reviews of Psychology*, **54**, 403–25.

Drevets, W.C., Price, J.L., Simpson, J.R., *et al.* (1997). Subgenual prefrontal cortex abnormalities in mood disorders. *Nature*, **386**, 824–7.

Everitt, B.J. and Robbins, T.W. (2005). Neural systems of reinforcement for drug addiction: from actions to habits to compulsion. *Nature Neuroscience*, **8**, 1481–9.

Fair, D.A., Cohen, A.L., Dosenbach, N.U., *et al.* (2008). The maturing architecture of the brain's default network. *Proceedings of the National Academy of Sciences United States of America*, **105**, 4028–32.

Feldman Barrett, L. and Wager, T.D. (2006). The structure of emotion: evidence from neuroimaging studies. *Current Directions in Psychological Science*, **15**, 79–83.

Fransson, P., Skiold, B., Horsch, S., *et al.* (2007). Resting-state networks in the infant brain. *Proceedings of the National Academy of Sciences United States of America*, **104**, 15531–6.

Fredrickson, B.L., Cohn, M.A., Coffey, K.A., Pek, J., and Finkel, S.M. (2008). Open hearts build lives: positive emotions, induced through loving-kindness meditation, build consequential personal resources. *Journal of Personality and Social Psychology*, **95**, 1045–62.

Freud, S. and Riviere, J. (1930). *Civilization and its Discontents*. New York: J. Cape & H. Smith.

Frijda, N. (2010). On the nature and function of pleasure. In M.L. Kringelbach and K.C. Berridge (eds.) *Pleasures of the Brain*, pp. 99–112. New York: Oxford University Press.

Georgiadis, J.R., Kortekaas, R., Kuipers, R., *et al.* (2006). Regional cerebral blood flow changes associated with clitorally induced orgasm in healthy women. *The European Journal of Neuroscience*, **24**, 3305–16.

Gilbert, D.T. and Wilson, T.D. (2007). Prospection: experiencing the future. *Science*, **317**, 1351–4.

Gildenberg, P.L. (2005). Evolution of neuromodulation. *Stereotactic and Functional Neurosurgery*, **83**, 71–9.

Gorwood, P. (2008). Neurobiological mechanisms of anhedonia. *Dialogues in Clinical Neuroscience*, **10**, 291–9.

Gottfried, J.A. (2010). Olfaction and its pleasures: human neuroimaging perspectives. In M.L. Kringelbach and K.C. Berridge (ed.) *Pleasures of the Brain*, pp. 125–45. New York: Oxford University Press.

Green, A.L., Pereira, E.A., and Aziz, T.Z. (2010). Deep brain stimulation and pleasure. In M.L. Kringelbach and K.C. Berridge (eds.) *Pleasures of the Brain*, pp. 302–19. New York: Oxford University Press.

Green, A.L., Wang, S., Stein, J.F., *et al.* (2009). Neural signatures in patients with neuropathic pain. *Neurology*, **72**, 569–71.

Gusnard, D.A. and Raichle, M.E. (2001). Searching for a baseline: functional imaging and the resting human brain. *Nature Reviews Neuroscience*, **2**, 685–94.

Haisken-De New, J.P. and Frick, R. (2005). *Desktop Companion to the German Socio-Economic Panel Study (GSOEP)*. Berlin: German Institute for Economic Research (DIW).

Heath, R.G. (1972). Pleasure and brain activity in man. Deep and surface electroencephalograms during orgasm. *Journal of Nervous and Mental Disease*, **154**, 3–18.

Hornak, J., Bramham, J., Rolls, E.T., *et al.* (2003). Changes in emotion after circumscribed surgical lesions of the orbitofrontal and cingulate cortices. *Brain*, **126**, 1671–712.

Hornak, J., O'Doherty, J., Bramham, J., *et al.* (2004). Reward-related reversal learning after surgical excisions in orbitofrontal and dorsolateral prefrontal cortex in humans. *Journal of Cognitive Neuroscience*, **16**, 463–78.

Iversen, S.D. and Mishkin, M. (1970). Perseverative interference in monkeys following selective lesions of the inferior prefrontal convexity. *Experimental Brain Research*, **11**, 376–86.

James, W. (1920). To Miss Frances R. Morse. Nanheim, July 10 1901. In H. James (ed.) *Letters of William James*. Boston, MA: Atlantic Monthly Press.

Kahneman, D. (1999). Objective happiness. In D. Kahneman, E. Diener, and N. Schwartz (eds.) *Foundations of Hedonic Psychology: Scientific Perspectives on Enjoyment and Suffering*, pp. 3–25. New York: Sage.

Kahneman, D. (2000). Experienced utility and objective happiness: A moment-based approach. In D. Kahneman, and A. Tversky (eds.) *Choices, Values, and Frames*, pp. 673–92. New York: Cambridge University Press.

Kahneman, D., Krueger, A.B., Schkade, D.A., Schwarz, N., and Stone, A.A. (2004). A survey method for characterizing daily life experience: the day reconstruction method. *Science*, **306**, 1776–80.

Kesebir, P. and Diener, E. (2008). In pursuit of happiness: Empirical answers to philosophical questions. *Perspectives on Psychological Science*, **3**, 117–25.

Kosel, M., Sturm, V., Frick, C., *et al.* (2007). Mood improvement after deep brain stimulation of the internal globus pallidus for tardive dyskinesia in a patient suffering from major depression. *Journal of Psychiatric Research*, **41**, 801–3.

Kringelbach, M.L. (2004a). Emotion. In R.L. Gregory (ed.) *The Oxford Companion to the Mind* (2nd edition), pp. 287–90. Oxford: Oxford University Press.

Kringelbach, M.L. (2004b). Food for thought: hedonic experience beyond homeostasis in the human brain. *Neuroscience*, **126**, 807–19.

Kringelbach, M.L. (2005). The human orbitofrontal cortex: linking reward to hedonic experience. *Nature Reviews Neuroscience*, **6**, 691–702.

Kringelbach, M.L. (2009). *The Pleasure Center. Trust Your Animal Instincts*. New York: Oxford University Press.

Kringelbach, M.L. (2010). The hedonic brain: A functional neuroanatomy of human pleasure. In M.L. Kringelbach and K.C. Berridge (eds.) *Pleasures of the Brain*, pp. 202–21. Oxford: Oxford University Press.

Kringelbach, M.L. and Berridge, K.C. (2009). Towards a functional neuroanatomy of pleasure and happiness. *Trends in Cognitive Sciences*, **13**, 479–87.

Kringelbach, M.L. and Berridge, K.C. (2010). *Pleasures of the Brain*. New York: Oxford University Press.

Kringelbach, M.L., Berridge, K.C., Frijda, N., *et al.* (2010). Short answers to fundamental questions about pleasure. In M.L. Kringelbach and K.C. Berridge (eds.) *Pleasures of the Brain*, pp. 7–23. Oxford: Oxford University Press.

Kringelbach, M.L., Jenkinson, N., Green, A.L., *et al.* (2007a). Deep brain stimulation for chronic pain investigated with magnetoencephalography. *Neuroreport*, **18**, 223–8.

Kringelbach, M.L., Jenkinson, N., Owen, S.L.F., and Aziz, T.Z. (2007b). Translational principles of deep brain stimulation. *Nature Reviews Neuroscience*, **8**, 623–35.

Kringelbach, M.L., Lehtonen, A., Squire, S., *et al.* (2008). A specific and rapid neural signature for parental instinct. *PLoS ONE*, **3**, e1664. doi:1610.1371/journal.pone .0001664.

Kringelbach, M.L., O'Doherty, J., Rolls, E.T., and Andrews, C. (2003). Activation of the human orbitofrontal cortex to a liquid food stimulus is correlated with its subjective pleasantness. *Cerebral Cortex*, **13**, 1064–71.

Kringelbach, M.L. and Rolls, E.T. (2003). Neural correlates of rapid context-dependent reversal learning in a simple model of human social interaction. *Neuroimage*, **20**, 1371–83.

Kringelbach, M.L. and Rolls, E.T. (2004). The functional neuroanatomy of the human orbitofrontal cortex: evidence from neuroimaging and neuropsychology. *Progress in Neurobiology*, **72**, 341–72.

Kuppens, P., Realo, A., and Diener, E. (2008). The role of positive and negative emotions in life satisfaction judgment across nations. *Journal of Personality and Social Psychology*, **95**, 66–75.

Laureys, S., Owen, A.M., and Schiff, N.D. (2004). Brain function in coma, vegetative state, and related disorders. *Lancet Neurology*, **3**, 537–46.

Leknes, S. and Tracey, I. (2008). A common neurobiology for pain and pleasure. *Nature Reviews Neuroscience*, **9**, 314–20.

Lou, H.C., Kjaer, T.W., Friberg, L., Wildschiodtz, G., Holm, S., and Nowak, M. (1999). A 15O-H2O PET study of meditation and the resting state of normal consciousness. *Human Brain Mapping*, **7**, 98–105.

Mayberg, H.S., Lozano, A.M., Voon, V., *et al.* (2005). Deep brain stimulation for treatment-resistant depression. *Neuron*, **45**, 651–60.

Miller, J.M., Vorel, S.R., Tranguch, A.J., *et al.* (2006). Anhedonia after a selective bilateral lesion of the globus pallidus. *American Journal of Psychiatry*, **163**, 786–8.

Nauta, W.J. (1971). The problem of the frontal lobe: a reinterpretation. *Journal of Psychiatric Research*, **8**, 167–87.

Nesse, R.M. (2004). Natural selection and the elusiveness of happiness. *Philosophical Transactions of the Royal Society of London B Biological Sciences*, **359**, 1333–47.

O'Doherty, J., Kringelbach, M.L., Rolls, E.T., Hornak, J., and Andrews, C. (2001). Abstract reward and punishment representations in the human orbitofrontal cortex. *Nature Neuroscience*, **4**, 95–102.

Oishi, S., Diener, E., and Lucas, R.E. (2007). The optimal level of well-being: Can we be too happy? *Perspectives on Psychological Science*, **2**, 346–60.

Olds, J. and Milner, P. (1954). Positive reinforcement produced by electrical stimulation of septal area and other regions of rat brain. *Journal of Comparative and Physiological Psychology*, **47**, 419–27.

Öngür, D. and Price, J.L. (2000). The organization of networks within the orbital and medial prefrontal cortex of rats, monkeys and humans. *Cerebral Cortex*, **10**, 206–19.

Parkin, S. G., Gregory, R. P., Scott, R., *et al.* (2002). Unilateral and bilateral pallidotomy for idiopathic Parkinson's disease: a case series of 115 patients. *Movement Disorders*, **17**, 682–92.

Peciña, S., Smith, K.S., and Berridge, K.C. (2006). Hedonic hot spots in the brain. *Neuroscientist*, **12**, 500–11.

Pickens, C.L., Saddoris, M.P., Gallagher, M., and Holland, P.C. (2005). Orbitofrontal lesions impair use of cue-outcome associations in a devaluation task. *Behavioral Neuroscience*, **119**, 317–22.

Pickens, C.L., Setlow, B., Saddoris, M.P., Gallagher, M., Holland, P.C., and Schoenbaum, G. (2003). Different roles for orbitofrontal cortex and basolateral amygdala in a reinforcer devaluation task. *Journal of Neuroscience*, **23**, 11078–84.

Robinson, T.E. and Berridge, K.C. (1993). The neural basis of drug craving: an incentive-sensitization theory of addiction. *Brain Research. Brain Research Reviews*, **18**, 247–91.

Robinson, T.E. and Berridge, K.C. (2003). Addiction. *Annual Review of Psychology*, **54**, 25–53.

Ryan, R.M. and Deci, E.L. (2001). On happiness and human potentials: a review of research on hedonic and eudaimonic well-being. *Annual Review of Psychology*, **52**, 141–66.

Ryff, C.D., Dienberg Love, G., Urry, H.L., *et al.* (2006). Psychological well-being and ill-being: do they have distinct or mirrored biological correlates? *Psychotherapy and Psychosomatics*, **75**, 85–95.

Schlaepfer, T.E., Cohen, M.X., Frick, C., *et al.* (2008). Deep brain stimulation to reward circuitry alleviates anhedonia in refractory major depression. *Neuropsychopharmacology*, **33**, 368–77.

Schnider, A. (2003). Spontaneous confabulation and the adaptation of thought to ongoing reality. *Nature Reviews Neuroscience*, **4**, 662–71.

Seligman, M.E., Steen, T.A., Park, N., and Peterson, C. (2005). Positive psychology progress: empirical validation of interventions. *American Psychologist*, **60**, 410–21.

Skov, M. (2010). The pleasures of art. In M.L. Kringelbach and K.C. Berridge (eds.) *Pleasures of the Brain*, pp. 270–83. New York: Oxford University Press.

Small, D.M., Zatorre, R.J., Dagher, A., Evans, A.C., and Jones-Gotman, M. (2001). Changes in brain activity related to eating chocolate: From pleasure to aversion. *Brain*, **124**, 1720–33.

Smith, K.S. and Berridge, K.C. (2007). Opioid limbic circuit for reward: interaction between hedonic hotspots of nucleus accumbens and ventral pallidum. *Journal of Neuroscience*, **27**, 1594–1605.

Smith, K.S., Mahler, S.V., Pecina, S., and Berridge, K.C. (2010). Hedonic hotspots: generating sensory pleasure in the brain. In M.L. Kringelbach and K.C. Berridge (eds.) *Pleasures of the Brain*, pp. 27–49. New York: Oxford University Press.

Steele, J.D., Christmas, D., Eljamel, M.S., and Matthews, K. (2008). Anterior cingulotomy for major depression: clinical outcome and relationship to lesion characteristics. *Biological Psychiatry*, **63**, 670–7.

Steiner, J.E., Glaser, D., Hawilo, M.E., and Berridge, K.C. (2001). Comparative expression of hedonic impact: affective reactions to taste by human infants and other primates. *Neuroscience and Biobehavioral Reviews*, **25**, 53–74.

Teasdale, J.D., Segal, Z.V., Williams, J.M., Ridgeway, V.A., Soulsby, J.M., and Lau, M.A. (2000). Prevention of relapse/recurrence in major depression by mindfulness-based cognitive therapy. *Journal of Consulting and Clinical Psychology*, **68**, 615–23.

Veldhuizen, M.G., Rudenga, K.J., and Small, D.M. (2010). The pleasure of taste, flavor and food. In M.L. Kringelbach and K.C. Berridge (eds.) *Pleasures of the Brain*, pp. 146–68. New York: Oxford University Press.

Völlm, B.A., de Araujo, I.E.T., Cowen, P.J., *et al.* (2004). Methamphetamine activates reward circuitry in drug naïve human subjects. *Neuropsychopharmacology*, **29**, 1715–22.

Vuust, P. and Kringelbach, M.L. (2010). The pleasure of music. In M.L. Kringelbach, and K.C. Berridge (eds.) *Pleasures of the Brain*, pp. 255–69. New York: Oxford University Press.

Waterman, A.S. (1993). Two conceptions of happiness: contrasts of personal expressiveness (eudaimonia) and hedonic enjoyment. *Journal of Personality and Social Psychology*, **64**, 678–91.

Watson, K.K., Shepherd, S.V., and Platt, M.L. (2010). Neuroethology of pleasure. In M.L. Kringelbach, and K.C. Berridge (eds.) *Pleasures of the Brain*, pp. 85–95. New York: Oxford University Press.

Williams, J.M., Ellis, N.C., Tyers, C., Healy, H., Rose, G., and MacLeod, A.K. (1996). The specificity of autobiographical memory and imageability of the future. *Memory & Cognition*, **24**, 116–25.

Willoch, F., Schindler, F., Wester, H.J., *et al.* (2004). Central poststroke pain and reduced opioid receptor binding within pain processing circuitries: a [11C]diprenorphine PET study. *Pain*, **108**, 213–20.

CHAPTER 3

....

THE NEUROBIOLOGICAL
BASIS OF MORALITY

....

CHRISTOPHER SUHLER AND
PATRICIA CHURCHLAND

INTRODUCTION

....

THE study of morality, once the proprietary domain of philosophers, is increasingly an interdisciplinary endeavor spanning the cognitive, social, and biological sciences. While philosophers do still have a role to play in this project, they must now share the stage (and, perhaps, collaborate) with researchers from fields including psychology, neuroscience, experimental economics, anthropology, and evolutionary biology. Our aim in this chapter is to provide an overview and synthesis of recent work in these and other fields relevant to the scientific understanding of morality, with a focus on how moral judgment and behavior are rooted in the functioning, development, and evolution of the brain.

We acknowledge at the outset that although there have been great advances in the scientific understanding of morality in recent years, much is still unknown. Despite the growing trend toward interdisciplinary collaboration and toward studies explicitly investigating morality, the relevant evidence remains somewhat fragmented across disciplines. Moreover, this evidence is often indirect or its implications not fully worked out, coming in the course of studies not undertaken with the stated goal of examining morality. Consequently, our discussion will be organized as a series of sections on various, relatively discrete, lines of work that shed light on the neurobiological basis—or, better, *bases*—of morality.

We further acknowledge that although one major project in the years ahead will be to develop a unified theory of morality and its neurobiological underpinnings, we do not intend to develop such a theory here. While a handful of such theories have been proposed in recent years, they are generally less than satisfactory, resting on and accounting for a relatively small subset of the relevant data (see Moll *et al.* 2005; Monin *et al.* 2007 for recent overviews of some prominent theoretical approaches and their shortcomings). Instead, we will be content to call attention to some important themes running through the work discussed, themes that, we believe, should in one form or another figure in a unified account of morality.

The organization of the chapter will be as follows. We will begin by describing empirical work in so-called "moral psychology." Our discussion of this field will be divided into two smaller sections. In the first, we will present a short overview of themes that have emerged from studies examining the cognitive (but not neural) processes involved in morality. In the second, we will look at the relatively small—but growing—body of studies that directly investigate the neural substrates of morality using modern brain imaging techniques. The next section will examine work from experimental economics, a discipline that, in contrast to moral psychology, is relatively large and mature. Experiments in this field rarely target morality explicitly, but they are highly relevant nonetheless because they frequently involve behaviors and decisions that qualify as moral, such as whether to punish a wrongdoer or reciprocate a partner's trust. We will pay particular attention to studies drawn from "neuro-economics," a subfield of experimental economics that seeks to understand the neurobiological processes underlying decision-making.

In these sections, a number of brain regions and systems will be identified—notably those having to do with affect and with reward—that appear to be essential for normal moral behavior. In the next section of the chapter, we will look at what happens when these systems are compromised. Our focus will be on two clinical conditions: lesions to the prefrontal cortex (specifically the ventromedial subregion) and psychopathy. Studies of populations with these conditions not only corroborate findings from moral psychology and experimental economics, but also provide novel insight into the brain regions and processes involved in morality and, importantly, into moral development and the features of the nervous system necessary for its normal progression.

In the last major section of the chapter, we will turn to a different level of explanation—neuroendocrinology and evolutionary neurobiology—that is relevant to understanding the development of morality. Our focus will be on the evolutionary history and functions of two neuropeptides, oxytocin and vasopressin, in the mammalian brain and their effects on behavior. Generally speaking, these functions relate to attachment, bonding, and affiliative behavior, and thus understanding their evolution may help to explain the expanding sphere of caring and valuation characteristic of much of morality. We will close the chapter by summarizing the major themes that have emerged from the work discussed and highlighting a number of questions that remain to be addressed by future research.

MORAL PSYCHOLOGY (PART I)

The advent of functional magnetic resonance imaging (fMRI) as a tool for neuroscientific inquiry has been a boon to the investigation of the neural substrates of morality. The moral psychology studies using this technique are, however, somewhat varied in their designs and relatively small in number. As such, there is a risk associated with interpreting and generalizing from their findings. With an eye to reducing this risk and placing these studies in their proper context, we will open by sketching some of the general findings of moral psychological work employing techniques other than brain imaging.

One of the principal methods used in moral psychology involves presenting experimental subjects with hypothetical scenarios (typically in written form) and asking them to judge whether or not some action in a given scenario is morally permissible. This approach has its antecedents in the thought-experimental method employed in much of moral philosophy, notably normative ethics, where one major project aims to extract from people's moral intuitions a system of principles, or moral theory, that specifies what people ought to do. Thought experiments are meant to test the adequacy of a proposed system of principles, and to motivate refinements or alternative systems where that system is found wanting. For instance, a utilitarian may devise a hypothetical example which undermines a Kantian theory by showing that the theory delivers a verdict in the case that is deemed unacceptably counterintuitive. (An enduring problem, not surprisingly, is that people's moral intuitions, taken as a whole, rarely line up in a philosophically convenient way.)

These methods, as well as many of the thought experimental cases themselves, have been appropriated by moral psychologists. But whereas the primary aim of ethicists using such cases is to construct theories about how people *should* judge and behave in the moral domain, moral psychologists' principal goal is to understand and explain why people judge and behave as they *do*. The distinction, put simply, is thus between normative and descriptive projects. That is, although data from moral psychology may be used to argue for one or another normative ethical position (see, e.g. Casebeer 2003; Greene 2008), the principal purpose for which they are gathered is to illuminate the cognitive processes that actually are involved in morality.

In an ironic twist, one of the major findings of empirical moral psychology has been that, contrary to the assumptions of many philosophers (most prominently Immanuel Kant and his modern-day followers—see, e.g. Korsgaard 1996, 1999), emotion appears to play an indispensable role in moral judgment. Furthermore, and again in sharp contrast to philosophical idealizations, many moral judgments appear to be the result of cognitive processes that are non-conscious and automatic (Greene and Haidt 2002).

Some of the strongest evidence that moral judgment is not generally the result of conscious reasoning comes from the work of Jonathan Haidt (for a fairly recent review, see Haidt 2001). In an early study, Haidt and colleagues (1993) presented subjects with descriptions of actions that were harmless but likely to trigger an affective response (e.g. eating one's pet dog after it was killed by a car, using the national flag to clean one's toilet). They found—as expected, given that the scenarios were designed to be offensive—that subjects often judged the actions described to be wrong. However, the justifications subjects provided when pressed, which typically focused on (non-existent) harms associated with the actions, were poor predictors of their judgments of wrongness. Instead, subjects' moral judgments were best predicted by their affective responses to the stories (Haidt *et al.* 1993). Similarly, Haidt and Hersh (2001) described a phenomenon that they termed "moral dumbfounding," which occurs when a person shows "marked confusion and incoherence" (Haidt and Hersh 2001, p. 200) or simply admits to being dumbfounded upon being asked to explain a moral judgment (yet, remarkably, refuses to change that judgment). Paralleling the results of the earlier study (Haidt *et al.* 1993), Haidt and Hersh (2001) found that affective reactions were better predictors of moral judgment than were perceptions of harmfulness and that moral dumbfounding was most likely to occur when participants had strong affective reactions to a case.

Further evidence for the automatic, non-conscious nature of (at least some) moral judgments comes from two recent studies by Marc Hauser and colleagues. In one (Cushman *et al.* 2006), Hauser's team presented subjects with moral dilemmas closely based on those from the philosophical literature. Participants were asked not only to judge whether or not a particular course of action was morally permissible but also to provide a justification for their judgment. The researchers then examined whether these justifications mapped onto three principles, which they called the "action principle" (bringing about a harm by action is worse than bringing about the same harm by omission), the "intention principle" (a harm brought about as a means to a goal is worse than the same harm brought about as a side effect of a goal), and the "contact principle" (bringing about a harm through physical contact is worse than the same harm brought about without physical contact) (Cushman *et al.* 2006). (These principles were predefined by the researchers but were not provided to subjects for use during the experiment.) The team found that although subjects were usually able to articulate sufficient justifications mapping onto the first and third principles, they were not able to do so for the second principle, despite the fact that their patterns of judgments were consistent with this principle. From this, the researchers concluded that although the intention principle (or, we would add, at least some combination of cognitive processes approximating it) is operative in moral judgment, it is not consciously accessible (Cushman *et al.* 2006).

This finding was corroborated by a second study (Hauser *et al.* 2007) that used an Internet-based design to obtain access to a particularly large and diverse (in terms of education, religion, nationality, etc.) subject pool. Subjects across these demographic dimensions made very similar judgments about the rightness and wrongness of the hypothetical cases with which they were presented. Moreover, as in the earlier study (Cushman *et al.* 2006), although these judgments were generally consistent with the intention principle (also known, as it was in this study, as the "principle of double effect"), a majority of participants were unable to articulate a sufficient justification in terms of this principle (Hauser *et al.* 2007).

One of our aims in describing these studies is to provide background for the section that follows. Another important aim, however, is to help clear the way for an understanding of the work discussed throughout this paper untainted by philosophical or folk psychological assumptions that moral judgment simply *must* be the result of something like conscious, deductive reasoning. Rather, affect often plays a substantial role in moral judgment, and its role (and that of other factors) is often automatic and something of which the individual making the judgment is not consciously aware. In this way, moral behavior and moral judgment are similar to many other complex behaviors and abilities that are an integral part of our effective daily functioning (see, e.g. Wilson 2002; Wegner 2002; Dijksterhuis 2004; Johansson *et al.* 2005; Suhler and Churchland 2009).

MORAL PSYCHOLOGY (PART II)

Perhaps the best-known study directly investigating the neural correlates of moral judgment was conducted by Joshua Greene and colleagues in 2001. Greene and his team (2001) hypothesized that certain patterns in people's judgments about hypothetical cases from normative ethics—patterns that have long resisted satisfactory explanation by philosophers— are caused by differences in the emotional salience of the actions described. Specifically, they predicted that cases involving "personal" harms to other individuals (e.g. pushing a person into the path of a runaway trolley in order to stop the trolley, thereby saving five others on the track) would cause a larger negative emotional response than cases in which the harms were "impersonal" (e.g. flipping a switch that diverts the runaway trolley onto a track that has one person on it, again saving five on the main track). This large negative emotional response, according to their hypothesis, would make people more likely to judge the action that triggered it morally wrong (Greene *et al.* 2001).

Greene and his collaborators (2001) presented subjects with a battery of personal and impersonal moral dilemmas (as well as non-moral control cases) while the subjects' brains were scanned using fMRI. The scanning data generally supported their hypothesis: when presented with personal moral dilemmas, subjects tended (compared to the impersonal and non-moral cases) to judge that the actions described were wrong and to exhibit greater activity in brain areas associated with emotion and social cognition, namely the medial frontal gyrus, posterior cingulate gyrus, and bilateral superior temporal sulcus (Greene *et al.* 2001; Greene and Haidt 2002). That these emotional responses contributed to, rather than resulted from, subjects' moral judgments was supported by reaction-time data gathered in a second experiment reported by Greene and colleagues (2001). (See also Greene *et al.* 2004.)

Another very active research group studying the neural substrates of morality is led by Jorge Moll. The experimental paradigm used in many of Moll and colleagues' studies involves presenting subjects with both moral and non-moral stimuli, and using fMRI to determine which brain areas, if any, exhibit differential activity in response to the moral stimuli. In one study, Moll and his collaborators (2002a) presented subjects with emotion-ally charged moral and non-moral written statements. Their aim in using emotionally charged non-moral statements was to see whether there were brain areas that were active in response to moral statements as such, independent of any increased emotional salience that such statements might have. The researchers found that the moral statements elicited increased activity in the medial orbitofrontal cortex, left temporal pole, and superior temporal sulcus, compared to the non-moral statements (Moll *et al.* 2002a).

Similar results were obtained in another study (Moll *et al.* 2002b) comparing the brain areas associated with basic emotions and moral emotions. Moll and his team (2002b) pre-sented subjects in an fMRI scanner with pictures containing emotionally charged moral content (assumed to evoke moral emotions), emotionally charged non-moral content (assumed to evoke basic emotions), and emotionally neutral content. There were, not sur-prisingly, brain areas that were found to be associated with both basic and moral emotions, including the amygdala, thalamus, and upper midbrain. Additionally, however, there were areas that exhibited increased activation specific to the moral emotions: the medial orbitof-rontal cortex, medial frontal gyrus, and right posterior superior temporal sulcus (Moll *et al.* 2002b). Drawing on prior work associating the orbitofrontal cortex with automatic emo-tional appraisals, Moll and colleagues (2002b) interpreted these findings as evidence that automatic, emotion-based moral assessments may play an important role in guiding rapid, effective behavioral responses to one's social environment. This accords well with the behav-ioral data on the automaticity and affect-dependence of moral judgment described earlier, as well as with the large body of work suggesting that valuation is endemic to perception across a variety of domains (see, e.g. Panksepp 1998; Damasio 1999; Thompson *et al.* 2006).

The studies just reviewed do not exhaust the literature on neuroimaging investigations of morality. Nor, given the relatively young state of the field and the limits on what can be inferred from imaging data alone, should they be taken as the final word on the subject. But despite these limitations, the findings described do give a flavor of the work that is being done on the subject and of the brain regions that may be important to moral judgment. They also support (and are supported by) findings from behavioral investigations of morality suggesting, contrary to philosophical orthodoxy, that moral judgment is often an emotional, automatic process.

Nevertheless, one complaint that can be (and often has been—see, e.g. Casebeer 2003; Casebeer and Churchland 2003; Moll *et al.* 2005) lodged against the moral psychology literature as a whole is that the stimuli and methods it uses are of dubious ecological validity. That is, presenting subjects with contrived, behaviorally inconsequential scenarios in highly artificial environments, while a reasonable way to satisfy the constraints of rigorous experimental design, may fail to give an accurate picture of an inherently social phenomenon like morality (see, e.g. Monin *et al.* 2007). In the remaining sections of this chapter, we will look at evidence from other areas of cognitive scientific research that are relevant to the study of morality and help to address the concerns about ecological validity associated with work in moral psychology proper.

EXPERIMENTAL ECONOMICS

The concern of ecological invalidity emphasizes that the method of presenting subjects with hypothetical cases (or other stimuli such as declarative statements or pictures) may fail to track real-world moral judgment and behavior. Knowing that their responses will not have any real consequences, subjects may not reach or report judgments that reflect how they actually would judge or behave if they believed the situation to be real or encountered it in real life. For instance, few people, when asked if they would administer increasingly severe electric shocks to another individual as punishment for getting wrong answers on a test, would say that they would do so, let alone that they would continue administering these shocks until they reached the most severe possible shock. But as Stanley Milgram showed in his famous series of experiments on obedience (see Milgram 1974 for a review), a large proportion of participants—65% in the original experiment (Milgram 1963)—indeed did continue increasing the shocks up to the maximum level when asked to do so by the experimenter. (The "victim" was in fact a confederate of the experimenter, and the "shocks" and the victim's "agony" in response to them were feigned.)

Studies from experimental economics go some way toward addressing this concern. While the tasks and experimental environments of these studies are still rather artificial— typically involving playing strategic games drawn from the game theory literature while in a laboratory or an fMRI scanner—participants' choices in these games usually result in actual gains or losses to themselves and other individuals in the game. (Participants are typically given the opportunity to convert their experimental credits into real currency at the end of the experiment.) Importantly for our purposes, the game theoretic tasks used present opportunities to engage in various types of moral behavior: showing generosity, reciprocating or breaching trust, punishing wrongdoers, and so on. As such, they may provide a more ecologically valid way of examining the psychological and neural bases of moral judgment and behavior than do studies relying primarily on responses to hypothetical cases.

One prominent strand of research in experimental economics investigates people's decisions about whether or not to punish other individuals for violations and the effect that this punishment (or the possibility of it) has on behavior, specifically cooperative behavior. The economic game often used in these experiments is the "public goods game," which is played by two or more individuals and is structured as follows. Each player begins with a private endowment of experimental credits and each round chooses how much of this, if anything, to contribute to a public fund. The amount contributed to the public fund is multiplied by some number (greater than one, with a multipliee of 1.6 used in most of the studies described later), and the resulting amount is divided evenly among the players, who get to keep this amount plus whatever they did not contribute to the fund. Because of the multiplier, the group does best (i.e. the total pool of credits is maximized) when everyone contributes. However, the game theoretic rational strategy for a given individual is to be a "free rider" or "defector" by contributing nothing at all, since this will maximize the individual's payoff regardless of what others contribute. But, of course, if everyone follows this strategy, all will end up worse off than if they had cooperated by contributing to the public fund. In this way, and as suggested by its name, the public goods game mirrors situations often encountered by nations and other aggregates of individuals trying to determine who will bear the costs of some project or policy the benefits of which can be enjoyed even by those who manage to avoid paying the costs.

In an early experiment, Fehr and Gächter (2000) compared participants' behavior in a public goods game in two conditions: one with punishment and one without. Importantly, punishment in these experiments was costly for the individual doing the punishing; a player had to pay a fee using her own experimental credits in order to punish another player by reducing that person's credits. The game was played in groups of four individuals, and in order to prevent the development of individual reputation over the course of the ten rounds of the game, subjects were anonymous and the composition of the groups randomly changed from round to round.

Fehr and Gächter (2000) found, in line with previous studies not incorporating punishment, that in the non-punishment condition, initial contributions were moderate and decreased in subsequent rounds until free-riding (zero contribution) was the dominant strategy. In sessions in which punishment was available, they found that subjects were willing to punish other individuals who contributed little or nothing to the public fund. Subjects did this even though they incurred a cost by doing so and despite the fact that, due to the randomized, anonymized design of the game, they might not interact with the punished individual again (and would not know it even if they did). The availability of punishment had a dramatic effect on cooperation: average contributions were two to four times higher in the punishment condition than in the non-punishment condition, with contributions in the final rounds being six to seven and a half times higher when punishment was available (Fehr and Gächter 2000). Moreover, even the mere possibility of punishment was effective as a means of increasing cooperation. In one experimental session, subjects played a 20-round game in which punishment was not available for the first ten rounds; here, the standard pattern of contributions decreasing from an initial modest level was observed. But when punishment became available in round 11, contributions immediately jumped to almost four times their round ten level and continued increasing through the twentieth and final round (Fehr and Gächter 2000).

By itself, this study can say little about the psychological or neural mechanisms underlying people's willingness to incur a cost to punish others even when no monetary benefit, whether short- or long-term, is likely to accrue from doing so. Other studies, however, do shed light on the causes of the pattern of punishment behavior just described. We will begin by looking at the possible psychological mechanisms behind punishment before moving on to the neural mechanisms.

Fehr and Gächter (2002) conducted a study suggesting that the relevant psychological mechanism of so-called "altruistic punishment" is negative emotion directed toward defectors. (The punishment is "altruistic" because, as noted previously, it is costly and does not yield any material benefit to the punisher. Indeed, people will pay a cost to punish defectors even when they are "third parties," individuals who are merely observing an economic game rather than playing in it themselves—see Fehr and Fischbacher 2004.) The design and behavioral results of this study were very similar to those of the previous study (Fehr and Gächter 2000). Participants played a randomized, anonymized public goods game in punishment and non-punishment conditions. Contributions were again significantly higher in the punishment condition, and the mere switch from punishment to non-punishment or vice versa resulted in an immediate change in average contribution levels. When the option of punishment became available, contributions immediately jumped and continued to increase; when it was removed, contributions immediately dropped and continued to decrease. Once more, the frequency of punishment was high despite its costliness: in a typical six-round game, 84.3% of subjects punished at least once, and 34.4% punished more than five times (Fehr and Gächter 2002). Defectors were by far the most frequent targets of acts of punishment, receiving 74.2% of the total, and cooperators (those who contributed above-average amounts) tended to be the ones doing the punishing.

Now comes the interesting part. Fehr and Gächter (2002) hypothesized that negative emotions toward defectors might be the proximate mechanism behind altruistic punishment. To test this, they presented subjects who had just finished playing the games with written descriptions of hypothetical scenarios. A sample scenario is as follows:

> You decide to invest 16 francs to the project. The second group member invests 14 and the third 18 francs. Suppose the fourth member invests 2 francs to the project. You now accidentally meet this member. Please indicate your feeling towards this person. (Fehr and Gächter 2002, p. 139)

Subjects indicated how much anger, if any, they would feel using a seven-point scale, with seven representing the highest level of anger. In the version of the scenario reprinted here, in which the individual had contributed a high amount relative to the defector, 47% selected an anger level of six or seven, and a further 37% selected an anger level of five (Fehr and Gächter 2002). Moreover, when subjects were instead presented with a hypothetical scenario in which they were the defector (and the other individuals were high contributors) and asked to rate how angry they expected the others would be, they again gave very high anger ratings, with 74.5% choosing six or seven and a further 22.5% choosing five).

In sum, behavioral and self-report evidence suggests that anger is a powerful driver of a canonical moral behavior, namely the punishing of wrongdoers. Moreover, most people are aware of this, as indicated by their ratings of the anger they would expect others to feel toward them if they defected. This latter fact may help explain the immediate jump in contributions observed upon the switch from non-punishment to punishment conditions. Accordingly, the emotions probably have an important role not only in the actual process of making moral judgments (see, e.g. Greene *et al.* 2001; Haidt 2001; Moll *et al.* 2002b) but also in motivating behavioral responses to these judgments and, through the anticipation of such emotion-driven responses, in deterring people from behaving immorally in the first place.

Given the shortcomings of self-reports in response to hypothetical scenarios noted previously, it would be unwise to rely solely on this type of data in the present case. Luckily, researchers in the field of neuroeconomics have taken advantage of a variety of methods from the cognitive sciences—including, but not limited to, fMRI—in an effort to better understand the neural bases of punishment, cooperation, and other behaviors that are both economically and morally significant.

Most directly relevant to Fehr and Gächter's (2002) anger hypothesis are studies examining decision-making in the "ultimatum game." This is a simple economic game in which one player (the "proposer") unilaterally proposes a division of an allotment of credits between herself and a second player (the "responder"); the responder then decides whether to accept or reject the offer. If the responder accepts, the players get credits according to the proposed division. But if she rejects the offer, neither player gets anything. Game theory predicts that rational responders should be willing to accept any non-zero offer and that rational proposers, knowing this, should offer the smallest possible non-zero amount to the responder. When people actually play the game, however, proposers tend to be far more generous than predicted by game theory, offering 40–50% of the total allotment (Nowak *et al.* 2000). Responders, too, deviate from the game theoretic prediction, tending to reject offers of less than 30% of the total allotment (Nowak *et al.* 2000).

The neural basis of responders' behavior has been the primary object of neuroeconomic study of the ultimatum game. (Our later discussion of studies on cooperation will shed light on what, in addition to anticipation of the responder's anger, might cause proposers to offer relatively generous splits.) In one study, Sanfey and colleagues (2003) used fMRI to scan subjects' brains while they played the role of the responder. They found that the rejection of unfair offers, as well as the degree of an offer's unfairness, was associated with increased activity in the anterior insula, an area of the brain associated with negative emotional states, particularly anger and disgust (Sanfey *et al.* 2003). Moreover, insula activation was higher when the unfair offer was made by a human partner as opposed to a computer partner. This suggests that being treated unfairly by another person—an act that, unlike being treated unfairly by a computer, has a moral dimension—is something to which the brain is particularly emotionally responsive. Similar results were obtained in a study by van't Wout and colleagues (2006) that used skin conductance responses (SCRs) to measure autonomic arousal in response to unfair ultimatum game offers. Increased emotional arousal, as measured by SCRs, was associated with rejection of unfair offers. Moreover, this increased arousal was selective, being observed in response to unfair offers made by human partners but not by computer partners (van't Wout *et al.* 2006).

Anger and other negative states are not, however, the whole story. Additional neuroeconomic studies suggest that areas of the brain implicated in positive states, specifically those associated with reward, also play an important role in guiding decisions about punishment, cooperation, and so forth. Before describing the studies themselves, we will set out the basic rules of two economic games often used in them.

The first is the so-called "trust game." This game is played by two individuals, each of whom begins with an initial allotment of credits. One player (the "investor") is given the opportunity to send some of her own credits to the second player (the "trustee"). This amount is multiplied by some amount (a multiplier of three is often used) and added to the trustee's fund. The trustee is then given the opportunity to return an amount of credits of her choosing (including zero) to the investor. As in the public goods game, the rational strategy according to game theory is for the trustee (in the absence of punishment) to defect by not returning any credits to the investor, since this maximizes the trustee's own return. But a rational investor, knowing this, will not send any credits to the trustee in the first place, with the result that both players, by adopting the "rational" strategy, are left worse off than if they had cooperated.

The second game is known as the "prisoner's dilemma game." This game is played by two individuals and consists of each player choosing, without communicating with the other, one of two actions: cooperate or defect. Each player's facing a binary choice yields four possible combinations of responses. The highest payoff for an individual comes when she defects and her partner cooperates, and the lowest payoff comes when the reverse occurs. If both players cooperate, each receives the same payoff; this payoff is the second-highest available. Mutual defection too results in the same payoff for each, and this payoff is the third-highest. As in the other games, the game theoretic rational strategy for a given individual is to defect, since this will yield the highest payoff regardless of what one's partner does. But once more, each player pursuing this strategy results in a lower payoff than would have been attained had both cooperated.

In one study, de Quervain and colleagues (2004) used positron emission tomography (PET) to scan subjects' brains while they played the trust game. Subjects were given the opportunity to punish defectors (i.e. trustees who did not reciprocate trust) by assigning "punishment points" to them. Two punishment conditions were tested: "symbolic punishment" (subjects could assign punishment points, but these points would not reduce the monetary payoff of either player) and "effective punishment" (subjects could pay a cost of one credit for every two that would be deducted from the other player's fund). The researchers found that effective punishment, as compared to symbolic punishment, was associated with increased activation in the caudate nucleus (de Quervain *et al.* 2004). This brain area is part of the dorsal striatum, itself part of the midbrain dopamine system and thus crucial to reward processing. Moreover, higher caudate activation was associated with increased investment in punishment, a finding the researchers interpreted as evidence that the anticipation of satisfaction derived from punishing a defector drives decisions about whether to punish and how much one is willing to pay to do so (de Quervain *et al.* 2004). This study therefore suggests that at least part of the neural basis for one type of moral behavior, the punishment of perceived wrongdoers, is that punishing is anticipated to be (and actually is) rewarding because it increases activity in dopamine-rich areas of the punisher's brain.

The role of the striatum and other reward-processing areas is not limited to interactions involving punishment. This is indicated by a number of recent studies implicating these areas in various forms of cooperative and prosocial behavior. For instance, Rilling and colleagues (2002) found that mutual cooperation in the prisoner's dilemma game was associated with increased activation in a number of areas associated with reward. One of these was the area de Quervain and colleagues (2004) found to be involved in punishment behavior, the caudate nucleus (Rilling *et al.* 2002). Other reward-processing areas that exhibited increased activation in response to cooperation were the nucleus accumbens, the ventromedial frontal and orbitofrontal cortices, and the rostral anterior cingulate cortex. The researchers interpreted these findings as evidence that, as in the case of punishment, activity in reward areas helps reinforce and motivate the decision to cooperate (Rilling *et al.* 2002).

This interpretation is corroborated by a later fMRI study by Rilling and colleagues (2004), in which the ventral striatum and the ventromedial prefrontal cortex (VMPFC, a brain area associated with affect and affect-driven learning) exhibited increased activity in response to reciprocated cooperation in the prisoner's dilemma game. Echoing the studies of the ultimatum game described earlier (Sanfey et al. 2003; van't Wout et al. 2006), the increased activity in these two areas was observed when participants cooperated with a human partner but not when they cooperated with a computer partner (Rilling et al. 2004). Further support for the view that activity in reward areas reinforces and motivates cooperation comes from work by King-Casas and colleagues (2005). These researchers found that activity in the caudate nucleus (measured using fMRI) was associated with subjects' intention to trust their partner in the trust game. Notably, this study used a multiround variant of the trust game, and the "intention to trust" response in the caudate moved progressively earlier as trust developed between the partners as a result of reciprocated cooperation (King-Casas et al. 2005).

Perhaps the most dramatic experimental economic evidence for the involvement of affect- and reward-associated brain regions in morality comes from studies of charitable donation. Moll and colleagues (2006) gave participants the opportunity to donate (or refuse to donate) to actual charitable organizations with a variety of missions while their brains were scanned using fMRI. They found that the decision to donate to a charity, even when costly to the subject, was associated with increased activity in the midbrain dopamine system, specifically the ventral tegmental area, dorsal striatum, and ventral striatum (Moll et al. 2006). Consistent with their general role in reward, these areas were also active in a condition in which subjects received a direct monetary reward. Strikingly, however, the ventral striatum exhibited *greater* activity in response to charitable donation than to direct monetary reward.

Moll and his team (2006) also examined the neural correlates of subjects' choice to oppose particular charitable causes—some of which had missions concerned with controversial issues such as abortion and the death penalty—by refusing to donate to them. They found that the decision to oppose a cause was associated with increased activity in the lateral orbitofrontal cortex, an area associated with, among other things, negative affective states such as anger and disgust (Moll et al. 2006).

These findings were extended by Harbaugh and colleagues (2007), who found that reward-associated brain areas, including the ventral striatum, exhibited increased activation not only when participants voluntarily chose to donate to a charity, but also when they observed a mandatory transfer from their personal fund to the charity's. Notably, however, the increase in activity was greater in the voluntary condition, suggesting that not only an outcome itself but also the way it is brought about is an important determinant of how rewarding it is (Harbaugh et al. 2007; Sanfey 2007). This accords well with the weight that many people, as well as many normative ethical theories, give to the intentions behind an action and to how a given outcome occurs when assessing its moral status (see, e.g. Greene et al. 2001; Cushman et al. 2006; Hauser et al. 2007).

In sum, a wide range of recent work in experimental economics has substantially enhanced our understanding of the neural bases of decision-making in general and moral decision-making in particular. One notable theme of this work echoes a theme encountered in our discussion of moral psychology, the importance of affect in moral decisions and behaviors. Another theme is the importance of the brain's reward system, notably the striatum and other parts of the midbrain dopamine system, in reinforcing and motivating people to behave cooperatively or generously toward others rather than taking advantage of them for immediate selfish gain.

Notably, all of the studies discussed so far have used neurologically normal subjects. In the next section, we will look at work on two types of clinical subjects, individuals with prefrontal cortex damage and psychopathy, that provides additional support for a substantial role for affect and reward systems in morality. Crucially, this work also provides novel insight into the role of these systems, and in particular into the importance of their normal functioning for normal moral development.

CLINICAL EVIDENCE

Much of what is known about the effects of damage to the prefrontal cortex, especially the ventromedial aspect of the prefrontal cortex, comes from the trailblazing work of Antonio Damasio and his collaborators. In an early study, Damasio and colleagues (1990) demonstrated that patients with VMPFC damage, unlike healthy controls and patients with non-VMPFC brain damage, did not exhibit increased autonomic arousal (as measured by SCRs) in response to emotionally charged stimuli. This, the researchers suggested, provides a possible neurobiological explanation for the dramatic deficits in decision-making and planning abilities exhibited by VMPFC patients. Specifically, they proposed that such individuals are unable to activate anticipatory somatic states associated with punishment and reward that have been previously encountered in a given type of situation. In the absence of these states, VMPFC patients would be missing an important source of information about the outcomes associated with different courses of action in the situation (Damasio et al. 1990).

Dramatic support for this hypothesis was provided by a series of follow-up studies using a novel experimental task—the Iowa Gambling Task—that involved learning and making decisions about the merits of different possible options (Bechara et al. 1994). In this task, subjects began with an initial allotment of (fake) currency and were presented with four decks of cards. Each round of the game consisted of the subject choosing a card from any of the four decks. All of the decks contained both reward and penalty cards. Unbeknownst to subjects, however, two of the decks were "good" in that they had low rewards but also low penalties; if subjects drew primarily from these decks, they would gain money in the long run. The other two decks were "bad" in that they had higher rewards but also very high penalties; drawing primarily from these decks would cause subjects to lose money in the long run. Subjects' objective was to earn as much (or lose as little) money as possible (Bechara et al. 1994; Damasio 1996).

Damasio and his colleagues found that VMPFC patients, unlike normal or non-VMPFC brain-damaged controls, drew primarily from the bad decks throughout the task (Bechara et al. 1994; Bechara et al. 1996). In other words, they failed to learn (in the sense of being able to act on) the punishment and reward contingencies of the different decks, in contrast to controls, who eventually drew almost exclusively from the good decks. The reason for this, in line with the team's hypothesis, was the failure of VMPFC patients to activate anticipatory feelings, positive or negative, when trying to decide which deck they would draw from. Although the VMPFC patients, like controls, generated SCRs in response to gains or losses encountered *after* drawing a card, they did not generate *anticipatory* SCRs when contemplating which deck to draw from (Bechara et al. 1996).

To connect this work on VMPFC patients to morality, three additional pieces of information are needed. First, the patients used in the studies just described sustained their VMPFC
damage in adulthood; before that, they presumably were able to learn from past experiences
of punishment and reward and guide their decisions accordingly. Second, although adult-
onset VMPFC patients often cause significant (albeit unintentional) harm to themselves due
to their decision-making deficits, they typically do not harm others or otherwise behave
immorally (Anderson et al. 1999). The third, critical piece of information comes from a
study by Damasio and colleagues (Anderson et al. 1999) that examined two subjects with
early VMPFC damage. In contrast to the adult-onset patients, these individuals' moral and
social behavior was extremely poor. One subject, a female, was, among other things, a
chronic liar, verbally and physically abusive, and a strikingly indifferent mother to the child
she had at age 18. Moreover, she "never expressed guilt or remorse for her behavior," and
"[t]here was little or no evidence that she experienced empathy" (Anderson et al. 1999, p.
1032). The story was similar for the second individual studied by the team, a male.

The contrast between the moral behavior of early- and adult-onset VMPFC patients
suggests that the brain's affect and reward systems play a critical role not only in learning,
reinforcing, and motivating moral patterns of behavior over the short timescales found, for
example, in experimental economics studies, but also in the basic acquisition of such
patterns of behavior beginning in childhood. When the ability to associate past affect and
reward signals with the situation or action that led to them (e.g. associating punishment
with harming another individual) is compromised, individuals lack a crucial source of motivation to behave morally. This has dramatic consequences for behavior; indeed, Damasio
and colleagues go so far as to suggest that early VMPFC damage results in a syndrome that
resembles psychopathy (Anderson et al. 1999). This is the condition to which we now turn.

The standard tool for the diagnosis of psychopathy is the Hare Psychopathy Checklist-
Revised (PCL-R) (Hare 1991). This consists of 20 items, each of which is assigned a score of
zero (does not apply), one (applies somewhat), or two (definitely applies) on the basis of a
subject's institutional records and an extended interview with the individual; a score of 30 or
above typically results in a diagnosis of psychopathy (Hare 1991, 2003; Kiehl 2006). Among
the four "factors" into which the second edition of the PCL-R is divided is an affective factor,
which encompasses four items: "shallow affect," "lack of remorse or guilt," "callous/lack of
empathy," and "failure to accept responsibility" (Hare 2003).

The affective deficits of psychopaths are therefore recognized as a standard part of the
behavioral diagnosis of the condition. They are also manifested in a number of physiological
measures of affective functioning. For instance, psychopaths exhibit significantly lower
SCRs than normal subjects in response to aversive stimuli such as slides of mutilated faces
(Mathis 1970; Kiehl 2006), the insertion of a needle (Hare 1972), and loud tones (Hare et al.
1978). Additionally, and in a notable parallel to the case of individuals with VMPFC damage,
psychopaths do not exhibit anticipatory SCR increases when they are about to receive painful stimuli (Hare 1965; Hare and Quinn 1971). Researchers have also begun to use fMRI to
investigate the neural bases of the psychopathy more directly. Kiehl and colleagues (2001),
for example, scanned subjects' brains while they performed an affective memory task. They
found that psychopaths, as compared to non-psychopathic criminals and normal subjects,
exhibited lower activity in a number of brain regions associated with affect and reward,
including the amygdala, ventral striatum, anterior cingulate, and posterior cingulate (Kiehl
et al. 2001; Kiehl 2006).

Coupled with psychopaths' well-established patterns of harmful, criminal, and otherwise antisocial behavior (Hare 1991, 2003; Kiehl 2006), as well as with evidence that this condition has a genetic component (see, e.g. Viding *et al.* 2005; Blonigen *et al.* 2005), these findings point, like those previously discussed, toward a central role for neural systems associated with affect and reward in morality in normal individuals. Although there are certain differences between psychopaths and early-onset VMPFC patients (see Kiehl 2006), both clinical populations exhibit a failure to develop anticipatory affect- and reward-related responses to previously encountered stimuli (e.g. punishment, monetary loss), and the existence of this deficit throughout life seems to have particularly deleterious consequences for the development of normal moral behavior and motivation.

This last point leads to one important remark we would like to make about our general project in this chapter. Our focus is on the neurobiological bases of morality, but this should not be taken to imply that morality, and the behaviors, values, motives, principles, and so forth that comprise it, is innate. It is now widely understood that genes and environment interact, and that many neurobiological systems must be "tuned up" by experience in order to reinforce and motivate normal behavior, including moral behavior. That morality is the result of both genetic and environmental factors is suggested not only by the clinical evidence just discussed, but also by a variety of other findings. For instance, social dispositions in many species, including moral dispositions in humans, can be seriously compromised by early severe deprivation (Beckett *et al.* 2006; Kreppner *et al.* 2007) and other socioenvironmental factors (Bowes *et al.* 2009), genetic variations (Bellugi *et al.* 1999; Blonigen *et al.* 2005; Viding *et al.* 2005; Dai *et al.* 2009), and by the interaction of genes and deprived or abusive experience (Champagne *et al.* 2001; Meaney 2001; Caspi *et al.* 2002; Cameron *et al.* 2005).

Neuroendocrinology and evolutionary neurobiology

The studies described thus far have focused on the general brain systems implicated in various types of moral judgment and behavior, including behaviors such as altruistic punishment (Fehr and Fischbacher 2004) and charitable giving (Moll *et al.* 2006; Harbaugh *et al.* 2007). Clinical work on individuals with early-onset VMPFC damage (Anderson *et al.* 1999) and psychopathy (e.g. Kiehl *et al.* 2001; Kiehl 2006) provided further evidence for the importance of these systems by suggesting that their dysfunction can result in patterns of pronounced harmful and immoral behavior toward others.

This account is not complete, however, for two principal reasons. First, it does not address the role, in brain function and thus in behavior, of the levels of various neurochemicals, nor the densities or distributions of their corresponding receptors. And second, it says relatively little about why, at the evolutionary level of explanation, the brain mechanisms for robust social and moral behavior might have come to exist. Also desired, therefore, is an explanation of how the circuitry that regulates mammalian social behavior came to exist at all, and hence how social values, in the most basic sense, came to be expressed by mammalian nervous systems. Because evolution is highly conservative, typically modifying existing structures for new purposes rather than designing whole structures *de novo*, the complexity seen in human social and moral behavior and value systems is unlikely to have been an unprecedented novelty. Rather, it likely depends on mammalian brain structures serving simpler social purposes, which in their turn are probably adaptations of pre-mammalian circuitry serving basic self-survival functions.

Our focus here will be on the neurobiological details of the evolution of prosocial behavior. We note, however, that important—and potentially complementary—work has been done on the broader evolutionary dynamics that may have led to the high levels of prosocial behavior seen in species such as humans. Couched in the vocabulary of evolutionary game theory, this work concerns how seemingly maladaptive cooperative, punitive, and other such behaviors could in fact have been what Maynard Smith and Price (1973) termed an "evolutionarily stable strategy" (see, e.g. Bowles and Gintis 1998, 2004; Boyd *et al.* 2003; Gintis *et al.* 2003; Boyd and Mathews 2007; Hrdy 2000).

To establish the general contours of a circuit-level evolutionary contribution to sociality and morality, this section will draw on both neuroendocrinology and evolutionary neurobiology. Neuroendocrinology adds critical pieces of the puzzle because of the central role of various hormones with ancient lineages, including the neuropeptides oxytocin and vasopressin (as well as the endogenous opiates), in various forms of attachment, affiliative, and social behaviors (for reviews, see Carter 2003; Carter *et al.* 2008). These hormones were put to new uses in the development and reorganization of the mammalian brainstem and limbic brain to accommodate viviparity—the internal gestation and live birth of offspring that are often initially helpless. Evolutionary neurobiology, meanwhile, documents the expansion of the prefrontal cortex, and thus makes sense of the contrasts between small-brained mammals such as rats whose social lives are relatively simple and whose behavior patterns are tightly linked to subcortical structures, and large-brained mammals such as primates whose social lives involve much more sophisticated executive control, increased abilities to plan and evaluate, and a vastly expanded capacity to learn both social skills and the idiosyncrasies of individuals in the group (Keverne *et al.* 1996; Keverne 2004). (The neuroendocrine basis of the sociality of birds will not be discussed here, since although there are similarities in behavior between avian and mammalian social species, their evolutionary histories are quite different—see Goodson *et al.* 2005a,b for reviews. Nevertheless, although much is still unknown about its role, a hypothesis well worth investigating is that mesotocin—the avian homolog of oxytocin—may, like its mammalian counterpart, have been recruited in attachment and affiliative behavior.)

Oxytocin and vasopressin are simple peptides, with a roughly 700 million-year history wherein they, or, more accurately, their ancestral homologs, played various roles in osmoregulation and in reproductive processes such as egg-laying, sperm ejection, and spawning stimulation (Donaldson and Young 2008). In mammals, their role in both the body and the brain was expanded and modified, mainly to ensure that dependent offspring are cared for until they are capable of fending for themselves. The expression of fetal genes in the placenta results in the release of hormones (e.g. progesterone, prolactin, estrogen) into the mother's blood. This release causes an upregulation of the level of oxytocin in neurons in her hypothalamus. When progesterone levels drop sharply just before parturition, the density and sensitivity of oxytocin receptors in the hypothalamus increases, and sequestered oxytocin is massively released in the hypothalamus. Oxytocin is released in the body during birth, facilitating uterine contractions, and also during lactation to cause milk ejection. It is also released in the brain of both mother and infant during suckling (see Carter 1998; Brunton and Russell 2008 for overviews of the neuroendocrine events associated with pregnancy, birth, and the postpartum period). (Also critical to maternal behavior—although beyond the scope of our present discussion—are the endogenous opiates, which if blocked also disrupt or block maternal behavior, an effect observed, for example, in rats, sheep, and rhesus monkeys—see Martel *et al.* 1993; Keverne 2004; Broad *et al.* 2006.)

Basic maternal behavior in mammals after parturition is organized around ensuring that the offspring are kept warm, fed, clean, and safe. The changes in mammalian limbic circuitry ensuring infant care appear to be extensions of the jobs of more ancient circuitry that organizes self-care—that is, keeping *oneself* warm, fed, clean, and safe (Keverne *et al.* 1996; Panksepp 1998; Damasio 1999; Keverne 2004). The ancient brainstem–limbic organization serves self-preservation functions by monitoring internal glucose and carbon dioxide levels, body temperature, and so on, and triggering appropriate seeking behavior when discomfort or pain is registered. And pain, and the prediction of possible pain, is a critical part of the attachment and bonding story in mammals (Tucker *et al.* 2005). Nociceptive circuitry that served self-preservation functions in the pre-mammalian brain has been modified in the mammalian brainstem-limbic structures to respond to separation from juveniles and to conditions that threaten their safety. In turn, juveniles, dependent as they are on the mother, experience pain at separation and make distress calls to which the mother's nociceptive circuitry responds (Tucker *et al.* 2005). In effect, "my pain" expands to include social pain—the pain of separation, disapproval, and more generally, distress during conditions perceived to be unsafe.

These considerations lead to the following realization: that anything has value *at all* and is motivating *at all* ultimately depends on the very ancient neural organization serving well-being and its maintenance. That is, the rudimentary "caring organization" consisting of, among other neurobiological factors, oxytocin, vasopressin, and the endogenous opiates, serves to extend the basic value of being alive and well to selected others (Panksepp 1998; Damasio 1999). Put slightly differently, the nature of the neuroendocrine adaptations seen in mammals implies that the brainstem–limbic organization for self-maintenance and self-care has been "exapted" to serve attachment functions and to feeling pain at separation or distress, and thus to caring about the presence and well-being of others. The hypothesis on offer therefore sees the expanding circles of caring characteristic of humans and many other mammals as expansions of the magic circle of "me-and-mine." It entails widening the range of individuals who are valued, extending care beyond the individual to include offspring, mates, kin, and affiliates. These others may, in consequence, receive aid, defense, comfort, warmth, or whatever else conditions call for. Just as a threat to self-survival causes physical and/or psychological discomfort and motivates action, so too do threats to offspring- or kin-survival, although exactly how much risk is taken for these others' sake will of course depend on many additional factors.

Assuming this general platform for valuing, we can now examine some specific experimental work that sheds light on the relation between the neuroendocrine system and social and moral behavior. A particularly detailed and fruitful program of study on the role of oxytocin/vasopressin in the brain and behavior has focused on three species of vole: the montane vole (*Microtus montanus*) and meadow vole (*Microtus pennsylvanicus*), which are polygamous, and the prairie vole (*Microtus ochrogaster*), which is monogamous. Researchers have found that modest changes in the genes for oxytocin and vasopressin receptors in these species, as well as changes in these receptors' patterns of expression in the brain, are responsible for substantial differences in their social and mating systems (Donaldson and Young 2008). For example, in prairie voles these genetic and epigenetic changes enable long-term attachment of mates after the first mating and a high degree of sociability, behaviors which are absent in montane and meadow voles (Carter *et al.* 1995; Young *et al.* 1998; Donaldson and Young 2008).

More broadly, approximately 3% of mammals, including prairie voles, pine voles, California deer mice, beavers, titi monkeys, and marmosets show strong mate bonding (Kleiman 1977; Carter *et al.* 1995; Carter 2003). For these mammals, caring and valuing extend not only to offspring but to mates: they prefer to be with their mate rather than another adult, and males typically help to rear the offspring and guard the nest against intruders. Prairie voles exhibit a substantial stress response if they are separated from their mates (Carter *et al.* 1995) or if they are isolated from their kin (Kim and Kirkpatrick 1996). Moreover, in marmosets, but not in rats, attachment continues to exist even for offspring who have matured, and these mature offspring remaining in their natal group may help their parents feed and tend the next litter of baby marmosets (Roberts *et al.* 2001). The tendency by siblings or other non-parental individuals to exhibit alloparenting may therefore be another behavior that can emerge as a result of relatively minor changes to the genes for and distribution of receptors for oxytocin and vasopressin, given ecological conditions conducive to this trait's manifestation.

It would, of course, be misleading to refer to oxytocin, as popular science writers sometimes do, as a molecule "for" morality or love. Nevertheless, there *is* a connection between neurochemicals such as oxytocin, vasopressin, endogenous opiates, and dopamine on the one hand, and social behavior, including that subdomain of social behavior we call moral behavior, on the other. Because oxytocin is associated with downregulation of amygdala activity and with the parasympathetic component of the autonomic responses controlled by the brainstem, Sue Carter and colleagues (2009) have described it as being associated with an increased sense of safety. For example, levels of corticotropin releasing factor (CRF), associated with anxiety and sympathetic arousal, decrease when prairie voles are with a familiar partner, offspring, and other affiliated conspecifics; by contrast, CRF levels increase in the face of isolation or threats (Carter 2003; Ruscio *et al.* 2007). Results such as these imply that social animals that are near to others they trust are comfortable and relaxed. They also provide a neurobiological explanation for why, in highly social species (including humans), shunning and isolation are a potent form of punishment, just as inclusion and touching are potent sources of pleasure (Bekoff and Pierce 2009).

The foregoing constitutes a very brief overview of some of the roles of oxytocin and vasopressin in mammalian behavior. One puzzling question, however, is this: what is the link between oxytocin's role in the maternal behavior of early mammals, on the one hand, and its wider role in sociality, for instance as a signal of safety, on the other? These seem like very different sorts of operations. Probably, however, these superficial differences mask important deep relationships. Supporting this contention is work by Stephen Porges (e.g. 2007), who suggests that evolutionary changes in the brainstem circuitry involving the vagus nerve allowed for the transition from the common reptilian "freezing in fear" to the quite different "immobility without fear." Anatomically, the locus of these changes is the periaqueductal gray (PAG), which coordinates freezing behavior, and the emergence in mammals of the ventrolateral region of the PAG (vlPAG), which is rich in oxytocin receptors and is connected to the new myelinated branch of the vagus nerve. As Porges (2007) points out, small changes can signal a shift from *safe* to *unsafe*, and the close interconnections of the circuitry regulating aggression, freezing, and immobility-without-fear allow for fast responses.

In light of this, a plausible evolutionary connection between oxytocin and parasympathetic responses in early, small-brained mammals was the advantage gained by mothers who were content to remain "immobile without fear" for relatively long periods while the infants suckled. Unlike a female frog that just drops her eggs in a chosen spot and hops on her way, the female mammal needs to spend a lot of her time in the nest, much of it awake but lying still so that her offspring can feed. If she feels comfortable and content—if her autonomic system is in a resting or non-defensive mode and her endogenous opiates in ample supply—it is more likely she will find the suckling business and contact with her offspring rewarding.

As a result of these advantages, the rudiments of attachment emerged through evolution by natural selection, and further modifications embellished and diversified these rudiments so that attachments utilizing oxytocin/vasopressin/opiate mechanisms could form without the need for suckling itself. Consequently, attachment may extend beyond suckling-age offspring to include mates, older offspring, non-offspring kin, and even unrelated individuals. For instance, humans, unlike rats, may become spontaneously attached to infants even without pregnancy and parturition (Keverne 2004).

Additional modifications to these attachment mechanisms would also have motivated larger and more complex mammals, such as bears and monkeys, to continue tending their young after weaning; some, such as baboons and humans, may remain attached in varying degrees for life. Adaptations to the neurohormone system that are specific to primates, and in particular humans, will thus probably be relevant to explanations of some specific features of primate and human sociality, although many details are not yet known. But in spite of this relative dearth of available details, there are some general explanatory possibilities that the foregoing discussion suggests, and it is to these that we now turn.

We will begin with a bit of additional evolutionary and theoretical background. When ecological conditions make living in groups advantageous, as in baboons, chimpanzees, or humans, additional adaptations—probably including changes in circuitry involving oxytocin, vasopressin, and the endogenous opiates—allow for valuing kin, affiliates, and friends. In group-living species, learning local conventions and personality traits of individuals, knowing who is related to whom, and tending one's own reputation become increasingly important. The development of a large forebrain highly interconnected to limbic structures allows for synaptic distance between instincts and behavior, permitting flexibility in planning, evaluation of consequences, impulse control, and innovative social strategies (Panksepp 1998; Tucker *et al.* 2005). As Tucker and colleagues (2005) point out, control by prefrontal structures makes use of feelings of general pain associated with the anterior cingulate in the anticipation of a possible painful situation, so that plans for evasive action or aggressive forestalling can be made. And given the role of pain in separation and disapproval, it is not surprising that shunning and rejection are common solutions to problems of potentially damaging anti-social behavior. Also relevant to what follows is the notion that social problem-solving is probably an instance of a more general capacity for problem solving, and is directed toward finding suitable ways to cope with challenges such as instability, conflict, and resource scarcity (Churchland 2008). From this perspective, moral problem-solving is, in its turn, likely a special instance of social problem-solving more broadly.

Our suggestion is that in humans, as in other highly social mammals, social values are anchored by circuitry in the brainstem-limbic system that supports self-caring and kin-caring. Like other large-brained mammals, human young learn social skills and local practices, which, by engaging the reward and pain systems, can become largely automatic, and thus often seem intuitively obvious and absolutely inviolable. Roughly within the last 40,000 years of *Homo sapiens'* approximately 200,000-year existence on the planet, human cultures have developed in uniquely rich ways. Consequently, cultural and social institutions have changed the ecological conditions for modern humans, whose social lives are very different from those of humans who lived, say, 100,000 years ago. Groups have grown large, and inter-action has expanded far beyond the occasional gatherings where small groups could meet and exchange tools. "Niche construction" by humans has changed the species' ecology in many ways, altering social organizations and leading to the formulation of specific institu-tions, laws, and rules. Consequently, social behavior—including what we would now identify as moral behavior—has changed accordingly (Hrdy 2000; Laland *et al.* 2000; Nesse 2007). (Differences in social practices between human groups are, of course, also observed and will reflect differences in ecological conditions, as well as historical accidents.)

Among the responses to these changing ecological conditions, and to group living more generally, are an expanding sphere of attachment, the internalization of rules, and the devel-opment of institutions structuring social behavior including cooperation and punishment. These cognitive and behavioral responses have, in turn, been enabled by expansions in the functions of a number of preexisting brain systems, notably the oxytocin/vasopressin/opiate and affect/reward systems. (These systems also interact in important ways. For instance, there is evidence suggesting that a major reason for the affiliation- and attachment-promoting effects of oxytocin and vasopressin is their activation of reward mechanisms in the brain—see Curley and Keverne 2005.)

A philosophical objection to the approach outlined here, hinted at in our earlier discus-sion of moral psychology, is that social behavior anchored by the brainstem–limbic system and shaped by reward-based learning and problem-solving cannot be genuinely moral behavior, for such must be grounded solely in moral reasons (e.g. moral duties to others) that are consciously acknowledged and reasoned about. One response to this objection is simply that the "traditional" philosophical picture of morality is psychologically highly unrealistic, at odds with what a substantial body of scientific research reveals. This negative response to the objection, while forceful on its own, is further strengthened when paired with a more positive response. While a full development of this response would require a lengthy disquisition, a brief sketch may help to give an idea of how it would go.

The essence of the positive response is that moral behaviors, sentiments, motives, judg-ments, and so forth—the love felt by a parent for a child or by mates for one another, for example—are completely real, not lacking in moral worth merely because they have a neu-robiological mechanism or because that mechanism has an evolutionary history. Consider an analogy to the trichromatic color vision possessed by humans and a number of other primate species. Evolutionarily, trichromacy is rooted in monochromatic and dichromatic vision; mutations for trichromacy were, according to one prominent hypothesis, selected for in certain primates due to the advantages trichromats have over monochromats and dichro-mats in spotting ripe fruit against a background of leaves (see Regan *et al.* 2001; Surridge *et al.* 2003). Understanding the evolutionary history of our color vision does not, however, entail that appreciating the hues of a painting or sunset is somehow a counterfeit experience or that so-called "color" vision is somehow just seeing shades of gray or of colors seen by dichromats (e.g. blue/yellow, red/green) and pretending it is something more experientially rich.

Likewise, mammals are not just frogs with a few bells and whistles, behaviorally and cognitively unsophisticated and dominated by self-regard. Caring about the well-being of kith and kin is not just "as if" caring; it is a complex, powerful force in our social and psychological lives, and the greater our understanding of the neurobiology of sociality, the more evident its complexity and power becomes. To require of "real morality" that our moral behavior be autonomous with respect to our evolutionary history and our brains' portfolio of oxytocin, vasopressin, endorphins, and their receptors, as well as the activity of systems for pain, pleasure, emotion, and reward, is to put morality out of reach entirely.

That these neurobiological mechanisms are highly relevant to morality is further brought out by recent work investigating the effects of oxytocin on trusting behavior in economic games. Although much less is known about the details of oxytocin's role in humans than in voles and other non-human species, we believe that this is a fitting conclusion to the section since it directly links work in neuroendocrinology and evolutionary neurobiology to human moral behavior and to our earlier discussion of experimental economics.

Very briefly, the research in question asked whether elevating oxytocin levels in humans through intranasal administration of the neuropeptide (see Born *et al.* 2002) would influence behavior by investors in the trust game. Kosfeld and colleagues (2005) hypothesized, on the basis of previous work demonstrating the importance of oxytocin in attachment and affiliation (see earlier), that artificially increasing levels of this hormone would increase subjects' willingness to invest money with their trust game partner. Their experimental results supported this hypothesis: the average transfer from investor to trustee was 17% higher in the oxytocin group as compared to the placebo group, a statistically significant difference (Kosfeld *et al.* 2005). Additionally, a far higher percentage of subjects in the oxytocin group made the maximum possible transfer to the trustee (45% versus 21% in the placebo group).

Still more interestingly, the researchers established that the higher average transfer of subjects given oxytocin was not due to a general decrease in risk aversion. They did this by examining whether oxytocin would lead to increased transfers when the subject's "partner" in the game was a random mechanism rather than another individual; in this case, the average transfer was identical in the oxytocin and placebo groups (Kosfeld *et al.* 2005). Thus, the trust-increasing effects of oxytocin appear to be specific to interactions with other humans, a notable parallel to the results described earlier concerning selective or heightened affect and reward responses while playing economic games with human as compared to computer partners (e.g. Sanfey *et al.* 2003; Rilling *et al.* 2004; van't Wout *et al.* 2006).

SUMMARY AND FUTURE DIRECTIONS

In this chapter, we have reviewed evidence from a variety of areas of cognitive science—moral psychology, experimental economics, clinical neurology, neuroendocrinology, and evolutionary neurobiology—that shed light on the neurobiological bases of morality. Taken together, findings from these fields point toward a substantial role for brain systems associated with affect and reward, as well as neuroendocrine mechanisms including oxytocin and vasopressin, in morality.

Notably, much of the moral learning, judgment, motivation, and behavior underwritten by affect, reward, and neuroendocrine processes need not be mediated by conscious reasoning. An individual contemplating donating to a charity whose mission she supports, or punishing someone perceived to have acted unfairly, is often simply motivated to do these things because she, as a result of how the relevant systems in her brain work, finds them rewarding and emotionally satisfying. She does not, in other words, need to go through a quasi-deductive process of moral reasoning to determine, for example, that she should donate to charity because the obligation to do so follows from some general moral rule she accepts plus additional premises describing her situation. In this way, morality is like a complex skill—playing chess or performing brain surgery, say—which, despite its sophistication, need not (and indeed often should not) be subject to continuous conscious oversight to operate effectively.

This is not to say that conscious reasoning has no role to play in morality, but rather that its role may be less substantial than many philosophers are wont to assume. Determining exactly what role conscious reasoning, explicit moral rules, higher-order beliefs, and so on play in the development and exercise of normal moral capacities will be an important project for future research. Also crucial will be gaining a more detailed understanding of the neurobiological substrates of the various cognitive processes involved in morality, as well as the ways these processes interact. One important aspect of this will involve examining how the neuroendocrine system, particularly oxytocin and vasopressin, modulates affective and reward responses to moral situations, actions, and the like (see Curley and Keverne 2005 for a review of some suggestive data from non-human species). Progress in this area may be expedited by improvements in the spatial and temporal resolution of brain imaging techniques, by utilizing data from multiple recording and imaging techniques (e.g. fMRI, electroencephalography, SCR), by combining experimental interventions (e.g. administering intranasal oxytocin before an fMRI-based task), and by further neurobiological and behavioral studies of non-human species, especially primates. A further question for future research concerns the precise density and distribution of receptors for oxytocin and vasopressin in the human brain. This is not known at present but will probably be addressed with the improvement of non-invasive techniques such as magnetic resonance spectroscopy. Finally, as always, there is much scope for creative experimental designs and technological advances that will allow more ecologically valid investigations of moral judgment and behavior without compromising the requirements of controlled and ethical experimentation.

These are but a few of the general lines of inquiry that we believe will prove important and illuminating in the years ahead. As should be apparent, there is substantial work to be done. Even so, as this chapter has aimed to show, there have also been substantial advances in our knowledge of the neurobiological bases of morality in a relatively short period of time. This rapid progress, combined with the tantalizing prospects for future progress, is one of many reasons that the study of morality is one of the most exciting and dynamic areas of cognitive science today.

Acknowledgements

We thank Sue Carter and Barry Keverne for helpful feedback on an earlier draft of this chapter.

References

Anderson, S.W., Bechara, A., Damasio, H., Tranel, D., and Damasio, A.R. (1999). Impairment of social and moral behavior related to early damage in human prefrontal cortex. *Nature Neuroscience*, 2, 1032–7.

Bales, K.L., Pfeifer, L.A., and Carter, C.S. (2004). Sex differences and developmental effects of manipulations of oxytocin on alloparenting and anxiety in prairie voles. *Developmental Psychobiology*, 44, 123–31.

Bechara, A., Damasio, A.R., Damasio, H., and Anderson, S.W. (1994). Insensitivity to future consequences following damage to human prefrontal cortex. *Cognition*, 50, 7–12.

Bechara, A., Tranel, D., Damasio, H., and Damasio, A.R. (1996). Failure to respond autonomically to anticipated future outcomes following damage to prefrontal cortex. *Cerebral Cortex*, 6, 215–25.

Beckett, C., Maughan, B., Rutter, M., *et al.* (2006). Do the effects of early severe deprivation on cognition persist into early adolescence? Findings from the English and Romanian adoptees study. *Child Development*, 77, 696–711.

Bekoff, M. and Pierce, J. (2009). *Wild justice: the moral lives of animals*. Chicago, IL: The University of Chicago Press.

Bellugi, U., Lichtenberger, L., Mills, D., Galaburda, A., and Korenberg, J.R. (1999). Bridging cognition, the brain and molecular genetics: evidence from Williams syndrome. *Trends in Neurosciences*, 22, 197–207.

Blonigen, D.M., Hicks, B.M., Krueger, R.F., Patrick, C.J., and Iacono, W.G. (2005). Psychopathic personality traits: heritability and genetic overlap with internalizing and externalizing psychopathology. *Psychological Medicine*, 35, 637–48.

Born, J., Lange T., Kern, W., McGregor, G.P., Bickel, U., and Fehm, H.L. (2002). Sniffing neuropeptides: a transnasal approach to the human brain. *Nature Neuroscience*, 5, 514–16.

Bowes, L., Arseneault, L., Maughan, B., Taylor, A., Caspi, A., and Moffitt T.E. (2009). School, neighborhood, and family factors are associated with children's bullying involvement: a nationally representative longitudinal study. *Journal of the American Academy of Child & Adolescent Psychiatry*, 48, 543–5.

Bowles, S. and Gintis, H. (1998). The moral economy of communities: structured populations and the evolution of pro-social norms. *Evolution and Human Behavior*, 19, 3–25.

Bowles, S. and Gintis, H. (2004). The evolution of strong reciprocity: cooperation in heterogeneous populations. *Theoretical Population Biology*, 65, 17–28.

Boyd, R. and Mathew, S. (2007). A narrow road to cooperation. *Science*, 316, 1858–9.

Boyd, R., Gintis, H., Bowles, S., and Richerson, P.J. (2003). The evolution of altruistic punishment. *Proceedings of the National Academy of Sciences of the United States of America*, 100, 3531–5.

Broad, K.D. Curley, J.P., and Keverne, E.B. (2006). Mother–infant bonding and the evolution of mammalian social relationships. *Philosophical Transactions of the Royal Society of London B: Biological Sciences*, 361, 2199–214.

Brunton, P.J. and Russell, J.A. (2008). Keeping oxytocin neurons under control during stress in pregnancy. *Progress in Brain Research*, 170, 365–77.

Cameron, N.M., Champagne, F.A., Parent, C., Fish, E.W., Ozaki-Kuroda, K., and Meaney, M.J. (2005). The programming of individual differences in defensive responses and reproductive strategies in the rat through variations in maternal care. *Neuroscience and Biobehavioral Reviews*, 29, 843–65.

Carter, C.S. (1998). Neuroendocrine perspectives on social attachment and love. *Psychoneuroendocrinology*, **23**, 779–818.

Carter, C.S. (2003). Developmental consequences of oxytocin. *Physiology & Behavior*, **79**, 383–97.

Carter, C.S., DeVries, A.C., and Getz, L.L. (1995). Physiological substrates of mammalian monogamy: the prairie vole model. *Neuroscience and Biobehavioral Reviews*, **19**, 303–14.

Carter, C.S., Grippo, A.J., Pournajafi-Nazarloo, H., Ruscio, M.G., and Porges, S.W. (2008). Oxytocin, vasopressin and sociality. In I. Neumann and R. Landgraf (eds.) *Progress in Brain Research 170: Advances in Vasopressin and Oxytocin: From Genes to Behaviour to Disease*, pp. 331–6. New York: Elsevier.

Carter, C.S., Harris, J., and Porges, S.W. (2009). Neural and evolutionary perspectives on empathy. In J. Decety and W. Ickes (eds.) *The Social Neuroscience of Empathy*, pp. 169–82. Cambridge, MA: MIT Press.

Casebeer, W.D. (2003). Moral cognition and its neural constituents. *Nature Reviews Neuroscience*, **4**, 841–6.

Casebeer, W.D. and Churchland, P.S. (2003). The neural mechanisms of moral cognition: a multiple-aspect approach to moral judgment and decision-making. *Biology and Philosophy*, **18**, 169–94.

Caspi, A., McClay, J., Moffitt, T.E., *et al.* (2002). Role of genotype in the cycle of violence in maltreated children. *Science*, **297**, 851–4.

Champagne, F., Diorio, J., Sharma, S., and Meaney, M.J. (2001). Variations in maternal care in the rat are associated with differences in estrogen-related changes in oxytocin receptor levels. *Proceedings of the National Academy of Sciences of the United States of America*, **98**, 12736–41.

Churchland, P.S. (2008). The impact of neuroscience on philosophy. *Neuron*, **60**, 409–11.

Curley, J.P. and Keverne, E.B. (2005). Genes, brains and mammalian social bonds. *Trends in Ecology and Evolution*, **20**, 561–67.

Cushman, F., Young, L., and Hauser, M.D. (2006). The role of conscious reasoning and intuition in moral judgment: testing three principles of harm. *Psychological Science*, **17**, 1082–9.

Dai, L., Bellugi, U., Chen, X.-N., *et al.* (2009). Is it Williams syndrome? *GTF2IRD1* Implicated in visual-spatial construction and *GTF2I* in sociability revealed by high resolution arrays. *American Journal of Medical Genetics* Part A, **149A**, 302–14.

Damasio, A.R. (1996). The somatic marker hypothesis and the possible functions of the prefrontal cortex. *Philosophical Transactions of the Royal Society of London: Biological Sciences*, **351**, 1413–20.

Damasio, A.R. (1999). *The Feeling of What Happens*. New York: Harcourt Brace.

Damasio, A.R., Tranel, D., and Damasio, H. (1990). Individuals with sociopathic behavior caused by frontal damage fail to respond autonomically to social stimuli. *Behavioural Brain Research*, **41**, 81–94.

Dijksterhuis, A. (2004). I like myself but I don't know why: enhancing implicit self-esteem by subliminal evaluative conditioning. *Journal of Personality and Social Psychology*, **86**, 345–55.

Donaldson, Z.R. and Young, L.J. (2008). Oxytocin, vasopressin, and the neurogenetics of sociality. *Science*, **322**, 900–4.

Fehr, E. and Fischbacher, U. (2004). Third-party punishment and social norms. *Evolution and Human Behavior*, **25**, 63–87.

Fehr, E. and Gächter, S. (2000). Cooperation and punishment in public goods experiments. *The American Economic Review*, **90**, 980–94.

Fehr, E. and Gächter, S. (2002). Altruistic punishment in humans. *Nature*, **415**, 137–40.

Gintis, H., Bowles, S., Boyd, R., and Fehr, E. (2003). Explaining altruistic behavior in humans. *Evolution and Human Behavior*, **24**, 153–72.

Goodson, J.L., Evans, A.K., Lindberg, L., and Allen, C.A. (2005a). Neuro-evolutionary patterning of sociality. *Proceedings of the Royal Society of London B: Biological Sciences*, **272**, 227–35.

Goodson, J.L., Saldanha, C.J., Hahn, T.P., and Soma, K.K. (2005b). Recent advances in behavioral neuroendocrinology: Insights from studies on birds. *Hormones and Behavior*, **48**, 461–73.

Greene, J.D. (2008). The secret joke of Kant's soul. In W. Sinnott-Armstrong (ed.) *Moral Psychology, Vol. 3: The Neuroscience of Morality: Emotion, Brain Disorders, and Development*, pp. 35–79. Cambridge, MA: MIT Press.

Greene, J. and Haidt, J. (2002). How (and where) does moral judgment work? *Trends in Cognitive Sciences*, **6**, 517–23.

Greene, J.D., Sommerville, R.B., Nystrom, L., Darley, J., and Cohen, J.D. (2001). An fMRI investigation of emotional engagement in moral judgment. *Science*, **293**, 2105–8.

Greene, J.D., Nystrom, L.E., Engell, A.D., Darley, J.M., and Cohen, J.D. (2004). The neural bases of cognitive conflict and control in moral judgment. *Neuron*, **44**, 389–400.

Haidt, J. (2001). The emotional dog and its rational tail: A social intuitionist approach to moral judgment. *Psychological Review*, **108**, 814–34.

Haidt, J. and Hersh, M.A. (2001). Sexual morality: the cultures and emotions of conservatives and liberals. *Journal of Applied Social Psychology*, **31**, 191–221.

Haidt, J., Koller, S., and Dias, M. (1993). Affect, culture and morality. *Journal of Personality and Social Psychology*, **65**, 613–28.

Harbaugh, W.T., Mayr, U., and Burghart, D.R. (2007). Neural responses to taxation and voluntary giving reveal motives for charitable donations. *Science*, **316**, 1622–5.

Hare, R.D. (1965). Psychopathy, fear arousal and anticipated pain. *Psychological Reports*, **162**, 499–502.

Hare, R.D. (1972). Psychopathy and physiological responses to adrenalin. *Journal of Abnormal Psychology*, **792**, 138–47.

Hare, R.D. (1991). *Manual for the Hare Psychopathy Checklist-Revised*. Toronto: Multi-Health Systems.

Hare, R.D. (2003). *Manual for the Hare Psychopathy Checklist-Revised, 2nd ed.* Toronto: Multi-Health Systems.

Hare, R.D., Frazelle, J., and Cox, D.N. (1978). Psychopathy and physiological responses to threat of an aversive stimulus. *Psychophysiology*, **152**, 165–72.

Hare, R.D. and Quinn, M.J. (1971). Psychopathy and autonomic conditioning. *Journal of Abnormal Psychology*, **773**, 223–35.

Hauser, M., Cushman, F., Young, L., Jin, R.K., and Mikhail, J. (2007). A dissociation between moral judgments and justifications. *Mind & Language*, **22**, 1–21.

Hrdy, S.B. (2000). *Mother Nature: Maternal Instincts and How they Shape the Human Species*. New York: Ballantine Books.

Johansson, P., Hall, L., Sikström, S., and Olsson, A. (2005). Failure to detect mismatches between intention and outcome in a simple decision task. *Science*, **310**, 116–19.

Keverne, E.B. (2004). Understanding well-being in the evolutionary context of brain development. *Philosophical Transactions of the Royal Society of London B: Biological Sciences*, **359**, 1349–58.

Keverne, E.B., Martel, F.L., and Nevison, C.M. (1996). Primate brain evolution: genetic and functional considerations. *Proceedings of the Royal Society of London B: Biological Sciences*, **263**, 689–96.

Kiehl, K.A. (2006). A cognitive neuroscience perspective on psychopathy: evidence for paralimbic system dysfunction. *Psychiatry Research*, **142**, 107–28.

Kiehl, K.A., Smith, A.M., Hare, R.D., *et al.* (2001). Limbic abnormalities in affective processing by criminal psychopaths as revealed by functional magnetic resonance imaging. *Biological Psychiatry*, **50**, 677–84.

Kim, J.W. and Kirkpatrick, B. (1996). Social isolation in animal models of relevance to neuropsychiatric disorders. *Biological Psychiatry*, **40**, 918–22.

King-Casas, B., Tomlin, D., Anen, C., Camerer, C.F., Quartz, S.R., and Montague, P.R. (2005). Getting to know you: reputation and trust in a two-person economic exchange. *Science*, **308**, 78–83.

Kleiman, D.G. (1977). Monogamy in mammals. *The Quarterly Review of Biology*, **52**, 39–69.

Korsgaard, C. (1996). *The Sources of Normativity*. Cambridge: Cambridge University Press.

Korsgaard, C. (1999). Self-constitution in the ethics of Plato and Kant. *The Journal of Ethics*, **3**, 1–29.

Kosfeld, M., Heinrichs, M., Zak, P.J., Fischbacher, U., and Fehr, E. (2005). Oxytocin increases trust in humans. *Nature*, **435**, 673–6.

Kreppner, J.M., Rutter, M., Beckett, C., *et al.* (2007). Normality and impairment following profound early institutional deprivation: a longitudinal follow-up into early adolescence. *Developmental Psychology*, **43**, 931–46.

Laland, K.N., Odling-Smee, J., and Feldman, M.W. (2000). Niche construction, biological evolution, and cultural change. *Behavioral and Brain Sciences*, **23**, 131–46.

Martel, F.L., Nevison, C.M., Rayment, F.D., Simpson, M.J.A., and Keverne, E.B. (1993). Opioid receptor blockade reduces maternal affect and social grooming in rhesus monkeys. *Psychoneuroendocrinology*, **18**, 307–21.

Mathis, H. (1970). *Emotional responsivity in the antisocial personality*. Unpublished Doctoral Dissertation. Washington, DC: George Washington University.

Maynard Smith, J. and Price, G.R. (1973). The logic of animal conflict. *Nature*, **246**, 15–18.

Meaney, M.J. (2001). Maternal care, gene expression, and the transmission of individual differences in stress reactivity across generations. *Annual Review of Neuroscience*, **24**, 1161–92.

Milgram, S. (1963). Behavioral study of obedience. *Journal of Abnormal and Social Psychology*, **67**, 371–8.

Milgram, S. (1974). *Obedience to authority: An experimental view*. New York: Harper & Row.

Moll, J., de Oliveira-Souza, R., Bramati, I.E. and Grafman, J. (2002a). Functional networks in emotional moral and nonmoral social judgments. *NeuroImage*, **16**, 696–703.

Moll, J., de Oliveira-Souza, R., Eslinger, P.J., *et al.* (2002b). The neural correlates of moral sensitivity: a functional magnetic resonance imaging investigation of basic and moral emotions. *Journal of Neuroscience*, **22**, 2730–6.

Moll, J., Zahn, R., de Oliveira-Souza, R., Krueger, F., and Grafman, J. (2005). The neural basis of human moral cognition. *Nature Reviews Neuroscience*, **6**, 799–809.

Moll, J., Krueger, F., Zahn, R., Pardini, M., de Oliveira-Souza, R., and Grafman, J. (2006). Human fronto-mesolimbic networks guide decisions about charitable donation. *Proceedings of the National Academy of Sciences*, **103**, 15623–8.

Monin, B., Pizarro, D.A., and Beer, J.S. (2007). Deciding versus reacting: conceptions of moral judgment and the reason-affect debate. *Review of General Psychology*, **11**, 99–111.

Nesse, R.M. (2007). Runaway social selection for displays of partner value and altruism. *Biological Theory*, 2, 143–55.

Nowak, M.A., Page, K.M., and Sigmund, K. (2000). Fairness versus reason in the Ultimatum Game. *Science*, 289, 1773–5.

Panksepp, J. (1998). *Affective Neuroscience: The Foundations of Human and Animal Emotions*. New York: Oxford University Press.

Porges, S.W. (2007). The polyvagal perspective. *Biological Psychology*, 74, 116–43.

de Quervain J., Fischbacher, U., Treyer, V., *et al.* (2004). The neural basis of altruistic punishment. *Science*, 305, 1254–8.

Regan, B.C., Julliot, C., Simmen, B., Vienot, F., Charles-Dominique, P., and Mollon, J.D. (2001). Fruits, foliage and the evolution of primate colour vision. *Philosophical Transactions of the Royal Society of London B: Biological Sciences*, 356, 229–83.

Rilling, J.K., Gutman, D.A., Zeh, T.R., Pagnoni, G., Berns, G.S., and Kilts, K.D. (2002). A neural basis for social cooperation. *Neuron*, 35, 395–405.

Rilling, J.K., Sanfey, A.G., Aronson, J.A., Nystrom, L.E., and Cohen, J.D. (2004). Opposing BOLD responses to reciprocated and unreciprocated altruism in putative reward pathways. *NeuroReport*, 15, 2539–43.

Roberts, R.L., Jenkins, K.T., Lawler, T., *et al.* (2001). Prolactin levels are elevated after infant carrying in parentally inexperienced common marmosets. *Physiology & Behavior*, 72, 713–20.

Ruscio, M.G., Sweeny, T., Hazelton, J., Suppatkul, P., and Carter, C.S. (2007). Social environment regulates corticotropin releasing factor, corticosterone and vasopressin in juvenile prairie voles. *Hormones and Behavior*, 51, 54–61.

Sanfey, A.G. (2007). Social decision-making: insights from game theory and neuroscience. *Science*, 318, 598–602.

Sanfey, A.G., Rilling, J.K., Aronson, J.A., Nystrom, L.E., and Cohen, J.D. (2003). The neural basis of economic decision-making in the ultimatum game. *Science*, 300, 1755–8.

Suhler, C.L. and Churchland, P.S. (2009). Control: conscious and otherwise. *Trends in Cognitive Sciences*, 13, 341–7.

Surridge, A.K., Osorio, D., and Mundy, N.I. (2003). Evolution and selection of trichromatic vision in primates. *Trends in Ecology and Evolution*, 18, 198–205.

Thompson, R.R., George, K., Walton, J.C., Orr, S.P., and Benson, J. (2006). Sex-specific influences of vasopressin on human social communication. *Proceedings of the National Academy of Sciences of the United States of America*, 103, 7889–94.

Tucker, D.M., Luu, P., and Derryberry, D. (2005). Love hurts: the evolution of empathic concern through the encephalization of nociceptive capacity. *Developmental Psychopathology*, 17, 699–713.

Viding, E., Blair, R.J.R., Moffitt, T.E., and Plomin, R. (2005). Evidence for substantial genetic risk for psychopathy in 7-year-olds. *Journal of Child Psychology and Psychiatry*, 46, 592–7.

van't Wout, M., Kahn, R.S., Sanfey, A.G., and Aleman, A. (2006). Affective state and decision-making in the Ultimatum Game. *Experimental Brain Research*, 169, 564–8.

Wegner, D.M. (2002). *The Illusion of Conscious Will*. Cambridge, MA: MIT Press.

Wilson, T.D. (2002). *Strangers to Ourselves: Discovering the Adaptive Unconscious*. Cambridge, MA: Harvard University Press.

Young, L.J., Wang, Z., and Insel, T.R. (1998). Neuroendocrine bases of monogamy. *Trends in Neurosciences*, 21, 71–5.

CHAPTER 4

DEVELOPMENT OF THE ADOLESCENT BRAIN: NEUROETHICAL IMPLICATIONS FOR THE UNDERSTANDING OF EXECUTIVE FUNCTION AND SOCIAL COGNITION

MONICA LUCIANA

INTRODUCTION

Current conceptualizations of adolescence focus on this period as one of "storm and stress" (Arnett 1992), as one where risk-taking accelerates to an alarming degree (Arnett 1992; Steinberg 2008) and where mortality increases, primarily due to accidental deaths (presumably due to risk-taking). The popular press conveys adolescence largely in terms of this behavioral storm with the implicit (if not explicit) assertion that otherwise easy-to-manage children will turn into out-of-control strangers during this period, leaving parents and teachers ill-prepared to cope with the alien that their child has become. Evidence suggests that adolescent risk-taking leads to vulnerability to externalizing psychopathology, such as substance abuse, and that teens are impervious to educational interventions designed to prevent such outcomes (Steinberg 2008). The tone within the literature is unambiguously negative. As a group, adolescents are characterized as having difficulties with behavioral regulation and it is suggested that these difficulties have a basis in neural function (or dysfunction). Specifically, immaturity of the prefrontal cortex (PFC) may account for the problematic constellation of behaviors that characterize adolescence given the PFC's role in behavioral regulation. Adolescents are likened in some sense to frontal lobe lesion patients; such patients have been known for decades to exhibit deficits in judgment, decision-making, behavioral control, and high-level cognition (Bechara *et al.* 1994; Milner 1963; Shallice 1982).

The implications of these assertions have only infrequently been examined from a neuro-ethical standpoint.

Neuroethics is the consideration of what is good versus bad or right versus wrong in the consequences of brain research (Safire 2007). Brain research has informed many recent studies of adolescent development either through direct measures of brain structure and activity in neuroimaging studies or through behavioral studies where laboratory tasks are selected on the basis of their links to brain function. This body of work has led to a popular understanding of adolescence as a time period when risk-taking behavior escalates to extreme levels due to brain-based immaturities. This chapter will consider what neurobehavioral studies allow us to conclude about executive functions in adolescence, what studies of brain development indicate about the status of the adolescent brain, and then, importantly, if these research domains cohere. That is, can it be said that brain-based substrates clearly underlie the immaturities in executive function observed in adolescence? The practical and ethical implications of these findings, in theory as well as practice, will be discussed using legal decisions as a prominent example.

EXECUTIVE FUNCTIONS AND SOCIAL COGNITION IN ADOLESCENCE

The concept of executive function broadly refers to *"capacities that enable a person to engage successfully in independent, purposive, self-serving behavior"* (Lezak et al. 2004, p. 35). Executive function difficulties impact an individual's ability to approach and carry out tasks that are important for adaptive functioning and impact an individual's control over, and monitoring of, ongoing behavior. Tasks and behaviors that are impacted can be purely cognitive ones or can represent aspects of social and emotional functioning. As a construct, *executive function* is a brain-neutral term in the sense that there is no explicit link with functioning in any one brain region. However, decades of brain research indicate reliable associations between the intact functioning of the prefrontal cortex and capacities that allow for self-organized future-directed behavior. These capacities are numerous, including working memory (the ability to actively represent information in mind as one works toward a goal (Goldman-Rakic 1987)), inhibitory control (the ability to withhold inappropriate but compelling responses (Fuster 1997)), behavioral flexibility (the ability to switch behavior away from a given response based on environmental feedback (Rosenkilde 1979)), conflict monitoring (the ability to monitor and execute responses that conflict with others that are salient at a given point in time (Braver *et al.* 2001)), probabilistic decision-making (the ability to make and execute decisions adaptively when potential choice options vary according to their probabilities of success), and the related construct of motivated decision-making, the ability to adaptively consider probabilities associated with potential choices even when those probabilities might conflict with an immediate motivation (Bechara *et al.* 1994). A key executive ability concerns the extent to which an individual can fluidly problem-solve under novel, ambiguous, or stressful circumstances. As this brief description suggests, these many processes are interrelated, particularly as situational complexity increases, requiring the integration of multiple information-processing tasks.

From a developmental standpoint, rudimentary executive functions that have been linked to prefrontal substrates are evident in infancy (Bell and Fox 1992; Diamond 1990a,b; Diamond and Goldman-Rakic 1989), coincident with the capacity for independent locomotion. These functions include mnemonically-guided approaches to salient objects following short delay intervals (an early manifestation of working memory) as well as the ability to reach around a clear barrier to reach a desired object (inhibitory control) and behavioral flexibility. These functions show a steady rate of improvement through early and middle childhood as assessed by set-shifting, conflict-monitoring, working memory, and inhibitory control tasks (Diamond and Taylor 1996; Gerstadt et al. 1994; Kerr and Zelazo 2004; Levin et al. 1991; Luciana and Nelson 1998, 2002; Passler et al. 1985; Ridderinkhof et al. 1997; Welsh and Pennington 1991; Zelazo et al. 1996). Thus, throughout childhood, executive functions become increasingly well-developed, although those items and/or tasks that differentiate among children of different ages demand relatively little as viewed from an adult perspective. As children mature, they become capable of processing increasingly larger amounts of information and integrating that information to achieve behavioral goals. This observation led our group to suggest that a primary aspect of what is developing is a form of informational multi-tasking, the ability to hold multiple sources of information in mind simultaneously and to use that information to work toward future goals (Luciana et al. 2005). Importantly, this information includes internal motivational cues/drives as well as externally cued social signals that must be integrated with other information in the context of ongoing behavior.

Many early studies concluded that adolescence was a period of continued executive function development, because pre-adolescents (generally including individuals under the age of 12 years) differed from young adults (individuals over the age of 18 years) in their behavioral performance (Levin et al. 1991; Luciana and Nelson 2002; Welsh et al. 1991). For example, using the Cambridge Neuropsychological Testing Automated Battery (CANTAB) (Sahakian and Owen 1982), Luciana and Nelson (2002) found, among other things, that 11–12-year-olds were statistically inferior to 18-year-olds in their ability to hold multiple spatial locations in mind and reproduce a spatial sequence in the correct order. They reported that 11–12-year-olds were successful on average when 6.1 items had to be recalled in order, while 18–30-year-olds were, on average, successful when 7.4 items had to be recalled. This example illustrates an important feature of executive function development as assessed in this age range using laboratory tasks: the absolute difference between adolescents' and adults' performance is often small in magnitude when considered from a practical perspective, although the groups statistically differ. Over the past 10 years, the field has experienced a surge in studies that have examined the adolescent period more directly through the study of 12–17-year-olds.

These studies confirm that adolescence is a time of continued development of planning skills (Tower of London task performance (Asato et al. 2006; Luciana et al. 2009)), working memory (De Luca et al. 2003; Luciana et al. 2005; Luna et al. 2004), and inhibitory control (go/no-go and flanker tasks (Hooper et al. 2004; Luna et al. 2004, 2010)). The upper limit or apparent developmental plateau varies across studies depending on the task employed. For instance, in our lab's work with healthy pre-teens, teenagers, and young adults, we have found that recognition memory for non-verbal items developmentally asymptotes sometime before the age of 9 years. In contrast, very young adolescents (ages 9–11) are still developing the working memory skills allowing them to recall a single piece of information after a short delay. After age 11, that ability seems to developmentally asymptote. The ability to hold several items in mind and to repeat them in a prescribed sequential order apparently matures by age 14. The ability to use and manipulate several pieces of information to self-organize behavior continues to mature until the age of approximately 17 years. A general conclusion from this body of work is that as task demands become more and more complex, age-related improvements continue to be observed particularly on measures that require memory and attention skills in the service of behavioral self-organization (Luciana *et al.* 2005).

It is rare for studies that have focused on similar cognitive aspects of executive function to observe age-related improvements after the ages of 16–17 in healthy individuals. Summarizing data from a recent cross-sectional study of over 900 adolescents representative of the United States population, Steinberg *et al.* (2009) report that general cognitive capacities that are important for executive function mature until the age of 16 and are stable thereafter up to the age of 30 years. The measure of cognitive capacity in their summary included a composite index that combined standardized scores on verbal fluency, digit span memory, and resistance-to-interference working memory tasks. Similarly, we (Luciana *et al.* 2009) recently reported the development of planning skills as measured by a computerized Tower of London paradigm in healthy 9–20-year-olds. Our sample was grouped into 9–11-, 12–14-, 15–17-, and 18–20-year-olds. We found that age effects were moderated by task difficulty and were most pronounced on the task's most challenging problems. Performance on these problems improved until the age of 15 years. In contrast, the number of perfect task solutions across the entire range of problems showed a trend toward increasing development until the age of 17 years. When we examined deliberation times, we found that a longer deliberation prior to starting a problem was associated overall with better performance. Furthermore, age impacted the relative amount of time allotted to planning versus execution across problem sets. For each problem, a ratio was calculated, dividing initial deliberation times by total problem solution times. These scores indicated that more than half of a problem's overall solution time reflected planning with a difficulty by age group interaction, $\eta_p^2 = 0.10$. Age impacted four-move problems ($\eta_p^2 = 0.07$), with 9–14-year-olds both spending relatively less time planning relative to 15–20-year-olds. Age also impacted five-move problems ($\eta_p^2 = 0.19$). The 9–11-year-olds spent less relative time planning than did all other groups; the 12–14-year-olds spent less time planning than 15–20-year-olds. We also considered the slope of this performance feature, that is, the extent to which the proportion of time devoted to planning versus execution increased linearly from two-to-five-move problems. This variable has not typically been analyzed in the context of this task. The slope showed a strong age effect, $\eta_p^2 = 0.19$, with 9–14-year-olds exhibiting lower values than 15–20-year-olds. What this suggests overall is that early-to-middle adolescence is a time period when individuals have difficulty *modulating* their performance within the overall task context, that is, determining how much time should be spent on deliberation as the context (problem difficulty) shifts. Interestingly, there are individual differences in this pattern when age is controlled, such that those who are better able to modulate their performance are individuals with higher IQs, with better developed working memory skills, and better levels of response control, as measured by a go/no-go task. This finding coheres with other interpretations of behavioral control functions in adolescents where it has been noted that many adolescents are highly capable of adult levels of executive function even though they do not always behave accordingly (see Luna *et al.* 2010 for discussion). In the Steinberg *et al.* (2009) study, for example, 45% of individuals above the age of 16–17 scored above the adult mean on the composite measure of cognitive executive function; less than 15% of individuals under the age of 14 did so. What seems to be the case, then, is that there is a rapid acceleration of executive capacity between the ages of 13–15, but these capacities are not invoked uniformly or reliably across individuals or situations.

This observation has inspired interest in factors that impact how adolescents make decisions under varying circumstances, since the threshold defining when performance is compromised may vary between individuals or in the context of certain motivational contingencies. Accordingly, affective decision-making as measured by gambling tasks and similar measures of reward processing has been used as an index to determine how adolescents make decisions under conditions of ambiguity or risk, particularly when there is a potential for personal gain or loss (Crone and van der Molen 2004; Hooper *et al.* 2004; Overman *et al.* 2004). These studies generally indicate that even 14–17-year-olds are deficient relative to adults in their abilities to make decisions based on long-term rather than immediate consequences. Moreover, this tendency to be swayed by "in the moment" contingencies as opposed to the potential for longer-term gains or losses may be exacerbated by the presence of peers, as elegantly illustrated in a risk behavior paradigm (Gardener and Steinberg 2005). Adolescent participants were more likely to take risks (directing a car to run a yellow light in the context of a video game) in the presence of their peers as opposed to when they were alone; adults do not show this pattern. Steinberg *et al.* (2009) have suggested that a lack of psychosocial maturity is, in part, responsible for the behavioral dysregulation that is often observed in adolescence. Data from their laboratory supports this assertion. They created a composite index based on selected questions from self-report measures of impulsivity, sensation-seeking, resistance to peer influence, and future orientation in the same large sample of subjects that contributed to the cognitive capacity study. Self-reported psychosocial maturity was indistinct among individuals ages 10–11, 12–13, 14–15 and 16–17. In contrast, 16–17- and 18–21-year-olds achieved lower scores than individuals in their mid-twenties and older. By the age of 21, only approximately 25% of individuals scored above the 26–30-year-old mean in their psychosocial maturity scores. Notably, these findings are impervious to gains that would otherwise be predicted by high intelligence. Concordantly, in our studies, which generally include adolescents who are, as a group, performing in the high average range of general intelligence, we observe less-than-adult levels of adaptive future-directed decision-making when individuals have the opportunity for personal gain (Hooper *et al.* 2004). Thus, high intellect does not *necessarily* predict sound decision-making.

An exhaustive review of this literature is outside the scope of this chapter, but it is clear from this sampling of studies that executive functions continue to show age-related improvements during adolescence as evidenced by laboratory research. On most laboratory measures of executive function that require working memory, inhibitory control and other "cold" cognitive functions, performance reaches an asymptote before the age of 17 years. However, as situational complexity increases even on measures that could be described as purely "cognitive" and as cognitive performance is demanded in the context of compelling personal and social motivations (where so-called "hot" cognition is demanded), stable adult levels of performance may not be reached until the early to mid-twenties.

Adolescent brain development: current status of knowledge

To complement these behavioral studies and in the wake of neuroimaging technology, a great deal has been learned about the relative status of the adolescent brain from a structural standpoint. In evaluating brain structure, researchers employ techniques to quantify the volumes of various tissue classes. These quantifications can include total brain measures or regional analyses. Tissue classes and characteristics that have been examined include gray matter volume, cortical thickness, white matter volume, the microstructural properties of white matter that reflect myelination and fiber tract organization, and gyrification (also called cortical complexity).

Gray matter volume

Gray matter refers neuronal cell bodies, neuropil (primarily dendrites), and glial cells. Its name is derived from its notably grayish appearance. Gray matter is concentrated in the cortex, the basal ganglia, thalamus, and outer layers of the cerebellum. Gray matter volume accelerates throughout infancy and early childhood, after which it reaches a plateau. There are consistently-observed decreases in gray matter during adolescence, a finding that has been observed by several developmental laboratories (Giedd 2004; Giedd *et al.* 1999; Gogtay and Thompson 2010; Gogtay *et al.* 2004; Jernigan *et al.* 1991; Luders *et al.* 2005; Sowell *et al.* 2003; Thompson *et al.* 2005). Collectively, these studies indicate that the total volume of cortical gray matter increases in the age range prior to puberty with an apparent post-pubertal decline. (A caveat to this summary is that pubertal status is difficult to precisely quantify and has been inferred on the basis of age or, less often, on the basis of self-report questionnaire data.) The post-pubertal changes in gray matter are non-linear and vary with respect to brain region. For instance, gray matter volume peaks in the frontal lobe several years before it peaks in anterior temporal regions. Peaks in posterior (occipital and parietal) regions occur even earlier. A recent longitudinal study conducted by Gogtay and colleagues has provided more detail on the time-course of gray matter change during adolescence. This study indicates, through time-lapsed images obtained from a small sample that was repeatedly studied, that the primary sensorimotor cortices and the frontal and occipital poles mature first. The remainder of the cortex develops in a parietal-to-frontal (posterior to anterior) direction with the superior temporal cortex maturing last (Gogtay *et al.* 2004). Moreover, there are sex differences in that gray matter volumes appear to peak earlier in males versus females in the frontal, temporal and parietal regions (Lenroot and Giedd 2010). Examinations of cortical thickness have yielded similar findings (Shaw *et al.* 2006).

White matter volume

There are also increases in white matter volume and density (Bartzokis *et al.* 2010; Giedd *et al.* 1999; Paus 1999, 2001; Pfefferbaum *et al.* 1994). White matter is nerve tissue that is pale in color and comprised of nerve fibers (axons), some of which contain large amounts of insulating material (myelin). White matter does not contain nerve cell bodies. Accordingly, white matter connects cell bodies with one another via fiber pathways. White matter increases have been observed during adolescence. These increases occur across regions and are more linear with increasing age as compared to the non-linear changes in gray matter volumes. As with gray matter, there is sexual dimorphism, with evidence that males exhibit steeper increases in white matter volume across adolescence as compared to females (Lenroot *et al.* 2007).

White matter organization

In addition to the assessment of white matter volumes, increases in the directional organization of white matter, as assessed through diffusion tensor imaging, have been observed (Ashtari *et al.* 2007; Barnea-Goraly *et al.* 2005; Ben Bashat *et al.* 2005; Bonekamp *et al.* 2007; Eluvathingal *et al.* 2007; Klingberg *et al.* 2000; Hasan *et al.* 2007; Lebel *et al.* 2008; Li and Noseworthy 2002; Muetzel *et al.* 2008; Qiu *et al.* 2008; Schmithorst and Yuan 2010; Schneider *et al.* 2004; Snook *et al.* 2005, 2007; Zhang *et al.* 2005). Diffusion tensor imaging (DTI) is an imaging method that quantifies the degree and direction of the random movement of water molecules over fixed time periods. These movement patterns are described as *diffusion*. If there are no obstacles to movement, water molecules diffuse uniformly in three-dimensional space, a pattern referred to as *isotropic* diffusion. If the molecules encounter structural barriers, then diffusion is not uniform in all directions, a pattern referred to as *anisotropic*. Based on the spatial patterns of observed anisotropy, the extent and type of structural barriers can be reconstructed (Basser and Jones 2002). The diffusion tensor is a 3-by-3 matrix that captures the movement of water molecules in each voxel along three axes. The measurements along each axis are fit to a three-dimensional ellipsoid that characterizes the direction of water motion. The eigenvalues of the tensor ($\lambda_1, \lambda_2, \lambda_3$) reflect the length of the three axes. The eigenvectors of the tensor (V_1, V_2, V_3) reflect the orientations of the axes. If gradients are applied in at least six different directions, these values can be calculated to compute the diffusion tensor. Frequently used measures in DTI research include trace diffusion ($\lambda_1 + \lambda_2 + \lambda_3$), a measurement of the overall amount of water diffusion in the voxel (in all three directions), mean diffusivity (MD: ($\lambda_1 + \lambda_2 + \lambda_3$)/3), an averaged measurement of the amount of water diffusion in the voxel, and fractional anisotropy (FA) (Pierpaoli and Basser 1996), the sum of the squared differences of the eigenvalues, reflecting the extent to which there are differences between them. FA will be high in cases where there is anisotropic diffusion, presumably due to fiber structures' relatively ellipsoid shapes, and low when there is isotropic diffusion, reflecting fiber structure with more spherical shapes. It has generally been found that FA increases in major fiber tracts with age in adolescent samples, while MD decreases (see Schmithorst and Yuan 2010 for review). Regional comparisons suggest that tracts connecting the frontal lobe to other regions may be among the last to mature in terms of increasing levels of FA (Eluvathingal *et al.* 2007; Schmithorst and Yuan 2010). Developmental changes in DTI indices of white matter microstructure are often inferred to reflect, at least in part, increased myelination of neural fibers. Increased myelin improves the conduction velocity of neural signals.

Gyrification/cortical complexity

Gyrification refers to the process by which the brain develops its characteristic convolutions (gyri) and grooves (sulci). Much of this process is complete by the third trimester of pregnancy in humans, although gyrification is impacted by changes in synaptic structure. Accordingly, it could be that as synaptic pruning occurs during adolescence, gyrification is altered in response as a function of the changes in cortical connectivity that result (White et al. 2010).

Overall, these studies support the notion that during adolescence, functional networks are being remodeled in a manner that may lead to increases in information processing efficiency. Redundant or unused synaptic connections are eliminated through pruning. Those that remain become more organized in terms of the directional organization of fiber pathways, increases in myelin, and possibly, increases in axonal caliber (Paus 2010). Moreover, with increasing development, frontal systems become increasingly capable from a functional neuroanatomical perspective of assuming greater regulation over subcortical and primary sensory and motor processing. This patterning suggests that we should observe associations between adolescent-limited changes in brain structure and the concomitant development of executive skills.

Indeed, structure–function associations are relatively sparse as reported in the extant literature but are of increasing interest. DTI studies have shown associations between indices of white matter microstructure and a range of behavioral processes and functions including general intelligence (Schmithorst et al. 2005; Shaw et al. 2006), delay discounting (Olson et al. 2009), interhemispheric transfer (Muetzel et al. 2008), working memory (Nagy et al. 2004; Olesen et al. 2003), inhibitory control (Liston et al. 2006), and reading ability (Qiu et al. 2008). Gray matter volumes and cortical thickness measures have also been associated with aspects of memory function and general intelligence (Shaw et al. 2006; Sowell et al. 2003). Overall, these studies suggest regional associations between changes in tissue composition and behavior, providing some support for the notion that the structural integrity of broadly distributed functional networks supports behavioral development. However, it should be emphasized that age effects are, in a relative sense, generally small in magnitude particularly in later adolescence (see Olson et al. 2009 for an example).

Finally, several groups have used functional magnetic resonance imaging techniques to document developmental differences in brain activation patterns during the completion of behavioral tasks. With respect to more purely cognitive functions, adolescents as compared to adults show inefficient patterns of neural activation during the performance of cognitive control tasks (see Luna et al. 2010 for a comprehensive review). Bunge et al. (2002) were one of the first groups to examine patterns of brain activation in children, as compared to adults, who were administered measures of cognitive control, including a flanker task. Flankers are arrows that point either to the left or to the right. On each trial, participants viewed five stimuli (arrows) arranged in a row. The middle stimulus was a flanker that pointed right or left, and the general task was to look at the middle arrow to decide whether to push a response button that was on the left or right. The other stimuli served as distracters. On congruent trials, a ride-sided button was pressed if the arrow pointed right, and a left-sided button was pressed if the arrow pointed left. On incongruent trials, the task was to respond in the direction opposite to where the arrow pointed. Finally, on no-go trials, subjects were asked to refrain from responding. Bunge et al. (2002) reported inferior performance in

8–12-year-old children as compared to adults on no-go and incongruent trials. In addition, children demonstrated a greater interference effect as indicated by slower response times across all task conditions. Adults and children also showed different patterns of neural activation. In adults, response inhibition activated a number of PFC regions including the bilateral ventrolateral and dorsolateral regions as well as the anterior and posterior cingulate, but these areas were not significantly activated in children as a whole. However, children who performed particularly well activated a subset of the same regions that were activated in adults.

Other studies have demonstrated robust activation of the lateral PFC in prepubescent children during response inhibition (Casey *et al.* 1997; Vaidya *et al.* 1998). Because the study by Bunge *et al.* (2002) found substantial differences in 8–12-year-olds versus young adults, it suggested that a major transition in the capacity for cognitive control occurs between the ages of 12–19. Similarly, Tamm *et al.* (2002) studied go/no-go performance in a small (n = 19) sample of 8–20-year-olds and found that while age did not predict absolute accuracy of performance, it was related to performance speed or efficiency in inhibitory control. Moreover, as compared to younger subjects who activated extensive regions of the dorsolateral PFC while they performed the task, older ones showed a more focal and more restricted pattern of activation (Luna *et al.* 2010).

More recently, similar comparisons of children, adolescents, and young adults have compared brain activation patterns in response to stimuli or tasks that have a more motivational component. These studies have found age-related differences in orbitofrontal cortex and ventral striatum activation with the general pattern of heightened activity during adolescence (Ernst *et al.* 2005; Galvan *et al.* 2006; May *et al.* 2004; Van Leijenhorst *et al.* 2010). Additionally, adolescents exhibit unique patterns of amygdala activation when emotional facial expressions are viewed (Baird *et al.* 1999; Thomas *et al.* 2001). There is controversy regarding how more versus less focal patterns of activation should be interpreted (see Luna *et al.* 2010 for discussion), since more focal activation could be interpreted as a reflection of decreased overall activation or as a reflection of more efficient processing. It is also the case within imaging studies as a whole that the nature of the findings can dramatically change with differences in methodology, when different analytic techniques are applied to the same dataset, and when different threshold values are applied to determine statistical significance. There is not a universal standard within the field.

INTEGRATION OF FINDINGS

Behavioral studies lead to the obvious conclusion that adolescents are not capable of the same level of executive control as young adults, particularly under conditions that require a high information processing demand, when motivational stakes are high, and/or when decisions must be made quickly. These findings are most pronounced for individuals under the age of 16. Structural neuroimaging suggests that the dynamics of neural networks are being altered, particularly in early to mid-adolescence as a consequence of synaptic pruning. These alterations may or may not have a basis in pubertal timing (see Forbes and Dahl 2010 for discussion). Structure–function associations are weak at best and have been disappointing in allowing us to conclude that adolescent risk-taking is *unequivocally* due to changing patterns of synaptic architecture. An interpretive leap has been made by most researchers in this area on the basis of the temporal correlation between the two sets of events (structural change and behavioral maturation). Functional imaging studies are more compelling to the extent that they suggest unique patterns of neural engagement in the context of behavioral performance during adolescence.

Based on this work, "dual system" models have been recently invoked to explain adolescent behavior (Fareri *et al*. 2008). These models advocate that there is poor regulatory control exerted by cortical structures, particularly the PFC, due to immaturity while at the same time there is unrestrained activity within limbic and striatal circuits. Core limbic system structures such as the amygdala, septum, hippocampus, nucleus accumbens (ventral striatum), and ventral portions of the frontal lobe are involved in reward evaluation and reward-related decision-making, while the dorsal and ventral striatum modulate the flow of information to the cortex and participate in response modulation. Whether limbic and striatal circuitry is developmentally overactive (and thereby difficult to control even in the presence of a fully functional PFC) or whether it is normal in tone but poorly regulated is a matter of debate. Minimally, dual system models cohere regarding the potential importance of PFC underdevelopment as a cause of adolescent risk-taking and deficient behavioral regulation.

Another view, more behaviorally based, is that there is a maturational dissociation between cognitive and social/emotional functioning between late childhood and early adulthood (Steinberg *et al*. 2009). Accordingly, adolescents may be able to logically reason through decisions in an adult-like manner when they have time to deliberate. In contrast, their abilities to make psychosocially mature decisions in less deliberative, more rapidly-occurring, contexts mature later. In other words, it has been suggested that a uniform age cannot necessarily be applied to all domains of executive function in terms of when the age of maturation is achieved and that these different domains may differentially relate to real-world behavioral contexts (Steinberg *et al*. 2009).

This conclusion, if accurate, creates a host of dilemmas regarding the treatment of adolescents in legal and public policy contexts, since it could be argued that each domain of function that is assessed in the laboratory should be thoroughly analyzed to determine its age of maturation and then which "real-world" decisions or behaviors are most reliably associated with it. The answers to those questions are not clear at the present time. Importantly, there is no laboratory measure that yields definitive executive weaknesses in all adolescents who complete it or in the same adolescent when tested repeatedly (although it should be acknowledged that there are few, if any, large-scale longitudinal studies available). Performance on many measures is state-dependent. Thus, in understanding adolescents' deficiencies in executive control, we make probabilistic judgments based on statistical findings to infer that in the absence of any other source of influence, youthful age biases behavior so that there is a likelihood of poor judgment or deficient behavioral control in the face of risk or uncertainty.

ADOLESCENT BRAIN DEVELOPMENT, PARENTING, AND PUBLIC POLICY

Interpretive complexities aside, these findings have a rapt audience in parents, educators, public health advocates, and the legal system. Consider the following recent book titles obtained through a search of the amazon.com website, entering the term "adolescent brain": *The Adolescent Brain: Reaching for Autonomy* (Sylwester 2007), *Why do they act that way: A survival guide to the adolescent brain for you and your teen* (Walsh 2005), *The primal teen: What the new discoveries about the adolescent brain tell us about our kids* (Strauch 2004), *Yes, Your Teen is Crazy!: Loving Your Kid Without Losing Your Mind* (Bradley 2003), *Secrets of the Teenage Brain: Research-Based Strategies for Reaching and Teaching Today's Adolescents* (Feinstein 2009). Parents are obviously searching for understanding as their children navigate the transition through the teen years; science is being called upon to provide that understanding.

Adolescents' limitations are recognized on national levels in terms of public policy decisions. As a society, we limit (or attempt to limit) adolescents' access to behaviors that are considered "privileged," including the ability to vote in public elections, to serve on juries, to marry without parental consent, to engage in consensual sexual activity, to drive a motor vehicle, to consume alcohol, to enlist in the military, to seek medical care without parental knowledge, and to engage in various recreational activities, for instance, the purchase of tickets to gain entry to films that are rated as having a high level of mature, violent, or sexual content. From the vantage point of the individual teen, access to these experiences typically represents a much-anticipated rite of passage in the transition to adulthood. From the vantage point of parents and educators, allowing their children access to these experiences is generally fraught with anxiety about what is appropriate or not given the fear that adolescents are inferior to adults in their information-processing capacities. Moreover, when adolescents violate parental or societal rules, questions and doubts are raised about their culpability (the "my brain made me do it" defense (Gazzaniga 2007)). At the most extreme, some wonder if the scientific data indicate that adolescents' capacities for free will are diminished on the basis of brain-based immaturities or if poor judgment and risk-taking are predetermined outcomes. Are adolescents' executive capacities impaired to the extent that they are less responsible than adults for their actions? For the answer to this question to be positive, one would need to prove that bad behavior is somehow inevitable, automatic, or initiated without awareness.

In a provocative neuroscientific analysis of free will, Gazzaniga (2007) presented a summary of findings that addressed the question of whether the brain initiates behavior before one becomes consciously aware of it. Several psychophysiological paradigms exist to permit the measurement of the time-course of movement initiation potentials in relation to conscious awareness of control over those impulses. Gazzaniga described a study by Libet (1999) through which it was demonstrated in an electrophysiological paradigm that there is a window of approximately 500–1000ms between the brain's initiation of a readiness potential and a voluntary hand movement. The conscious awareness of the decision to make the movement came 300ms into that window of time, suggesting that the brain initiates behavioral responses outside of awareness, a finding that is not surprising to most neuroscientists. Given the temporal aspects of neural dynamics, an individual would have approximately 100ms to make a decision to inhibit the initiated response before it is executed. Similarly, behavioral paradigms such as the stop-signal task, which records how quickly an individual can inhibit a response once initiated, are relevant in showing that this ability is mediated by a region of the inferior frontal cortex in concert with other structures (Aron *et al.* 2003). Another electrophysiological potential, the error-related negativity (ERN) occurs after an error response has been made in the context of an ongoing behavioral sequence but before an individual is aware of having made an error (Davies *et al.* 2004). Within this context, then, willful behavior could be construed as more a matter of inhibitory control than deliberately making a choice to do X versus Y, a phenomenon described by Gazzaniga (2007) as "free won't" versus "free will."

While it is not necessarily appropriate to generalize these findings to more complex situations, they do suggest, via simple behaviors, that a person may be better able to exert conscious control if s/he can process neural signals rapidly to overcome more prepotent or automatic tendencies. Given the changes in white matter development and organization that are occurring during adolescence, it stands to reason that even minor changes in the efficiency through which information is processed would lead to measurable increments in the ability to volitionally control behavior and increases in the consistency through which this control can be achieved. The opposite is also true. As there is more information to manage, it is likely that "stop" signals cannot be generated rapidly enough to consistently impact behavior. Accordingly, while it would be extreme and indeed, erroneous, to conclude that free will is *absent* in the typical adolescent on the basis of his/her age, one could convincingly argue that the capacity may be diminished in certain contexts, particularly those in which decisions to act are rapidly made and executed.

There are numerous legal ramifications in accepting that adolescents are inferior to adults in these processing skills. Psychology has entered these debates by presenting data to the courts regarding adolescents' rights under various legal contexts. Consider, for instance, the question of whether female adolescents should be allowed to receive abortions without parental consent. Many youth advocates are in favor of such policies, since the requirement for parental consent may place an undue burden upon adolescent girls in need or who are vulnerable within their rearing environments. On the other hand, the evidence summarized within this chapter regarding adolescents' executive functioning would suggest that teens are too immature to make such life-altering decisions without parental approval. It is arguably inconsistent to prevent teens from viewing R-rated movies, for instance, but allowing them to make abortion decisions on their own. In a brief filed in *Hodgson v. Minnesota* (1990), adolescents' rights to seek abortions without parental approval were upheld. In support of this decision, the American Psychological Association (APA) presented research regarding cognitive abilities that bear on medical choices, suggesting that adolescents are as mature as adults in their logical reasoning skills. On the one hand, much of the research on cognitive capacity would support this approach given that many adolescents perform at adult levels of competence on measures of executive function when these measures are purely "cognitive" and when they are administered in a laboratory setting. On the other hand, few would argue that the decision to have an abortion is a purely cognitive one; such decisions, whether faced by adolescents or adults, are likely to occur within highly stressful emotional contexts and may be made without long-term deliberation. These contexts are those that we know to be the ones in which executive functions can be derailed. Steinberg *et al.* (2009) have considered whether the APA has been inconsistent in their use of the scientific data to support legal decisions using this abortion rights debate as one example. The second example follows.

In apparent contrast to the previously discussed legal decision and citing brain development research, the United States Supreme Court made a decision on March 1, 2005, in *Roper v. Simmons*, abolishing the death penalty for crimes committed by adolescents under the age of 18. This latter ruling explicitly distinguished adolescents from adults. Writing for the majority, Justice Anthony Kennedy cited scientific research to conclude that juveniles have a lack of maturity and sense of responsibility as compared to adults. The court noted that adolescents are overrepresented in virtually every category of reckless behavior, that most states and many countries recognize the comparative immaturity and irresponsibility of juveniles, that juveniles are vulnerable to peer pressure, and that they have less control over their environments. Yet, the impact of this ruling has not been as far-reaching as it may intuitively seem. In many states, 16–17-year-olds can be prosecuted as adults in criminal cases. Some states have transfer policies that allow judges and prosecutors to transfer even younger individuals to the adult system for certain offenses. One might imagine that these policies apply exclusively to relatively heinous violent crimes, but they apply in some cases to less violent offenses as well.

As this chapter is being prepared, the United States Supreme Court is in the process of evaluating two cases concerning the constitutionality of sentencing juveniles to life without the possibility of parole. The APA has filed an amicus curiae brief in those cases presenting relevant research on adolescent brain development in support of the notion that juveniles are immature and that this immaturity should be considered as a mitigating factor in sentencing decisions. As a society, are we trying to have it both ways? Or are youth advocates such as Steinberg *et al.* (2009) correct when they imply that different age standards legitimately apply to different forms of otherwise adult-like privileges? What is certainly the case is that a 13-year-old who commits a crime or behaves in a way that shows poor judgment and is then sentenced or punished for it will have a different brain, on the basis of intrinsic maturational signals, at the age of 21. This fact alone would seem to argue for leniency in how courts and parents handle these situations.

Another issue that relates to legal rulings concerns the extent to which adolescents can comprehend the complexities of the legal process. For instance, Grisso *et al.* (2003) studied a representative sample of individuals recruited across four states. Half were in jail or in juvenile detention and half had no contact with correction agencies. The sample ranged in age from 11–24 years. The data were analyzed by grouping the sample into age bins. As compared to older adolescents and young adults, adolescents who were 11–13 years of age were three times more likely to have trouble understanding the legal process and applying sound reasoning to their legal decisions. This finding bears a striking parallel to the data presented earlier in this chapter regarding developmental improvements in executive cognition. Participants in the Grisso study who were aged 16 and older did not differ from adults in their understanding and reasoning skills. The impairments in understanding and reasoning that characterized younger adolescents were present regardless of whether the individual was part of the community sample or a detainee.

It is tempting to generate broad conclusions regarding the need to protect adolescents, particularly younger ones, from the legal process based on studies such as this one. However, Grisso *et al.* also reported that as compared to youth in the community who had no justice system contact, detainees were lower in measured intelligence, had higher rates of learning disorders and other psychological difficulties including symptoms of thought disorder. This finding supports the idea that individual difference factors, in addition to age, impact which teens engage in problem behaviors to the extent that legal action is necessary and then how these individuals react to the legal process once detained. This work raises the question of whether legal decisions should be made on the basis of individual capacities or on the basis of normative data within age groups.

Another complexity in considering such decisions is that there are cross-cultural and cross-country differences with respect to how public policy decisions are handled. Consider, for example, the age of legal alcohol consumption. In the United States, most states mandate that the legal age of alcohol consumption is 21 years. In countries such as China, Belgium, Italy, France, and the Netherlands, it is 16–18 years. In Canada, it is 18–19 years (International Center for Alcohol Policies 2009: http://www.icap.org). Worldwide and throughout history, there are differences in responsibilities assigned to adolescents. Even more interesting is that adolescents across different cultures are seemingly able to react to meet the demands of their particular cultures. In some locales, it is not uncommon for youth to be married and parents of young children as they, themselves, are navigating the adolescent years as we define them based on the majority in industrialized cultures. These observations raise a number of questions regarding the importance of neurobehavioral findings, whether experience is able to alter the course of brain and behavioral development, and/or whether the process of brain development is invariant such that there are contexts in which individuals with immature brains and associated behavioral limitations are being thrust ill-prepared into adult roles. Cross-cultural studies of executive function would be helpful in addressing the extent to which neurobehavioral data can be generalized.

Summary and conclusions

The body of knowledge related to adolescent brain development and the maturation of executive skills raises the following issues for ethical and interpretive consideration. At the most basic level, those of us who do work in this area must consider the practical implications of our findings and how these findings will be interpreted by the media, by parents, and by the legal system. We have a duty to accurately inform the public (Blakemore 2007). The media renders this task difficult. A personal experience illustrating this difficulty occurred several years ago after the publication of Luciana *et al.* (2005), a paper in which it was reported that adolescents reach maturity of cognitive function in a graded fashion according to the multi-tasking demands imposed by a task. The website http://www.livescience.com "rewrote" the findings with the slant "Why are teens lousy at chores?" (an issue that was never discussed in the scientific paper). Multiple media interviews were invited to explain why teens cannot help out at home, parents sent hate mail suggesting that this was just another example of poor science conducted by a clueless investigator, and even some adolescents weighed in to protest that they have more abilities than are recognized. At the most basic level, the paper was misunderstood by this particular outlet, although the writers were most likely commended for generating the interest that they did. What was frustrating was that no one seemed interested in an accurate description of the findings.

Moreover, in the face of interpretive complexities, conclusions are inconsistently drawn from available data. Take the recent case of a paper by Berns *et al.* (2009), in which it was reported that increased risk-taking in adolescents was associated with relative increases in fractional anisotropy in the frontal lobe in a DTI study. High levels of fractional anisotropy are typically interpreted as reflecting a better directional organization to white matter pathways in a region. Accordingly, the findings were interpreted to suggest that risk-takers have more mature brains. This interpretation contradicts nearly every prominent theory of adolescent neurological and neurocognitive development. Yet, it received a great deal of media attention. One critique that can be applied to the paper, which otherwise appears to be very well done, is that it does not present data in a sufficient enough fashion to conclude that the sample studied exhibited anything beyond tentative risk-taking behavior. Minimally, this study is important in suggesting to us, as scientists, that the meaning of high versus low fractional anisotropy within a region such as the frontal lobe may be different or at least more complex than has been conceptualized. Perhaps an apparently more connected brain is not always a more mature or *better* brain. The average consumer rarely consults primary sources in evaluating these sorts of details and is unprepared to place single findings in a broad context.

Second, in assessing executive capacity and social influences over behavior, it is not clear how adolescence should be defined. Although it is tempting to use pubertal onset as a marker, this strategy is difficult because of the complexities associated with assessing individuals' hormonal status. Thus, a given age (e.g. age 12) cannot be prescribed as the onset of adolescence, nor do we know how to define the offset of this period. There is variability cross-culturally in the expectations for responsible conduct at a given age. Generally, individuals in those cultures meet those expectations. Should adolescence be defined on the basis of biological events that occur through this period in the lifespan or on the basis of cultural/experiential ones? The answer to this question has profound public policy implications.

Third, while it is reasonably clear that adolescents differ statistically from older adults in their executive skills, it is not clear when the age of maturation is reached or indeed, if there is a uniform age of maturation that characterizes all executive processes. Moreover, many adolescents at various ages perform as well as adults on laboratory tasks, suggesting that individual difference factors in combination with age should be considered in structuring policy implications that are based on such data.

While the brain is also showing evidence of subtle change in neuronal architecture during this time, there are few studies that show a reliable coherence between the two sets of processes. Thus, we cannot conclude with absolute certainty that insufficiencies in executive function during adolescence are "due to" structural immaturity of the brain. We do know that patterns of brain activation are different in adolescents than in children and adults as they perform behavioral tasks. However, this patterning could be due to factors other than structural brain development, such as neurochemistry or even to methodological confounds that limit interpretations between adults and children or adolescents. Given that we cannot predict which *brains* are vulnerable in the absence of any behavioral assessment, can brain science be used to support public policy decisions related to responsibility for behavior and culpability when norms are violated? Is it accurate to conclude that adolescence is a risk period on the basis of age alone?

In a provocative paper regarding ways in which brain science should or should not inform the legal process, scholar Stephen Morse asserts in his opening sentence that "Brains do not commit crimes; people commit crimes." (Morse 2006). In some sense, this can be viewed as a provocative statement, since it would seem to imply dualism of mind versus brain (though Morse is careful to state that he is not a dualist). In neuroscience, we do not make a distinction at the *theoretical level* between brain activity and behavioral actions. People cannot exist as functional agents without their brains; in that sense, agency is an emergent property of brain function. Because activity in our nervous systems underlies everything that we do, as well as internal emotions and thoughts, it is the nervous system that registers stimuli in the environment, relays that information to the brain, moves it through various brain circuits allowing perceptions to form, and ultimately, a judgment is made regarding whether a behavioral response should be initiated. Sometimes this pathway is so efficient that the behavioral response appears to be automatic or instinctive. In these cases, responses that have been initiated may be difficult to stop if an individual reaches conscious awareness of a desire to inhibit his/her actions after response initiation. However, in humans, decisions to act are typically more deliberate, occurring over minutes, hours, or days. Given this deliberation time, there are seemingly several "decision points" where a tendency or desire to act can be altered or controlled. This possibility for control suggests that people can stop or regulate their actions in a way that does not involve the brain, but in fact, this is a circular argument. The brain allows control to occur regardless of its time course. Ultimately, then, brains are the mediators of all actions, and brains are the filters through which each of us understands the world around us, so at some level, it can be said that they do indeed commit crimes. No two brains are equal, and if we could fully understand neurophysiology at this individual level, we could confidently assert an equivalence between a person and his/her brain. We are not there yet, but in theory, neuroscience can provide us with information pertaining to individual cases (was the brain damaged after a head injury?) as well as groups of people.

It is broadly accepted that all other things being equal, the healthy adolescent's brain is different from the adult's brain. These differences are thought to be particularly pronounced in networks of neurons that include the prefrontal cortex, the part of the brain that regulates our highest levels of reasoning and—most important to this discussion—behavioral control. It is worth mentioning, too, that achieving control is made even more difficult by the fact that neurochemical systems—especially those that facilitate responding to rewards—are in overdrive during adolescence. Thus, at a normative level, the adolescent's brain is different from the adult's. It is less efficient under conditions of high demand, and it permits a lower threshold for the loss of behavioral control. For these reasons, even the typically-developing adolescent may be biologically vulnerable to "crimes of passion" in ways that typical adults are not. Put another way, the threshold for loss of control is lowered in the adolescent and for biological reasons that, as far as we know, cannot be altered. But even so, it is a tall order to demonstrate on the basis of brain science alone that adolescents are less intentional, less conscious, and without the same *capacity* for rationality as adults. The behavioral evidence is much stronger and more consistent.

The healthy adolescent's behavior is markedly distinct from that of adults. Even without neuroscience, we have acknowledged as a society that these differences are salient and should structure public policy. Many of us who study the behaviors of adolescents are in possession of data to support these public policy measures. Many of us study teenagers who are relatively risk-free. These groups show all of the earlier-mentioned indications of neural immaturity as evidenced by brain imaging. In addition, they are behaviorally more impulsive than adults. They weigh the negative consequences of their actions differently than adults and respond physiologically to those actions in a distinct manner. Their information-processing circuits become "overloaded" at a lower threshold of demand than those of adults. Their sense of time is different. When an adult thinks about an outcome that might occur 5 years from now, he or she has a different perspective on that timeframe than does a teenager. Neuroscience guides much of the behavioral work that has been conducted, because tests are selected that are derived from animal and human brain-based experiments. Together, this evidence from neurobehavioral testing, bolstered by what we know about the course of prefrontal development, suggests that teenagers, as a group, do not view consequences through the same lens as adults. One might reasonably expect, given the cohesiveness of this evidence, that the behavioral data and brain findings would be strongly correlated.

Unfortunately, the observed correlations between laboratory measures of behavior and brain-based evidence, typically derived from neuroimaging, are not strong in magnitude, which may be due to non-linear trends that obscure associations that are present, to methodological factors in quantifying the imaging data, or the intrusion of individual differences that outweigh age-related trends. What, then, is the value of neuroscientific evidence?

We have identified extremely reliable group-based processes that tell us how the brain regions that control reasoning processes continue to develop into adulthood, but we are still looking for the unambiguous neural "signature" that will tell us whose individual brain is impulsive, whose brain is unintelligent, whose brain is criminal. To date, our confidence in group-based findings—normative data—is stronger than our confidence in individual differences at the neural level. Thus, it is difficult to use brain-based data, in and of itself, to support legal decisions that apply to individual cases. Such data can rarely be introduced as exculpatory evidence in court proceedings. Courts are unlikely to be impressed by correlational group-based evidence. Parents may be similarly skeptical of neuroscience, if they think of it at all, when considering how to manage an adolescent who shows poor judgment but who has not committed a crime.

In legal contexts, an individual is judged to be criminally responsible if that person acts intentionally and with a mental state required by the specific defense (for instance, purpose knowledge, recklessness, or negligence) (Morse 2006, p. 397). An act is considered to be an intentional bodily movement performed by a person who has reasonably intact consciousness. An individual is not responsible for his/her actions if he or she behaves unintentionally, if he or she is not fully conscious, if the person has a defect in rationality such as caused by a mental illness, or if the individual acted under great duress (Morse 2006). Unless we want to go so far as to say that adolescents are in some sense *disordered* simply by virtue of age, there is little basis for concluding that an otherwise healthy individual over the age of 16 has any defect in rationality. Adolescents, despite their inconsistencies in using their executive capacities in emotionally challenging contexts, are not frontal lobe patients.

On the positive side, a developing brain is a more malleable brain. In the context of that development, it is more likely than not that adolescents who show poor judgment, make poor decisions, and behave impulsively will nonetheless go on to contribute in a meaningful way to society as adults. In summary, the neurobehavioral study of executive functioning in adolescence is being increasingly brought into the public domain to structure public policy, educational programs, and parenting strategies. Because of situational complexities that vary from case to case, it is not possible to predict if or when any particular individual might exhibit executive impairment, notably deficient behavioral control. Flexible public policies that allow cases to be evaluated on the basis of their distinct characteristics may represent the best use of currently available neuroscientific and neurobehavioral data regarding whether free will and responsibility are diminished in adolescence on the basis of brain-based constraints and how those constraints impact behavior.

Acknowledgments

The preparation of this chapter was supported in part by grant DA017843-05 awarded to Monica Luciana from the National Institute on Drug Abuse.

References

Arnett, J. (1992). Reckless behavior in adolescence: a developmental perspective. *Developmental Reviews*, **12**, 112–63.

Aron, A.R., Fletcher, P.C., Bullmore, E.T., Sahakian, B.J., and Robbins, T.W. (2003). Stop-signal inhibition disrupted by damage to right inferior frontal gyrus in humans. *Nature Neuroscience*, **6**, 115–16.

Asato, M.R., Sweeney, J.A., and Luna, B. (2006). Cognitive processes in the development of TOL performance. *Neuropsychologia*, **44**, 2259–69.

Ashtari, M., Cervellione, K.L., Hasan, K.M., *et al.* (2007). White matter development during late adolescence in healthy males: a cross-sectional diffusion tensor imaging study. *Neuroimage*, **35**, 501–10.

Baird, A.A., Gruber, S.A., Fein, D.A., *et al.* (1999). Functional magnetic resonance imaging of facial affect recognition in children and adolescents. *Journal of the American Academy of Child and Adolescent Psychiatry*, **38**, 195–9.

Barnea-Goraly, N., Menon, V., Eckert, M., *et al.* (2005). White matter development during childhood and adolescence: a cross-sectional diffusion tensor imaging study. *Cerebral Cortex*, **15**, 1848–54.

Bartzokis, G., Lu, P.H., Tingus, K., *et al.* (2010). Lifespan trajectory of myelin integrity and maximum motor speed. *Neurobiology of Aging*, **31**, 1554–62.

Bechara, A., Damasio, A.R., Damasio, H., and Anderson, S.W. (1994). Insensitivity to future consequences following damage to human prefrontal cortex. *Cognition*, **50**, 7–15.

Ben Bashat, D., Ben Sira, L., Graif, M., *et al.* (2005). Normal white matter development from infancy to adulthood: comparing diffusion tensor and high b value diffusion weighted MR images. *Journal of Magnetic Resonance Imaging*, **21**, 503–11.

Bonekamp, D., Nagae, L.M., Degaonkar, M., *et al.* (2007). Diffusion tensor imaging in children and adolescents: reproducibility, hemispheric, and age-related differences. *Neuroimage*, **34**, 733–42.

Basser, P.J. and Jones, D.K. (2002). Diffusion-tensor MRI: theory, experimental design and data analysis - a technical review. *NMR Biomed*, **15**, 456–67.

Bell, M.A. and Fox, N.A. (1992). The relations between frontal brain electrical activity and cognitive development during infancy. *Child Development*, **63**, 1142–63.

Bell, M.A. and Fox, N.A. (1997). Individual differences in object permanence performance at 8 months: Locomotor experience and brain electrical activity. *Developmental Psychobiology*, **31**, 287–97.

Berns, G., Moore, S., and Capra, C. (2009). Adolescent engagement in dangerous behaviors is associated with increased white matter maturity of frontal cortex. *PLoS ONE*, **4**, e6773.

Blakemore, C. (2007). From the "public understanding of science" to scientists' understanding of the public, In W. Glannon (ed.) *Defining right and wrong in brain science: Essential readings in neuroethics*, pp. 67–74. New York: Dana Press.

Bradley, M.J. (2003). *Yes, your teen is crazy: Loving your kids without losing your mind*. Gig Harbor, WA: Harbor Press, Inc.

Braver, T.S., Barch, D.M., Gray, J.R., Molfese, D.L., and Snyder, A. (2001). Anterior cingulate cortex and response conflict: effects of frequency, inhibition and errors. *Cerebral Cortex*, **11**, 825–36.

Bunge, S.A., Dudukovic, N.M., Thomason, M.E., Vaidya, C.J., and Gabrieli, J.D.E. (2002). Development of frontal lobe contributions to cognitive control in children: Evidence from fMRI. *Neuron*, **33**, 301–11.

Casey, B.J., Trainor, R.J., Orendi, J.L., *et al.* (1997). A developmental functional MRI study of prefrontal activation during performance on a go no-go task. *Journal of Cognitive Neuroscience*, **9**, 835–47.

Crone, E.A. and van der Molen, M.W. (2004). Developmental changes in real-life decision-making performance on a gambling task previously shown to depend on the ventromedial prefrontal cortex. *Developmental Neuropsychology*, **25**, 251–79.

Dahl, R.E. and Spear, L.P. (2004). Adolescent brain development. *Annals of the New York Academy of Sciences*, **1021**, 1–22.

Davies, P.L., Segalowitz, S.J., and Gavin, W.J. (2004). Development of response-monitoring ERPs in 7- to 25-year-olds. *Developmental Neuropsychology*, **25**, 355–76.

De Luca, C.R., Wood, S.J., Anderson, V., *et al.* (2003). Normative data from the CANTAB. I: Development of executive function over the lifespan. *Journal of Clinical and Experimental Neuropsychology*, **25**, 242–54.

Diamond, A. (1990a). The development and neural bases of memory functions as indexed by the AB and delayed response tasks in human infants and infant monkeys. In A. Diamond (ed.) *The Development and Neural Basis of Higher Cognitive Functions*. Vol. 608, pp. 267–317. New York: New York Academy of Sciences Press.

Diamond, A. (1990b). Developmental time course in human infants and infant monkeys and the neural basis of inhibitory control in reaching, In A. Diamond (ed.) *The Development and Neural Basis of Higher Cognitive Functions*. Vol. 608, pp. 637–76. New York: New York Academy of Sciences Press.

Diamond, A. and Goldman-Rakic, P.S. (1989). Comparison of human infants and rhesus monkeys on Piaget's AB task: Evidence for dependence on dorsolateral prefrontal cortex. *Experimental Brain Research*, **74**, 24–40.

Diamond, A., and Taylor, C. (1996). Development of an aspect of executive control: development of the abilities to remember what I said and to "do as I say, not as I do". *Developmental Psychobiology*, **29**, 315–34.

Dias, R., Robbins, T.W., and Roberts, A.C. (1996). Dissociation in prefrontal cortex of affective and attentional shifts. *Nature*, **380**, 69–72.

Eluvathingal, T.J., Hasan, K.M., Kramer, L., Fletcher, J.M., and Ewing-Cobbs, L. (2007). Quantitative diffusion tensor tractography of association and projection fibers in normally developing children and adolescents. *Cerebral Cortex*, **17**, 2760–8.

Ernst, M., Nelson, E.E., Jazbec, S.P., *et al.* (2005). Amygdala and nucleus accumbens in responses to receipt and omission of gains in adults and adolescents. *Neuroimage*, **25**, 1279–91.

Fareri, D.S., Martin, L.N., and Delgado, M.R. (2008). Reward-related processing in the human brain: developmental considerations. *Development and Psychopathogy*, **20**, 1191–211.

Feinstein, S. (2009). Secrets of the teenage brain: Research-based strategies for reaching and teaching today's adolescents. Thousand Oaks, CA: Corwin Press.

Forbes, E.E. and Dahl, R.E. (2010). Pubertal development and behavior: Hormonal activation of social and motivational tendencies. *Brain and Cognition*, 72, 66–72.

Fuster, J.M. (1997). *The prefrontal cortex: Anatomy, physiology, and neuropsychology of the frontal lobe, 3rd edition*. Philadelphia, PA: Lippincott-Raven Press.

Galvan, A., Hare, T.A., Parra, C.E., *et al.* (2006). Earlier development of the accumbens relative to orbitofrontal cortex might underlie risk-taking behavior in adolescents. *Journal of Neuroscience*, 26, 6885–92.

Gardener, M. and Steinberg, L. (2005). Peer influence on risk taking, risk preference, and risky decision making in adolescence and adulthood: an experimental study. *Developmental Psychology*, 41, 625–35.

Gazzaniga, M. (2007). My brain made me do it. In W. Glannon (ed.) *Defining Right and Wrong in Brain Science: Essential Readings in Neuroethics*, pp. 183–94. New York: Dana Press.

Gerstadt, C., Hong, Y., and Diamond, A. (1994). The relationship between cognition and action: performance of 3.5–7 year-old children on a Stroop-like day-night test. *Cognition*, 53, 129–53.

Giedd, J.N. (2004). Structural magnetic resonance imaging of the adolescent brain. *Annals of the New York Academy of Sciences*, 1021, 77–85.

Giedd, J.N., Blumenthal, J., Jeffries, N.O., *et al.* (1999). Brain development during childhood and adolescence: a longitudinal MRI study. *Nature Neuroscience*, 2, 861–3.

Gogtay, N. and Thompson, P.M. (2010). Mapping gray matter development: Implications for typical development and vulnerability to psychopathology. *Brain and Cognition*, 72, 6–15.

Gogtay, N., Giedd, J.N., Lusk, L., *et al.* (2004). Dynamic mapping of human cortical development during childhood through early adulthood. *Proceedings of the National Academy of Sciences U S A*, 101, 8174–9.

Goldman-Rakic, P.S. (1987). Circuitry of primate prefrontal cortex and regulation of behavior by representational memory. *Handbook of Physiology: The Nervous System*, vol 5, pp. 373–417. Bethesda, MD: American Physiological Society.

Grisso, T., Steinberg, L., Woolard, J., *et al.* (2003). Juveniles' competences to stand trial: A comparison of adolescents' and adults' capacities as trial defendants. *Law and Human Behavior*, 27, 333–63.

Hasan, K.M., Sankar, A., Halphen, C., *et al.* (2007). Development and organization of the human brain tissue compartments across the lifespan using diffusion tensor imaging. *Neuroreport*, 18, 1735–9.

Hooper, C.J., Luciana, M., Conklin, H.M., and Yarger, R.S. (2004). Adolescents' performance on the Iowa Gambling Task: implications for the development of decision making and ventromedial prefrontal cortex. *Developmental Psychology*, 40, 1148–58.

Jernigan, T.L., Trauner, D.A., Hesselink, J.R., and Tallal, P.A. (1991). Maturation of human cerebrum observed in vivo during adolescence. *Brain*, 114, 2037–49.

Kerr, A. and Zelazo, P.D. (2004). Development of "hot" executive function: The children's gambling task. *Brain and Cognition*, 55, 148–57.

Kessler, R.C., Berglund, P., Demler, O., Jin, R., Merikangas, K.R., and Walters, E.E. (2005). Life-time prevalence and age-of-onset distributions of DSM-IV disorders in the National Comorbidity Survey Replication. *Archives of General Psychiatry*, 62, 593–602.

Klingberg, T., Hedehus, M., Temple, E., *et al.* (2000). Microstructure of temporo-parietal white matter as a basis for reading ability: evidence from diffusion tensor magnetic resonance imaging. *Neuron*, 25, 493–500.

Lebel, C., Walker, L., Leemans, A., Phillips, L., and Beaulieu, C. (2008). Microstructural maturation of the human brain from childhood to adulthood. *Neuroimage, 40*, 1044–55.

Lenroot, R.K. and Giedd, J.N. (2010). Sex differences in the adolescent brain. *Brain and Cognition, 72*, 46–55.

Lenroot, R.K., Gogtay, N., Greenstein, D.K., *et al.* (2007). Sexual dimorphism of brain developmental trajectories during childhood and adolescence. *Neuroimage, 36*, 1065–73.

Levin, H.S., Culhane, K.A., Hartman, J., *et al.* (1991). Developmental changes in performance on tests of purported frontal lobe functioning. *Developmental Neuropsychology, 7*, 377–95.

Lezak, M.D., Howieson, D.B., and Loring, D.W. (2004). *Neuropsychological Assessment, 4th Edition*. Oxford: Oxford University Press.

Li, T.Q. and Noseworthy, M.D. (2002). Mapping the development of white matter tracts with diffusion tensor imaging. *Developmental Science, 5*, 293–300.

Libet, B. (1999). Do we have free will? *Journal of Consciousness Studies, 6*, 8–9.

Liston, C., Watts, R., Tottenham, N., *et al.* (2006). Frontostriatal microstructure modulates efficient recruitment of cognitive control. *Cerebral Cortex, 16*, 553–60.

Luciana, M. and Nelson, C.A. (1998). The functional emergence of prefrontally-guided working memory systems in four-to-eight year-old children. *Neuropsychologia, 36*, 273–93.

Luciana, M. and Nelson, C.A. (2000). Neurodevelopmental assessment of cognitive function using the Cambridge Neuropsychological Testing Automated Battery (Cantab): Validation and future goals. In M. Ernst and J.M. Rumsey (eds.) *Functional Neuroimaging in Child Psychiatry*, pp. 379–97. Cambridge: Cambridge University Press.

Luciana, M. and Nelson, C.A. (2002). Assessment of neuropsychological function through use of the Cambridge Neuropsychological Testing Automated Battery: performance in 4- to 12-year-old children. *Developmental Neuropsychology, 22*, 595–624.

Luciana, M., Conklin, H.M., Hooper, C.J., and Yarger, R.S. (2005). The development of nonverbal working memory and executive control processes in adolescents. *Child Development, 76*, 697–712.

Luciana, M., Collins, P.F., Olson, E.A., and Schissel, A.M. (2009). Tower of London performance in healthy adolescents: The development of planning skills and associations with self-reported inattention and impulsivity. *Developmental Neuropsychology, 34*, 461–75.

Luders, E., Narr, K.L., Thompson, P.M., *et al.* (2005). Mapping cortical gray matter in the young adult brain: effects of gender. *Neuroimage, 26*, 493–501.

Luna, B., Garver, K.E., Urban, T.A., Lazar, N.A., and Sweeney, J.A. (2004). Maturation of cognitive processes from late childhood to adulthood. *Child Development, 75*, 1357–72.

Luna, B., Padmanabhan, A., and O'Hearn, K. (2010). What has fMRI told us about the development of cognitive control through adolescence? *Brain and Cognition, 72*, 101–13.

May, J.C., Delgado, M.R., Dahl, R.E., *et al.* (2004). Event-related functional magnetic resonance imaging of reward-related brain circuitry in children and adolescents. *Biological Psychiatry, 55*, 359–66.

Milner, B. (1963). Effects of different brain lesions on card sorting: the role of the frontal lobe. *Archives of Neurology, 9*, 90–100.

Morse, S.J. (2006). Brain overclaim syndrome and criminal responsibility: A diagnostic note. *Ohio State Journal of Criminal Law, 3*, 397–411.

Muetzel, R.L., Collins, P.F., Mueller, B.A., Schissel, A.M., Lim, K.O., and Luciana, M. (2008). The development of corpus callosum microstructure and associations with bimanual task performance in healthy adolescents. *Neuroimage, 39*, 1918–25.

Nagy, Z., Westerberg, H., and Klingberg, T. (2004). Maturation of white matter is associated with the development of cognitive functions during childhood. *Journal of Cognitive Neuroscience*, **16**, 1227–33.

Olesen, P.J., Nagy, Z., Westerberg, H., and Klingberg, T. (2003). Combined analysis of DTI and fMRI data reveals a joint maturation of white and grey matter in a fronto-parietal network. *Brain Research Cognitive Brain Research*, **18**, 48–57.

Olson, E.A., Collins, P.F., Hooper, C.J., Muetzel, R., Lim, K.O., and Luciana, M. (2009). White matter integrity predicts delay discounting behavior in adolescents: a diffusion tensor imaging study. *Journal of Cognitive Neuroscience*, **21**, 1406–21.

Overman, W.H., Frassrand, K., Ansel, S., Trawalter, S., Bies, B., and Redmond, A. (2004). Performance on the Iowa card task by adolescents and adults. *Neuropsychologia*, **42**, 1838–51.

Passler, P.A., Isaac, W., and Hynd, G.W. (1985). Neuropsychological development of behavior attributed to frontal lobe functioning in children. *Developmental Neuropsychology*, **4**, 349–70.

Paus, T. (2005). Mapping brain maturation and cognitive development during adolescence. *Trends in Cognitive Sciences*, **9**, 60–8.

Paus, T. (2010). Growth of white matter in the adolescent brain: Myelin or axon? *Brain and Cognition*, **72**, 26–35.

Paus, T., Zijdenbos, A., Worsley, K., *et al.* (1999). Structural maturation of neural pathways in children and adolescents: in vivo study. *Science*, **283**, 1908–11.

Paus, T., Collins, D.L., Evans, A.C., Leonard, G., Pike, B., and Zijdenbos, A. (2001). Maturation of white matter in the human brain: a review of magnetic resonance studies. *Brain Research Bulletin*, **54**, 255–66.

Paus, T., Keshavan, M., and Giedd, J.N. (2008). Why do many psychiatric disorders emerge during adolescence? *Nature Reviews Neuroscience*, **9**, 947–57.

Petrides, M. (1995). Functional organization of the human frontal cortex for mnemonic processing. Evidence from neuroimaging studies. *Annals of the New York Academy of Sciences*, **769**, 85–96.

Petrides, M. and Milner, B. (1982). Deficits in subject-ordered tasks after frontal and temporal-lobe lesions in man. *Neuropsychologia*, **20**, 249–62.

Pfefferbaum, A., Mathalon, D.H., Sullivan, E.V., Rawles, J.M., Zipursky, R.B., and Lim, K.O. (1994). A quantitative magnetic resonance imaging study of changes in brain morphology from infancy to late adulthood. *Archives of Neurology*, **51**, 874–87.

Pierpaoli, C.J., and Basser, P.J. (1996). Toward a quantitative assessment of diffusion anisotropy. *Magnetic Resonance Medicine*, **36**, 893–906.

Qiu, D., Tan, L.H., Zhou, K., and Khong, P.L. (2008). Diffusion tensor imaging of normal white matter maturation from late childhood to young adulthood: voxel-wise evaluation of mean diffusivity, fractional anisotropy, radial and axial diffusivities, and correlation with reading development. *Neuroimage*, **41**, 223–32.

Ridderinkhof, K.R. and van der Molen, M.W. (1997). Mental resources, processing speed, and inhibitory control: a developmental perspective. *Biological Psychology*, **45**, 241–61.

Rosenkilde, C.E. (1979). Functional heterogeneity of the prefrontal cortex in the monkey: a review. *Behavioral and Neural Biology*, **25**, 301–45.

Sahakian, B.J. and Owen, A.M. (1992). Computerised assessment in neuropsychiatry using CANTAB. *Journal of the Royal Society of Medicine*, **85**, 399–402.

Safire, W. (2007). Visions for a new field of neuroethics. In W. Glannon (ed.) *Defining Right and Wrong in Brain Science: Essential Readings in Neuroethics*, pp. 7–11. New York: Dana Press.

Schmithorst, V.J. and Yuan, W.Y. (2010). White matter development during adolescence as shown by diffusion MRI. *Brain and Cognition*, **72**, 16–25.

Schmithorst, V.J., Wilke, M., Dardzinski, B.J., and Holland, S.K. (2005). Cognitive functions correlate with white matter architecture in a normal pediatric population: A diffusion tensor MRI study. *Human Brain Mapping*, **26**, 139–47.

Schneider, J.F., Il'yasov, K.A., Hennig, J., and Martin, E. (2004). Fast quantitative diffusion-tensor imaging of cerebral white matter from the neonatal period to adolescence. *Neuroradiology*, **46**, 258–66.

Shallice, T. (1982). Specific impairments in planning. *Philosophical Transactions of the Royal Society of London B*, **298**, 199–209.

Shaw, P., Greenstein, D., Lerch, J., *et al.* (2006). Intellectual ability and cortical development in children and adolescents. *Nature*, **440**, 676–9.

Snook, L., Paulson, L.A., Roy, D., Phillips, L., and Beaulieu, C. (2005). Diffusion tensor imaging of neurodevelopment in children and young adults. *Neuroimage*, **26**, 1164–73.

Snook, L., Plewes, C., and Beaulieu, C. (2007). Voxel based versus region of interest analysis in diffusion tensor imaging of neurodevelopment. *Neuroimage*, **34**, 243–52.

Sowell, E.R., Peterson, B.S., Thompson, P.M., Welcome, S.E., Henkenius, A.L., and Toga, A.W. (2003). Mapping cortical change across the human life span. *Nature Neuroscience*, **6**, 309–15.

Steinberg, L. (2008). A social neuroscience perspective on adolescent risk-taking. *Developmental Review*, **28**, 78–106.

Steinberg, L., Cauffman, E., Woolard, J., Graham, S., and Banich, M. (2009). Are adolescents less mature than adults? Minors' access to abortion, the juvenile death penalty, and the alleged APA "flip-flop". *American Psychologist*, **64**, 583–94.

Strauch, B. (2004). *The primal teen: What the new discoveries about the teenage brain tell us about our kids*. New York: Anchor Books.

Sylwester, R. (2007). *The Adolescent Brain: Reaching for Autonomy*. Thousand Oaks, CA: Corwin Press.

Tamm, L., Menon, V., and Reiss, A. (2002). Maturation of brain function associated with response inhibition. *Journal of the American Academy of Child and Adolescent Psychiatry*, **41**, 1231–8.

Thomas, K.M., Drevets, W.C., Whalen, P.J., *et al.* (2001). Amygdala response to facial expressions in children and adults. *Biological Psychiatry*, **49**, 309–16.

Thompson, P.M., Sowell, E.R., Gogtay, N., *et al.* (2005). Structural MRI and brain development. *International Review of Neurobiology*, **67**, 285–323.

Vaidya, C.J., Austin, G., Kirkorian, G., *et al.* (1998). Selective effects of methylphenidate in attention deficit hyperactivity disorder: a functional magnetic resonance study. *Proceedings of the National Academy of Sciences USA*, **95**, 14494–9.

Van Leijenhorst, L., Zanolie, K., Van Meel, C.S., Westenberg, P.M., Rombouts, S.A.R.B., and Crone, E.A. (2010). What motivates the adolescent? Brain regions mediating reward sensitivity across adolescence, *Cerebral Cortex*, **20**, 61–9.

Walsh, D. (2005). *Why do they act that way? A survival guide to the adolescent brain for you and your teen*. New York: Free Press.

Welsh, M.C., Pennington, B.F. and Groisser, D.B. (1991). A normative-developmental study of executive function: a window on prefrontal function in children. *Developmental Neuropsychology*, 7, 131–49.

White, T., Su, S., Schmidt, M., Kao, C.Y. and Sapiro, G. (2010). The development of gyrification in childhood and adolescence. *Brain and Cognition*, 72, 36–45.

Zelazo, P.D., Frye, D. and Rapus, T. (1996). An age-related dissociation between knowing rules and using them. *Cognitive Development*, 11, 37–63.

Zhang, L., Thomas, K.M., Davidson, M.C., Casey, B.J., Heier, L.A. and Ulug, A.M. (2005). MR quantitation of volume and diffusion changes in the developing brain. *American Journal of Neuroradiology*, 26, 45–9.

CHAPTER 5

NEURAL FOUNDATIONS TO CONSCIOUS AND VOLITIONAL CONTROL OF EMOTIONAL BEHAVIOR: A MENTALISTIC PERSPECTIVE

MARIO BEAUREGARD

INTRODUCTION

One of the central tenets of evolutionary psychology is that primary and secondary (social) emotions represent efficient modes of adaptation to changing environmental demands (Tooby and Cosmides 1990; Levenson 1994). Emotions, however, are not always the most appropriate answer to the diverse situations encountered in daily life. Indeed, negative emotional states represent one of the main causes of human suffering. This is why it is paramount for human beings to properly control and modulate their emotional reactions using their cognitive abilities. Fortunately, humans are capable of emotional self-regulation, i.e. they can change the way they feel by changing the way they think. Without this cognitive capacity, they would be slaves of their emotional impulses and thus unable to interact socially in an adequate and harmonious manner (Knoch and Fehr 2007).

Emotional self-regulation refers to the heterogeneous set of cognitive processes by which emotions are self-regulated, i.e. the ways individuals influence which emotions they have, when they have them, and how they experience and express these emotions (Gross 1999). This capacity is closely related to self-consciousness, metacognition, and self-agency. This form of self-regulation involves conscious and volitional changes in one or more of the various components (cognitive, experiential, physiological, and behavioral) of emotion (Gross 1999). These changes imply modifications in what Thompson (1990) has termed "emotion dynamics," i.e. the magnitude, rise time, duration, and offset of responses in the diverse components of emotion (Gross 1999). The cognitive strategies used to self-regulate emotion are numerous and include, among others, reappraisal and cognitive distancing. A growing body of literature indicates that successful regulation of emotion is critical to maintaining physical and mental health (Dennolet *et al.* 2007).

Several functional neuroimaging studies of emotional self-regulation have been conducted during the last decade. The main objective of this chapter is to demonstrate that these studies strongly support the mentalistic perspective that the subjective nature and the intentional content (what they are "about" from a first-person perspective) of the mental processes (e.g. volitions, thoughts, feelings) involved in emotional self-regulation significantly influence the functioning of the brain.

In this chapter, I review the findings of functional neuroimaging studies carried out with regard to the self-regulation of sexual arousal, sadness in adults and children, and negative emotion. In the last section, I discuss the theoretical implications of these neuroimaging studies regarding the relationships between subjective experience, mental processes, neurophysiological processes, and human behavior.

VOLITIONAL CONTROL OF SEXUAL AROUSAL

In the first neuroimaging study of conscious and volitional regulation of an emotional state (Beauregard *et al.* 2001), my group used functional magnetic resonance imaging (fMRI) to identify the neural correlates of the self-regulation of sexual arousal. Ten healthy male volunteers (university students) were scanned during two experimental conditions, i.e. a sexual arousal condition and a down-regulation condition. In the sexual arousal condition, volunteers viewed a series of erotic film excerpts. They were instructed to react normally to these stimuli, i.e. they had to allow themselves to become sexually aroused during the viewing of the erotic film excerpts. In the down-regulation condition, volunteers were instructed to use cognitive distancing, that is, to become a detached observer of comparable erotic film excerpts and the sexual arousal induced by these stimuli. This metacognitive strategy shares some similarity with mindfulness, a central mental state in Buddhist forms of meditation (Thera 2000). To assess the emotional reactions of the volunteers to the film excerpts, they were asked at the outset of each condition to rate on a numerical (analog) rating scale the intensity of primary emotions felt during the viewing of the film segments.

Phenomenologically, the viewing of the erotic film excerpts during both conditions induced a state of sexual arousal in all volunteers. In the down-regulation condition, most volunteers reported having been successful at distancing themselves from the erotic film excerpts and the sexual arousal induced by these stimuli. Consistent with this, the mean level of sexual arousal was significantly higher in the sexual arousal condition than in the down-regulation condition. Additionally, in line with the results of a previous study (Karama *et al.* 2002), the viewing of the erotic film excerpts in the sexual arousal condition produced a significant activation of the right amygdala, right anterior temporal pole (Brodmann area (BA) 38) and hypothalamus (Figure 5.1). In the down-regulation condition, activation peaks were noted in BA 10 of the right lateral prefrontal cortex (LPFC) and BA 32 of the right rostroventral anterior cingulate cortex (ACC). Interestingly, no significant loci of blood

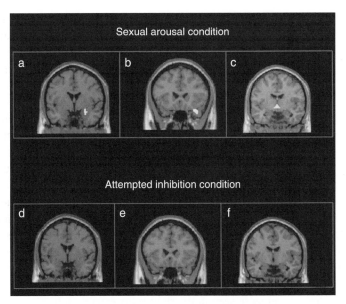

FIG. 5.1 (Also see Plate 4). Statistical activation maps showing limbic–paralimbic structures defined a priori. In the sexual arousal condition, greater activation during the viewing of erotic film excerpts relative to the viewing of emotionally neutral film excerpts was noted in the right amygdala (a), right anterior temporal pole (b), and the hypothalamus (c). In the suppression condition, no significant loci of activation were seen in the amygdalae (d), the anterior temporal polar region (e), and the hypothalamus (f). Reproduced with permission of the Society for Neuroscience from Beauregard, M. *et al.* (2001). Neural correlates of the conscious self-regulation of emotion. *Journal of Neuroscience,* **21,** 1–6.

oxygenation level-dependent (BOLD) activation were measured in the amygdala, anterior temporal pole and hypothalamus.

These results provided robust evidence for the view previously proposed that emotional self-regulation depends on a brain system in which prefrontal cortical areas mediate the cognitive modulation of emotional responses (Nauta 1971; Tucker *et al.* 1995; Davidson *et al.* 2000). Moreover, these results are consistent with studies indicating that the LPFC is involved in metacognitive/executive top-down processes (these processes refer to the ability to monitor and control the information processing necessary to produce voluntary action (Flavell 1979)). This prefrontal cortical region has been implicated in the selection and control of behavioral strategies and action (Fuster 1999), especially in the inhibition of inherent response tendency (Goldman-Rakic 1987; Damasio 1995; Frith and Dolan 1996; Fuster 1997). These results also support the hypothesis that by virtue of its anatomic connections with brain regions implicated in the modulation of autonomic and endocrine functions such as the amygdala, hypothalamus and orbitofrontal cortex (OFC), the rostroventral subdivision of the ACC plays a key role in the regulation of the autonomic aspect of emotional responses (Vogt *et al.* 1992; Devinsky *et al.* 1995; Bush *et al.* 2000). The fact that this portion of the ACC has both afferent and efferent connections with neural structures mediating autonomic functions such as the periaqueductal gray, the dorsal motor nucleus of the vagus, and the preganglionic sympathetic neurons in the intermediolateral cell column of the spinal cord (Benes 1997) supports this hypothesis.

SELF-REGULATION OF SADNESS IN ADULTS

A protocol similar to that used in the Beauregard *et al.* (2001) study was utilized in another fMRI study carried out by our research group (Lévesque *et al.* 2003). This study sought to delineate the neural substrates of conscious and voluntary regulation of sadness, a primary emotion with a negative valence (Plutchik 1994). Twenty healthy female volunteers were scanned during a sad condition and a down-regulation condition. Experientially, the mean level of reported sadness was significantly higher in the sad condition than in the down-regulation condition. Neurally, significant bilateral loci of activation were measured during the sad condition in the anterior temporal pole (BA 21 and BA 38) and midbrain. Significant BOLD signal increases were also seen in the right ventrolateral prefrontal cortex (VLPFC) (BA 47), left amygdala and left insula. In the down-regulation condition, significant loci of BOLD activations were detected in the right orbitofrontal cortex (OFC, BA 11) and right LPFC (BA 9).

The right LPFC activation measured during the down-regulation condition demonstrated that in addition to being involved in the volitional modulation of a positive emotional state such as sexual arousal (Beauregard *et al.* 2001), this prefrontal cortical region is also associated with the voluntary regulation of a negative emotion such as sadness. These results are in keeping with a variety of evidence indicating that the LPFC plays a crucial role in willed actions (Frith and Dolan 1996) and with the holding in mind of information on which an action is to be based (Goldman-Rakic 1987; Fuster 1999; Roberts and Wallis 2000).

Robust activation of the right OFC (BA 11) was also noted during down-regulation of sad feelings. This brain structure is located at the junction of the prefrontal associative cortex and the so-called limbic system. Given the fact that this cortical area sends projections to the amygdala, diencephalon, brainstem, and spinal cord, it has been associated with the integration of visceral-autonomic processes with cognitive and behavioral processes (Ongür *et al.* 1998; Rempel-Clower and Barbas 1998; Eslinger 1999a). It has been also proposed that this portion of the OFC plays a central role in the adaptation to complex changing environments (Eslinger 1999b) and the regulation of socioemotional behavior in settings involving social affiliation and social judgment, self-consciousness, inhibition, and the self-guidance of behavior through judgments and decisions about one's actions (Mesulam 1986; Damasio *et al.* 1990; Elliott 1990; Cummings 1993; Bechara *et al.* 1994; Giancola and Zeichner 1994; Damasio 1995; Lapierre *et al.* 1995; Grafman *et al.* 1996; Zald and Kim 1996; Dolan 1999; Eslinger 1999b; Fuster 1997; Grafman and Litvan 1999). The OFC is the only PFC region richly connected to the amygdala. The central nucleus of the amygdala is the main source of efferent connections to brainstem and hypothalamic structures modulating a wide range of endocrine and autonomic responses (Davis 1992). The caudal OFC receives information from the central nucleus of the amygdala and, in return, projects directly to this nucleus, procuring thereby a circuit through which the OFC may directly modulate the activity of the amygdala. Furthermore, the medial and lateral OFC send extensive connections to the lateral hypothalamus, suggesting that these OFC areas are particularly involved in the regulation of visceral responses to stimuli and events. The OFC has also strong links with the anterior temporal pole, the insular cortex and the LPFC (Morecraft *et al.* 1992; Cavada *et al.* 2000).

Clinical neuropsychological studies indicate that the OFC exerts an inhibitory control to protect goal-directed behavior from interference (Fuster 1999; Roberts and Wallis 2000). Damage to the OFC leads to a *frontal lobe syndrome* (Silver and Yudofsky 1987) or *pseudopsychopathic syndrome* (Stuss and Benson 1984) that is characterized by distractibility, impulsivity, emotional outbursts, shallowness, argumentativeness, verbal and physical aggressiveness, hypersexuality, hyperphagia, lack of concern of consequences of behavior, failure to observe social and moral rules, and risky decision-making behavior. Individuals with OFC lesions tend to be unpredictable, their humor is labile, and they often display inappropriate and childish humor. Remarkably, these individuals show abnormal autonomic responses to emotional elicitors, difficulty to experience emotion related to situations that would normally evoke emotion, and impaired understanding of the adverse consequences of detrimental social behaviors (Damasio *et al.* 1990).

SELF-REGULATION OF SADNESS IN CHILDREN

To be able to consciously and voluntarily self-regulate emotion, a child must first be aware of having an emotional experience, that is, the child must interpret and evaluate his/her perceived emotional state (Lewis 1998). To have an emotional experience, the child must be cognitively able to make reference to the fact that it is "I" to whom these internal events are happening. The child must also interpret these events in the context of the meaning systems that he/she has acquired through interactions with others. Indeed, children learn strategies for controlling their emotional responses in agreement with the social rules of their culture. These capacities involve the development of self-consciousness (Lewis 1995). There is some evidence that self-consciousness emerges at around 15–18 months (Lewis 1995). It is the emergence of this referencing self which allows the child to monitor and react to his/her emotional state, i.e. to self-reflect on his/her thoughts, emotions, and behavior. Cognitive development and social development thus play a pivotal role in the evolution of the capacity to self-regulate emotion (Cole *et al.* 1994).

Emotional self-regulation begins with the control of distress. Infants aged 8–18 months respond with distress and negative affect to brief separation from the mother. Between 19 and 24 months, there is a significant reduction of negative emotional responses to brief maternal separation (Mangelsdorf *et al.* 1996). Fox *et al.* (2001) speculated that changes in response to this event during the second year of life may be the result of an infant's increasing capacity to recognize, define, and represent the cause of distress; to appraise the contextual features of the emotion elicitor; to maintain a cognitive representation of his/her mother during her absence; and to form a plan for a sequence of actions in order to change the situation so that distress is diminished. Results of electroencephalography studies conducted by Fox and colleagues (2001) evidenced an important role for the PFC in the regulation of negative affect and emotional distress. Fox and Bell (1990) hypothesized that a combination of neurobiological maturation in the PFC and social learning experiences underlie the emergence of emotional self-regulation. Regarding this issue, during the first 6 months, the young infant's emotional regulatory capacity advances from a primarily reflexive response to physiological stimuli (e.g. thirst, hunger, pain, fatigue) to a nascent awareness of internal state and the ability to temporally associate emotional states with specific external stimuli (Kopp 1989). By 6–8 months of age, emotional regulation begins to involve typical PFC functions such as selective attention to stimuli and perception of temporal contingent sequences implicating the infant's own actions and external stimuli. These functions allow the infant to regulate states of emotional arousal, for instance, by signaling to caregivers to act in response to his/her emotional states. With the emergence of self-consciousness and intentionality (or goal-directedness), emotional regulatory capacities augment markedly during the second half of the first year of life. Emotion regulation then becomes truly emotional *self*-regulation, i.e. more conscious and self-guided. At this stage, the infant acquires new cognitive executive capacities (e.g. representational thought, self-monitoring, working memory, goal formulation, flexibility of responding internalization of rules to guide behavior, response inhibition, attentional control, planning) that critically depend on PFC development and allow him/her to engage in intentional self-regulatory behaviors (Dawson *et al.* 1992).

Phylogenetically as well as ontogenetically, the PFC is one of the last neocortical regions to develop. Evolutionarily, the PFC achieves maximal relative growth in the human brain, where it represents approximately one-third of the total volume of the neocortex. In the normal human individual, full PFC maturation is not reached until late adolescence/early adulthood (Fuster 1999). Myelination and dendritic development occur later in the human PFC than in other cortical regions. Synaptogenesis reaches a plateau between the ages of 1–7 years and declines through adolescence to the adult level (Bourgeois *et al.* 1994; Huttenlocher 1994; Rakic *et al.* 1994). This decrease in synaptic number coincides with the continued development of cognitive capacities (Caviness *et al.* 1996). Further, cortical gray matter volume achieves its peak at around 5 years of age and decreases from that time forward, while the white matter volume increases continuously until the age of 20 years (Pfefferbaum *et al.* 1994). It is noteworthy that Fox *et al.* (2001) emphasized the obvious similarities between the disinhibited behaviors of adults following damage to the PFC and the emotional reactions and behaviors of normal infants and young children. The cognitive and emotional changes following PFC damage have been attributed to a disruption in the inhibitory control normally exerted by the PFC on subcortical limbic structures. In accordance with this, Posner and Rothbart (1998) postulated that emotional self-regulation in childhood likely involves the interaction of the midfrontal ACC region with the amygdala.

Within a neurodevelopmental perspective, the fMRI protocol described in the preceding section was used to study the neural correlates of self-regulation of sadness in 14 healthy girls (age range: 8–10) (Lévesque *et al.* 2004). As in the Lévesque *et al.* (2003) study, the mean level of reported sadness was significantly higher in the sad condition than in the down-regulation condition. As for brain activity, significant loci of BOLD activation were seen, in the sad condition, in the left VLPFC (BA 47) and, bilaterally, in the midbrain and anterior temporal pole (BA 21). In the down-regulation condition, significant loci of activation were noted, bilaterally, in the LPFC (BA 9 and 10), OFC (BA 11), medial prefrontal cortex (MPFC) (BA 10), and rostral ACC (BA 24).

A certain portion of the rostral ACC is connected to the OFC (Devinsky *et al.* 1995) and has outflow to autonomic, visceromotor, and endocrine systems. The co-activation of the rostral ACC and the OFC, while children were attempting to down-regulate sadness, provided further evidence that these prefrontal regions are part of a brain system involved in the self-regulation of primary emotions. It is also worth mentioning that a region of the MPFC close to that identified in the Lévesque *et al.* (2004) study, during the down-regulation condition, has previously been postulated to be implicated in theory-of-mind tasks (Fletcher *et al.* 1995) and metacognitive representation of one's own emotional state (Reiman *et al.* 1997; Lane 2000). This cortical region receives sensory information from the body and the external environment via the OFC (Barbas 1993; Carmichael and Price 1995), and is heavily interconnected with limbic structures such as the amygdala, ventral striatum, hypothalamus, midbrain periaqueductal gray region, and brainstem autonomic nuclei (Barbas 1993; Carmichael and Price 1995). Such anatomical relationships suggest a role for this area of the MPFC in the integration of the visceromotor aspects of emotional processing with information gathered from the internal and external environments. It thus seems plausible that the MPFC activation noted in children, during the down-regulation task, was related to "reflective conscious awareness" (awareness of awareness) (Farthing 1992).

Down-regulation of sadness was experientially more difficult for children than adults (Lévesque *et al.* 2003). As for the brain regions activated in both studies, the down-regulation task recruited more prefrontal areas in children than in adults. Additionally, the spatial extent of the LPFC activation was fivefold greater in children than in adults. These differences suggest that volitional down-regulation of a primary emotion requires more prefrontal work in children than in adults. Accordingly, it has been demonstrated that children show greater volume of PFC activity than adults when performing tasks requiring active maintenance and/or suppression of different types of information (e.g. go/no-go paradigm) (Cohen *et al.* 1994; Casey *et al.* 1995). Casey and colleagues (1995) have proposed that such differences may reflect maturational differences with respect to the PFC. Along the same lines, it appears conceivable that conscious and volitional self-regulation of emotion is more challenging, cognitively and affectively, in children than in adults because the maturation of the PFC is not yet completed.

CONSCIOUS AND VOLITIONAL REGULATION
OF NEGATIVE EMOTION

To date a number of fMRI studies have been carried out regarding the neural substrates of self-regulation of negative emotion. In one of these studies, Schaefer *et al.* (2002) used an event-related design to test the hypothesis that volitional down-regulation of emotionally negative pictures is associated with changes in neural activity within the amygdala, a cardinal component of emotion perception. Negative and emotionally neutral pictures selected from the International Affective Picture System (IAPS) (Lang *et al.* 1998) were presented to seven healthy female volunteers. Volunteers were instructed to either maintain the initial emotional response induced by the picture throughout its presentation or passively view the picture without self-regulating the emotional reaction. After each picture presentation, volunteers indicated how they currently felt using a Likert-type scale. Volunteers reported feeling more negative during negative picture trials than neutral picture trials. Volunteers also reported feeling more negative on maintain trials than view trials. In keeping with previous functional neuroimaging studies having shown increased activation in the amygdala in response to emotionally negative stimuli (Phan *et al.* 2002), greater amygdalar signal change was noted during the presentation of negative pictures compared to neutral pictures. Increased activation in the amygdala was associated with maintenance of negative emotion compared to the passive viewing condition. Furthermore, a prolonged BOLD signal increase was found in the amygdala when volunteers maintained the negative emotional state during the presentation of negative pictures. This amygdalar signal increase was significantly correlated with volunteers' self-reported levels of negative emotion. These findings suggest that the conscious cognitive processes that modulated the emotional responses of the volunteers to the negative pictures were associated with an alteration of the degree of neural activity within the amygdala, i.e. the degree of amygdalar activity can be consciously and volitionally regulated. In keeping with this, Hariri *et al.* (2003) demonstrated that whereas perceptual processing of threatening and fearful non-face (IAPS) stimuli was associated with a bilateral amygdala response, cognitive appraisal of the same stimuli was associated with a reduction of this amygdala response and a concomitant increase in response of the right prefrontal and anterior cingulate cortices.

In another event-related fMRI study, Ochsner *et al.* (2002) used reappraisal as a cognitive strategy to modulate emotional experience (reappraisal consists of altering the trajectory of an unfolding emotional response by cognitively reinterpreting/transforming the meaning of the emotion-eliciting stimulus/event to change one's emotional response to it). Ochsner and colleagues (2002) hypothesized that the neural circuits and processing dynamics implicated in the cognitive control of emotion would be similar to those involved in other forms of cognitive control. In their study, negative and neutral pictures from the IAPS were presented to 15 healthy female volunteers. For each trial volunteers were instructed to view the picture and allow themselves to experience/feel any emotional response it might elicit. The picture remained on the screen for an additional period of time with an instruction either to attend or reappraise. On attend trials, volunteers were requested to attend to and be aware of, but not to try to modify, any feelings induced by negative or neutral pictures. On reappraise trials, volunteers were instructed to reinterpret the negative pictures so that they no longer generated a negative emotional response. After the presentation of each picture volunteers had to rate on a four-point scale the strength of current negative emotion. Behaviorally, reappraisal of negative pictures successfully lessened negative emotion. The average ratings of the strength of negative emotion were significantly lower on reappraise trials than on attend trials. Neurofunctionally, reappraisal was associated with a significant activation of the dorsal and ventral regions of the left LPFC (BA 6, 8, 10, 44, 46) as well as the dorsal MPFC (BA 8). Moreover, the right amygdala was significantly more activated on attend than reappraise trials. Interestingly, the medial orbitofrontal cortex (MOFC) (BA 11) displayed greater activation to most negative pictures on attend than on reappraise trials, whereas activated areas of the LPFC showed the opposite trend. For one of these areas, the ventral LPFC (VLPFC), increased activation during reappraisal was correlated across volunteers with decreased activation in amygdala.

For Ochsner *et al.* (2002), these results provide good evidence that reappraisal may modulate the emotion processes implemented in the amygdala and MOFC and involved in the evaluation of the emotional significance and contextual relevance of a stimulus (or event). The specific LPFC and MPFC areas found associated with reappraisal were comparable to the prefrontal areas frequently seen activated in diverse working memory and response-selection tasks that entail resisting to interference from competing stimuli and maintaining information in awareness (Courtney et al. 1998; Smith and Jonides 1999; Cabeza and Nyberg 2000). This similitude supports the view that a common ensemble of LPFC and MPFC areas underlies the cognitive regulation of both feelings and thoughts (Knight et al. 1999; Smith and Jonides 1999; Miller and Cohen 2001; Ochsner and Feldman Barrett 2001). The fact that the VLPFC activation was inversely correlated with the activation of the amygdala and MOFC indicates that the VLPFC may play an important role in the conscious and volitional regulation of emotional processes. Further, the modulation of the neural activity within the amygdala and the MOFC supports the view that reappraisal can influence processes involved in the evaluation of the emotional significance of a stimulus (Whalen et al. 1998; Anderson and Phelps 2001), as well as those implicated in the evaluation of the significance of that stimulus with reference to current contextual meaning (Elliott et al. 1997; Bechara et al. 2000; Kawasaki et al. 2001; Ochsner and Feldman Barrett 2001; O'Doherty et al. 2001). Ochsner et al. (2002) also claimed that the reappraisal processes implemented by lateral and medial prefrontal regions may play an important role in the regulation of evaluation processes associated with the OFC. This cortical region may be responsible for the selection of appropriate, and the transient suppression of inappropriate, emotional responses. Because the LPFC and the amygdala have few direct anatomical connections, Ochsner et al. (2002) further contended that the LPFC could influence the amygdala via the MOFC, which has reciprocal connections with both structures (Cavada et al. 2000). By directly modulating the representations of the emotional salience of a stimulus in the MOFC, activation in the LPFC could indirectly down-regulate processing in the amygdala.

Ochsner et al. (2004) performed another fMRI study in 24 healthy female volunteers to compare the neural systems supporting down- and up-regulation with reappraisal of negative emotion induced by IAPS pictures. Results indicated that amygdala activation was modulated up or down in agreement with the regulatory goal. Up-regulation recruited the ACC (BA 32), MPFC (BA 9, 32), left LPFC (BA 9), and left amygdala whereas down-regulation recruited the left LPFC (BA 8, 9) and the left lateral OFC (BA 47). For Ochsner et al. (2004), these results suggest that both common and distinct neural systems underlie various forms of reappraisal. These results further indicate that which specific prefrontal systems modulate the amygdala is contingent on the regulatory goal and strategy used.

More recently, Phan et al. (2005) scanned 14 healthy male and female volunteers while they down-regulated via reappraisal negative IAPS pictures. Online subjective ratings of intensity of negative emotion were used as covariates of brain activity. Down-regulation of negative emotion was associated with activation of dorsal ACC (BA 32), right dorsal MPFC (BA 9), and right LPFC (BA 9), and attenuation of brain activity within the left amygdala vicinity. Furthermore, activity within right dorsal ACC (BA 32) was negatively correlated with intensity of negative emotion, whereas activation of the amygdala was positively correlated with intensity of negative emotion. These findings highlight a functional dissociation of corticolimbic brain responses implicating enhanced activation of PFC and attenuation of limbic areas during down-regulation of negative emotion.

Other fMRI studies (Kim and Hamann 2007; Goldin et al. 2008) have confirmed the implication of the LPFC (BA 9, 10), ACC (BA 24, 32), MPFC (BA 9, 10), and OFC (BA 11) in the reappraisal of negative pictures or film clips. These data corroborate the view that several prefrontal cortical areas are involved in the cognitive regulation of emotion.

We previously proposed (Beauregard *et al.* 2004) a neurocognitive model according to which specific areas of the PFC participate in the neural mediation of the various top-down processes underlying conscious and volitional self-regulation of emotions (Figure 5.2). In this model the LPFC (BA 9, 10) is implicated in the selection of the appropriate cognitive operations in order to produce the desired outcome (e.g. down-regulation of the emotional response induced by film excerpts). To accomplish that role, the LPFC sends an executive command to the OFC (BA 11), which is involved in the modulation of the diverse aspects of emotion (e.g. physiological, experiential). In turn the OFC sends a message to the amygdala, which is implicated in the reframing of the stimuli presented. The OFC is informed about this cognitive "reframing" by virtue of the anatomic projections that the amygdala sends back to this cortical region. The OFC also informs the rostroventral ACC (BA 24, 32) to modulate activity in brain structures implicated in autonomic, visceral, and endocrine functioning (e.g. hypothalamus, insula, midbrain, brainstem nuclei). The rostroventral ACC conveys information related to the physiological state of the organism back to the OFC. Moreover, the OFC informs the MPFC (BA 10), which is involved in emotional self-consciousness, of the diverse changes related to the individual's feeling state.

Importantly, this rather mechanistic and reductionistic model (and other models of the same type) can be useful only to the extent that we keep in mind that the whole person, not only the brain, is implicated in conscious and volitional control of emotional behavior.

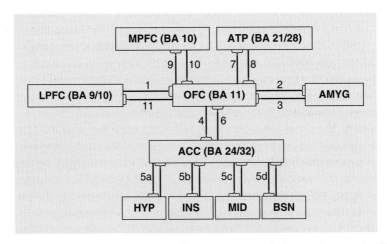

FIG. 5.2 Schematic diagram of a putative brain system underlying emotional self-regulation. The numbers refer to the temporal sequence of connection between the various components of the system. ACC: anterior cingulate cortex; AMYG: amygdala; ATP: anterior temporal pole; BA: Brodmann area; BSN: brainstem nuclei; HYP: hypothalamus; INS: insula; LPFC: lateral prefrontal cortex; MID: midbrain; MPFC: medial prefrontal cortex; OFC: orbitofrontal cortex. Reproduced with permission of John Benjamins Publishing Company from Beauregard, M. *et al.* (2004).

Theoretical implications of the neuroimaging studies of emotional self-regulation

The results of the neuroimaging studies of emotional self-regulation reviewed in this chapter indicate that the conscious and voluntary use of cognitive distancing and reappraisal selectively modulates the way the brain responds to emotional stimuli. In agreement with this, other neuroimaging studies suggest that the diverse mental processes and states implicated in various forms of psychotherapy exert a significant influence on the activity of specific brain regions and networks (Beauregard 2007). In addition, there is increasing evidence from neuroimaging investigations of the placebo effect in healthy individuals and patients with Parkinson's disease or unipolar major depressive disorder that beliefs and expectations can markedly modulate neurophysiological and neurochemical activity in brain structures involved in perception, movement, pain, and various aspects of emotion processing (Beauregard 2007).

Taken together, these neuroimaging data strongly support the view that the subjective nature and the intentional content of mental processes and states significantly influence the functioning and plasticity of the brain. In other words, mental variables can be causally efficacious and explanatory and have to be considered as much as neurophysiological variables to reach a correct understanding of human behavior. Such a mentalistic outlook is supported by the high explanatory and predictive value of agentic factors like volitions, goals, beliefs, and expectations (Bandura 2001).

Findings from neuroimaging studies of emotional self-regulation, psychotherapy, and placebo effect call into question the psychophysical identity theory and epiphenomenalism. For the psychophysical identity theory, mental processes are identical with neural processes (Feigl 1958) whereas for epiphenomenalism, mental processes are causally inert epiphenomena (i.e. by-products) of neural processes. These findings also challenge eliminative materialism (or eliminativism). According to this view, mental processes, which are prescientific concepts belonging to unsophisticated ideas of how the brain works, can be reduced entirely to brain processes. Eliminative materialism further proposes that all common language or "folk psychology" descriptions of mental experience should be eliminated and replaced by descriptions using neuroscientific language (Churchland 1981). For these materialist views, physically describable brain mechanisms represent the core and final explanatory vehicle for every kind of psychologically described data. These views are extremely counterintuitive since our most basic experience teaches us that our choice of perspective about how we apprehend our mental processes and states makes a huge difference in how we respond to them (Schwartz *et al.* 2005).

I stand firmly against the inclination of certain neuroscientists and philosophers toward neuroreductionism, i.e. the reduction of human beings to their brains (a form of "neural anthropomorphism"), and posit that the brain is necessary but not sufficient to explicate all the human psychological features. This position is shared by Fuchs (2008), Glannon (2009), and others. Indeed, persons are conscious, perceive, think, feel emotion, interpret, believe, and make decisions, not parts of their brains. To attribute such capacities to brains is to commit a philosophical mistake that Bennett and Hacker (2003) identified as "the mereo-logical fallacy" in neuroscience, i.e. the fallacy of attributing to parts of the brain attributes that are properties of the whole human person.

With the emergence of self-consciousness, self-agency, and metacognitive capacities, evolution has enabled human beings to consciously and volitionally shape the functioning of their brains. These advanced capacities allow humans to be driven not only by survival and reproduction but also by complex sets of insights, goals, and beliefs. For example, the ethical values associated with a given spiritual tradition help certain individuals to keep in check some of their emotional impulses and behave in an altruistic fashion. In this particular instance, moral conscience replaces innate programming as behavioral regulator, and allows emancipation from "selfish" genes and the primitive dictates of the mammalian brain.

References

Anderson, A.K. and Phelps, E.A. (2001). Lesions of the human amygdala impair enhanced perception of emotionally salient events. *Nature,* **17,** 305–9.

Bandura, A. (2001). Social cognitive theory: an agentic perspective. *Annual Review of Psychology,* **52,** 1–26.

Barbas, H. (1993). Organization of cortical afferent input to the orbitofrontal area in the rhesus monkey. *Neuroscience,* **56,** 841–64.

Beauregard, M., Lévesque, J., and Bourgouin, P. (2001). Neural correlates of the conscious self-regulation of emotion. *Journal of Neuroscience,* **21,** 1–6.

Beauregard, M., Lévesque, J., and Paquette, V. (2004). Neural basis of conscious and voluntary self-regulation of emotion. In M Beauregard (ed.) *Consciousness, Emotional Self-Regulation and the Brain,* pp. 163–94. Amsterdam: John Benjamins Publishing Company.

Beauregard, M. (2007). Mind does really matter: evidence from neuroimaging studies of emotional self-regulation, psychotherapy, and placebo effect. *Progress in Neurobiology,* **81,** 218–36.

Bechara, A., Damasio, A.R., Damasio, H., and Anderson, S.W. (1994). Insensitivity to future consequences following damage to human prefrontal cortex. *Cognition,* **50,** 7–12.

Bechara, A., Tranel, D., and Damasio, H. (2000). Characterization of the decision-making deficit of patients with ventromedial prefrontal cortex lesions. *Brain,* **123,** 2189–202.

Benes, F. (1997). Corticolimbic circuitry and the development of psychopathology during childhood and adolescence. In N.A. Krasnegor, G. Reid Lyon, and P.S. Goldman-Rakic (eds.) *Development of the Prefrontal Cortex,* pp. 211–40. Baltimore, MD: Paul H. Brookes Publishing Co., Inc.

Bennett, M.R. and Hacker, P.M.S. (2003). *Philosophical Foundations of Neuroscience.* New York: Blackwell Publishing.

Bourgeois J.-P., Goldman-Rakic, P.S., and Rakic P. (1994). Synaptogenesis in the prefrontal cortex of rhesus monkeys. *Progress in Brain Research,* **102,** 227–43.

Bush, G., Luu, P., and Posner, M.I. (2000). Cognitive and emotional influences in anterior cingulate cortex. *Trends in Cognitive Science,* **4,** 215–22.

Cabeza, R. and Nyberg, L. (2000). Neural bases of learning and memory: functional neuroimaging evidence. *Current Opinion in Neurology,* **13,** 415–21.

Carmichael, S.T. and Price, J.L. (1995). Limbic connections of the orbital and medial prefrontal cortex in macaque monkeys. *Journal of Comparative Neurology*, **25**, 615–41.

Casey, B.J., Cohen, J.D., Jezzard, P., *et al.* (1995). Activation of prefrontal cortex in children during a nonspatial working memory task with functional MRI. *Neuroimage*, **2**, 221–9.

Cavada, C., Company, T., Tejedor, J., Cruz-Rizzolo, R.J., and Reinoso-Suarez, F. (2000). The anatomical connections of the macaque monkey orbitofrontal cortex. A review. *Cerebral Cortex*, **10**, 220–42.

Caviness, V.S. Jr., Kennedy, D.N., Richelme, C., Rademacher, J., and Filipek, P.A. (1996). The human brain age 7–11 years: a volumetric analysis based on magnetic resonance images. *Cerebral Cortex*, **6**, 726–36.

Churchland, P.M. (1981). Eliminative materialism and the propositional attitudes. *Journal of Philosophy*, **78**, 67–90.

Cohen, J.D., Forman, S.D., Braver, T.S., Casey, B.J., Servan-Schreiber, D., and Noll, D.C. (1994). Activation of prefrontal cortex in a nonspatial working memory task with functional MRI. *Human Brain Mapping*, **1**, 293–304.

Cole, P.M., Michel, M.K. and Teti, L.O. (1994). The development of emotion regulation and dysregulation: a clinical perspective. *Monograph of the Society for Research on Child Development*, **59**, 73–100.

Courtney, S.M., Petit, L., Maisog, J.M., Ungerleider, L.G., and Haxby, J.V. (1998). An area specialized for spatial working memory in human frontal cortex. *Science*, **279**, 1347–51.

Cummings, J.L. (1993). Frontal-subcortical circuits and human behavior. *Archives of Neurology*, **50**, 873–80.

Damasio, A.R. (1995). On some functions of the human prefrontal cortex. *Annals of the New York Academy of Sciences*, **769**, 241–51.

Damasio, A.R., Tranel, D., and Damasio, H. (1990). Individuals with sociopathic behavior caused by frontal damage fail to respond autonomically to social stimuli. *Behavioural Brain Research*, **41**, 81–94.

Davidson, R.J., Putnam, K.M., and Larson, C.L. (2000). Dysfunction in the neural circuitry of emotion regulation – A possible prelude to violence. *Science*, **289**, 591–4.

Davis, M. (1992). The role of the amygdala in fear and anxiety. *Annual Review of Neuroscience*, **15**, 353–75.

Dawson, G., Panagiotides, H., Grofer Klinger, L., and Hill, D. (1992). The role of frontal lobe functioning in the development of infant self-regulatory behavior. *Brain and Cognition*, **20**, 152–75.

Dennolet, J., Nyklicek, I., and Vingerhoets, A. (2007). *Emotion, emotion regulation, and health*. New York: Springer.

Devinsky, O., Morrell, M.J., and Vogt, B.A. (1995). Contributions of anterior cingulate cortex to behaviour. *Brain*, **118**, 279–306.

Dolan, R.J. (1999). On the neurology of morals. *Nature Neuroscience*, **11**, 927–9.

Elliott, F.A. (1990). Neurology of aggression and episodic dyscontrol. *Seminars in Neurology*, **10**, 303–12.

Elliott, R., Frith, C.D., and Dolan, R.J. (1997). Differential neural response to positive and negative feedback in planning and guessing tasks. *Neuropsychologia*, **35**, 1395–404.

Eslinger, P.J. (1999a). Orbital frontal cortex: historical and contemporary views about its behavioral and physiological significance (Part I). *Neurocase*, **5**, 225–9.

Eslinger, P.J. (1999b). Orbital frontal cortex: behavioral and physiological significance (Part II). *Neurocase*, **5**, 299–300.

Farthing, W.G. (1992). *The Psychology of Consciousness*. Englewood Cliffs, NJ: Prentice Hall.

Feigl, H. (1958). The "mental" and the "physical". In: H. Feigl, M. Scriven, and G. Maxwell (eds.) *Concepts, Theories and the Mind-Body Problem*, pp. 320–492. Minneapolis, MN: Minnesota Studies in the Philosophy of Science.

Flavell, J.H. (1979). Metacognition and cognitive monitoring: A new area of cognitive development inquiry. *American Psychologist*, **34**, 906–11.

Fletcher, P.C., Happe, F., Frith, U., Dolan, R.J., Frackowiak, R.S., and Frith, C.D. (1995). Other minds in the brain: a functional imaging study of "theory of mind" in story comprehension. *Cognition*, **57**, 109–28.

Fox, N.A. and Bell, M.A. (1990). Electrophysiological indices of frontal lobe development. *Annals of the New York Academy of Sciences*, **608**, 677–704.

Fox, N.A., Henderson, H.A., and Marshall, P.J. (2001). The biology of temperament: An integrative approach. In C.A. Nelson and M. Luciana (eds.) *Handbook of Developmental Cognitive Neuroscience*, pp. 631–45. Cambridge, MA: MIT Press.

Frith, C. and Dolan, R. (1996). The prefrontal cortex in higher cognitive functions. *Cognitive Brain Research*, **5**, 175–81.

Fuchs, T. (2008). *Das Gehirn – Ein Beziehungsorgan*. Berlin: Springer.

Fuster, J.M. (1997). *The Prefrontal Cortex: Anatomy, Physiology and Neuropsychology of the Frontal Lobe*, 3rd edition. Philadelphia, PA: Lippincott-Raven.

Fuster, J.M. (1999). Synopsis of function and dysfunction of the frontal lobe. *Acta Psychiatrica Scandinava*, **99**, 51–7.

Giancola, P.R. and Zeichner, A. (1994). Neuropsychological performance on tests of frontal-lobe functioning and aggressive behavior in men. *Journal of Abnormal Psychology*, **103**, 832–5.

Glannon, W. (2009). Our brains are not us. *Bioethics*, **23**, 321–9.

Goldin, P.R., McRae, K., Ramel, W., and Gross, J.J. (2008). The neural bases of emotion regulation: reappraisal and suppression of negative emotion. *Biological Psychiatry*, **15**, 577–86.

Goldman-Rakic, P.S. (1987). Circuitry of primate prefrontal cortex and regulation of behavior by representational memory. In V.B. Mountcastle, F. Plum, F. and S.R. Geiger (eds.) *Handbook of Physiology*, Vol. 5, pp. 373–417. Bethesda, MD: American Physiological Society.

Grafman, J., Schwab, K., Warden, D., Pridgen, A., Brown, H.R., and Salazar, A.M. (1996). Frontal lobe injuries, violence, and aggression: a report of the Vietnam Head Injury Study. *Neurology*, **46**, 1231–8.

Grafman, J. and Litvan, I. (1999). Importance of deficits in executive functions. *Lancet*, **354**, 1921–3.

Gross, J.J. (1999). Emotion regulation: past, present, future. *Cognition and Emotion*, **13**, 551–73.

Hariri, A.R., Mattay, V.S., Tessitore, A., Fera, F., and Weinberger, D.R. (2003). Neocortical modulation of the amygdala response to fearful stimuli. *Biological Psychiatry*, **53**, 494–501.

Huttenlocher, P.R. (1994). Synaptogenesis, synapse elimination, and neural plasticity in human cerebral cortex. In C.A. Nelson (ed.) *Threats to optimal development: Integrating, biological, psychological, and social risk factors*, Vol. 27, pp. 35–54. Minnesota Symposia on Child Psychology. Hillsdale, NJ: Lawrence Erlbaum Associates.

Karama, S., Lecours, A.R., Leroux, J.-M., *et al.* (2002). Areas of brain activation in males and females during viewing of erotic film excerpts. *Human Brain Mapping*, **16**, 1–13.

Kawasaki, H., Kaufman, O., Damasio, H., *et al.* (2001). Single-neuron responses to emotional visual stimuli recorded in human ventral prefrontal cortex. *Nature Neuroscience,* **4,** 15–6.

Kim, S.H. and Hamann, S.J. (2007). Neural correlates of positive and negative emotion regulation. *Journal of Cognitive Neuroscience,* **19,** 776–98.

Knight, R.T., Staines, W.R., Swick, D., and Chao, L.L. (1999). Prefrontal cortex regulates inhibition and excitation in distributed neural networks. *Acta Psychologica,* **101,** 159–78.

Knoch, D. and Fehr, E. (2007). Resisting the power of temptations: the right prefrontal cortex and self-control. *Annals of the New York Academy of Sciences,* **1104,** 123–34.

Kopp, C.B. (1989). Regulation of distress and negative emotions: A developmental view. *Developmental Psychology,* **25,** 343–54.

Lane, R.D. (2000). Neural correlates of conscious emotional experience. In R.D. Lane, and L. Nadel (eds.) *Cognitive neuroscience of emotion,* pp. 345–70. New York: Oxford University Press.

Lang, P.J., Bradley, M.M., and Cuthbert, B.N. (1998). Emotion and motivation: measuring affective perception. *Journal of Clinical Neurophysiology,* **15,** 397–408.

Lapierre, D., Braun, C.M.J., and Hodgings, S. (1995). Ventral frontal deficits in psychopathy: neuropsychological test findings. *Neuropsychologia,* **33,** 139–51.

Levenson, C.A. (1994). Human emotion: a functional view. In P. Ekman and R.J. Davidson (eds.) *Fundamental questions about the nature of emotion,* pp. 123–26. New York: Oxford University Press.

Lévesque, J., Eugène, F., Joanette, Y., *et al.* (2003). Neural circuitry underlying voluntary self-regulation of sadness. *Biological Psychiatry,* **53,** 502–10.

Lévesque, J., Joanette, Y., Mensour, B., *et al.* (2004). Neural basis of emotional self-regulation in children. *Neuroscience,* **129,** 361–9.

Lewis, M. (1995). Aspects of self: From systems to ideas. In P. Rochat (ed.) *The Self in Infancy: Theory and Research. Advances in Psychology,* pp. 95–115. North Holland: Elsevier Science Publishers.

Lewis, M. (1998). The development and structure of emotions. In M.F. Mascolo and S. Griffin (eds.) *What develops in emotional development?,* pp. 29–50. New York: Plenum Press.

Mangelsdorf, S.C., Shapiro, J.R., and Marzolf, D. (1996). Developmental and temperamental differences in emotional regulation in infancy. *Child Development,* **66,** 1817–28.

Mesulam, M.-M. (1986). Frontal cortex and behavior. *Annals of Neurology,* **19,** 320–5.

Miller, E.K. and Cohen, J.D. (2001). An integrative theory of prefrontal cortex function. *Annual Review of Neuroscience,* **24,** 167–202.

Morecraft, R.J., Geula, C., and Mesulam, M.-M. (1992). Cytoarchitecture and neural afferents of orbitofrontal cortex in the brain of the monkey. *Journal of Comparative Neurology,* **323,** 341–58.

Nauta, W.J.H. (1971). The problem of the frontal lobe: A reinterpretation. *Journal of Psychiatry Research,* **8,** 167–87.

Thera, N. (2000). *The vision of Dhamma: Buddhist writings of Nyanaponika Thera.* Seattle, WA: BPS Pariyatti Editions.

Ochsner, K.N. and Feldman Barrett, L. (2001). A multiprocess perspective on the neuroscience of emotion. In T.J. Mayne and G. Bonanno (eds.) *Emotions: Currrent Issues and Future Directions,* pp. 38–81. New York: The Guilford Press.

Ochsner, K.N., Bunge, S.A., Gross, J.J., and Gabrieli, J.D. (2002). Rethinking feelings: an FMRI study of the cognitive regulation of emotion. *Journal of Cognitive Neuroscience,* **14,** 1215–29.

Ochsner, K.N., Ray, R.D., Cooper, J.C., *et al.* (2004). For better or for worse: neural systems supporting the cognitive down- and up-regulation of negative emotion. *NeuroImage*, **23**, 483–99.

O'Doherty, J., Kringelbach, M.L., Rolls, E.T., Hornak, J., and Andrews, C. (2001). Abstract reward and punishment representations in the human orbitofrontal cortex. *Nature Neuroscience*, **4**, 95–102.

Ongür, D., An, X. and Price, J.L. (1998). Prefrontal cortical projections to the hypothalamus in macaque monkeys. *Journal of Comparative Neurology*, **401**, 480–505.

Pfefferbaum, A., Mathalon, D.H., Sullivan, E.V., Rawles, J.M., Zipursky, R.B., and Lim, K. O. (1994). A quantitative magnetic resonance imaging study of changes in brain morphology from infancy to late adulthood. *Archives of Neurology*, **51**, 874–87.

Phan, K.L., Wager, T., Taylor, S.F., and Liberzon, I. (2002). Functional neuroanatomy of emotion: a meta-analysis of emotion activation studies in PET and fMRI. *Neuroimage*, **16**, 331–48.

Phan, K.L., Fitzgerald, D.A., Nathan, P.J., Moore, G.J., Uhde, T.W., and Tancer, M.E. (2005). Neural substrates for voluntary suppression of negative affect: a functional magnetic resonance imaging study. *Biological Psychiatry*, **57**, 210– 19.

Plutchik, R. (1994). *The Psychology and Biology of Emotion*. New York: Harper Collins College Publishers.

Posner, M.I. and Rothbart, M.K. (1998). Attention, self-regulation and consciousness. *Philosophical Transactions of the Royal Society of London B Biological Sciences*, **353**, 1915–27.

Rakic, P., Bourgeois, J.P., and Goldman-Rakic, P.S. (1994). Synaptic development of the cerebral cortex: implications for learning, memory, and mental illness. *Progress in Brain Research*, **102**, 227–43.

Reiman, E.M., Lane, R.D., Ahern, G.L., *et al.* (1997). Neuroanatomical correlates of externally and internally generated human emotion. *American Journal of Psychiatry*, **154**, 918–25.

Rempel-Clower, N.L., and Barbas, H. (1998). Topographic organization of connections between the hypothalamus and prefrontal cortex in the rhesus monkey. *Journal of Comparative Neurology*, **398**, 393–419.

Roberts, A.C. and Wallis, J.D. (2000). Inhibitory control and affective processing in the prefrontal cortex: neuropsychological studies in the common marmoset. *Cerebral Cortex*, **10**, 252–62.

Schaefer, S.M., Jackson, D.C., Davidson, R.J., Aguirre, G.K., Kimberg, D.Y., and Thompson-Schill, S.L. (2002). Modulation of amygdalar activity by the conscious regulation of negative emotion. *Journal of Cognitive Neuroscience*, **14**, 913–21.

Schwartz, J.M., Stapp, H., and Beauregard, M. (2005). Quantum theory in neuroscience and psychology: a neurophysical model of mind/brain interaction. *Philosophical Transactions of the Royal Society of London B Biological Sciences*, **360**, 1309–27.

Silver, J.M. and Yudofsky, S.C. (1987). Aggressive behavior in patients with neuropsychiatric disorders. *Psychiatric Annals*, **17**, 367–70.

Smith, E.E. and Jonides, J. (1999). Storage and executive processes in the frontal lobes. *Science*, **283**, 1657–61.

Stuss, D.T. and Benson, D.F. (1984). Neuropsychological studies of the frontal lobes. *Psychological Bulletin*, **95**, 3–28.

Thompson, R.A. (1990). Emotion and self-regulation. In R.A. Thompson (ed.) *Socioemotional Development: Nebraska Symposium on Motivation*, pp. 367–467, Lincoln, Nebraska: University of Nebraska Press.

Tooby, J. and Cosmides, L. (1990). On the universality of human nature and the uniqueness of the individual: the role of genetics and adaptation. *Journal of Personality*, **58**, 17–67.

Tucker, D.M., Luu, P., and Pribram, K.H. (1995). Social and emotional self-regulation. *Annals of New York Academy of Sciences*, **769**, 213–39.

Vogt, B.A., Finch, D.M., and Olson, C.R. (1992). Functional heterogeneity in cingulate cortex: the anterior executive and posterior evaluative regions. *Cerebral Cortex*, **2**, 435–43.

Whalen, P.J., Rauch, S.L., Etcoff, N.L., McInerney, S.C., Lee, M.B., and Jenike M.A. (1998). Masked presentations of emotional facial expressions modulate amygdala activity without explicit knowledge. *Journal of Neuroscience*, **18**, 411–18.

Zald, D.H. and Kim, S.W. (1996). The anatomy and function of the orbito-frontal cortex I: Anatomy, neurocircuitry, and obsessive-compulsive disorder. *Journal of Neuropsychiatry and Clinical Neuroscience*, **8**, 125–38.

CHAPTER 6

....

NEURAL CORRELATES
OF DECEPTION

....

GIORGIO GANIS AND J. PETER ROSENFELD

INTRODUCTION

....

DECEPTION can be defined in more than one way (Vrij 2008). Here, we define it as the attempt by someone to convince someone else of something the prevaricator knows is false. This definition can be stretched to include cases of concealed knowledge in which one attempts to convince others one does not have knowledge about an event of interest (e.g. some detail of a crime). Due to the potentially negative consequences associated with deceptive behavior, it is not surprising that societies have attempted to devise ways to detect its occurrence (Vrij 2008). Of course, the most direct way to determine if one is lying is to find objective evidence that contradicts one's claims (e.g. of not having certain knowledge). However, such direct evidence often is not available and so it is necessary to rely on indirect evidence. The oldest methods to infer deception relied on observing people's behavior and on trying to detect cues that would be diagnostic of deception, for instance, various forms of fidgeting or voice pitch. Unfortunately, although some behavioral cues are correlated with deception, none of them are diagnostic (DePaulo *et al.* 2003). Arousal theories of deception assume that many of these behavioral cues are associated with increased anxiety and emotional arousal during deception, for example due to fear of getting caught (National Research Council 2003). This logic led to the next class of methods, based on measuring subtler changes in the level of arousal, which are not visible to the naked eye. These methods focused on changes in peripheral psychophysiological variables, such as heart rate and skin conductance and resulted in the development of the polygraph, which is still the instrument most widely used for deception detection. However, despite their widespread application, this arousal-based approach also proved to be unreliable because the link between deception and emotional arousal is not very strong (National Research Council 2003). Recently, in an attempt to find variables more closely linked to deception, researchers have focused on the brain, the biological system that generates lies. The core idea is to try to determine the neural correlates of deceptive behavior in the hope of finding reliable brain signatures of such behavior (Ganis *et al.* 2003; Ganis and Keenan 2009).

This chapter has three aims: (1) to describe key paradigms employed to assess deception, (2) to review the main neuroscience-based technologies that have been employed to investigate the neural correlates of deception: electroencephalography (EEG), functional magnetic resonance imaging (fMRI), and transcranial direct current stimulation (tDCS), and (3) to briefly outline some of the ethical issues associated with these technologies to detect deceptive behavior.

DECEPTION PARADIGMS

As mentioned earlier, deception detection methods do not have direct access to deception processes per se, and can only infer deception by measuring processes that are associated with deception. Although neuroscience-based techniques provide new measures and variables, they cannot get around this basic logical constraint. Different deception paradigms and methods vary in the type of the associated processes and phenomena they measure. Three classes of paradigms have been used in most studies that have examined the neural correlates of deception (Table 6.1). The first class of paradigms is based on the "Control Question Test" (CQT). The CQT, preferred by "polygraphers" in North America and elsewhere, but adopted also by some neuroimaging work, involves asking "Did you do it?" type questions, e.g. "Did you take that $5000?" or "Did you kill your wife?" etc. This test is preferred by polygraph professionals because it is relatively easy to set up and apply in various situations, and because it tends to elicit confessions. On the other hand, this procedure has been criticized by the scientific research community because of the lack of standardization and because of the problems in devising suitable control questions (Ben-Shakhar *et al.* 2002; National Research Council 2003). The second class of paradigms is based on the Concealed Information Test (CIT), formerly called the guilty knowledge test (GKT), developed by Lykken (1959) as an alternative deception detection procedure to the CQT. This test relies on the oddball effect in which one class of stimuli stands out as rare and meaningful, giving rise to an orienting response that can be measured and detected with many techniques (Lykken 1974). As will be described later in more detail, people with knowledge about an item of interest (e.g. a detail from a crime scene) would exhibit signs of recognition when they see such item (usually referred to as "probe" item), even if they lie and deny recognizing it, relative to other unfamiliar items of the same type (e.g. items that could have plausibly been present at a crime scene but were not, usually referred to as "irrelevant" items). In contrast, individuals without such knowledge would respond equally to all items, including the probe item, since they are equally unfamiliar with all of them. Besides providing a tool to investigate the neural correlates of deception, this paradigm is thought by prominent researchers in the field to have the potential to become admissible in criminal court (Ben-Shakhar *et al.* 2002). The third class is based on the "differentiation of deception" idea and participants are instructed to produce deceptive responses on about half the trials and to tell the truth on the remaining trials (Furedy *et al.* 1988). In some cases, the same items are used in both conditions (counterbalanced across participants), so that they can be compared directly. Whereas differentiation of deception paradigms have usually been employed to address theoretical questions about deception, CQT and CIT paradigms have been used primarily for the purpose of actually trying to detect deception in single individuals.

Table 6.1 Summary of the main deception paradigms

Deception paradigm	Main features	Main use
Control Question Test (CQT)	Paradigm compares responses to crime-relevant questions of the type "Did you do it?" and control questions	Real-life polygraphic examinations
Concealed Information Test (CIT)	Paradigm relies on the orienting response subjects exhibit to items that are meaningful to them (e.g. because the were present at a crime scene) in order to infer concealed knowledge about such items	Laboratory studies of concealed information
Differentiation of Deception (DD)	Paradigm requires subjects to lie about half of the time. Same stimuli may be used in deceptive and honest conditions to maximize comparability	Laboratory studies of deception

NEURAL CORRELATES OF DECEPTION AND THEIR USE FOR DECEPTION DETECTION

In this section, we will describe briefly the recent use of EEG, fMRI, and tDCS to determine the neural correlates of deception. Additional neuroscience-based technologies that have only been employed very occasionally (or not at all) for this purpose, such as magnetoencephalography (Seth *et al.* 2006), near-infrared spectroscopy (Tian *et al.* 2009), positron emission tomography (Abe *et al.* 2006), and transcranial magnetic stimulation, will not be discussed.

EEG measures of deception

A time-varying voltage can be measured between an electrode placed on the scalp surface directly over the brain and another electrode connected to an electrically neutral part of the head (i.e. remote from neurons, such as the earlobe). These voltages comprise the spontaneously ongoing electroencephalogram (EEG), due to electrical activity taking place in large populations of pyramidal neurons, and are commonly known as brain waves (Ganis and Kosslyn 2002). If during the recording of EEG, a discrete stimulus such as a light flash occurs, the EEG breaks into a series of larger peaks and valleys lasting up to 2s after the stimulus. These waves, signaling the arrival in the cerebral cortex of neural activity elicited by the stimulus, comprise the wave series called the event-related potential (ERP). Modern EEG equipment can sample these signals every millisecond or faster, providing a non-invasive way of tracking brain processes with remarkable temporal resolution.

The ERP "rides on" the ongoing EEG, by which it is usually obscured in single trials (Ganis and Kosslyn 2002). Thus, one typically averages the EEG samples of many repeated presentation trials of either the same stimulus or stimulus category (e.g. female names, weapon types, etc.), and the resulting averaged stimulus-related activity is revealed as the ERP, while the non-stimulus-related features of the EEG tend to average out. Most of the literature on deception has focused on a specific ERP component, the P300, a positive going potential with a latency of about 300ms or longer, depending on the condition (Johnson 1986). Although other ERP components have been used to study deception, for example medial frontal negativities (MFNs) (Johnson *et al.* 2004), these ERP components have not been used systematically to determine whether they can be used to classify deceptive and honest responses in single individuals, and so we will focus on the P300. The P300 component results, among other situations, when a *meaningful* piece of information is *rarely* presented as a special stimulus among a random series of non-meaningful stimuli of the same category as the meaningful stimulus. For example, Figure 6.1 shows a set of three pairs of superimposed ERP averages from three scalp sites (called Fz, Cz, and Pz) on one subject, who was viewing a series of test items on a display (Rosenfeld *et al.* 2004). On 17% of the trials, a meaningful item (e.g. the participant's birth date) was presented, and on the remaining 83%

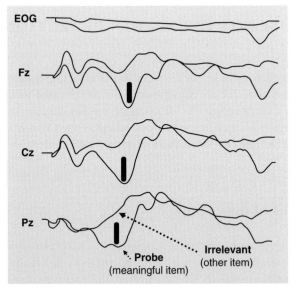

FIG. 6.1 ERPs from scalp sites Fz (frontal), Cz (central), and Pz (parietal) obtained during a 3-stimulus CIT paradigm. The sweeps are 2048ms long. P300 peaks are downgoing and indicated with thick vertical lines. They are in response to meaningful information items. They are superimposed on responses to meaningless items. Given that the sweeps are about 2s long, the P300s begin around 400ms and end around 900ms. Positive is plotted down by convention. The trace labeled "EOG" is a simultaneous recording of eye-movement activity. As required for sound EEG recording technique, EOG is flat during the segment of time when P300 occurs, indicating that no artifacts due to eye movements are occurring.

of the randomly occurring trials, other items with no meaning to the participant (e.g. other dates) were presented. The two superimposed waveforms at each scalp site represent averages of ERPs to (1) meaningful items and to (2) other items. In response to the meaningful items, a large down-going P300, indicated with thick vertical lines, is seen, which is absent in the superimposed other waveforms. Clearly, the *rare, recognized, meaningful* items elicit a P300, the other items do not. It should be evident that the ability of the P300 to signal the involuntary recognition of meaningful information suggests that this component could be used to signal the recognition of "concealed information" in CIT tests.

The first P300-based CIT studies (Allen *et al.* 1992; Farwell and Donchin 1991; Rosenfeld *et al.* 1988, 1991) utilized what we now refer to as the "3-stimulus protocol." On a given trial, subjects are presented with either a probe item, or several irrelevant other items from the same category as the probe. Participants may also be presented with a special irrelevant item called a *target*, an irrelevant item to which a unique response is assigned. Indeed the subject is instructed that on each trial, the presented stimulus must be classified as either a target or a non-target, a category that includes non-target irrelevant items and the probe. The probe and target are each presented rarely (about 10–20% of the trials) and the irrelevants (usually between 4 and 10) are presented frequently. Although probes and non-target irrelevants are responded to in the same (non-target) way, it is expected that the probe, because of its rareness and meaningfulness, will elicit P300, but the irrelevant will not. The rare target is also meaningful due to its special task relevance, and so it should also elicit a P300. The absence of the target P300 indicates that the subject is not attending the stimuli. The early studies utilizing this protocol were accurate in detecting personally relevant information, as well as well-rehearsed information relevant to mock crimes. These studies typically presented stimuli as text words on display screens, though some studies have shown that these older protocols also work with pictorial stimuli, (Lefebvre *et al.* 2007; Meijer *et al.* 2007). A more recent version of the CIT (Rosenfeld *et al.* 2008) will be described in the section on the performance of CIT paradigms.

Functional magnetic resonance imaging

FMRI is a particular type of magnetic resonance imaging scan that monitors some of the hemodynamic consequences of neural activity, rather than neural activity itself. Most fMRI research uses the blood oxygen level-dependent (BOLD) signal, which is based on local increases in cerebral blood flow due to neural activation that surpass changes in oxygen consumption. FMRI has very good spatial resolution, and so it can localize brain processes with great precision in space, which is why researchers have begun to use it to study the neural correlates of deception. However, the temporal resolution of the technique is intrinsically poor because the BOLD signal is very slow (several seconds) compared to the timecourse of neural activity (tens of milliseconds), and so it is difficult to directly relate fMRI findings with ERP findings (Ganis and Kosslyn 2002). Over the last few years, numerous laboratory studies have shown that deceptive and honest responses can be discriminated at the group level using hemodynamic signals measured with fMRI (e.g. Abe *et al.* 2006, 2007, 2008; Bhatt *et al.* 2008; Davatzikos *et al.* 2005; Gamer *et al.* 2007, 2009; Ganis and Keenan 2009; Ganis *et al.* 2003, 2011; Kozel *et al.* 2004, 2005; Langleben *et al.* 2002, 2005; Lee *et al.* 2002, 2005, 2008; Mohamed *et al.* 2006; Monteleone *et al.* 2008; Nose *et al.* 2009; Nunez *et al.*

2005; Spence *et al.* 2001, 2008). Most of these studies have used variants of CIT paradigms, but some have used differentiation of deception paradigms and also a version of the CQT paradigm. However, probably because of relatively small sample sizes, individual variability, and the broad range of stimuli/paradigms, the precise foci of activation have not been entirely consistent across studies. Figure 6.2 shows an example of typical activations in prefrontal cortex found when comparing activation to probes and irrelevants in 3-stimulus CIT protocols.

A recent meta-analysis of a subset of these studies attempted to find consistencies in the pattern of neural activation underlying generating deceptive responses (Christ *et al.* 2009). This meta-analysis also tried to determine some of the neurocognitive processes associated with deception by looking at the overlap between brain activation elicited by generating deceptive responses and by three classes of executive control processes thought to be recruited during deception (working memory, inhibitory control, and task switching). Regions that were more engaged during deceptive than honest responses included ventrolateral and dorsolateral prefrontal cortex, the anterior insula, medial prefrontal cortex, posterior parietal cortex, and bilateral inferior parietal lobule. The dorsolateral prefrontal and posterior parietal cortices overlapped with regions recruited by working memory tasks. The ventrolateral prefrontal cortex, the insula, and the medial prefrontal cortex (including the anterior cingulate) overlapped with regions also recruited by multiple executive control tasks. In contrast, regions in bilateral inferior parietal lobule did not overlap with regions engaged by any of the executive control tasks. These results are consistent with the idea that deception is a complex neurocognitive activity and that it relies upon many executive control processes.

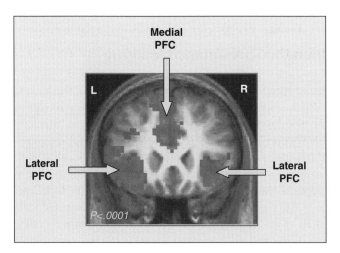

FIG. 6.2 (Also see Plate 5). Coronal section through the prefrontal cortex (y = 20) of a single subject, showing lateral and medial prefrontal regions in which stronger activation (*p* <0.0001, with a minimum cluster size of 15 voxels) was elicited by the subject's date of birth (probe) than by other dates not familiar to the subject (irrelevants) in a group of 14 subjects. A 3-item CIT paradigm was employed. The left side of the brain is on the left.

Transcranial direct current stimulation

Although ERPs and fMRI can measure some of the neural correlates of deception, they cannot determine whether such correlates are causally related to deception. The only way to show that a certain neural signature is also causally related to deception is to employ stimulation methods that can alter neural activity and document resulting changes in some aspects of deception performance. TDCS is a technique based on injecting a constant, weak current (usually around 1mA) into the brain, by means of electrodes placed on the scalp. The affected areas depend on the location of the electrodes and the effects depend on current intensity and polarity. TDCS has been shown to affect various perceptual and cognitive processes (Floel *et al.* 2008; Nitsche and Paulus 2000; Reis *et al.* 2009), although the exact mechanism of action is not known. A working hypothesis is that tDCS can alter the resting membrane potential of neurons, therefore increasing or decreasing their chance of firing, depending on the polarity of the stimulation (anodal is thought to increase the excitability of neurons, whereas cathodal is thought to decrease it). To date, only two studies have been published using this technique to affect deception processes, but the results are not very consistent with each other. The first study (Priori *et al.* 2008) used a differentiation of deception paradigm and showed that anodal tDCS stimulation of the dorsolateral prefrontal cortex (DLPFC) increased the response times for some deceptive responses, relative to truthful responses and to control stimulation conditions. The second study (Karim *et al.* 2009) used a CIT paradigm and reported that cathodal stimulation of the anterior prefrontal cortex resulted in faster deceptive response and in subjects feeling less guilty about lying. In contrast, anodal stimulation had no effect on deceptive responses. Clearly, additional studies will be required to determine if these results will replicate and, if so, why stimulating nearby parts of the prefrontal cortex can have opposite effects on deceptive responses.

PERFORMANCE OF NEUROSCIENCE-BASED METHODS FOR DECEPTION DETECTION

Any potential use of neuroscience-based methods to detect deception in real-life situations requires successful classification in single subjects. In this section, we will describe findings on the single subject performance of these methods and address the effects of two factors that are problematic for all deception detection methods, including neuroscience-based ones: (1) the potential use of countermeasures, strategies used by subjects to defeat the deception detection tests, and (2) the potential role of false memories and of incidental encoding.

Single subject performance

To quantify the performance of deception detection paradigms and methods, typically researchers have used sensitivity and specificity measures from signal detection theory (Wickens 2002). Sensitivity refers to the percentage of deceptive cases classified as such (when a deceptive cases is incorrectly classified as honest, then one has a false negative case), whereas specificity refers to the percentage of honest cases classified as such (when an honest cases is incorrectly classified as deceptive, then one has a false positive case).

Most work on single subject classification has been conducted with ERPs, and virtually all the ERP studies on single subject classification have been conducted using CIT paradigms using the P300 potential. Early studies employing 3-stimulus paradigms showed high accuracy in detecting when subjects lied about recognizing critical items. For example, in one such study about 88% of participants were classified correctly while 12% were classified as inconclusive (Farwell and Donchin 1991), with neither false positives nor false negatives. Another study using a similar paradigm showed a sensitivity of 94% and a specificity of 96% (Allen *et al.* 1992). Numerous publications by Rosenfeld and collaborators using these paradigms have reported accuracy rates between 80% and 95%, and a comparison of methods for ERP assessment in the P300-based CIT paradigms reported average accuracy rates between 74% and 80% (Abootalebi *et al.* 2006). Single subject detection rates with more recent variants of the CIT paradigm, described later, are typically over 90% (Rosenfeld *et al.* 2008; Rosenfeld and Labkovsky, 2010).

A few fMRI studies have conducted analyses at the single individual level, using data from a single region, a few regions, or the entire brain (e.g. Davatzikos *et al.* 2005; Ganis et al., 2011; Kozel *et al.* 2005, 2009; Langleben *et al.* 2005; Monteleone *et al.* 2008; Nose *et al.* 2009), with average detection accuracy rates of about 85%. The fMRI study of deception that is methodologically closest to a clinical trial is the one conducted by Kozel and collaborators (Kozel *et al.* 2009). This double blind study used a mock crime scenario in which participants damaged compact discs containing incriminating video footage and later lied about it. For a set of carefully selected participants, this study reported 100% sensitivity, but only 33% specificity.

With regard to tDCS, to date, no single subject analyses have been performed on datasets collected using this technique.

Countermeasures

It was hoped that, unlike CIT paradigms based on autonomic measures (Elaad and Ben-Shakhar 1991), P300 CIT paradigms would resist countermeasures. Indeed, it was assumed for years that the original P300 CIT would be unbeatable because the stimuli were presented so rapidly (every 2–4s) and responded to by the brain so quickly (300–600ms) that subjects would have no way to utilize countermeasures. Lykken put it this way: "Because such potentials are derived from brain signals that occur only a few hundred milliseconds after the GKT alternatives are presented…it is unlikely that countermeasures could be used successfully to defeat a GKT derived from the recording of cerebral signals" (Lykken 1998). Unfortunately, however, these early 3-stimulus CIT paradigms were shown to be vulnerable to countermeasures (Mertens and Allen 2008; Rosenfeld *et al.* 2004).

Rosenfeld and collaborators (2004) reasoned that if subjects could be instructed by the experimenter to explicitly respond uniquely to targets, then they could also instruct themselves to respond covertly to selected irrelevants, converting them into secret targets with enhanced P300s. Since the P300-based CIT typically detects concealed knowledge by comparing probe and irrelevant P300s, with the expectation that probe responses will be larger than irrelevant ones, enhancement of irrelevant P300s with these types of countermeasures destroys the probe-irrelevant distinction, making subjects with concealed knowledge about the probe look like subjects without such knowledge. For instance, in one study, these countermeasures caused sensitivity to drop from 92% to 50% (Rosenfeld *et al.* 2004). Rosenfeld and collaborators examined the reason for this vulnerability to countermeasures of the classic P300 protocol, with the aim of developing a modified paradigm resistant to countermeasures. In the original 3-stimulus P300 CIT, there were two tasks occurring on each trial, and dual-task protocols tend to reduce the P300 that may be elicited by one of the tasks (Donchin *et al.* 1986). In the 3-stimulus protocol, subjects have the explicit task of discriminating targets. However, involuntarily and implicitly, they also perform the probe recognition task, if they possess concealed knowledge about the probe. Although this recognition event is not explicitly assigned, it is an ongoing cognitive event requiring conscious attention; otherwise, the probe would not elicit P300. Thus, even though a subject with concealed knowledge will show an enhanced P300 to the recognized probe in comparison to the P300 elicited by unrecognized irrelevant, this P300 is not as large as it could be without the simultaneous, attention-diverting target discrimination task. These considerations led to the Complex Trial Protocol (CTP), which attempts to separate the two tasks into different phases of a trial (Rosenfeld *et al.* 2008). In the CTP, the implicit probe versus irrelevant recognition is separated in time by a randomly varying interval (1200–1800ms) from the explicit target discrimination task. As shown in Figure 6.3, a date stimulus, either a subject's birth date

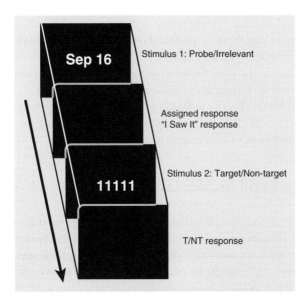

FIG. 6.3 Schematic of a trial used in the Complex Trial Protocol employed to decouple critical item processing from the target discrimination task. The first stimulus is either an infrequent probe or a frequent irrelevant item (a date, in this case) requiring a simple "I saw it" response. The second stimulus is either a target (T, a string of five ones) or a non-target (NT, a string of other numbers), requiring the corresponding judgment.

(probe) or an irrelevant stimulus, may be presented as stimulus 1 or S1 (just as in the study described in Figure 6.1). Then during the subsequent blank screen of random duration, the subject must press a single button (Response 1 or R1) acknowledging perception (no matter whether probe or irrelevant was presented) as soon as possible after S1 onset. We call this R1 the "I saw it" response. When the random dark interval expires, either a target, T (a string of five ones, 11111) or a non-target, NT, (a string of other numbers, 22222 through 55555) is presented, and the subject makes the T/NT target discrimination response (Response 2 or R2) to this Stimulus 2. The protocol is called complex because there are two separate tasks (S1/R1 and S2/R2) on each trial. This protocol is the most accurate ever reported for detecting self-referring (birth date) stimuli (Rosenfeld *et al.* 2008).

Detection rates with variants of the CTP protocols are consistently over 92% (Labkovsky and Rosenfeld 2009). This new CTP protocol seems very promising against any number of countermeasures, mental and physical, in detection of any kind of concealed information in the forensic situation in which the concealed knowledge items are known in advance. Most recently, these methods have been applied to the anti-terror scenario in which concealed knowledge stimuli are not known a priori. In this study, 10 of 12 mock terrorist agents were detected with no false positives. In these 10 subjects, we correctly detected 20 of 30 possible details of their planned terrorist acts (Meixner and Rosenfeld 2011).

The first evidence on the effect of countermeasures on fMRI methods, briefly mentioned in a study by Kozel and collaborators (Kozel *et al.* 2005), was anecdotal. Subjects were asked after the study if they had tried to use means to beat the test and no correlation was found between this variable and whether a subject could be correctly classified as deceptive or not based on fMRI activation. However, it is unclear whether subjects tried to use these measures systematically throughout the study (which would be the case for anybody trying to beat the test in a real situation). More recent and systematic fMRI evidence has indicated that countermeasures can have a profound effect at least on some CIT paradigms. Specifically, well-learned countermeasures of the type employed by Rosenfeld and collaborators (Rosenfeld *et al.* 2004) were shown to decrease the accuracy of single subject classification in a 3-stimulus CIT paradigm from 100% to 33% (Ganis *et al.* 2011). Most likely, these countermeasures are effective in fMRI paradigms for the same reasons they are in ERP paradigms. To date, no fMRI study has investigated the CTP paradigm, in part because of the required presentation of pairs of stimuli in rapid succession.

False memories and incidental encoding

The logic of virtually all deception detection paradigms assumes that information in memory is perfectly reliable. However, research has shown that memory is a constructive process and that there are many memory distortion phenomena, resulting, for instance, in false memories (e.g. Loftus 1996). CIT paradigms probe one's memories to infer the presence of concealed knowledge about an event. Hence, the reliability of memory is critical for the logic of these paradigms. Researchers have begun to address the issue of whether true and false recognition can be distinguished with ERPs (Miller *et al.* 2001; Allen and Mertens 2009). False memories, leading to false recognition, are typically induced by using the Deese–Roediger–McDermott paradigm (Roediger *et al.* 2001). In this paradigm, studying a list of words (e.g. bed, rest, blanket, and so on) that are strongly associated with a critical item that is never presented (e.g. sleep), results in high rates of false recognition of the critical item in subsequent recognition tests. Thus, one can compare ERPs to falsely and correctly recognized items. The results of a recent study using full head recordings (Allen and Mertens 2009) indicated that ERPs, in particular P300 amplitude and latency, could not distinguish between true and false memories during the recognition test. In contrast, a previous study using shorter delays between study and test (Miller et al., 2001) documented latency differences between the P300 elicited by true and false memories. This suggests that in some cases, both true and false memories elicit similar ERPs that index recognition processes. Although it is unknown whether these results hold with more realistic scenarios, the findings illustrate the type of difficulties that need to be overcome before one can use these methods in real-life situations.

A recent fMRI study used a similar paradigm to determine whether deceptive responses and false recognition could be distinguished (Abe *et al.* 2008). The results of this study indicated that, at least in the group, differences could be found between pretending to know and false recognition. For example, the right anterior hippocampus was more active during false recognition, relative to pretending to know. These results indicate that fMRI may be able to detect differences in brain activity between deception and false memories despite the fact that subjects deny recognition in both cases. More research will be needed to determine whether these group differences are robust enough to be measured reliably in single individuals.

No studies on the differential effects of tDCS on deceptive responses and false memories have been conducted so far.

Another assumption of most deception detection paradigms is that subjects have adequately encoded items of interest in memory. However, simply because one is present during an event does not mean that one automatically encodes all details of the event. Laboratories studies usually ensure that this assumption is satisfied by introducing various rehearsal procedures for the experimental items. However, in real life this assumption is often violated. Indeed, ERP evidence suggests that the accuracy of CIT tests is low with incidentally acquired or not well-rehearsed information and/or field-like crime scenarios; (Mertens and Allen 2008; Miyake *et al.* 1993; Rosenfeld *et al.* 2006, 2007). No fMRI or tDCS studies have assessed this factor.

Ethical issues associated with using neuroscience-based technologies to detect deception

Over the last decade, there has been growing discussion about neuroethics (e.g. Farah 2002, 2005; Illes and Raffin 2002), as documented extensively by this book. In this section, we will not address the broader ethical issues raised by the use of neurotechnologies nor their potential legal implications, such as potential violation of the Fifth Amendment (Stoller and Wolpe 2007), but only mention briefly some ethical issues specifically associated with the potential use of neuroscience-based methods to detect deception. In general, these issues are not entirely new, since they are in large part present also with more traditional deception detection methods (Farah 2005). Furthermore, given that there is little evidence that the accuracy of neuroscience-based methods is sufficiently high for field-like applications, many of these ethical issues are likely to be only theoretical and have to do with hypothetical future scenarios that may never occur. Nonetheless, in our opinion, two ethical issues need to be considered at the present moment.

The most pressing ethical issue associated with neuroscience-based techniques to detect deception is the risk of their premature use and adoption by society or by the legal system

(Greely and Illes 2007). Neuroscience-based data, and especially brain imaging pictures, are typically perceived by non-experts as being more "real" and compelling than other types of data (Dumit 2004; Weisberg *et al.* 2008), even when they have nothing to do with the question at hand. For example, brain maps showing regions that are more activated by deceptive than honest responses tend to convey a false impression of objectivity, that is, the impression that we now have a reliable "lie detector." This bias has contributed to the creation of for-profit companies that sell "lie detection" services based on fMRI (Greely and Illes 2007), increasing the urgency of addressing this ethical issue. As discussed earlier, the reality of the field is that the research conducted so far does not show deception detection accuracy rates that are sufficiently high or reliable for actual forensic use. One possible way to address this issue by legal means would be to tightly regulate the use of deception detection neurotechnologies for non-research purposes, as suggested by some researchers and lawyers (Greely and Illes 2007).

Another potential ethical issue raised by the use of neuroscience-based technologies to detect deception, is the one of privacy. Specifically, the results of a brain scan carried out for the purpose of detecting deception may contain additional information that is irrelevant to the situation and that the subject may not want to know about or to reveal. For example, one such brain scan may reveal the presence of a brain tumor or some brain features that are likely to be associated with future complications. This issue is not new, because it is present with traditional techniques to detect deception as well. For example, measuring variables such as blood pressure and heart rate with the polygraph could reveal information about cardiovascular abnormalities and diseases. One way to partially deal with this issue could be to employ automated analyses such that only processed variables relevant to whether the subject is being deceptive regarding the topic being examined can become available to the person administering the test.

TDCS and related non-invasive brain stimulation techniques pose a set of somewhat different ethical questions related to the important bioethical principle of autonomy (Luber *et al.* 2009), since they do not just monitor neural activity, but they may be able to alter temporarily cognitive, affective, and social processes, including those related to self-perception. For instance, as mentioned earlier, subjects in the study by Karim and collaborators (2009) felt less guilty about lying during tDCS stimulation. Similar ethical questions are associated with pharmacological methods with similar effects, for example using oxytocin to increase feelings of trust toward others (Theodoridou *et al.* 2009), or with other methods to transiently modify cognition (Farah 2005). Although it is not clear that non-invasive brain stimulation techniques will be useful for veracity assessment in the future, their potential use in this field needs to be closely monitored.

Summary and conclusions

In this chapter we have reviewed paradigms and methods used to determine some of the neural correlates of deception that could be employed to assess veracity. Although these methods provide rich variables closely linked to brain states and may lead to a better understanding of deception processes, it is not known whether they can produce accurate methods of detecting deception in real-life situations. For example, it is not clear whether it will be possible to find general procedures to get around the key problem of memory distortions. Furthermore, the impact of important factors such as various types of individual differences (Ganis and Keenan 2009; Ganis *et al.* 2009b), social context (Sip *et al.* 2008), and instructions to lie (Spence *et al.* 2008) on the reliability of deception detection in single subjects has been almost completely unexplored. It is likely that multiple paradigms and methods, with different strengths and weaknesses, may need to be used for different veracity assessment situations.

Despite much progress in neuroscience-based laboratory paradigms and methods, much more theoretical development, research, and replication of results will be needed before we can determine the extent to which these paradigms and methods can be employed in the field.

References

Abe, N., Suzuki, M., Tsukiura, T., *et al.* (2006). Dissociable roles of prefrontal and anterior cingulate cortices in deception. *Cerebral Cortex,* 16, 192–9.

Abe, N., Suzuki, M., Mori, E., Itoh, M., and Fujii, T. (2007). Deceiving others: distinct neural responses of the prefrontal cortex and amygdala in simple fabrication and deception with social interactions. *Journal of Cognitive Neuroscience,* 19, 287–95.

Abe, N., Okuda, J., Suzuki, M., *et al.* (2008). Neural correlates of true memory, false memory, and deception. *Cerebral Cortex,* 18, 2811–19.

Abootalebi, V., Moradi, M.H., and Khalilzadeh, M.A. (2006). A comparison of methods for ERP assessment in a P300-based GKT. *International Journal of Psychophysiology,* 62, 309–20.

Allen, J.J. and Mertens, R. (2009). Limitations to the detection of deception: true and false recollections are poorly distinguished using an event-related potential procedure. *Social Neuroscience,* 4, 473–90.

Allen, J.J., Iacono, W.G., and Danielson, K.D. (1992). The identification of concealed memories using the event-related potential and implicit behavioral measures: a methodology for prediction in the face of individual differences. *Psychophysiology,* 29, 504–22.

Ben-Shakhar, G., Bar-Hillel, M., and Kremnitzer, M. (2002). Trial by polygraph: reconsidering the use of the guilty knowledge technique in court. *Law and Human Behavior,* 26, 527–41.

Bhatt, S., Mbwana, J., Adeyemo, A., Sawyer, A., Hailu, A., and Vanmeter, J. (2008). Lying about facial recognition: An fMRI study. *Brain and Cognition,* 69, 382–90.

Christ, S.E., Van Essen, D.C., Watson, J.M., Brubaker, L.E., and McDermott, K.B. (2009). The contributions of prefrontal cortex and executive control to deception: evidence from activation likelihood estimate meta-analyses. *Cerebral Cortex,* 19, 1557–66.

Davatzikos, C., Ruparel, K., Fan, Y., *et al.* (2005). Classifying spatial patterns of brain activity with machine learning methods: application to lie detection. *Neuroimage,* 28, 663–8.

DePaulo, B.M., Lindsay, J.J., Malone, B.E., Muhlenbruck, L., Charlton, K., and Cooper, H. (2003). Cues to deception. *Psychological Bulletin,* 129, 74–118.

Donchin, E., Kramer, A., and Wickens, C. (1986). The Guilty Knowledge Test (GKT) as an application of psychophysiology: Future prospects and obstacles. In M. Coles, S. Porges, and E. Donchin (eds.) *Psychophysiology: Systems, Processes and Applications,* pp. 702–10. New York: Guilford.

Dumit, J. (2004). *Picturing Personhood: Brain Scans and Biomedical Identity*. Princeton, NJ: Princeton University Press.

Elaad, E. and Ben-Shakhar, G. (1991). Effects of mental countermeasures on psychophysiological detection in the guilty knowledge test. *International Journal of Psychophysiology*, **11**, 99–108.

Farah, M.J. (2002). Emerging ethical issues in neuroscience. *Nature Neuroscience*, **5**, 1123–9.

Farah, M.J. (2005). Neuroethics: the practical and the philosophical. *Trends in Cognitive Sciences*, **9**, 34–40.

Farwell, L.A. and Donchin, E. (1991). The truth will out: interrogative polygraphy ("lie detection") with event-related brain potentials. *Psychophysiology*, **28**, 531–47.

Floel, A., Rosser, N., Michka, O., Knecht, S., and Breitenstein, C. (2008). Noninvasive brain stimulation improves language learning. *Journal of Cognitive Neuroscience*, **20**, 1415–22.

Furedy, J.J., Davis, C., and Gurevich, M. (1988). Differentiation of deception as a psychological process: a psychophysiological approach. *Psychophysiology*, **25**, 683–8.

Gamer, M., Bauermann, T., Stoeter, P., and Vossel, G. (2007). Covariations among fMRI, skin conductance, and behavioral data during processing of concealed information. *Human Brain Mapping*, **28**, 1287–301.

Gamer, M., Klimecki, O., Bauermann, T., Stoeter, P., and Vossel, G. (2009). fMRI-activation patterns in the detection of concealed information rely on memory-related effects. *Social Cognitive and Affective Neuroscience* [EPub March 3, 2009].

Ganis, G. and Keenan, J.P. (2009). The cognitive neuroscience of deception. *Social Neuroscience*, **4**, 465–72.

Ganis, G. and Kosslyn, S.M. (2002). Neuroimaging. In V.S. Ramachandran (ed.) *Encyclopedia of the Human Brain*, pp. 493–505. San Diego, CA: Academic Press.

Ganis, G., Kosslyn, S.M., Stose, S., Thompson, W.L., and Yurgelun-Todd, D.A. (2003). Neural correlates of different types of deception: an fMRI investigation. *Cerebral Cortex*, **13**, 830–6.

Ganis, G., Rosenfeld, J.P., Meixner, J.B., Kievit, R.A., and Schendan, H.E. (2011). Lying in the scanner: Covert countermeasures disrupt deception detection by functional magnetic resonance imaging. *Neuroimage*, **55**, 312–9.

Ganis, G., Morris, R., and Kosslyn, S.M. (2009b). Neural processes underlying self- and other-related lies: An individual difference approach using fMRI. *Social Neuroscience*, **4**, 539–53.

Greely, H.T. and Illes, J. (2007). Neuroscience-based lie detection: the urgent need for regulation. *American Journal of Law and Medicine*, **33**, 377–431.

Illes, J. and Raffin, T.A. (2002). Neuroethics: an emerging new discipline in the study of brain and cognition. *Brain and Cognition*, **50**, 341–4.

Johnson, R., Jr. (1986). A triarchic model of P300 amplitude. *Psychophysiology*, **23**, 367–84.

Johnson, R., Jr., Barnhardt, J., and Zhu, J. (2004). The contribution of executive processes to deceptive responding. *Neuropsychologia*, **42**, 878–901.

Karim, A.A., Schneider, M., Lotze, M., *et al.* (2009). The Truth about Lying: Inhibition of the Anterior Prefrontal Cortex Improves Deceptive Behavior. *Cerebral Cortex*, **20**, 205–13.

Kozel, F.A., Padgett, T.M., and George, M.S. (2004). A replication study of the neural correlates of deception. *Behavioral Neuroscience*, **118**, 852–6.

Kozel, F.A., Johnson, K.A., Mu, Q., Grenesko, E.L., Laken, S.J., and George, M.S. (2005). Detecting deception using functional magnetic resonance imaging. *Biological Psychiatry*, **58**, 605–13.

Kozel, F.A., Johnson, K.A., Grenesko, E.L., *et al.* (2009). Functional MRI detection of deception after committing a mock sabotage crime. *Journal of Forensic Sciences,* **54**, 220–31.

Langleben, D.D., Schroeder, L., Maldjian, J.A., *et al.* (2002). Brain Activity during simulated deception: an event-related functional magnetic resonance study. *Neuroimage,* **15**, 727–32.

Langleben, D.D., Loughead, J.W., Bilker, W.B., *et al.* (2005). Telling truth from lie in individual subjects with fast event-related fMRI. *Human Brain Mapping,* **26**, 262–72.

Lee, T.M.C., Liu, H.-L., Tan, L.-H., *et al.* (2002). Lie detection by functional magnetic resonance imaging. *Human Brain Mapping,* **15**, 157–64.

Lee, T.M.C., Liu, H.L., Chan, C.C., Ng, Y.B., Fox, P.T., and Gao, J.H. (2005). Neural correlates of feigned memory impairment. *Neuroimage,* **28**, 305–13.

Lee, T.M.C., Au, R.K., Liu, H.L., Ting, K.H., Huang, C.M., and Chan, C.C. (2008). Are errors differentiable from deceptive responses when feigning memory impairment? An fMRI study. *Brain and Cognition,* **69**, 406–12.

Lefebvre, C.D., Marchand, Y., Smith, S.M., and Connolly, J.F. (2007). Determining eyewitness identification accuracy using event-related brain potentials (ERPs). *Psychophysiology,* **44**, 894–904.

Loftus, E.F. (1996). Memory distortion and false memory creation. *Bulletin of the American Academy of Psychiatry and the Law,* **24**, 281–95.

Luber, B., Fisher, C., Appelbaum, P.S., Ploesser, M., and Lisanby, S.H. (2009). Non-invasive brain stimulation in the detection of deception: scientific challenges and ethical consequences. *Behavioral Science and the Law,* **27**, 191–208.

Lykken, D. (1959). The GSR in the detection of guilt. *Journal of Applied Psychology,* **43**, 385–8.

Lykken, D. (1974). Psychology and the lie detector industry. *American Psychologist,* **29**, 725–39.

Lykken, D. (1998). *A tremor in the blood: Uses and abuses of the lie detector.* New York: Plenum.

Meijer, E.H., Smulders, F.T., Merckelbach, H.L., and Wolf, A.G. (2007). The P300 is sensitive to concealed face recognition. *International Journal of Psychophysiology,* **66**, 231–7.

Meixner, J.B. and Rosenfeld, J.P. (in press). A mock terrorism application of the P300-based concealed information test. *Psychophysiology,* **48**, 149–54.

Mertens, R. and Allen, J.J. (2008). The role of psychophysiology in forensic assessments: deception detection, ERPs, and virtual reality mock crime scenarios. *Psychophysiology,* **45**, 286–98.

Miller, A.R., Baratta, C., Wynveen, C., and Rosenfeld, J.P. (2001). P300 Latency, but not amplitude or topography, distinguished Between true and false recognition. *Journal of Experimental Psychology: Learning, Memory and Cognition,* **27**, 354–361.

Miyake, Y., Mizutanti, M., and Yamahura, T. (1993). Event related potentials as an indicator of detecting information in field polygraph examinations. *Polygraph,* **22**, 131–49.

Mohamed, F.B., Faro, S.H., Gordon, N.J., Platek, S.M., Ahmad, H., and Williams, J.M. (2006). Brain mapping of deception and truth telling about an ecologically valid situation: functional MR imaging and polygraph investigation – initial experience. *Radiology,* **238**, 679–88.

Monteleone, G.T., Phan, K.L., Nusbaum, H.C., *et al.* (2008). Detection of deception using fMRI: Better than chance, but well below perfection. *Social Neuroscience,* **4**, 528–38.

National Research Council. (2003). *The polygraph and lie detection.* Washington, DC: National Academies Press.

Nitsche, M.A. and Paulus, W. (2000). Excitability changes induced in the human motor cortex by weak transcranial direct current stimulation. *Journal of Physiology*, **527**, 633–9.

Nose, I., Murai, J., and Taira, M. (2009). Disclosing concealed information on the basis of cortical activations. *Neuroimage*, **44**, 1380–6.

Nunez, J.M., Casey, B.J., Egner, T., Hare, T., and Hirsch, J. (2005). Intentional false responding shares neural substrates with response conflict and cognitive control. *Neuroimage*, **25**, 267–77.

Priori, A., Mameli, F., Cogiamanian, F., *et al.* (2008). Lie-specific involvement of dorsolateral prefrontal cortex in deception. *Cerebral Cortex*, **18**, 451–5.

Reis, J., Schambra, H.M., Cohen, L.G., *et al.* (2009). Noninvasive cortical stimulation enhances motor skill acquisition over multiple days through an effect on consolidation. *Proceedings of the National Academy of Sciences, U S A*, **106**, 1590–5.

Roediger, H.L., 3rd, Watson, J.M., McDermott, K.B., and Gallo, D.A. (2001). Factors that determine false recall: a multiple regression analysis. *Psychonomic Bulletin and Review*, **8**, 385–407.

Rosenfeld, J.P., Cantwell, B., Nasman, V.T., Wojdac, V., Ivanov, S., and Mazzeri, L. (1988). A modified, event-related potential-based guilty knowledge test. *International Journal of Neuroscience*, **42**, 157–61.

Rosenfeld, J.P., Angell, A., Johnson, M., and Qian, J.H. (1991). An ERP-based, control-question lie detector analog: algorithms for discriminating effects within individuals' average waveforms. *Psychophysiology*, **28**, 319–35.

Rosenfeld, J.P., Soskins, M., Bosh, G., and Ryan, A. (2004). Simple, effective countermeasures to P300-based tests of detection of concealed information. *Psychophysiology*, **41**, 205–19.

Rosenfeld, J.P., Biroschak, J.R., and Furedy, J.J. (2006). P300-based detection of concealed autobiographical versus incidentally acquired information in target and non-target paradigms. *International Journal of Psychophysiology*, **60**, 251–9.

Rosenfeld, J.P., Shue, E., and Singer, E. (2007). Single versus multiple probe blocks of P300-based concealed information tests for self-referring versus incidentally obtained information. *Biological Psychology*, **74**, 396–404.

Rosenfeld, J. P., Labkovsky, E., Winograd, M., Lui, M.A., Vandenboom, C., and Chedid, E. (2008). The Complex Trial Protocol (CTP): a new, countermeasure-resistant, accurate, P300-based method for detection of concealed information. *Psychophysiology*, **45**, 906–19.

Rosenfeld, J. P. and Labkovsky, E (2010). New P300-based protocol to detect concealed information: Resistance to mental countermeasures against only half the irrelevant stimuli and a possible ERP indicator of countermeasures. *Psychophysiology*, **47**, 1002–10.

Seth, A.K., Iversen, J.R., and Edelman, G.M. (2006). Single-trial discrimination of truthful from deceptive responses during a game of financial risk using alpha-band MEG signals. *Neuroimage*, **32**, 465–76.

Sip, K.E., Roepstorff, A., McGregor, W., and Frith, C.D. (2008). Detecting deception: the scope and limits. *Trends in Cognitive Sciences*, **12**, 48–53.

Spence, S.A., Farrow, T.F., Herford, A.E., Wilkinson, I.D., Zheng, Y., and Woodruff, P.W. (2001). Behavioural and functional anatomical correlates of deception in humans. *Neuroreport*, **12**, 2849–53.

Spence, S.A., Kaylor-Hughes, C., Farrow, T.F., and Wilkinson, I.D. (2008). Speaking of secrets and lies: the contribution of ventrolateral prefrontal cortex to vocal deception. *Neuroimage*, **40**, 1411–18.

Stoller, S.E. and Wolpe, P.R. (2007). Emerging neurotechnologies for lie detection and the fifth amendment. *American Journal of Law and Medicine,* **33,** 359–75.

Theodoridou, A., Rowe, A.C., Penton-Voak, I.S., and Rogers, P.J. (2009). Oxytocin and social perception: oxytocin increases perceived facial trustworthiness and attractiveness. *Hormones and Behavior,* **56,** 128–32.

Tian, F., Sharma, V., Kozel, F.A., and Liu, H. (2009). Functional near-infrared spectroscopy to investigate hemodynamic responses to deception in the prefrontal cortex. *Brain Research,* **1303,** 120–30.

Vrij, A. (2008). *Detecting Lies and Deceit,* 2nd edition. Chichester: Wiley.

Weisberg, D.S., Keil, F.C., Goodstein, J., Rawson, E., and Gray, J.R. (2008). The seductive allure of neuroscience explanations. *Journal of Cognitive Neuroscience,* **20,** 470–7.

Wickens, T. D. (2002). *Elementary Signal Detection Theory.* New York: Oxford University Press.

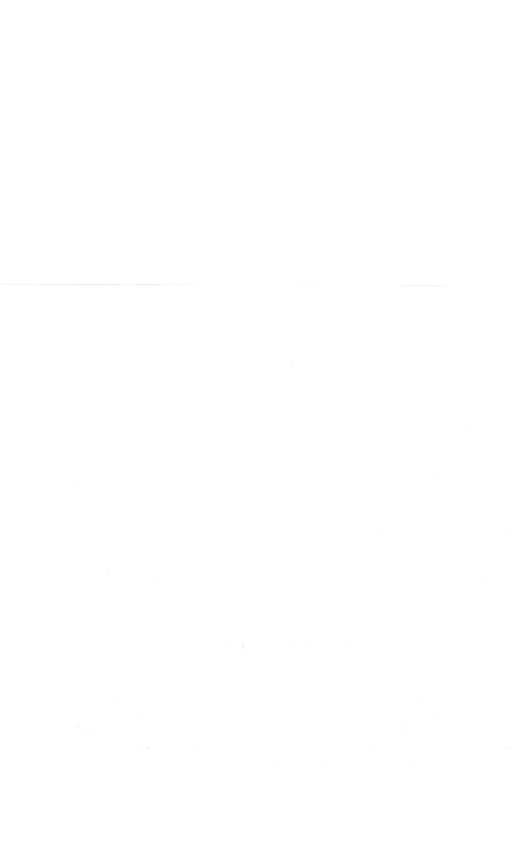

CHAPTER 7

UNDERSTANDING DISORDERS OF CONSCIOUSNESS

CAMILLE CHATELLE AND STEVEN LAUREYS

PROGRESS in medical and intensive care has led to an increased number of patients who survive severe brain damage. In most cases, these patients rapidly recover from coma in the first days after injury. Nevertheless, some of them permanently lose their brain functions (i.e. may evolve to brain death). Often, in cases of slower recovery, patients will go through different states of consciousness. This implies that patients may enter an awake but unaware state (i.e. vegetative state) sometimes followed by a partly conscious state (i.e. minimally conscious state) before recovering normal consciousness. But some patients may remain in a chronic or permanent vegetative or minimally conscious state. Clinical assessment of consciousness is based on motor responsiveness; however, the fact that many patients suffer from motor incapacities (e.g. spastic quadriplegia) and fluctuating levels of arousal makes the clinical evaluation of consciousness challenging. For that reason, more objective diagnostic tools are needed. Neuroimaging and electrophysiology are promising approaches to disentangle the different disorders of consciousness. At present, treatment options (pharmacologic and non-pharmacologic) exist but lack evidence-based recommendations.

CLINICAL ENTITIES

Consciousness consists of two major components: arousal and awareness (Figure 7.1) (Laureys *et al.* 2002a). Clinically, arousal is manifested by spontaneous eye opening. Awareness, on the other hand, is assessed by looking for responses to external stimuli (e.g. non-reflex movements or command following). Awareness requires arousal, but preserved arousal levels do not necessarily imply awareness.

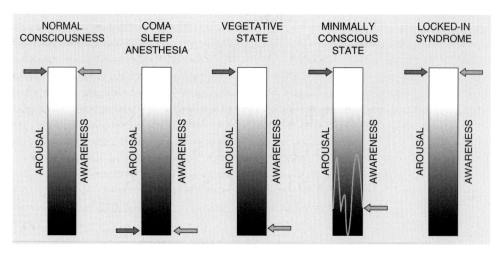

FIG. 7.1 Arousal (i.e. eye opening) and awareness (i.e. command following), the two components of consciousness in coma and related conditions. Adapted from Laureys S. et al. (2004). Brain function in coma, vegetative state and related disorders. *The Lancet Neurology*, 3, 537–46.

Brain death

Brain death means human death determined by neurological criteria. It is an unfortunate term as it misleadingly suggests that there are two types of death: brain death and "regular" death (Bernat 2002). There is, however, only one type of death which can be measured in two ways: by cardiorespiratory and by neurological criteria. The brain-centered definition of human death has three formulations called whole brain, brainstem, and neocortical death (Laureys 2005). Whole brain and brainstem death are both defined as the irreversible cessation of the organism as a whole but differ in their anatomic interpretation instantiating this concept. Because many of the areas of the supratentorial brain (including the neocortex, thalami, and basal ganglia) cannot be tested for clinical functions accurately in a comatose patient, most of the bedside tests for brain death (such as cranial nerve reflexes and apnea testing) directly measure functions of only the brainstem (Bernat 2002). The neocortical formulation of death, already proposed since the early days of the brain death debate (Dehaene and Changeux 2005), advocates a fundamentally different concept of death: the irreversible loss of the capacity for consciousness and social interaction. By application of this consciousness or personhood-centered definition of death, its proponents classify patients in a permanent vegetative state and anencephalic infants as dead but legal scholars endorsing the neocortical definition of death (Smith 1986; Stacy 1992) have never convinced legislatures or courts.

Coma

Patients in coma are neither aroused, nor aware (Figure 7.1); indeed, their eyes are constantly closed and they do not manifest voluntary behavioral responses. Generally, patients emerge

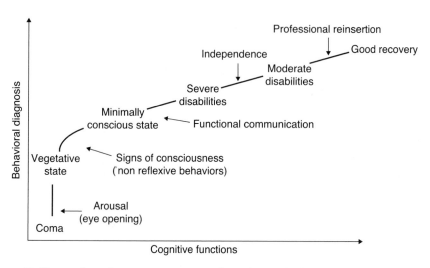

FIG. 7.2 Different clinical entities encountered on the gradual recovery from coma, illustrated as a function of cognitive and motor capacity. Restoration of spontaneous or elicited eye-opening, in the absence of voluntary motor activity, marks the transition from coma to vegetative state. The passage from the vegetative state to the minimally conscious state is marked by reproducible evidence of 'voluntary behavior' defined as (1) non-reflex behavior or simple command following, (2) gestural or verbal yes/no responses (regardless of accuracy), (3) intelligible verbalization, or (4) motor activity occurring in contingent relation to relevant, often emotional, stimuli (also including pursuit eye movement or sustained fixation). Emergence from the minimally conscious state is signaled by the return of functional communication or object use. The locked-in syndrome is the extreme example of intact cognition with nearly complete motor deficit (only permitting eye-coded communication). Adapted from Vanhaudenhuyse A, Boly, M, and Laureys, S (2009). Vegetative state. Scholarpedia 4:4163.

from their comatose state within days to weeks (Posner *et al.* 2007; Figure 7.2). The prognosis is influenced by different factors such as etiology, the patient's general medical condition and age. Outcome is known to be bad if, after 3 days of observation, there are no pupillary or corneal reflexes, stereotyped or absent motor response to noxious stimulation, iso-electrical or burst suppression pattern electroencephalogram (EEG), bilateral absent cortical responses on somatosensory evoked-potentials, and (for anoxic coma) biochemical markers such as serum neuron-specific enolase are increased. Prognosis in traumatic coma survivors is better than in anoxic cases (Laureys *et al.* 2008). Recovery from coma may lead to a vegetative state, a minimally conscious state, or, more rarely, to a locked-in syndrome (Laureys 2007; Posner *et al.* 2007) (Figure 7.3).

Vegetative state

The vegetative state (VS) was defined by Plum and Jennet in 1972 to describe "an organic body capable of growth and development but devoid of sensation and thought" (Jennett and

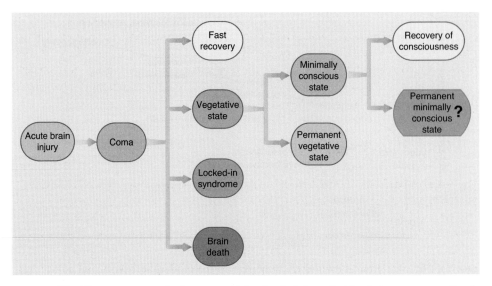

FIG. 7.3 Timeline encountered after coma. After brain injury that leads to coma, a patient's progress may follow one of several paths (left). If the patient does not die or quickly recover, he or she will most likely transition to the vegetative state. In rare cases, a person may develop locked-in syndrome, a complete paralysis of the body's voluntary muscles. The patient may then evolve to the minimally conscious state and often further recovery of consciousness or remain in the vegetative state permanently. Compared with people in other mental states (*right*), vegetative patients have a high level of wakefulness—unlike comatose individuals, they have sleep/wake cycles—but none of the awareness that characterizes normal conscious wakefulness. Adapted from Laureys, S. (2007). Eyes open, brain shut: the vegetative state. *Scientific American*, 4, 32–7.

Plum 1972). It is very important to stress the difference between persistent and permanent vegetative state which are, unfortunately, too often abbreviated identically as PVS, causing unnecessary confusion (Laureys *et al.* 2000a). When the term "persistent vegetative state" was first described (Jennett and Plum 1972), it was emphasized that persistent didn't mean permanent and it is now recommended to *omit "persistent"* and to describe a patient as having been vegetative for a certain time. When there is no recovery after a specified period—depending on etiology; 3 months (for non-traumatic) to 12 months (for traumatic cases)—the state can be declared permanent and only then do the ethical and legal issues around withdrawal of treatment arise (American Congress of Rehabilitation Medicine 1995; Jennett 2005).

Minimally conscious state

Patients in a minimally conscious state (MCS) are aroused and show fluctuating but reproducible signs of awareness (Giacino *et al.* 2002). These patients can manifest, even if inconsistently, oriented behavioral and emotional responses such as response to verbal order, object manipulation, oriented responses to noxious stimulation, visual pursuit or fixation. However, if visual fixation is considered as a sign of consciousness by the US Aspen Workgroup (Giacino *et al.* 2002), it is not the case in the UK (Royal College of Physicians 2003). Recovery from the MCS is defined by the return of functional communication and/or functional use of objects (Giacino *et al.* 2002).

Locked-in syndrome

The locked-in syndrome (LIS) is "a state in which selective supranuclear motor de-efferentation produces paralysis of all four limbs and the last cranial nerves without interfering with consciousness. The motor paralysis prevents the subjects from communicating by word or body movement" (Plum and Posner 1983). LIS patients are able to use vertical eye movements and blinking to communicate with their surroundings. A recent study reported intact cognitive functions of LIS patients by adapting standard neuropsychological testing (Schnakers *et al.* 2005b). However, as LIS and VS patients may superficially show similar behavioral patterns, differential diagnosis may be difficult (Cairns *et al.* 1941; American Congress of Rehabilitation Medicine 1995). According to Bauer *et al.* (1979), different categories of LIS can be based on the extent of motor impairment (Bauer *et al.* 1979): *Classical* LIS consists of a total immobility but preserved vertical eye movements and blinking; *Incomplete* LIS is characterized by remnant non-ocular voluntary motions; *total* LIS patients are completely immobile, unable to control any eye movements.

It has been shown that more than half of the time it is the family and not the physician who first realized that the patient was aware (Laureys *et al.* 2005a). Once a LIS patient becomes medically stable, and given appropriate medical care, life expectancy increases to several decades. Even if the chances of good motor recovery are very limited, existing eye-controlled, computer-based communication technology currently allows the patient to control his/her environment, use a word processor coupled to a speech synthesizer, and access the worldwide net. Healthy individuals and medical professionals sometimes assume that the quality of life of an LIS patient is so poor that it is not worth living (Bruno *et al.* 2008). On the contrary, chronic LIS patients typically self-report meaningful quality of life and their demand for euthanasia is surprisingly infrequent (Lule *et al.* 2009). Biased clinicians might provide less aggressive medical treatment and influence the family in inappropriate ways, especially in children (Bruno *et al.* 2009). In our view, only the medically stabilized, informed LIS patient is competent to consent to or refuse life-sustaining treatment. Patients suffering from LIS should not be denied the right to die—and to die with dignity—but also they should not be denied the right to live—and to live with dignity and the best possible revalidation, and pain and symptom management.

Diagnostic challenges

Behavioral assessment remains the classical way to assess consciousness in severely brain-damaged patients. It has been recently shown that, even with the integration of new criteria of consciousness (Giacino *et al.* 2002), there remains a high rate of misdiagnosis (Schnakers *et al.* 2009a). In a group of patients diagnosed as being in VS, 30–40% were actually conscious according to this study. Numerous standardized scales have been created to facilitate the consciousness assessment of these patients; the Glasgow Coma Scale (GCS) (Teasdale and Jennett 1974) is widely used to detect any sign of consciousness (Sternbach 2000) but if it is useful to detect a recovery from coma, it is not sensitive to detect emergence from VS to MCS (Schnakers *et al.* 2006). Canedo *et al.* (2002) reported the need of scales scoring behavioral responses to multimodal stimulation in order to increase the probability to detect any sign of consciousness, and by extension decreasing the high rate of misdiagnosis. Currently, more adapted scales have been proposed for the assessment of chronic post-comatose states such as the Sensory Modality Assessment and Rehabilitation Technique (SMART) (Gill-Thwaites 1997; Chatelle *et al.* submitted), the Wessex Head Injury Matrix (Shiel *et al.* 2000), and the Coma Recovery Scale-Revised (CRS-R) (Giacino *et al.* 2004; Schnakers *et al.* 2008a). These scales will, for example, assess visual pursuit, a behavior considered as the first sign of consciousness heralding recovery from VS (Giacino *et al.* 2002). Vanhaudenhuyse *et al.* (2008a) showed that evaluation of visual pursuit should employ autoreferential stimuli. The CRS-R currently is the only scale which requires a mirror in the assessment of eye-tracking.

Objective measures of brain function

Functional neuroimaging

Positron emission tomography (PET) studies have shown reduced global cerebral metabolism in coma, VS, and MCS patients (about 40–50% of normal values (Laureys *et al.* 1999a,b; Schiff *et al.* 2002)). It was shown that the relationship between global levels of brain function and the presence or absence of awareness is not absolute; rather, some areas in the brain seem more important than other for the emergence of awareness. Regional changes in the frontoparietal network of associative cortices, more so than global changes in cerebral metabolism, are a better correlate of awareness in severely brain damaged non-communicative patients (Laureys *et al.* 2004). Another hallmark of VS is the relative metabolic sparing of the pedunculopontine reticular formation, hypothalamus, and basal forebrain—allowing for the maintenance of patients' vegetative functions. Awareness is not exclusively related to activity in the frontoparietal "global workspace" (Baars *et al.* 2003) but, as importantly, to the functional connectivity within this network and the thalami. Long-range corticocortical (between laterofrontal and midline-posterior areas) and corticothalamocortical (between non-specific thalamic nuclei and midline-posterior cortices) "functional disconnections" could be identified in the vegetative state. Moreover, recovery from the vegetative state is paralleled by a functional restoration of the frontoparietal network and part of its corticothalamocortical connections (Laureys *et al.* 2000b). Metabolic activity in the medial parietal cortex (precuneus) and adjacent posterior cingulate cortex has been reported to disentangle MCS from VS (Laureys *et al.* 2003) (Figure 7.4). These areas are also the most active during conscious waking (Andreasen *et al.* 1995; Maquet *et al.* 1997; Gusnard and Raichle 2001), and show a decreased activation in altered state of consciousness such as general anesthesia (Maquet *et al.* 2005; Boveroux *et al.* 2008), and hypnotic state (Kupers *et al.* 2005). These results suggest that this multimodal posteromedial associative area may serve as a critical hub in the consciousness neural network.

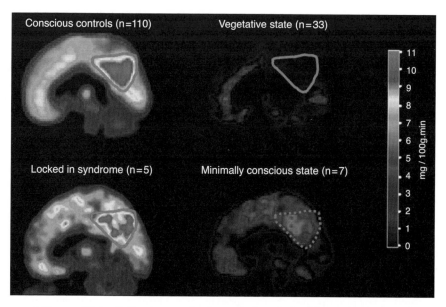

FIG. 7.4 (Also see Plate 6). Resting cerebral metabolism in healthy individuals and patients in a vegetative state, locked-in syndrome, and minimally conscious state. In healthy conscious individuals and locked-in patients the medial posterior cortex (encompassing the precuneus and adjacent posterior cingulate cortex, red line) is the most metabolically active region of the brain; in patients in vegetative state, this same area is the most dysfunctional (blue line). The precuneus and posterior cingulate cortex of patients in a minimally conscious state shows an intermediate metabolism, higher than in a vegetative state, but lower than in healthy subjects. Colors represent how much mg of glucose is consumed per mg of brain tissue per minute (adapted from Laureys S. et al. (2004). Brain function in coma, vegetative state and related disorders. *The Lancet Neurology*, 3, 537–46.

In response to auditory and nociceptive stimulation, VS patients show limited brain activation whereas MCS have an activity similar to controls (Laureys et al. 2000c; Boly et al. 2005, 2008). Cerebral activation induced by noxious stimulation seems limited to the primary cortex in VS (Laureys et al. 2002b). However, a dysfunction in associative areas and more importantly a thalamocortical disconnection have also been reported suggesting the key role of these areas in conscious processing. In MCS patients, auditory stimuli with emotional valence or nociceptive stimulations lead to more widespread activation, involving associative cortices considered as hierarchically superior in the treatment of the sensory information (Schnakers et al. 2004; Boly et al. 2008).

Pain management in severely brain-damaged patients constitutes a clinical and ethical stake. At the bedside, assessing the presence of pain and suffering is challenging due both to patients' physical condition and inherent limitations of clinical assessment (Laureys and Boly 2007). A European survey on over 2000 medical and paramedical professionals' beliefs on possible pain perception in patients with disorders of consciousness showed very divergent answers to the question "Do you think that patients in a vegetative state can feel pain?" Interestingly, healthcare givers' opinions varied according to religious beliefs, gender, and professional expertise (Demertzi *et al.* 2009). Recently, Boly *et al.* (2008) reported a near-normal brain activation to pain in MCS patients. Conversely, VS patients showed no higher-order cortical activation when the same methodology was employed. In addition, this study reported preserved functional connectivity between primary sensory cortex and a large set of associative cortices in MCS, including frontoparietal cortices and anterior cingulate cortex (important in the affective emotional perception of pain (Vanhaudenhuyse *et al.* 2009), never observed in VS patients. We interpret these findings as providing objective evidence of pain perception capacity in MCS, supporting the idea that these patients need analgesic treatment and monitoring by means of "pain" scales adapted to non-communicative coma survivors (Schnakers *et al.* 2010).

In addition to "passive" functional neuroimaging studies using external sensory stimulation, Owen and colleagues reported the interest of "active" paradigms showing motor-independent command-following (see Chapter 8 in this volume). In brief, a young woman considered as being clinically in a VS showed a brain activation indistinguishable to that observed in healthy subjects when asked to imagine playing tennis or visiting her house (Owen *et al.* 2006, 2007). A few months later, she recovered to MCS. Monti *et al.* (2010) using an "active" functional magnetic resonance imaging (fMRI) paradigm in 53 VS and MCS patients studied in Liège and Cambridge, showed that about 15% of VS patients may have fMRI based signs of consciousness inaccessible to bedside clinical evaluation.

Di *et al.* (2007) used fMRI to explore the brain activation with the patient's own name paradigm (as compared to other names). Results showed that five out of seven VS patients activated only lower level auditory cortex whereas MCS patients showed a more widespread activation including higher-level associative areas. Interestingly, the two VS who showed an activity in more extended areas recovered to MCS 3 months later, suggesting that neuroimaging may precede the clinic. Following this study, Di *et al.* (2008) and Coleman *et al.* (2009) showed in a larger cohort of patients that fMRI and PET activation studies may indeed have prognostic value.

Electroencephalography and evoked potentials

The bispectral index (BIS) of the EEG is an empirical, statistically derived variable (ranging from 0 (isoelectric) to 100 ("fully conscious")) that was designed as a measure of depth of anesthesia. Schnakers and colleagues showed a correlation between the BIS and the level of consciousness as assessed by means of the CRS-R. An empirically defined BIS cut-off value of 50 differentiated unconscious patients (coma or VS) from conscious patients (MCS or emergence from MCS) with a sensitivity of 75% and specificity of 75% (Schnakers *et al.* 2005a). Moreover, patients with higher BIS levels showed significantly higher chances of recovery of consciousness at 1-year follow-up (Schnakers *et al.* 2008b).

Auditory cognitive event-related potentials (ERPs) are useful to investigate residual cognitive functions, such as echoic memory (mismatch negativity, MMN), acoustical and semantic discrimination (P300), and incongruent language detection (N400). While early ERPs (such as the absence of cortical responses on somatosensory-evoked potentials) predict bad outcome, cognitive ERPs (MMN and P300) are indicative of recovery of consciousness. In coma survivors, cognitive potentials are more frequently obtained when using stimuli that are more ecologic or have an emotional content than when using classical sine tones (for a review, see Vanhaudenhuyse *et al.* 2008b). Using ERPs, the integrity of detection of the patients' own name—a potent "attention-grabbing" self-related stimulus—has been studied in VS, MCS, and LIS patients (Perrin *et al.* 2006). Surprisingly, some behaviorally well-documented VS patients who never recovered consciousness emitted a differential response (P300 wave) to their own name and not to other names. Hence, a P300 response does not necessarily reflect conscious perception and cannot be used to reliably differentiate individuals in VS from a MCS (Perrin *et al.* 2006). Therefore, Schnakers *et al.* (2008c) developed a new active ERP paradigm where the participant is instructed to voluntarily direct her or his attention to a target stimulus and to ignore other stimuli. They showed command-following (and hence consciousness) based on electrophysiological recordings in patients not showing any behavioral (motor) signs of command-following. So far, no P300 differences between passive and active conditions were observed for any patient in VS. However, in MCS patients only showing eye tracking a P300 response to target stimuli was shown to be higher in the active than in the passive condition as seen in healthy controls (and LIS patients, see Figure 7.5), illustrating voluntary compliance to task instructions and hence consciousness (Schnakers *et al.* 2008c)—similar (but easier and cheaper to obtain) than the fMRI active paradigm where patients imagine playing tennis (Boly *et al.* 2007).

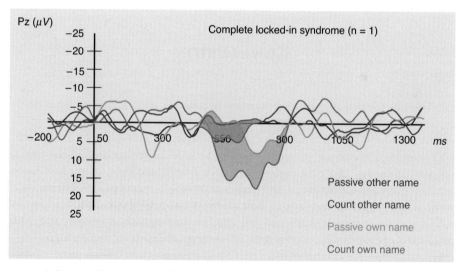

FIG. 7.5 (Also see Plate 7). Grand-averaged event-related potentials in a LIS patient at Pz. Response to the subject's own name (SON) in the passive condition (listened target SON; in green) and in the active condition (counted target SON; in pink) vs. unfamiliar names in passive (listened non-targets UN; in blue) and active condition (counted target UN, in red). Adapted from Schnakers C. *et al.* (2009). Detecting consciousness in a total locked-in syndrome. *Neurocase*, **15**, 271–7. Reprinted with permission of the publisher (Taylor and Francis Group http://www/informaworld.com).

TREATMENT

At present, no evidence-based recommendations can be made for the pharmacological or non-pharmacological treatment of patients with disorders of consciousness (Demertzi *et al.* 2008). Amantadine, a dopaminergic agent, has been reported to induce some cognitive improvement (Whyte *et al.* 2005; Laureys *et al.* 2006; Sawyer *et al.* 2008). A recent PET study showed amantadine-related metabolic increases in frontoparietal cortices in MCS (Schnakers *et al.* 2008d). Other pharmacologic treatments have also been reported as possibly efficient in disorders of consciousness such as levodopa and bromocriptine (also dopaminergic agents (Passler and Riggs 2001)), baclofen (a GABA agonist, mainly administered against spasticity (Taira and Hori 2007)), and finally zolpidem (a non-benzodiazepine sedative drug normally used as sleeping pill). Number of patients need to be made to confirm the effectiveness of the different drugs.

Deep brain stimulation (DBS) has putatively been shown to enhance arousal in VS (Yamamoto and Katayama 2005), but its effect seems limited. Schiff and Fins (2007) recently showed the interest of bilateral thalamic DBS in selected MCS patients (Schiff *et al.* 2007). Sensory stimulation techniques (Tolle and Reimer 2003) and occupational therapy (creativity and productivity (Reed and Sanderson 1992; Munday 2005)) are also suggested as means to prevent complications and enhance recovery. However, the effectiveness of these treatment options remains debated (Lombardi 2002; Giacino 2005). Physical therapy that includes postural changes, hygienic management and prevention of joint contractures should be part of the routine care in disorders of consciousness (Shiel *et al.* 2001; Oh and Seo 2003).

CONCLUSION

At the bedside, the evaluation of consciousness in coma survivors is challenging and sometimes erroneous. Understanding the state of awareness in such patients is of major medical and ethical interest. The alarming rate of misdiagnosis shows how difficult it is to disentangle VS from MCS and should prompt the routine bedside use of standardized and validated "consciousness scales." Objective methods such as PET, fMRI, and EEG studies can objectively describe the cerebral activity at rest, and under various conditions of passive stimulation and during "active" mental imagery tasks. These studies are increasing our understanding of the neural correlates of consciousness and will improve the diagnosis, prognosis, and clinical management of disorders of consciousness encountered after severe brain damage.

Neuroimaging and EEG studies in severely brain-damaged, non-communicative patients raise several methodological and ethical concerns (Giacino *et al.* 2006; Fins *et al.* 2008). Ongoing international collaborative studies and the standardization of validated experimental imaging protocols are aiming to bring the much-awaited evidence-based medicine permitting to improve our care for patients with disorders of consciousness. We feel that caring for severely brain damaged patients represents such an immense humane, affective, and social problem that it warrants further research to better understand the underlying cerebral dysfunction of their condition. Unconscious, minimally conscious, and locked-in patients are very vulnerable and deserve special procedural protections but they are also vulnerable to being denied potential access to research and new technology (Fins *et al.* 2008).

REFERENCES

American Congress of Rehabilitation Medicine (1995). Recommendations for use of uniform nomenclature pertinent to patient with severe alterations of consciousness. *Archives of Physical Medicine and Rehabilitation*, 76, 205–9.

Andreasen, N., O'Leary, D., Cizadlo, T., *et al.* (1995). Remembering the past: two facets of episodic memory explored with positron emission tomography. *American Journal of Psychiatry*, 152, 1576–85.

Baars, B., Ramsoy, T., and Laureys, S. (2003). Brain, conscious experience and the observing self. *Trends in Neurosciences*, 26, 671–5.

Bauer, G., Gerstenbrand, F., and Rumpl, E. (1979). Varieties of the locked-in syndrome. *Journal of Neurology*, 221, 77–91.

Bernat, J.L. (2002). *Ethical Issues in Neurology*, pp. 243–81. Boston, MA: Butterworth Heinemann.

Boly, M., Faymonville, M.E., Peigneux, P., *et al.* (2005). Cerebral processing of auditory and noxious stimuli in severely brain injured patients: Differences between VS and MCS. *Neuropsychological Rehabilitation*, 15, 283–9.

Boly, M., Coleman, M.R., Davis, M.H., *et al.* (2007). When thoughts become action: an fMRI paradigm to study volitional brain activity in non-communicative brain injured patients. *Neuroimage*, 36, 979–92.

Boly, M., Faymonville, M.E., Schnakers, C., *et al.* (2008). Perception of pain in the minimally conscious state with PET activation: an observational study. *The Lancet Neurology*, 7, 1013–20.

Boveroux, P., Bonhomme, V., Boly, M., Vanhaudenhuyse, A., Maquet, P., and Laureys, S. (2008). Brain function in physiologically, pharmacologically, and pathologically altered states of consciousness. *International Anesthesiology Clinics*, 46, 131–46.

Bruno, M., Bernheim, J.L., Schnakers, C., and Laureys, S. (2008). Locked-in: don't judge a book by its cover. *Journal of Neurology, Neurosurgery and Psychiatry*, 79, 2.

Bruno, M.A., Schnakers, C., Damas, F., *et al.* (2009). Locked-in syndrome in children: report of five cases and review of the literature. *Pediatric Neurology*, 41, 237–46.

Cairns, H., Oldfield, R.C., Pennybacker, J.B., and Whitteridge, D. (1941). Akinetic mutism with an epidermoid cyst at the third ventricle. *Brain*, 64, 273–90.

Canedo, A., Grix, M.C., and Nicoletti, J. (2002). An analysis of assessment instruments for the minimally responsive patient (MRP): clinical observations. *Brain Injury*, 16, 453–61.

Chatelle, C., Vanhaudenhuyse, A., and Laureys, S. (Submitted). La Sensory Modality Assessment and Rehabilitation Technique (SMART) : une échelle comportementale d' de la conscience et un traitement. *La Revue neurologique*.

Coleman, M.R., Davis, M.H., Rodd, J.M., *et al.* (2009). Towards the routine use of brain imaging to aid the clinical diagnosis of disorders of consciousness. *Brain*, 132, 2541–52.

Dehaene, S. and Changeux, J.P. (2005). Ongoing spontaneous activity controls access ton consciousness: a neuronal model for inattentional blindness. *PLoS Biology*, 3, e141.

Demertzi, A., Vanhaudenhuyse, A., Bruno, M.A., *et al.* (2008). Is there anybody in there? Detecting awareness in disorders of consciousness. *Expert Review of Neurotherapeutics*, 8, 1719–30.

Demertzi, A., Schnakers, C., Ledoux, D., *et al.* (2009). Different beliefs about pain perception in the vegetative and minimally conscious states: a European survey of medical and paramedical professionals. *Progress in Brain Research*, 177, 329–38.

Di, H.B., Yu, S.M., Weng, X.C., *et al.* (2007). Cerebral response to patient's own name in the vegetative and minimally conscious states. *Neurology*, 68, 895–9.

Di, H.B., Boly, M., Weng, X., Ledoux, D., and Laureys, S. (2008). Neuroimaging activation studies in the vegetative state: predictors of recovery? *Clinical Medicine*, 8, 502–7.

Fins, J.J., Illes, J., Bernat, J.L., Hirsch, J., Laureys, S., and Murphy, E. (2008). Neuroimaging and disorders of consciousness: envisioning an ethical research agenda. *American Journal of Bioethics*, 8, 3–12.

Giacino, J. (ed.) (2005). *Rehabilitation for traumatic brain injury*. New York: Oxford University Press.

Giacino, J., Ashwal, S., Childs, N., *et al.* (2002). The minimally conscious state: Definition and diagnostic criteria. *Neurology*, 58, 349–53.

Giacino, J., Kalmar, K., and Whyte, J. (2004). The JFK Coma Recovery Scale-Revised: measurement characteristics and diagnostic utility. *Archives of Physical Medicine and Rehabilitation*, 85, 2020–9.

Giacino, J.T., Hirsch, J., Schiff, N., and Laureys, S. (2006). Functional neuroimaging applications for assessment and rehabilitation planning in patients with disorders of consciousness. *Archives of Physical Medicine and Rehabilitation*, 87, S67–76.

Gill-Thwaites, H. (1997). The Sensory Modality Assessment Rehabilitation Technique - a tool for assessment and treatment of patients with severe brain injury in a vegetative state. *Brain Injury*, 11, 723–34.

Gusnard, D.A. and Raichle, M.E. (2001). Searching for a baseline: functional imaging and the resting human brain. *Nature Reviews Neuroscience*, 2, 685–94.

Jennett, B. (2005). The assessment and rehabilitation of vegetative and minimally conscious patients: Definitions, diagnosis, prevalence and ethics. *Neuropsychological Rehabilitation*, 15, 163–5.

Jennett, B. and Plum, F. (1972). Persistent vegetative state after brain damage. A syndrome in search of a name. *Lancet*, 1, 734–7.

Kupers, R., Faymonville, M.E., and Laureys, S. (2005). The cognitive modulation of pain: hypnosis- and placebo-induced analgesia. *Progress in Brain Research*, 150, 251–69.

Laureys, S. (2005). Science and society: death, unconsciousness and the brain. *Nature Reviews Neuroscience*, 6, 899–909.

Laureys, S. (2007). Eyes open, brain shut: the vegetative state. *Scientific American*, 4, 32–7.

Laureys, S. and Boly, M. (2007). What is it like to be vegetative or minimally conscious. *Current Opinion in Neurology*, 20, 609–13.

Laureys, S., Goldman, S., Phillips, C., *et al.* (1999). Impaired effective cortical connectivity in vegetative state: preliminary investigation using PET. *Neuroimage*, 9, 377–82.

Laureys, S., Lemaire, C., Maquet, P., Phillips, C., and Franck, G. (1999). Cerebral metabolism during vegetative state and after recovery to consciousness. *Journal of Neurology, Neurosurgery and Psychiatry*, 67, 121.

Laureys, S., Faymonville, M.E., and Berre, J. (2000a). Permanent vegetative state and persistent vegetative state are not interchangeable terms. *British Medical Journal*.

Laureys, S., Faymonville, M.E., Luxen, A., Lamy, M., Franck, G., and Maquet, P. (2000b). Restoration of thalamocortical connectivity after recovery from persistent vegetative state. *Lancet*, 355, 1790–1.

Laureys, S., Faymonville, M., and Maquet, P. (2002a). Quelle conscience durant le coma? *Pour la science*, 302, 122–8.

Laureys, S., Faymonville, M.E., Peigneux, P., *et al.* (2002b). Cortical processing of noxious somatosensory stimuli in the persistent vegetative state. *Neuroimage*, 17, 732–41.

Laureys, S., Faymonville, M. E., Degueldre, C., *et al.* (2000c). Auditory processing in the vegetative state. *Brain*, 123, 1589–601.

Laureys, S., Faymonville, M.E., Ferring, M., *et al.* (2003). Differences in brain metabolism between patients in coma, vegetative state, minimally conscious state and locked-in syndrome. 7th Congress of the European Federation of Neurological Societies (FENS). Helsinki, Finland. *European Journal of Neurology*, 10, 224.

Laureys, S., Owen, A., and Schiff, D. (2004). Brain function in coma, vegetative state and related disorders. *The Lancet Neurology*, 3, 537–46.

Laureys, S., Pellas, F., Van Eeckhout, P., *et al.* (2005a). The locked-in syndrome : what is it like to be conscious but paralyzed and voiceless? *Progress in Brain Research*, 150, 495–511.

Laureys, S., Perrin, F., Schnakers, C., Boly, M., and Majerus, S. (2005b). Residual cognitive function in comatose, vegetative and minimally conscious states. *Current opinion in neurology*, 18, 726–33.

Laureys, S., Giacino, J.T., Schiff, N.D., Schabus, M., and Owen, A.M. (2006). How should functional imaging of patients with disorders of consciousness contribute to their clinical rehabilitation needs? *Current Opinion in Neurology*, 19, 520–7.

Laureys, S., Boly, M., Moonen, G., and Maquet, P. (2008). Arousal and awareness in coma and post-comatose states. In L. Squire (ed.) *New Encyclopedia of Neuroscience*, pp. 1133–42. Oxford: Academic Press.

Lombardi, F., Taricco, M., De Tanti, A., Telaro, E., Liberati, A. (2002). Sensory stimulation of brain-injured individuals in coma or vegetative state: results of a Cochrane systematic review. *Clinical Rehabilitation*, 16, 464–72.

Lule, D., Zickler, C., Hacker, S., *et al.* (2009). Life can be worth living in locked-in syndrome. *Progress in Brain Research*, 177, 339–51.

Maquet, P., Degueldre, C., Delfiore, G., *et al.* (1997). Functional neuroanatomy of human slow wave sleep. *Journal of Neuroscience*, 17, 2807–12.

Maquet, P., Ruby, P., Maudoux, A., *et al.* (2005). Human cognition during REM sleep and the activity profile within frontal and parietal cortices: a reappraisal of functional neuroimaging data. *Progress in Brain Research*, 150, 219–27.

Monti, M.M., Vanhaudenhuyse, A., Coleman, M.R., *et al.* (2010). Willful modulation of brain activity in disorders of consciousness. *New England Journal of Medicine*, 362, 579–89.

Munday, R. (2005). Vegetative and minimally conscious states: how can occupational therapists help? *Neuropsychological Rehabilitation*, 15, 503–13.

Oh, H. and Seo, W. (2003). Sensory stimulation programme to improve recovery in comatose patients. *Journal of clinical nursing*, 12, 394–404.

Owen, A.M., Coleman, M.R., Boly, M., Davis, M.H., Laureys, S., and Pickard, J.D. (2006). Detecting awareness in the vegetative state. *Science*, 313, 1402.

Owen, A.M., Coleman, M.R., Boly, M., Davis, M.H., Laureys, S., and Pickard, J.D. (2007). Using functional magnetic resonance imaging to detect covert awareness in the vegetative state. *Archives of Neurology*, 64, 1098–102.

Passler, M.A. and Riggs, R.V. (2001). Positive outcomes in traumatic brain injury-vegetative state: patients treated with bromocriptine. *Archives of Physical Medicine and Rehabilitation*, 82, 311–15.

Perrin, F., Schnakers, C., Schabus, M., *et al.* (2006). Brain response to one's own name in vegetative state, minimally conscious state, and locked-in syndrome. *Archives of Neurology*, 63, 562–9.

Plum, F. and Posner, J.B. (1983). *The Diagnosis of Stupor and Coma*. Philadelphia, PA: FA Davis.

Posner, J., Saper, C., Schiff, N., and Plum, F. (2007). *Plum and Posner's Diagnosis of Stupor and Coma*. New York: Oxford University Press.

Reed, K. and Sanderson, S. (eds.) (1992). *Concepts of Occupational Therapy*. Baltimore, MD: Williams and Wilkins.

Royal College of Physicians (2003). *The vegetative state: guidance on diagnosis and management. (Report of a working party)*. London: Royal College of Physicians.

Sawyer, E., Mauro, L.S., and Ohlinger, M.J. (2008). Amantadine enhancement of arousal and cognition after traumatic brain injury. *The Annals of Pharmacotherapy*, 42, 247–52.

Schiff, N.D. and Fins, J.J. (2007). Deep brain stimulation and cognition: moving from animal to patient. *Current Opinion in Neurology*, 20, 638–42.

Schiff, N.D., Ribary, U., Moreno, R., *et al.* (2002). Residual cerebral activity and behavioural fragments can remain in the persistently vegetative brain. *Brain*, 125, 1210–34.

Schiff, N.D., Giacino, J.T., Kalmar, K., *et al.* (2007). Behavioural improvements with thalamic stimulation after severe traumatic brain injury. *Nature*, 448, 600–3.

Schnakers, C., Majerus, S., and Laureys, S. (2004). Diagnostic et évaluation des états de conscience altérée. *Réanimation*, 13, 368–75.

Schnakers, C., Majerus, S., and Laureys, S. (2005a). Bispectral analysis of electroencephalogram signals during recovery from coma: Preliminary findings. *Neuropsychological Rehabilitation*, 15, 381–8.

Schnakers, C., Majerus, S., Laureys, S., Van Eeckhout, P., Peigneux, P., and Goldman, S. (2005b). Neuropsychological testing in chronic locked-in syndrome. Psyche. *Abstracts from the Eighth Conference of the Association for the Scientific Study of Consciousness (ASSC8)*, pp. 11, University of Antwerp, Belgium.

Schnakers, C., Giacino, J., Kalmar, K., *et al.* (2006). Does the FOUR score correctly diagnose the vegetative and minimally conscious states? *Annals of Neurology*, 60, 744–5.

Schnakers, C., Majerus, S., Giacino, J., *et al.* (2008a). A French validation study of the Coma Recovery Scale-Revised (CRS-R). *Brain Injury*, 22, 786–92.

Schnakers, C., Ledoux, D., Majerus, S., *et al.* (2008b). Diagnostic and prognostic use of bispectral index in coma, vegetative state and related disorders. *Brain Injury*, 22, 926–31.

Schnakers, C., Perrin, F., Schabus, M., *et al.* (2008c). Voluntary brain processing in disorders of consciousness. *Neurology*, 71, 1614–20.

Schnakers, C., Hustinx, R., Vandewalle, G., *et al.* (2008d). Measuring the effect of amantadine in chronic anoxic minimally conscious state. *Journal of Neurology, Neurosurgery and Psychiatry*, 79, 225–7.

Schnakers, C., Vanhaudenhuyse, A., Giacino, J., *et al.* (2009a). Diagnostic accuracy of the vegetative and minimally conscious state: Clinical consensus versus standardized neurobehavioral assessment. *BMC Neurology*, 9, 35.

Schnakers, C., Perrin, F., Schabus, M., *et al.* (2009b). Detecting consciousness in a total locked-in syndrome: An active event-related paradigm. *Neurocase*, 15, 271–7.

Schnakers, C., Chatelle, C., Vanhaudenhuyse, A., *et al.* (2010). The nociception coma scale: A new tool to assess nociception in disorders of consciousness. *Pain,* **148**, 215–19.

Shiel, A., Horn, S.A., Wilson, B.A., Watson, M.J., Campbell, M.J., and McLellan, D.L. (2000). The Wessex Head Injury Matrix (WHIM) main scale: a preliminary report on a scale to assess and monitor patient recovery after severe head injury. *Clinical Rehabilitation,* **14**, 408–16.

Shiel, A., Burn, J.P., Henry, D., *et al.* (2001). The effects of increased rehabilitation therapy after brain injury: results of a prospective controlled trial. *Clinical Rehabilitation,* **15**, 501–14.

Smith, D.R. (1986). Legal recognition of neocortical death. *Cornell Law Review,* **71**, 850–88.

Stacy, T. (1992). Death, privacy, and the free exercise of religion. *Cornell Law Review,* **77**, 490–595.

Sternbach, G.L. (2000). The Glasgow coma scale. *Journal of Emergency Medicine,* **19**, 67–71.

Taira, T. and Hori, T. (2007). Intrathecal baclofen in the treatment of post-stroke central pain, dystonia, and persistent vegetative state. *Acta Neurochirurgica Supplement,* **97**, 227–9.

Teasdale, G. and Jennett, B. (1974). Assessment of coma and impaired consciousness. A practical scale. *Lancet,* **2**, 81–4.

Tolle, P. and Reimer, M. (2003). Do we need stimulation programs as a part of nursing care for patients in "persistent vegetative state"? A conceptual analysis. *Axone,* **25**, 20–6.

Vanhaudenhuyse, A., Schnakers, C., Brédart, S., and Laureys, S. (2008a). Assessment of visual pursuit in post comatose sates: use a mirror. *Journal of Neurology, Neurosurgery and Psychiatry,* **79**, 223.

Vanhaudenhuyse, A., Laureys, S., and Perrin, F. (2008b). Cognitive event-related potentials in comatose and post-comatose states. *Neurocritical Care,* **8**, 262–70.

Vanhaudenhuyse, A., Boly, M., Balteau, E., *et al.* (2009). Pain and non-pain processing during hypnosis: a thulium-YAG event-related fMRI study. *Neuroimage,* **47**, 1047–54.

Vanhaudenhuyse, A., Boly, M., and Laureys, S. (2009). Vegetative state. *Scholarpedia,* **4**, 4163.

Whyte, J., Katz, D., Long, D., *et al.* (2005). Predictors of outcome in prolonged posttraumatic disorders of consciousness and assessment of medication effects: A multicenter study. *Archive of Physical Medicine and Rehabilitation,* **86**, 453–62.

Yamamoto, T. and Katayama, Y. (2005). Deep brain stimulation therapy for the vegetative state. *Neuropsychological Rehabilitation,* **15**, 406–13.

....

CHAPTER 8

FUNCTIONAL MAGNETIC RESONANCE IMAGING, COVERT AWARENESS, AND BRAIN INJURY

....

ADRIAN M. OWEN

INTRODUCTION

....

The limits of consciousness are hard to define satisfactorily and we can only infer the self-awareness of others by their appearance and their acts

(Plum and Posner 1966)

In recent years, rapid technological advances have produced a variety of novel techniques that allow a comprehensive assessment of brain function (e.g. cognitive performance) to be combined with detailed information about brain structure (e.g. anatomy) and connectivity. So-called "event-related" studies, using functional magnetic resonance imaging (fMRI), are now used routinely to combine high-resolution anatomical imaging with sophisticated psychological paradigms. Until recently, such methods were used primarily as a correlational tool to map the cerebral changes that are associated with a particular cognitive process or function, be it an action, a reaction (e.g. to some kind of external stimulation), or a thought. But recent advances in imaging technology and, in particular, the ability of fMRI to detect reliable neural responses in individual participants in real time, are beginning to reveal thoughts, actions, and intentions based solely on the pattern of activity that is observed in the brain. One area where significant progress has been made is in the assessment of covert awareness, or consciousness, following acute brain injury. In recent years, improvements in intensive care have lead to an increase in the number of patients who survive severe brain injury. Although some of these patients go on to make a good recovery, many do not, and some of these individuals progress to a condition known as the vegetative state. Central to the description of this complex condition is the concept of "wakefulness without awareness," according to which vegetative patients are assumed to be entirely unaware, despite showing clear signs of wakefulness (Jennet and Plum 1972). However, the assessment of these patients is extremely difficult and relies heavily on subjective interpretation of observed behavior at rest and in response to stimulation. A diagnosis is made after repeated examinations have yielded no evidence of sustained, reproducible, purposeful, or voluntary behavioral response to visual, auditory, tactile, or noxious stimuli. Thus, a positive diagnosis (of vegetative state) is ultimately dependent on a negative finding (no signs of awareness) and is therefore inherently vulnerable to a Type II error or a *false negative* result. Indeed, internationally agreed diagnostic criteria for the vegetative state repeatedly emphasize the notion of *"no evidence of awareness of environment or self"*—in this instance, absence of evidence does appear to be considered adequate evidence of absence. Indeed, any assessment that is based on exhibited behavior after brain injury will be prone to error for a number of reasons. First, an inability to move and speak is a frequent outcome of chronic brain injury and does not necessarily imply a lack of awareness. Second, the behavioral assessment is highly subjective: behaviors such as smiling and crying are typically reflexive and automatic, but in certain contexts they may be the only means of communication available to a patient and therefore reflect a willful, volitional act of intention. These difficulties, coupled with inadequate experience and knowledge engendered through the relative rarity of these complex conditions, contribute to an alarmingly high rate of misdiagnosis (up to 43%) in this patient group (Childs *et al.* 1993; Andrews *et al.* 1996; Schnakers *et al.* 2006).

These issues expose a central conundrum in the study of covert awareness in general and, in particular, how it relates to conditions such as the vegetative state. Historically, the only reliable method that we have had for determining if another being is consciously aware is to ask him/her. The answer may take the form of a spoken response or a non-verbal signal (which may be a movement as simple as the blink of an eye), but it is this answer, and only this answer, that allows us to infer awareness. Thus, while *wakefulness* can be measured and monitored accurately using techniques such as electroencephalography (EEG), *awareness* is an internal state of being that can only be measured via some form of self-report. Put simply, our ability to know unequivocally that another being is consciously aware is ultimately determined, not by whether they are aware or not, but by their ability to communicate that fact through a recognized behavioral response. But what if the ability to speak, or blink an eye, or move a hand is lost, yet conscious awareness remains? Following the logic described, in a case where every opportunity for self-report has been lost, it would be impossible to determine whether any level of awareness remains. Of course, cases of locked-in syndrome following acute brain injury or disease have been reported for many years, but where such cases are unexpectedly identified it is always through the (sometimes chance) detection of a minor residual motor response. Against this background it is an unfortunate, but inevitable, fact that a population of patients will exist who retain at least some level of residual conscious awareness, yet remain entirely unable to convey that fact to those around them.

Recent advances in neuroimaging technology may provide a solution to this problem. If measurable brain responses could be marshaled and used as a proxy for a motor response then a patient who is entirely unable to move may be able to signal awareness by generating a pattern of brain activity that is indicative of a specific thought or intention. Of course, this possibility raises many ethical issues and has profound implications for the prolongation, or otherwise, of life after severe brain injury. In what circumstances should imaging be used to look for evidence of covert awareness? What sorts of brain responses should be admissible as evidence of covert awareness and, in the absence of any possibility for behavioral verification, how much weight should be given to such evidence? In this chapter, these questions will be explored in the context of recent studies in both healthy populations and brain-injured patients that have sought to investigate covert awareness through the use of functional neuroimaging. Those circumstances in which fMRI data can be used to infer awareness in the absence of a behavioral response will be contrasted with those circumstances in which it cannot. This distinction is fundamental for understanding and interpreting patterns of brain activity following acute brain injury and has implications for clinical care, diagnosis, prognosis, and medicolegal decision-making after serious brain injury.

An historical perspective

There now exists substantial evidence to suggest that so-called "activation" methods, such as $H_2^{15}O$ positron emission tomography (PET) and fMRI can be used to link changes in regional cerebral blood flow to specific cognitive processes without the need for any overt response (e.g. a motor action or a verbal response) (for review, see Owen *et al.* 2001). In the first study of its kind, de Jong *et al.* (1997) measured regional cerebral blood flow in a post-traumatic vegetative patient during an auditorily-presented story told by his mother. Compared to non-word sounds, activation was observed in the anterior cingulate and temporal cortices, possibly reflecting emotional processing of the contents, or tone, of the mother's speech. A year later, PET was used in another patient diagnosed as vegetative to study visual processing in response to familiar faces (Menon *et al.* 1998). Robust activity was observed in the right fusiform gyrus, the so-called human face area (or fusiform face area, FFA). In both of these early cases, normal brain activation was observed in the absence of any behavioral responses to the external sensory stimulation.

A significant development in this rapidly evolving field has been the relative shift of emphasis from PET activation studies using $H_2^{15}O$ methodology, to fMRI. Not only is fMRI more widely available than PET, it offers increased statistical power, improved spatial and temporal resolution, and does not involve radiation (Owen *et al.* 2001). However, the use of fMRI in this context is not without difficulties—in particular, the design of paradigms that allow the unambiguous interpretation of positive results (when they occur) in non-behaviorally responsive patients is extremely complex. In the largest study to date, 41 patients with disorders of consciousness were graded according to their brain activation on a hierarchical series of language paradigms (Coleman *et al.* 2009). The tasks increased in complexity systematically from basic acoustic processing (a non-specific response to sound) to more complex aspects of language comprehension and semantics. At the highest level, responses to sentences containing semantically ambiguous words (e.g. the *creak/creek* came from a *beam* in the *ceiling/ sealing*) are compared to sentences containing no ambiguous words (e.g. her secrets were written in her diary), in order to reveal brain activity associated with spoken language *comprehension* (Owen *et al.* 2005a,b; Rodd *et al.* 2005; Coleman *et al.* 2007, 2009). Nineteen of the patients (almost 50%), who had been diagnosed as either vegetative or minimally conscious showed normal or near normal temporal-lobe responses in the low-level auditory contrast (sound responses) and in the mid-level speech perception contrast (a specific response to speech over and above the more general response to sounds). Four patients, including two who had been diagnosed as behaviorally vegetative were also shown to exhibit normal fMRI activity during the highest-level speech comprehension task, suggesting that the neural processes involved in *understanding* speech were also intact (Coleman *et al.* 2009). What is most remarkable about these fMRI findings is that the imaging results were found to have no association with the patients' behavioral presentation at the time of investigation and thus provide additional diagnostic information beyond the traditional clinical assessment. Moreover, the level of auditory processing revealed by the fMRI results *did* correlate strongly with the patients' subsequent behavioral recovery (assessed 6 months after the scan), suggesting that brain imaging may also provide valuable prognostic information not evident through bedside testing. These results provide compelling evidence for intact high-level residual linguistic processing in some patients who behaviorally meet the clinical criteria for vegetative and minimally conscious states.

On the relationship between brain activity and awareness

Does the presence of normal brain activation in behaviorally non-responsive patients indicate awareness? In most of the cases discussed earlier and elsewhere in the literature, the answer is probably no. Many types of stimuli, including faces, speech, and pain, will elicit relatively automatic responses from the brain; that is to say, they will occur without the need for active (i.e. conscious) intervention on the part of the participant (e.g. you can not choose to not recognize a face, or to not understand speech that is presented clearly in your native language). In addition, a wealth of data in healthy volunteers, from studies of implicit learning and the effects of priming (see Schacter 1994 for review) to studies of learning and speech perception during anaesthesia (e.g. Bonebakker *et al.* 1996; Davis *et al.* 2007) have demonstrated that many aspects of human cognition can go on in the absence of awareness. Even the semantic content of masked information can be primed to affect subsequent behavior without the explicit knowledge of the participant, suggesting that some aspects of semantic processing may occur without conscious awareness (Dehaene *et al.* 1998). By the same argument, normal neural responses in patients who are diagnosed as vegetative do not necessarily indicate that these patients have any conscious experience associated with processing those same types of stimuli. To investigate this issue directly, Davis *et al.* (2007) recently used fMRI in sedated healthy volunteers and exposed them to exactly the same speech stimuli that have been shown to elicit normal patterns of brain activity in some vegetative and minimally conscious patients (Owen *et al.* 2005a,b; Coleman *et al.* 2007, 2009). During three scanning sessions, the participants were non-sedated (awake), lightly sedated (a slowed response to conversation) and deeply sedated (no conversational response, rousable by loud command). In each session, they were exposed to sentences containing ambiguous words, matched sentences without ambiguous words, and signal-correlated noise. Equivalent temporal-lobe responses for normal speech sentences compared to signal-correlated noise were observed, bilaterally, at all three levels of sedation, suggesting that a normal brain response to speech sounds is not a reliable correlate of awareness. This result suggests that extreme caution needs to be exercised when interpreting normal responses to speech in patients who are diagnosed as vegetative, a problem of interpretation that applies to many of the activation studies that have been conducted in vegetative patients to date. However, when Davis *et al.* (2007) examined the effects of anaesthesia on ambiguous sentences, the frontal-lobe and posterior temporal-lobe activity that occurs in the awake individual (and is assumed to be a neural marker for semantic processing) was markedly absent, even during light sedation. This finding suggests that vegetative patients who show this specific pattern of neural activity during the presentation of ambiguous semantic material *may* be consciously aware (e.g. Owen *et al.* 2005a,b; Coleman *et al.* 2007, 2009). However, as tantalizing as such conclusions might be, they are entirely speculative; the fact that awareness is *associated* with the activity changes that are thought to reflect sentence comprehension does not mean that it is *necessary* for them to occur (by simple analogy, the fact that amygdala activity is often observed during fMRI studies of fear, does not mean that in all studies that have reported amygdala activity, the participants were fearful).

BRAIN ACTIVITY AS A FORM OF RESPONSE

The studies described earlier in this chapter confirm that many of the brain responses that have been observed to date using fMRI in brain damaged patients *could* have occurred automatically; that is, they could have occurred in the absence of any awareness of self (or others) on the part of the patient. But let us now consider an entirely different type of brain imaging experiment in which the responses observed *cannot* occur in the absence of awareness, because they are necessarily guided by a conscious choice, or *decision*, on the part of the participant. For example, in one recent study, Haynes *et al.* (2007) asked healthy volunteers to freely decide which of two mental tasks to perform (to add or subtract two numbers) and to covertly hold onto that decision during a delay. After the delay they actually performed the chosen task, the result being used to confirm which task they had previously been intending to do. A classifier (a mathematical algorithm used to categorize data in some complex feature space into one of a number of groups or classes) was trained to recognize the characteristic fMRI signatures associated with the two mental states and in 80% of trials was able to decode from activity in medial and lateral regions of prefrontal cortex which of the two tasks the volunteers were intending to perform, *before they actually performed it*. The principle employed in that study was that certain types of thought are associated with a unique brain activation pattern that can be used as a signature for that specific thought. If a classifier is trained to recognize these characteristic signatures, a volunteer's thoughts can be decoded (within the constraints of the experimental design), using their brain activity alone. In this case, the brain response cannot possibly be automatic as it is entirely unspecified by any external stimulus and is chosen by the volunteers according to their own free will. Such feats of rudimentary mind-reading involving reproducible and robust task-dependent fMRI responses suggest a novel method by which both healthy participants and patients may be able to communicate their thoughts to those around them by simply modulating their own neural activity. Indeed, another recent study has shown that fMRI can be used in this way as a brain–computer interface (BCI), allowing real-time communication of thoughts using changes in brain activity alone (Weiskopf *et al.* 2004). In that study, healthy volunteers learned to regulate the fMRI signal in a particular brain area using their own fMRI signal as feedback and in this manner were able to convey one of two thoughts through voluntary activation of the corresponding brain states. Crucially, these paradigms differ from all of the passive tasks described previously (e.g. speech or face perception) because normal patterns of fMRI activity are only observed when the participant makes a conscious choice to exert a specific willful, or voluntary, response. In this sense, awareness can be measured using such responses, simply because awareness is necessary for them to occur.

This contrast, between the responses observed in passive fMRI tasks that are (or at least *could be*) elicited automatically by an external stimulus and active tasks in which the response itself represents a conscious choice (and is therefore, by definition, a measure of conscious awareness), is absolutely central to the debate about the use of functional neuroimaging to measure covert awareness. A significant recent addition to this field, therefore, has been the development of fMRI paradigms that render awareness reportable in the absence of an overt behavioral (e.g. motor or speech) response in patients who are entirely behaviorally non-responsive (Owen *et al.* 2006; Boly *et al.* 2007; Owen and Coleman, 2008b; Monti *et al.* 2010). Some of these techniques make use of the general principle that imagining performing a particular task generates a robust and reliable pattern of brain activity in the fMRI scanner that is similar to actually performing the activity itself. For example, imagining moving or squeezing the hands will generate activity in the motor and premotor cortices (Jeannerod and Frak 1999), while imagining navigating from one location to another will activate the same regions of the parahippocampal gyrus and the posterior parietal cortex that have been widely implicated in map-reading and other so-called spatial navigation tasks (Aguirre *et al.* 1996).

In one recent study (Boly *et al.* 2007), 34 healthy volunteers were asked to imagine hitting a tennis ball back and forth to an imaginary coach when they heard the word "tennis" (thereby eliciting vigorous imaginary arm movements) and to imagine walking from room to room in their house when they heard the word "house" (thereby eliciting imaginary spatial navigation). Imagining playing tennis was associated with robust activity in the supplementary motor area in each and every one of the participants scanned. In contrast, imagining moving from room to room in a house activated the parahippocampal cortices, the posterior parietal lobe, and the lateral premotor cortices; all regions that have been shown to contribute to imaginary, or real, spatial navigation (Aguirre *et al.* 1996; Boly *et al.* 2007).

The robustness and reliability of these fMRI responses across individuals means that activity in these regions can be used as a neural proxy for behavior, confirming that the participant retains the ability to understand instructions, to carry out different mental tasks in response to those instructions, and, therefore, is able to exhibit willed, voluntary behavior in the absence of any overt action. On this basis, they permit the identification of awareness at the single-subject level, without the need for a motor response (for discussion, see Owen and Coleman 2008a; Monti *et al.* 2009). In severe brain injury, when the request to move a hand or a finger is followed by an appropriate motor response, the diagnosis can change from vegetative state (no evidence of awareness) to minimally conscious state (some evidence of awareness). By analogy then, if the request to activate, say, the supplementary motor area of the brain by imagining moving the hand was followed by an appropriate brain response, shouldn't we give that response the very same weight? Skeptics may argue that brain responses are somehow less physical, reliable, or immediate than motor responses but, as is the case with motor responses, all of these arguments can be dispelled with careful measurement, replication, and objective verification. For example, if a patient who was assumed to be unaware raised his/her hand to command on just one occasion, there would remain some doubt about the presence of awareness given the possibility that this movement was a chance occurrence, coincident with the instruction. However, if that same patient were able to repeat this response to command on ten occasions, there would remain little doubt that the patient was aware. By the same token, if that patient was able to activate his/her supplementary motor area in response to command (e.g. by being told to imagine hand movements), and was able to do this on every one of ten trials, would we not have to accept that this patient was consciously aware?

This same logic was used recently to demonstrate that a young woman who fulfilled all internationally agreed criteria for the vegetative state was, in fact, consciously aware and able to make responses of this sort using her brain activity (Owen *et al.* 2006, 2007). Prior to the fMRI scan, the patient was instructed to perform the two mental imagery tasks described earlier in this section. When she was asked to imagine playing tennis, significant activity was observed in the supplementary motor area (Owen *et al.* 2006) that was indistinguishable from that observed in the healthy volunteers scanned by Boly *et al.* (2007). Moreover, when she was asked to imagine walking through her home, significant activity was observed in the parahippocampal gyrus, the posterior parietal cortex, and the lateral premotor cortex which was, again, indistinguishable from those observed in healthy volunteers (Owen *et al.* 2006, 2007). On this basis, it was concluded that, despite fulfilling all of the clinical criteria for a diagnosis of vegetative state, this patient retained the ability to understand spoken commands and to respond to them through her brain activity, rather than through speech or movement, confirming beyond any doubt that she was consciously aware of herself and her surroundings. In a follow-up study of 23 patients who were behaviorally diagnosed as vegetative, Monti and colleagues (2010) showed that four (17%) were able to generate reliable responses of this sort in the fMRI scanner.

Owen and Coleman (2008b) extended the general principle described earlier, by which active mental rehearsal is used to signify awareness, to show that communication of "yes" and "no" responses was possible using the same approach. Thus, a healthy volunteer was able to reliably convey a "yes" response by imaging playing tennis and a "no" response by imaging moving around a house, thereby providing the answers to simple questions posed by the experimenters using only their brain activity. This technique was further refined by Monti and colleagues (2010) who successfully decoded the "yes" and "no" responses of 16 healthy participants with 100% accuracy using only their real-time changes in the supplementary motor area (during tennis imagery) and the parahippocampal place area (during spatial navigation). Moreover, in one traumatic brain injury patient, who had been repeatedly diagnosed as vegetative over a 5-year period, similar questions were posed and successfully decoded using the same approach (Monti *et al.* 2010). In contrast, and despite a reclassification to minimally conscious state following the fMRI scan, it remained impossible to establish any form of communication with this patient at the bedside.

Another approach to detecting covert awareness after brain injury is to target processes that require the willful adoption of mind-sets in carefully matched (perceptually identical) experimental and control conditions. For example, Monti and colleagues (2009) presented healthy volunteers with a series of neutral words, and alternatively instructed them to just listen, or to count, the number of times a given word was repeated. As predicted, the counting task revealed the frontoparietal network that has been previously associated with target detection and working memory. When tested on this same procedure, a minimally conscious patient produced a very similar pattern of activity, confirming that he could willfully adopt differential mind-sets as a function of the task condition and could actively maintain these mind-sets across time. As in the tennis/spatial navigation example described in detail earlier, because the external stimuli were identical in the two conditions (count words and listen to words), any difference in brain activity observed cannot reflect an automatic brain response (i.e. one that can occur in the absence of consciousness). Rather, the activity must reflect the fact that the patient has performed a particular action (albeit a brain action) in response to the stimuli on one (but not the other) presentation; in this sense, the brain response is entirely analogous to a (motor) response to command and should carry the same weight as evidence of awareness.

These types of approach all illustrate a paradigmatic shift away from passive (e.g. perceptual) tasks to more active (e.g. willful) tasks in the assessment of covert awareness after serious brain injury. What sets such tasks apart is that the neural responses required are not produced *automatically* by the eliciting stimulus, but, rather, depend on time-dependent and sustained responses generated by the participant. Such behavior (albeit neural behavior) provides a proxy for a motor action and is, therefore, an appropriate vehicle for reportable awareness (Zeman 2009).

IMPLICATIONS FOR NEUROETHICS

The possibility of using fMRI for the detection of awareness in the vegetative state raises a number of issues for legal decision-making relating to the prolongation, or otherwise, of life after severe brain injury. Foremost is the concern that diagnostic and prognostic accuracy is assured, as treatment decisions often include the possibility of withdrawal of life-support. In an excellent discussion of these issues, Joseph Fins notes "the utter and fixed futility of the vegetative state became the ethical and legal justification for the genesis of the right-to-die movement in the United States" (Fins 2003, 2006). At present, decisions concerning life support (nutrition and hydration) are only made once a diagnosis of *permanent* vegetative state has been made. In cases in which the critical threshold for a diagnosis of permanent vegetative state has passed, the medical team formally reviews the evidence and discuss this with those closest to the patient. In England and Wales the courts require that a decision to withdraw nutrition and hydration should be referred to them before any action is taken (Royal College of Physicians 1996). On the other hand, decisions not to use resuscitation in the case of cardiac arrest, or not to use antibiotics or dialysis, can be taken by the doctor in the best interests of the patient after full discussion with all those concerned. Interestingly, according to the same working party, "one cannot ever be certain that a patient in the vegetative state is wholly unaware…in view of this small but undeniable element of uncertainty, it is reasonable to administer sedation when hydration and nutrition are withdrawn to eliminate the possibility of suffering, however remote" (Royal College of Physicians 1996).

With the emergence of novel neuroimaging techniques that permit the identification of covert awareness in the absence of any behavioral response (Owen *et al.* 2006), the wording of the Royal College of Physicians 1996 statement ("one cannot ever be certain that a patient in the vegetative state is wholly unaware") acquires renewed resonance. Unfortunately, at present, although several of the neuroimaging approaches discussed in this chapter hold great promise for improving both diagnostic and prognostic accuracy in behaviorally non-responsive patients, the accepted assessment procedure continues to be based on standard behavioral criteria and a careful and repeated neurological exam by a trained examiner. However, in an increasing number of cases, neuroimaging findings have been reported that are entirely inconsistent with the formal clinical diagnosis. For example, the patient described by Owen *et al.* (2006), was clearly able to produce voluntary responses to command (albeit neural responses), yet was unable to match this with any form of motor response at the bedside. Paradoxically therefore, this patient's (motor) behavior was consistent with a diagnosis of vegetative state (an absence of evidence of awareness or purposeful response), yet her brain imaging data confirmed that the alternative hypothesis was correct, i.e. that she was entirely aware during the scanning procedure. Clearly the clinical diagnosis of vegetative state based on behavioral assessment was inaccurate in the sense that it did not accurately reflect her internal state of awareness. On the other hand, she was not *misdiagnosed* in the sense that no behavioral marker of awareness was missed. Likewise, the patient described recently by Monti *et al.* (2010) was clearly not vegetative because he could generate "yes" and "no" responses in real time by willfully modulating his brain activity. In fact, these consistent "responses to command" which allowed him to *functionally communicate* suggest a level of residual cognitive function that would actually place this patient beyond the minimally conscious state and (at least) into the severely disabled category. Similarly, the minimally conscious patient described by Monti *et al.* (2009) was able to perform a complex working memory task in the scanner, in the sense that his brain activity revealed consistent and repeatable command following. While this behavior does not necessarily alter the patient's formal diagnosis (from low MCS) it certainly demonstrated a level of responsively that was not evident from the behavioral examination. These findings suggest an urgent need for a re-evaluation of the existing diagnostic guidelines for the vegetative state and related disorders of consciousness and for the development and formal inclusion of validated, standardized neuroimaging procedures into those guidelines.

A related issue concerns the implications that emerging neuroimaging approaches may have for prognosis in this patient group. It is of interest that in the case described by Owen and colleagues (2006), the patient began to emerge from her vegetative state to demonstrate diagnostically relevant behavioral markers before the prognostically important 12-month threshold was reached (for a diagnosis of permanent vegetative state), suggesting that early evidence of awareness acquired with functional neuroimaging may have important prognostic value. Indeed, with a marked increase in the number of studies using neuroimaging techniques in patients with disorders of consciousness, a consistent pattern is beginning to emerge. Di *et al.* (2008) reviewed 15 separate $H_2^{15}O$ PET and fMRI studies involving 48 published cases which were classified as "absent cortical activity," "typical activity" (involving low level primary sensory cortices), and "atypical activity" (corresponding to higher level associative cortices). The results suggest that atypical activity patterns appear to predict recovery from vegetative state with 93% specificity and 69% sensitivity. That is to say, nine of 11 patients exhibiting atypical activity patterns recovered consciousness, whereas 21 of 25 patient with typical primary cortical activity patterns and four out of four patients with absent activity failed to recover. This important review strongly suggests that functional neuroimaging data can provide important prognostic information beyond that available from bedside examination alone. Similarly, in the large recent study of 41 patients with disorders of consciousness described in detail earlier, Coleman *et al.* (2009) also found direct evidence of prognostically important information from the neuroimaging data that was at odds with the behavioral assessment at the time of scanning. Thus, contrary to the clinical impression of a specialist team using behavioral assessment tools, two patients who had been referred to the study with a diagnosis of vegetative state, did in fact demonstrate clear signs of speech comprehension when assessed using fMRI. More importantly, however, across the whole group of patients, the fMRI data were found to have no association with the behavioral presentation at the time of the investigation, but correlated significantly with subsequent behavioral recovery, 6 months after the scan. In this case, the fMRI data predicted subsequent recovery in a way that a specialist behavioral assessment could not.

In summary, although it is not yet the case that fMRI data forms part of the diagnostic and prognostic assessment of behaviorally non-responsive patients, more evidence to support its formal inclusion is being published each year (Owen and Coleman 2007) The prevailing view is not that brain imaging should replace behavioral assessments, but rather that it should be used, wherever possible, to acquire further information about the patient. In doing so, and on the basis of the evidence reviewed here, one can reasonably expect that the current rate of misdiagnosis will fall. Patients will be examined with all available tools and thus be given the greatest opportunity to respond. Likewise, care teams will have the best possible information for planning and monitoring interventions to facilitate recovery. Although behavioral markers and brain imaging will undoubtedly reveal inconsistencies, it is these inconsistencies that will ultimately improve the accuracy of diagnosis and prognosis in this patient group.

Returning to the issue of the continuation, or otherwise, of life support in behaviorally non-responsive patients, in the case described by Owen and colleagues (2006), and in most of the similar cases that have appeared in the subsequent literature (e.g. Owen and Coleman 2008a; Monti *et al.* 2010), as noted earlier, the scans that revealed awareness were acquired before the time at which the decision-making process governing withdrawal of life-support is legally permitted to begin (i.e. the patients had not yet reached the threshold for a diagnosis of *permanent* vegetative state). Therefore, even if the neuroimaging evidence had been admissible as part of the formal diagnostic and prognostic evaluation, it would not have influenced the decision-making in those particular cases. The same is not true of the patient described recently by Monti and colleagues (2010) who was able to communicate using his fMRI responses despite being repeatedly diagnosed as vegetative over a 5-year period. In that case, the scan that revealed awareness and, indeed, the ability to functionally communicate, was acquired several years after the critical threshold had been reached. Even so, it is likely to be a number of years before such evidence could ever be used in the context of end-of-life decision-making and significant legal, ethical, and technical hurdles will need to be overcome beforehand. For example, in principle it would be possible to ask the patient described by Monti *et al.* (2010) whether he wanted to continue living in his current situation (subject to an appropriate ethical framework being put into place), but would a "yes" or a "no" response be sufficient to be sure that the patient retained the necessary cognitive and emotional capacity to make such a complex decision? Clearly much more work would need to be done and many more questions asked of the patient (involving considerable time in the scanner), before one could be sure that this was the case and, even then, new ethical and legal frameworks will need to be introduced to determine exactly how such situations are managed and by whom. In the short term, it is more likely that this approach will be used to address less ethically challenging issue such as whether or not any patients who are in this situation are experiencing any pain. For example, using this technique patients who are aware, but cannot move or speak, could be asked if they are feeling any pain, guiding the administration of analgesics where appropriate.

On the other hand, it is important to point out that neuroimaging of covert awareness is unlikely to influence legal proceedings where negative findings have been acquired. False negative findings in functional neuroimaging studies are common, even in healthy volunteers, and they present particular difficulties in this patient population. For example, a patient may fall asleep during the scan or may not have properly heard or understood the task instructions, leading to an erroneous negative result. Indeed, in the recent study by Monti *et al.* (2010) no willful fMRI responses were observed in 19 of 23 patients—whether these are *true* negative findings (i.e. those 19 patients were indeed vegetative) or *false negative* findings (i.e. some of those patients were conscious, but this was not detected on the day of the scan) can not be determined. Accordingly, negative fMRI findings in patients should never be used as evidence for impaired cognitive function or lack of awareness.

Finally, ethical concerns are also sometimes raised concerning the participation of severely brain injured patients in functional neuroimaging studies (for example, to assess pain perception), studies that require invasive procedures (e.g. intra-arterial or jugular lines required for quantification of PET data or modeling), or the use of neuromuscular paralytics (for an excellent discussion of this topic, see Fins and Illes *et al.* 2008). By definition, unconscious or minimally conscious patients cannot give informed consent to participate in clinical research and written approval is typically obtained from family or legal representatives depending on governmental and hospital guidelines in each country. Any proposed ethical framework must balance access to research and medical advances with protection for vulnerable patient populations. In the summer of 2007, a working party of leading investigators in neuroimaging, disorders of consciousness, and neuroethics was convened at Stanford University to consider how best such a balance might be maintained. The resulting recommendations (Fins and Illes *et al.* 2008) provide the only existing comprehensive ethical framework through which investigative neuroimaging techniques could mature into useful clinical tools for the diagnosis and treatment of those with disorders of consciousness. Severe brain injury represents an immense social and economic problem that warrants further research. Unconscious, minimally conscious, and locked-in patients are very vulnerable and deserve special procedural protections. However, it is important to stress that they are also vulnerable to being denied potentially life-saving therapy if clinical research cannot be performed adequately (for further discussion, see Fins 2009).

ACKNOWLEDGEMENTS

I would like to thank the James S. McDonnell Foundation and the Medical Research Council, UK for their generous funding of my research program.

REFERENCES

Aguirre, G.K., Detre, J.A., Alsop, D.C., and D'Esposito, M. (1996). The parahippocampus subserves topographical learning in man. *Cerebral Cortex*, **6**, 823–9.

Andrews, K., Murphy, L., Munday, R., and Littlewood, C. (1996). Misdiagnosis of the vegetative state: retrospective study in a rehabilitation unit. *British Medical Journal*, **313**, 13–16.

Boly, M., Coleman, M.R., Davis, M.H., *et al.* (2007). When thoughts become action: an fMRI paradigm to study volitional brain activity in non-communicative brain injured patients. *Neuroimage*, **36**, 979–92.

Bonebakker, A., Bonke, B., Klein, J., *et al.* (1996). Information processing during general anaesthesia: Evidence for unconscious memory. In B. Bonke, J.G.W. Bovill, and N. Moerman (eds.) *Memory and Awareness in Anaesthesia*, pp. 101–9. Lisse, Amsterdam: Swets and Zeitlinger.

Childs, N.L., Mercer, W.N., and Childs, H.W. (1993). Accuracy of diagnosis of persistent vegetative state. *Neurology*, **43**, 1465–7.

Coleman, M.R., Rodd, J.M., Davis, M.H., *et al.* (2007). Do vegetative patients retain aspects of language: Evidence from fMRI. *Brain*, **130**, 2494–507.

Coleman, M.R., Davis, M.H., Rodd, J.M., *et al.* (2009). Towards the routine use of brain imaging to aid the clinical diagnosis of disorders of consciousness. *Brain*, **132**, 2541–52.

Davis, M.H., Coleman, M.R., Absalom, A.R., *et al.* (2007). Dissociating speech perception and comprehension at reduced levels of awareness. *Proceedings of the National Academy of Sciences*, **104**, 16032–7.

de Jong, B., Willemsen, A.T., and Paans, A.M. (1997). Regional cerebral blood flow changes related to affective speech presentation in persistent vegetative state. *Clinical Neurology and Neurosurgery*, **99**, 213–16.

Dehaene, S., Naccache, L., Le Clec'H, G., *et al.* (1998). Imaging unconscious semantic priming. *Nature*, **395**, 597–600.

Di, H., Boly, M., Weng, X., Ledoux, D., and Laureys, S. (2008). Neuroimaging activation studies in the vegetative state: predictors of recovery? *Clinical Medicine*, **8**, 502–7.

Fins, J.J. (2003). Constructing an ethical stereotaxy for severe brain injury: balancing risks, benefits and access. *Nature Reviews Neuroscience*, **4**, 323–7.

Fins, J.J. (2006). *A Palliative Ethic of Care: Clinical Wisdom at Life's End*. Sudbury, MA: Jones and Bartlett.

Fins, J.J. (2009). The ethics of measuring and modulating consciousness: the imperative of minding time. In S. Laureys, N.D. Schiff, and A.M. Owen (eds.) *Coma science: Clinical and ethical implications – Progress in Brain Research*, pp. 371–82. Oxford: Elsevier.

Fins, J.*, Illes, J.*, Bernat, J.L., Hirsch, J., Laureys, S., and Murphy, E.R. (*lead authors) (2008). Neuroimaging and disorders of consciousness: Envisioning an ethical research agenda. *American Journal of Bioethics – Neuroscience*, **8**, 3–12.

Giacino, J.T., Schnakers, C., Rodriguez-Moreno, D., Schiff, N.D., and Kalmar, K., (2009). Behavioral assessment in patients with disorders of consciousness: Gold standard or fool's gold? In S. Laureys, N.D. Schiff, and A.M. Owen (eds.) *Coma Science: Clinical and Ethical Implications – Progress in Brain Research*, pp. 33–48. Oxford: Elsevier.

Haynes, J.D., Sakai, K., Rees, G. *et al.* (2007). Reading hidden intentions in the human brain. *Current Biology*, **17**, 323–8.

Jeannerod, M. and Frak, V. (1999). Mental imaging of motor activity in humans. *Current Opinion in Neurobiology*, **9**, 735–9.

Jennett, B. and Plum, F. (1972). Persistent vegetative state after brain damage. *Lancet*, **1**, 734–7.

Menon, D.K., Owen, A.M., Williams, E.J., *et al.* (1998). Cortical processing in persistent vegetative state. *Lancet*, **352**, 200.

Monti, M.M., Coleman, M.R., and Owen, A.M. (2009). Executive functions in the absence of behavior: functional imaging of the minimally conscious state. In S. Laureys, N.D. Schiff, and A.M. Owen (eds.) *Coma Science: Clinical and Ethical Implications – Progress in Brain Research*, pp. 249–60. Oxford: Elsevier.

Monti, M.M., Vanhaudenhuyse, A., Coleman, M.R., *et al.* (2010). Willful modulation of brain activity and communication in disorders of consciousness. *New England Journal of Medicine*, **362**, 579–89.

Owen, A.M. and Coleman M.R. (2007). Functional MRI in disorders of consciousness: advantages and limitations. *Current Opinion in Neurology*, **20**, 632–7.

Owen, A.M. and Coleman, M. (2008a). Functional imaging in the vegetative state. *Nature Reviews Neuroscience*, **9**, 235–43.

Owen, A.M. and Coleman M.R. (2008b). Detecting awareness in the vegetative state. In D. Pfaff (ed.) Molecular and Biophysical Mechanisms of Arousal, Alertness and Attention. *Annals of the New York Academy of Sciences*, **1129**, 130–40.

Owen, A.M., Epstein, R., and Johnsrude, I.S. (2001). fMRI: Applications to cognitive neuroscience. In P. Jezzard, P.M. Mathews, and S. M. Smith (eds.) *Functional Magnetic Resonance Imaging. An Introduction to Methods* pp. 311–28. Oxford: Oxford University Press.

Owen, A.M., Menon, D.K., Johnsrude, I.S., *et al.* (2002). Detecting residual cognitive function in persistent vegetative state. *Neurocase*, **8**, 394–403.

Owen, A.M., Coleman, M.R., Menon, D.K., *et al.* (2005a). Using a heirarchical approach to investigate residual auditory cognition in persistent vegetative state. In S. Laureys (ed), The boundaries of consciousness: neurobiology and neuropathology. *Progress in Brain Research*, **150**, 461–76.

Owen, A. M., Coleman, M.R., Menon, D. K., *et al.* (2005b). Residual auditory function in persistent vegetative state: a combined PET and fMRI study. *Neuropsychological Rehabilitation*, **15**, 290–306.

Owen, A.M., Coleman, M.R., Davis, M.H., Boly, M., Laureys, S., and Pickard, J.D. (2006). Detecting awareness in the vegetative state. *Science*, **313**, 1402.

Owen, A.M., Coleman, M.R., Davis, M.H., *et al.* (2007). Response to comments on "Detecting awareness in the vegetative state". *Science*, **315**, 1221c.

Plum F. and Posner J.B. (1966). *The diagnosis of stupor and coma*. Philadelphia, PA: F.A. Davis Co.

Rodd, J.M., Davis, M.H., and Johnsrude, I.S. (2005). The neural mechanisms of speech comprehension: fMRI studies of semantic ambiguity. *Cerebral Cortex*, **15**, 1261–9.

Royal College of Physicians Working Group. (1996). The permanent vegetative state. *Journal of the Royal College of Physicians of London*, **30**, 119–21.

Schacter, D.L. (1994). Priming and multiple memory systems: Perceptual mechanisms of implicit memory. In D.L. Schacter and E. Tulving (eds.) *Memory Systems*, pp. 233–68. Cambridge, MA: MIT Press.

Schnakers, C., Giacino, J., Kalmar, K., *et al.* (2006). Does the FOUR score correctly diagnose the vegetative and minimally conscious states? *Annals of Neurology*, **60**, 744–5.

Weiskopf, N., Mathiak, K., Bock, S.W., *et al.* (2004). Principles of a brain-computer interface (BCI) based on real-time functional magnetic resonance imaging (fMRI). *IEEE Transactions on Biomedical Engineering*, **51**, 966–70.

Zeman, A. (2009). The problem of unreportable awareness. In S. Laureys, N.D. Schiff, and A.M. Owen (eds.) *Coma Science: Clinical and Ethical Implications – Progress in Brain Research*, pp. 1–10. Oxford: Elsevier.

PART II

RESPONSIBILITY
AND
DETERMINISM

CHAPTER 9

GENETIC DETERMINISM, NEURONAL DETERMINISM, AND DETERMINISM *TOUT COURT*

BERNARD BAERTSCHI AND ALEXANDRE MAURON

INTRODUCTION

FOR a long time, human beings have noticed that particular events follow regularly from other ones. Philosophers and scientists have expressed this observation with the notion of "causality": if an event *A* is the cause of an event *B*, then *B* follows necessarily from *A*, or *B* is produced by the power of *A*. As causality is a pervasive relation, the world has consequently been conceived as a huge web of causal relations. Quantum mechanics has made the matter more complex, but the general picture of the world as a causal nexus remains.

Human beings live in this world, they are a part of it. Does this mean that they are imprisoned in this web or do they have some slack? This question can be answered at two different levels. The first is the metaphysical level, and the two main answers are hard determinism and libertarianism: for the first, human beings are subject to the very same regularities we observe in the natural world, because they are completely natural beings. This the libertarian denies, arguing for human free will. The second level is more mundane and focuses on human actions, which are very different from physical movements since they are conscious and intentional. Yet sometimes they are not, and the agent is constrained by various factors. The list is rather long, but comprises mainly sociological, psychological, genetic, and neuronal influences. Each of those factors underpins a qualified determinism, as opposed to determinism *tout court* (i.e. determinism as part of a metaphysical view).

In this chapter, our aim is to place neuronal determinism (neurodeterminism) in its right place. At first sight it appears to be a type of qualified determinism, but, in the end, we shall see that this is not exactly the case: neurodeterminism is better conceived as determinism *tout court* when it is applied to human beings. In this sense, neuronal determinism differs importantly from genetic determinism, two views that are often regarded as similar in form if not in content.

After clarifying the two types of determinisms (the two levels of answers), we examine the question of genetic determinism, because it is a paradigm of qualified determinism and because it has generated many confusions. We then explain the meaning of determinism *tout court*, its relation with the notions of "free will" and "responsibility," and the debate about their alleged incompatibility. With those distinctions in mind, we will be able to adequately understand what neurodeterminism consists of, and to show that it should be conceived as determinism *tout court* when it is applied to human beings, imparting an empirical turn to a very old metaphysical conundrum.

QUALIFIED DETERMINISMS

For much of history, describing and explaining *human behavior* was the province of religious myth and literature. Epic poets, storytellers, novelists, and historiographers all availed themselves of the common-sense explanatory framework of reasons and motives. These categories provided an understanding of the deliberations, actions, and choices of deities, mythical heroes, political rulers, and common people. Most philosophers adopted this conception of human behavior as well. On the other hand, philosophy and pre-scientific thought were reflecting the *world* in terms of causes and effects, i.e. some form of determinism. Occasionally philosophers wondered whether human behavior might be deterministic in some ultimate sense. Could it be the case that "reasons" and "motives" are just superficial concepts, which are actually underpinned at some deeper level by the same sort of causation that operates throughout nature, including all living things and inanimate objects? A strand of Western thought from the Stoics to Spinoza, all the way to contemporary determinists, has persistently asked that question. We might call this the problem of determinism *tout court*.

The story becomes more complicated when taking on board the accelerating progress of science during the 19th century and its complex effects on deterministic explanations. On the one hand, the success of Newtonian physics gave credence to determinism in physics and in biology. Furthermore, the Darwinian revolution strengthened the basic commonality of humans and the living world, which are all part of the same evolutionary history. It also gave plausibility to causal, biological explanations of behaviors that would apply both to humans and to non-human animals (Darwin 1873). But while the zeitgeist became more congenial to causal explanations of human behavior, the scientific contenders poised to provide such causal accounts became more numerous. Psychology, sociology, and anthropology declared independence from philosophy, and to a large extent from one another as well. It is indeed striking how the fledgling social sciences' early self-definitions were often exclusionary and attempted to state some form of fundamental, "atomic" object, in terms of which all genuinely scientific explanations within their remit had to be formulated. Relevant examples are the "social fact" of Durkheimian sociology or the stimulus-response of behavioristic psychology. The resulting predicament is a coexistence of competing causal accounts of human behavior coming from the various social sciences, that until relatively recently seemed to have but one thing in common, namely their distrust of biological explanations. The diversification of scientific approaches towards human nature generated several qualified determinisms, or determinisms "with an adjective" such as social determinism, cultural determinism, the determinism of individual psychology (however understood) on one side, biological determinism, genetic determinism on another side. In recent decades, the last two, and especially the last one, seem to have been treated as ugly ducklings and generated polemical debates (for a history of the controversies around sociobiology, see Segerstråle 2001).

GENETIC DETERMINISM

First, we need to point out the ambivalence in the very concept of genetic determinism, a problem which largely affects other qualified determinisms as well. On the one hand, among the possible meanings of "genetic determinism," one is trivially correct and one trivially wrong. If genetic determinism refers to the fact that genes have some causal influence on human behavior, then that is a statement of an obvious truth. There is a highly successful behavioral genetics of worms, of *Drosophila*, and of mice, hence it is hard to see how the behavior of *Homo sapiens* could be utterly disconnected from human genetics (for a general treatment of human behavioral genetics, see Plomin *et al.* 2008). On the other hand, defining genetic determinism as the belief that every possible behavior of an individual is somehow encoded in that person's genome is obviously silly. It is true that genes are destiny in the very special and limited sense that, to take a hackneyed example, a person knowing that she has the Huntington's disease (HD) gene may reasonably feel predestined to suffer HD. But there is an enormous gap between such special cases and the notion the humans are like a piece of hardware passively doing the bidding of the genetic software within their genome, as if the genome was a human's true essence (Mauron 2001).

Nevertheless, genetic determinism is often treated as a straw man in the literature, as the belief that genes dictate entirely how a human individual develops and comes to exhibit its entire range of phenotypic characteristics and typical behaviors. Clearly, for genetic determinism to be a concept that reasonable people can discuss and have disagreements about, it has to mean something less simplistic. Roughly speaking, it has to mean either that genetic explanations of behavior have some sort of privileged epistemic status, maybe undeservedly (Oyama 1985), or that genetic factors are predominant (as compared to various acquired characteristics) amongst the different causal influences impinging on human behavior, and that this idea could be wrong.

Discussing the first meaning would lead us into the morass of alternative theoretical accounts of the role of genes in development (Oyama *et al.* 2001), which we will not do. We will, however, discuss the second point briefly, with a view to showing that the question of whether some human behavior or trait is predominantly genetic or environmental is beset with serious misunderstandings. But first, we will focus on the supposed unfortunate moral implications of genetic determinism. Indeed, it is striking how many critics of genetic determinism consider it not only as a mistaken opinion to be corrected, but as an evil way of thinking that ought to be exorcised. "… arguing against genetic determinism is like battling the undead: no matter how many times you stab them, they keep coming at you." (De Melo-Martin 2005, p.526). In the heyday of the sociobiology controversy, objections to genetic determinism were quite stridently political (Rose *et al.* 1984). There was an underlying assumption that the Right votes for the genes and the Left votes for the environment. In other words, conservative thought was supposed to embrace the notion of innate inequalities as an unavoidable fact of human nature, whereas progressives would want human nature to be sufficiently malleable to effect changes directed towards more social justice and equality.

These political assumptions are less prominent today. The objections to genetic determinism are mainly expressed in moral terms and seem to fall into two broad categories (De Melo-Martin 2005). The first is closely linked to healthcare policy and claims that an over-emphasis on the genetic causation of disease may misdirect the healthcare system away from prevention, lifestyle interventions, and social reform with a view to correcting the social determinants of disease. The second objection is more basic and argues that genetic determinism induces a fatalist belief that human behaviors, characteristics, and health and disease states, are accounted for by genetics alone and that, as a result, there is nothing that can be done to change them. The underlying assumption seems to be that "genetic determinism" is the one really hard and inflexible determinism, whereas changes in human behaviors, characteristics, health and disease states, that work through environmental influences, education, social reform, and the like are soft and more compatible with a degree of human freedom.

There are two (related) problems with this line of thought. The first originated from debates on the inheritance of quantitative traits such as intelligence quotient (IQ), but it has broader implications. The problem is that it is easy to confuse (1) the question whether genes determine the quantitative value of a particular phenotypic trait and (2) the question whether the *variability* in a phenotypic trait in a given population and a given environment is mostly accounted for by *genetic variability*. To see the difference, consider the number of fingers humans typically have. There is no doubt that the fact that most of us have ten fingers is genetically determined (question no. 1). If, however, we ask about the cause of the variability in the number of fingers in a human population, it is clear that it is mostly environmental. In most individuals whose finger number differs from ten, the explanation refers to some environmental, usually accidental cause, although for a small minority it denotes a genetic anomaly (polydactyly, syndactyly). Therefore, although the answer to question no. 1 falls entirely on the side of the genes, when we turn to question no. 2, the environment wins over genetics. In the language of population genetics, the heritability of finger number is low, and yet at the same time the involvement of genes in determining finger number is very high.

Heritability is an important concept for population geneticists because high heritability is one of several factors that render a particular phenotype susceptible to evolutionary change through selective pressure. But it has no relevance to what is really on the mind of those who worry about genetic determinism, i.e. that genetic causation equals inevitability. This is simply wrong. High heritability of a trait implies nothing about whether that trait can be changed by environmental, or any other, interventions. This is one lesson we (should) have learned from the controversies on the heritability of IQ. In fact, this error also applies to non-quantitative, all-or-none, phenotypes, such as having or not having a monogenic disease. These are diseases in which a single genetic abnormality is the necessary cause of the disease phenotype, such as HD or phenylketonuria (PKU). If an individual person is homozygous for the PKU mutation, that person will suffer the disease unless diagnosed as a newborn and fed a phenylalanine-poor diet early on, i.e. unless that child's environment is changed appropriately. Unlike for PKU, no prevention or cure of HD has been discovered so far, but that is a matter of historical contingency, not an essential feature of diseases that are described as monogenic. In summary, saying that the explanation of some human trait lies in the genes is a vague statement that may or may not have some meaningful content. In any event, it says little about whether and how that trait could be influenced, or corrected in the case of undesirable characteristics or behaviors.

The second problem with the critique described earlier is that there is nothing special about the potential of genetic determinism to inspire a fatalistic, "laissez-faire" attitude towards a particular human problem. We have seen that genetic determinism is basically an ill-constructed concept based on over-simplifications and downright errors. If one is allowed to be similarly fuzzy about other determinisms with an adjective, the same fatalistic and disheartening discourses could be constructed about those. For instance, psychological determinism, suitably oversimplified, can be made to be just as "hard" as genetic determinism. In the middle of last century, psychoanalysis in its heyday was often interpreted in popular culture as concluding that everything in a child's development is determined before the age of 3 or 4 years. If you are a neurotic and unhappy adult, something must have gone awry with your Oedipus complex during your early childhood and nothing but the arduous, lengthy, and expensive process of psychoanalysis might just possibly make your life less miserable. The same could be said of social determinism and in actuality, the founders of sociology such as Emile Durkheim had to defend themselves from being deterministic in a similar manner (Bourdieu *et al.* 1991).

Having a clear-cut view of the qualified determinisms impinging on human problems and debating which is more powerful or relevant than the other; that may be a more difficult and less interesting endeavor than is often assumed. In addition determinisms with an adjective basically belong to semi-empirical disputes that attempt to compare and rank different causal schemes. They do not even begin to address the fundamental philosophical issue, which is that of determinism *tout court*, i.e. the causal closure of the sphere of human action.

DETERMINISM *TOUT COURT*

If, conceptually, qualified determinisms stand alone on their feet, it is not the case with determinism *tout court*. It can only be understood with a contrasting notion: free will. Traditionally, free will has been conceptualized as the capacity possessed by persons to decide and act in accordance with an unimpeded will of their own. The criterion of an unimpeded will is the possibility for it to choose between different alternatives: if a person decide to do something, she is free as long as it is possible for her to choose A or to choose B; and when she has decided, she was free inasmuch as it would have been possible for her to choose otherwise (Fischer 2002). To thwart such a will is to make it absolutely unable to choose any alternative to a certain determinate course of actions—an inability for a matter of principle, not due to some accidental circumstance. What could cause such an inability? Not the usual constraints that are typical of qualified determinisms. God could cause it, because as an all-knowing and eternal being, he knows everything in advance from the beginning of time (*divine prescience*), and because as an omnipotent being, he has decided from the beginning of the times which courses of actions will be chosen by all of us (and, consequently, if we will go to hell or heaven: this is the doctrine of *predestination*). It was no accident that Martin Luther wrote in 1525 a book named *De servo arbitrio* to counter the arguments put forth one year before by Erasmus in his *De libero arbitrio*. More interestingly for our topic, nature could cause it, too. From the 17th century onwards—and particularly with the success of Newtonian physics, as it was said before—a new concept of nature emerged, superseding the Aristotelian perspective. In this new conception, the world is causally closed: every event is caused by another event of the same ontological kind, and there is no place for an event that would not be imprisoned in the causal network of the world. In short, every event in the world is caused, and causes and effects are of the same material nature, their interaction being regulated by the laws of nature. This is physical determinism or determinism *tout court*.

By itself, physical determinism is not necessarily antagonistic to free will. Descartes was able to believe in the truth of physical determinism and of free will, because for him, free will was not a feature of the natural world; it was a faculty of the soul. But this position became soon untenable, as it was impossible for it to explain the interaction between the soul and the body (e.g. the action of the will on the limbs, for instance, when I decide to move my arm) without violating the causal closure of the world: when the will raises the arm, the former must create the latter's movement from nothing, because the soul is an unmoved being that cannot lose the quantity of movement it gives to the arm. Leibniz was very aware of this fact, and the Enlightenment philosophers of the following century too (Baertschi 2005). There are several ways out if this conundrum. The solution that has prevailed in post-enlightened philosophy and science (with *Idéologistes* like Cabanis and Lamarck, with Karl Vogt and Charles Darwin, and with the majority of contemporary scientists) is the following: human actions and decisions ought to be accounted for in the frame of the new science: like physical events, they are submitted to the laws of nature, and therefore to physical determinism (Kim 1998). Of course, our decisions and actions are not caused by pure material movements; they are preceded by deliberation, where motives and reasons are examined and discovered. But for this account, motives and reasons are causes, too—more precisely, they are causes of actions that are the effects of brain events (and are themselves brain events). As Cabanis said in 1802, an assertion repeated by Vogt and Darwin: the brain digests the impressions, thought being an organic secretion of the brain (Cabanis 1980).

Accordingly, free will as traditionally conceived and determinism exclude each other. Since determinism is the upshot of our best conception of the world (i.e. the scientific conception), free will ought to be given up. But this renunciation has its price, because, traditionally too, free will is linked with moral and legal responsibility. The argument goes this way:

1) If an agent A is morally responsible for an act B, then A could have refrained from doing B.

2) If B hangs uniquely on the previous state of the world E, then B is inescapable.

3) If B is inescapable, then A could not have eschewed doing B.

4) Therefore A is responsible for B only if B does not uniquely hang on E.

5) B does not uniquely hangs on E only if it additionally depends on a causal power independent of E.

6) Free will is such a causal power.

7) Therefore A is morally responsible for B only if A possesses free will.

8) Free will is incompatible with the truth of physical determinism.

9) Therefore A does not possess free will, and consequently A could not have eschewed doing B.

10) Conclusion: A is not morally responsible for B (and is never responsible for any decision or act of its own).

For many authors, this conclusion is not acceptable: we cannot give up responsibility, because it is basic to all our practical institutions (notably morality and law). How to get out of this dilemma (responsibility versus determinism)? When two propositions p and q are contradictory, it is logically possible to reject p or to reject q. So, we can logically reject determinism or free will. Those who accept the conclusion (i.e. propositions 1 to 10) reject free will; they are called *hard determinists*, a conception first proposed by Spinoza and the French materialists like Diderot. *Libertarians* keep free will and reject determinism (Kane 2002). Hard determinists usually think that responsibility is an illusion and that we ought to change our moral and legal practices accordingly. Libertarians deny propositions 9 and 10 and, consequently, must weaken the causal closure of the world, usually by appealing to quantum mechanics (Eccles in Popper and Eccles 1977; Searle 2008).

But hard determinism and libertarianism are not the only options. When two propositions p and q are contradictory, it is still possible to modify p or q, in order for them to become compatible. *Compatibilists* adopt this strategy, denying proposition 8. Conceding the truth of determinism, they modify the meaning of free will accordingly. In their conception, free will no longer is the power to decide and choose without being impeded *tout court*, but without being hindered by certain causes rather than others. Coercion is such a cause, so a coerced act is not free and implies no responsibility; but the previous state of the world is not such a cause and usual acts are free, implying responsibility (Churchland 2002).

Neurodeterminism

Neurodeterminism belongs to the family of qualified determinisms: it is in effect brain determinism. So it is not determinism *tout court*. Brain is on a par with genes, social and psychological conditioning. Consequently, it does not have any impact on the question of free will, but possesses, for instance, its entire weight as possible excusing conditions in Courts (insanity defense). So, if you are a hard determinist, neurodeterminism is only one particular aspect of an already deterministic conception of nature; if you are a libertarian, neurodeterminism is one of the multiple problems a person can encounter since her freedom is not absolute; and if you are a compatibilist, you will follow the argument of the libertarian, giving only a different meaning to the words free will.

But is neurodeterminism merely one qualified determinism among others? Consider the following thought experiment. A serial killer is standing trial and her attorney is considering various possible defenses aimed at diminishing the defendant's responsibility on the basis of various qualified determinisms. The lawyer imagines different statements that the defendant could make:

> "Your Honor:
> —My genes made me do it.
> —My unresolved childhood complexes made me do it.
> —My terrible childhood circumstances, marred by neglect and violence made me do it..."

Even if we put aside the confusions alluded to in our first paragraph, something goes awry here. What is odd in these utterances is that they attribute agency to some outside element, a kind of master puppeteer, pulling the strings behind the scenes and controlling the criminal's behavior. The strangeness of such explanation is especially obvious when genes are invoked. The genome seems to be conceived of as a ghost in the machine causing behaviors directly, bypassing the will of the agent. But in reality, to the extent that genes influence behavior, they do it in a highly indirect fashion through genetic control of developmental and biochemical processes implicated in the formation and functioning of various brain areas. Similarly, other determinisms of a broadly biographical nature (invoking, for example, psychology, societal conditioning, culture) are efficacious if and only if they influence brain structure and function in some way. So the defendant should perhaps say: "Your Honor, my brain made me do it," while her attorney adds: "Please consider my client's fMRI brain scan. Doesn't that prefrontal cortex look kind of messed up?"Arthur Caplan made this prediction some years ago: "In ten years there will be a show called *My Brain Made Me Do It.*" (in Marcus 2002).

Nevertheless, a clever judge might retort: "Well of course your brain made you do it! But why should that be an excuse? After all, you admit that you did it, not someone else. Furthermore, if, as the best materialist philosophers have shown, the brain IS the mind, so it is your guilty brain, which is the same thing as your guilty mind—*mens rea!*—who made you do it. You are not commandeered by your brain, because your brain is YOU. Therefore YOU are guilty." Of course, the defense lawyer could still pursue an insanity defense i.e., a "diseased brain" argument, but except for the more biological focus of his plea (invoking neuroimaging data, for instance), there would not seem to be anything conceptually new in the logic of his argument, as compared to how a traditional insanity defense might have been mounted decades ago.

As a result, we could be tempted to think that involving neurodeterminism into this discussion was merely a detour leading us back to the traditional problem of legal and moral responsibility, without changing the basic configuration of the issue. Properly understood, neurodeterminism would be a kind of particular determinism, without any effect on the free will debate (the problem of determinism *tout court*). Neurodeterminism only adds a set of factors that sometimes constrain our decisions and behavior, when our brain is abnormal.

Nevertheless, this understanding of the situation is not correct, as the judge saw clearly: in reality, we did gather an interesting result along the way, namely that all determinisms "with an adjective" converge on the brain, as it were. They cannot be considered efficient causes if they do not impinge on the human brain in some way. In summary, it turns out that neurodeterminism is indeed special in the sense that other qualified determinisms are simply different pathways leading to it. Consequently it is special in a second sense, in that it appears to be a reformulation in modern scientific terms of the traditional doctrine of determinism *tout court* when it is applied to human beings. If every event that has an influence on our behavior can only have an effect through some brain events, if all brain events are determined by causal chains of events, and if every mental state is a brain state, then neurodeterminism is determinism *tout court* applied to human actions. Accordingly, for the first time in history, we are able to observe determinism *tout court* at work in our mental life. It follows that if you deny the truth of determinism *tout court* because you are a libertarian, you must deny the truth of neurodeterminism or confine it to the status of qualified determinism. So, the status you are ready to give to neurodeterminism parallels the status you are ready to give to free will.

Actually that conclusion may well be controversial but this controversy converges with the general philosophical debate about neuroscience and responsibility. More importantly perhaps, this debate tends to become less philosophical and more empirical: contemporary neurosciences and brain imaging allow us explore the functional machinery of the brain and we hope to become more and more acquainted with this machinery. We can now see particular determinisms at work, and we will see more of them in the future, observing what is going on in our brain and the mental effects it has. Advocates of determinism *tout court* claim that these advances will, in the end, give us a complete picture of the functioning of the mind; advocates of libertarian free will must deny this and claim that some mental states or events are not causally related to brain states or events. This antagonism is well-known; what is now new is that we have the idea of an empirical test of those metaphysical positions by the neurosciences (the discovery an uncaused mental event will falsify determinism, the continuing failure to discover such an event will corroborate determinism *tout court*).

The neurosciences will thus strengthen a particular concept of the human being. Will they modify accordingly our conception of human *action*? Joshua Greene and Jonathan Cohen have claimed that, for the Law, neurosciences change nothing for some authors (compatibilists such as Stephen Morse) and everything for others (hard determinists such as they) (Greene and Cohen 2004; see Morse 2006). According to them, neurosciences should change our notion of responsibility and force us to adopt a hard determinist stance together with a consequentialist concept of punishment, and logically to abandon the compatibilist stance. Are they right? Possibly, but we believe their conclusion to be premature: neurosciences are not compelling enough as yet, more empirical work will be necessary. And for the moment, the data concern the debate for and against determinism *tout court*, not the battle between hard determinism and compatibilism, since they both accept determinism *tout court*.

REFERENCES

Baertschi, B. (2005). Diderot, Cabanis and Lamarck on psycho-physical causality. *History and Philosophy of the Life Sciences*, **27**, 451–63.

Bourdieu, P., Chamboredon, J.C., and Passeron J.C. (1991). *The Craft of Sociology: Epistemological Preliminaries*. Berlin: De Gruyter.

Cabanis, P.J.G. (1980). *Rapports du physique et du moral de l'homme*. Genève: Slatkine.

Churchland, P. (2002). *Brain-Wise*. Cambridge MA: MIT Press.

Darwin, C. (1873). *The expression of the emotions in man and animals*. London: John Murray.

De Melo-Martin, I. (2005). Firing up the nature/nurture controversy: bioethics and genetic determinism. *Journal of Medical Ethics*, 31, 526–30.

Fischer, J.M. (2002). Frankfurt-type examples and semi-compatibilism. In R. Kane (ed.) *The Oxford Handbook of Free Will*, pp. 281–307. Oxford: Oxford University Press.

Greene, J. and Cohen, J. (2004). For the law, neuroscience changes nothing and everything. *Philosophical Transactions of the Royal Society B*, 358, 1451. Available at http://www.wjh. harvard.edu/~jgreene/GreeneWJH/GreeneCohenPhilTrans-04.pdf (accessed 5 September 2009).

Kane, R. (ed.) (2002). *The Oxford Handbook of Free Will*. Oxford: Oxford University Press.

Kim, J. (1998). *Mind in a Physical World*. Cambridge Mass.: MIT Press.

Marcus, S.J. (ed.) (2002). *Neuroethics, Mapping the Field*. New York: Dana Foundation.

Mauron, A. (2001). Is the genome the secular equivalent of the soul? *Science*, 291, 831–2.

Morse, S.J. (2006). Moral and legal responsibility and the new neuroscience. In J. Illes (ed.) *Neuroethics*, pp. 33–50. Oxford: Oxford University Press.

Oyama, S. (1985). *The Ontogeny of Information: Developmental Systems and Evolution*. Cambridge: Cambridge University Press.

Oyama, S., Griffiths, P.E. and Gray, R.D. (eds.) (2001). *Cycles of Contingency: Developmental Systems and Evolution*. Cambridge, MA: MIT Press.

Plomin, R., DeFries, J.C., McClearn, G.E., and McGuffin, P. (2008). *Behavioural Genetics*, 5th edition. New York: Worth Publishers.

Popper, K.R. and Eccles J.C. (1977). *The Self and its Brain*. Berlin: Springer.

Rose, S., Kamin, L.J., and Lewontin R.C. (1984). *Not in Our Genes: Biology, Ideology and Human Nature*. New York: Pantheon Books.

Searle, J.R. (2008). *Freedom and Neurobiology*. New York: Columbia University Press.

Segerstråle, U. (2001). *Defenders of the Truth: the Sociobiology Debate*. Oxford: Oxford University Press.

CHAPTER 10

THE RISE OF
NEUROESSENTIALISM

PETER B. REINER

INTRODUCTION

NEUROESSENTIALISM is the position that, for all intents and purposes, we *are* our brains (Roskies 2002). It is not so much that we are not also our genes, our bodies, members of social groups, and so on, but rather that when we conceive of ourselves, when we think of who we are as beings interacting in the world, the *we* that we think of primarily resides in our brains. The goals of this chapter are to review the scientific advances and cultural trends that have resulted in the rise of neuroessentialism, to provide a portrait of the varieties of neuroessentialist thought that draws on our current understanding of brain function, and then to use these insights to see how neuroessentialist thinking might alter the mores of society. I will argue that there are domains of modern life in which neuroessentialist thinking supports the development of policies that can be viewed as progressive and prosocial, supporting the objective of aligning innovations in the neurosciences with societal and individual values. At the same time, I shall highlight instances in which neuroessentialist thinking may have nuanced but important unintended consequences, and that proponents of this worldview should thoroughly consider the ramifications of neuroessentialist thought becoming a cultural meme.

THE RISE OF NEUROESSENTIALISM

The dawn of neuroessentialism began as long ago as the mid-1600s when Elisabeth of Bohemia posed a daunting question to Descartes as part of their long correspondence (Shapiro 2007). An early and robust challenge to dualism, her question went something like this: if there is an immaterial soul, how might it communicate with the material brain? In the succeeding 400 years, and in particular in the last 50 years as the research program of the neurosciences has matured, the weight of evidence in favor of neuroessentialism has grown considerably. Today, amongst those steeped in the neurosciences, there is little debate about the merits of neuroessentialist thinking. As one draws concentric circles around this core group, clarity on the topic gives way in some circles to folk-psychology and in others to deep philosophical discourse. It is not just that folk-psychology and its kissing cousin substance dualism are comforting, but rather that these conceptions of the world suffuse modern culture in so many ways that they are unlikely to be easily displaced.

There are serious scholars of the mind who heartily reject dualism but nonetheless disagree with neuroessentialist thinking (Bennett and Hacker 2003; Glannon 2009; Pardo and Patterson, in press). The debate as to whether neuroessentialism represents a defensible position or not is outside the scope of this chapter. Rather, the question that I wish to pursue is, "If there were widespread adoption of neuroessentialist thinking, what might be the implications for society at large?" I will argue that in some instances neuroessentialism is likely to lead to a more just society, while in others it may raise concerns. As with advances in technology, changing the worldview of humans is not to be entered into lightly.

One of the most compelling accounts of the consequences of neuroessentialist thinking is Josh Greene and Jonathan Cohen's broadside on the impact that neuroscience may have upon the law (Greene and Cohen 2004, reprinted in this volume). After making (what neuroessentialists might view to be) a credible case that discoveries in the neurosciences are increasingly chipping away at folk-intuitions about how the brain works, Greene and Cohen conclude by stating,

> ...advances in neuroscience are likely to change the way people think about human action and criminal responsibility by vividly illustrating lessons that some people appreciated long ago. Free will as we ordinarily understand it is an illusion generated by our cognitive architecture. Retributivist notions of criminal responsibility ultimately depend on this illusion, and, if we are lucky, they will give way to consequentialist ones, thus radically transforming our approach to criminal justice. At this time, the law deals firmly but mercifully with individuals whose behaviour is obviously the product of forces that are ultimately beyond their control. Some day, the law may treat all convicted criminals this way. That is, humanely. (Greene and Cohen 2004, p. 1784)

Ending on this decisive note, Greene and Cohen suggest that the relentless rise of neuroessentialist thinking will lead us away from practices that were perhaps well-intentioned but are clearly indefensible in light of modern understanding of the brain. Moreover, in this newly enlightened age, society will be guided not by the wishful thinking of folk-psychology but rather by the clear-eyed rationality of neuroessentialism.

The public is not (yet) marching in lock-step with the neuroessentialists, but there is little doubt that recent years have witnessed a groundswell of popular fascination with the workings of the human brain, with academics, journalists, and artists taking note of the trend. The cultural historian Fernando Vidal collaborating with the philosopher Francisco Ortega states that, "[f]rom public policy to the arts, from the neurosciences to theology, humans are often treated as reducible to their brains." (Ortega and Vidal 2007, p. 255). More recently, Vidal has described a phenomenon that he terms "the cerebral subject" which embodies "the ascendancy, throughout industrialized and highly medicalized societies, of a certain view of the human being." (Vidal 2009, p .6). Sociologist Scott Vrecko suggests that "explanations of the neurosciences are changing the understandings that lay individuals have of themselves and their worlds" (Vrecko 2006, p. 300). Utilizing cognitive semantic analysis of ordinary language and cultural images, Paul Rodriguez argues that, "the impact of neuroscience is an emerging, modern, common sense understanding about the reduction of behavior and mental phenomena (e.g. thoughts, desires, memories, feelings, etc.) to brain entities or processes." (Rodriguez 2006, p. 302). In a similar vein, Giovanni Frazzetto and Suzanne Anker have established a neuroculture project whose aims include documenting images and concepts associated with 21st century brain science in an explicit effort to examine their penetration in contemporary culture. In a recent paper they have argued that "we are witnessing the rise of a neuroculture (or neurocultures), in which neuroscience knowledge partakes in our daily lives, social practices and intellectual discourses" (Frazzetto and Anker 2009). Finally, journalist Marco Roth argues that in literature there has been a new trend towards the *neuronovel* that "follows a cultural (and, in psychology proper, a disciplinary) shift away from environmental and relational theories of personality back to the study of brains themselves, as the source of who we are." (Roth 2009, pp. 139–40).

In an attempt to provide quantitative support for the claim that neuroessentialist thinking is on the rise, Roland Nadler, a research intern at the National Core for Neuroethics, and I investigated the frequency of the word *neuroscience* or *neuroscientist* in the popular press (see Appendix). As can be seen in Figure 10.1, there was a 31-fold rise in the number of articles that utilized this term between 1985 and 2009.

We also considered the hypothesis that there was a general upswing in interest on the part of the public in articles about science in general, and that our data might reflect this trend rather than a specific increase in interest in the neurosciences. To test this hypothesis, we searched the same database for the term "biology," finding that there was a 5.8-fold increase in mention of this term over the time period 1985–2009. When we divided the neuroscience data by the biology data (Figure 10.2), there was still a 5.5-fold increase in the number of neuroscience articles when normalized to the increase in biology articles. Thus, the increase in neuroscience articles outstrips the overall increase in articles referring to biology.

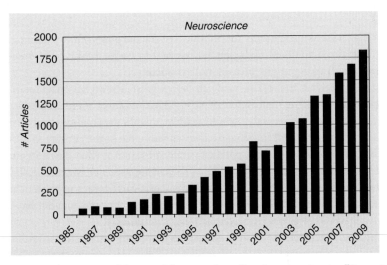

FIG. 10.1 Annual frequency of the word "neuroscience" or "neuroscientists" in major world English language newspapers for the years 1985–2009.

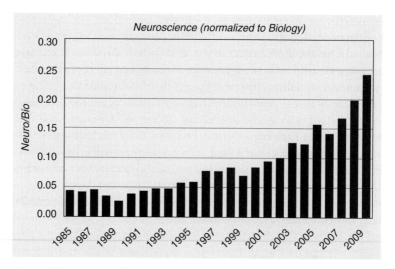

FIG. 10.2 Annual frequency of the word "neuroscience" or "neuroscientists" normalized to the occurrence of the word "biology" in major world English language newspapers for the years 1985–2009.

These data provide a measure of the incursion of neuroessentialist thinking into modern thought. It seems reasonable to conclude that, at least in certain circles, the world around us is indeed moving towards neuroessentialism as an important paradigm by which people view themselves.

THE VARIETIES OF NEUROESSENTIALISM

Neuroessentialist thinking is hardly monolithic. For the purposes of the present discussion, I will highlight three points of view that are relevant to understanding the trajectory that neuroessentialist thinking might have on modern society.

The first perspective is that of the *hard neuroessentialist*. The archetypical member of this group might be a practicing neuroscientist, steeped in the canon of modern neuroscientific thought. The hard neuroessentialist would readily provide explanations for all manner of behavior, from catching a ball to falling in love, as reducible to the activity of neuronal circuits in the brain. The hard neuroessentialist would subscribe to what Barry Stroud refers to as *naturalism* (Stroud 1996), and Owen Flanagan clarifies as *scientific naturalism* (Flanagan 2008): utter rejection of anything that hints of supernatural forces in understanding the world around us. In the realm of neuroessentialist thinking, I would suggest that this philosophical stance would best be termed *neuroscientific naturalism*.

The second perspective that I wish to describe is that of the *soft neuroessentialist*. Imagine an individual who is inquisitive, reasonably well read, and interested in human behavior—a member of the informed public, but hardly an expert in the workings of the brain. While acknowledging that the brain is the primary seat of behavior, the soft neuroessentialist remains somewhat uncomfortable in ascribing all of human behavior to the workings of the brain. When pressed, the soft neuroessentialist might agree with the logical position that the brain is the ultimate seat of behavior, but they also harbor intuitions, consciously or unconsciously, at variance with neuroscientific naturalism. These intuitions may be the result of general enculturation, religious beliefs in such non-material phenomena as a divinity, an afterlife, etc., or even skepticism with the program of modern scientific progress. This hypothetical conflicted soft neuroessentialist dominates the cultural audience whose worldview might be expected to be modified by the images and concepts of modern neuroscience, such as those curated in the neuroculture project (Frazzetto and Anker 2009).

The final example in our hypothetical triad is that of a *neuroessentialist naïf* who has not only had no exposure to modern neuroscience, but has not considered the contribution that brains make to behavior. It is not so much that the naïf denies the role of brain in behavior; rather, the issue lies outside of his or her worldview.

Towards a neurobiology of neuroessentialist thought

In thinking about the impact that the rise of neuroessentialist thinking has upon society, and in particular what impact it might have on soft neuroessentialists, it is worth briefly reviewing a few salient observations regarding the neurobiology of decision-making in the brain. It is now well-established that our brains integrate information from disparate sources, and it is this integrative activity that ultimately results in the decisions that govern behavior. At the top of the hierarchy is the prefrontal cortex, a key structure that orchestrates thought in alignment with internal goals (Miller and Cohen 2001). The prefrontal cortex is often invoked as the region in the brain responsible for top-down control of behavior, integrating information from both cortical regions and subcortical structures. In many ways, the prefrontal cortex is the ultimate locus for logical thought.

An important conceptual advance in thinking about the neurobiology of decision-making came with the elucidation of Antonio Damasio's somatic marker hypothesis (Damasio 1996) which suggests that prior experience leads to the development of undeliberated responses to events. These responses, often but not exclusively expressed as emotions, provide important contextual information about a given situation. By so doing they provide useful constraints to the options available to the logical machinery of the prefrontal cortex. According to Haidt's social intuitionist model of moral decision-making (Haidt 2001), a particularly noteworthy feature of these inputs is that they provide *rapid* access to relevant contextual information, resulting in the sorts of intuitions that humans regularly experience in the course of everyday social cognition. Thus, one can coarsely divide decision-making in the human brain into two camps: *deliberative thought* which is relatively slow and is carried out by cortical structures such as the prefrontal cortex, and *intuitions* which provide rapid access to preconceived notions about the state of the world. Both modes of thinking are highly adaptive: deliberative thought allows us to use our intellect to assess the world around us, while intuitions allow us to react quickly to situations that merit brisk responses.

It is not just the speed of processing that distinguishes deliberative thought from intuitions. It turns out that intuitions, which have been formally studied as *implicit attitudes*

(Devos and Banaji 2003), are largely unavailable to conscious perception (Greenwald and Banaji 1995) in marked contrast to deliberative processes that primarily occur in what Stanislas Dehaene has championed as the conscious global workspace (Dehaene and Naccache 2001). Finally, while under certain conditions implicit attitudes can be demonstrated to change (Gawronski and Bodenhausen 2006), the dominant observation is that implicit attitudes are stable and resistant to modification (Wilson *et al.* 2000).

Summarizing, we find that there is a distinction between deliberative thought which involves relatively slow processing, is available to conscious perception, and is highly plastic, and intuitive implicit attitudes that provide rapid access to preconceived deductions, to a substantial degree are devoid of conscious reasoning, and are generally resistant to change.

In considering the incursion of neuroessentialist thinking upon the modern mind, these observations are relevant. Hard neuroessentialists, by definition, are those individuals who have long incorporated the neuroscientific naturalist perspective. I would further suggest that for many hard neuroessentialists, this manner of thinking would be manifest not only in their deliberative thought processes but also, to a greater or lesser degree, in their intuitive, implicit attitudes. The naïf, living outside of the realm of neuroscientific naturalism, is essentially agnostic on the issues that concern us here.

Most relevant to the present discussion is the brain of the soft neuroessentialist, the individual who I have argued is most likely to be affected by the rise of neuroessentialist thinking in popular culture. To the soft neuroessentialist, these ideas are new and intellectually challenging, and require the sort of deliberative processing exemplified by prefrontal cortical circuits. At the same time, within the brain of the soft neuroessentialist, these new ideas must compete with the long-standing, culturally imposed, and highly adaptive perspectives that have formed their implicit attitudes about the world around them. The tension between these two ways of thinking about the world will likely determine the social impact of the rise of neuroessentialist thinking.

THE NEUROBIOLOGY OF NEUROESSENTIALISM PREDICTS EFFECTS ON SOCIAL MORES

My claim is that for those categories of human behavior which allow sufficient time to consider issues in a reflective manner, neuroessentialist thinking will have an ever increasing impact upon social mores, while for those behaviors which are dominated by emotional responses, the rise of neuroessentialism will have little or no impact. Furthermore, the underlying neurobiology of decision-making by the hypothetical triad of naïf, soft, and hard neuroessentialist suggests that the effects will be most marked on those individuals who might be characterized as soft neuroessentialists. A few illustrative cases are provided next.

Retributive justice

In considering the impact that neuroscience will have on the law, Greene and Cohen argue that modern neuroscience suggests that free will "is an illusion generated by our cognitive architecture. Retributivist notions of criminal responsibility ultimately depend on this illusion" (Greene and Cohen 2004). Proponents of retributive justice argue that neuroscience has little impact upon the issue, as responsibility persists regardless of what evidence neuroscience offers (Morse 2008). It is not so much the propriety of the consequentialist or retributivist arguments that concern us here, but rather the manner in which people will evaluate the positions put forward by these two camps.

The hard neuroessentialist will readily accept the neuroscience argument about the illusion of free will (Wegner 2002), and would likely side with Greene and Cohen in this debate. Soft neuroessentialists, on the other hand, will be put in a position where they must weigh the arguments carefully, arriving at their own conclusion on the topic. Because the issue is subject to careful deliberation, I would suggest that this is precisely the sort of topic where the rise of neuroessentialism might indeed have a substantial impact. After all, the process by which jurists, legal scholars, and even jurors consider issues such as the value of retribution is one in which there is ample time for informed debate.

As optimistic as Greene and Cohen may be about the move towards a more humane manner of treating criminals, it is not clear that soft neuroessentialists, whether part of the judicial system or not, will be swayed by consequentialist arguments. Culturally inscribed intuitions about free will and moral responsibility are deeply ingrained, and it may be wishful thinking to imagine that mores will change on the basis of arguments alone. In a thoughtful essay on neuroscience and the law, David Eagleman suggests other ways in which neuroscience might alter this equation: by developing new neurotechnologies that increase the criminal justice system's ability to predict recidivism, and to develop new drugs and behavioral techniques that promote rehabilitation by modifying the brains of criminals (Eagleman 2008).

Behavioral economics

One arena of modern life in which we can expect neuroessentialist thinking to play an important role is the field of behavioral economics. As comprehensively documented by Richard Thaler and Cass Sunstein in their book *Nudge*, humans in the real world bring a range of biases to their economic decision-making and consequently behave in ways that are contrary to the frictionless behavior of classical economics (Thaler and Sunstein 2008). Drawing upon the seminal work of Tversky and Kahneman (1981), they describe the myriad ways in which underlying unconscious biases affect decisions in the economic sphere. It is noteworthy that these biases fit very nicely under the rubric of intuitions as described earlier, as they represent shorthand approaches to problem solving that are traditionally adaptive, but put the individual at a disadvantage in the world of modern economic activity.

To take but one example, most individuals will opt to receive a smaller reward today than a modestly larger reward at some future time point (Frederick *et al.* 2002). The phenomenon is called *temporal discounting* and has been extensively studied by psychologists who suggest that it is intimately related to issues of impulse control (Ainslie 1975). The dominant hypothesis is that the impetus to accept the modest reward today is driven by intuitive reasoning, even when logic suggests that waiting for the larger reward will produce a greater gain for the individual. Consistent with this hypothesis, functional magnetic resonance imaging studies have demonstrated that when people are presented with the prospect of an immediate reward, parts of the limbic system associated with the midbrain dopamine system are preferentially activated, while the prefrontal cortex is activated regardless of the temporal delay offered (McClure *et al.* 2004). One way of thinking about these data is that the immediate reward activates both the rapid response, intuitive circuitry of the brainstem (which urges us to take the reward) as well as the deliberative architecture of the prefrontal cortex (which weighs the options carefully); the delayed reward only activates the "logical" deliberative areas of the cerebral cortex. The empirical observation is that unless the delayed reward is very much greater than the near-term reward, we opt for immediate gratification. Thus, the activation of different regions of the brain provides a neurobiological explanation for temporal discounting in humans.

Understanding biases inherent in our neural circuitry, that is *neuroessentializing* our economic world, provides an opportunity to modify the economic landscape in ways that minimize the errors that humans brains are likely to make. Consider for a moment the use of credit cards. A variant of temporal discounting allows a person to maximize the value of a reward today while at the same time minimizing the increased deferred cost that interest charges add to the cost of the object. What Thaler and Sunstein (2008) suggest is that if we consider these biases in establishing the rules by which economic activity is coordinated, we can construct a more equitable society. Although they do not state it as such, what they are really saying is that if we take a neuroessentialist view of economic activity, we can "nudge" people to behave more in line with the considered reasoning of their prefrontal cortical circuitry and be less influenced by their intuitive biases.

This is not just a justification for adopting a neuroessentialist view of the world, but also an important issue of distributive justice. It is hardly the case that hard neuroessentialists are immune from the influence of unconscious biases in the economic sphere, but I would argue that these individuals are in a strong position to utilize their deliberative cortical architecture to minimize such biases. In like manner, soft neuroessentialists are reasonably well positioned to understand and mitigate these intuitive biases, although we might expect that their ability to do so would be less than that of hard neuroessentialists. On the other hand, naïfs are least equipped to analyze the situation logically, and therefore would be most helped by the sorts of nudges that Thaler and Sunstein (2008) suggest. Thus, application of neuroessentialist thinking to the world of behavioral economics is likely to make the economic sphere fairer to all.

Stigma

There is a school of thought that suggests that increased understanding of the neural basis of mental illness and addiction will reduce stigma (Rüsch *et al.* 2005). The idea is that once one understands that these maladies are caused by changes in brain chemistry, they will be viewed in a manner similar to other somatic diseases of the body. It is easy to see how this idea is, at its core, advocacy for the value of neuroessentialist thinking. Promoting the idea that brain disease is a result of altered chemistry is grounded in beneficent and utilitarian thinking, and is intended to promote enlightened social and legal policies. However, as we have argued elsewhere (Buchman *et al.*, 2010), such claims may reduce blame while paradoxically resulting in increased social distance, inscribing individuals suffering from mental illness and addiction with the mark of being *neurobiologically other*, yielding the unintended consequence of fostering discrimination.

In order to understand how this process works, it is worth remembering that at least part of the biological basis of stigma is *moral revulsion* towards individuals with infectious disease (Chapman *et al.* 2009). These intuitions presumably served an adaptive value during the millennia when humans lived as a social species and social distance prevented infection (Kurzban and Leary 2001; Schaller *et al.* 2003). This perspective dovetails very nicely with our outline of the neurobiology of neuroessentialist thought (see earlier) with intuitive processing being predominantly subcortical, quick and relatively automatic, and generally less available to conscious perception than introspective deliberation which involves relatively slow cortical processing. Together, these two cognitive processes contribute to an individual's decision about how to evaluate people with mental illness and addiction, and play an important role in the phenomenon that is commonly characterized as stigma.

How might depictions of the neural basis of mental illness and addiction affect the spectrum of neuroessentialists that we have described? I would suggest that hard neuroessentialists would readily agree with the premise that these maladies are the result of altered brain chemistry and would support compassionate treatment of these "afflicted" individuals. That is not to say that hard neuroessentialists are immune from stigma: like everyone else, they harbor implicit attitudes, and these might still result in subconscious feelings of moral disgust. Given time to consider the matter however, hard neuroessentialists would be the most likely of our triad to quell whatever feelings of moral disgust they may entertain, but if pressed to decide on the matter quickly, might well respond with behaviors consistent with traditional stigmatizing attitudes. Soft neuroessentialists might be a bit more hesitant in accepting the premise that mental illness and addiction arise secondary to a change in brain chemistry, but again, if given sufficient time and education, would likely agree; when pressed to decide quickly, they, like the hard neuroessentialists, might respond by stigmatizing the target group. Naïfs are the least likely to be swayed by the argument that mental illness and addiction are due to a change in brain chemistry, and would have the most difficult time of the three overcoming their subcortical attitudes of moral disgust. Of course, there are many individuals, be they naïfs, soft or hard neuroessentialists, who are compassionate and able to overcome inherent biases in the absence of knowledge about the neurochemical underpinnings of behavior irrespective of their views on neuroessentialism; our discussion merely highlights that fact that neuroessentialist thinking about mental illness and addiction may have unintended consequences, and that these may paradoxically increase some aspects of stigma.

These conclusions are in accord with what has been observed when individuals have been educated about the genetic attributions of mental illness and then subsequently queried on their attitudes towards the mentally ill. Jo Phelan and her colleagues have investigated the effects of describing schizophrenia as having a genetic cause upon stigma and found that while blame was indeed reduced, measures of social distance were strengthened (Phelan *et al.* 2002; Phelan 2005), and similar conclusions have emerged from the work of others (Lam and Salkovskis 2007; Bennett *et al.* 2008; Jorm and Griffiths 2008; Schnittker 2008). These observations suggest caution when attempting to modify public perception of the biological basis of mental illness and addiction via educational campaigns (Corrigan and Watson 2004; Lincoln *et al.* 2008; Henderson and Thornicroft 2009). Whether these attempts to expand neuroessentialist thinking about mental illness and stigma to the public succeed or not may depend upon the basic structure of our brains, and the ways in which moral intuitions intrude upon the decision-making process itself.

THE RISE OF NEUROESSENTIALISM AND
THE FUTURE OF SOCIETY

One of the most important functions of the field of neuroethics is to follow advances in the neurosciences and discern their potential implications for society before they have widespread impact. The rise of neuroessentialism fits well into this purview, and the current analysis provides a framework for examining not only the range of neuroessentialist thinking that appears to be emerging but also provides some guidance as to the impact that such a shift in public perception may have on society at large.

The data in Figures 10.1 and 10.2 imply that neuroessentialist thinking is indeed on the rise. An important question is whether widespread adoption of a neuroessentialist perspective may be nihilating (Roskies 2006, 2007; Doucet 2007; Farah and Heberlein 2007; Kaposy 2009). Supporting this view are two particularly noteworthy experiments in which it was demonstrated that merely reading a text which suggested that free will did not exist resulted in an increase in cheating behavior and aggression (Vohs and Schooler 2008; Baumeister *et al.* 2009). Fearing just such an outcome, there have been calls in some circles for the adoption of "necessary illusions" to forestall the emergence of an existential crisis in response to neuroessentialist thinking (Smilansky 2001; Nadelhoffer and Feltz 2007).

There is merit in this view, and certainly considering these issues carefully is worthwhile, but at the same time I would recommend that we approach the matter without undue hyperbole. As we have seen in examining the implications of neuroessentialist thinking upon three domains of modern life, retributive justice, behavioral economics, and stigma, under some circumstances there are substantial prosocial effects of expanding the impact of neuroessentialist thinking to the public at large.

The key issue is how best to strengthen the moral compass in the face of the potentially nihilating influence of neuroessentialism. It is worth recalling that neuroscientific materialism and normative ethics are distinct issues. In his treatment of this topic, Owen Flanagan helpfully points out that, "the ends of creatures constrain what is good for them" (Flanagan 2008, p. 15). That is to say that we remain social beings, and that the mores that we collectively decide to accept are ones that advance individual and collective aspirations for living well. These mores are codified in our legal system, which, for better or worse, provides guidance on such lofty issues as human rights and liberty, and more mundane issues such as property theft and illegal parking. Moreover, the mores of society are widely discussed in the news media, sometimes when a prominent figure exhibits a lapse in ethical behavior but also in the vigorous public debate of the "culture wars" (Jensen 1997). One useful suggestion would be for neuroessentialists to join social theorists and educators in calling for improvements in moral and character education (Gardner *et al.* 2002; Narvaez 2008), thereby aligning social policy with the rise of neuroessentialism.

ACKNOWLEDGEMENTS

This work is supported by a grant from the Canadian Institutes of Health Research to PBR. I thank Roland Nadler for help in preparing the data in Figures 10.1 and 10.2, members of the

Table 10.1 Major world newspapers searched

ABIX - Australasian Business Intelligence	The Canberra Times
Belfast Telegraph	The Courier Mail/The Sunday Mail (Australia)
Brisbane News	The Daily Mail and Mail on Sunday (London)
BRW Abstracts (Australia)	The Daily Star and Sunday Star
Business Day (South Africa)	The Daily Telegraph (London)
Countryman	The Daily Yomiuri (Tokyo)
Daily News (New York)	The Dominion (Wellington)
Daily Record & Sunday Mail	The Dominion Post (Wellington, New Zealand)
Daily Telegraph and Sunday Telegraph (Sydney, Australia)	The Express
	The Globe and Mail (Canada)
Financial Mail (South Africa)	The Guardian (London)
Financial Post Investing	The Herald (Glasgow)
Global News Wire	The Independent (London)
Herald Sun/Sunday Herald Sun (Melbourne, Australia)	The Irish Times
	The Japan Times
Het Financieele Dagblad (English)	The Jerusalem Post
Independent on Sunday	The Jerusalem Report
Information Bank Abstracts	The Kalgoorlie Miner
International Herald Tribune	The Mercury/Sunday Tasmanian (Australia)
Kiplinger Publications	The Mirror (The Daily Mirror and The Sunday Mirror)
Korea Herald	
Korea Times	The Moscow Times
Los Angeles Times (most recent 6 months)	The Nation (Thailand)
Moscow News	The News of the World
Newsday (most recent 6 months)	The New York Times
New Straits Times (Malaysia)	The New York Times - Biographical Materials
Northern Territory News (Australia)	The New York Times - Government Biographical Materials
South China Morning Post	
Sunday Times (South Africa)	The New Zealand Herald
Sunday Tribune	The Observer
The Advertiser/Sunday Mail (Adelaide, South Australia)	The Philadelphia Inquirer
	The Prague Post
The Age (Melbourne, Australia)	The Press (Christchurch, New Zealand)
The Australian	The Scotsman & Scotland on Sunday
The Australian Financial Review Abstracts	The Straits Times (Singapore)
The Business	The Sun
The Business Times Singapore	The Sunday Express

continued

Table 10.1 (*continued*) Major world newspapers searched

The Sunday Telegraph (London)	The Washington Post Biographical Stories
The Sunday Times (London)	The Washington Times
The Sydney Morning Herald (Australia)	The Weekender (South Africa)
The Times (London)	The West Australian
The Toronto Star	USA Today
The Toronto Sun	Wall Street Journal Abstracts
The Washington Post	Xtreme Information

National Core for Neuroethics, in particular Daniel Buchman, for many spirited discussions on the topic of neuroessentialism, and Judy Illes for her insightful comments on an earlier draft.

APPENDIX

Methods

The LexisNexis Academic Database's power search function was used (to allow us to restrict our search to major world newspapers; for full list of searched newspapers, see Table 10.1) to search for the word "neuroscience" or "neuroscientists" in English, year by year from 1985 through 2009. [The term "neuroscientists" returns results for both the singular and plural forms of the word.] We rejected terms such as brain, as preliminary searches indicated that they were more likely to deliver results related to brain diseases than interest in neuroscience per se, as well as more technical terms such as "neuroessentialism" which rarely appeared in the database. In order to test the degree to which the search term "neuroscience" or "neuroscientists" acted as a proxy for the rise of neuroessentialist thinking in newspaper articles, we examined the content of the 20 least relevant articles (defined by fewest mentions of the search term) for each year, manually scoring them for their bearing on neuroessentialist thought. The results indicated that 74% of the least relevant articles dealt with issues that could readily be attributed to neuroessentialist thinking. Given that these were the *least* relevant articles retrieved by the database search, we interpret these data as suggesting that greater than 74% of the articles included in our analysis were directly relevant to the rise of neuroessentialism.

In order to investigate whether the increase in the use of the term "neuroscience" or "neuroscientists" was secondary to a general increase in science reporting in major world newspapers, we carried out a second search using as our search term "biology." The data confirmed our hypothesis that science reporting in general increased over the time period being studied, with an observed 5.8-fold increase in the frequency of the term "biology" between 1985 and 2009. Normalizing the "neuroscience" or "neuroscientists" data to the "biology" data provided a measure of the relative rise of neuroessentialist thinking in the face of a generalized increase in science reporting.

REFERENCES

Ainslie, G. (1975). Specious reward: A behavioral theory of impulsiveness and impulse control. *Psychological Bulletin, 82,* 463–96.

Baumeister R.F., Masicampo E.J. and Dewall C.N. (2009). Prosocial benefits of feeling free: disbelief in free will increases aggression and reduces helpfulness. *Personality and Social Psychology Bulletin, 35,* 260–8.

Bennett, L., Thirlaway, K. and Murray, A. (2008). The stigmatising implications of presenting schizophrenia as a genetic disease. *Journal of Genetic Counseling, 17,* 550–9.

Bennett, M.R. and Hacker, P.M.S., (2003). *Philosophical Foundations of Neuroscience.* Malden, MA: Blackwell Publishing.

Buchman, D.Z., Illes, J. and Reiner, P.B. (2010). The paradox of addiction neuroscience. *Neuroscience* [EPub June 22, 2010]. *Neuroethics.*

Chapman H.A., Kim D.A., Susskind J.M. and Anderson, A.K. (2009). In bad taste: evidence for the oral origins of moral disgust. *Science, 323,* 1222–6.

Corrigan, P., and Watson, A. (2004). At issue: stop the stigma: call mental illness a brain disease. *Schizophrenia Bulletin, 30,* 477–9.

Damasio, A. (1996). The somatic marker hypothesis and the possible functions of the prefrontal cortex. *Philosophical Transactions of the Royal Society B, 351,* 1413–20.

Dehaene, S. and Naccache, L. (2001). Towards a cognitive neuroscience of consciousness: basic evidence and a workspace framework. *Cognition, 79,* 1–37.

Devos, T. and Banaji, M. (2003). Implicit self and identity. *Annals of the New York Academy of Sciences, 1001,* 177–211.

Doucet, H. (2007). Anthropological challenges raised by neuroscience: some ethical reflections. *Cambridge Quarterly of Healthcare Ethics, 16,* 1–8.

Eagleman, D.M. (2008). Neuroscience and the law. *Houston Lawyer, 16,* 36–40.

Farah, M. and Heberlein, A. (2007). Personhood and neuroscience: naturalizing or nihilating? *American Journal of Bioethics, 7,* 37–48.

Flanagan, O. (2007). *The Really Hard Problem: Finding Meaning in a Material World.* Cambridge, MA: MIT Press.

Flanagan, O., Sarkissian, H. and Wong, D. (2007). Naturalizing ethics. In W. Sinnott-Armstrong (ed.) *Moral Psychology: The Evolution of Morality,* pp. 1–26. Cambridge, MA: MIT Press.

Frazzetto, G. and Anker, S. (2009). Neuroculture. *Nature Reviews Neuroscience, 10,* 815–21.

Frederick S., Loewenstein, G. and O'Donoghue, T. (2002). Time discounting and time preference: a critical review. *Journal of Economic Literature, 40,* 351–401.

Gardner, H., Csikszentmihalyi, M., and Damon, D. (2001). *Good Work: When Excellence and Ethics Meet.* New York: Basic Books.

Gawronski, B. and Bodenhausen, G.V. (2006). Associative and propositional processes in evaluation: an integrative review of implicit and explicit attitude change. *Psychological Bulletin, 132,* 692–731.

Glannon, W. (2009). Our brains are not us. *Bioethics, 23,* 321–9.

Greene, J., and Cohen, J. (2004). For the law, neuroscience changes nothing and everything. *Philosophical Transactions of the Royal Society B, 359,* 1775–85.

Greenwald, A.G. and Banaji, M.R. (1995). Implicit social cognition: attitudes, self-esteem, and stereotypes. *Psychological Review,* **102,** 4–27.

Haidt, J. (2001). The emotional dog and its rational tail: A social intuitionist approach to moral judgment. *Psychological Review,* **108,** 814–34.

Henderson, C. and Thornicroft, G. (2009). Stigma and discrimination in mental illness: time to change. *Lancet,* **373,** 1928–30.

Jensen, L.A. (1997). Different worldviews, different morals: America's culture war divide. *Human Development,* **40,** 325–44.

Jorm, A.F. and Griffiths, K.M. (2008). The public's stigmatizing attitudes towards people with mental disorders: how important are biomedical conceptualizations? *Acta Psychiatrica Scandinavica,* **118,** 315–21.

Kaposy, C. (2009). Will neuroscientific discoveries about free will and selfhood change our ethical practices? *Neuroethics,* **2,** 51–9.

Kurzban, R. and Leary, M. (2001). Evolutionary origins of stigmatization: the functions of social exclusion. *Psychological Bulletin,* **2,** 187–208.

Lam, D., and Salkovskis, P. (2007). An experimental investigation of the impact of biological and psychological causal explanations on anxious and depressed patients' perception of a person with panic disorder. *Behaviour Research and Therapy,* **45,** 405–11.

Lincoln, T.M., Arens, E., Berger, C. and Rief, W. (2008). Can antistigma campaigns be improved? A test of the impact of biogenetic vs. psychosocial causal explanations on implicit and explicit attitudes to schizophrenia. *Schizophrenia Bulletin,* **34,** 984–94.

McClure S.M., Laibson D.I., Loewenstein G. and Cohen J.D. (2004). Separate neural systems value immediate and delayed monetary rewards. *Science,* **306,** 503–7.

Miller, E.K. and Cohen, J.D. (2001). An integrative theory of prefrontal cortex function. *Annual Review of Neuroscience,* **24,** 167–202.

Morse, S. (2008). Determinism and the death of folk psychology: two challenges to responsibility from neuroscience. *Minnesota Journal of Law, Science and Technology,* **9,** 1–35.

Nadelhoffer, T. and Feltz, A. (2007). Folk intuitions, slippery slopes, and necessary fictions: an essay on Saul Smilansky's free will illusionism. *Midwest Studies in Philosophy,* **31,** 202–13.

Narvaez, D. (2008). Human flourishing and moral development: cognitive science and neurobiological perspectives on virtue development. In L. Nucci and D. Narvaez (ed.) *Handbook of Moral and Character Education,* pp. 310–27. Mahwah, NJ: Erlbaum.

Ortega, F. and Vidal, S. (2007). Mapping the cerebral subject in contemporary culture. *Electronic Journal of Communication Information and Innovation Health,* **1,** 255–9.

Pardo, M. and Patterson, D. (in press). Minds, Brains, and Norms. *Neuroethics.*

Phelan, J.C. (2005). Geneticization of deviant behavior and consequences for stigma: the case of mental illness. *Journal of Health and Social Behavior,* **46,** 307–21.

Phelan, J., Cruz-Rojas, R. and Reiff, M. (2002). Genes and stigma: the connection between perceived genetic etiology and attitudes and beliefs about mental illness. *American Journal of Psychiatric Rehabilitation,* **6,** 159–85.

Rodriguez, P. (2006). Talking brains: a cognitive semantic analysis of an emerging folk neuropsychology. *Public Understanding of Science,* **15,** 301–30.

Roskies, A. (2002). Neuroethics for the new millenium. *Neuron,* **35,** 21–3.

Roskies, A. (2006). Neuroscientific challenges to free will and responsibility. *Trends in Cognitive Sciences,* **10,** 419–23.

Roskies, A.L. (2007). Neuroethics beyond genethics. Despite the overlap between the ethics of neuroscience and genetics, there are important areas where the two diverge. *EMBO Reports*, 8, S52–S56.

Roth, M. (2009). The rise of the neuronovel. *N+1*, 8, 139–48.

Rüsch, N., Angermeyer, M.C. and Corrigan, P.W. (2005). Mental illness stigma: concepts, consequences, and initiatives to reduce stigma. *European Psychiatry*, 20, 529–39.

Schaller M., Park, J. and Faulkner, J. (2003). Prehistoric dangers and contemporary prejudices. *European Review of Social Psychology*, 14, 105–37.

Schnittker, J. (2008). An uncertain revolution: why the rise of a genetic model of mental illness has not increased tolerance. *Social Science and Medicine*, 67, 1370–81.

Shapiro, L. (ed. and trans.) (2007). *The Correspondence between Princess Elisabeth of Bohemia and Rene Descartes*. Chicago, IL: University of Chicago Press.

Smilansky, S. (2001). Free will: from nature to illusion. *Proceedings of the Aristotelian Society*, 101, 71–95.

Stroud, B. (1996). The charm of naturalism. *Proceedings and Addresses of the American Philosophical Association*, 70, 43–55.

Thaler, R.H. and Sunstein, C.R. (2008). *Nudge*. New York: Penguin Press.

Tversky, A. and Kahneman, D. (1981). The framing of decisions and the psychology of choice. *Science*, 211, 453–8.

Vidal, F. (2009). Brainhood, anthropological figure of modernity. *History of the Human Sciences*, 22, 5–36.

Vohs, K.D. and Schooler, J.W. (2008). The value of believing in free will: encouraging a belief in determinism increases cheating. *Psychological Science*, 19, 49–54.

Vrecko, S. (2006). Folk neurology and the remaking of identity. *Molecular Interventions*, 6, 300–3.

Wegner, D.M. (2002). *The Illusion of Conscious Will*. Cambridge, MA: MIT Press.

Wilson, T.D., Lindsey, S. and Schooler, T.Y. (2000). A model of dual attitudes. *Psychological Review*, 107, 101–26.

CHAPTER 11

A NEUROSCIENTIFIC APPROACH TO ADDICTION: ETHICAL CONCERNS

MARTINA RESKE AND MARTIN P. PAULUS

PREFACE

NEUROPSYCHOLOGY and, more recently neuroimaging, have added most valuable insights into the neurophysiological basis of drug addiction. This knowledge needs to be integrated into current models on drug use to achieve neuroscientists' and clinicians' goals to improve both early detection and the therapeutic process by developing more effective intervention tools. A joint effort of researchers and clinicians is needed to determine whether cerebral dysfunctions are pre-existing and therewith predisposing or an effect of cumulative drug use. However, identifying neuropsychological and new biological markers of susceptibility to drug addiction or drug relapse raise important ethical concerns, e.g. "what does it mean to be at risk for drug addiction?," "should an individual be aware of its increased risk or could that add the pressure needed to put him over the edge to consume drugs?," or "how should we approach an individual in treatment who is very likely to relapse?"

We can only begin to address these concerns if we have a clear status of the current scientific knowledge. The goal of this chapter is to outline the current status of drug addiction research as it relates to the susceptibility to drug addiction. The specific emphasis is put on the neuropsychological and neurofunctional characteristics of drug use and their relation to personality and other modulating variables.

DRUG USE: RELEVANCE, BASIS, AND
MODULATING FACTORS

Among 15–64-year-olds, the most recent World Drug Report describes annual prevalence rates of up to 17% for marijuana (Canada 17%, USA 12%, Italy and Spain 11%, UK 8%) and considerably lower rates for opiates and psychostimulants (amphetamines: Australia 3%, USA 1.6%, UK 1.3%; cocaine: USA and Spain 3%, UK 2.6%). Other studies have found that as many as 1 in 10 young Americans aged 16–25 years reported misuse of stimulants in their lifetime (Wu *et al.* 2007) and past-year prevalence of non-medical use of prescription stimulants, which has raised significant concern (Wilens *et al.* 2002), has been estimated at about 5% among those aged 18–25 years. Facing high cognitive demands in vulnerable ages, college students are known to misuse psychostimulants and were reported to have used amphetamines non-medically in the past year in 7% or in 8% in their lifetime (Teter *et al.* 2003). In addition, 5% reported past-year non-medical use of methylphenidate, and 3% reported past-year use of methamphetamine. In general, 17% of male and 11% of female US undergraduates reported lifetime non-medical prescription stimulant use (Hall *et al.* 2005). About 7 million people in the US consume marijuana at least weekly. In 2000, an estimated 76% of America's 14.8 million illicit drug users (more than 11 million people) used marijuana either alone (59%) or in conjunction with other illicit drugs (17%), and about 7 million Americans used at least once weekly (US Department of Health and Human Services Substance Abuse and Mental Health Services Administration Office of Applied Studies 1999).

Factors affecting the risk for addiction

Substance use disorders (SUDs) are both phenotypically and genetically heterogeneous, which implies that different neurobiological mechanisms contribute to the development of the disease (Wong and Schumann 2008). For instance, there is a strong genetic association between parents with SUDs and the offspring's risk for such disorders. Parental alcohol dependence and parental drug dependence are similarly associated with increased risks for nearly all offspring disorders, with offspring of alcohol and drug-dependent parents having approximately 2–3 times the odds for developing a disorder by late adolescence compared to low-risk offspring (Marmorstein *et al.* 2008). Exposure to parental smoking represents an environmental risk for substance use in adolescent offspring (Keyes *et al.* 2008). There appear to be sex-related differences in genetic versus environmental risk for substance use disorders. Specifically, whereas girls showed greater genetic risks, the risk for substance use disorders in boys was more determined by the shared environment, which typically reflects family dysfunction and deviant peers (Silberg *et al.* 2003).

On the other hand, children of parents with SUDs do not necessarily develop problem use and children without a genetic/familiar risk may show severe substance disorders. Recently, a number of externalizing or internalizing factors have been identified to be highly associated with substance use. The prevalence of *attention deficit hyperactivity disorder* (ADHD) for instance, is higher among individuals with SUDs (Arias *et al.* 2008), for review see Kalbag and Levin (2005), with estimated prevalences being up to three times higher than for the non-ADHD population. Rates of SUDs among ADHD subjects are as high as 40% (Kalbag and Levin 2005) as compared to the general public showing a ratio of about 15% and adults with a history of ADHD hold a doubled risk for developing SUDs compared to adults without ADHD (Biederman *et al.* 1998). Clear evidence for a causal relationship between ADHD and SUDs has not been stated. Among others, Kalbag and Levin (2005) proposed that ADHD and SUDs may be based on common genetic risk factors and similar personality factors and psychosocial environmental factors and that the co-occurrence of ADHD and SUDs may derive from self-medication of ADHD symptoms. *Externalizing behavior*, i.e. an increased frequency of aggressive behavior, delinquency, and hyperactivity, is well known to constitute a risk factor for alcohol-related problems (for review see Zucker 2008) and SUDs (for review see Kendler *et al.* 2003) for the transition from adolescent to adult substance use (Lansford *et al.* 2008) as well as for poor treatment outcome (Winters *et al.* 2008). Although the construct of externalizing behavior is comprised of a set of different facets ranging from dishonesty, aggression, to illegal activities (Krueger *et al.* 2007), to be summarized as conduct symptoms in modern diagnostic classification systems, the effect of these behaviors may be due to a number of independent factors, which also include behavioral disinhibition (McGue *et al.* 2006; Iacono *et al.* 2008). For boys and girls, hyperactivity/impulsivity predicted initiation of all types of substance use, nicotine dependence, and cannabis abuse/dependence even when controlling for conduct symptoms. By contrast, relationships between inattention and substance outcomes disappeared when hyperactivity/impulsivity and conduct symptoms were controlled for. A categorical diagnosis of ADHD significantly predicted tobacco and illicit drug use only and a diagnosis of conduct disorder between the ages of 11–14 years was a powerful predictor of substance disorders at age 18 (Elkins *et al.* 2007).

Negative emotionality, i.e. the tendency to exhibit a stress response, interpersonal alienation, and aggressive behavior (Harkness *et al.* 1995), has also been shown to be related to increased use of alcohol (McGue *et al.* 1997) and other drugs (Lilienfeld and Penna 2001; Conway *et al.* 2002). However, whereas some investigators have found an increase in negative emotionality prior to use of drugs (Elkins *et al.* 2004), others did not show an increase in this construct among high-risk individuals (Swendsen *et al.* 2002) or found that the relationship did not hold up after controlling for evidence of an independent mood disorder (Riehman *et al.* 2002). These discrepancies may be due to complex gene–environment interactions, which have recently been reported for negative emotionality (Krueger *et al.* 2008). In particular, exposure to stressful live events in the presence of high negative emotionality resulted in an increased risk for subsequent drug use (King and Chassin 2008). For example, depressed mood and negative emotionality has been associated with stimulant use (Poulin 2007) and women with higher levels of depressive symptoms were more likely to use methamphetamine during a subsequent follow-up period (Semple *et al.* 2007). Moreover, individuals abusing methamphetamine were found to also report higher self-ratings of depression and anxiety (London *et al.* 2004).

Sensation seeking, i.e. the tendency to seek novel, varied, complex, and intense sensations and experiences (Zuckerman 1990), is another construct that has consistently been associated with an increased likelihood of drug use (Galizio *et al.* 1983; Jaffe and Archer 1987). Furthermore, individual differences in impulsivity and related constructs are consistently identified as key factors in the initiation and later problematic use of substances. Some authors have recently attempted to reframe thinking on adolescent impulsivity to include the positive as well as negative aspects of impulsivity as it relates to drug addiction (Gullo and Dawe 2008).

High prevalences of these psychiatric syndromes and personality traits in substance users suggest either a causal or modulating relationship. These factors may contribute both to the initial seeking out of psychoactive drugs as well as the continued use or could, as proposed for ADHD, be two expressions of the same, underlying genetic disposition or physiological basis. For example, individuals who scored high on impulsive sensation seeking reported significantly greater subjective effects following an acute administration of d-amphetamine (Kelly *et al.* 2006) but did not differ on inhibitory performance or risk-taking. Some have argued that this is mediated by the different experience high sensation seeking individuals report when using stimulants (Hutchison *et al.* 1999). These findings may relate to genetic differences across individuals. Genetic variation of the norepinephrine transporter gene for instance was found to be associated with increases in positive mood and elation after acute administration of amphetamine (Dlugos *et al.* 2007).

Large longitudinal studies carried out from early adolescence through adulthood would enable researchers to chronologically describe the development of both substance initiation, use, and problem use on the one hand and manifestations of such associated externalizing and internalizing factors on the other hand. The knowledge about the sequential development, however, would not necessarily reflect a causal relationship as one joint and underlying pathomechanism may be expressed. Huge samples and appropriate statistical approaches will be needed to further elucidate this question which can be of major impact for treatment planning. Psychoeducation and cognitive behavioral strategies could, for example, be indicated in high-risk adolescent subjects to prevent the development of substance use disorders.

Neuropsychological impairments in drug use: premorbid and predisposing or resulting from drug use?

Key symptoms of drug addiction are compulsive intake and the intense impulse to use drugs at the expense of other behaviors that could be more advantageous in the short or long term. Substance users show deficits in all three related components: (1) the expectation component based on reward predictions, the (2) compulsive "drive" component which is a motivational state, and the (3) decision-making component which is based on the motivational properties of the stimulus and the relative importance given to the expectation of immediate reward over possible long-term losses. These deficits suggest a deterioration of executive functioning, with executive functioning referring to a group of superior cognitive abilities of organization and integration. Executive functions are a flexible system performing and coordinating higher-order cognitive processes including anticipating and establishing goals, designing plans and programs, manipulation of memories, switching tasks, selective attention, self-regulation and monitoring of tasks, executive execution, and feedback and are associated with prefrontal brain functioning. They can directly contribute to drug use; they can, for example, increase the probability of drug-seeking behaviors and the vulnerability to relapse, even after long periods of abstinence. For example, response inhibition deficits are related to difficulties in controlling attentional biases and impulsive responses to drug stimuli (Hester *et al.* 2006). Further, executive dysfunctions may interfere with psychosocial behavioral treatment (Baicy and London 2007) such as cognitive behavioral therapy, currently the most effective treatments for stimulant dependence. Aharononich and colleagues (Aharonovich *et al.* 2003, 2006), for instance, reported negative correlations between cognitive performance and number of weeks in cognitive behavioral treatment or program drop-out rate. Prediction models for treatment compliance in cocaine-dependent subjects taking performance on the Stroop test , a measure for interference processing, into consideration outperformed models focusing on mood only (Streeter *et al.* 2008).

The nature of these neuropsychological deficits in substance users point towards disruptions in frontal, temporal, parietal, and basal ganglia systems. However, there is also a marked heterogeneity within dependent or abusing subjects, which may be due to both drug-related factors such as drug use patterns, e.g. drug type, duration, dosage, and drug-unrelated factors such as demography, education, psychiatric, or neurological comorbidities. Studies on neuropsychological functioning in cocaine users for instance present inconsistent results, either showing severe (Gillen *et al.* 1998) or mild deficits (Goldstein *et al.* 2004; Woicik *et al.* 2008) or a lack of neuropsychological impairments (Hoff *et al.* 1996). The majority of studies, however, reports higher-order cognitive impairments (e.g. inhibitory dysregulation), impairment on tasks involving executive control, visuoperception, psychomotor speed, verbal learning and memory (for review see Yucel *et al.* 2007) in cocaine users.

The problem of whether neuropsychological dysfunctions are pre-existing or predisposing to drug use or a consequence of cumulative drug use has not been fully solved yet. Experimentally challenging longitudinal studies would be needed to examine neuropsychological functioning through adolescence. We recently gave evidence for impaired verbal learning and memory (Reske et al. 2010a) and verbal fluency capacities (Reske et al. 2010b) in young *occasional users* of prescription stimulants and/or cocaine, thus in individuals that have not developed stimulant-related problems. These results point to potentially pre-existing cognitive dysfunctions which may have led to stimulant initiation in the first place. A few prediction-based studies, have been carried out in children at high and low risk of substance use and found that deficits in behavioral regulation (referred to as "neurobehavioral inhibition," deriving from primarily prefrontal tests) at age 16 predicted SUDs at age 19 with a 85% accuracy (Tarter *et al.* 2003; Kirisci *et al.* 2004). While both executive functioning and hyperactivity have been linked to substance abuse, childhood executive functioning served as a more salient predictor of drug use in early adolescence (Aytaclar *et al.* 1999). A series of cross-sectional neuropsychological studies has shown that cognitive performance of cocaine users depends on the length of use (Ardila *et al.* 1991; Rosselli and Ardila 1996). Others (Bolla *et al.* 2002) describe a persistent dose-related association between increasing number of joints per week and greater neurocognitive impairments (Medina *et al.* 2007) and an influence of lifetime marijuana use on psychomotor speed, complex attention, verbal memory, and sequencing. Chronic cannabis abusers in the non-toxicated state have shown impaired performance on a variety of attention, memory and executive function tasks (for review see Yucel *et al.* 2007) with deficits being attributed to duration and frequency of cannabis use and performance on cognitive tasks deteriorating with increasing years of heavy frequent cannabis use (Messinis *et al.* 2006).

Taken together, although definite conclusions as to whether neuropsychological impairments contribute to drug use cannot be drawn at this stage, it seems likely that at least subtle impairments exist prior to and potentially promote drug initiation. The emergence of neuroimaging techniques are now able to identify subtle brain dysfunctions in early drug users even in absence of subjective or neuropsychological test performance impairments. Thus, neuroimaging tools may soon help researchers and clinicians to solve this chicken and egg question. In the end, this knowledge will lead to a better understanding of the physiological basis of substance use disorders and, with practical relevance for diagnosis and treatment, to more effective and sensitive early detection tools.

Current drug use models

Drug addiction is characterized by several key characteristics: (1) chronicity; (2) compulsive, habitual use of a substance; (3) difficulty in desisting use despite recognizing the harmful consequences; and (4) high probability of relapse even if attempts at abstinence are successful (Koob and Kreek 2007). As pointed out by Rachlin, the irrationality of drug addiction can be defined as the inability to appropriately predict ones own future behavior and acting upon those predictions to maximize reinforcement in the long run (Rachlin 2007).

Several theoretical approaches have conceptualized drug addiction:

- *Incentive sensitization* The incentive sensitization model was first proposed by Robinson and Berridge in 1993 (Robinson and Berridge 1993). In its original formulation, it stated that drug-using individuals experience a sensitization or hypersensitivity to the incentive motivational effects of drugs and drug-associated stimuli, which has been paraphrased as increased "wanting" of drugs and drug-related stimuli (Robinson and Berridge 2008). Several animal studies have implicated subcortical systems and, in particular, the ventral striatum and pallidum in the sensitization of hedonic dysregulation (Pecina and Berridge 2005).

- *Allostatic dysregulation* The allostatic regulation model is an extension of the stress regulation model (McEwen 1998), which states that allostasis is an unstable state of stress in which the brain and hypothalamic, pituitary, adrenal axis are chronically dysregulated (Koob and Kreek 2007). This model, developed by Koob and Le Moal (1997), was originally based on the opponent process theory (Solomon 1980). Drugs have profound effects on the reward–stress circuit and impair the ability to maintain a homeostatic equilibrium. Thus, repeated use drives a transition of behavioral processes from an impulsive mode of action, which is driven by pleasure relief and gratification, i.e. maintained by positive reinforcement, towards a compulsive mode of action, which is driven by relief of anxiety or stress, i.e. maintained by negative reinforcement. As addiction develops, individuals engage a cue-induced reinstatement or craving circuit that maintains compulsive use and promotes relapse during attempts at abstinence (Le Moal and Koob 2007). These authors have proposed that the ventral striatum, amygdala, and top-down modulatory structures such as corticothalamic feedback loops play important roles in the maintenance of drug-taking behavior via negative reinforcement.

- *Habit formation* Robbins and Everitt (Robbins and Everitt 1999) have proposed a transition from goal-directed action to habitual behavior during the development of drug addiction. In particular, these authors hypothesize that the transition from voluntary drug-related behaviors, which are regulated by outcomes, to a habitual mode of drug-motivated responding reflects a transition from prefrontal cortical to striatal control over responding as well as a transition from ventral to more dorsal striatal subregions (Everitt and Robbins 2005). Moreover, this transition is driven by instrumental learning via action-outcome contingencies of the control over interoceptive and exteroceptive states associated with drugs. This model involves different regions of the striatum, the amygdala, as well as top-down cortical control systems.

- *Top-down and bottom-up, multi-stage failure models* Redish and colleagues (2008) recently proposed a series of decision-related vulnerabilities that break down in addiction, following a two-systems conceptualization of processing with a top-down cognitive planning system (presumed cortical) and an associative habit network (presumed striatal). Among the failure modes is an increased sensitivity to associations between stimuli and available choices. Several other important related models include that of Kalivas and colleagues, in which addiction is viewed as pathological assignment of the salience of drug stimuli and neural regulation of behavioral output in response to those stimuli (Kalivas and Volkow 2005). Bechara similarly has conceptualized addiction as an instability as well as a disrupted equilibrium between a top-down control system and a bottom-up impulsive system that results in an increased propensity to engage in short-term reward seeking behavior (Bechara 2005).

- *Interoceptive models* Several authors (Naqvi and Bechara 2008; Verdejo-Garcia and Bechara 2008) have integrated recent findings implicating the insular cortex in addiction and concluded that there are at least two types of dysfunction in addiction. First, a hyperactivity in the amygdala or impulsive system, which exaggerates the rewarding impact of available incentives; and second a hypoactivity in the prefrontal cortex or reflective system, which forecasts the long-term consequences of a given action. As a consequence, overwhelming interoceptive input may act to maintain drug-taking behavior. These authors stress the importance of the interoceptive cues associated with drug use or with conditioned stimuli that elicit specific interoceptive responses.

- *Dual-process model* Some investigators have proposed a dual-process model whereby early adolescent problem behavior is associated with an increased risk of adult psychopathology because both are indicators of a common inherited liability and because early adolescent problem behavior increases the likelihood an adolescent is exposed to high-risk environments (McGue and Iacono 2008). Iacono and colleagues have proposed that a common genetic liability to behavioral disinhibition underlies the co-occurrence of these externalizing attributes, which may be expressed as altered processing of cognitive control, impulsivity and sensitivity to reward. In addition, exposure to various environmental risks further amplifies the risk associated with the common liability, increasing the likelihood of addiction generally (Iacono *et al.* 2008). Maturation-related suboptimal executive capacities in conjunction with inefficient behavioral control and emotional dysregulation are supposed to increase the risk for substance abuse and a developmental model proposes that dysfunctions of the prefrontal cortex (PFC) may at least partially, if not predominately underlie the liability for substance use disorders (see, e.g. Ivanov *et al.* 2008; Goldstein and Volkow 2002). Altered PFC activation is also found in youth with positive family history for SUD (Fryer *et al.* 2007). Others have suggested that SUDs are consequences of imbalances between overactive "impulsive" amygdala systems, which signal pain or pleasure of immediate prospect, and weakened "reflective" prefrontal cortex system for signaling pain or pleasure of future prospect (Bechara 2005). In particular, drugs and/or conditioned stimuli associated with the availability of drug are thought to overwhelm the goal-driven cognitive resources important for exercising the willpower to resist drugs (Bechara 2005).

In summary, these models stress the importance of (1) transition from positive reinforcement or voluntary, reward-related behavior to negative reinforcement, habitual or even compulsive use; (2) delineate a circuitry that involves the striatum, amygdala, insula, and prefrontal cortex; (3) and emphasize that homeostatic nature of drug addiction and its relationship to stress-related processes.

THE FUNCTIONAL NEUROIMAGING VIEW ON SUBSTANCE USE DISORDERS

Neuroimaging is useful in linking psychologically defined processes to implementation in specific neural substrates of substance users. The following sections describe recent achievements of neuroimaging for addiction. First, recent imaging findings on relevant neuropsychological constructs such as decision making and inhibition shall be discussed in light of their implications for the understanding of the underlying processing dysfunction. Moreover, we propose that the degree of dysfunction in substance users can be more comprehensively assessed using neuroimaging, as neuroscientists are already able to assemble a picture of the physiological basis of addiction with different imaging techniques adding valuable information on the molecular, structural, and functional level, vastly exceeding the acquisition of one behavioral or experience-based measure like reaction time or craving. Neuroimaging can already be used to objectively measure symptom severity and to predict relapse which, reversely, should impact treatment planning.

Imaging neurocognitive impairments

Decision making is among the central dysfunctional behaviors in drug dependent individuals (Monterosso *et al.* 2001; Bechara *et al.* 2002; Bechara and Damasio 2002; Paulus 2007). Decision making consists of the process of transforming options into actions according to the individual's preference, which may result in experiencing an outcome that leads to a different psychological and physiological state of the decision-maker. Operationally, one can divide decision making into three stages that occur over time (Ernst and Paulus 2005): (1) the assessment and formation of preferences among possible options, (2) the selection and execution of an action (and inhibition of inappropriate actions), and (3) the experience or evaluation of an outcome. An important aspect during the first stage—assessment and formation of preferences among possible options—is to assign value or utility to each of its available options (Kahneman and Tversky 1984), which determines the preference structure within the decision-making situation. In particular, the brain must not only evaluate what is occurring now, but also what may or may not occur in the future (Montague *et al.* 2006). Examining the behavioral and brain processes underlying decision-making provides an experimental window to understand whether drugs of abuse exacerbate an individual's pre-existing inefficiency to function adaptively in everyday life. In particular, decisions by methamphetamine-dependent individuals are more influenced by the immediately preceding choice (Paulus *et al.* 2002), show a more rigid stimulus–response relationship (Paulus *et al.* 2003), and methamphetamine users are less well able to adjust their decision making to short-term versus long-term gains (Gonzalez *et al.* 2007). Neuroimaging helped identifying associated brain mechanisms. Methamphetamine users, for instance, performed a two-choice prediction task and, relative to control participants and the control task (two-choice response task), failed to activate, or activated less, regions within the dorsolateral, orbitofrontal, and right inferior cortices (Paulus *et al.* 2002). In addition, stimulant use duration could be predicted by orbitofrontal cortex activation with subjects with a shorter duration of methamphetamine use activating more within this region than subjects with a longer use history. These results hint at a progression in brain dysfunction and implications for behavior, which was supported by a follow-up study (Paulus *et al.* 2003), where days of sobriety were correlated with more activation in the left medial frontal gyrus (see later for more detail).

Inhibition, the process that overrides and reverses the execution of predominant thoughts, actions, or emotions, involves monitoring and stopping a planned or already ongoing behavior and presents one of the highest evolved human cognitive functions. It is closely linked to error processing, for example, during failed inhibition and a deficient capacity to control and inhibit behavior, psychologically manifested as irritability, reactive aggression, impulsivity, and sensation seeking, has been associated with the liability for early age onset of substance use disorders. From a theoretical point of view, inhibitory control is understood to encompass cognitive, affective, and behavioral processes modulated by the prefrontal cortex (Ivanov *et al.* 2008), which, as a top-down process, interacts with subcortical and posterior-cortical regions. Besides being found in a broad spectrum of psychiatric disorders, impaired inhibitory control is prominent in drug abuse. The majority of reports indicates that acute (de Wit *et al.* 2002b; Fillmore *et al.* 2002, 2006; Garavan *et al.* 2008), recreational (Colzato *et al.* 2007), and chronic cocaine use (Fillmore and Rush 2002; Kaufman *et al.* 2003; Li *et al.* 2006) as well as chronic methamphetamine use (Monterosso *et al.* 2005) have a negative impact on motor inhibitory control tasks. Specifically, stimulant users require more time to inhibit responses to stop-signals and show a lower probability of inhibiting responses, while response execution performance, measured via reaction times to go stimuli, did not differ (Fillmore and Rush 2002; Colzato *et al.* 2007; Li *et al.* 2008). D-amphetamine on the other hand, can improve performance on the stop task (decreasing stop times but not affecting go-times), particularly in slow stopping subjects (de Wit *et al.* 2000, 2002). Reviewing 41 brain imaging studies, Dom and colleagues (2005) documented consistent differential activation in prefrontal areas in subjects with SUD on tasks of cognitive inhibition, supporting the relevance of prefrontal structures in SUD. Along with prefrontal dysfunctions, inhibitory processing in chronic cocaine use has been associated with diminished activation of anterior cingulate (Kaufman *et al.* 2003; Li *et al.* 2008) and insular regions (Kaufman *et al.* 2003), where measures of self-reported impulse control and emotion regulation were inversely correlated to anterior cingulate (ACC) blood oxygenation level-dependent (BOLD) signal (Li *et al.* 2008). Leland and colleagues (Leland *et al.* 2008) could show that abstinent methamphetamine dependent subjects activate the ACC to cues predicting the need to inhibit responses and that subsequent inhibition success increased with ACC activation.

Imaging symptom severity

Neuroimaging has been used recently to add an objective component to evaluations of symptom severity which previously relied on patients' self reports or diagnostic assessments, which, again, depend on patients' adequate descriptions. Substance abuse and dependence are often considered an all-or-none condition which is either present or absent with dependence and abuse assumed to arise once an individual reaches a defined threshold. This categorical model which is implemented in current classification systems contradicts clinical reality, where basic elements of the dependence process may be prominent in early stages of substance use but may quantitatively change during the development of abuse or dependence. Substance use disorders are not sufficiently quantified by presence or absence of abuse or dependence (Neale *et al.* 2006). Others proposed a severity index of drug use, which takes into account the number of uses and duration of use (Verdejo-Garcia *et al.* 2004), which was shown to be negatively correlated with performance on some executive functioning measures. For example, the severity of cocaine use was inversely related to performance on the Stroop-interference test (Verdejo-Garcia *et al.* 2005) and predicted greater disinhibition behavior (Verdejo-Garcia *et al.* 2006). A series of neuropsychological studies acknowledged this matter of debate and has shown that cognitive performance of cocaine users is related to the amount of recent use (Bolla *et al.* 2000), the duration of use (Ardila *et al.* 1991; Rosselli and Ardila 1996) as well as to the recency of use (Berry *et al.* 1993; Strickland *et al.* 1993). Some (Bolla *et al.* 2002) have reported a dose-related association between increasing number of joints per week and greater neurocognitive impairments. Recent brain imaging studies aimed at the neurofunctional characterization of symptom severity. Modeling nicotine dependence parametrically, Smolka and colleagues (2006), for instance, tested the hypothesis whether brain activation elicited by smoking cues increases with severity of nicotine dependence and report significant associations of dependence measures and ACC, parahippocampal, and parietal activation. ACC activation was also reported to be related to severity of nicotine dependence (McClernon *et al.* 2008). Hong *et al.* (2009) extended the focus beyond the ACC and showed that the severity of nicotine dependence is inversely correlated with connectivity between dorsal ACC and striatum. Even short-term nicotine challenge did not abolish this relation. Subjective measures such as experienced craving were also found to be correlated with neurofunctional measures (Bonson *et al.* 2002; Brody *et al.* 2002; Smolka *et al.* 2006).

Prediction of treatment success and relapse

A central characteristic of addictive behaviors is their chronically relapsing nature (Miller *et al.* 1996). However, "relapse" represents a somewhat arbitrary binary judgment imposed on a complex clinical condition. Moreover, the use of the term "relapse" has been criticized because it connotes an unrealistic and inaccurate conception of how successful change can occur over time (Miller 1996). Relapse is a complex process and includes multiple dimensions such as the process prior to re-use of the drug, the event of using the drug, the level to which the use returns, and the consequences associated with use (Donovan 1996). Several models that stress cognitive behavioral (Marlatt and Gordon 1985), person-situation interactional (Litman *et al.* 1984), cognitive appraisal (Sanchez-Craig 1976), and outcome expectation factors (Rollnick and Heather 1982; Annis 1991) have been put forth to explain the process of relapse. On the other hand, psychobiological models of relapse have been based on opponent process and acquired motivation theories (Solomon 1980), craving or loss of control (Ludwig *et al.* 1974), urges or craving (Wise 1988), withdrawal (Mossberg *et al.* 1985; Crosby *et al.* 1991), and kindling processes (Crosby *et al.* 1991). These models focus on the fact that brain reward systems become sensitized to drugs and drug-associated stimuli (Robinson and Berridge 2000) resulting in increased "drug-wanting," which increases the susceptibility to relapse. Some investigators have suggested that relapse is best understood as having multiple and interactive determinants that vary in their temporal proximity from and their relative influence on relapse.

Several factors can predict outcomes: severity of dependence or withdrawal; psychiatric comorbidity; substance-related problems; motivation (abstinence commitment); length of treatment; negative affective states; cognitive factors; personality traits and disorders; coping skills; multiple substance abuse; contingency contracting or coercion; genetic factors; sleep architecture; urges and craving; self-efficacy; and economic and social factors (Ciraulo *et al.* 2003). Decision making, for example, has been proposed to represent an essential ingredient for understanding relapse (Allsop 1990). Performance on two tests of decision-making, but not on tests of planning, motor inhibition, reflection impulsivity, or delay discounting, was found to predict abstinence from illicit drugs at 3 months with high specificity and moderate sensitivity (Passetti *et al.* 2008). Surprisingly little research has been conducted to relate neurobiological variables to relapse susceptibility. In a longitudinal study of methamphetamine dependent individuals we used a two-choice prediction task to probe simple decision-related processing. By comparing brain activation during a two-choice response task relative to a two-choice prediction condition, we were able to separate sensorimotor processing from prediction and decision making. Individuals who engage in this task show bilateral activation of prefrontal cortex, striatum, posterior parietal cortex, and anterior insula during decision making (Paulus *et al.* 2001). Individuals who relapsed later on, but not those who did not, showed attenuated or reversed activation patterns in prefrontal, parietal, and insular cortical regions. Optimized prediction calculations based on step-wise discriminant function analyses revealed that right insula, right posterior cingulate, and right middle temporal gyrus response best differentiated between relapsing and non-relapsing methamphetamine-dependent subjects. In combination, we obtained 94% sensitivity, with 86% specificity using this approach. Using Cox regression analyses, we were also able to predict time to relapse. This study demonstrated that the attenuated activation patterns during decision making may play a critical role in processes that "set the stage" for relapse (Donovan 1996).

Drug cue-induced brain activation can also distinguish between subjects subsequently abstinent or relapsing (McClernon *et al.* 2007) and can be a better predictor of relapse than subjective reports of craving (Kosten *et al.* 2006). Focusing on striatum, ACC, and medial prefrontal cortex (mPFC), Grusser *at al.* (2004) showed that cue-induced brain activation was a better predictor of subsequent relapse in abstinent alcoholics than overt craving. Preliminary results specifically highlight roles for the medial prefrontal and sensory cortex, the anterior and posterior cingulate gyri, the insula, and the right middle temporal gyrus in relapse processes. Other studies combined initial brain scans with psychopathological and neuropsychological re-assessments in abstinent stimulant (Paulus *et al.* 2005) and cocaine (Sinha *et al.* 2005; Kosten *et al.* 2006) users, and a small sample of abstinent alcoholics (Grusser *et al.* 2004). These authors were also able to differentiate brain activation patterns of patients with subsequent drug use from those of abstinent patients.

The value of functional neuroimaging on its own compared to clinical, socio-demographical, and neuropsychological variables for the prediction of relapse in substance abuse has not been clearly delineated. A combination of data from all those modalities, however, may soon enable clinicians to deduce individual predictions, even though current imaging studies rely on group analyses. Further, other functional brain imaging techniques such as positron emission tomography (PET), single photon emission computed tomography (SPECT), and magnetoencephalography (MEG) have already proven their relevance in predicting mild cognitive impairment (Matsuda 2007) and depression (Gemar *et al.* 2007) and may also be useful for the prediction of relapse to substance use.

Treatment selection and monitoring

Clinicians recognize that psychological interventions can profoundly alter patients' sets of belief, ways of thinking, or behavior, but the putative mechanisms and underlying changes in the brain have only recently attracted the attention they deserve. Extending the initial use of functional magnetic resonance imaging (fMRI) to characterize the neural correlates of major psychiatric symptoms, researchers have now begun to develop study designs that incorporate fMRI into the treatment process directly. Indirectly or unintentionally, most substance treatments already employ paradigms that target brain areas crucial for addictive behavior. For example, prefrontal cortex functioning will be addressed by improvement of response selection by exploring advantages and disadvantages of continued drug use and the development of drug-refusal skills and coping mechanisms to overcome craving will improve dorsal ACC functioning. It has been reliably shown that training- and learning-related changes in the brain can be detected with fMRI. So far, addiction medicine, however, has only rarely integrated brain imaging in such ways but researchers recognize this necessity and usefulness (Volkow *et al.* 2004; Etkin *et al.* 2005; Moras 2006; Yucel and Lubman 2007).

Kosten and colleagues (2006) presented videotapes showing cocaine smoking to recently abstinent cocaine dependent subjects while acquiring BOLD fMRI and assessing craving. Activation in sensory, posterior cingulate, and superior temporal cortical as well as lingual and occipital gyri showed significant correlations with treatment effectiveness. Subsequent relapsers and abstinent patients differed in their activation in right temporal and precentral, left occipital, and posterior cingulate cortical regions.

Applying a Stroop test during fMRI, Brewer *et al.* (2008) found self-reported longest durations of cocaine abstinence following treatment correlated with activation of the right putamen, left ventromedial prefrontal cortex extending into the orbitofrontal cortex and ventral ACC, as well as the posterior cingulate cortex. Inverse correlations between abstinence and activation emerged for the left dorsolateral prefrontal cortex (DLPFC).

Despite these obvious findings neuroimaging can add to the diagnostic and treatment processes in addiction medicine, resistance to the idea of integrating neuroscience and psychological/pharmacological treatment can be observed among practitioners and even among neuroscientists. Efficacy of treatment, though, is more likely to be based on brain functional differences than on how a patient is diagnosed and visionaries already picture cognitive emotional stress tests to predict treatment responsiveness (Etkin *et al.* 2005). One valuable application of brain imaging to aid in the diagnostic process may be its ability to differentiate among heterogeneous substance users according to distinct etiologies, which—in turn—could help to trigger more individualized clinical interventions. Thus, neuroimaging may in the end lead to the development of a more predictive severity measure of the disease. Neuroimaging may also one day help identifying the best treatment regime for individuals with substance use disorders, for instance cognitive behavioral strategies aiming at brain areas particularly deficient or hyperactive in a given patient. Results from neuroimaging studies are promising, but more research is needed to prove specificity and selectivity.

SUBSTANCE USE IN ADOLESCENTS: THE MATURING BRAIN

Substance use typically evolves in early to mid-adolescence, a neurodevelopmentally most vulnerable and crucial point in life. The temporal and causal association between substance use and brain development is still a matter of debate, but adolescent drug use clearly needs special consideration, both clinically and scientifically, to understand involved dysfunctions, to offer treatment at early stages, and to deduce to adult drug-use problems. We here give a brief overview about drug use in adolescence and its implications for adult use.

Alcohol use is consistently high among youth in the UK, with 91% of 15–16-year-olds reporting past year drinking (Hibell *et al.* 2004), and more significantly, 68% reported past-year drunkenness. Thirty-eight per cent of 15–16-year-olds describe having tried cannabis at least once. Other drugs are used by 9% of UK adolescents, with most of the other drugs being inhalants (12%), and ecstasy (5%). The onset of substance use typically coincides with a critical maturation period of the human brain. Two key processes of brain maturation continue into adolescence and are particularly vulnerable to substance abuse: (1) synaptic refinement and (2) myelination. Synaptic refinement refers to the elimination of neural connectivity occurring after the ages of 9–11 years, when the peak number of synaptic connections is attained (Shaw *et al.* 2006). While overall brain size only changes slightly beyond early school-age (Giedd 2004), gray matter volume begins to decrease around puberty, largely due to synaptic refinement (Huttenlocher 1990) in subcortical and frontal regions which ends with the DLPFC (Gogtay *et al.* 2004). The DLPFC plays a key role in planning, organization, emotional regulation, response inhibition, and decision making, which, in return, are tightly connected to substance use. Volume increases in the hippocampus, a critical structure for encoding new information (Jernigan and Gamst 2005), and decreases in the thalamus (sensory integration) and nucleus accumbens (reward) also continue into young adulthood, concurrent with continuing myelination of the underlying white matter in this region (Jernigan and Gamst 2005). Myelination, the coating of axons of brain cells with myelin, results in the faster transmission of electrical signals along the axon shaft and causes an increase in size (or volume) of white brain matter until at least the second decade of life (Jernigan and Gamst 2005). White matter integrity in subcortical regions continues to improve until young adulthood (Snook *et al.* 2005).

Recent studies have shown that adolescence may be a period of heightened brain vulnerability for substance effects, such as alcohol (Spear and Varlinskaya 2005). Heavy drinking adolescents have been characterized with smaller volumes of the hippocampus (Medina *et al.* 2007) and prefrontal cortex (De Bellis *et al.* 2005) than age-matched non-drinkers. To date, no studies investigated effects of cannabis on neuromaturation. In reverse, however, adults who used cannabis before age 17 were shown to have smaller gray matter and larger white matter volumes than later-onset users (Wilson *et al.* 2000), suggesting abnormal progression of normal adolescent brain development. Taken together, these results emphasize the possibility that heavy drinking and early cannabis use significantly counteract adolescent neuromaturation. If substance abuse continues throughout adolescence, the brain may eventually not be able to compensate due to subtle neuronal damage, and task performance may begin to deteriorate. Female adolescents appear more vulnerable to deleterious effects of heavy drinking on brain function than males (Caldwell *et al.* 2005), suggesting an at least additional hormonal modulation.

Associated with effects on brain structural integrity, substances like alcohol, marijuana, and other drugs can have profound effects on neural substrates that are important for cognition and emotion. For example, adolescents exhibit distinct patterns of risk-taking behavior and evaluate rewards and punishments different from adults. Heavy alcohol use in adolescents is further associated with poorer scores on tests of information retrieval (Brown *et al.* 2000), attention (Tapert *et al.* 2002), and visuospatial functioning (Tapert *et al.* 2002) with impairments persisting even after extended periods of reduced or halted use (Brown *et al.* 2000; Tapert *et al.* 2002). Heavy nicotine use in adolescence has been associated with increased risk-taking propensity (Lejuez *et al.* 2003), and a longitudinal study (Tapert *et al.* 2002) of substance dependent youth suggested that more frequent adolescent stimulant use was associated with poorer attention, speeded psychomotor processing, and working memory in young adulthood. The fact that substance abuse strongly effects neuropsychological functioning is reflected by an inverse predictive association of cannabis use and follow-up attention functioning between the ages of 16–24 years (Tapert *et al.* 2002). However, some studies report no correlations between cannabis use and cognition (Teichner *et al.* 2000), and some abnormalities may predate use (Aytaclar *et al.* 1999), keeping the debate about chicken and egg open. Longitudinal studies are critical to elucidate the extent to which abnormalities pre-date the onset of regular substance use and long-term prospective studies of youth at high-risk are still urgently needed to one day enable researchers and clinicians to achieve an individual outcome prediction and therewith early-intervention possibilities.

Neuroimaging studies have shown that adolescents, compared to children and adults, differently engage neural systems, for instance, the nucleus accumbens when processing rewards and punishments. Children's accumbens response to reward is linked to anticipating negative consequences while adults' accumbens response is mainly associated with anticipating positive consequences. As opposed to both, adolescents' nucleus accumbens activity relates to the anticipation of negative and positive consequences, and has been shown to be linked to the degree of risk-related behavior.

FMRI has also revealed that adolescent heavy drinkers show greatly enhanced response to alcohol cues in attention and reward-related brain regions (Tapert *et al.* 2003) and that abnormal brain response during spatial working memory (Tapert *et al.* 2004) in adolescent heavy drinkers as compared to non-drinkers exists despite intact task performance, suggesting reorganization and compensation for subtle neuronal injury. During nicotine withdrawal, cannabis-using adolescents showed poorer verbal recall, increased posterior activation, and disrupted frontoparietal connectivity than non-cannabis users, further implying that adolescent cannabis use may disrupt memory related substrates (Jacobsen *et al.* 2007). A long-lasting negative effect of cannabis has also been described in adolescent cannabis users where an increased brain processing effort during an inhibition task was present after a month of verified abstinence in dorsolateral prefrontal, parietal, and occipital regions (Tapert *et al.* 2007). Adolescent cannabis *and* nicotine users on the other hand performed less accurately on a working memory task than nicotine-only users and non-using controls, and showed greater fMRI response in the right hippocampus relative to other groups. This suggests that adolescent cannabis users might fail to inhibit hippocampal activity, perhaps due to changes in inhibitory neurotransmission (Jacobsen *et al.* 2004). Teenagers with comorbid alcohol and cannabis use disorders performed equally well but showed DLPFC responses increased over mono-substance users, which is consistent with the idea that these individuals need to expend an increased neural or computational effort to show appropriate levels of performance (Schweinsburg *et al.* 2005).

Taken together, neuropsychological and neuroimaging studies indicate that adolescent substance use is associated with neural disadvantages, particularly regarding executive functioning, attention, and learning. This will be based on negative effects on maturation of particularly frontal brain regions. On the other hand, pre-existing structural or functional brain abnormalities may themselves put adolescents at high risk for substance abuse. Longitudinal studies comparing substance naive youth with high-risk and problem users are necessary to better clarify the interaction between substance use, neuropsychological performance, and brain function.

ETHICAL IMPLICATIONS

As results from brain imaging gain more relevance for the diagnostic process, the planning of treatment, and for predictions of clinical outcomes, researchers and clinicians will need to better anticipate and evaluate implied ethical concerns. Neuroscientists will have to comment on the accuracy, validity, and reliability of functional neuroimaging. As long as those have not been proven, measures to guarantee confidentiality have to be implemented to protect individuals from premature conclusions.

Neuroscientists, clinicians, and ethicians will have to determine if, and how, to integrate neuroimaging results into diagnosis or the course of treatment. What, for instance, does it specifically mean to be at risk for drug addiction? Should an individual be made aware of its increased risk or could that add the pressure needed to put him/her over the edge to consume drugs? What shall be the next step after a subject at high risk has been identified? Should early intervention regimens be applied?

The predictive validity of functional imaging results has to be clearly demonstrated and the cost of imaging has to be weighed against its ability to generate better predictions. Recent results, however, clearly show that fMRI results outperform current prediction models.

The medical and social consequences of predicting drug dependency or relapse, based on functional brain images, have to be acknowledged and effects on health insurance and stigmatization are obvious issues to be addressed by researchers and clinicians. It will have to be determined how we should approach an individual in treatment who is very likely to relapse. Moreover, should providers—as a consequence—suggest that a high/low-risk individual attend more or less intense treatment programs? In other areas of psychiatry early interventions are increasingly being considered. It appears that we are at a critical threshold and addiction medicine will need to discuss, identify, and in the end develop specific training and treatment tools for both diagnosis and relapse prevention.

Can imaging results be used directly, thus, can neuroscience help to overcome characterized cerebral dysfunctions? New applications such as neurofeedback using fMRI signal are appealing, but their transfer into patients' lives outside the brain scanner have to be elaborated. On the other hand, cognitive behavioral therapy may develop trainings and treatments particularly addressing certain brain areas known to be deficient or overactive in drug users. While it seems unlikely, it cannot be ruled out that individuals at high risk or already-abusing subjects may be liable to increased stress of such neuroimaging testing. Along with results from neuroimaging investigations, it may add pressure or stress on the individual, potentially increasing risks involuntarily.

Lastly, neuroscientists along with clinicians and ethicians will need to discuss the legal responsibility and consequences of the identified neural basis of substance addiction. Is someone with substance addiction responsible for his/her actions? One popular philosophical view on drug use was originally formulated by Harry G. Frankfurt (1971) when elaborating his theory on the freedom of the will. Frankfurt discusses the concept of the free will, specifically drawing on examples of substance-dependent subjects. In his terms, a human, in contrast to most animals, has the peculiar characteristic of having "second-order desires." Besides the wanting (e.g. consuming a drug) and choosing and being moved to do this or that, which would be subsumed under "first-order desires" in Frankfurt's words, humans are also able to want to have (or not to have) certain desires and motives, thus, have the capacity for reflective self-evaluation. Individuals, however, who do have first-order desires but—independent of whether they have or not have second-order desires—have no second-order *volitions* (a person wants a certain desire to be his/her will), Frankfurt calls "*wantons*." The distinction between a person and a wanton is explained illustrating "two narcotic addicts," sharing the same physiological condition accounting for the addiction and both sharing a periodic desire for the drug. One of those dependent subjects hates his addiction and always struggles desperately, trying to overcome his addition. He has conflicting first-order desires as he wants to take the drug and to refrain from using it. In addition to these first-order desires, this dependent *person* has a second-order volition, namely to refrain from continuous use. The second, hypothetical user is a *wanton*. He uses the drug (according to his first-order desire) without being concerned whether those desires are desires by which he wants to be moved. He may have second-order desires, but he does not even reflect upon those. In Frankfurt's terms, this substance user is "not different from an animal." Further, is it supposed to be the wanton's lack of capacity for reflection or his mindless indifference to the enterprise of evaluating his own desires and motives? While the unwilling dependent person's will is not free (as the will to consume the drug is not the will he wants), this does not pose a problem to the wanton since he neither has the will he wants nor has the will that differs from the will he wants. He lacks the free will by default. Frankfurt, however, does not give an explanation as to why a substance user may be or become a person or a wanton. Philosophers and addiction medicine would need to cooperatively elaborate the practical, clinical, and legal relevance of this philosophical approach. Do certain (or all?) drugs affect second-order desires or volitions? Thus, does for instance cumulative use, whether initially wanted or not, lead to a deteriorating capacity for self-evaluation and reflection? Does continued use thus lead to dissolving a person's free will? Are those wantons responsible for their actions? Neuroscientists, clinicians, ethicians, and maybe lawyers will need to closely collaborate to solve pressing challenges deriving from recent neuroimaging findings, such as to which extent is it a substance dependent person responsible for his/her actions? If he is not, what are the consequences? Can neuroscientists and clinicians identify increased risks for deviant behaviors? Do neuroscientists and clinicians have the tools to prevent those or should the legal system be involved only? This dialogue should urgently be addressed and will be realizable if professional boundaries based on different theoretical constructs, communication strategies, and scientific backgrounds can be overcome.

SUMMARY/PROSPECTS

Although functional brain imaging has become a powerful tool to investigate the physiological basis of neuropsychiatric disorders, it has only very recently been integrated into the diagnosis and treatment of SUDs. Since MRI instruments are widely available, the use new developments in magnetic resonance technology for identifying subjects at high risk, for treatment monitoring, and predicting individual differences in treatment responses and relapses is particularly appealing. In order for neuroimaging to play a critical clinical role for SUDs, its sensitivity and specificity must be documented. Thus far, most imaging studies have revealed intriguing results at the level of groups of subjects. To become clinically and therapeutically relevant, modern brain imaging has to be taken to the next step: How should results from diffusion tensor imaging, high-resolution structural brain imaging, or functional brain imaging of cognitive or emotional tasks be integrated into the individual treatment planning? In order for this modality to be useful for defining diagnostic categories or monitoring treatment success, we need to push the limits of this technology to clearly show its ability to define clinically-relevant information on a single-subject basis. Thus, it is not sufficient to show that ill individuals differ from healthy subjects but also that recovered or asymptomatic individuals with SUDs have altered processing in specific brain structures when compared to those individuals without SUDs. Such consistent distinctions can enable us to make clinical predictions about individuals who are at high risk for experiencing exacerbation of substance use symptoms. On the other hand, most imaging studies have demonstrated surprisingly large effect sizes, which supports the idea that differences across individuals and across time within individuals may be large enough to provide meaningful results when measured on a subject-by-subject basis.

Combining neuroimaging approaches within medications studies of substance users could prove useful for targeting specific pharmacological agents to subgroups of patients, prediction of response to medication, and relapse to use. Clearly, functional neuroimaging started playing an important role in substance use disorder research.

REFERENCES

Aharonovich, E., Hasin, D.S., Brooks, A.C., Liu, X., Bisaga, A., and Nunes, E.V. (2006). Cognitive deficits predict low treatment retention in cocaine dependent patients. *Drug and Alcohol Dependence*, 81, 313–22.

Aharonovich, E., Nunes, E., and Hasin, D. (2003). Cognitive impairment, retention and abstinence among cocaine abusers in cognitive-behavioral treatment. *Drug and Alcohol Dependence*, 71, 207–11.

Allsop, S. (1990). Relapse prevention and management. *Drug and Alcohol Review*, 9, 143–53.

Annis, H.M. (1991). A cognitive-social learning approach to relapse: pharmacotherapy and relapse prevention counselling. *Alcohol Alcoholism*, 1, 527–30.

Ardila, A., Rosselli, M., and Strumwasser, S. (1991). Neuropsychological deficits in chronic cocaine abusers. *International Journal of Neuroscience*, 57, 73–9.

Arias, A.J., Gelernter, J., Chan, G., *et al.* (2008). Correlates of co-occurring ADHD in drug-dependent subjects: prevalence and features of substance dependence and psychiatric disorders. *Addiction Behaviors*, 33, 1199–207.

Aytaclar, S., Tarter, R.E., Kirisci, L., and Lu, S. (1999). Association between hyperactivity and executive cognitive functioning in childhood and substance use in early adolescence. *Journal of the American Academy of Child and Adolescent Psychiatry*, 38, 172–8.

Baicy, K. and London, E.D. (2007). Corticolimbic dysregulation and chronic methamphetamine abuse. *Addiction*, 102, 5–15.

Bechara, A. (2005). Decision making, impulse control and loss of willpower to resist drugs: a neurocognitive perspective. *Nature Neuroscience*, 8, 1458–63.

Bechara, A. and Damasio, H. (2002). Decision-making and addiction (part I): impaired activation of somatic states in substance dependent individuals when pondering decisions with negative future consequences. *Neuropsychologia*, 40, 1675–89.

Bechara, A., Dolan, S., and Hindes, A. (2002). Decision-making and addiction (part II): myopia for the future or hypersensitivity to reward? *Neuropsychologia*, 40, 1690–705.

Berry, J., van Gorp, W.G., Herzberg, D.S., *et al.* (1993). Neuropsychological deficits in abstinent cocaine abusers: preliminary findings after two weeks of abstinence. *Drug and Alcohol Dependence*, 32, 231–7.

Biederman, J., Wilens, T.E., Mick, E., Faraone, S.V., and Spencer, T. (1998). Does attention-deficit hyperactivity disorder impact the developmental course of drug and alcohol abuse and dependence? *Biological Psychiatry*, 44, 269–73.

Bolla, K.I., Funderburk, F.R., and Cadet, J.L. (2000). Differential effects of cocaine and cocaine alcohol on neurocognitive performance. *Neurology*, 54, 2285–92.

Bolla, K.I., Brown, K., Eldreth, D., Tate, K., and Cadet, J.L. (2002). Dose-related neurocognitive effects of marijuana use. *Neurology*, 59, 1337–43.

Bonson, K.R., Grant, S.J., Contoreggi, C.S., *et al.* (2002). Neural systems and cue-induced cocaine craving. *Neuropsychopharmacology*, 26, 376–86.

Brewer, J.A., Worhunsky, P.D., Carroll, K.M., Rounsaville, B.J., and Potenza, M.N. (2008). Pretreatment brain activation during stroop task is associated with outcomes in cocaine-dependent patients. *Biological Psychiatry*, 64, 998–1004.

Brody, A.L., Mandelkern, M.A., London, E.D., *et al.* (2002). Brain metabolic changes during cigarette craving. *Archives of General Psychiatry*, 59, 1162–72.

Brown, S. A., Tapert, S. F., Granholm, E. & Delis, D. C. (2000) Neurocognitive functioning of adolescents: Effects of protracted alcohol use. *Alcoholism: Clinical and Experimental Research*, 24, 164–71.

Caldwell, L.C., Schweinsburg, A.D., Nagel, B.J., Barlett, V.C., Brown, S.A. & Tapert, S.F. (2005) Gender and adolescent alcohol use disorders on BOLD (blood oxygen level dependent) response to spatial working memory. *Alcohol & Alcoholism*, 40, 194–200.

Ciraulo, D.A., Piechniczek-Buczek, J., and Iscan, E.N. (2003). Outcome predictors in substance use disorders. *Psychiatric Clinics of North America*, 26, 381–409.

Colzato, L.S., van den Wildenberg, W.P., and Hommel, B. (2007). Impaired inhibitory control in recreational cocaine users. *PLoSONE*, 2, e1143. ·

Conway, K.P., Swendsen, J.D., Rounsaville, B.J., and Merikangas, K.R. (2002). Personality, drug of choice, and comorbid psychopathology among substance abusers. *Drug and Alcohol Dependence*, 65, 225–34.

Crosby, R.D., Halikas, J.A., and Carlson, G. (1991). Pharmacotherapeutic interventions for cocaine abuse: present practices and future directions. *Journal Addictive Disorders*, 10, 13–30.

De Bellis, M.D., Narasimhan, A., Thatcher, D.L., Keshavan, M.S., Soloff, P. & Clark, D.B. (2005) *Prefrontal cortex, thalamus and cerebellar volumes in adolescents and young adults with adolescent onset alcohol use disorders and co-morbid mental disorders.* Alcoholism: Clinical and Experimental Research.

de Wit,W.H., Crean, J., and Richards, J.B. (2000). Effects of d-amphetamine and ethanol on a measure of behavioral inhibition in humans. *Behavioral Neuroscience*, 114, 830–7.

de Wit, W.H., Enggasser, J.L., and Richards, J.B. (2002). Acute administration of d-amphetamine decreases impulsivity in healthy volunteers. *Neuropsychopharmacology*, 27, 813–25.

Dlugos, A., Freitag, C., Hohoff, C., *et al.* (2007). Norepinephrine transporter gene variation modulates acute response to D-amphetamine. *Biological Psychiatry*, 61, 1296–305.

Dom, G., Sabbe, B., Hulstijn, W., and van den, B.W. (2005). Substance use disorders and the orbitofrontal cortex: systematic review of behavioural decision-making and neuroimaging studies. *British Journal of Psychiatry*, 187, 209–20.

Donovan, D.M. (1996). Assessment issues and domains in the prediction of relapse. *Addiction*, 91, 29–36.

Elkins, I.J., McGue, M., Malone, S., and Iacono, W.G. (2004). The effect of parental alcohol and drug disorders on adolescent personality. *American Journal of Psychiatry*, 161, 670–6.

Elkins, I.J., McGue, M., and Iacono, W.G. (2007). Prospective effects of attention-deficit/hyperactivity disorder, conduct disorder, and sex on adolescent substance use and abuse. *Archives of General Psychiatry*, 64, 1145–52.

Ernst, M. and Paulus, M.P. (2005). Neurobiology of decision making: a selective review from a neurocognitive and clinical perspective. *Biological Psychiatry*, 58, 596–604.

Etkin, A., Pittenger, C., Polan, H.J., and Kandel, E.R. (2005). Toward a neurobiology of psychotherapy: basic science and clinical applications. *Journal of Neuropsychiatry and Clinical Neuroscience*, 17, 145–58.

Everitt, B.J. and Robbins, T.W. (2005). Neural systems of reinforcement for drug addiction: from actions to habits to compulsion. *Nature Neuroscience*, 8, 1481–9.

Fillmore, M.T. and Rush, C.R. (2002). Impaired inhibitory control of behavior in chronic cocaine users. *Drug and Alcohol Dependence*, 66, 265–73.

Fillmore, M.T., Rush, C.R., and Hays, L. (2002). Acute effects of oral cocaine on inhibitory control of behavior in humans. *Drug and Alcohol Dependence*, 67, 157–67.

Fillmore, M.T., Rush, C.R., and Hays, L. (2006). Acute effects of cocaine in two models of inhibitory control: implications of non-linear dose effects. *Addiction*, 101, 1323–32.

Frankfurt, H.G. (1971). Freedom of the will and the concept of a person. *Journal of Philosophy*, 68, 5–20.

Fryer, S.L., Tapert, S.F., Mattson, S.N., Paulus, M.P., Spadoni, A.D., and Riley, E.P. (2007). Prenatal alcohol exposure affects frontal-striatal BOLD response during inhibitory control. *Alcoholism Clinical and Experimental Research*, 31, 1415–24.

Galizio, M., Rosenthal, D., and Stein, F.A. (1983). Sensation seeking, reinforcement, and student drug use. *Addictive Behaviors*, 8, 243–52.

Garavan, H., Kaufman, J.N., and Hester, R. (2008). Acute effects of cocaine on the neurobiology of cognitive control. *Philosophical Transactions of the Royal Society London B Biological Sciences*, 363, 3267–76.

Gemar, M.C., Segal, Z.V., Mayberg, H.S., Goldapple, K., and Carney, C. (2007). Changes in regional cerebral blood flow following mood challenge in drug-free, remitted patients with unipolar depression. *Depression and Anxiety*, 24, 597–601.

Giedd, J. N. (2004) Structural magnetic resonance imaging of the adolescent brain. *Annals of the New York Academy of Sciences*, 1021, 77–85.

Gillen, R.W., Kranzler, H.R., Bauer, L.O., Burleson, J.A., Samarel, D., and Morrison, D.J. (1998). Neuropsychologic findings in cocaine-dependent outpatients. *Progress in Neuropsychopharmacology Biological Psychiatry*, 22, 1061–76.

Goldstein, R.Z. and Volkow, N.D. (2002). Drug addiction and its underlying neurobiological basis: neuroimaging evidence for the involvement of the frontal cortex. *American Journal of Psychiatry*, 159, 1642–52.

Goldstein, R.Z., Leskovjan, A.C., Hoff, A.L., *et al.* (2004). Severity of neuropsychological impairment in cocaine and alcohol addiction: association with metabolism in the prefrontal cortex. *Neuropsychologia*, 42, 1447–58.

Gonzalez, R., Bechara, A., and Martin, E.M. (2007). Executive functions among individuals with methamphetamine or alcohol as drugs of choice: preliminary observations. *Journal of Clinical Experimental Neuropsychology*, 29, 155–9.

Gogtay, N., Giedd, J.N., Lusk, L., Hayashi, K. M., Greenstein, D., Vaituzis, A.C., Nugent, T. F., 3rd, Herman, D. H., Clasen, L.S., Toga, A.W., Rapoport, J. L. & Thompson, P. M. (2004) Dynamic mapping of human cortical development during childhood through early adulthood. *Proceedings of the National Academy of Sciences*, 101, 8174–9.

Grusser, S.M., Wrase, J., Klein, S., *et al.* (2004). Cue-induced activation of the striatum and medial prefrontal cortex is associated with subsequent relapse in abstinent alcoholics. *Psychopharmacology (Berl)*, 175, 296–302.

Gullo, M.J. and Dawe, S. (2008). Impulsivity and adolescent substance use: Rashly dismissed as "all-bad"? *Neuroscience and Biobehavioral Reviews*, 32, 1507–18.

Hall, K.M., Irwin, M.M., Bowman, K.A., Frankenberger, W., and Jewett, D.C. (2005). Illicit use of prescribed stimulant medication among college students. *Journal of American College Health*, 53, 167–74.

Harkness, A.R., Tellegen, A., and Waller, N. (1995). Differential convergence of self-report and informant data for multidimensional personality questionnaire traits: implications for the construct of negative emotionality. *Journal Personality Assessment*, 64, 185–204.

Hester, R., Dixon, V., and Garavan, H. (2006). A consistent attentional bias for drug-related material in active cocaine users across word and picture versions of the emotional Stroop task. *Drug and Alcohol Dependence*, 81, 251–7.

Hibell, B., Andersson, B., Bjarnason, T., Ahlström, S., Balakireva, O., Kokkevi, A. & Morgan, M. (2004) *The ESPAD Report 2003. Alcohol and Other Drug Use Among Students in 35 European Countries*. Stockholm: Sweden, The Swedish Council for Information on Alcohol and Other Drugs (CAN) and the Pompidou Group at the Council of Europe.

Hoff, A.L., Riordan, H., Morris, L., *et al.* (1996). Effects of crack cocaine on neurocognitive function. *Psychiatry Research*, **60**, 167–76.

Hong, L.E., Gu, H., Yang, Y., *et al.* (2009). Association of nicotine addiction and nicotine's actions with separate cingulate cortex functional circuits. *Archives of General Psychiatry*, **66**, 431–41.

Hutchison, K.E., Wood, M.D., and Swift, R. (1999). Personality factors moderate subjective and psychophysiological responses to d-amphetamine in humans. *Experimental and Clinical Psychopharmacology*, **7**, 493–501.

Huttenlocher, P. R. (1990) Morphometric study of human cerebral cortex development. *Neuropsychologia*, **28**, 517–527.

Iacono, W.G., Malone, S.M., and McGue, M. (2008). Behavioral disinhibition and the development of early-onset addiction: common and specific influences. *AnnualReviews Clinical Psychology*, **4**, 325–48.

Ivanov, I., Schulz, K.P., London, E.D., and Newcorn, J.H. (2008). Inhibitory control deficits in childhood and risk for substance use disorders: a review. *American Journal of Drug and Alcohol Abuse*, **34**, 239–58.

Jacobsen, L.K., Mencl, W.E., Westerveld, M. & Pugh, K.R. (2004) Impact of cannabis use on brain function in adolescents. *Annals of the New York Academy of Sciences*, **1021**, 384–90.

Jaffe, L.T. and Archer, R.P. (1987). The prediction of drug use among college students from MMPI, MCMI, and sensation seeking scales. *Journal Personality Assessmen*, **51**, 243–53.

Jernigan, T. & Gamst, A. (2005) Changes in volume with age: Consistency and interpretation of observed effects. *Neurobiology of Aging*, **26**, 1271–4.

Kahneman, D. and Tversky, A. (1984). Choices, values, and frames. *American Psychologist*, **39**, 341–50.

Kalbag, A.S. and Levin, F.R. (2005). Adult ADHD and substance abuse: diagnostic and treatment issues. *Substance Use and Misuse*, **40**, 1955–8.

Kalivas, P.W. and Volkow, N.D. (2005). The neural basis of addiction: a pathology of motivation and choice. *American Journal of Psychiatry*, **162**, 1403–13.

Kaufman, J.N., Ross, T.J., Stein, E.A., and Garavan, H. (2003). Cingulate hypoactivity in cocaine users during a GO-NOGO task as revealed by event-related functional magnetic resonance imaging. *Journal of Neuroscience*, **23**, 7839–43.

Kelly, T.H., Robbins, G., Martin, C.A., *et al.* (2006). Individual differences in drug abuse vulnerability: d-amphetamine and sensation-seeking status. *Psychopharmacology (Berl)*, **189**, 17–25.

Kendler, K.S., Prescott, C.A., Myers, J., and Neale, M.C. (2003). The structure of genetic and environmental risk factors for common psychiatric and substance use disorders in men and women. *Archives of General Psychiatry*, **60**, 929–37.

Keyes, M., Legrand, L.N., Iacono, W.G., and McGue, M. (2008). Parental smoking and adolescent problem behavior: an adoption study of general and specific effects. *American Journal of Psychiatry*, **165**, 1338–44.

King, K.M. and Chassin, L. (2008). Adolescent stressors, psychopathology, and young adult substance dependence: a prospective study. *Journal of Studies on Alcohol and Drugs*, **69**, 629–38.

Kirisci, L., Tarter, R.E., Vanyukov, M., Reynolds, M., and Habeych, M. (2004). Relation between cognitive distortions and neurobehavior disinhibition on the development of substance use during adolescence and substance use disorder by young adulthood: a prospective study. *Drug and Alcohol Dependence*, **76**, 125–33.

Koob, G. and Kreek, M.J. (2007). Stress, dysregulation of drug reward pathways, and the transition to drug dependence. *The American Journal of Psychiatry*, **164**, 1149–59.

Koob, G.F. and Le Moal, M. (1997). Drug abuse: hedonic homeostatic dysregulation. *Science*, **278**, 52–8.

Kosten, T.R., Scanley, B.E., Tucker, K., *et al.* (2006). Cue-induced brain activity changes and relapse in cocaine-dependent patients. *Neuropsychopharmacology*, **31**, 644–50.

Krueger, R.F., Markon, K.E., Patrick, C.J., Benning, S.D., and Kramer, M.D. (2007). Linking antisocial behavior, substance use, and personality: an integrative quantitative model of the adult externalizing spectrum. *Journal of Abnormal Psychology*, **116**, 645–66.

Krueger, R.F., South, S., Johnson, W., and Iacono, W. (2008). The heritability of personality is not always 50%: gene-environment interactions and correlations between personality and parenting. *Journal of Personality*, **76**, 1485–522.

Lansford, J.E., Erath, S., Yu, T., Pettit, G.S., Dodge, K.A., and Bates, J.E. (2008). The developmental course of illicit substance use from age 12 to 22: links with depressive, anxiety, and behavior disorders at age 18. *Journal of Child Psychology and Psychiatry*, **49**, 877–85.

Le Moal, M. and Koob, G.F. (2007). Drug addiction: pathways to the disease and pathophysiological perspectives. *European Neuropsychopharmacology*, **17**, 377–93.

Lejuez, C. W., Aklin, W. M., Jones, H. A., Richards, J. B., Strong, D. R., Kahler, C. W. & Read, J. P. (2003) The Balloon Analogue Risk Task (BART) differentiates smokers and nonsmokers. *Experimental and Clinical Psychopharmacology*, **11**, 26–33.

Leland, D.S., Arce, E., Miller, D.A., and Paulus, M.P. (2008). Anterior cingulate cortex and benefit of predictive cueing on response inhibition in stimulant dependent individuals. *Biological Psychiatry*, **63**, 184–90.

Li, C.S., Milivojevic, V., Kemp, K., Hong, K., and Sinha, R. (2006). Performance monitoring and stop signal inhibition in abstinent patients with cocaine dependence. *Drug and Alcohol Dependence*, **85**, 205–12.

Li, C.S., Huang, C., Yan, P., Bhagwagar, Z., Milivojevic, V., and Sinha, R. (2008). Neural correlates of impulse control during stop signal inhibition in cocaine-dependent men. *Neuropsychopharmacology*, **33**, 1798–806.

Lilienfeld, S.O. and Penna, S. (2001). Anxiety sensitivity: relations to psychopathy, DSM-IV personality disorder features, and personality traits. *Journal of Anxiety Disorders*, **15**, 367–93.

Litman, G.K., Stapleton, J., Oppenheim, A.N., Peleg, M. and Jackson, P. (1984). The relationship between coping behaviours, their effectiveness and alcoholism relapse and survival. *British Journal of Addiction*, **79**, 283–91.

London, E.D., Simon, S.L., Berman, S.L., *et al.* (2004). Mood disturbances and regional cerebral metabolic abnormalities in recently abstinent methamphetamine abusers. *Archives of General Psychiatry*, **61**, 73–84.

Ludwig, A.M., Wikler, A., and Stark, L.H. (1974). The first drink: psychobiological aspects of craving. *Archives of General Psychiatry*, **30**, 539–47.

Marlatt, G.A. and Gordon, J.R. (1985). Relapse prevention: maintenance strategies in the treatment of addictive behaviors. New York: Guilford Press.

Marmorstein, N.R., Iacono, W.G., and McGue, M. (2008). Alcohol and illicit drug dependence among parents: associations with offspring externalizing disorders. *Psychological Medicine*, 1–7.

Matsuda, H. (2007). The role of neuroimaging in mild cognitive impairment. *Neuropathology*, **27**, 570–7.

McClernon, F.J., Hiott, F.B., Liu, J., Salley, A.N., Behm, F.M., and Rose, J.E. (2007). Selectively reduced responses to smoking cues in amygdala following extinction-based smoking cessation: results of a preliminary functional magnetic resonance imaging study. *Addiction Biology*, **12**, 503–12.

McClernon, F.J., Kozink, R.V., and Rose, J.E. (2008). Individual differences in nicotine dependence, withdrawal symptoms, and sex predict transient fMRI-BOLD responses to smoking cues. *Neuropsychopharmacology*, **33**, 2148–57.

McEwen, B.S. (1998). Stress, adaptation, and disease. Allostasis and allostatic load. *Annals of the New York Academy of Sciences*, **840**, 33–44.

McGue, M. and Iacono, W.G. (2008). The adolescent origins of substance use disorders. *International Journal Methods in Psychiatry Research*, **17**, 30–8.

McGue, M., Slutske, W., Taylor, J., and Iacono, W.G. (1997). Personality and substance use disorders: I. Effects of gender and alcoholism subtype. *Alcoholism: Clinical and Experimental Research*, **21**, 513–20.

McGue, M., Iacono, W.G., and Krueger, R. (2006). The association of early adolescent problem behavior and adult psychopathology: a multivariate behavioral genetic perspective. *Behavior Genetics*, **36**, 591–602.

Medina, K.L., Hanson, K.L., Schweinsburg, A.D., Cohen-Zion, M., Nagel, B.J., and Tapert, S.F. (2007). Neuropsychological functioning in adolescent marijuana users: subtle deficits detectable after a month of abstinence. *Journal of the International Neuropsychological Society*, **13**, 807–20.

Messinis, L., Kyprianidou, A., Malefaki, S., and Papathanasopoulos, P. (2006). Neuropsychological deficits in long-term frequent cannabis users. *Neurology*, **66**, 737–9.

Miller, W.R. (1996). What is a relapse? Fifty ways to leave the wagon. *Addiction*, **91**(Suppl), 15–27.

Miller, W.R., Westerberg, V.S., Harris, R.J., and Tonigan, J.S. (1996). What predicts relapse? Prospective testing of antecedent models. *Addiction*, **91**(Suppl), 155–72.

Montague, P.R., King-Casas, B., and Cohen, J.D. (2006). Imaging valuation models in human choice. *Annual Reviews Neuroscience*, **29**, 417–48.

Monterosso, J., Ehrman, R., Napier, K.L., O'Brien, C.P., and Childress, A.R. (2001). Three decision-making tasks in cocaine-dependent patients: do they measure the same construct? *Addiction*, **96**, 1825–37.

Monterosso, J.R., Aron, A.R., Cordova, X., Xu, J., and London, E.D. (2005). Deficits in response inhibition associated with chronic methamphetamine abuse. *Drug and Alcohol Dependence*, **79**, 273–7.

Moras, K. (2006). The value of neuroscience strategies to accelerate progress in psychological treatment research. *Canadian Journal of Psychiatry*, **51**, 810–22.

Mossberg, D., Liljeberg, P., and Borg, S. (1985). Clinical conditions in alcoholics during long-term abstinence: a descriptive, longitudinal treatment study. *Alcohol*, **2**, 551–3.

Naqvi, N.H. and Bechara, A. (2008). The hidden island of addiction: the insula. *Trends in Neuroscience*, **32**, 56–67.

Neale, M.C., Aggen, S.H., Maes, H.H., Kubarych, T.S., and Schmitt, J.E. (2006). Methodological issues in the assessment of substance use phenotypes. *Addictive Behaviors*, **31**, 1010–34.

Passetti, F., Clark, L., Mehta, M.A., Joyce, E., and King, M. (2008). Neuropsychological predictors of clinical outcome in opiate addiction. *Drug and Alcohol Dependence*, **94**, 82–91.

Paulus, M.P. (2007). Decision-making dysfunctions in psychiatry–altered homeostatic processing? *Science*, **318**, 602–6.

Paulus, M.P., Hozack, N., Zauscher, B., *et al.* (2001). Prefrontal, parietal, and temporal cortex networks underlie decision-making in the presence of uncertainty. *Neuroimage*, **13**, 91–100.

Paulus, M.P., Hozack, N.E., Zauscher, B.E., *et al.* (2002). Behavioral and functional neuroimaging evidence for prefrontal dysfunction in methamphetamine-dependent subjects. *Neuropsychopharmacology*, **26**, 53–63.

Paulus, M.P., Hozack, N., Frank, L., Brown, G.G., and Schuckit, M.A. (2003). Decision making by methamphetamine-dependent subjects is associated with error-rate-independent decrease in prefrontal and parietal activation. *Biological Psychiatry*, **53**, 65–74.

Paulus, M.P., Tapert, S.F., and Schuckit, M.A. (2005). Neural activation patterns of methamphetamine-dependent subjects during decision making predict relapse. *Archives of General Psychiatry*, **62**, 761–68.

Pecina, S. and Berridge, K.C. (2005). Hedonic hot spot in nucleus accumbens shell: where do mu-opioids cause increased hedonic impact of sweetness? *Journal of Neuroscience*, **25**, 11777–86.

Poulin, C. (2007). From attention-deficit/hyperactivity disorder to medical stimulant use to the diversion of prescribed stimulants to non-medical stimulant use: connecting the dots. *Addiction*, **102**, 740–51.

Rachlin, H. (2007). In what sense are addicts irrational? *Drug and Alcohol Dependence*, **90**, 92–9.

Redish, A.D., Jensen, S., and Johnson, A. (2008). Addiction as vulnerabilities in the decision process. *Behavioral and Brain Sciences*, **31**, 461–87.

Riehman, K.S., Iguchi, M.Y., and Anglin, M.D. (2002). Depressive symptoms among amphetamine and cocaine users before and after substance abuse treatment. *Psychology in Addictive Behaviors*, **16**, 333–7.

Robbins, T.W. and Everitt, B.J. (1999). Drug addiction: bad habits add up [news]. *Nature*, **398**, 567–70.

Robinson, T.E. and Berridge, K.C. (1993). The neural basis of drug craving: an incentive-sensitization theory of addiction. *Brain Research Brain Research Reviews*, **18**, 247–91.

Robinson, T.E. and Berridge, K.C. (2000). The psychology and neurobiology of addiction: an incentive-sensitization view. *Addiction*, **95**, 91–117.

Robinson, T.E. and Berridge, K.C. (2008). Review. The incentive sensitization theory of addiction: some current issues. *Philosophical Transactions of the Royal Society London B Biological Sciences*, **363**, 3137–46.

Rollnick, S. and Heather, N. (1982). The application of Bandura's self-efficacy theory to abstinence-oriented alcoholism treatment. *Addictive Behaviors*, **7**, 243–50.

Rosselli, M. and Ardila, A. (1996). Cognitive effects of cocaine and polydrug abuse. *Journal of Clinical Experimental Neuropsychology*, **18**, 122–35.

Sanchez-Craig, B.M. (1976). Cognitive and behavioral coping strategies in the reappraisal of stressful social situations. *Journal of Counseling Psychology*, **23**, 7–12.

Schweinsburg, A. D., Schweinsburg, B. C., Cheung, E. H., Brown, G. G., Brown, S. A. & Tapert, S. F. (2005) fMRI response to spatial working memory in adolescents with comorbid marijuana and alcohol use disorders. *Drug and Alcohol Dependence*, **79**, 201–10.

Semple, S.J., Zians, J., Strathdee, S.A., and Patterson, T.L. (2007). Psychosocial and behavioral correlates of depressed mood among female methamphetamine users. *J Psychoactive Drugs*, **4**, 353–66.

Shaw, P., Greenstein, D., Lerch, J., Clasen, L., Lenroot, R., Gogtay, N., Evans, A., Rapoport, J. & Giedd, J. (2006) Intellectual ability and cortical development in children and adolescents. *Nature*, 440, 676–9.

Silberg, J., Rutter, M., D'Onofrio, B., and Eaves, L. (2003). Genetic and environmental risk factors in adolescent substance use. *Journal of Child Psychology and Psychiatry*, 44, 664–76.

Sinha, R., Lacadie, C., Skudlarski, P., *et al.* (2005). Neural activity associated with stress-induced cocaine craving: a functional magnetic resonance imaging study. *Psychopharmacology (Berl)*, 183, 171–80.

Smolka, M.N., Bühler, M., Klein, S., *et al.* (2006). Severity of nicotine dependence modulates cue-induced brain activity in regions involved in motor preparation and imagery. *Psychopharmacology (Berl)*, 184, 577–88.

Snook, L., Paulson, L. A., Roy, D., Phillips, L. & Beaulieu, C. (2005) Diffusion tensor imaging of neurodevelopment in children and young adults. *Neuroimage*, 26, 1164–73.

Solomon, R.L. (1980). The opponent-process theory of acquired motivation: the costs of pleasure and the benefits of pain. *American Psychology*, 35, 691–712.

Spear, L. P. & Varlinskaya, E. I. (2005) Adolescence. Alcohol sensitivity, tolerance, and intake. *Recent developments in alcoholism*, 17, 143–59.

Streeter, C.C., Terhune, D.B., Whitfield, T.H., *et al.* (2008). Performance on the Stroop predicts treatment compliance in cocaine-dependent individuals. *Neuropsychopharmacology*, 33, 827–36.

Strickland, T.L., Mena, I., Villanueva-Neyer, J., *et al.* (1993). Cerebral perfusion and neuropsychological consequences of chronic cocaine use. *Journal of Neuropsychiatry and Clinical Neuroscience*, 5, 419–27.

Swendsen, J.D., Conway, K.P., Rounsaville, B.J., and Merikangas, K.R. (2002). Are personality traits familial risk factors for substance use disorders? Results of a controlled family study. *American Journal of Psychiatry*, 159, 1760–6.

Tapert, S., Schweinsburg, A., Drummond, S., Paulus, M., Brown, S., Yang, T. & Frank, L. (2007) Functional MRI of inhibitory processing in abstinent adolescent marijuana users. *Psychopharmacology*.

Tapert, S.F., Granholm, E., Leedy, N.G. & Brown, S.A. (2002) Substance use and withdrawal: Neuropsychological functioning over 8 years in youth. *Journal of the International Neuropsychological Society*, 8, 873–83.

Tapert, S.F., Cheung, E.H., Brown, G.G., Frank, L.R., Paulus, M.P., Schweinsburg, A.D., Meloy, M.J. & Brown, S.A. (2003) Neural response to alcohol stimuli in adolescents with alcohol use disorder. *Archives of General Psychiatry*, 60, 727–35.

Tapert, S.F., Schweinsburg, A.D., Barlett, V.C., Brown, S.A., Frank, L.R., Brown, G.G. & Meloy, M.J. (2004) Blood oxygen level dependent response and spatial working memory in adolescents with alcohol use disorders. *Alcohol Clin Exp Res*, 28, 1577–86.

Teichner, G., Donohue, B., Crum, T.A., Azrin, N.H. & Golden, C.J. (2000) The relationship of neuropsychological functioning to measures of substance use in an adolescent drug abusing sample. *International Journal of Neuroscience*, 104, 113–24.

Tarter, R.E., Kirisci, L., Mezzich, A., *et al.* (2003). Neurobehavioral disinhibition in childhood predicts early age at onset of substance use disorder. *American Journal of Psychiatry*, 160, 1078–85.

Teter, C.J., McCabe, S.E., Boyd, C.J., and Guthrie, S.K. (2003). Illicit methylphenidate use in an undergraduate student sample: prevalence and risk factors. *Pharmacotherapy*, 23, 609–17.

U.S. Department of Health and Human Services Substance Abuse and Mental Health Services Administration Office of Applied Studies (1999). National household survey on drug abuse. Washington, DC: US Government Printing Office.

Verdejo-Garcia, A., and Bechara, A. (2008). A somatic marker theory of addiction. *Neuropharmacology*, 56, 48–62.

Verdejo-Garcia, A., Lopez-Torrecillas, F., Gimenez, C.O., and Perez-Garcia, M. (2004). Clinical implications and methodological challenges in the study of the neuropsychological correlates of cannabis, stimulant, and opioid abuse. *Neuropsychology Review*, 14, 1–41.

Verdejo-Garcia, A., Rivas-Perez, C., Lopez-Torrecillas, F., and Perez-Garcia, M. (2006). Differential impact of severity of drug use on frontal behavioral symptoms. *Addictive Behaviors*, 31, 1373–82.

Verdejo-Garcia, A.J., Lopez-Torrecillas, F., Guilar de, A.F., and Perez-Garcia, M. (2005). Differential effects of MDMA, cocaine, and cannabis use severity on distinctive components of the executive functions in polysubstance users: a multiple regression analysis. *Addictive Behaviors*, 30, 89–101.

Volkow, N.D., Fowler, J.S., and Wang, G.J. (2004). The addicted human brain viewed in the light of imaging studies: brain circuits and treatment strategies. *Neuropharmacology*, 47, 3–13.

Wilens, T.E., Spencer, T.J., and Biederman, J. (2002). A review of the pharmacotherapy of adults with attention-deficit/hyperactivity disorder. *Journal of Attention Disorders*, 5, 189–202.

Wilson, W., Mathew, R., Turkington, T., Hawk, T., Coleman, R.E. & Provenzale, J. (2000) Brain morphological changes and early marijuana use: a magnetic resonance and positron emission tomography study. *Journal of addictive diseases*, 19, 1–22. Winters, K.C., Stinchfield, R.D., Latimer, W.W., and Stone, A. (2008). Internalizing and externalizing behaviors and their association with the treatment of adolescents with substance use disorder. *Journal of Substance Abuse and Treatment*, 35, 269–78.

Wise, R.A. (1988). The neurobiology of craving: implications for the understanding and treatment of addiction. *Journal of Abnormal Psychology*, 97, 118–32.

Woicik, P.A., *et al.* (2008). The neuropsychology of cocaine addiction: recent cocaine use masks impairment. *Neuropsychopharmacology*, 34, 1112–22.

Wong, C.C. and Schumann, G. (2008). Review. Genetics of addictions: strategies for addressing heterogeneity and polygenicity of substance use disorders. *Philosophical Transactions of the Royal Society London B Biological Sciences*, 363, 3213–22.

Wu, L.T., Pilowsky, D.J., Schlenger, W.E., and Galvin, D.M. (2007). Misuse of methamphetamine and prescription stimulants among youths and young adults in the community. *Drug and Alcohol Dependence*, 89, 195–205.

Yucel, M. and Lubman, D.I. (2007). Neurocognitive and neuroimaging evidence of behavioural dysregulation in human drug addiction: implications for diagnosis, treatment and prevention. *Drug and Alcohol Review*, 26, 33–9.

Yucel, M., Lubman, D.I., Solowij, N., and Brewer, W.J. (2007). Understanding drug addiction: a neuropsychological perspective. *Australian and New Zealand Journal of Psychiatry*, 41, 957–68.

Zucker, R.A. (2008). Anticipating problem alcohol use developmentally from childhood into middle adulthood: what have we learned? *Addiction*, 103, 100–8.

Zuckerman, M. (1990). The psychophysiology of sensation seeking. *Journal of Personality*, 58, 313–45.

CHAPTER 12

THE NEUROBIOLOGY OF ADDICTION: IMPLICATIONS FOR VOLUNTARY CONTROL OF BEHAVIOR

STEVEN E. HYMAN

INTRODUCTION

A foundational assumption of most modern systems of morality and law is that human beings can voluntarily regulate their behavior in accord with freely chosen goals, and, when necessary, inhibit unbidden (prepotent) behavioral responses. In judicial proceedings there is a high bar for excusing illegal acts due to the perpetrator's mental state—perhaps advanced dementia, some (but not all) cases of severe psychosis, or a powerfully compelling external force such as acting with a gun pointed at one's head. It is widely understood that people are influenced by prior experience, by their biological makeup, and by the context in which they find themselves. Under most circumstances, however, such influences are not thought to extirpate free choice and behavioral control. Yet neurobiology is beginning to close the gap between diverse forms of influence and behavioral outputs with ever tighter mechanistic explanations. As a result, a central problem at the intersection of neuroscience with ethics, law, and policy is whether scientific progress has begun to erode the basis for believing that, for the most part, human behavior is under free and voluntary control, and thus whether new thinking is warranted concerning justifications for moral outrage, punishment, and policies directed toward diverse problematic behaviors. I believe that progress can be made on such ethical and policy implications of neuroscience independently of age-old philosophical discussions of free will and determinism. New findings concerning the neural mechanisms that underpin human behavior can be interpreted and applied independently of questions concerning chance and determinism in our universe. At a metaphysical level, neuroscience is less of a challenge to the concept of free will than that of an omnipotent and omniscient God, which had been at the heart of such discussions for centuries

(Roskies 2006). What is currently at stake here is a more worldly set of issues related to the moral status of individuals who transgress social conventions and laws as well as significant questions about justice (Green and Cohen 2004).

In recent years, theories of decision-making and behavioral control derived from cognitive neuroscience and other branches of neurobiology have become increasingly prominent in policy debates. The influence of such theories can be seen in diverse discussions ranging from the possible utility of mildly paternalistic applications of behavioral economics (Thaler and Sunstein 2008), to debates over involuntary treatment for drug addiction (Caplan 2008; Hall *et al.* 2008), to disagreements about the moral underpinnings of retributive justice (Greene and Cohen 2004; Snead 2008). A salient example is found in arguments made in a US Supreme Court case, Roper v. Simmons (2005). The court found it unconstitutional to impose capital punishment if a defendant was under the age of 18 at the time of the crime because that would represent a cruel and unusual punishment that is impermissible under the 8th amendment to the Constitution. The American Psychological Association and the American Medical Association argued in influential *amicus curiae* briefs, based largely on neuroimaging evidence, that the adolescent prefrontal cortex is anatomically and functionally immature, thus limiting the capacity for decision-making and impulse control. As the broad sweep of these several examples suggest, it is timely to discuss the long-term implications of research on decision-making and behavioral control. It is also important, given the excitement that often surrounds new technologies and scientific findings, to forestall a premature embrace of interim conclusions.

In this chapter I have chosen addiction as the lens through which to examine the issues of decision-making and behavioral control and their ethical implications. I have chosen to focus on addiction for several reasons. Addicted people habitually engage in apparently voluntary behaviors, such as drug seeking and drug use, that are by standard definitions of addiction, compulsive or beyond the person's control (World Health Organization 1992; American Psychiatric Association 2000). It is useful to consider what it means to engage in voluntary behaviors that one might not have intended or that one cannot control. In the case of putative behavioral addictions such as compulsive gambling, shopping, eating, or Internet use (Potenza 2006; Volkow *et al.* 2008), the question of what is meant by loss of control is even more pointed: lacking even the action of drugs, it is especially unlikely that such behavior is caused by a brain lesion (such as frontal lobe damage) or by biochemical toxicity. Such compulsions are more likely to result from the effects of normal brain mechanisms, such as experience-dependent neural plasticity, taken to an extreme.

Addiction also provides a useful window because there has been made substantial progress toward understanding its neural mechanisms, even if somewhat divergent perspectives remain (Berke and Hyman 2000; Everitt and Robbins 2005; Koob and LeMoal 2005; Hyman *et al.* 2006). At the same time, the topic of addiction directly raises significant ethical and policy issues related to autonomy and personal responsibility. If, for example, addicted people have lost control of their behavior, and thus put themselves and others at risk of harm, might involuntary treatment be ethically acceptable (Caplan 2008; Hall *et al.* 2008)? If loss of control is so severe as to be considered a symptom of a disorder or disease (World Health Organization 1992; American Psychiatric Association 2000), is punishment still justifiable for violations of the law, such as drug possession, that are direct consequences of the disorder? Do mechanistic understandings or acceptance of a disease model

(Leshner 1997) diminish the moral opprobrium that has historically attached to addicted individuals? If so, is this a societally beneficial or damaging result (Satel 1999)?

CHALLENGES TO NEUROSCIENCE

It will prove extraordinarily difficult to discover the precise mechanisms by which human beings make choices, use those choices to regulate their behavior, and conform to laws and to social norms. Without claiming too much, progress is being made. The basis for this progress includes new technologies that make it possible to investigate the human brain at work and the integration of results from multiple subdisciplines of neuroscience. Relevant neurobiological approaches include invasive physiological experiments in animals (Sugrue *et al.* 2005; Kable and Glimcher 2009), neuropsychological analysis of humans who have suffered brain lesions (Wallis 2007), cognitive neuroscience (Koechlin and Hyafil 2007; Haggard 2008; Soon *et al.* 2008), pharmacology (Robbins and Arnsten 2009), and computational neuroscience (Gold and Shadlen 2007). Nonetheless significant obstacles remain, especially for those aspects of human brain function, such as "volition" or "will," that are difficult to model in animals. Indeed agreed scientific definitions for slippery concepts such as "autonomy," "volition," and "will" remain elusive (Roskies 2010).

For both ethical and technological reasons, most current experiments in human neurobiology, including many based on functional magnetic resonance imaging (fMRI), yield correlative information rather than direct tests of causal mechanisms. That said, current methods have yielded many important new observations, and can test hypotheses concerning the spatiotemporal substrates of neural processes. For example, neuroimaging can determine which circuits are, or are not activated by a certain stimulus or cognitive task. Based on pattern analysis, it is possible, within significant constraints, to predict actions from brain imaging, even before the subject is conscious of his intentions (Haynes and Rees 2006; Norman *et al.* 2006). That said, until ethically acceptable experiments can be performed that directly and precisely examine causal mechanisms underlying cognition, we will have only limited understandings of human decision-making and behavioral control, among other aspects of cognition. Current tools to activate or inactivate human neural circuits, such as deep brain stimulation (DBS) (Mayberg *et al.* 2005) or repetitive transcranial magnetic stimulation (rTMS) (Knoch *et al.* 2009) are either limited to particular patient populations (DBS) for ethical reasons or to relatively broad swaths of cerebral cortex (rTMS) for technical reasons. In addition, DBS and rTMS may activate or inhibit circuits several synapses away from the pathways that are the direct targets of investigation. Pharmacologic tools to activate or block specific neurotransmitter or hormone receptors (Kosfeld *et al.* 2005) or other molecular targets are quite useful. Their precision is limited, however, by issues of selectivity, toxicity, and perhaps most importantly, by the distribution of the molecular target in the nervous system. Particular receptors have, as a general rule, been used by evolution for divergent functions on diverse cells and circuits. Thus it is likely that deep mechanistic understandings will only be achieved slowly and iteratively as new technologies emerge that can be applied safely to study the neural representations of human cognition and action.

Despite these current limitations, progress has been made in understanding how internally represented goals and both external and interoceptive stimuli regulate human behavior (Schultz *et al.* 1997; Miller and Cohen 2001; Montague *et al.* 2004; Wallis 2007). Much data converges on the idea that even healthy people under ordinary conditions have less control of their choices and actions than is generally believed based on introspection. Insight is also being gained into how neuropsychiatric disorders such as schizophrenia or attention deficit hyperactivity disorder degrade "top down" or "cognitive" control of behavior (Barch 2005; Gilbert and Sigman 2007; Vaidya *et al.* 2005). Perhaps the largest such body of research has focused on addiction. As described earlier, given that obtaining and taking drugs represents a series of voluntary acts, this research has not only contributed to understandings of pathogenesis and treatment, but has fueled a vibrant discussion of the degree to which addicted people can be treated as moral agents, responsible for their drug-taking behavior (Morse 2004, 2007; Hyman 2007; Caplan 2008; Hall *et al.* 2008).

Definition of addiction

The core feature of current mainstream definitions of drug addiction (World Health Organization 1992; American Psychiatric Association 2000) is compulsive drug or substance use, despite serious negative consequences. Compulsive drug use means that the affected person cannot control use for a significant period of time, despite powerful reasons to do so, such as significant drug-related health problems, family disruption, threatened job loss, or arrest. The focus on compulsive drug use as the cardinal feature of addiction improves upon older views that had focused on dependence and withdrawal. This older view proved inadequate because some highly addictive drugs such as the psychostimulants, cocaine and amphetamine, may produce mild withdrawal symptoms if any. In addition, a focus on dependence and withdrawal fails to explain why late relapses may occur long after detoxification, and may be initiated by specific drug-associated cues (O'Brien *et al.* 1998; Hyman *et al.* 2006) or by stress (Koob 2008). Finally, the focus on compulsion leaves open the possibility that behavioral states, such as compulsive gambling, might plausibly share mechanisms with drug addiction. While some severe problem gamblers describe withdrawal-like symptoms, these are far from universal; what is most salient is loss of control characterized by continued gambling despite significant debt and other negative consequences (Potenza 2006).

Stages of drug use and risk factors

Addiction is, perforce, preceded by drug experimentation, followed by a period of variable length in which use becomes regular, but is not yet compulsive. During this period of regular use, tolerance, dependence, and withdrawal symptoms may occur. With continued regular use, a subset of individuals find that they can no longer cut back without feeling intense drug urges and discover that drug seeking and drug taking are now beyond their control. Not everyone who tries drugs, whether tobacco, cocaine, or heroin, ultimately becomes a regular user or becomes addicted. Of those who become addicted, some can cease drug use without outside help, perhaps because of a change in life circumstance or perhaps as an act of will. Some who eventually find their way to treatment respond rapidly. Yet many others continue to relapse despite many attempts at treatment and remain compulsive users for decades (Hser *et al.* 2001).

Risk factors both for initiating drug use and for becoming addicted include male sex (across countries and cultures), family history, and availability of drugs in the person's environment and culture. Twin and adoption studies have demonstrated that familial risk is explained by genes rather than by shared environment. Twin studies consistently show higher rates of concordance for heavy drug use and addiction within monozygotic twin pairs than within dizygotic twin pairs (Tsuang *et al.* 1996; Merikangas *et al.* 1998). Adoption studies that have been performed in several Scandinavian countries and in the United States have focused mostly on alcoholism (Sigvardsson *et al.* 1996). These studies demonstrate that individuals adopted early in life resemble their biological rather than their adoptive parents with respect to patterns of alcohol use.

Although genes play a substantial role in vulnerability to addiction, few of the specific genetic variants that confer risk have been identified to date. Like all common neuropsychiatric disorders, addiction risk is highly genetically complex (Goldman *et al.* 2005); evidence from linkage and association studies is consistent with contributions to both risk and resilience from a very large number of allelic variants. Moreover, based on family and twin studies, there appear to be both shared and unshared genetic risk factors underlying a propensity to addiction in general, and underlying preferences for specific drugs.

It is often argued out that even if attributions of personal responsibility for drug use might be relaxed once a state of addiction has set in, individuals must be accounted responsible during earlier periods of experimentation and use. At one level this is straightforwardly the case. No matter what the temptations, the early stage drug user must have some notion of the risk, including illegality for many drugs, and should retain the capacity for impulse control. In some contexts, however, the case for simple attribution of responsibility and moral opprobrium becomes somewhat murkier. For example, within some peer cultures, for example in some colleges, approximately 80% of the students may use alcohol. After a period of years that may include periods of heavy drinking, the majority of these young people emerge as social drinkers. Perhaps one in ten of those in the initial cohort may find themselves addicted to alcohol. It would not be an easy argument to make that the majority, who do not become alcoholic, are morally superior to those who become alcoholic. They may have fewer risk factors or better luck than those who become addicted. While more of those who develop alcoholism may have alcoholic close relatives than those who settle into healthy patterns of social drinking, it is not at present possible to predict future alcoholism (Vaillant 1996).

EMOTION, MOTIVATION, AND BRAIN REWARD CIRCUITRY

Emotions are critical to the survival of individuals and species. Constituting far more than subjective feelings, emotions are transient physiological, cognitive, and behavioral responses to potentially survival-relevant stimuli. Primary emotions can be crudely divided into two broad categories by their valence. Negative emotions, such as fear, anger, and disgust may be elicited by threat, present danger, pain, or foul tastes and smells. These result in avoidance or protective behaviors. Positive emotions may be elicited by food, drink, safety, comfort, or sexual opportunities and lead to approach and consummatory behaviors. Physiological responses to either threatening or life-enhancing stimuli may include increased arousal and activation of the sympathetic nervous system. Threat may also cause release of stress hormones such as corticotropin releasing hormone, adrenocorticotropin, and cortisol. Cognitive responses include alterations in attentional state, and significantly, memory formation. Learning to predict danger may save precious seconds on a future occasion that can be the margin between life and death. Learning the circumstances under which food, water, or safety can be obtained might, in a competitive world, be the difference, e.g. between eating and starvation. Thus experiences and predictive cues learned under conditions of strong negative or positive emotion, are learned rapidly (i.e. without need for much repetition), and are relatively resistant to forgetting. Neural circuits that have been highly conserved in evolution underlie these survival functions. A "fear circuit," centered on the amygdala regulates responses to threats, and a "reward circuit" that involves dopamine-releasing neurons that project from the ventral tegmental area (VTA) of the midbrain to the nucleus accumbens (NAc), prefrontal cortex, and other forebrain structures, regulates the pursuit of positive goals.

Goals with positive survival value such as food, water, safety, and sexual opportunities act as "rewards" (Kelley and Berridge 2002). A simple operational definition of a reward is a stimulus that elicits approach and appetitive behaviors. Rewards are experienced as pleasurable, but more significantly from the point of view of survival, they are imbued with motivational or incentive properties. They are desired and activate physiological, cognitive, and behavioral responses that promote acquisition and consumption or consummation. Environmental cues that predict the availability of rewards also become imbued with motivational properties or "incentive salience" (Robinson and Berridge 2003). Such cues, like the rewards themselves, induce desire and activate responses aimed at obtaining the associated goal. Desire is intensified by motivational states of the organism, such as hunger, thirst, or perhaps, drug withdrawal symptoms. Behaviors required to obtain rewards tend to be repeated (i.e. they are reinforced), and to become automatic and highly efficient.

Natural rewards cause firing of VTA neurons and release of dopamine in the NAc and other forebrain regions. When dopamine action is blocked, whether by experimental lesions of dopamine neurons, blockade of post-synaptic dopamine receptors, or inhibition of dopamine synthesis, rewards no longer motivate approach behaviors. Dopamine release in the NAc plays the central role in binding reward-associated stimuli to reward-seeking responses including reinforcement. Dopamine release in the orbital prefrontal cortex is involved in updating of internal representations of rewards and assignment of relative values compared to other possible goals (Montague *et al.* 2004; Schoenbaum *et al.* 2006).

Dopamine neuron firing and dopamine release in response to rewards and predictive cues involves not only VTA neurons, which project to the NAc, prefrontal cortex, hippocampus, and amygdala, but also substantia nigra (SN) neurons, which project to the caudate and putamen. While dopamine is acting in the NAc to associate incentive salience with specific cues, it is acting in parallel in the caudate and putamen to consolidate programs of action aimed at efficiently obtaining rewards. Because reward seeking, a pleasurable experience if successful, tends to be repeated, associated motor programs become deeply ingrained (or overlearned) under the guidance of dopamine. Ultimately reward-seeking behaviors become automatic and come under the control of predictive cues. Under natural conditions, speed and efficiency in gaining food, water, and shelter improve the probability of survival. Over time responses to strong predictors of highly valued rewards can be characterized as stimulus-response habits (Everitt and Robbins 2005).

New insights into the role of dopamine have emerged from studies of patients with Parkinson's disease (PD) (Dagher and Robbins 2009). PD results from the death of midbrain dopamine neurons. Neurons within the SN, which project to the caudate and putamen, are more severely affected than neurons within the VTA. L-DOPA, a dopamine precursor, is an effective neurotransmitter replacement therapy early in the illness. As the disease progresses, however, there are no longer enough SN neurons to take up the L-DOPA, convert it to dopamine, and release it in the caudate and putamen. Thus drugs that can directly bind postsynaptic dopamine receptors, such as selective D_2 dopamine receptor agonists, may become necessary. A minority of patients who are treated with D_2 dopamine receptor agonists, develop striking, new risky, goal directed behaviors such as compulsive gambling or compulsive shopping. These behaviors generally cease when the D_2 agonist is withdrawn. It has been hypothesized that selective D_2 dopamine receptor agonists act within the dopamine depleted caudate and putamen to produce therapeutic effects on motor behavior. However, when combined with dopamine from preserved VTA neurons, these drugs may overstimulate the NAc and other components of reward circuitry. These observations not only underscore the role of dopamine in motivation and reward seeking, but also are consistent with the idea that compulsive gambling and related behaviors are dependent on brain reward circuitry.

THE FUNCTION OF DOPAMINE

Current theories of dopamine action in the forebrain were initially based on electrophysiological recordings from midbrain dopamine neurons in monkeys (Schultz *et al.* 1997; Schultz 2006). Similar results have subsequently been obtained in human subjects using diverse rewards, including monetary rewards combined with functional magnetic resonance imaging (fMRI). Contrary to earlier ideas, dopamine does not function as the neural representation of pleasure; rather it serves as a learning signal in diverse forebrain circuits to shape behavior so as to maximize future success in obtaining rewards. Other neurotransmitters, perhaps endogenous opioid peptides, may act as hedonic signals (i.e. signaling pleasure). Additional evidence that dissociates dopamine from hedonic signaling is the action of nicotine, a substance that causes dopamine release, and is highly addictive, but does not produce significant euphoria of the sort produced by cocaine or heroin.

The shaping of behavior to maximize future reward is dependent on the precise pattern of dopamine release. Transient changes in dopamine neuron firing send a signal to the forebrain that there is a discrepancy between expectations and actual rewards. When the test animal (or test subject) is in a resting state, dopamine neurons exhibit a slow basal rate of firing, referred to as a "tonic" firing pattern. When a reward is encountered that is not expected or greater than expected (based on already learned cues), a transient or "phasic" burst of firing occurs, causing a transient increase in synaptic dopamine. Once a particular cue predictive of reward is fully learned, dopamine neurons produce a phasic burst when that cue appears unexpectedly, but produce no additional phasic bursts if the predicted reward appears at the time expected. If, however, the predicted reward is omitted at the time when it would have been expected, there is a pause in dopamine neuron firing. Finally, once a cue is fully learned, dopamine neurons stop responding to it if it is, in turn, predicted by a prior cue. Overall, dopamine neurons fire at the earliest reliable predictor of reward and thus influence behavior to maximize future consumption of rewards. Phasic increases in firing, and thus synaptic dopamine, signify that the world is better than expected, facilitate learning of new predictive information, and to bind the newly learned predictive cues to action. Pauses signify that the world is worse than expected.

ADDICTIVE DRUGS

Addictive drugs are chemically diverse and interact with different molecular targets in the nervous system (Nestler *et al.* 2009). Unlike natural rewards, addictive drugs have no homeostatic, reproductive, or other survival value. Given their chemical differences, it is not surprising that addictive drugs exert diverse physiological and behavioral effects. For example, cocaine and amphetamines are stimulants: they increase arousal, at lower doses they enhance cognitive performance, and at higher doses they may cause anxiety and insomnia. Alcohol, in contrast, is a depressant; it is anxiolytic at low doses, and degrades cognitive and motor performance. Despite their differences, addictive drugs share the pharmacologic property of releasing dopamine in the forebrain. They share the behavioral property of being able to cause compulsive use.

Addictive drugs can be likened to Trojan horses in the brain. All addictive drugs mimic one or another of the endogenous neurotransmitters and thus interact with neurotransmitter receptors, transporters, and other signaling proteins in the brain. Cocaine, for example, resembles dopamine in such a manner that it binds to—and blocks—the dopamine transporter (DAT), which normally clears dopamine from synapses, but does not interact with dopamine receptors. Because cocaine blocks the DAT, dopamine builds up to very high levels in synapses. Opiates, nicotine, alcohol, and cannabinoids act on different receptors in the brain, but by diverse mechanisms, all ultimately cause dopamine release (Nestler *et al.* 2009; Tang and Dani 2009). (Opiates and other drugs also influence reward by other mechanisms, but this is a level of detail beyond the scope of this chapter.) Psychotropic drugs, such as tricyclic or selective serotonin reuptake inhibitor (SSRI) antidepressants that do not release dopamine, are neither rewarding nor addictive.

Because of their direct pharmacologic action, addictive drugs always cause dopamine release and can cause a false reward prediction signal that cannot be corrected by experience: upon consumption, addictive drugs invariably signal that the world is better than expected, thus reinforcing further drug taking (Redish 2004). Moreover, drug-induced dopamine release masks any potential pauses in dopamine neuron firing, even when drug use proves less pleasurable than expected or even aversive. For example, when the inhalation of tobacco smoke causes painful coughing or shortness of breath in an ill smoker, it might seem that the brain would signal an experience that is worse than expected, with a resulting decrement in VTA neuron firing rate. Because, however, nicotine causes dopamine release pharmacologically, independent of the smoker's actual experience, forebrain circuits, still receive a signal that reinforces tobacco use. Among other effects, this grossly abnormal dopamine signal acts in the orbital prefrontal cortex to value drug use above all other rewards (Montague *et al.* 2004), thus the life of the addicted person often becomes narrowed to obtaining, using, and recovering from drugs. These actions of addictive drugs within the reward circuit begin to explain why drug use continues despite negative consequences. Such mechanisms also are consistent with the notion that decision-making in addicted people is highly deranged. Instead of making choices freely, addicted individuals are powerfully influenced by a reward circuit that has been usurped by false (i.e. direct pharmacologic) signals. Because dopamine projections across the forebrain have the critical role, under normal circumstances, of directing and integrating a critical survival function, the maximization of future reward, addicted individuals finds drugs to be the chief objects of their desire and their most valued goal among all other goals. In addition to impairments in decision-making, addicted people are subject to abnormal prepotent behaviors. Cues that had previously been associated with drug use active automatic drug seeking (Berke and Hyman 2000; Everitt and Robbins 2005). If drug seeking cannot proceed to completion because of some obstacle or because the addicted person is attempting to cut down, intense drug craving is likely to result (Tiffany 1990).

Research that has compared individuals with established drug addiction to healthy control subjects has found impairments in cognitive control. Given tasks requiring cognitive control of thought or behavior, addicted people fare worse than healthy subjects, and, as ascertained by fMRI, fail to recruit their prefrontal cortex. These impairments are thought to reflect abnormalities in glutamatergic excitatory neurotransmission that develop late in the course of addiction (Kalivas and Volkow, 2005). The implication is that the ability to exert executive control over impulses is weakened just at the time when an addicted person is also experiencing powerful drives to seek and consume drugs. This research suggests that in addiction, not only is decision-making impaired as discussed earlier, but also the ability to control behavior is undermined resulting from the combination of subcortically-based drug-seeking with failures of top-down cortical control.

THE PERSISTENCE OF ADDICTION

One of the most significant features of drug addiction is its persistence. While addicted individuals may recover even after years of smoking, long periods of alcoholism, or regular heroin or cocaine use, a large fraction of individuals do not. Many profoundly addicted individuals derive only brief periods of respite during repeated episodes of treatment followed by relapse. The persistence of addiction is thought to reflect several long-lived biological processes. Some of the biological mechanisms that contribute to addiction may represent homeostatic responses to drug stimulation. These include well-documented alterations in the levels of expression of certain genes within the nervous system (Nestler *et al.* 2009). Some persistent drug-induced changes in gene expression are now thought to reflect epigenetic modifications of chromatin (Kumar *et al.* 2005), the histones, and other proteins that bind DNA in the cell nucleus and render genes either silent or available for transcription.

Perhaps the longest-lived neural mechanism underlying addiction is the synaptic plasticity that is thought to be the substrate for associative memories. Associative memories are the key mechanisms by which specific drug-associated cues activate drug seeking and drug urges. By altering the strength of connections between neurons, drug-induced synaptic plasticity that has been documented in reward circuits, including long-term potentiation (LTP) and long-term depression (LTD), produce persistent changes in information processing (Hyman and Malenka 2001; Hyman *et al.* 2006). Physiologic processes such LTP and LTD are ultimately associated with alterations in the number of dendritic spines that are the critical substrates for synapse formation. The persistence of addiction is thought to reflect, in part, the drug-induced remodeling of the nervous system that results from synaptic plasticity.

IMPLICATIONS FOR VOLUNTARY
CONTROL OF BEHAVIOR

In the addicted state, neural mechanisms that evolved to motivate survival behaviors, such as the pursuit and consumption of food and water, the pursuit of safety, and of opportunities for mating, are usurped by the potent dopamine signals produced by addictive drugs. The result is a person who pathologically overvalues drugs, for whom drug cues activate drug seeking, whose impulse control is weakened, and for whom hard-won attempts to suppress drug-seeking may result in little more than intense drug craving. With respect to compulsive gambling, shopping, or other putative behavioral addictions, it must be acknowledged that far too little is known to draw firm conclusions. Early experiments, however, conducted mostly with gambling tasks that are conducive to study with fMRI, suggest that gambling situations cause dopamine release and activate brain reward circuitry (Clark 2009). Although the dopamine signals activated by gambling or other risky behaviors are not likely to be as reliable or as strong as those that occur with addictive drugs, the result may still plausibly be some degree of loss of control.

The view of addiction described here can explain how individuals continue to use drugs (and perhaps engage in other maladaptive behaviors) despite powerful health-related, social, legal, and economic disincentives, and why they remain at high risk of relapse even long after detoxification. This model helps explicate one of the questions posed at the beginning of this chapter: how can a protracted series of voluntary behaviors, such as finding money, seeking and buying drugs, preparing them, and then using them, be described as out of control? The answer lies in the remodeling of neural circuits under the influence of dopamine (and undoubtedly other neurotransmitters) so that drug associated cues come reliably to activate deeply ingrained programs of behavior (Everitt and Robbins 2005) in a person who also has impaired prefrontal cortical mechanisms of impulse control (Kalivas and Volkow 2005). This bleak picture notwithstanding, this model does not reduce addicted individuals to zombies permanently at the mercy of drug cues or stress (Hyman 2007). The function of reward circuits is to facilitate adaptive responses to external cues and bodily states (ranging from hunger and thirst to symptoms of drug withdrawal). In the addicted state, these responses are no longer adaptive, but perverted by the pathological dopamine signal produced by addicted drugs. Nonetheless, even the most severely addicted person has settings and times free of drug seeking, drug craving, or drug-related bodily sensations. True, even at such times and places, the addicted person's system of valuation remains highly skewed toward drugs. Nevertheless these may represent windows of greater self-control during which treatment recommendations or other adaptive goals can be weighed more rationally than at other times when drug-related goals invariably win out. In such windows of at least modest lucidity, perhaps with a good measure of initial coercion, perhaps with family, friends, physicians, and employers acting as cognitive and emotional "prostheses" to aid in decision-making and to shore up damaged mechanisms of cognitive control, addicted individuals can commit to plans for detoxification and treatment. Because there may be many false starts, caregivers must be both patient and implacable. The caregiver role for a severely addicted person may be frustrating and exhausting, but in this role there is no place for blame or moral opprobrium that might drive the addicted person away. Help rejection and relapse cannot be accepted as a final answer, but an understanding of addiction makes help rejection and relapse understandable.

The study of addiction suggests that some apparently voluntary behaviors may not be as freely planned and executed as they first appear. While addicted individuals may not be zombies, their decision-making and behavioral control are undoubtedly severely impaired. Beyond the stance, described earlier, assumed by many experienced clinicians, of caring but implacable confrontation of maladaptive behaviors, the impairments that are central to addiction raise the question of whether an even more paternalistic approach might be appropriate. There is little question that for severely demented individuals, a significantly paternalistic approach to care is warranted. Such an approach might mandate treatment if it is safe and effective and would limit freedom in the interests of preventing self-harm. Unlike dementia, however, in which deficits are fixed and often progressive, addiction permits windows of relative lucidity that would seem, in Western societies, to make an excessive abrogation of freedom repugnant. Thus, I would argue, that treatment ethically demands the consent of an addicted person, even if it is known to be safe and effective. The need for consent is heightened when it comes to invasive treatments, such as implantation of a long-acting opiate antagonist drug such as naltrexone into the bodies of opiate addicts (Hulse *et al.* 2009). An important situation arises when an addicted person is convicted of a non-violent drug offense, such as possession. Much has been written about the ethics and efficacy of mandated treatment (whether behavioral or pharmacologic) in such contexts. Many ideas about mandated treatment have been implemented, often without adequate long-term information, in the growing number of drug courts in the US (Belenko 2001). This is a topic that warrants a long discussion. Here it must suffice to say that I believe it a highly defensible position, knowing what we do about addiction, to argue that a judge can ethically give a convicted offender a choice between a punishment, such as incarceration, and mandated treatment, but ethically, I believe that a choice must be offered.

Ideas emerging from cognitive neuroscience suggest that even healthy individuals exert far less control over their behavior than folk psychology recognizes or is obvious upon introspection. As a result, some scientists have argued that retribution makes little sense as a justification for punishment (Greene and Cohen 2004). Punishments such as incarceration could still be justified by the desire to incapacitate criminals, for deterrence, and for rehabilitation. For the addicted individual, with substantial impairment in decision-making and control of behavior, the justification for moral outrage (independent of criminal acts) and retribution would seem to be pressing questions. I agree with Morse (2004, 2007) that at this stage of knowledge, it is premature to use neuroscience as an excuse for crimes committed by addicted individuals. The open question, however, is whether the mechanistic explanations of neuroscience should cause society to retire moral outrage and retribution as justifications for punishment, at least of addicts who have committed nonviolent crimes. Strong arguments can be made that long mandatory sentences for non-violent drug crimes, likely driven in recent decades by anger and moral outrage among US legislators were neither just in proportion to punishments for other crimes, nor good policy with respect to cost and the goal of rehabilitation. The response to this historical error does not, however, mean that moral outrage and retribution have no place in justifications for punishment. Indeed, insofar as a goal of punishment is deterrence of future crimes, including non-violent drug-related crimes, a good argument can be made that moral outrage, if kept within proportion, is an important component of the instructive environment.

I have argued here, that for caregivers, a moralizing stance is neither useful nor appropriate with respect to addicted individuals. I would not argue, however, that a moral stance should be eschewed by the entire society as long as it is kept in proportion. Addicts are highly impaired, but, as I have stated, they are not zombies. If an important societal goal is to rehabilitate currently addicted people and to prevent harmful drug use and addiction in the future, it may be wise and ethically defensible for some components of society to retain a moral rather than a mechanistic, scientific stance concerning unwanted behaviors. Without demanding too much of addicted individuals, it may be wise to err, if only slightly, on the side of holding them responsible for their behavior, and to act as if they can exert at least somewhat more control than perhaps they can.

References

American Psychiatric Association (2000). *Diagnostic and Statistical Manual of Mental Disorders, 4th Edition, Text Revision.* Washington, DC: American Psychiatric Association.

Barch, D.M. (2005). The cognitive neuroscience of schizophrenia. *Annual Review of Clinical Psychology,* 1, 321–53.

Belenko, S. (2001). *Research on Drug Courts. A Critical Review. 2001 Update.* New York: The National Center on Addiction and Substance Abuse at Columbia University.

Berke J.D. and Hyman, S.E. (2000). Addiction, dopamine, and the molecular mechanisms of memory. *Neuron,* 25, 515–32.

Caplan, A. (2008). Denying autonomy in order to create it: the paradox of forcing treatment upon addicts. *Addiction,* 103, 1919–21.

Clark L., Lawrence A.J., Astley-Jones F., and Gray, N. (2009). Gambling near-misses enhance motivation to gamble and recruit win-related brain circuitry. *Neuron,* 61, 481–90.

Dagher A. and Robbins T.W., (2009). Personality, addiction, dopamine: insights from Parkinson's disease. *Neuron,* 61, 502–10.

Everitt, B.J. and Robbins, T.W. (2005). Neural systems of reinforcement for drug addiction: from actions to habits to compulsion. *Nature Neuroscience,* 8, 1481–9.

Gilbert, C.D. and Sigman, M. (2007). Brain states: Top-down influences in sensory processing. *Neuron,* 54, 677–96.

Gold, J.I. and Shadlen, M. N. (2007). The neural basis of decision making. *Annual Review of Neuroscience,* 30, 535–74.

Goldman, D., Oroszi, G., and Ducci, F. (2005). The genetics of addictions: uncovering the genes. *Nature Reviews Genetics*, **6**, 521–32.

Greene, J. and Cohen, J. (2004). For the law, neuroscience changes nothing and everything. *Philosophical Transactions of the Royal Society B. Biological Sciences*, **359**, 1775–85.

Greene, J.D., Nystrom, L.E., Engell, A.D., Darley, J.M., and Cohen, J.D. (2004). The neural bases of cognitive conflict and control of moral judgment. *Neuron*, **44**, 389–400.

Haggard, P. (2008). Human volition: towards a neuroscience of will. *Nature Reviews Neuroscience*, **9**, 934–46.

Hall, W., Capps, B., and Carter, A. (2008). The use of depot naltrexone under legal coercion: the case for caution. *Addiction*, **103**, 1922–4.

Haynes, J-D. and Rees, G. (2006). Decoding mental states from brain activity in humans. *Nature Reviews Neuroscience*, **7**, 523–34.

Hser, Y.I., Hoffman, V., Grella, C.E., and Anglin, M.D. (2001). A 33-year follow-up of narcotics addicts. *Archives of General Psychiatry*, **58**, 503–8.

Hulse, G.K., Morris, N., Arnold-Reed, D., and Tait, R.J. (2009). Improving clinical outcomes in treating heroin dependence. Randomized, controlled trial of oral or implant naltrexone. *Archives of General Psychiatry*, **66**, 1108–15.

Hyman, S.E. (2007). The neurobiology of addiction: Implications for voluntary control of behavior. *American Journal of Bioethics*, **7**, 8–11.

Hyman, S.E. and Malenka, R.C. (2001). Addiction and the brain: the neurobiology of compulsion and its persistence. *Nature Reviews Neuroscience*, **2**, 695–703.

Hyman, S.E., Malenka, R.C. and Nestler, E.J. (2006). Neural mechanisms of addiction: The role of reward-related learning and memory. *Annual Review of Neuroscience*, **21**, 565–98.

Kable, J.W. and Glimcher, P.W. (2009). The neurobiology of decision: consensus and controversy. *Neuron*, **24**, 733–45.

Kalivas, P.W. and Volkow, N.D. (2005). The neural basis of addiction: a pathology of motivation and choice. *American Journal of Psychiatry*, **162**, 1403–13.

Kelley, A.E. and Berridge, K.C. (2002). The neuroscience of natural rewards: relevance to addictive drugs. *The Journal of Neuroscience*, **22**, 3306–11.

Koechlin, E. and Hyafil, A. (2007). Anterior prefrontal function and the limits of human decision-making. *Science*, **318**, 594–8.

Koob, G. (2008). A role for brain stress systems in addiction. *Neuron*, **59**, 11–14.

Koob, G.F and Le Moal, M. (2005). *Neurobiology of Addiction*. New York: Academic Press.

Knoch, D., Schneider, F., Schunk, D., Hohmann, M. and Fehr, E. (2009). Disrupting the prefrontal cortex diminishes the human ability to build a good reputation. *Proceedings of the National Academy of Sciences*, **106**, 20895–99.

Kosfeld, M., Heinrichs, M., Zak, P.J., Fischbacher, U. and Fehr, E. (2005). Oxytocin increases trust in humans. Nature, **435**, 673–6.

Kumar, A., Choi, K.-H., Renthal, W., *et al.* (2005). Chromatin remodeling is a key mechanism underlying cocaine-induced plasticity in striatum. *Neuron*, **48**, 303–14.

Leshner, A.I. (1997). Addiction is a brain disease, and it matters. *Science*, **278**, 45–7.

Mayberg, H.S., Lozano, A.M., Voon, V., *et al.* (2005). Deep brain stimulation for treatment-resistant depression. *Neuron*, **45**, 651–60.

Merikangas, K.R., Stolar, M., Stevens, D.E., *et al.* (1998). Familial transmission of substance use disorders. *Archives of General Psychiatry*, **55**, 973–9.

Miller, E.K. and Cohen, J.D. (2001). An integrative theory of prefrontal cortex function. *Annual Review of Neuroscience*, **24**, 167–202.

Montague, P.R., Hyman, S.E. and Cohen, J.D. (2004). Computational roles for dopamine in behavioural control. *Nature*, **431**, 760–7.

Morse, S.J. (2004). Medicine and morals, craving and compulsion. *Substance Use & Misuse*, **39**, 437–60.

Morse, S.J. (2007). Voluntary control of behavior and responsibility. *The American Journal of Bioethics*, **7**, 12–14.

Nestler, E.J., Hyman, S.E. and Malenka, R.J. (2009). *Molecular Neuropharmacology: Foundation for Clinical Neuroscience*, Chapter 15. New York: McGraw-Hill.

Norman, K.S., Polyn, S.M., Detre, G.J. and Haxby, J.V. (2006). Beyond mind-reading: multi-voxel pattern analysis of fMRI data. *Trends in Cognitive Sciences*, **10**, 424–30.

O'Brien, C.P., Childress, A.R., Ehrman, R. and Robbins, S.J. (1998). Conditioning factors in drug abuse: Can they explain compulsion? *Journal of Psychopharmacology*, **12**, 15–22.

Potenza, M.N. (2006). Should addictive disorders include non-substance-related conditions? *Addiction*, **101**(Suppl 1), 142–51.

Redish, A.D. (2004). Addiction as a computational process gone awry. *Science*, **306**, 1944–7.

Robbins, T.W. and Arnsten, A.F.T. (2009). The neuropsychopharmacology of fronto-executive function: monoaminergic modulation. *Annual Review of Neuroscience*, **32**, 267–87.

Robinson, T.E. and Berridge, K.C. (2003). Addiction. *Annual Review of Psychology*, **54**, 25–53.

Roskies, A. (2006). Neuroscientific challenges to free will and responsibility. *Trends in Cognitive Sciences*, **10**, 419–23.

Roskies, A. (2010). How does neuroscience affect our concept of volition? *Annual Review of Neuroscience*, **33**, 109–30.

Satel, S.L., (1999). What should we expect from drug abusers? *Psychiatric Services*, **50**, 861.

Schoenbaum, G., Roesch, M.R. and Stalnaker, T.A. (2006). Orbitofrontal cortex, decision-making and drug addiction. *Trends in Neurosciences*, **29**, 116–24.

Schultz, W. (2006). Behavioral theories and the neurophysiology of reward. *Annual Review of Psychology*, **57**, 87–115.

Schultz, W., Dayan, P. and Montague, P.R. (1997). A neural substrate of prediction and reward. *Science*, **275**, 1593–9.

Sigvardsson, S., Bohman, M. and Cloninger, C.R. (1996). Replication of the Stockholm adoption study of alcoholism confirmatory cross-fostering analysis. *Archives of General Psychiatry*, **53**, 681–7.

Snead, C. (2008). Neuroimaging and capital punishment. *The New Atlantis*, **19**, 35–63.

Soon, C.S., Brass, M., Heinze, H-J. and Haynes, J-D. (2008). *Nature Neuroscience*, **11**, 543–5.

Sugrue, L.P., Corrado, G.S. and Newsome, W.T. (2005). Choosing the greater of two goods: neural currencies for valuation and decision making. *Nature Reviews Neuroscience*, **6**, 363–75.

Tang, J. and Dani, J.A. (2009). Dopamine enables in vivo synaptic plasticity associated with the addictive drug nicotine. *Neuron*, **63**, 673–82.

Thaler, R.H. and Sunstein, C.R. (2008). *Nudge: Improving Decisions about Health, Wealth, and Happiness*. New Haven, CT: Yale University Press.

Tiffany, S.T. (1990). A cognitive model of drug urges and drug-use behavior: Role of automatic and nonautomatic processes. *Psychological Review*, **97**, 147–68.

Tsuang, M.T., Lyons, M.J., Eisen, S.A., *et al.* (1996). Genetic influences on DSM-III-R drug abuse and dependence: a study of 3,372 twin pairs. *American Journal of Medical Genetics*, **67**, 473–7.

Vaidya, C.J., Bunge, S.A., Dudukovic, N.M., Zalecki, C.A., Elliott, G.R. and Gabrieli, J.D. (2005). Altered neural substrates of cognitive control in childhood ADHD: Evidence from functional magnetic resonance imaging. *American Journal of Psychiatry*, **162**, 1605–13.

Vaillant, G.E. (1996). A long-term follow-up of male alcohol abuse. *Archives of General Psychiatry*, **53**, 243–9.

Volkow, D.D., Want, G.-J, Fowler, J.D. and Telang, F. (2008). Overlapping neuronal circuits in addiction and obesity: evidence of systems pathology. *Philosophical Transactions of the Royal Society B. Biological Sciences*, **363**, 3191–200.

Wallis, J.D. (2007). Orbitofrontal cortex and its contribution to decision-making. *Annual Review of Neuroscience*, **30**, 31–56.

World Health Organization (1992). *The ICD-10 Classification of Mental and Behavioural Disorders*. Geneva: World Health Organization.

CHAPTER 13

NEUROETHICS OF FREE WILL

PATRICK HAGGARD

INTRODUCTION

In this piece, I will first set out the reasons why scientific questions regarding free will have important ethical and social consequences. I will then consider the neuroscientific debate over whether a conscious experience of volition does or does not precede the brain's preparation for action. I will outline Benjamin Libet's evidence that conscious volition is a consequence of brain activity, perhaps linked to the capacity to inhibit ongoing actions. A major objection to this view is reviewed, based on social psychological studies of unconscious determinants of behavior, and of attribution theory. Finally, some specific issues for neuroethical debate are suggested.

ETHICAL IMPLICATIONS OF "FREE WILL"

The debate over "free will" involves a series of several questions about the origin of human actions, and their resulting social, legal, and ethical implications. The idea that individuals have the power to choose and perform actions, and that they can exercise this power freely, is deeply entrenched in human cultures. This view of the individual as a free agent leads directly to the idea that people are responsible for their actions, since a person's actions depend on their conscious decisions and their conscious intentions. All human societies have a concept of responsibility for action and for the effects of action along these lines. Social practices and legal codes both express and enforce the concept of personal responsibility. For example, systems of law deriving from Roman law require that two components be present in order to constitute a crime. The first is *actus reus*, or a physical action. Thus, thought alone is not generally a crime. The second component is *mens rea*, or a conscious intention to perform the action. Thus, a person may not be responsible for actions performed unconsciously (e.g. while sleepwalking), or for unintended an unforeseeable consequences of an intentional action.

In recent years, the debate over free will and responsibility has become a neuroscientific debate, as well as a sociological, philosophical, and legal one. The standard view of free will and responsibility outlined previously sees a person's conscious decisions and conscious intentions as the causes of their actions. In contrast, the neuroscientific view is materialist. The brain follows causal laws, which in turn depend on the basic laws of physics. On this view, actions result from physiological processes in the brain, rather than from conscious decisions or conscious intentions. This raises two immediate problems for the concepts of free will and responsibility. First, the law-like causal nature of brain processes seem to leave no place for freedom. In philosophy, an action is often considered free if the person could have acted otherwise. However, if the action directly results from a set of law-like events in the person's brain, as claimed by neuroscience, the person presumably could not have acted otherwise, and is therefore not free. Second, the material nature of the brain seems to leave no room for conscious decision. The standard everyday concept of free will suggests that people consciously choose a particular action, and then consciously cause the action by an act of conscious will. Neuroscience, however, rejects the idea of person-level, brain-independent consciousness. For neuroscience, conscious choice and conscious will can only be brain processes. Therefore, if conscious thought is conceived as brain-independent, it cannot cause actions or any other neural or physical event.

LIBET'S EXPERIMENT

A powerful and influential demonstration of the gulf between the everyday concepts of free will and the neuroscientific view of the brain comes from Libet *et al.*'s famous experiment (Libet *et al.* 1983). In this experiment, the participant is asked to make a voluntary action at a time of their own choosing. In the original experiment the action was a brisk wrist flexion, but the case of pressing a button with the finger may offer a simpler example. At the same time, the participant watched a gradually rotating spot, similar to a clock hand, on a screen. After making the movement, they reported the position of the clock hand at which they had first "felt the urge to act." It remains unclear how participants interpreted this instruction, and what phenomenology they actually identified by it. However, the aim was to identify the moment at which people experience consciously willing or intending an action. For these reasons, Libet referred to this moment as the moment of "W judgment." In his original data, the moment of conscious will averaged 206ms prior to action itself, though there was considerable variability both within and between individuals. Libet also measured the brain activity preceding voluntary action, using scalp electrodes over the motor areas of the frontal lobe. These recordings showed the characteristic readiness potential (Kornhuber and Deecke 1965). This is an increasing ramp-like negativity, which begins at least several hundred milliseconds prior to voluntary action, and rapidly reverses around the time of movement itself. In Libet's own data, the readiness potential began around 700ms, and sometimes more than 900ms prior to action. This is clearly several hundred ms before the moment that participants report an experience of conscious will or intention to make the action. In Libet's view, the temporal precedence of brain activity over conscious will ruled out the idea that conscious will caused brain activity and thus action. A cause must precede, and cannot follow its effects. Therefore, conscious will cannot be the cause of our actions.

Libet's result seems to raise profound problems for the concept of human voluntary action by which we live our everyday lives. In particular, if "I" do not cause my actions by my conscious decisions and intentions, but rather my actions are determined by unconscious brain processes, how can I be held responsible for what I do?

Although the experiment has been heavily criticized on several grounds (for examples, see the replies to Libet's (1985) target article in *Behavioural and Brain Sciences*), the basic result has been replicated (Haggard and Eimer 1999; Sirigu *et al.* 2004). Indeed, recent work using more sophisticated experimental and neurophysiological techniques suggests an even longer gap between brain activity and conscious will (Matsuhashi and Hallett 2008; Soon *et al.* 2008). However, for neuroscience, the basic concept of volition that emerges from the Libet experiment is uncontroversial. Materialist neuroscience holds that conscious experiences are products of brain activity, rather than causes of brain activity. The notion of a brain-independent consciousness with causal powers is not consistent with neuroscience.

Since Libet's work, empirical work on free will has moved in two different directions. Both aim at rescuing a concept of personal responsibility for action, though the meaning and value of responsibility that emerges is quite different in the two cases.

FREE WILL AND FREE WON'T

The first approach is broadly libertarian. It holds that people can, in fact, make free choices about action. On one view, the truly free choice is not the choice to act that Libet purports to study, but rather the choice to volunteer in the experiment in the first place. On another view, shared by Libet himself, the unconscious initiation of action conceals an implicit free choice to continue with an action after its initiation, as opposed to canceling it. Libet argued that the short interval between the moment of conscious intention and action might be sufficient for a "conscious veto" to prevent the impending action. Thus, while we clearly do not have free will, we might conceivably have "free won't."

The veto idea has attracted much discussion. First, a veto process of this kind has recently been identified in the human brain. Brass and Haggard (2007) asked participants to prepare a voluntary keypress action, but withhold it at the last possible moment on some trials which they freely chose. Crucially, subjects reported the moment of conscious intention on every trial, even on trials where the conscious intention was subsequently inhibited. Event-related functional magnetic resonance imaging locked to the time of conscious intention showed an activation in the medial prefrontal cortex on inhibition trials which was absent on action trials. A second activation in the insula was interpreted as coding the experience of frustration that frequently accompanies failing to execute a prepared action. Recently, Walsh *et al.* (2010) used scalp electroencephalography (EEG) recording in an identical experiment. They identified the well-known decrease in beta-band power that precedes voluntary actions. However, on trials where participants intentionally inhibited a prepared voluntary action, a significant increase in beta band power over frontal electrodes was found around the time that subjects reported experiencing the conscious intention which they subsequently cancelled.

The human brain, then, contains a mechanism for intentionally inhibiting a voluntary action whose preparation is already underway. Indeed, it would be strange if it were not so.

It is clear that the brain monitors ongoing movements to check if some adjustment is required. Similarly, there would be a clear advantage in checking whether a prepared action is still appropriate and should really be executed. The action would then be cancelled it should it prove unsuitable. However, there is no convincing evidence that this intentional inhibition is a "*conscious* veto," in the sense of a brain-independent conscious cause. Just as the experience of conscious will is in fact a consequence of preceding brain activity, our sense of "conscious veto" must presumably also be a consequence of unconscious brain activity. Intentional inhibition therefore involves a specific set of brain processes, which both prevent the prepared action, and produce the conscious experience of inhibition. The conscious experience itself, however, does not cause anything.

Psychology of attribution

In the last decade or so, a second tradition of work on responsibility has arisen in social psychology. Whereas neuroscientists have identified brain processes occurring before action, and their conscious correlates, social psychologists have generally focused on the identifying factors that influence whether people *experience* or *attribute* responsibility for causing an external event. One classic example is the I-Spy experiment of Wegner and Wheatley (1999). In this experiment, a participant and a confederate play a competitive computer game in which keypress actions cause changes in the objects displayed on a computer screen. In some trials, the participant's action causes the change, while in others the confederate's action is responsible. Interestingly, participants felt that they were responsible for the change in the display even when the action was in fact made by the confederate, provided they had themselves been thinking about making the action, and provided the change occurred in close proximity to the action.

Wegner used these results, and others, to develop a general theory of authorship of actions. For present purposes, authorship can be taken as equivalent to responsibility. According to Wegner, we do not feel, or even know that we are the authors of our actions. Rather, we *infer* that we are the authors of our actions, if the action fits with our prior conscious thought, if it occurs in appropriate time-window relative to the thought, and if there is no other obvious candidate cause. In essence, these are the same principles that Hume argued to underlie the experience of causation and volition. Importantly, this line of thinking leads Wegner to reject the idea of conscious will as an illusion (Wegner 2003): we have no direct experience of willing actions, and no direct evidence that we control our actions at all. Instead, we make a postdictive inference that our action is the consequence of our prior conscious thought. Personal responsibility is something that we attribute to ourselves because of the way the mind works, rather than a fundamental causal truth.

Both the neuroscientific view and the attributional view therefore agree in rejecting the concept of "conscious free will" that underlies our everyday notions of personal responsibility and social behavior. Both views explain that the feeling of conscious will is not an example of mental, person-level control over actions as it seems to be, but is actually something else. However, the two views adopt quite different positions regarding what the feeling of conscious will really is. Moreover, these different positions have important consequences for both ethics and views of human nature.

The materialist neuroscientist holds that brain processes cause behavior." Conscious decision," "conscious intention," and other such states cannot possibly cause our actions, but are rather reflections of the underlying brain processes that *do* cause our actions. Conscious intention would therefore be a perception linked to preparatory brain activity, just as a phosphene is a perception linked to visual cortex activity (Hallett 2007). What, then, is the role of conscious intention? Materialist neuroscience feels uncomfortable with conscious having a direct causal role in the control of current action. However, conscious experience may act as a reinforcing marker for learning to control future actions. For example, if a very clear conscious experience of preparing and executing a particular action leads to a desirable outcome, a person might be motivated to repeat the action.

The attributional view also holds that behavior is determined largely unconsciously. However, the attributionist emphasis on postdictive inference makes free will seem perhaps even more illusory than under a neuroscientific view. The attributional view sees human behavior as unconsciously determined by environmental events. The human mind then produces narrative confabulations to provide explanations of one's own behavior. On this view, the doctrine of personal responsibility for action is effectively just a myth. It may be a quite convenient myth by which to organize society, since it can encourages everyone to use the same narratives to explain their behavior, and seems to work. But the myth of responsibility could not be a basis for either naturalized ethics, or for a scientific view of human nature.

Neuroethical challenges

Both of the dominant views in modern cognitive science, namely the materialist neuroscientific view and the attributional view, seem incompatible with the basic assumption of personal responsibility on which most ethical and legal systems are founded. This incompatibility raises an important metascientific question. If current neuroscientific and psychological thinking invalidates existing ethical codes, four possibilities exist. First, one could abandon existing ethical codes as being mere irrational foibles and arbitrary social conventions, superseded by new scientific knowledge. Second, one could dismiss the experimental evidence as being mere inconclusive, inadequate, pseudoscience. Third, one could accept the incompatibility, and agree to adhere to use ethical codes as a convenient way of life which nevertheless lacks a scientific basis. Our neuroscientific and psychological understanding of volition is still in its infancy, so it is perhaps too soon to say which route will be taken in the future. However, the second and third possibilities seem, prima facie, unlikely: legal and ethical arguments can and should be in touch with reality, by according an important role to scientific evidence.

In the meantime, we can consider several specific questions that a neuroethics of volition will have to deal with.

First, recent neuroscientific work associates a specific brain network, focused on the pre-supplementary motor area (pre-SMA) and the parietal cortex, with the conscious experience of voluntary action. For example, direct stimulation of both these areas in neurosurgical patients creates an experience which has been described as an "urge to move" (Fried *et al.* 1991; Desmurget *et al.* 2009). As might be expected, lesions in these areas produce a deficit in conscious intention and voluntary control. For example, patients with pre-SMA lesions may exhibit an "alien hand syndrome" in which one hand makes compulsive actions which the patient has not intended (Della Sala *et al.* 1991). Patients with parietal lesions appear to experience a conscious intention to press a key only some 50–60ms before the keypress itself, by which time the relevant muscles are presumably already active (Sirigu *et al.* 2004). Given this scientific evidence, one might pose the following ethical question: is an individual with documented damage to one or both of these brain areas truly responsible for their actions? One can imagine a situation where a person with a brain lesion in these areas commits a criminal action, and claims to have had no conscious intention to act. Holding the person responsible for this action would seem to violate the principle of *mens rea*. On the other hand, the person's argument might seem dubious, because of the great difficulty of proving whether they did or did not have conscious intention preceding the action. For example, the defense of automatism or sleepwalking effectively requires third parties to judge whether an individual did or did not have any conscious experience of their action. Neuroscientific evidence about the functioning of pre-SMA and parietal cortex might be brought to prove or disprove this point. However, this evidence should be treated with the greatest caution. A healthy actor who was appropriately trained by a neuroscientist could probably produce voluntarily the kinds of brain activity and behavior consistent with someone who had genuinely reduced function of these areas. Neuroscientific data alone may not be sufficiently reliable to judge whether a person does or does not have *mens rea* for their actions in general, let alone for a specific past action. Further research on this point would be invaluable. In the meantime, judgments about whether a person did or did not consciously intend a particular action need to be based on a general assessment of their cognitive function, and the plausibility of *mens rea* being absent for the specific action under discussion.

A final neuroethical consideration arises from the assumption, common to both the materialist neuroscientist and the attributionist, that our actions are determined by unconscious causes such as brain events, and not by our conscious thought. On this assumption, most of our actions must "just happen" as either as a direct result of immediate stimulation, or as a result of our previous reinforcement history. For example, we may be unconsciously caused to perform again an action that is rewarded, and to refrain from performing again an action that is punished. If, therefore, a person performs a wrong action, and is punished for it, they are effectively being punished for having been inappropriately reinforced in the past, since their present action was determined by the previous history or reinforcement. Greene and Cohen (2004) point out that we are often inclined to say that someone is not responsible for their actions when we know the causal and reinforcement history that determined the action. They therefore reject the idea of a retributive justice, since it depends on a notion of responsibility that is incompatible with materialist neuroscience. In their view, punishment should be justified because of the future benefits it brings to society, notably by deterring potential wrongdoers.

Another concept of responsibility *can* be reconciled with neurobiological determinism. However, this is a much more socially conservative form of responsibility than many people might like. In brief, when society holds someone responsible for an action, it may effectively be passing a normative judgment on the practices, values and reinforcement history that lead to the action. On this view, judging an individual guilty may not mean that they are personally responsible for a particular action, but rather that society disapproves of the rules they have learned for governing the action.

CONCLUSION

The concept of individual free will by which we live our daily lives is difficult to reconcile with a materialist view of the brain. Recent psychology treats our behaviors as unconsciously determined, and dismisses the conscious experience of will as a mere retrospective illusion. This view tends to lead to the position that people are not responsible for their actions, at least not in the dualistic way envisaged by current law. However, this conclusion may be premature for two reasons. First, there are reliable correlations between specific brain events and pre-movement experiences of conscious volition, suggesting that an illusory view is too strong. Second, the determinist view, like many other views of volition, neglects the obvious fact that the human will can be trained. Societies require individuals to limit the targets that their will aims at, and to inhibit the will where appropriate. Individuals learn these functions of the will through family and peer reinforcement, and through formal education. To that extent, our responsibility for action depends on prior training regarding what actions are appropriate and which are not.

REFERENCES

Brass, M. and Haggard, P. (2007). To do or not to do: the neural signature of self-control. *Journal of Neuroscience*, 27, 9141–5.

Della Sala, S., Marchetti, C. and Spinnler, H. (1991). Right-sided anarchic (alien) hand: a longitudinal study. *Neuropsychologia*, 29, 1113–27.

Desmurget, M., Reilly, K., Richard, N., Szathmari, A., Mottolese, C., and Sirigu, A. (2009). Movement intention after parietal cortex stimulation in humans. *Science*, 324, 811–13.

Fried, I., Katz, A., McCarthy, G., *et al.* (1991). Functional organization of human supplementary motor cortex studied by electrical stimulation. *Journal of Neuroscience*, 11, 3656–66.

Greene, J. and Cohen, J. (2004). For the law, neuroscience changes nothing and everything. *Philosophical Transactions of the Royal Society of London. Series B, Biological Sciences*, 359, 1775–85.

Haggard, P. and Eimer, M. (1999). On the relation between brain potentials and the awareness of voluntary movements. *Experimental Brain Research. Experimentelle Hirnforschung. Expérimentation Cérébrale*, 126, 128–33.

Hallett, M. (2007). Volitional control of movement: the physiology of free will. *Clinical Neurophysiology*, 118, 1179–92.

Kornhuber, H.H. and Deecke, L. (1965). [Changes in the brain potential in voluntary movements and passive movements in man: readiness potential and reafferent potentials.] *Pflügers Archiv Für Die Gesamte Physiologie Des Menschen Und Der Tiere*, 284, 1–17.

Libet, B., Gleason, C.A., Wright, E.W., and Pearl, D.K. (1983). Time of conscious intention to act in relation to onset of cerebral activity (readiness-potential). The unconscious initiation of a freely voluntary act. *Brain*, 106, 623–42.

Matsuhashi, M. and Hallett, M. (2008). The timing of the conscious intention to move. *European Journal of Neuroscience*, 28, 2344–51.

Sirigu, A., Daprati, E., Ciancia, S., *et al.* (2004). Altered awareness of voluntary action after damage to the parietal cortex. *Nature Neuroscience*, 7, 80–4.

Soon, C.S., Brass, M., Heinze, H.J., and Haynes, J.D. (2008). Unconscious determinants of free decisions in the human brain. *Nature Neuroscience*, **11**, 543–5.

Walsh, E., Kühn, S., Brass, M., Wenke, D., and Haggard, P. (2010). EEG activations during intentional inhibition of voluntary action: an electrophysiological correlate of self-control? *Neuropsychologia*, **48**, 619–26.

Wegner, D.M. (2003). *The Illusion of Conscious Will*. Cambridge, MA: MIT Press.

Wegner, D.M. and Wheatley, T. (1999). Apparent mental causation. Sources of the experience of will. *American Psychologist*, **54**, 480–92.

PART III

MIND AND BODY

CHAPTER 14

··

PHARMACEUTICAL
COGNITIVE
ENHANCEMENT

··

SHARON MOREIN-ZAMIR AND
BARBARA J. SAHAKIAN

THE drive to alleviate human cognitive deficits has given rise to multiple interventions. One of these is pharmaceutical cognitive enhancers (PCEs), or drugs that are aimed at improving cognition and everyday performance in individuals who suffer from impaired cognition due to brain injury or neuropsychiatric disorders (Sahakian and Morein-Zamir 2010). The goal for better cognition in such individuals is to improve functional outcome and quality of life (Beddington *et al.* 2008). While the link between cognition and well-being in the elderly population is established (Beddington *et al.* 2008; Whalley and Deary 2001), the popularity of substances such as caffeine in enhancing alertness and concentration highlights the central role of cognition to functionality in healthy adults. This chapter will first consider current scientific research into PCEs and likely future directions. Then we will discuss the trends in use of PCEs within patients groups for whom they were intended, as well as in those for whom they were not originally intended, including healthy adults and children. Finally, we will provide an overview of current and future ethical considerations.

We conclude that the use of PCE will likely continue both within patient and healthy individuals in the foreseeable future. Information regarding actual use, benefits, and harms in various populations is severely lacking. Therefore, more emphasis should be placed on obtaining the relevant empirical data, for example, by long-term monitoring of effectiveness and side effects, and by accurate large-scale surveys to assess actual usage. Mechanisms to obtain this information should be put in place. We propose careful consideration is essential of the short- and long-term benefits and risks for each group and each drug, and that over-generalization due to insufficient information should be avoided. Likewise, some mechanisms should be in place for informing healthcare providers and potential users of the trade-offs and of the present lack of long-term conclusive information. In addition, other forms of enhancing cognition such as education and physical exercise should be promoted (Beddington *et al.* 2008).

THE PHARMACOLOGY OF COGNITION IN PCEs: CURRENT RESEARCH

Pharmacological substances used to improve cognition and brain function range from dietary supplements and caffeine to drugs targeted at altering particular neurochemical concentrations in the brain. Pharmacological interventions influence the concentration and action of chemicals called neurotransmitters in the brain, which relay, amplify, or modulate neuronal activity. The effects of pharmacological substances on cognition are complex, as cognition is a multifaceted construct encompassing numerous mental functions including attention, executive functioning (e.g. planning, problem-solving, and inhibition), and spatial and verbal learning and memory. This chapter does not review all PCEs available (cf. Jones *et al.* 2005), but rather uses some prominent examples to illustrate general principles and trends. Current pharmacological influences on cognition are largely non-specific, in part due to the overlapping and complex interdependence of different cognitive processes and of neurotransmitter systems. Methylphenidate (Ritalin®) and atomoxetine (Strattera®), for example, may improve inhibitory control and impulsive responding in attention deficit hyperactivity disorder (ADHD). Whereas methylphenidate increases the synaptic concentration of the neurotransmitters dopamine and noradrenaline by blocking their reuptake, atomoxetine, is a relatively selective noradrenaline reuptake inhibitor (SNRI) (Stahl 2008). Modafinil (Provigil®) can also improve attention and executive function difficulties but its neurochemical underpinnings are presently unclear, with evidence pointing to numerous neurotransmitters including noradrenaline and dopamine (Minzenberg and Carter 2008; Minzenberg *et al.* 2008; Volkow *et al.* 2009).

Academic studies into the effects of PCE on cognition typically use double-blind placebo-control studies where participants undergo objective cognitive tasks targeted at measuring the various aspects of cognition. Often acute or short-term administrations of the drug are given and performance is compared across various doses and placebo. Studies using this methodology in patients have demonstrated that atomoxetine improves response inhibition in ADHD patients (Chamberlain *et al.* 2007). Similarly, modafinil improved short-term memory and attentional shifting in schizophrenia (Turner *et al.* 2004). Moreover, both drugs also produced better performance on some tests in healthy volunteers, with atomoxetine improving response inhibition (Chamberlain *et al.* 2006), and modafinil improving spatial planning, response inhibition, visual recognition, short-term memory (Turner *et al.* 2003a), and demanding attentional shifting (Marchant *et al.* 2009). Studies using concurrent neuroimaging techniques such as positron emission tomography (PET) or functional magnetic resonance imaging (fMRI) can offer some insight into the neural substrates involved in mediating the drug effects. For example, methylphenidate improved both performance and efficiency in the neural network mediating spatial working memory involving the dorsolateral prefrontal cortex and posterior parietal cortex in healthy volunteers (Mehta *et al.* 2000).

Such results demonstrate the potential of drugs to enhance certain cognitive domains. At the same time, psychopharmacological research entails the consideration of several complex factors (Morein-Zamir *et al.* 2010). These include neurotransmitter function at times following an inverted U-shaped curve, with deviations from optimal level in either direction impairing performance (e.g. Ramos and Arnsten 2007; Tannock *et al.* 1995), also known as the Yerkes–Dodson principle. Some drugs have simultaneous linear and inverted-U effects on different elements of cognition. For example, as the dose of methylphenidate is increased, performance on sustained attention tasks improves in a linear fashion in children with ADHD, but at high doses, response inhibition is worse than at low doses (Konrad *et al.* 2004). Likewise, different neurotransmitter levels can be found across brain regions, suggesting a complex interplay between baseline levels and drug administration. Taken together, this suggests that while some cognitive functions may improve following drug administration, others may worsen, as they depend on different optimum neurotransmitter levels (Cools and Robbins 2004). Hence it remains uncertain how enhancing one cognitive domain could come at the expense of another. For instance, dopaminergic medications can assist in some cognitive aspects but impair others, as evidenced in Parkinson's disease (Cools *et al.* 2003; Swainson *et al.* 2000).

These and related findings further suggest that drug-induced neurotransmitter increases may improve functioning in some groups but have no effect or even impair performance in others, already at optimum. In accordance, it is not uncommon for PCEs to improve performance primarily or exclusively in individuals with greater impairment (e.g. Mehta *et al.* 2000). Individual differences in response to drugs may also be mediated in part by genetic variation, though to date, single genes generally account for only small percentages of the population variance (Diaz-Asper *et al.* 2006). Thus, the response to conventional cholinesterase inhibitors in Alzheimer's disease (AD) appears to be genotype-specific, with APOE-4/4 carriers as the worst responders to conventional treatments (Cacabelos 2005). Cognition is influenced by additional group-level factors that remain to be explored. PCE effectiveness in various groups is important as some drugs may be less or more effective in particular populations. For example, the role of age, gender, and ethnic groups in both drug efficacy and safety is far from clear, though such factors account for reliable differences in the neurotransmitter systems (Apud and Weinberger 2006; Turner *et al.* 2003b; Wong 2008).

Despite the research dedicated to the development and understanding of various cognitive enhancers, knowledge of how neurotransmitters and PCEs modulate cognitive functions remains limited. In fact, pharmacological intervention is further modulated by complex interactions between neurotransmitters, such as cortical interactions between noradrenaline and dopamine (Arnsten 2000), or serotonin and dopamine (Apud and Weinberger 2006). Unsurprisingly then, the exact roles of the neurotransmitters dopamine and noradrenaline in mediating the effects of methylphenidate remains unclear (Swanson and Volkow 2009). Nevertheless, neurochemical specialization is also apparent, with pharmacological double dissociations being found for cognitive functions (Chamberlain *et al.* 2006).

There are additional important considerations regarding the function of PCEs on cognition that require systematic investigation. First, the extension of enhancement from the controlled laboratory environment to daily life remains controversial. This results in part from the extreme difficulty of conducting long-term controlled studies in patients but virtual impossibility of comparable research in healthy individuals. Thus, the influence of dosage, frequency, and pattern of use is far from clear. A second consideration is the effect sizes found, their stability, and relation to everyday efficacy (Morein-Zamir *et al.* 2010). Effect sizes are generally modest in healthy individuals, and in many patients the effects are small to moderate. Nevertheless, even small percentage increments in performance can lead to significant improvements in function outcome (Academy of Medical Sciences 2008). The size of the effects can also vary depending on the state of the individual, such as stress or fatigue. Third, with the increasing appreciation of the complex relationship between emotion and cognition, the possible role of antidepressants, such as serotonin reuptake inhibitors (SSRIs) and beta-blockers, in cognition remain to be further clarified (see also de Jongh et al. 2008). Similarly, the relationship between mood and cognition in everyday functionality and the pharmacological modulation of various aspects of both remain as yet uncertain.

On the one hand such considerations pose practical problems for the effective and safe use of PCEs. Nevertheless, technological advances in understanding neurotransmitter systems at the cellular level, together with brain imaging techniques, animal models, and the development of sophisticated testing of cognitive functions, have all facilitated our understanding of the neurochemistry of cognition (Morein-Zamir et al. 2010). Though current PCEs are far from specific interventions, with this increasing understanding of the brain's neurochemistry, genetics, the complex roles of factors such as pre-existing baseline levels, drug dosage, and individual differences, improved and more specific compounds can be better understood (Morein-Zamir et al. 2010; see also Lee and Silva 2009). Presently, the brain's complexity is being harnessed to influence cognition in increasingly sophisticated and targeted ways.

USE OF PCEs: CURRENT TRENDS AND LIKELY DETERMINANTS

Any neuroethical discussion of PCE must be conducted against the backdrop of who uses them at present and who is likely to use them in future. This cannot be considered without one of the most central issues regarding any drug: analysis of the risks and benefits, which is specific to a particular indication. Thus, for individuals in particular circumstances only, beneficial effects may outweigh the risks and side effects. Side effects can range from mild, such as dry mouth and insomnia, to more significant, such as addiction or cardiovascular effects with long-term use (as in the case of methylphenidate).

The harm–benefit ratio for PCEs is likely to be markedly different for various patient and non-patient groups. Moreover, it will be influenced by individual motivations for use and even by the circumstances of acquirement. PCE may be obtained in several ways for a variety of purposes: as part of approved treatment for a given neuropsychiatric or neurological condition, off-label administration by a healthcare practitioner for alleviating a recognized condition or for other reasons, within the course of occupational activities as is the case in the military, or via other means such as friends, self-purchase from individuals or the Internet, typically for enhancement purposes to allow one to study, work, or even party better (Sahakian and Morein-Zamir 2010).

The PCEs considered in this chapter have generally been approved as therapy for various disorders and this has governed their use in society. For treatment purposes, PCEs must undergo approval from regulatory bodies (e.g. the Food and Drug Administration (FDA) in the US; the European Medicines Agency in Europe). Authorization by the FDA, for instance, requires large-scale studies to test for safety and efficacy of each drug. The final label details

the approved indications, dosage, method of administration, and use in specific populations. Following approval for an intended use, physicians and other authorized practitioners
may prescribe the drug for uses not covered by the approved label. This off-label use is
common, particularly in the case of psychiatric drugs and in children and is not closely
regulated or monitored (Dresser 2007; Evans 2007; Zito *et al.* 2008).

Past and present trends of PCE use are another important consideration. In some
neuropsychiatric and neurodegenerative disorders there has been a dramatic increase in use
over the past decades, but the underlying reasons in each case differ. In the case of ADHD in
the US, prescriptions of stimulant medication have been increasing from the 1990s until the
present (Mayes *et al.* 2008). Mayes and colleagues identified a confluence of trends from that
time (clinical, economic, educational, and political), and alignment of incentives (among
clinicians, educators, policymakers, health insurers, the pharmaceutical industry) and the
sizable growth in scientific knowledge about ADHD and stimulants (Mayes *et al.* 2008). This
was accompanied by more sophisticated pharmacological formulations (Swanson and
Volkow 2009). Another contributing factor has been the recent recognition of adult ADHD.
Individuals first prescribed stimulant medications for ADHD as children are continuing to
take them during high school and beyond, and the number of prescriptions given to adult
ADHD patients in the US has increased dramatically (Okie 2006). The general trends are
not controversy free, and have raised concerns about the possibility of many children with a
"shadow" of ADHD who have easy access to medications (Mayes *et al.* 2008; see also
Swanson *et al.* 2007).

In the case of neurodegenerative dementias such as AD and acetylcholinesterase inhibitors, such as donepezil, their rising use has stemmed from a different set of trends largely
relating to the increasing aging population and the pressure to find treatments at various
stages of dysfunction (Knapp and Prince 2007). In the UK, recent National Institute for
Health and Clinical Excellence (NICE) guidelines have actively tried to decrease the use of
donepezil, galantamine, and rivastigmine as well as the glutamatergic NMDA (N-methyl-
D-aspartic acid) receptor antagonist memantine for dementia purportedly due to cost-
effectiveness considerations (NICE implementation uptake report 2009), the accuracy of
which have been contested. Interestingly, though the guidelines did not recommend these
treatments for mild (until very recently) or severe AD, in primary care their use continues to
increase. The same report noted that 60% of those prescribed the drugs did not have a diagnosis of AD in their records despite donepezil galatamine, and memantine only being used
to treat AD, suggesting pervasive off-label use, probably for individuals who likely have mild
cognitive impairment, and inconsistent diagnosis reporting in older adults (NICE 2009).

Ongoing research also suggests cognitive impairment in other neuropsychiatric diseases
where cognitive dysfunction is less prominent may be targeted for treatment using existing
PCEs. For instance, evidence indicates cognitive dysfunction in schizophrenia is associated
both with impaired functional and subjective outcomes (Morein-Zamir *et al.* 2007).
Preliminary evidence suggests that additional patient groups may benefit from PCE including multiple sclerosis patients, stroke patients, and those experiencing cognitive impairment
following traumatic brain injury (Christodoulou *et al.* 2006; Mehta and Riedel 2006; Porcel
and Montalban 2006; Salmond *et al.* 2005; Tenovuo 2006).

Trends of use are also influenced by label expansion, where treatment is sought for
additional disorders beyond the original use for which a drug was approved. For example, in
the case of modafinil—originally approved for narcolepsy—additional conditions such as

excessive sleepiness due to shift-work sleep disorder can now be treated. This can lead to additional off-label use as reported by the media for modafinil and jetlag. There has been some concern that trends for rising use of various PCEs results from labeling formerly "normal" states as disorders or diseases, allowing them to become legitimate goals of pharmacotherapy (Schermer *et al.* 2009). On the other hand, increasing use can be attributed in part to more sensitive diagnostic tools and less associated stigma (Mayes *et al.* 2008).

Information about the use of PCEs for purposes other than medical treatment is considerably more difficult to ascertain. In the US military, stimulants have been employed for decades, and more recently modafinil and donepezil use have also been examined (e.g. Caldwell *et al.* 2000). Though much research has been conducted with healthy individuals, such as sleep-deprived pilots, understandably only a minority of the research on these broadly-termed "cogniceuticals" (Russo 2007) may reach public domain. Nevertheless, off-label PCE are increasingly being employed on battlefields (Russo *et al.* 2008). Obviously, the risk–benefit ratio is markedly different under such circumstances and may include the risks and safety of other individuals directly dependent on the individual taking a PCE (see later).

Non-prescription use where PCE are obtained via means other than healthcare providers is by far the most difficult to monitor. Surveys of college students in the US suggest that between 1993 and 2001 there was a clear increase in the lifetime and 12-month prevalence rates of non-medical use of prescription drugs (McCabe *et al.* 2007). Similar studies indicate that up to 16% of students in some colleges use stimulants (Babcock and Byrne 2000; McCabe *et al.* 2005), while in others 8% of university undergraduates report having illegally used prescription stimulants (Teter *et al.* 2005). Most illicit uses of prescription stimulants in such surveys involved amphetamine/dextroamphetamine agents with higher use amongst Caucasians and Hispanics compared to African-Americans and Asians and considerable variations between colleges (Teter *et al.* 2006).

The evidence regarding general academic use of PCE and students in other countries is very limited and at times suffers from inadequate sampling. In an online voluntary poll by the journal *Nature*, based on data from 1400 respondents from 60 countries, one in five respondents reportedly used drugs for non-medical reasons as cognitive enhancers (Maher 2008). Of those, 52% obtained cognitive enhancing drugs by prescription, 34% by the Internet, and 14% by pharmacy. In the UK, a student newspaper revealed that in an informal survey of 1000 students, one in ten claimed to have taken a prescription drug for cognitive enhancement (Lennard 2009). The survey found large differences between students of different colleges within the university, as well as between areas of study. Though suggestive, such surveys are likely to suffer from selection bias and so should be interpreted with caution. Nevertheless, together with the large variations in use between colleges in the US (Teter *et al.* 2006), such results point to the importance of local sociological factors that likely govern the use in the healthy population. Currently there appear to be several surveys underway in European countries which point to lower but still existent use of non-prescription psychostimulants among students (Schermer *et al.* 2009).

At present we are unaware of reliable data on psychostimulants and PCE use in other sections of the population. One can presume that improvements in cognitive skills such as memory would appeal to middle-aged and elderly people facing a decline in memory and other cognitive functions. It is probable that PCE are used by some long-haul trucking, shift-workers, hi-tech, business, and other white-collar professionals. Further research should

investigate current use of cognitive enhancing drugs in the various sections of the population. Usage is also likely to be influenced by various socioeconomic and demographic
characteristics such as age and gender. Additional factors likely influence PCE use, such as
whether a single dose is sufficient (e.g. methylphenidate or modafinil) or prolonged administration is necessary (e.g. donepezil).

Attitudes towards the use of PCEs in the general population should inform neuroethical
discussion. There is also a dearth of information on these, though attitudes are likely influenced by factors that are similar to those that govern usage. Preliminary evidence from the
Nature poll described earlier indicated that 96% of all respondents thought people with neuropsychiatric disorders should be given cognitive enhancing drugs. In marked contrast, 86%
of respondents thought healthy children should be restricted from taking cognitive enhancing drugs. However, 33% of respondents said they would feel pressure to give their children
PCE if other children at school were taking them. Moreover, as scientific and public understanding of PCE as medical and non-medical interventions continues to develop, attitudes
will likely change.

In sum, the discussion about PCEs is fractionated by the different yet overlapping
purposes, methods, and circumstances of obtainment. It is evident that rising use in patients
often exists amid controversy, at times heated discussion, and opposing pressures for and
against PCEs as treatment. Further, there is a lack of consensus and in many cases insufficient information regarding actual and perceived risks and benefits in different populations.
Long-term effects with chronic administration are particularly unclear, though they may
differ from short-term effects (Swanson *et al.* 2007; Yesavage *et al.* 2008). Thus, while some
embrace or even fight for PCE, others reject them outright and still others remain unde-
cided. The present situation is exacerbated by relatively little reliable information about
off-label and non-prescription pervasiveness and their overlap with the use of various PCE
by healthy individuals for enhancement purposes.

PRESENT AND UPCOMING NEUROETHICAL CONSIDERATIONS

Neuroethical considerations are pertinent for PCE as treatments for neuropsychiatric disorders and brain injury, as well as for enhancement purposes in healthy adults (see Chapter 15
by Hildt and Metzinger for discussion of the notions of normality and enhancement). The
following discussions are grounded in current empirical evidence with a view towards
potential upcoming developments. First and foremost, risk–benefit analyses reflect safety
considerations versus efficacy. Safe in essence means safe enough, as no drugs are free of side
effects and the risk of adverse effects is weighed against probable benefits (Harris 2009). The
trade-off can also be examined at the level of society, which may benefit from more functional or productive individuals and from the achievements stemming from enhanced individuals. On the other hand, society must also bear the cost to individuals suffering from
adverse consequences (e.g. addiction), and potentially in future to general norms relating to
individual freedom, accepted productivity levels, etc. Nevertheless, society as a whole
already tolerates a certain amount of risk for an expected utility.

As evident from discussions here, long-term use remains relatively poorly understood with some PCEs, though in others long-term monitoring is adequate and suggests the benefits continue to outweigh the risks for some populations. For example, guidelines issued in 2002 by the American Academy of Child and Adolescent Psychiatry on stimulant use in children, adolescents, and adults recommend monitoring medicated adult blood pressure and pulse every 3 months (Okie 2006). In the case of healthy individuals, however, it is unclear whether the benefits outweigh the risks. As long-term reliable data is generally not available on healthy individuals, efficacy versus safety considerations remain a significant concern and are continuously debated (Chatterjee 2009; Harris 2009). Additional risks exist for individuals who acquire PCEs from sources other than healthcare providers. When a drug is provided on- or off-label, healthcare providers can monitor for possible drug-related complications and counter-indications such as risks from existing medical conditions (e.g. high blood pressure) and from drug–drug interaction. Obtaining PCE from unregulated sources, such as the Internet, leads to even greater risks as the content of pills remains uncertain (Califano 2008).

The relative efficacy for different sections of the population also remains poorly understood (e.g. Turner *et al.* 2003b). Further, efficacy has implications on the possible relationships between therapy and enhancement (Wolpe 2002) and possibly on some doctors who may be required or expected to subsume new roles rather than treatment providers (Chatterjee 2004). Moreover, expectations about the efficacy of PCE may be unrealistic in some groups such as the elderly which typically suffer from normal decline in some cognitive domains and may expect complete reversal of these age-related changes. Neither is it clear whether or not any enhancements observed will come at the expense of other cognitive abilities, mood, or personality traits (Farah 2005) or even social skills; (though see Bolt and Schermer 2009). Improvements in cognitive skills are believed to increase both an individual's quality of life and ability to contribute to society (Beddington *et al.* 2008). Using PCEs may indeed lead to better functionality, more efficiency, and even better fulfillment of potential. Evidence supporting this can be found in the case of some patients (Davidson and Keefe 1995), though additional research is required to examine this in healthy individuals. In fact, measurement of efficacy is also far from straightforward in healthy individuals where no clear deficits can be measured. Though self-report and one's personal view would be primary in determining use, it would not be considered conclusive evidence for effectiveness. Objective measurements of cognitive performance at a discrete time and place is important but also would ideally translate into quantifiable improvements of daily performance at work or in other environments.

From a practical perspective, usage information suggests healthy individuals will continue to use PCE as well as other pharmaceutical enhancers (e.g. mood). The drive for self-enhancement of cognition is likely to be as strong if not stronger than in the realms of beauty, physical, and sexual performance. Thus, the pertinent questions are what can be done within the present reality/conditions in terms of regulation, education, and other means to both inform but also monitor. Empirical data is needed to ascertain who is being monitored and whether there are drug-related complications ascribed to off-label or non-prescribed use. The issues of safety and harm–benefit analyses become particularly pertinent when children are concerned. Though children with disorders such as ADHD and depression are routinely given pharmaceuticals, very little empirical data is available and in healthy children there is even less information (Parens and Johnston 2008; Zito *et al.* 2008). Some of the concerns overlap with those relevant to adults, such as abuse and addiction; however, the implications of these are more pronounced given the limited liberty of children, their limited capacity for decision-making, and the fact that they are at the beginning of their life span. There are additional specific concerns, not present in adults, such as influence on growth rates and brain development (Swanson et al. 2007; see also Moll et al. 2001). The consideration of trade-offs and arguments for safety does not necessarily preclude PCEs, but they do necessitate caution and careful individual assessment and monitoring.

Further neuroethical considerations pertain to direct and indirect coercion and personal freedom. The ethical discussion of coercion in the treatment for neuropsychiatric and neurodegenerative disorders is ongoing and complex (Kallert 2008) and will not be considered here. Coercion of PCEs in non-medical cases encompasses many potential situations. The military is a current example where occupational coercion may exist (Wolfendale 2008). Though clear guidelines have been suggested for the ethical use of PCEs in the military and they are dispensed under medical supervision (Russo 2007; Russo et al. 2008), indirect coercion remains a concern given the forces of conformity and peer pressure, and the fact that military members often operate in small close-knit units dependent on one another for their individual and collective survival (Russo et al. 2008). The discussion of these guidelines has also highlighted the differences amongst various Western countries, and suggests that cultural and legislative differences play a key role in PCE use worldwide (Russo 2007).

Clear guidelines and ensuring individual awareness of their own benefit–risk ratio is important not only in organizations such as the military. PCE usage requires very little effort and can at times be viewed by some as a viable replacement for seemingly more costly measures such as sleep—though see Russo (2007). In the near future, coercion could become a greater concern for civil occupations that entail cognitive demands in the face of lack of sleep or high pressure with great responsibility (e.g. surgeons, air traffic controllers). Coercion may be explicit and codified in regulations (e.g. shift-work requirements) or implicit (e.g. manifested in incentive schemes). The guidelines for ethical use of PCE in the military (Russo 2007) may prove a useful starting point if this became widespread. More subtle but no less powerful coercion is also likely to be found outside the work environment, as individuals ascribe better scholastic performance and overall better functioning to better cognition and are pressured to perform better in competitive environments. In all cases there is the possibility of a gradual drift in the performance standards routinely expected of individuals by themselves and others. This may be accompanied by real or misperceived new social norms, together with extensive and often hyped media coverage (Sahakian and Morein-Zamir 2010). Already individuals believe the use of PCE is more pervasive than it actually is (McCabe 2008). Coercion together with a shift in norms would be an even greater concern in cases where any perceived benefits were outweighed by adverse effects on the self and performance. In addition, such concerns apply doubly so for children who often experience strong peer pressure to conform, and self and parental pressure to succeed at school. Given the safety concerns, any steps taken to inform and monitor use in adults (see below) would not be sufficient by themselves in children.

Neuroethical considerations about personal identity and authenticity (Farah et al. 2004) can also be informed by empirical research. Even at present, with PCEs of modest effects, the full gamut of possible relations between the self and PCEs can be found. Taking ADHD as an example, some individuals perceive their true self on drugs, while others perceive their true self as off drugs and others still finding no relationship between the drug and their view of self (Bolt and Schermer 2009). More importantly, individual characteristics and circumstances also dictate how each person addresses any issues relating to unintended influences of PCE on their behavior and even personality traits (Bolt and Schermer 2009). Though at present, issues regarding authenticity appear premature, given that PCE effectiveness will likely increase in future, concerns about motivation and hard work and the possibility of a homogeneous society will likely receive more attention (for additional discussion please see Chatterjee 2004; Greely *et al.* 2008; and Wolpe 2002).

Considerations of fairness in use and equity in access largely hinge on current and future efficacy of PCE. PCE may ameliorate cognitive deficits in those particularly impaired and may play a beneficial role in the removal of unfair disparities. Both pharmaceutical and non-pharmaceutical cognitive enhancers may help mitigate the negative effects of poverty on brain development and cognition. Many individuals find themselves under strains to perform in a suboptimal state, such as parents of young children and other suffering from sleep deprivation. Under such conditions, PCE may be an alternative to self-medications or the use of other substances such as nicotine, caffeine, or alcohol. At the same time, for cognition to influence functionality the individual must still invest time and effort to express their cognitive abilities via learning and actual performance. However, concerns over cheating and PCE conveying an unfair advantage over others highlight the complexity of everyday situations where competitiveness plays a role (Farah 2005). The press has already reported negative opinions of some college students against their peers who use PCEs when studying for exams.

Previous discussions have underlined the fact that fairness in access is not a concern specific to PCE (e.g. see Chapter 16 by Harris in this volume). Fairness is largely dictated by equality in availability which already is heavily influenced by education and socioeconomic status, but in addition some social, religious, and ethnic factors may preclude the use of PCEs in some groups. The risk–benefit ratio may also be markedly different as a result of some of these factors, making their use more or less fair in other groups. For example, if a particular PCE would lead to marked benefits in one ethnic group in particular, would it provide them with an unfair advantage? These general considerations are true both within societies but also between societies (Sahakian and Morein-Zamir 2010). At the level of the individual, unclear regulations governing access may also lead to situations where individuals and groups put undue pressure on healthcare providers for provision of off-label PCE (Chatterjee 2002). Thus, in the future, off-label heathcare providers may be influenced by opposing pressures such as on the one hand users seeking PCEs under medical supervision (e.g. leading to doctor-shopping) and on the other hand legislative concerns (e.g. lawsuits). In sum, there are grounds for both optimism and caution about future PCE use, with PCEs likely playing a role in reducing some disparities while increasing others. In any case, generalizations across PCEs, populations, and circumstances must be avoided.

CONCLUDING REMARKS

Where does this discussion leave us? Within the context of an accelerating modern society and the consideration of the work–life balance it is useful to consider other methods of enhancing cognitive function (e.g. education, neurocognitive activation or cognitive training, exercise). Cognition, of course, cannot be viewed in isolation as mood, social skills, and all other forms of enhancement likely involve overlapping considerations, which may interact with each other in complex ways (e.g. could PCEs interact with effects of diet or education?). Though invasive, PCEs will be particularly attractive for those searching for a rapid and temporary boost which requires relatively little effort. We believe that future use will ultimately be determined by three key factors: efficacy versus risks of new drugs, commercial forces, and, as yet, still developing social norms. Previously we have argued for the responsible and rational use of PCEs (Greely *et al.* 2008; Sahakian and Morein-Zamir 2007, 2010). It is evident that for this to occur, more information is required about the risks and benefits in all sections of the population. Ideally, information about the profile of cognitive effects of each drug on specific populations should be obtained, along with its short- and long-term risks and benefits. Thus PCEs found to be effective and safe in the elderly would still require empirical evidence supporting similar effects in middle-aged or young adults. Incentives and changes in regulation may be necessary to obtain some of this information (e.g. consistent and inclusive reporting of all adverse events in emergency rooms and drop-in clinics).

The gathering of information is not sufficient by itself. Scientists, physicians, and policy-makers must also ensure that easy access to information about the advantages and dangers of using PCEs is available to the public (Sahakian and Morein-Zamir 2007). However, access to the information is also not enough, as humans do not generally make rational decisions about relative risk (Fischoff *et al.* 1981). Thus, treatment providers and monitors must ensure that additional guidance is available. Guidance must also refer to the non-pharmacological viable alternatives to improve cognition such as those mentioned earlier including exercise, nutrition, and sleep, which have all been shown to induce beneficial neural changes (Cooper *et al.* 2010). Training for healthcare providers and educators should be available so that they may offer such guidance where necessary.

At the same time, current monitoring policies should be critically examined and updated in light of existing trends in PCE use. Mechanisms must be in place for consistent monitoring of off-label and non-prescription use. Enforceable guidelines and regulatory discussion concerning the use of PCEs to support fairness, protect individuals from coercion, and minimize enhancement-related socioeconomic disparities are critical (Foresight Mental Capital and Wellbeing Project 2008; Greely *et al.* 2008). However, should future PCE offering large and desirable effects become available, regulating individual use may prove challenging regardless of safety concerns.

Commercial interests and social norms have previously played an important role in the popularity of other enhancers (e.g. caffeine), including some once used exclusively for treatment (e.g. plastic surgery), and are likely to play a substantial role in future trends of use and policy making. The role of the popular media, which can be very subtle at times as with celebrity culture, may also change as it is currently largely impassive. Should PCEs become fashionable or publicized, except for extreme cases, considerations of efficacy versus risks as discussed earlier may run the risk of being ignored by some sections of society. It is outside the scope of this chapter to discuss how social norms develop and change, but undoubtedly such processes could be relevant to the use of PCEs in future and should be better understood and anticipated.

Neuroethical discussion of PCEs depends largely on the PCEs currently available and current regulations and norms. Engagement of the public on PCEs is important to ensure maximum benefits and minimal harms for both the individual and society (Morein-Zamir and Sahakian 2010). The advent of future PCEs (Robbins 2009) together with increasing pressures in modern society will likely accelerate debate about cognitive enhancing drugs in upcoming years. At the same time, the discussion should remain grounded in the evidence and empirical trends to avoid both inflated expectations and fears.

ACKNOWLEDGEMENTS

The authors are funded in part by Wellcome Trust Programme Grant (076274/Z/04/Z) to BJS, Trevor Robbins, Barry Everitt, and Angela Roberts. The Behavioural and Clinical Neuroscience Institute is supported by a joint award from the Medical Research Council and Wellcome Trust. BJS consults for Cambridge Cognition and a number of pharmaceutical companies.

REFERENCES

Academy of Medical Sciences. (2008). *Brain science, addiction and drugs.* Working group report chaired by Professor Sir Gabriel Horn. Foresight Brain Science, Addiction and Drugs Project. London: Office of Science and Technology.

Apud, J.A. and Weinberger, D.R. (2006). Pharmacogenetic tools for the development of target-oriented cognitive-enhancing drugs. *NeuroRx,* **3**, 106–16.

Arnsten, A.F. (2000). Stress impairs prefrontal cortical function in rats and monkeys: role of dopamine D1 and norepinephrine alpha-1 receptor mechanisms. *Progress in Brain Research,* **126**, 183–92.

Babcock, Q. and Byrne, T. (2000). Student perceptions of methylphenidate abuse at a public liberal arts college. *Journal of American College Health,* **49**, 143–5.

Beddington, J., Cooper, C.L., Field, J., *et al.* (2008). The mental wealth of nations. *Nature,* **455**, 1057–60.

Bolt, I. and Schermer, M. (2009). Psychopharmaceutical enhancers: Enhancing identity? *Neuroethics,* **2**, 103–11.

Cacabelos, R. (2005). Pharmacogenomics and therapeutic prospects in Alzheimer's disease. *Expert Opinion in Pharmacotherpy,* **6**, 1967–87.

Caldwell, J.A., Jr., Caldwell, J.L., Smythe, N.K., 3rd, and Hall, K.K. (2000). A double-blind, placebo-controlled investigation of the efficacy of modafinil for sustaining the alertness and performance of aviators: a helicopter simulator study. *Psychopharmacology (Berl),* **150**, 272–82.

Califano, J. (2008). *"You've got drugs!" Prescription drug pushers on the Internet.* The National Center on Addiction and Substance Abuse. New York, Columbia University.

Chamberlain, S.R., Muller, U., Blackwell, A.D., Clark, L., Robbins, T.W., and Sahakian, B.J. (2006). Neurochemical modulation of response inhibition and probabilistic learning in humans. *Science,* **311**, 861–3.

Chamberlain, S.R., Del Campo, N., Dowson, J., *et al.* (2007). Atomoxetine improved response inhibition in adults with attention deficit/hyperactivity disorder. *Biological Psychiatry,* **62**, 977–84.

Chatterjee, A. (2004). Cosmetic neurology: the controversy over enhancing movement, mentation, and mood. *Neurology*, **28**, 968–74.

Chatterjee, A. (2009). Is it acceptable for people to take methylphenidate to enhance performance? No. *BMJ*, **338**, b1956.

Christodoulou, C., Melville, P., Scherl, W.F., Macallister, W.S., Elkins, L.E., and Krupp, L.B. (2006). Effects of donepezil on memory and cognition in multiple sclerosis. *Journal of Neurological Science*, **245**, 127–36.

Cools, R. and Robbins, T.W. (2004). Chemistry of the adaptive mind. *Philosophical Transactions A Math Phys Eng Sci*, **362**, 2871–88.

Cools, R., Barker, R.A., Sahakian, B.J., and Robbins, T.W. (2003). L-Dopa medication remediates cognitive inflexibility, but increases impulsivity in patients with Parkinson's disease. *Neuropsychologia*, **41**, 1431–41.

Cooper, C.L., Field, J., Goswami, U., Jenkins, R., and Sahakian, B.J. (2010). *Mental Capital and Wellbeing*. Oxford: Wiley-Blackwell.

Davidson, M. and Keefe, R.S. (1995). Cognitive impairment as a target for pharmacological treatment in schizophrenia. *Schizophrenia Research*, **17**, 123–9.

de Jongh, R., Bolt, I., Schermer, M., and Olivier, B. (2008). Botox for the brain: enhancement of cognition, mood and pro-social behavior and blunting of unwanted memories. *Neuroscience and Biobehavioral Reviews*, **32**, 760–6.

Diaz-Asper, C.M., Weinberger, D.R., and Goldberg, T.E. (2006). Catechol-O-methyltransferase polymorphisms and some implications for cognitive therapeutics. *NeuroRx*, **3**, 97–105.

Dresser, R. (2007). The curious case of off-label use. *Hastings Centre Report*, **37**, 9–11.

Evans, B.J. (2007). Distinguishing product and practice regulation in personalized medicine. *Clinical Pharmacology and Therapeutics*, **81**, 288–93.

Farah, M.J. (2005). Neuroethics: the practical and the philosophical. *Trends in Cognitive Science*, **9**, 34–40.

Fischoff, B., Lichtenstein, S., Slovic, P., Derby, S.L., and Keeney, R.L. (1981). *Acceptable Risk*. Cambridge, MA: Cambridge University Press.

Foresight Mental Capital and Wellbeing Project (2008). *Final Project Report*. London: The Government Office for Science.

Greely, H., Sahakian, B., Harris, J., *et al.* (2008). Towards responsible use of cognitive enhancing drugs in the healthy. *Nature*, **456**, 702–5.

Harris, J. (2009). Is it acceptable for people to take methylphenidate to enhance performance? Yes. *British Medical Journal*, **338**, b1955.

Johnston, L.D., O'Malley, P.M., Bachman, J.G., and Schulenberg, J.E. (2006). *Monitoring the Future national results on adolescent drug use: Overview of key findings, 2005* (NIH Publication No. 06-5882). Bethesda, MD: National Institute on Drug Abuse.

Jones, R.W., Morris, K., and Nutt, D. (2005). *Cognition Enhancers. Foresight Brain Science Addiction and Drugs Project*. London: Office of Science and Technology.

Kallert, T.W. (2008). Coercion in psychiatry. *Current Opinion in Psychiatry*, **21**(5), 485–9.

Knapp, M. and Prince, M. (2007). *Dementia UK: Summary of key findings*. London, UK: Alzheimer's Society.

Konrad, K., Gunther, T., Hanisch, C., and Herpertz-Dahlmann, B. (2004). Differential effects of methylphenidate on attentional functions in children with attention-deficit/hyperactivity disorder. *J Am Acad Child Adolesc Psychiatry*, **43**, 191–8.

Lee, Y.S. and Silva, A.J. (2009). The molecular and cellular biology of enhanced cognition. *Nature Reviews Neuroscience*, **10**, 126–40.

Lennard, N. (2009, March 6th). One in ten takes drugs to study. *Varsity*, **693**, 1.

Maher, B. (2008). Poll results: look who's doping. *Nature*, **452**, 674–5.

Marchant, N.L., Kamel, F., Echlin, K., Grice, J., Lewis, M., and Rusted, J.M. (2009). Modafinil improves rapid shifts of attention. *Psychopharmacology (Berl)*, **202**, 487–95.

Mayes, R., Bagwell, C., and Erkulwater, J. (2008). ADHD and the rise in stimulant use among children. *Harvard Review of Psychiatry*, **16**, 151–66.

McCabe, S.E. (2008). Misperceptions of non-medical prescription drug use: a web survey of college students. *Addictive Behaviors*, **33**, 713–24.

McCabe, S.E., Knight, J.R., Teter, C.J., and Wechsler, H. (2005). Non-medical use of prescription stimulants among US college students: prevalence and correlates from a national survey. *Addiction*, **100**, 96–106.

McCabe, S.E., West, B.T., and Wechsler, H. (2007). Trends and college-level characteristics associated with the non-medical use of prescription drugs among US college students from 1993 to 2001. *Addiction*, **102**, 455–65.

Mehta, M.A. and Riedel, W.J. (2006). Dopaminergic enhancement of cognitive function. *Current Pharmaceutical Design*, **12**, 2487–500.

Mehta, M.A., Owen, A.M., Sahakian, B.J., Mavaddat, N., Pickard, J.D., and Robbins, T.W. (2000). Methylphenidate enhances working memory by modulating discrete frontal and parietal lobe regions in the human brain. *Journal of Neuroscience*, **20**, RC65.

Minzenberg, M.J. and Carter, C.S. (2008). Modafinil: a review of neurochemical actions and effects on cognition. *Neuropsychopharmacology*, **33**, 1477–502.

Minzenberg, M.J., Watrous, A.J., Yoon, J.H., Ursu, S., and Carter, C.S. (2008). Modafinil shifts human locus coeruleus to low-tonic, high-phasic activity during functional MRI. *Science*, **322**, 1700–2.

Moll, G.H., Hause, S., Ruther, E., Rothenberger, A., and Huether, G. (2001). Early methylphenidate administration to young rats causes a persistent reduction in the density of striatal dopamine transporters. *Journal of Child and Adolescent Psychopharmacology*, **11**, 15–24.

Morein-Zamir, S. and Sahakian, B.J. (2010). Neuroethics and public engagement training needed for neuroscientists. *Trends in Cognitive Science*, **14**, 49–51.

Morein-Zamir, S., Turner, D.C., and Sahakian, B.J. (2007). A review of the effects of modafinil on cognition in schizophrenia. *Schizophrenia Bulletin*, **33**, 1298–306.

Morein-Zamir, S., Robbins, T.W., Turner, D.C., and Sahakian, B.J. (2010). Pharmacological cognitive enhancement. In C. L. Cooper, J. Field, U. Goswami, R. Jenkins, and B. J. Sahakian (eds.) *Mental Capital and Mental Wellbeing Project*, pp. 129–38. Oxford, UK: Wiley-Blackwell.

National Institute for Health and Clinical Excellence (2009). *NICE implementation uptake report: Donepezil, galantamine, rivastigmine and memantine for the treatment of Alzheimer's disease*. London: NICE.

National Institute for Health and Clinical Excellence: National Collaborating Centre for Mental Health (2007). *Dementia: A NICE-SCIE guideline on supporting people with dementia and their carers in health and social care*. Commissioned by the National Institute for Health and Clinical Excellence: The British Psychological Society and Gaskell. London: NICE.

Okie, S. (2006). ADHD in adults. *New England Journal of Medicine*, **354**, 2637–41.

Parens, E. and Johnston, J. (2008). Understanding the agreements and controversies surrounding childhood psychopharmacology. *Child and Adolescent Psychiatry and Mental Health*, **2**, 5.

Porcel, J., and Montalban, X. (2006). Anticholinesterasics in the treatment of cognitive impairment in multiple sclerosis. *Journal of Neurological Science*, **245**, 177–181.

Ramos, B.P. and Arnsten, A.F. (2007). Adrenergic pharmacology and cognition: focus on the prefrontal cortex. *Pharmacology and Therapeutics*, **113**, 523–36.

Robbins, T.W. (2009). Special issue on cognitive enhancers. *Psychopharmacology (Berl)*, **202**, 1–2.

Russo, M.B. (2007). Recommendations for the ethical use of pharmacologic fatigue counter-measures in the U.S. military. *Aviation, Space and Environmental Medicine*, **78**, B119–127; discussion B128–37.

Russo, M.B., Arnett, M.V., Thomas, M.L., and Caldwell, J.A. (2008). Ethical use of cogniceu-ticals in the militaries of democratic nations. *American Journal of Bioethics*, **8**, 39–41; discussion W34–6.

Sahakian, B. and Morein-Zamir, S. (2007). Professor's little helper. *Nature*, **450**, 1157–9.

Sahakian, B. and Morein-Zamir, S. (2010). Neuroethical issues in cognitive enhancement. *Journal of Psychopharmacology*. [Epub 8 March 2010]

Salmond, C.H., Chatfield, D.A., Menon, D.K., Pickard, J.D., and Sahakian, B.J. (2005). Cognitive sequelae of head injury: involvement of basal forebrain and associated structures. *Brain*, **128**, 189–200.

Schermer, M., Bolt, I., de Jongh, R., and Olivier, B. (2009). The future of psychopharmaco-logical enhancements: expectations and policies. *Neuroethics*, **2**, 75–87.

Stahl, S.M. (2008). *Stahl's Essential Psychopharmacology*, 3rd edition. New York: Cambridge University Press.

Swainson, R., Rogers, R.D., Sahakian, B.J., Summers, B.A., Polkey, C.E., and Robbins, T.W. (2000). Probabilistic learning and reversal deficits in patients with Parkinson's disease or frontal or temporal lobe lesions: possible adverse effects of dopaminergic medication. *Neuropsychologia*, **38**, 596–612.

Swanson, J.M., Elliott, G.R., Greenhill, L.L., *et al.* (2007). Effects of stimulant medication on growth rates across 3 years in the MTA follow-up. *Journal of the American Academy of Child and Adolescent Psychiatry*, **46**, 1015–27.

Swanson, J.M. and Volkow, N.D. (2009). Psychopharmacology: concepts and opinions about the use of stimulant medications. *Journal of Child Psychology and Psychiatry*, **50**, 180–93.

Tannock, R., Schachar, R. and Logan, G.D. (1995). Methylphenidate and cognitive flexibility: Dissociated dose effects in hyperactive children. *Journal of Abnormal Child Psychology*, **23**, 235–66.

Tenovuo, O. (2006). Pharmacological enhancement of cognitive and behavioral deficits after traumatic brain injury. *Current Opinion in Neurology*, **19**, 528–33.

Teter, C.J., McCabe, S.E., Cranford, J.A., Boyd, C.J., and Guthrie, S.K. (2005). Prevalence and motives for illicit use of prescription stimulants in an undergraduate student sample. *Journal of American College Health*, **53**, 253–62.

Teter, C.J., McCabe, S.E., LaGrange, K., Cranford, J.A., and Boyd, C.J. (2006). Illicit use of specific prescription stimulants among college students: prevalence, motives, and routes of administration. *Pharmacotherapy*, **26**, 1501–10.

Turner, D.C., Robbins, T.W., Clark, L., Aron, A.R., Dowson, J., and Sahakian, B.J. (2003a). Cognitive enhancing effects of modafinil in healthy volunteers. *Psychopharmacology*, **165**, 260–9.

Turner, D.C., Robbins, T.W., Clark, L., Aron, A.R., Dowson, J., and Sahakian, B.J. (2003b). Relative lack of cognitive effects of methylphenidate in elderly male volunteers. *Psychopharmacology*, **168**, 455–64.

Turner, D.C., Clark, L., Pomarol-Clotet, E., McKenna, P., Robbins, T.W., and Sahakian, B.J. (2004). Modafinil improves cognition and attentional set shifting in patients with chronic schizophrenia. *Neuropsychopharmacology, 29*, 1363–73.

Volkow, N.D., Fowler, J.S., Logan, J., *et al.* (2009). Effects of modafinil on dopamine and dopamine transporters in the male human brain: clinical implications. *Journal of the American Medical Association, 301*, 1148–54.

Wolfendale, J. (2008). Performance-enhancing technologies and moral responsibility in the military. *American Journal of Bioethics, 8*, 28–38.

Wolpe, P.R. (2002). Treatment, enhancement, and the ethics of neurotherapeutics. *Brain and Cognition, 50*, 387–95.

Wong, D.F. (2008). Is getting older all that rewarding? *Proceedings of the National Academy of Sciences, 105*, 14751–2.

Yesavage, J.A., Friedman, L., Ashford, J.W., *et al.* (2008). Acetylcholinesterase inhibitor in combination with cognitive training in older adults. *Journal of Gerontology: Psychological Sciences, 63*, P288–94.

Zito, J.M., Derivan, A.T., Kratochvil, C.J., Safer, D.J., Fegert, J.M., and Greenhill, L.L. (2008). Off-label psychopharmacologic prescribing for children: History supports close clinical monitoring. *Child and Adolescent Psychiatry and Mental Health, 2*, 24.

CHAPTER 15

....

COGNITIVE
ENHANCEMENT

....

THOMAS METZINGER AND ELISABETH HILDT

INTRODUCTION

....

THIS chapter deals with ethical issues in cognitive enhancement (CE). We will begin by discussing some standard conceptual issues related to the notion of "cognitive enhancement" and then continue from a purely descriptive point of view by briefly reviewing some empirical aspects and sketching the current situation. Then we will offer some reflections on the treatment/enhancement distinction. In the second half of this contribution, we will turn to normative issues by first describing standard topics in current debates, then highlighting three examples of what we take to be relevant novel questions under an ethical perspective. We will end by making some general proposals for policy makers.

CONCEPTUAL ISSUES: WHAT IS
"COGNITIVE ENHANCEMENT"?

....

CE is a technology. It aims at optimizing a specific class of information-processing functions: *cognitive* functions, physically realized by the human brain. The human brain, however, not only possesses a long evolutionary history, but it also changes over a lifetime. Importantly, it is embodied as well as embedded in a dense network of environmental interactions, many of which are of a distinctly cultural and social nature. Indeed, human cognition might be a process that extends into the world, beyond skin and skull (see Menary 2010). With regard to CE, the first problem seems to consist in finding a suitable definition of "cognition" in order to discern the *domain* in which CE takes place, as well as clarifying the notion of "enhancement." But this might be a harder project than it might seem.

There are many different cognitive functions, and to date there is no standardized working definition of "cognition" on which neuroethicists could draw. Obvious examples of seemingly distinct cognitive functions are: concept formation, mental abstraction, language acquisition, text comprehension, higher linguistic abilities, inference, learning, symbolic reasoning, planning, decision making, and metacognition (i.e. thinking about thinking). But what about unconscious or entirely subsymbolic phenomena, like low-level perceptual processing, procedural memory, focal attention, introspection, or empathy-based forms of social cognition? To give just one example: a mood-enhancing antidepressant drug may improve our capacities for reasoning and planning, just as physical exercise certainly does. Should this drug then count as a "cognitive enhancer," or is the causal route it takes in influencing its target phenomenon too indirect? What about physical exercise, like jogging or swimming? Is there a decisive difference between optimizing one's cognitive functions through the right kind of athletic activity and "emotional enhancement"? What makes modern day (i.e. pharmacological) CE special is its functional "level of granularity": it presents us with a technology that very directly influences the *core realizers* of certain cognitive functions, on the molecular level of brain chemistry itself. However, for many such functions it is not at all clear if they are actually *constituted* by their local correlates in the brain and their neurocomputational properties. Often, the neural/molecular-level core realizer will be just one central aspect of a cognitive process that is much more extended—a complex process which can only be understood if we take additional higher-level levels of description into account, levels perhaps including symbolic representation, personal-level cognitive agency, and social interaction.

Neuroethics cannot wait for philosophers of mind and cognitive scientists to come up with a clear-cut and commonly shared definition for the concept of "cognition" or indeed "cognitive function." What neuroethicists can and should do, however, is use existing conceptual tools to describe *what* is being enhanced by a specific psychoactive substance (or perhaps by some other new technology not operating on the molecular level), and they should do so as precisely as possible. Does a given substance perhaps only increase vigilance, leading to a placebo effect and a self-fulfilling prophecy of increased insight in certain subjects? Does it perhaps selectively improve the capacity of working-memory? Which aspects of attentional processing are strengthened, and is there a specific type of memory recall that is optimized? Or are we actually seeing an enhancement in the capacity for abstract, symbolic thought? Does this come at a price, say, a lack in impulse control? The point is that making broad statements about "cognition" per se will not help. Neuroethics needs an empirically plausible, fine-grained description of potential *action goals* in CE before it can proceed to any proper ethical assessment. Part of the difficulty consists in the fact that what it actually means to describe a certain cognitive domain and the targeted mental function "as precisely as possible" is itself continuously changing: rapid empirical progress and the emergence of cognitive neurotechnology go hand in hand. Notwithstanding the considerable relevance of a conceptual clarification of "cognitive," the conceptual analysis of "enhancement" may be viewed as more useful for a neuroethics of CE than a conceptual analysis of "cognitive." For what is really important in the latter case is the social and ethical context of various affected functions, rather than whatever it might be about these functions that licenses describing them as cognitive. In particular, describing something as an enhancement has normative consequences that are deeply entangled with a range of poignant issues for policy making.

The second major conceptual issue is to define the notion of "enhancement" as clearly as possible. Here, the central philosophical problem is that *normative* elements are already built into the concept itself. In bioethics, the term "enhancement" is "usually used […] to characterize interventions designed to improve human form or functioning beyond what is necessary to sustain or restore good health." (Juengst 1998, p. 29). As opposed to medical treatments or therapies, enhancements modify physical or mental characteristics in healthy individuals. These include fields such as cosmetic surgery, the increase of physical performance in sports, or psychopharmacological enhancement (Parens 1998; President's Council on Bioethics 2003). In psychopharmacological enhancement, psychoactive drugs that have been devised as a therapy for specified diseases are used off-label or illicitly by normal, healthy individuals in order to modify brain functioning.

Who counts as a "healthy individual"? The trivial point is that concepts like "normal mental functioning" or, say, "normal age-related cognitive decline" possess a statistical and a normative reading (for an overview, see Murphy 2009). The semantics of both types of concepts change over time. For example, the statistical and descriptive features of "normal mental functioning" or "normal age-related cognitive decline" change as science progresses, as the predictive success of our theories improves, and as textbook definitions are adapted. Our concepts become richer in content, and more differentiated. But if a specific society suddenly has new tools and new potentials for action at hand—say, to alter certain cognitive functions in the elderly—then the statistical distribution of even those objective properties underlying a purely statistical notion of what is normal may also change. CE is a technology, and technologies change the objective world. Objective changes are subjectively perceived, and may lead to correlated shifts in value judgements.

The second reading of concepts like "healthy individual," "normal mental functioning," or "normal age-related cognitive decline" is normative, because it appears in statements about how human beings *should* be. Is it really necessary to suffer from memory loss or a decreasing attention span after the age of 55? If one writes a PhD thesis at 25, and if one is honestly interested in making a substantial contribution to research, is one not even morally obliged to optimize one's capacities for concentration and sustained intellectual achievement? Or is there anything sacred about the natural human condition, something that should never be touched? If other options are actually on the table, does this turn passively succumbing to age-related cognitive decline or certain, individually given limitations in high-level, abstract thought into a form of unkemptness and dishevelment?

A central point many neuroethicists often ignore (or perhaps deliberately avoid) is that, from a more rigorous philosophical perspective, it is not at all obvious that moral judgments are capable of being objectively true, because they describe some feature of the world—there may simply be no moral facts (van Roojen 2009). One logical possibility is that normative statements are not true or false at all, because there is no distinct kind of ethical *knowledge* they might express. Philosophical keywords are "moral anti-realism" and "non-cognitivism." It is beyond the scope of this short entry to penetrate into such metaethical issues, or to even give a very short introduction. But our first conclusion about the concept of "enhancement" is threefold, if quite obvious and self-evident: First, there is a statistical and normative reading of what counts as "normal cognitive functioning." Second, the normative reading may be epistemologically unfounded, that is, we must face the possibility that it might not express any form of knowledge in a strong, ethically interesting, sense. And third, making the distinction between "therapy" and "enhancement" is itself a normative act.

The not-so-trivial challenge lies in understanding the dynamic interaction between "normality" (in the descriptive sense) and "normalization" (in the normative sense). The theoretical and social dynamics linking both concepts and their interpretation is highly complex.

It involves scientific theories (in cognitive neuroscience, molecular neurobiology, and psychopharmacology), applied philosophical ethics, changing cultural contexts, globalization, policy-making, and industrial lobbies trying to influence the historical change of our very own concepts and their meaning. Normalization is a complex sociocultural process by which certain new norms become accepted in societal practice. This process is of a more obvious political nature, because it typically involves powerful forces, like the pharmaceutical industry's continuous attempt to control the implementation and the marketing of new enhancement technologies in society, for example, by changing the medical taxonomy or inventing new diseases and theoretical entities. The scientific process—say, of optimizing textbook definitions, predictions, and therapeutical success—is highly political as well. It attempts to firmly anchor theoretical entities like "normal mental functioning" or "normal age-related cognitive decline" in empirical data, but it is also driven by individual career interests, influenced by funding agencies, media coverage, and so on. In addition, it may well be that concepts like that of a "cognitively healthy individual" will always possess an *irreducibly* normative component.

However, this is not a tragedy: As soon as we have clearly understood that there *is* a dynamic interaction between "normality" (in the descriptive sense) and "normalization" (in the normative sense) we can make this interaction itself the object of a rigorous, rational approach. We can base our search for temporary solutions in the applied ethics of CE on available empirical data and rational arguments. We can try to reduce the signal-to-noise ratio in public debates, and we can gradually improve the conceptual clarity and the rationality underlying practical decisions in the neuroethics of CE. We will not achieve certainty or any form of absolute knowledge about what is a good action. But we can certainly improve the *coherence* between the way we act ethically on the level of society as a whole and what we actually know—including our knowledge about what we *don't* know.

COGNITIVE ENHANCEMENT: THE CURRENT SITUATION

Currently, several enhancement strategies are being tested, used, and discussed (Chatterjee 2004; Farah *et al.* 2004; Glannon 2008; de Jongh *et al.* 2008). One of the most prominent is the use of antidepressants such as fluoxetine (Prozac®), a selective serotonin reuptake inhibitor (SSRI), for mood-brightening. Since the 1990s, in particular in the US, these psychoactive substances have been widely utilized for mood enhancement, i.e. in order to modulate mood, attain mental well-being, and positively influence social behavior (cf. Kramer 1993; Elliott 2000; Pieters and Snelders 2009). Another approach aims at preventing the consolidation or reconsolidation of unwanted, problematic or traumatic memories through beta-blockers such as propranolol, which has been shown to have therapeutic effects in post-traumatic stress disorder (PTSD) (Pitman 2002; Marshall 2004; Miller 2004; Glannon 2006; Bell 2008). At present, this strategy is still in an experimental phase, however.

In contrast to mood enhancement or memory blocking, CE seeks to improve mental performance by increasing cognitive functions such as concentration, memory, or alertness (Whitehouse *et al.* 1997; Farah 2002; Chatterjee 2004; Farah *et al.* 2004). Psychoactive substances currently being used as cognitive enhancers include psychostimulants such as methylphenidate (Ritalin®) and Adderall® (a combination of dextroamphetamine and racemic DL-amphetamine salts) normally prescribed for the treatment of attention deficit hyperactivity disorder (ADHD), and modafinil (Provigil®) which is approved as a treatment for narcolepsy, excessive sleepiness associated with obstructive sleep apnea/hypopnea syndrome and shift-work sleep disorder (Turner *et al.* 2003; Minzenberg and Carter 2008). There are also studies indicating some positive effects of donepezil (Arizept®) on memory functioning in healthy individuals. Donepezil is an acetylcholinesterase inhibitor prescribed as a treatment in Alzheimer's disease (Yesavage *et al.* 2002; Grön *et al.* 2005; Glannon 2006; Dekkers and Rikkert 2007). *Ginkgo biloba* is often used to improve memory or prevent memory decline, despite the fact that there is no conclusive evidence of its putative cognition-enhancing effects (Canter and Ernst 2007). And several pharmaceutical companies are aiming to develop memory-enhancing drugs that either target glutamate receptors or increase the function of the cAMP response element binding protein (CREB) (Marshall 2004; Glannon 2006).

According to recent reports, psychostimulants such as methylphenidate or modafinil are increasingly being used in offices, schools, and universities. Users aim at augmenting mental fitness in order to better cope with intellectual challenges and time pressure, shift work (doctors, nurses), school or university exams, or jetlag (Sahakian and Morein-Zamir 2007; Maher 2008; DAK 2009). According to studies carried out so far among US college students, illicit use of prescription drugs seems to be quite widespread: data on non-medical stimulant use varies, but between 5% and 35% of college students—in most studies under 20%—report having misused prescription stimulants in order to improve academic output by increasing alertness or concentration, but also for partying or experimentation. Data indicate that there is a correlation between use of cognitive enhancers and abuse of other (illicit) drugs (McCabe *et al.* 2005; Teter *et al.* 2006; Wilens *et al.* 2008). However, at least currently, there are considerable differences between societies. Whereas cognitive enhancers seem to be used quite widely in some societies such as the US, in others only few people actively seek them at present. For example, according to preliminary results of research carried out at the University of Mainz, 3% of a group of 18/19-year-old pupils at German secondary schools and vocational schools have ever used psychostimulants (amphetamines or methylphenidate) for cognition enhancement (Franke *et al.* 2009).

The effects of psychostimulants in healthy individuals seem to be moderate and include improvements in alertness, cognitive performance, and concentration. Among the reported side effects are sleeplessness, jitteriness, anxiety, headaches, nausea, vertigo, and dizziness (Caldwell *et al.* 2000; Turner *et al.* 2003; Sahakian and Morein-Zamir 2007; Maher 2008; for a detailed review of the effects and side effects of cognition-enhancing drugs cf.: Sahakian and Morein-Zamir 2010; and Chapter 14 in this volume).

It is important to stress that there is a considerable lack of empirical data on the actual spread and extent of the circulation of cognitive enhancers among the general population, as well as on the safety and efficacy of cognition-enhancing drugs in healthy individuals. This is particularly true in view of the covert use of these drugs, and the flourishing and almost uncontrollable internet market. Especially, the impacts of cognition-enhancing drugs on everyday life, for example, on academic output, as well as their long-term effects, need further investigation.

In spite of the current lack of empirical data, however, there seems to be not only a considerable number of individuals willing to boost their brain power, but also substantial commercial interest in cognitive enhancers. If some cognitive enhancer should prove to be effective at an acceptable risk-benefit ratio, a rapidly growing use of cognition-enhancing drugs can be expected in the future.

HEALTH, DISEASE, AND NORMALITY

As described earlier, the concept of enhancement is a "moral boundary concept" (Juengst 1998) with descriptive and normative roles. On the descriptive level, enhancement characterizes an improvement, whereas on the normative level, enhancements are considered to be measures that go beyond medical requirement. Typically, the concept of enhancement is used to delineate the limits of medicine's proper domain of practice, which consists in restoring health and preventing disease. In other words, enhancement serves to characterize the limits of professional obligations to provide and finance medical interventions. As D.M. Frankford stresses, the term "enhancement" already implies a normative statement, because to label an intervention an "enhancement" means to position it outside the medical realm. According to Frankford, "[T]he treatment/enhancement distinction is not a foundation for moral justification but the result of the justification itself" (Frankford 1998, p. 72; see also section "Conceptual issues: What is "cognitive enhancement"?" of this chapter).

For the distinction between treatment and enhancement, the concepts of health and disease are crucial. Notwithstanding its broad use, a clear and unequivocal distinction between treatment and enhancement is difficult, however, for two reasons: The concepts of health and disease are very general and allow a wide range of definitions; drawing clear lines is difficult (President's Council on Bioethics 2003; Caplan et al. 2004; Flower 2004). It makes a considerable difference whether you consider "health" to be a state that can be characterized by the absence of disease; whether health is depicted as a condition characterized by biostatistical normality or normal species-typical functioning (Boorse 1977; Daniels 1985); or whether health is defined as "a state of complete physical, mental and social well-being and not merely the absence of disease or infirmity" (World Health Organization 1958). According to the famous World Health Organization definition, almost any measurement that serves to promote well-being—and this includes various enhancements—can be considered a "therapy" in some sense. In contrast, other definitions consider legitimate medical measures to be those that counteract some specified abnormality or disease, and thus view the situation quite differently.

In addition, disease categories are quite flexible and undergo various changes, as can be seen from the revisions and updates that classifications such as the International Classification of Diseases (ICD) and the Diagnostic and Statistical Manual of Mental Disorders (DSM) have undergone in the past. In these modifications, medical and scientific developments, but also technical and social aspects play a role. Furthermore, a current certain tendency to enlarge categories of "disease" can be observed (Bostrom 2008; Schermer et al. 2009). By expanding diagnostic categories or creating new pathological conditions, conditions that were previously considered normal come to be labeled as diseases. In the context of CE, relevant examples include ADHD and mild cognitive impairment

(MCI)—conditions characterized by broad gray zones. Last but not least, the broadening of disease categories implies an extension and facilitation of access to public funding, health-care, and drugs.

Instead of bearing on the concepts of health and disease, another line of argumentation refers to the concept of normality in order to distinguish between treatment and enhance-ment: According to this distinction, measures aiming to restore individuals to normality are considered medical therapies, whereas those aiming to provide individuals with abilities they would not otherwise have are enhancements (Jones 2006; Synofzik 2009). What complicates this distinction is that the term "normal" is far from being well-defined (cf. section Conceptual issues: What is cognitive enhancement? in this chapter). On the one hand, the term "normal" can be purely descriptive in the sense of being the statistical average, on the other hand it often involves a normative component. This can be seen from authors who use concepts such as biostatistical normality or normal species-typical functioning as a basis for defining the concepts of health and disease and for defining the limits of healthcare provision (Boorse 1977; Daniels 1985; Sabin and Daniels 1994). In Norman Daniels' reflections, normal species-typical functioning serves as a criterion for determining what is necessary from a medical point of view, what is covered by just healthcare. Accordingly, interventions that serve to extend an individual's range of functional capacities beyond what is typical for mem-bers of his or her reference class (age, gender, etc.), i.e. enhancements, would be considered medically unnecessary and therefore not socially underwritten (Daniels 1985; Sabin and Daniels 1994; Whitehouse *et al.* 1997; Daniels 2000; Schleim and Walter 2007).

STANDARD ISSUES IN THE NEUROETHICS OF COGNITIVE ENHANCEMENT

CE in healthy individuals raises a considerable number of issues at the individual, social, ethical, and legal level that require careful interdisciplinary discussion (Whitehouse *et al.* 1997; Farah 2002; President's Council on Bioethics 2003; Chatterjee 2004; Farah *et al.* 2004; Flower 2004; Glannon 2008; Greely *et al.* 2008; de Jongh *et al.* 2008; Galert *et al.* 2009; Schermer *et al.* 2009). Regarding the use of cognition-enhancing drugs, safety aspects undoubtedly are central. To what extent are risks and side effects acceptable in using psy-choactive substances in healthy individuals? At the individual level, issues to be discussed include individual autonomy, authenticity, and personal identity. At the social level, issues concerning indirect coercion, equal opportunities, and distributive justice arise.

Cognitive liberty and autonomy

One of the main arguments in favor of CE concerns autonomy: it is up to the individual person to shape his or her life and make decisions concerning his or her health and well-being. For reasons of autonomy, individuals ought to be free to decide for themselves whether or not to make use of cognitive enhancers. Based on this type of argument, many authors call for free access to cognition-enhancing drugs (cf. Sententia 2004; Greely *et al.* 2008;

Galert *et al.* 2009; Metzinger 2009). The underlying idea seems to be something like "cognitive liberty," a notion Wrye Sententia characterizes as follows:

> Cognitive liberty is a term that updates notions of "freedom of thought" for the 21st century by taking into account the power we now have, and increasingly will have, to monitor and manipulate cognitive function. Cognitive liberty is every person's fundamental right to think independently, to use the full spectrum of his or her mind, and to have autonomy over his or her own brain chemistry. Cognitive liberty concerns the ethics and legality of safeguarding one's own thought processes, and by necessity, one's electrochemical brain states. The individual, not corporate or government interests, should have sole jurisdiction over the control and/or modulation of his or her brain states and mental processes. (Sententia 2004, pp. 222–3)

According to this line of reasoning, individuals should be free to actively choose their brain states and modulate brain functioning through the use of cognition-enhancing substances; as long as other persons are not harmed, the use of cognitive enhancers should not be prohibited; and individuals who use cognition-enhancing substances should not be criminalized for using them. While it is adequate to claim that the individual person should have autonomy over her mental states and that no other person should be allowed to tamper with one's brain, it is another question, however, whether the use of cognition-enhancing substances in fact *serves* cognitive liberty or individual autonomy. For there are various factors limiting autonomy.

Autonomous control over one's brain chemistry undoubtedly presupposes free and well-informed decision making. In order to be able to make autonomous decisions concerning his or her brain chemistry, a person has to be thoroughly informed of the relevant aspects, as well as of the effects and side effects of cognitive enhancers. Currently, reliable information on the effects and side effects of cognition-enhancing drugs in healthy individuals is scarce. The second problematic aspect relates to freedom in decision making: in many situations, it is questionable whether individuals freely choose to boost their brain power. Instead, it seems that for many individuals, academic and workplace requirements, indirect social pressure in competitive situations and the desire to conform to social expectations play a central role. And special issues undoubtedly arise in cases in which cognition-enhancing drugs are administered to specific subject groups, i.e. soldiers, children, or adolescents. Here the individuals involved may not have the option or the capacity to decide whether or not to use cognitive enhancers (cf. "Indirect coercion" and "Military use" sections). Furthermore, fairness is tricky to balance with cognitive liberty. Consider not only the isolated individual, but also all individuals potentially affected in their social or professional environment: use of psychostimulants may confer negative effects or disadvantages to others. In most cases, people do not make use of cognitive enhancers to aim at contemplation, pure pleasure, or some altruistic goal, but because they seek a competitive advantage.

From the point of view of autonomy, the fundamental question concerns the *effects* of cognition-enhancing drugs: How far does the use of cognitive enhancers serve cognitive liberty, autonomy and individual well-being? How far does the use of cognition-enhancing substances allow for better self-creation, for a more autonomous way to determine the course of one's life, to fulfill one's plans and to reach one's goals? Some authors have questioned whether the use of cognition-enhancing substances is an adequate means to autonomously achieve one's ends. They argue that deliberate modifications in mental characteristics and individual personality involve inauthenticity because they interfere with the person's true self and result in a life that is not really one's own (Elliott 1998). In addition, they stress that enhancement involves cheating in so far as an individual does not achieve her goals and earn her success as a result of hard work and discipline, but rather relies on the support of a psychoactive substance (Cole-Turner 1998). Instead of genuine self-creation, enhancements serve to achieve something that cannot be achieved by "normal ways," they are "corrosive shortcuts" (Juengst 1998) that lead to an "erosion of character" (Maher 2008) and undermine the value of human effort.

By contrast, others have argued that self-creation implies using any means available, including modifications in mental characteristics and personality (Caplan 2002; DeGrazia 2000; Bublitz and Merkel 2009). But how far does the use of CE (and the presumable corollary increase in attention or memory) allow for better self-creation? It may be argued here that any change for the better and any additional option conferred by CE are of benefit. For example, better scores at school or university or increased job-related success may allow a person to have more and better options in life. There is a problem here, however: cognitive enhancers will only confer significant competitive advantages as long as brain-boosting drugs are not widely used in society. The more widespread the enhancement of cognition becomes, the less marked its positive effects will be for the individual. At the same time, social life will increasingly be dominated by the pressure for social conformism. It is highly questionable whether this is a situation worth aiming for. Instead of stressing the claim arguing in favor of free access to CE, it is important for each of us to reflect on the kind of person he or she wants to be. Autonomy and cognitive liberty involves much more than free access to some kind of drug.

Authenticity and personal identity

Whereas some authors stress that CE allows for self-creation and autonomy and enables people to effectively shape their lives, others point to the negative implications associated with modifications in cognition, behavior, or individual character traits brought about by psychoactive substances. Issues to be taken into account involve individuality, personal identity and individual authenticity. In this context, the question of whether CE alienates us from our true selves or rather helps us to become who we really are—or who we really want to be—plays an important role (Elliott 1998, 2000; deGrazia 2000; Parens 2005; Bell 2008; Bolt and Schermer 2009; Bublitz and Merkel 2009).

A widespread intuition says that CE is dangerous, because it could compromise the "authenticity" of human persons or even make them "lose their identity." The idea of an "authenticity" that one could lose seems to be based on an implicit assumption, which one might term "metaphysical essentialism": there is something in me which allows me to be the *real* me, it is a *necessary* property without which I would lose my identity, it makes me *genuine*, and it is something that can gradually disappear. Of course, it is possible that a given social environment will perceive persons under the influence of molecular-level CE as "different from what they were like in the past" or as "not genuine" any more. And there is a vague normative ideal that one should be true to oneself, as integrated as possible, and try to "realize oneself."

All of these ideas are conceptually fuzzy. But note the ethical difficulty that arises if there is a conflict between first-person and third-person ascriptions: If the patient or a given enhanced (but healthy) individual actually described herself as "more herself" or "more authentic," and the perception of their doctor or their social environment clearly diverged from this description, then we would have not only an unclear conceptual framework (which may always be the case in real-life situations), but also a conflict of interest. A second important aspect of this classical issue is the problem of self-deception and delusion: in principle, it is entirely conceivable that cognitively enhanced persons—just like some psychiatric patients or those with brain lesions but with a lack of insight into the ensuing deficit—may actually claim (and experience) a cognitive improvement or a heightened degree of "self-realization" when there is none to be discovered using objective, third-person criteria.

Then there is a common misunderstanding about the notion of identity: Identity is not a thing or a property which you can have, like a bicycle or the color of your eyes, but a relation. Identity is the relation in which an entity stands to itself. The canonical philosophical problem of "personal identity" involves issues having to do with criteria of identity relations for *persons*, for instance across time (transtemporal identity), or of sameness (numerical identity) as opposed to mere qualitative identity (Metzinger 2003, 2011). In neuroethical discussions "personal identity" often seems to be confused with the much simpler concept of a "personality," i.e. with a specific collection of properties, viz. personality traits. Saying that someone has "lost their identity," or that "their identity has changed" is really shorthand for saying that there are no identity relations holding between certain sets of traits at different times, or even only a weak similarity relation. The danger then becomes that this collection or set of psychological properties (one's *personality* identity if you will) might change over time, and in an undesirable manner.

Can one damage one's personality through CE? This is of course a real problem, and a risk that must be assessed carefully. What is often overlooked, however, is that the *alternative* to enhance or improve some characteristics, at least in medical contexts, is another, often much more serious change in one's personality traits—just think of senile anhedonia, loss of autobiographical memory, or dementia. In non-medical contexts, and if one views the choice between enhancement and non-enhancement as a choice between two desirable, yet mutually exclusive results, there is the possibility of an "opportunity cost," or indeed an "opportunity loss," as the value of the next best alternative is foregone as the result of making a decision. The question then becomes one of estimating how high the price is for the natural and perhaps slower changes in personality traits going along with not enhancing and just living a normal life, as compared to the price of having a fast and perhaps more unpredictable change in personality as the result of employing pharmacological enhancement techniques. Therefore, this issue also has to do with the ethics of risk-taking: In the specific domain of potential personality changes, how does one deal with future uncertainties in a rational and ethically coherent way?

Indirect coercion

In a competitive context, the emergence of new technologies boosting productivity typically presents an advantage to those who have access to them, and immediate disadvantage to those who have no access, or choose not to employ them. As soon as some people clearly benefit from CE, there undoubtedly will be a certain indirect pressure for others to use them as well in order to be able to compete with them.

Individuals may experience indirect social pressure to boost their brain power in order to better compete with their colleagues at the workplace, at school or at the university (McCabe *et al.* 2005; Greely *et al.* 2008; Warren *et al.* 2009; Wilens *et al.* 2008). In certain situations, e.g. in military service, people may even be directly coerced to use cognitive enhancers (Kautz *et al.* 2007; Russo 2007). In all of these situations, pressure to perform and the desire to better cope with intellectual challenges and competitive situations, to improve academic performance or to achieve higher socio-economic status undoubtedly play a role. Whereas up to now data on the use of psychostimulants in offices is sparse (cf. DAK 2009), studies carried out at high schools and colleges in the US indicate that there seems to be a positive correlation between the extent of cognitive enhancer use observed among adolescents and young adults at a certain institution and the competitiveness of the environment (McCabe *et al.* 2005; Wilens *et al.* 2008).

Particular problems arise when cognition-enhancing substances are given to healthy minors (Glannon 2008; Greely *et al.* 2008; Singh and Kelleher 2010). Parents may feel stimulated to give cognitive enhancers to their children in order to improve their compliance at school, to make them learn better or get better scores, or to enable them to attend prestigious education institutions. Besides issues concerning individual autonomy (cf. "Cognitive liberty and autonomy" section), note that currently the long-term effects of cognitive enhancers on the developing brains of children are unknown. And there is a comparable lacuna concerning the educational effect of a strategy like this on children and adolescents. For what the use of cognition enhancers teaches them directly is that what counts most is not the individual person's effort and discipline, but the exams passed and the scores achieved.

Arguably, the more adolescents or adults assume or experience that others might benefit from cognitive enhancers, the more likely they are to use them. This could be a plausible consequence of striking media reports on individuals who enormously benefit from CE: people worldwide might get the impression that cognition enhancement may confer significant advantages to their lives; and that their competitors might already be using them. A desire to not be left behind, at disadvantage, would result in a heightened tendency towards CE. Not least, this could incur increasing pressure upon medical doctors—important gatekeepers in this context—to prescribe some substance in this or that situation. Thus, widespread, overoptimistic and uncritical discussion in the public might contribute to intensify the use CE. Clearly then, it is very important to carry out empirical research on the effects, benefits and risks of cognitive enhancers, and on their dissemination in society, in order to confer a realistic picture of these aspects. Indeed, this may cause many dreams and nightmares to vanish.

Equal opportunities and distributive justice

With regard to CE, issues of relevance at the level of society undoubtedly relate to fairness, equal opportunity, and justice. A central aspect involves the question: How much does enhancement confer an unfair advantage to certain individuals in competitive situations? Here, a distinction can be made between usage in the competitive situation itself and usage in some related context. For example, with regard to a university exam, there is a significant difference between employing the substance directly during the exam situation, and employing the substance to facilitate better and more efficient learning during exam preparation. Whereas it may be argued that in both situations it is unfair if some individuals avail themselves of psychopharmacological substances and profit from enhanced mental capacities they otherwise would not have when others do not, only the first situation could involve *direct* cheating and fraud. There may be an analogy to doping in sports: in the competition itself, there must be the same conditions for all competitors. But in training, the situation may be different. For commonly, individuals are licensed a higher degree of individual choice in the training strategy they employ to better fulfill their potential.

Nevertheless, in all kinds of competitive situations, issues concerning fairness and justice are crucial, for not all members of society will have equal access to CE and its putative positive effects. First of all, it might be that only individuals who are financially better off would be able to afford effective CE, with an adequate risk-benefit ratio. This may confer additional advantages to the group of wealthier people within society, increasing social inequality. Indeed, the broad use of cognition-enhancing drugs might in certain respects be beneficial for a society as a whole, for instance by extending work productivity, and this might further increase inequality between richer and poorer nations. Interestingly though, some people may be disposed to benefit more from cognition-enhancing drugs than others: effects might be modest in individuals with high-level cognitive functioning, whereas people with lower baseline abilities might profit most. And this might also lead to a reduction of inequalities (Juengst 1998; Farah *et al.* 2004; de Jongh *et al.* 2008; Glannon 2008; Greely *et al.* 2008).

If we assume that functionally effective CE will be available anyway to some individuals, it may be argued that in the interest of distributive justice CE should be available to all in order to enable every individual to receive a fair share. The question of what counts as a fair share is far from being trivial, however. According to the principle of equality, justice requires the distribution of cognitive enhancers equally among all individuals. This implies either (literally) free access to psychostimulants, or access for no-one, i.e. a general ban on CE. According to the principle of need, fair distribution would imply that only those individuals who are disadvantaged for one reason or another should have access in order to reach a "normal" level of mental performance. With regard to CEs, this will imply a leveling of mental capacities among the members of the population, leading to a reduction of inequalities resulting from differences in "natural endowment." A disadvantage here, of course, is that it will be difficult to clearly define a cut-off point. Another criterion would be a principle of deserving, i.e. to distribute according to the role individuals have in society. Individuals whose performance has (or may in the future have) a high impact on society would accrue favored access to CE. Pilots come to mind, as do medical doctors, politicians, scientists, or individuals with laudable moral goals. Here, selection criteria would be difficult to justify.

Novel issues in the neuroethics of cognitive enhancement

In this section we will briefly highlight three examples of concrete problems faced by the neuroethics of CE today.

Studies in healthy volunteers

It is urgent to arrive at an empirically grounded ethical assessment for the use of cognitive enhancers by healthy individuals. In order to reach this goal, it will be of central importance to be able to draw on long-term studies yielding data on the benefits, risks and side-effects involved in the use of such substances over months and years. In many countries, however, an application of prescription drugs in healthy persons is prohibited by pharmaceutical law. This hampers an objective longitudinal analysis of long-term risks and side effects, while the actual illicit and off-label use of these substances in society is already increasing. While more and more individuals actually decide to take the risks in question, a rational, data-driven assessment of the risk-benefit ratio remains out of reach. The point can also be put differently: We currently describe and discuss something as "enhancement." But it is not at all clear if it actually *is* an enhancement, if we look into it through a longer time-window. If one were able to take scientific data on long-term side effects into consideration, one would perhaps stop speaking of the possibility of "cognition enhancement" altogether (Racine and Forlini 2010).

One obvious perspective one can take is to say that prescription drug abuse as such is an unethical activity, and that therefore it must remain illegal. Therefore, there is no need for longitudinal studies in healthy subjects, because the results of such studies would not lead to any conceivable policy-change. This slightly circular attitude is opposed by another view, which would say that in order to minimize future harm and suffering, one is ethically obliged to gain all information and gather all data necessary to arrive at a rational decision. As one of the major objectives of existing pharmaceutical law is exactly the minimization of harm and human suffering, and given the spreading illicit use of such substances (which may not yet be an objective fact in many societies outside of the US), it would seem irrational to have existing legal structures impeding actual progress on urgent neuroethical issues. We will not take any position here, because our sole aim is to sketch one concrete, and novel, problem for neuroethics.

Moral enhancement

In the first section in this chapter we saw how there are very different domains of cognitive functioning. One such domain, of course, is moral reasoning itself: all cognitive capacities relating to the proper mental representation and successful practical solution of ethical problems, i.e. insight into coherence and self-contradiction in normative contexts, moral judgment, and decision making, the capacity to respond to rational ethical arguments, and so on. There are also moral emotions like shame, guilt, embarrassment, but also moral pride, gratitude, the purely affective sense of responsibility, and the capacity for other-directed empathy. These guide human moral behavior much more effectively than high-level cognitive processes alone and have a long evolutionary history (many of them can be found in other animals as well).

Now consider: What if enhancement technologies became available that specifically optimized all or a subset of those cognitive functions underlying human moral behavior? What if there were specific molecular-level technologies to optimize prosocial behavior, by selectively enhancing certain moral emotions?

Again, we do not want to engage in an extended or detailed discussion here (see Douglas (2008) for an interesting starting point). There is an argument that makes the issue of moral enhancement particularly interesting, to which we will now briefly draw the reader's attention. Anyone considering ethical and moral issues relevant issues *at all*, and anyone who thinks that at least some progress can actually be made on these issues (like, e.g. most researchers in neuroethics), will also accept some sort of ethical standard for their own actions. Indeed, everyone who accepts at least *some* sort of normative dimension in their own life, who attempts to orient his or her actions according to a set of moral values or abstract ethical principles at all, ought to have the goal of continuously improving their own moral integrity as well. That is, anyone accepting the relevance of ethical considerations for their own personal life will also strive to continuously optimize the coherence between their own moral judgments or feelings and their actions. Ethically sensitive people will be aware of their own failures in achieving this coherence, and they will naturally strive for an improvement of their own moral insight, as well as of their overt behavior. If new and effective means become available to attain these goals more fully, then many ethically sensitive people will publicly argue in favor of the obligation to use moral enhancement technologies. Because the acceptance of moral values should cause a sense of commitment to the realization of these values, we might face historically unprecedented discussions if moral enhancement technologies with an acceptable risk-benefit ratio actually became available. More concretely: If prosocial behavior, increased capacity for empathy, better impulse control, altruistic feelings, or certain aspects of social cognition can be directly and reliably targeted with the help of new psychopharmacological instruments; if high-level moral cognition or any other mental capacity supporting a person's overall moral integrity could be improved by novel means of directly intervening in the human brain, then there will be voices pointing out how moral enhancement is just and reasonable. It would be a self-evident civic duty with regard to the stability, cohesion and improvement of the society he or she lives in. We should be prepared for public debates of this type.

Military use

Cognitive enhancers like modafinil were used in the Iraq war. Modern antidepressant drugs have been given pre-emptively to hundreds of soldiers in order to prevent PTSD following exposure to combat situations. CE is an obvious example of a neurotechnology which has obvious military applications (Kautz *et al.* 2007; Russo 2007). This results in ethical dilemmata beyond the level of medical treatment or the sociocultural effects of "lifestyle use."

First, research into CE is dual-use research, and dual-use research is often morally problematic. On the one hand, such research provides benefits (at least to potential future patients); on the other hand, there is the risk of misuse by states without any democratic legitimation, terrorists groups, and the like. That is, cognitively-enhancing psychoactive substances can also function as weapons in the hands of malevolent state actors, terrorist groups, criminal organizations, or individual criminals. This is a well-known problem in bioethics, and as such it is not qualitatively new.

What, however, presents a perhaps more novel challenge is the possibility of dampening or inhibiting certain aspects of natural moral emotions in soldiers. Think of soldiers fighting under the influence of modern antidepressants, but not being able to use their own naturally evolved moral emotions like shame or embarrassment in guiding their actions any more. In the previous section we asked: What if there were specific molecular-level technologies to optimize prosocial behavior, by selectively enhancing certain moral emotions? There is an obvious mirror-image of this question: What if we can selectively block or downregulate certain aspects of a soldier's moral personality, say, the capacity to be touched or emotionally hurt, to be ashamed of himself, to empathize? Imagine military personnel on an ethically dubious mission, but pharmacologically manipulated in a way that made them perhaps highly alert and focused, but at the same time emotionally unmoved, numbed, incapable of translating their perception and their moral insight into an emotional reaction that could cause a change of their behavior. We could call this "dissociative enhancement," and frequently it could be a case of indirect coercion as well (see earlier). Why "dissociative"? Whereas moral enhancement (as discussed in the previous section) would be an attempt to optimize not only moral insight, but also the *integrity* of persons (i.e. the degree to which their actions cohere with their judgments), one can of course envisage ways of pharmacologically blocking certain or inhibiting moral personality traits, say, by the use of antidepressants, with the result of *disintegrating* moral insight and behavioral profile, namely, by intervening on the emotional and motivational level. Obviously, this point also relates to the issues of authenticity, indirect coercion, and personality change discussed previously. For professional neuroethicists, the major problem with such potential military abuse of CE technologies obviously is that it will be very hard to gain reliable, objective information of newly emerging patterns of use in military contexts.

POLICY MAKING

In view of the numerous ethical implications of CE on the individual as well as on the socio-cultural level adequate regulations for the use of cognition-enhancing drugs have to be developed. In open, democratic societies such regulations must be based on rational arguments and available empirical data, and they should be guided by a general principle of liberalism: In principle, the individual citizen's freedom and autonomy in dealing with their own brain and in choosing their own desired states of mind (including all of their phenomenal and cognitive properties) should be maximized. However, once such a general "Principle of Phenomenal and Cognitive Liberty" has been clearly stated, the much more interesting and demanding task lies in *limiting* this freedom in an intelligent way, in minimizing potential individual suffering and the overall psychosocial cost to society as a whole (Metzinger 2009). In this, it is necessary to carefully take current risks and benefits, as well as future chances and problems into account, most importantly not only at the individual but also at the social level.

- With regard to policy making, the role of medicine and the aims of medicine are of central relevance in so far as (in the social context) they serve as a *legitimization* for a certain procedure, introducing new neurotechnologies into society. At the level of society, it is important to draw a line between the medical and non-medical uses of biotechnologies, even if a clear and unequivocal distinction between treatment and enhancement may prove difficult. At the level of society, the treatment/enhancement distinction is of central relevance with regard to healthcare coverage and public policy.

- Governments, medical associations, and other professional organizations in the field of medicine are obliged to *actively monitor* the process in which medical taxonomies, diagnosis manuals, etc., continuously evolve. It is in their direct responsibility to make sure that the process in which new theoretical and semantic entities (such as, e.g. "mild cognitive impairment") are introduced into medical practice is guided by rigorous scientific criteria alone, and not influenced by industrial lobbies, ideological pressure groups, etc.

- At the individual level, however, formal distinctions such as health versus disease or treatment versus enhancement are of limited value. For here, the point of view is quite different. At the individual level, the question is not so much whether a certain procedure is labeled as a treatment or an enhancement. Instead, what matters here are individual well-being, life-plans, and autonomy, as well as the question of how far people consider it desirable to avail themselves of certain measurements. This is not primarily a matter of policy or of concepts of health and disease, but of individual decision-making. Often, for the individual person seeking enhancement, the question is not so much whether she is objectively diseased or otherwise at a disadvantage, but whether enhancement is available and whether he or she is willing to take certain risks in order to improve herself and attain some putative advantage. Obviously, the individual and the social level are directly related, as is reflected by the various problematic aspects of CE concerning indirect coercion, fairness, and justice.

- Policy makers should stay clear of ideological debates: They face an optimization problem in harm reduction, risk assessment, and the maximization of benefit on two different levels. Their task is to solve this problem without discounting future values (e.g. the quality of life of future generations), and to find an adaptable trade-off between individual preferences and the interests of society as a whole.

- All decisions must be evidence-based. Additional empirical research must be carried out concerning, for example, the *actual* patterns of illicit and off-label use of cognitive enhancers as they develop in a specific sociocultural context.

- If it can be shown that uncontrolled, illicit, and off-label use by healthy individuals is already spreading in a given society, then governments are obliged to gather empirical data about the risks of long-term use in the healthy, for example by enabling longitudinal studies.

- It is necessary to thoroughly and *objectively* inform the public on the effects, side effects, chances, and risks of cognition-enhancing substances.

- All forms of direct-to-customer marketing should be prohibited.

- Even in those countries in which illicit and off-label CE is not yet widespread, it is necessary to carefully reflect on adequate regulations right now. Medical doctors, educational professionals and representatives of other social and professional groups should collaborate in order to seek clear and unequivocal regulations concerning CE at offices, schools, and universities.

- On the other hand, policy making must avoid playing a facilitating role in the uncontrolled use of cognition-enhancing drugs: Policy making should stick to evidence concerning the current social situation and should not hastily, or in some kind of anticipatory obedience, adjust to putative future scenarios of widespread use that might never materialize.

- Policy making cannot be confined to devising new regulations. There is a wider anthropological and ethical dimension, which cannot be ignored: in the special field of gradually introducing new, cognitive, and/or phenomenal neurotechnologies into society what is needed is the *setting of a cultural context* in which the overall development can unfold (Metzinger 2009). What are the states of mind we want to live our lives in? Put very simply, it may be necessary to stimulate individual citizens themselves to think about the kind of person he or she wants to be, about what a good life is, and about the general social conditions we all want to live in for the future. This includes reflections on the question of how far we are willing to adjust our personality and our mental life to external expectations, to the social and the performance pressures we face in competitive, secularized societies of the 21st century. Put even more simply, we should have good, convincing answers to the following question: Why, and in order to attain what goal, should one enhance one's cognitive function *at all?*

ACKNOWLEDGEMENTS

We wish to thank Jennifer M. Windt, Adrian J. T. Smith and Michael Madary for stimulating discussions and editorial help with the English version of this chapter.

REFERENCES

Bell, J. (2008). Propranolol, post-traumatic stress disorder and narrative identity. *Journal of Medical Ethics*, **34**, e23.

Bolt, I. and Schermer, M. (2008). Psychopharmaceutical enhancers: enhancing identity? *Neuroethics*, **2**, 103–11.

Boorse, C. (1977). Health as a theoretical concept. *Philosophy of Science*, **44**, 542–73.

Bostrom, N. (2008). Drugs can be used to treat more than disease. *Nature*, **451**, 520.

Bublitz, J.C. and Merkel, R. (2009). Autonomy and authenticity of enhanced personality traits. *Bioethics*, **23**, 360–74.

Caldwell, J.A. Jr, Caldwell, J.L., Smythe, N.K. 3rd, and Hall, K.K. (2000). A double-blind, placebo-controlled investigation of the efficacy of modafinil for sustaining the alertness and performance of aviators: a helicopter simulator study. *Psychopharmacology*, **150**, 272–82.

Canter, P.H. and Ernst, E. (2007). Ginkgo biloba is not a smart drug: an updated systematic review of randomised clinical trials testing the nootropic effects of G. biloba extracts in healthy people. *Human Psychopharmacology*, **22**, 265–78.

Caplan, A. (2002). No-brainer: can we cope with the ethical ramifications of new knowledge of the human brain? In S.J. Marcus (ed.) *Neuroethics: Mapping the Field*, pp. 95–106. Chicago, IL: University of Chicago Press.

Caplan, A.L., McCartney, J.J. and Sisti, D.A. (eds.) (2004). *Health, Disease and Illness. Concepts in Medicine*. Washington, DC: Georgetown University Press.

Chatterjee, A. (2004). Cosmetic neurology. The controversy over enhancing movement, mentation, and mood. *Neurology*, **63**, 968–74.

Cole-Turner, R. (1998). Do means matter?, In E. Parens (ed.) *Enhancing Human Traits: Ethical and Social Implications*, pp. 151–61. Washington, DC: Georgetown University Press.

DAK (Deutsche Angestellten-Krankenkasse) (2009): *Gesundheitsreport 2009. Analyse der Arbeitsunfähigkeitsdaten. Schwerpunktthema Doping am Arbeitsplatz*. Available at: http://www.dak.de/content/filesopen/Gesundheitsreport_2009.pdf (accessed 28 October 2009)

Daniels, N. (1985). *Just Health Care*. Cambridge: Cambridge University Press.

Daniels, N. (2000). Normal functioning and the treatment-enhancement distinction. *Cambridge Quarterly of Healthcare Ethics*, **9**, 309–22.

Dekkers, W. and Rikkert, M.O. (2007). Memory enhancing drugs and Alzheimer's disease: enhancing the self or preventing the loss of it? *Medicine, Health Care and Philosophy*, **10**, 141–51.

DeGrazia, D. (2000). Prozac, enhancement, and self-creation. *Hastings Center Report*, **30**, 34–40.

Douglas, T. (2008). Moral enhancement. *Journal of Applied Philosophy*, **25**, 228–45.

Elliott, C. (1998). The tyranny of happiness: ethics and cosmetic psychopharmacology. In E. Parens (ed.) *Enhancing Human Traits: Ethical and Social Implications*, pp. 177–188. Washington, DC: Georgetown University Press.

Elliott, C. (2000). Pursued by happiness and beaten senseless. Prozac and the American dream. *Hastings Center Report*, **30**, 7–12.

Farah, M.J. (2002). Emerging ethical issues in neuroscience. *Nature Neuroscience*, **5**, 1123–9.

Farah, M.J., Illes, J., Cook-Deegan, R., *et al.* (2004). Neurocognitive enhancement: what can we do and what should we do? *Nature Reviews Neuroscience*, **5**, 421–5.

Flower. R. (2004). Lifestyle drugs: pharmacology and the social agenda. *Trends in Pharmacological Science*, **25**, 182–5.

Franke, A.G., Bonertz, C., Christmann, M., Fellgiebel, A., and Lieb, K. (2009). Use of potential neurocognitive enhancing substances and attitudes towards them among pupils in Germany, Poster, Conference "Brain Matters," Sept. 24–26, 2009, Halifax, Nova Scotia, Canada.

Frankford, D.M. (1998). The treatment/enhancement distinction as an armament in the policy wars. In E. Parens (ed.) *Enhancing Human Traits: Ethical and Social Implications*, pp. 70–94. Washington DC: Georgetown University Press.

Galert, T., Bublitz, C., Heuser, I., *et al.* (2009). Das optimierte Gehirn. *Gehirn and Geist*, **11**, 40–49.

Glannon, W. (2006). Psychopharmacology and memory. *Journal of Medical Ethics*, **32**, 74–78.

Glannon, W. (2008). Psychopharmacological enhancement. *Neuroethics*, **1**, 45–54.

Greely, H., Sahakian, B., Harris, J., *et al.* (2008). Towards responsible use of cognitive-enhancing drugs by the healthy. *Nature*, **456**, 702–05.

Grön, G., Kirstein, M., Thielscher, A., Riepe, M.W., and Spitzer, M. (2005). Cholinergic enhancement of episodic memory in healthy young adults. *Psychopharmacology (Berl)*, **182**, 170–9.

Jones, D.G. (2006). Enhancement: are ethicists excessively influenced by baseless speculations? *Journal of Medical Ethics*, **32**, 77–81.

de Jongh, R., Bolt, I., Schermer, M., and Olivier, B. (2008). Botox for the brain: enhancement of cognition, mood and pro-social behavior and blunting of unwanted memories. *Neuroscience and Biobehavioral Reviews*, **32**, 760–76.

Juengst, E.T. (1998). What does enhancement mean? In E. Parens (ed.) *Enhancing Human Traits: Ethical and Social Implications*, pp. 29–47. Washington DC: Georgetown University Press.

Kautz, M.A., Thomas, M.L., and Caldwell, J.L. (2007). Considerations of pharmacology on fitness for duty in the operational environment. *Aviation, Space and Environmental Medicine*, 78, B107-12.

Kramer, P.D. (1993). *Listening to Prozac. A Psychiatrist Explores Antidepressant Drugs and the Remaking of the Self*. New York: Viking Press.

Maher, B. (2008). Poll results: look who's doping. *Nature*, 452, 674–75.

Marshall, E. (2004). A star-studded search for memory-enhancing drugs. *Science*, 304, 36–8.

McCabe, S.E., Knight, J.R., Teter, C.J., and Wechsler, H. (2005). Non-medical use of pre-scriptions stimulants among US college students: prevalence and correlates from a national survey. *Addiction*, 100, 96–106.

Menary, R. (ed.) (2010). *The Extendend Mind*. Cambridge, MA: MIT Press.

Metzinger, T. (2003). Being No One. The Self-Model Theory of Subjectivity. Cambridge, MA: MIT Press.

Metzinger, T. (2009). *The Ego Tunnel. The Science of the Mind and the Myth of the Self*. New York: Basic Books.

Metzinger, T. (20011). The no-self-alternative. In S. Gallagher *(ed.)*, *Oxford Handbook of the Self* (Chapter 11). Oxford, UK: Oxford University Press.

Miller, G. (2004). Learning to forget. *Science*, 304, 34–6.

Minzenberg, M. J. and Carter, C. S. (2008). Modafinil: a review of neurochemical actions and effects on cognition. *Neuropsychopharmacology*, 33, 1477–1502.

Murphy, D. *Concepts of Disease and Health*. In E. N. Zalta (ed.) *The Stanford Encyclopedia of Philosophy* (Fall 2009 edition). Available at: http://plato.stanford.edu/archives/sum2009/entries/health-disease/ (accessed 12 November 2009).

Parens, E. (1998). *Enhancing Human Traits: Ethical and Social Implications*. Washington, DC: Georgetown University Press.

Parens, E. (2005). Authenticity and ambivalence: toward understanding the enhancement debate. *Hastings Center Report*, 35, 34–41.

Pieters, T. and Snelders, S. (2009). Psychotropic drug use: between healing and enhancing the mind. *Neuroethics*, 2, 63–73.

Pitman, R.K. Sanders, K.M., Zusman, R.M., *et al.* (2002). Pilot study of secondary preven-tion of posttraumatic stress disorder with propranolol. *Biological Psychiatry*, 51, 189–92.

President's Council on Bioethics (2003). *Beyond Therapy. Biotechnology and the Pursuit of Happiness*. Washington, DC: Dana Press.

Racine, E. and Forlini, C. (2010). Cognitive enhancement – lifestyle choice or misuse of pprescription drugs? *Neuroethics*, 3, 1–4.

Russo, M.B. (2007). Recommendations for the ethical use of pharmacologic fatigue countermea-sures in the U.S. military. *Aviation, Space, and Environmental Medicine*, 78, Section II: B119–B127.

Sabin, J.E. and Daniels, N. (1994). Determining "medical necessity" in mental health practice. *Hastings Center Report*, 24, 5–13.

Sahakian, B.J. and Morein-Zamir, S. (2007). Professor's little helper. *Nature*, 450, 1157–59.

Sahakian, B.J. and Morein-Zamir, S. (2010). Neuroethical issues in cognitive enhancement. *Journal of Psychopharmacology*. [Epub 8 March 2010]

Schermer, M., Bolt, I., de Jongh, R., and Olivier, B. (2009). The future of psychopharmaco-logical enhancements: expectations and policies. *Neuroethics*, 2, 75–87.

Schleim, S. and Walter, H. (2007). Cognitive enhancement – Fakten und Mythen. *Nervenheilkunde*, 26, 83–87.

Sententia, W. (2004). Neuroethical considerations: cognitive liberty and converging technologies for improving human cognition. *Annals of the New York Academy of Sciences*, **1013**, 221–28.

Singh, I. and Kelleher, K.J. (2010). Neuroenhancement in young people: proposal for research, policy and clinical management. *American Journal of Bioethics – Neuroscience*, **1**, 3–16.

Synofzik, M. (2009). Ethically justified, clinically applicable criteria for physician decision-making in psychopharmacological enhancement. *Neuroethics*, **2**, 89–102.

Teter, C.J., McCabe, S.E., LaGrange, K., Cranford, J.A., and Boyd, C.J. (2006). Illicit use of specific prescription stimulants among college students: prevalence, motives, and routes of administration. *Pharmacotherapy*, **26**, 1501–10.

Turner, D.C., Robbins, T.W., Clark, L., Aron, A.R., Dowson, J., and Sahakian, B.J. (2003). Cognitive enhancing effects of modafinil in healthy volunteers. *Psychopharmacology*, **165**, 260–69.

van Roojen, M. *Moral Cognitivism vs. Non-Cognitivism.* In E. N. Zalta (ed.) *The Stanford Encyclopedia of Philosophy* (Fall 2009 edition). Available at: http://plato.stanford.edu/archives/fall2009/entries/moral-cognitivism/ (accessed 12 November 2009).

Warren, O.J., Leff, D.R., Athanasiou, T., Kennard, C., and Darzi, A. (2009). The neurocognitive enhancement of surgeons: an ethical perspective. *Journal of Surgical Research*, **152**, 167–72.

Whitehouse, P.J., Juengst, E., Mehlman, M., and Murray, T.M. (1997). Enhancing cognition in the intellectually intact. *Hastings Center Report*, **27**, 14–22.

Wilens, T.E., Adler, L.A., Adams, J., *et al.* (2008). Misuse and diversion of stimulants prescribed for ADHD: a systematic review of the literature. *Journal of the American Academy of Child and Adolescent Psychiatry*, **47**, 21–31.

World Health Organization (1958). *Constitution of the World Health Organization (preamble): The First Ten Years of the World Health Organization.* Geneva: WHO.

Yesavage, J.A., Mumenthaler, M.S., Taylor, J.L., *et al.* (2002). Donepezil and flight simulator performance: effects on retention of complex skills. *Neurology*, **59**, 123–5.

....

CHAPTER 16

CHEMICAL COGNITIVE ENHANCEMENT: IS IT UNFAIR, UNJUST, DISCRIMINATORY, OR CHEATING FOR HEALTHY ADULTS TO USE SMART DRUGS?

....

JOHN HARRIS

Selfishness is not living as one wishes to live, it is asking other people to live as one wishes to live.

Oscar Wilde.

H.H. Asquith, a Balliol undergraduate and British Prime Minister, allegedly described Balliol men as possessing "the tranquil consciousness of an effortless superiority."

SUPPOSE a university, perhaps the famous Ritalin College in Virginia, were to set out deliberately to improve the mental powers and capacities of its students; suppose its stated aims were to ensure that the students developed enhanced executive functioning, enhanced study skills, and improvement in the focusing of attention and in the manipulation of information. Suppose that a group of educationalists had actually worked out a method of achieving

Note: This paper builds on and to some extent repeats earlier work of mine, most notably in my Enhancing Evolution, Princeton University Press, Oxford and Princeton 2007 and Henry Greely, Barbara Sahakian, John Harris, Ron Kessler, Michael Gazzaniga, Philip Campbell, Martha Farah: Towards responsible use of cognitive enhancing drugs by the healthy Nature, Vol 456, 18/25 December 2008.

this, in the form, perhaps, of an educational and physical curriculum. What should our reaction be? Should we welcome such a breakthrough? Would we want to send our own children to this famous seat of learning, and if Ritalin College was too expensive would we be anxious for our local college to adopt the same revolutionary methods?

Now suppose that instead of an elaborate new curriculum and special teaching methods, we could use drugs to produce, if not more intelligent individuals, at least individuals with better cognitive functioning, what should our reaction be?

Would it be unethical to do so? Would it be ethical not to do so?

If the goal of enhanced: cognitive functioning is something that we might strive to produce through education, including of course the more general health education of the community; why should we not produce these goals, if we can do so safely enough, through enhancement technologies or procedures including chemical cognitive enhancers (Greely *et al.* 2008; Harris 2007a)?

If these are legitimate aims of education and the legitimate aspirations of parents and students, how would they be illegitimate as the aims or as the products of medical or life science, as opposed to educational science?

Enhancements of course are good if and only if those things we call enhancements do good, make us better, they are good if they make us better at doing some of the things we want to do including better at experiencing the world through all of the senses, better at assimilating and processing what we experience, better at remembering and understanding things, more competent, more of everything we want to be. Some of those things we might want to be and which others might want us to be are also better and more successful students and better and more rewarding employees. In short, better at our work and our play—including, of course, sports.

Chemical enhancement

There are numerous and varied candidates for chemical cognition enhancers, a recent report listed literally scores (Jones *et al.* 2007). Two of the most popular are: methylphenidate (Ritalin®) a cognition enhancer with a good evidence base widely used for improving various aspects of cognition in children and adults, and modafinil, which enhances wakefulness and alertness and is identified for possible enhancement of the functioning of pilots, long-distance drivers, and military personnel.

I would like to take as my point of departure a remark by the English biologist Steven Rose. Talking of the possible use of so-called smart drugs like Ritalin® asks:

> Is it cheating to pass a competitive examination under the influence of such a drug? Polls conducted among youngsters make it clear that they do regard it as cheating, *in the same way that* the use of steroids by athletes is considered to be cheating.

Of course Rose is wrong to think that taking cognitive enhancers could be cheating *in the same way that* the use of drugs by athletes is considered cheating. If we ask why athletes using steroids are considered to be cheats, one obvious answer is that because the use of performance-enhancing drugs in competitive sport is banned their use must be clandestine and it is cheating because it is a) contrary to the rules and b) an attempt to steal an unfair advantage. If however the rules permitted such use then the advantage would not be "unfair" because it would be an advantage available to all (e.g. Savulescu *et al.* 2004).

In the context of education many think: it is alright to buy educational privilege for one's children by paying for private tuition, but dubious to enhance their skills by feeding them drugs.

Buying educational privilege in a context in which not all can afford to do so is certainly unfair in some sense. But if we defend people's rights to do this it is because we see education as a good and we feel it is right to encourage people to provide good things for their children and indeed for themselves and wrong to deny them these goods even if not all can obtain them.

It is possible, of course, that people may be seeking an edge, a relative advantage for their children or themselves; but it is more likely (and perhaps more decent?) that they are simply seeking excellence, the best rather than seeking an unfair advantage over others. To seek excellence, to do the best for your kids when others cannot match your efforts, will probably also confer an advantage, but is it doubtful ethics to deny a benefit to any until it can be delivered to all? The same is true of many other goods that cannot be equally provided for all, I believe this despite many powerful arguments to the contrary. For more on the moral permissibility and impermissibility of advantage in education see Brighouse (1998, 2000, 2002, 2006) and Swift (2003, 2004a, 2004b). Though for a critique of Brighouse's arguments see Foster (2002) and Tooley (2003).

Access to performance-enhancing drugs is obviously unlike education in that it is not considered to be an intrinsic good; such an intrinsic good in terms of education is often termed "education for its own sake."

There is clearly no substitute for education, but for many there may also be no substitute for chemical cognitive enhancers. Education does not only, or even principally, increase the knowledge base, it develops transferable skills of all sorts. But some of those skills are also enabled or enhanced by drugs like Ritalin® or modafinil: benefits reported for these drugs include enhanced executive functioning, enhanced study skills, and improvement in the focusing of attention and in the manipulation of information (Greely *et al.* 2008).

Moreover, unlike formal education, access to these skills through drugs is instant and relatively low cost, certainly when compared to education or training. Let us now turn to the issue of justice and the question of whether or not it is unfair or unjust to permit the use of smart drugs.

POSITIONAL GOODS

Let me declare an interest and make a confession. I am a habitual drug-taker. I have for many years taken daily aspirin and statins. These drugs are widely available, but even if they were not, and I could afford them or access them when others could not, I would still take them. I do not take these drugs to get the better of my fellow men and women, as a so-called "positional good" (to improve my position relative to others) but to give to myself the best chance (in absolute terms) of a long and healthy life. If they are available to all I lose nothing.

True, taking aspirin is not straightforwardly, or perhaps one should say not "obviously" a means to a positional good in the same way that taking a performance enhancer before an exam, the results of which will mean that some will succeed while others fail. But this apparent obviousness is misleading. If my taking aspirin while others do not means that I live and they do not, I do seem to have a positional advantage in that I am here and they are…well… nowhere! Just as it is not wrong to save some lives when all cannot be saved, it is not wrong to advantage some in ways that also confer a positional advantage when all cannot be bettered in those ways.

Humans are creatures that result from an enhancement process called evolution and moreover are inveterate self-improvers in every conceivable way. Familiar cognitive enhancers include written language, formal education, physical exercise, and diet, and all of these create problems of justice as well as side effects of use and overuse.

Cognitive enhancements, improvements in brain functioning, are among the most important and most attractive of all forms of human enhancement. Beneficial neural changes have been reported for such familiar technologies as reading (Schlaggar *et al.* 2007), education (Draganski *et al.* 2004), physical exercise (Hillman *et al.* 2008), and diet (Almeida *et al.* 2002). How then are drugs ethically distinct from, for example, my other favorite enhancement technology—synthetic sunshine?

Synthetic sunshine

Before synthetic sunshine people slept when it was dark and worked in the light of day. With the advent of synthetic sunshine, firelight, candlelight, lamplight, and electric light, work, including study and other attempts to improve the mind, and indeed social life could continue into and through the night creating competitive pressures and incentives for those able or willing to use them to their advantage. The solution, however, was not to outlaw synthetic sunshine but, perhaps belatedly, to regulate working hours and improve access to the new technology and think hard about how to manage and control pressure.

Synthetic sunshine created two of the features that are most deplored today in the prospect of smart drugs: synthetic sunshine created positional advantage and competitive pressures. Should we, or rather our early ancestors, have turned their backs on synthetic sunshine and gone back to sleep…and said "thanks but no-thanks"? We have just looked at the issue of positional advantage and it seems to me, and I hope now to you, that the right response to things that confer significant benefits to humans individually and collectively is not to say "no thanks" but rather "yes please." Of course we must also work hard, tirelessly, and ceaselessly to make sure that the benefits or their effects are as widely and as fairly available as possible.

Kidney transplants

Kidney transplants are not universally available and yet they liberate those who can receive them from the imprisonment and pain of dialysis (when available) and deliver much enhanced and extremely cost-effective life extension. No one says we must ban kidney transplants to any until they are available to all. The therapy of choice is the therapy chosen in preference to others and to make that therapy as widely and as fairly available as possible is the goal of all people of good will and sound ethics.

Consider building a curriculum vitae

Curriculum vitae (CVs) are interesting because they are mostly used in competitive situations. It is true that some sad individuals (of whom I admit to being one), keep their CVs up-to-date less in the expectation that they will be useful in out-competing their fellows to great new jobs or opportunities, but more in the spirit of Oscar Wilde who explained (in *The Importance of being Ernest*) that it was important to keep a diary to "always have something sensational to read on the train!"

But while a CV, and the things on it, are classically competitive, a life is seldom created to fill a CV, rather a CV records the selected highlights (for a particular purpose) of a life to date; and usually tries to indicate future directions and future promise. A CV records the building of a career and perhaps even the building of a life. Sure, CVs are things that are useful in competition, but they are also characteristic, expressive of the person whose life they record. They detail her achievements, chosen because she wanted (or at least chose) to do the things which they record and because she could imagine and wish to live the sort of life of which they would be a part. A CV works because and in so far as it is testimony to wise choices, great and even modest achievements, and promise for the future; it is the record of a life to date. Of course it contains selected highlights, but it is testimony to (and works because it is) a life constructed according to, characterized by, and expressive of the choices, decisions, and achievements of that life. For most people (I hope some can detect irony here) the CV is a record of, rather than a blueprint for or indeed a wish list for, a life. And while some of the things on it will have been chosen for the expected positional advantage it is hoped they will confer, they are also (almost always) chosen because they are required to help build the sort of life the individual wants to lead.

If an individual had to forego those things in life that might, or would probably, confer positional advantage she could scarcely get out of bed in the morning, let alone have a life let alone a *curriculum vitae* which might in any sense be worth living.

Of course some of the things achieved will be unfair to others because, for example, there was no level playing field on which most others would stand a chance of doing the same or perhaps even similar things. Other items on the CV will be unfair because the individual is brighter, fitter, and better able than are others to exploit the opportunities she chooses or which come her way. But this is not for her or for you or for anyone, a reason not to capitalize on the opportunities she makes for herself or of which because perhaps of her "natural" endowments, she takes advantage. If society wishes to regulate opportunities in the public interest it can and probably it should. But it cannot and should not do so opportunistically or in ways inconsistent with other permitted choices. This is a large topic and one. A small corner of which, I have addressed elsewhere (Claxton and Culyer 2006; Harris 2005a, 2005b, 2006, 2007b; Holm 2006; Rawlins and Dillon 2005).

COMPETITIVE PRESSURES

It is often said that smart drugs create irresistible competitive pressures such that once they are used everyone is forced to follow in order to keep up, and this is coercive and corrosive.

Here the analogy with study for students or training in sport or simply with "hard work" is potent. If a student studies hard or an athlete trains exhaustively or exhaustingly, or an employee works "all hours" these things create pressures on others which may be hard to resist. (And so they should you might think!). The issue is, of course, that of what if any remedy is appropriate and surely the remedy in these and other cases is not to ban study, or training, or hard work.

This raises the question of setting limits on, for example, working hours. These are sometimes set in the interests of safety both of the worker and those she works with or on (perhaps in the case of doctors or pilots). Working hours directives may be just and justified but we should also remember the virtue of working above and beyond the call of duty and how and whether this should be regulated. I was recently at a conference in Italy talking to a famous transplant surgeon who performed one the of first xenotransplantations of a liver. The patient survived for 72 days and for every one of those days this dedicated young surgeon slept in the room next to the patient, never leaving the hospital in the whole of that time. We might not wish to require that sort of commitment from our doctors, but I am doubtful that we want to legislate against it or protect people from feeling the moral pressure, commitment, or benevolence that leads them to act in that way.

Some relevant questions might be:

- When and how am I coerced to follow the example of others?
- Am I free to refuse to do so?
- What does it take to resist?
- Are their rational motives for resistance?
- Are parents free to refuse to give smart drugs to their children?
- Would they be "good parents" if they do or if they don't?

I will not attempt to answer these questions specifically here although it will be obvious from the argument so far what my answers would be. I will note simply that the answers to such questions are far too often assumed to be clear without a shred of evidence or argument being offered for the assumptions made. We can simply note here that pressures are usually resistible or laws would never be broken; and that while there are good reasons to protect people from pressures to harm themselves or others there are usually no good reasons to protect people from pressures to do themselves good or benefit others. Indeed one could regard morality (let alone law) as a system designed to create irresistible pressures to do good, or at least such pressures which are hard to resist and in no way to be resisted.

Now is the moment to say something about how safe is "safe enough." It is a truism that all drugs have side effects and that there is little in life that is risk free. When we judge a drug to be safe we can only mean "safe enough" and the "enough" part of this conjunction means safe given the magnitude of the expected benefits and the dimensions of the risks it is worth running to secure those benefits. A final element is the degree to which we judge people to be free to make their own judgments about how this trade-off works out in their own case and to implement those judgments once made. Cancer drugs are currently notoriously toxic and would never be tested on healthy subjects in the way that many other drugs are tested (Jayson and Harris 2006; Rosa *et al.* 2006). However, it is rational for patients with severe cancer to accept toxicity risks which would be unacceptable to those with milder conditions. In the case of the cognitive enhancer Ritalin®, for example, we know that Ritalin® has been prescribed reasonably safely for hundreds of thousands of children below the age of consent with, for example, attention deficit hyperactivity disorder (ADHD) and other conditions for more than 30 years. ADHD is not life-threatening nor is it a painful condition. If it has been judged safe enough to give this drug to children incapable of consenting for themselves it is certainly "safe enough" to permit healthy adults including university students to make up their own minds as to whether or not to take it electively as a cognitive enhancer.

Cognitive enhancement that works is an opportunity that it is in the interests of society and government to take, since governments spend huge amounts on education and the evidence emerging is that cognitive enhancers improve educational attainment. Similarly, since "if it wasn't good for you it wouldn't be an enhancement" (Harris 2007a), parents act ethically when they try to do the best for their kids, and those of us who are autonomous enough to consider such questions, have good reasons to confer such benefits on ourselves (Harris 2001). Governments have prudential as well as moral reasons to support parental and individual choice in such matters because the more receptive our children are to education the better it works and the more cost-effective it becomes.

References

Almeida, S.S., Duntas, L.H., Dye, L., *et al.* (2002). Nutrition and brain function: A multidisciplinary virtual symposium. *Nutritional Neuroscience,* **5,** 311–20.

Brighouse, H. (1998). Why should states fund schools? *British Journal of Educational Studies,* **46,** 138–52.

Brighouse, H. (2000). *A level playing field: The reform of private schools.* London: Fabian Society.

Brighouse, H. (2002). A modest defence of school choice. *Journal of Philosophy of Education,* **36,** 653-59.

Brighouse, H. (2003). *School Choice and Social Justice.* New York: Oxford University Press.

Brighouse, H. (2006). *On Education.* London: Routledge.

Claxton, K. and Culyer, A.J. (2006). Wickedness or folly? The ethics of NICE's decisions. *Journal of Medical Ethics,* **32,** 373–7.

Claxton, K. and Culyer, A.J. (2007). Rights, responsibilities and nice: a rejoinder to Harris. *Journal of Medical Ethics,* **33,** 462–4.

Draganski, B., Gaser, C., Busch, V., Schuierer, G., Bogdahn, U., and May, A. (2004). Neuroplasticity: changes in grey matter induced by training. *Nature,* **427,** 311–12.

Foster, S.S. (2002). School choice and social injustice: a response to Harry Brighouse. *Journal of Philosophy Of Education,* **36,** 291-308.

Greely, H., Sahakian, B., Harris, J., *et al.* (2008). Towards responsible use of cognitive-enhancing drugs by the healthy. *Nature,* **456,** 702–5.

Harris, J. (2001). One principle and three fallacies of disability studies. *Journal Of Medical Ethics,* **27,** 383–8.

Harris, J. (2005a). It's not nice to discriminate. *British Medical Journal,* **31,** 373–5.

Harris, J. (2005b). Nice and not so nice. *Journal of Medical Ethics,* **31,** 685.

Harris, J. (2006). NICE is not cost effective. *Journal of Medical Ethics,* **32,** 378–80.

Harris, J. (2007a). *Enhancing Evolution: The Ethical Case for Making Better People.* Princeton, NJ: Princeton University Press.

Harris, J. (2007b). NICE rejoinder. *Journal of Medical Ethics,* **33,** 467.

Hillman, C.H., Erickson, K.I., and Kramer, A.F. (2008). Be smart, exercise your heart: exercise effects on brain and cognition. *Nature Reviews Neuroscience,* **9,** 58–65.

Holm, S. (2006). Self inflicted harm; NICE in ethical self destruct mode. *Journal of Medical Ethics,* **32,** 125.

Jayson, G.C. and Harris, J. (2006). Recruitment of research subjects: ethics and policy. *Nature Reviews Cancer,* **6,** 330–6.

Jones, R., Elderly, B., Morris, K., and Nutt, D. (2007). *Cognition Enhancers. Drugs and The Future: Brain Science, Addiction and Society.* Available at: http://www.foresight.gov.uk (Accessed 1 March 2006).

Rawlins, M. and Dillon, A. (2005). NICE discrimination. *British Medical Journal,* **31,** 683.

Rosa, D.D., Harris, J. and Jayson, G.C. (2006). The best guess approach to phase I trial design. *Journal of Clinical Oncology,* **24,** 206–8.

Savulescu, J., Foddy, B., and Clayton, M. (2004). Why we should allow performance enhancing drugs in sport. *British Journal of Sports Medicine,* **38,** 666–70.

Schlaggar, B.L. and McCandliss, B.D. (2007). Development of neural systems for reading. *Nature,* **30,** 475–503.

Swift, A. (2003). *How Not To Be a Hypocrite: School Choice for The Morally Perplexed Parent.* London: Routledge Falmer.

Swift, A. (2004a). The morality of school choice. *Theory and Research in Education,* **2,** 7–21.

Swift, A. (2004b). The morality of school choice reconsidered: a response. *Theory and Research in Education,* **2,** 323–42.

Tooley, J. (2003). Why Harry Brighouse is nearly right about the privatisation of education. *Journal of Philosophy of Education,* **37,** 427–47.

CHAPTER 17

COGNITIVE ENHANCEMENT IN COURTS

ANDERS SANDBERG, WALTER SINNOTT-ARMSTRONG, AND JULIAN SAVULESCU

HUMAN cognitive performance has crucial significance for legal process, often making the difference between fair and unfair imprisonment. Lawyers, judges, and jurors need to follow long and complex arguments. They need to understand technical language. They need to observe what happens during the trial.

Moreover, trials depend crucially on memory.[1] Eyewitnesses must remember what they saw. Expert witnesses must remember their fields and their data and analyses in this case. Lawyers must remember which points they and the other side made and what each of their witnesses is supposed to say. Judges must remember the law, including complex procedural rules. Jurors need to remember what happened during a long trial.

COGNITIVE CHALLENGES FOR JURORS

The demands imposed on jurors in particular are sizeable:

> The rules and procedures used to govern the conduct of jury trials reflect a great deal of faith in jurors' ability to understand and retain information over long periods of time, often with much intervening information. Jurors are expected to operate as passive recipients of information presented by the parties, and generally are prohibited from taking notes, asking questions, or using other potentially memory-enhancing tools. In addition, little opportunity is provided for review or elaboration of the concepts presented. From this impoverished learning environment, jurors are expected to recall the evidence and testimony presented at trial, recall the judge's instructions about the law applicable to the case, and reach a rational conclusion regarding the proper verdict in the case. (Johnson 1993)

---

[1] This is one reason why the statutes of limitations exist (Johnson 1993).

These memory demands likely affect real court cases. Johnson (1993) cites the experience of litigation consultants that test the comprehensibility and memorability of particular case presentations to surrogate jurors. These evaluations often find inaccurate recall of case information, especially in complex cases.

The legal process also assumes that jurors can accurately assess what they do and do not remember. However, in mock jury trials there was no link between how confident jurors were about their memory and their actual accuracy: the most confident (and hence most likely to sway uncertain fellow jurors) were not the most accurate. The same was true for individual estimates of memory for particular categories of evidence. The accuracy improved once the jurors answered questions about the evidence, suggesting that a proper jury deliberation can compensate for individual memory failure. Unfortunately this requires a careful review of all evidence, something that might be hard to achieve due to memory and communication limitations (Pritchard and Keenan 1999).

Jurors are often subjected to both tremendous decision complexity (because of intricate legal principles) and tremendous evidence complexity (because of high information load as well as low implicational clarity and comprehensibility). Lawyers sometimes intentionally obscure their opponents' points, such as by introducing red herrings or continuously objecting in order to break the flow of testimony. When asked, jurors report that increasing the quantity of information they have to consider decreases their ability to understand the issues and the confidence in their verdict (Heuer and Penrod 1994). Decisions of jurors in a simulated civil trial were affected by different levels of evidence complexity. In a high-information load situation, they attributed greater blameworthiness to the plaintiffs, contrary to the evidence, and were less able to distinguish between differently liable plaintiffs (Horowitz *et al.* 1996).

In general, the psychology of decision making has found that decision quality decreases as information load increases (Hwang and Lin 1999). To handle the information load the subject typically uses heuristics to rapidly weed out possibilities (Payne 1976), a process that seems likely to introduce some biases.

Learning and memory are strongly affected by other psychological factors, such as emotions, stress, alertness, and attention. The court environment is often stressful for jurors (The National Center for State Courts 2002), and this stress will likely affect their cognition. Equally, monotony, lack of stimulation, and active participation can also produce inattention and sleepiness that interfere with learning the evidence. Gruesome evidence may also arouse emotion and thereby bias recall through an emotional von Restorff effect (von Restorff 1933; Bradley *et al.* 1992).

For a trial to be fair, the jury needs to remember the details of the case, as well as their instructions from the judge, and to deliberate until they reach a consensus based on this information without being biased. Cognitive limitations might preclude bringing accurate memories to the deliberation, and they might affect the impartiality of the deliberation and the fairness of the trial. In some cases, jurors are asked to disregard evidence, which requires an additional high degree of mental control.[2]

---

[2] In this chapter, we will not deal with the implications of inherent cognitive limitations of jurors due to low IQ or mental disorder. If there is a 10% chance of a mental disorder per juror, there is only a 28% chance that a random jury will be entirely free of mental disorder.

Sleepiness in the courtroom is another cognitive problem. Judicial sleepiness is not uncommon, but mistrials due to sleeping judges appear to be rare. In White 589F.2d 1283 1289 (5th Circuit, 1979), the presiding judge fell asleep during the defense counsel's opening statement, but there was no mistrial because there was no evidence of prejudice to the defendant's case. Nonetheless, such somnolence is increasingly disparaged by the public and the profession.

In many ways, the evidence from these cases suggests that judges are now held to a high standard similar to those in the trucking industry or hospital medical staff. While potential consequences of fall-asleep errors by truck drivers and hospital medical staff often involve death or serious injury, fall-asleep episodes by judges could possibly lead to serious consequences such as a wrong conviction or incorrect sentence (Grunstein and Banerjee 2007).

Jurors are even more prone to sleep. In a survey of juror delinquency, 562 judges (69%) reported cases over the previous 3 years where jurors had fallen asleep. This would correspond to 2300 cases, approximately 5–10% of all cases (King 1996). There were probably many more cases where jurors were sleepy, perhaps very sleepy, but did not actually fall asleep. However, the number of new trials actually granted due to juror misconduct (of any kind) was very low: 51 cases out of 26,000.

Ways to enhance cognition

Some of these problems could be ameliorated if we could somehow enhance the cognitive capacities, including attention and memory, of various players in trials. There are multiple ways in which cognition can be improved either by external tools or by an increasing number of biomedical interventions that act directly on the brain.

External tools

Memory and cognition in general are not strictly located solely within the brain: we often employ parts of the environment as extensions of the mind, and hence external tools can enhance or extend their abilities (Clark and Chalmers 1998; Dror and Harnad 2008). Typical examples include counting on fingers or adding on calculators. There are many more possibilities for jurors, some of which indicated in Table 17.1.

Some external tools that enhance cognition are simple and obvious. Exercise (which is, strictly speaking, not external) can enhance attention and memory. One might suggest that courts allow jurors (as well as witnesses, etc.) to go for a run or brisk walk occasionally during trials, when time permits. Requiring jurors to sit still for long periods can reduce memory and cognition in general.

Memory can also be enhanced by manipulating the environment. People tend to remember more and more accurately when they recall in the same circumstances as when they first experienced an event. Jurors then might recall more of the evidence in a long trial and might make fewer recall mistakes during their deliberations if they deliberate inside the courtroom where they heard the evidence.

Table 17.1 External tools for cognitive enhancement in the courtroom

1. Exercise and environment
2. Instructions and procedures
3. Note-taking:
   a. Improve memory by making notes and using them as memory cues
   b. Increasingly but not always allowed
   c. Concerns:
      i.   Distract from testimony and observation
      ii. Overemphasize actually written information
      iii. Give literate people an advantage
   d. Studies:
      i.   Likely improve recall of trial events
      ii. May be less effective with ambiguous information
      iii. Helps handle information load
4. Access to transcripts and recordings:
   a. Less useful as memory cue

Instructions and procedures can improve memory as well. These tools might include mnemonics or merely repetition of important information.

Taking notes is an obvious external memory enhancer. Note-taking by jurors used to be forbidden in most US jurisdictions, partly out of fear that jurors who took notes would gain inordinate dominance over illiterate jurors. Today, it is reportedly allowed in most but still not all jurisdictions. Note-taking can enhance memory both by the process of recording notes and by providing memory cues for later recall. Even doodling might act as an indirect memory enhancer by reducing boredom (Andrade 2009). Several studies have found that jurors taking notes recalled more trial events than non-note takers, and this might increase juror competence in some circumstances (Forsterlee *et al.* 1994; Rosenha *et al.* 1994; Forsterlee and Horowitz 1997). However, other field studies have questioned the improvement of recall of trial information (Heuer and Penrod 1988, 1989), especially when the evidence was ambiguous (Forsterlee and Horowitz 1997). Note-taking may help the jury confront higher information loads: in an experiment with 6- and 12-member mock juries note-taking reduced the tendency for the smaller (and likely more overloaded) juries to give too high compensatory awards in high-complexity situations (Horowitz and Bordens 2002).

Pre-existing knowledge tends to aid recall of related information by providing a framework for assimilating the new information. Careful pre-instruction assists with juror recall of evidence (Elwork *et al.* 1977; Kassin and Wrightsman 1979). Note-takers, while showing better memory than non-note-takers, performed even better in terms of decision making when given effective pre-instructions (Forsterlee and Horowitz 1997).

When memory fails, jurors can ask for access to transcripts and recordings. However, the ability to ask for transcripts is useful only if jurors remember enough to know which parts to ask for. Moreover, some courts surprisingly suggest that jurors should put less weight on the transcript than on their memories of what was said. Courts could more strongly encourage jurors to refer to official records by making access easier.

In these and other ways, courts could enhance juror memory and performance by the use of external tools. Each of these methods raises legal, moral, and practical issues that might preclude its use in actual trials. Still, the cost of refusing to use these tools will be decreased cognitive performance by jurors (and other legal actors).

Biomedical cognition enhancement

Like external tools, biomedical cognitive enhancers could improve a wide variety of cognitive functions (Table 17.2):

- Wakefulness: caffeine, modafinil, stimulants in general.
- Attention: methylphenidate (Ritalin®), nicotine.
- Memory encoding: glucose, cholinergic drugs (eg. donepezil, nicotine, physiostigmine), levodopa, ampakines.
- Working memory: methylphenidate (Ritalin®), modafinil, dopaminergic drugs.
- Stress reduction: beta blockers (propranolol).
- Self-control: glucose.
- Executive inhibitory control: Modafinil.
- Empathy/prosocial behavior: oxytocin.

Some jurors already use some of these substances regularly. Glucose improves episodic memory and other cognitive abilities in middle-aged people, especially when the task is demanding (Riby *et al.* 2008). Many jurors use caffeine and nicotine while serving on a jury. Some take stronger energy drinks, such as 5-hour Energy™.

Other biomedical cognitive enhancers are used less often, but are still probably used by some jurors today. US sales of metylphenidate (Ritalin®) are growing so fast that many jury members probably already take it as a therapeutic medication. Cognitive enhancers are used deliberately by at least some professionals (Sahakian and Morein-Zamir 2007). Levodopa, a precursor to dopamine used in the treatment of Parkinson's disease, when given over 5 days improved learning of an artificial vocabulary in terms of speed of learning, correctness of answers (the effect was approximately 10% more correct responses in the levodopa condition). There was a decrease of false alarm responses (Knecht *et al.* 2004).

Much research has examined how to enhance sleep-deprived healthy subjects. Stimulants (modafinil, caffeine, and dextroamphetamine) improved general alertness, reaction speed, and other cognitive abilities, including the ability to discriminate and label complex emotional blends in pictures of faces (Huck *et al.* 2008). This ability can be crucial for assessing witnesses. However, modafinil and caffeine appear more efficacious for improving executive function (Wesensten *et al.* 2005). Modafinil is able to restore humor appreciation (a complex cognitive ability), unlike the other stimulants (Killgore *et al.* 2006). Modafinil also resulted in greater deliberation before making decisions than the use of amphetamines. Different stimulants are, thus, likely to have subtly different effects on cognitive subsystems (Killgore *et al.* 2009). In a court setting, the basic stimulant effect would allow jurors to remain awake and vigilant, while enhancing the higher cognitive abilities needed for making observations

Table 17.2 Some cognition–affecting substances and court–relevant cognitive effects

	Positive cognitive effects	Negative cognitive effects
Alcohol	Reduce persuasion? (Bostrom and White 1979)	Memory, attention, and wakefulness impairment, disinhibition (Weissenborn and Duka 2003)
Ampakines	Memory (Lynch 2002)	
Benzodiazepines	Stress reduction (Lydiard *et al.* 1988)	Memory impairment, alertness reduction (Gorissen *et al.* 1995; Stewart 2005)
Beta blockers	Stress reduction (Alexander *et al.* 2007)	Memory biasing (Callaway *et al.* 1991; Cahill and van Stegeren 2003)
Caffeine	Wakefulness (Smith 2002)	More easily persuaded? (Mintz and Mills 1971; Martin *et al.* 2005)
Cholinergic drugs (donepezil, physiostigmine)	Memory (Furey *et al.* 2000; Barch 2004)	
Glucose	Memory (Riby *et al.* 2008), self-control (Gailliot *et al.* 2007)	
Marijuana	Stress reduction (Hart *et al.* 2001)	Premature responses, learning impairment, working memory impairment, possibly memory bias (Hart *et al.* 2001; Lundqvist 2005)
Methylphenidate (Ritalin®)	Planning, working memory (Elliott *et al.* 1997)	
Modafinil	Wakefulness (Baranski *et al.* 2004), working memory, decisionmaking, inhibitory control (Turner *et al.* 2003)	
Nicotine	Attention (Rezvani and Levin 2001; Newhouse *et al.* 2004)	Withdrawal distraction, reduced recall (Kelemen and Fulton 2008)
Stimulants	Wakefulness, some memory encoding, emotional discrimination (Barch 2004; Huck *et al.* 2008)	Impulsivity (Ramaekers and Kuypers 2006)

of subtle evidence (e.g. witness testimony), following lines of argument, and avoiding rash decisions during deliberation.

However, some biomedical cognitive enhancers have worrying side effects that could impair legal decision making. Propranolol, used for the treatment of hypertension, reduces anxiety in subjects forced to give a speech, so it might reduce anxiety and its effects in witnesses and jurors, but it was also found to impair recall of difficult (but not easy) words in anxious subjects (Hartley *et al.* 1983). Again, some enhancers might improve memory performance among the worst performers but reduce it among the top performers (Kukolja *et al.* 2009). Enhancer effects might, for example, be larger among older jurors, since they may be suffering from neuromodulatory deficits; but the same enhancers might have detrimental side effects on younger jurors. Each biomedical enhancer must be tested separately and carefully for its costs as well as benefits to cognitive capacity.

THE ETHICS OF COGNITION ENHANCEMENT IN COURT

Should cognitive enhancers be allowed, made readily available, provided for free, encouraged, or required for jurors or other participants in the legal process? These moral and legal issues can be illuminated by comparing biomedical enhancers with note-taking. As we said, note-taking is allowed in most but not all jurisdictions. Where note-taking is not allowed, various objections are raised (though not based on empirical research) (Penrod and Heuer 1997). Only some of these objections apply to the use of cognitive enhancers:

- Note-taking is alleged to distract jurors.
  - No distraction occurs with the use of biomedical cognitive enhancers.
- Note-taking is assumed to consume too much trial time.
  - No trial time is taken by biomedical cognitive enhancers.
- Juror notes are often not accurate records of the trial.
  - Enhanced memories might be more accurate than non-enhanced memories, but accuracy is not guaranteed by any method.
- uror notes might favor one side or the other. For example, notes tend to trail off, so the side that goes first might get an unfair advantage if notes are allowed.
  - Biomedical cognitive enhancers give no such advantage to the side that starts, and might even reduce an unfair disadvantage to the side that goes last by counteracting detrimental effects of exhaustion, impatience, and boredom.
- Note-takers might have undue influence over non-note takers.
  - Biomedically enhanced jurors might become over-confident, and jurors who are not biomedically enhanced might become over-deferential.

This brief comparison suggests that biomedical cognitive enhancers are no more questionable than note-taking, unless they lead to excessive confidence by users and/or excessive deference by non-users. Greater confidence of those who use biomedical cognitive enhancers might be justified by their greater cognitive abilities, but they might become even more confident than is warranted. In any case, these dangers should be taken seriously and tested empirically.

Biasing effects

There would be a strong reason to forbid the use of biomedical cognitive enhancers in courts if they biased judgment in some unfair way. Drugs can produce effects that are not strictly memory failures yet influence what is remembered and how deliberation is conducted.

Drugs can, for example, influence how easily jurors are swayed by persuasive communication. Caffeine appears to facilitate persuasion (Mintz and Mills 1971; Martin *et al.* 2005). In a double-blind test, moderate amounts of caffeine (3.5mg/kg) led to greater agreement with a counter-attitudinal message. The effect may be mediated by the increased arousal, attention, and information processing due to the drug, which facilitates systematic thinking about the message and hence being convinced by it. More persuasive arguments showed a stronger effect in the caffeine condition than in the non-caffeine condition, while less persuasive arguments had similarly low effect (Martin *et al.* 2005). Contrary to common belief, alcohol appears to have the opposite effect (Bostrom and White 1979). It is not clear, however, whether these effects carry over to conditions of lengthy cross-examination and opposing arguments, as in real trials.

Some drugs can also affect memory in ways that might bias trials. The ability to recall information is influenced by the emotional valence and strength of the information at the time of encoding. Drugs may affect this. (Cahill and van Stegeren 2003) found a sex-related impairment of memory for emotional information by an adrenergic blockade. They gave test subjects the beta-blocker propranolol and showed them slides of an emotionally arousing story, afterwards asking central and peripheral questions. They found that in men the drug impaired memory for information central to the storyline but not peripheral details. Conversely, in women the effect was opposite: they recalled more of the central storyline and less of the peripheral details. These effects on emotional memory might be relevant to trials: trial testimony can have a strong emotional component, and recall of central and even peripheral details is relevant for making a correct decision.

Propranolol also affects how users deal with difficult memory tasks. In hypertensive patients given a memory task treatment with propranolol gave them a more conservative bias, that is, an increased tendency to answer "no" when uncertain about whether they recognized an item (Callaway *et al.* 1991). This effect appears similar to how depressed patients have a conservative bias in a word-recognition task, while manics have the opposite bias (i.e. more positives when uncertain) (Corwin *et al.* 1990). It is not implausible that this effect is mediated through noradrenergic mechanisms, making drugs that increase noradrenergic levels, such as amphetamine or atomoxetine, potential cognitive enhancers, have the positive biasing effect. Response bias effects may be relevant in juries, especially during deliberation. A conservative bias would generally favor the defense, whereas the opposite bias would favor the prosecution.

In conclusion, some drugs, such as propranolol, can bias judgment. Given that such beta-blockers are widely prescribed for cardiovascular disease and are used by many to relieve symptoms of stress (including reduction of stage-fright among music performers (Slomka 1992)), it is not unlikely that some jurors are using these drugs. These drugs may be used for medical or lifestyle reasons, but their potential biasing effects might be grounds to ban them from trials.

It is unlikely, however, that the use of cognition-affecting drugs would result in a mistrial. Defendants have a right to a competent and fair jury, which has led to concerns about juror drunkenness. In the US, 12 of the 562 judges surveyed in King (1996) reported jurors under the influence of drugs or alcohol. Over time the forms of juror drinking needed to grant a retrial has changed from a strict view in the 1800s to increasingly viewing it as a harmless form of misconduct, at least as long as it was the fault of the individual juror (King 1996). After investigations into the excessive use of drugs by a jury, the Supreme Court ruled,

> The same policy considerations supported the Supreme Court's decision in Tanner v. United States upholding the trial judge's refusal to conduct an investigation into broad allegations that a jury "was on one big party" and numerous claims alleging jurors' excessive use of

alcohol and drugs. The Court rejected the defendant's contention that substance abuse constituted an improper external influence. According to the Court, "drugs or alcohol voluntarily ingested by a juror seems no more an 'outside influence' than a virus, poorly prepared food, or lack of sleep." As an internal matter, ingestion of drugs and alcohol was within the rule prohibiting juror testimony to upset a verdict. (Gershman 2005)

If drunkenness and excessive use of illegal drugs is not enough to justify a mistrial, then it seems unlikely that the use of caffeine or propranolol would be enough for a mistrial, even if such enhancers did have some biasing effect.

Policy considerations

We have surveyed a range of beneficial and detrimental effects that substances can have on cognition. Some can adversely affect or bias deliberation, but their effects appear smaller than the biasing effects of jury deliberation itself (Sunstein 2006). Given the low requirements for juror competence, it is not consistent with current legal practice to ban such substances. Similarly, given the low bar required for juror competence, coupled with rights to control what goes into one's body, courts could not legally require consumption of even clearly safe cognition enhancing drugs.

Even if courts neither ban nor require biomedical cognitive enhancers in trials, other steps could be taken. An increasing number of agents that affect cognition are clearly entering use. Courts and jurors should be aware of the effects of these substances on cognition. Better information about how to deliberate more effectively, including interventions and strategies, should be made available prior to the court process. Courts should also consider deployment of simple strategies, such as breaks and exercise, to improve juror performance.

As our range and knowledge of cognitive enhancers increases, some enhancers should be provided, as we now provide coffee, if they are safe and do not bias judgment. Substances like modafinil may well meet this criterion. Given the stakes, we have a moral imperative to investigate ways to utilize these new technologies to improve cognitive performance in the courtroom. Innocent people's lives may well depend on them.

References

Alexander, J.K., Hillier, A., Smith, R.M., Tivarus, M.E., and Beversdorf, D.Q. (2007). Beta-adrenergic modulation of cognitive flexibility during stress. *Journal of Cognitive Neuroscience,* **19**, 468–78.

Andrade, J. (2009). What does doodling do? *Applied Cognitive Psychology,* **24**, 100–6.

Baranski, J.V., Pigeau, R., Dinich, P., and Jacobs, I. (2004). Effects of modafinil on cognitive and meta-cognitive performance. *Human Psychopharmacology – Clinical and Experimental,* **19**, 323–32.

Barch, D.M. (2004). Pharmacological manipulation of human working memory. *Psychopharmacology,* **174**, 126–35.

Bostrom, R.N. and White, N.D. (1979). Does drinking weaken resistance? *Journal of Communication,* **29**, 73–80.

Bradley, M.M., Greenwald, M.K., Petry, M.C., and Lang, P.J. (1992). Remembering pictures – pleasure and arousal in memory. *Journal of Experimental Psychology–Learning Memory and Cognition,* **18**, 379–90.

Cahill, L. and van Stegeren, A. (2003). Sex-related impairment of memory for emotional events with beta-adrenergic blockade. *Neurobiology of Learning and Memory*, 79, 81–8.

Callaway, E., Halliday, R., Perez-Stable, E.J., Coates, T.J., and Hauck, W.W. (1991). Propranolol and response bias – an extension of findings reported by Corwin *et al. Biological Psychiatry*, 30, 739–42.

Clark, A. and Chalmers, D. (1998). The extended mind (active externalism). *Analysis*, 58, 7–19.

Corwin, J., Peselow, E., Feenan, K., Rotrosen, J., and Fieve, R. (1990). Disorders of decision in affective disease – an effect of beta-adrenergic dysfunction. *Biological Psychiatry*, 27, 813–33.

Dror, I. and Harnad, S. (2008). Offloading cognition onto cognitive technology. In I. Dror and S. Harnad (eds.) *Cognition Distributed: How Cognitive Technology Extends Our Minds*, pp.1–23. Amsterdam: John Benjamins.

Elliott, R., Sahakian, B.J., Matthews, K., Bannerjea, A., Rimmer, J., and Robbins, T.W. (1997). Effects of methylphenidate on spatial working memory and planning in healthy young adults. *Psychopharmacology*, 131, 196–206.

Elwork, A., Sales, B.D., Alfini, J.J., Elwork, A., Sales, B.D., and Alfini, J.J. (1977). Juridic decisions: in ignorance of the law of in light of it? *Law and Human Behavior*, 1, 163–89.

Forsterlee, L. and Horowitz, I.A. (1997). Enhancing juror competence in a complex trial. *Applied Cognitive Psychology*, 11, 305–19.

Forsterlee, L., Horowitz, I.A., and Bourgeois, M. (1994). Effects of notetaking on verdicts and evidence processing in a civil trial. *Law and Human Behavior*, 18, 567–78.

Furey, M.L., Pietrini, P., and Haxby, J. V. (2000). Cholinergic enhancement and increased selectivity of perceptual processing during working memory. *Science*, 290, 2315–19.

Gailliot, M.T., Baumeister, R.F., DeWall, C.N., *et al.* (2007). Self-control relies on glucose as a limited energy source: Willpower is more than a metaphor. *Journal of Personality and Social Psychology*, 92, 325–36.

Gorissen, M., Eling, P., Van Luijtelaar, G., and Coenen, A. (1995). Effects of diazepam on encoding processes. *Journal of Psychopharmacology*, 9, 113–21.

Grunstein, R.R. and Banerjee, D. (2007). The case of "Judge Nodd" and other sleeping judges. Media, society, and judicial sleepiness. *Sleep*, 30, 625–32.

Hart, C.L., van Gorp, W., Haney, M., Foltin, F.W., and Fischman, M.W. (2001). Effects of acute smoked marijuana on complex cognitive performance. *Neuropsychopharmacology*, 25, 757–65.

Hartley, L.R., Ungapen, S., Davie, I., *et al.* (1983). The effect of beta-adrenergic blocking-drugs on speakers performance and memory. *British Journal of Psychiatry*, 142, 512–17.

Heuer, L. and Penrod, S. (1988). Increasing jurors participation in trials – a field experiment with jury notetaking and question asking. *Law and Human Behavior*, 12, 231–61.

Heuer, L. and Penrod, S.D. (1989). Instructing jurors – a field experiment with written and preliminary instructions. *Law and Human Behavior*, 13, 409–30.

Heuer, L. and Penrod, S. (1994). Trial complexity – a field investigation of its meaning and its effects. *Law and Human Behavior*, 18, 29–51.

Horowitz, I.A. and Bordens, K.S. (2002). The effects of jury size, evidence complexity, and note taking on jury process and performance in a civil trial. *Journal of Applied Psychology*, 87, 121–30.

Horowitz, I.A., ForsterLee, L., and Brolly, I. (1996). Effects of trial complexity on decision making. *Journal of Applied Psychology*, 81, 757–68.

Huck, N.O., McBride, S.A., Kendall, A.P., Grugle, N.L., and Killgore, W.D. (2008). The effects of modafinil, caffeine, and dextroamphetamine on judgments of simple versus complex emotional expressions following sleep deprivation. *International Journal of Neuroscience*, 118, 487–502.

Hwang, M.I. and Lin, J.W. (1999). Information dimension, information overload and decision quality. *Journal of Information Science*, 25, 213–18.

Johnson, M.T. (1993). Memory phenomena in the law. *Applied Cognitive Psychology*, 7, 603–18.

Kassin, S.M. and Wrightsman, L.S. (1979). Requirements of proof – timing of judicial instruction and mock juror verdicts. *Journal of Personality and Social Psychology* 37(10): 1877–87.

Kelemen, W.L. and Fulton, E.K. (2008). Cigarette abstinence impairs memory and metacognition despite administration of 2mg nicotine gum. *Experimental and Clinical Psychopharmacology*, 16, 521–31.

Killgore, W.D.S., Kahn-Greene, E.T., Grugle, N.L., Killgore, D.B., and Balkin T.J. (2009). Sustaining executive functions during sleep deprivation: a comparison of caffeine, dextroamphetamine, and modafinil. *Sleep*, 32, 205–16.

Killgore, W.D.S., McBride, S.A., Killgore, D.B., and Balkin, T.J. (2006). The effects of caffeine, dextroamphetamine, and modafinil on humor appreciation during sleep deprivation. *Sleep*, 29, 841–7.

King, N.J. (1996). Juror delinquency in criminal trials in America, 1796–1996. *Michigan Law Review*, 94, 2673–751.

Knecht, S., Breitenstein, C., Bushuven, S., *et al.* (2004). Levodopa: faster and better word learning in normal humans. *Annals of Neurology*, 56, 20–6.

Kukolja, J., Thiel, C.M., and Fink, G.R. (2009). Cholinergic stimulation enhances neural activity associated with encoding but reduces neural activity associated with retrieval in humans. *Journal of Neuroscience*, 29, 8119–28.

Lundqvist, T. (2005). Cognitive consequences of cannabis use: comparison with abuse of stimulants and heroin with regard to attention, memory and executive functions. *Pharmacology Biochemistry and Behavior*, 81, 319–30.

Lydiard, R.B., Roybyrne, P.P., and Ballenger, J.C. (1988). Recent advances in the psychopharmacological treatment of anxiety disorders. *Hospital and Community Psychiatry*, 39, 1157–65.

Lynch, G. (2002). Memory enhancement: the search for mechanism-based drugs. *Nature Neuroscience*, 5, 1035–8.

Martin, P.Y., Laing, J., and Mitchell, M. (2005). Caffeine, cognition, and persuasion: Evidence for caffeine increasing the systematic processing of persuasive messages. *Journal of Applied Social Psychology*, 35, 160–82.

Mintz, P.M. and Mills, J. (1971). Effects of arousal and information about its source upon attitude change. *Journal of Experimental Social Psychology*, 7, 561–70.

Newhouse, P.A., Potter, A., Singh, A. (2004). Effects of nicotinic stimulation on cognitive performance. *Current Opinion in Pharmacology*, 4, 36–46.

Payne, J.W. (1976). Task complexity and contingent processing in decision-making — information search and protocol analysis. *Organizational Behavior and Human Performance*, 16, 366–87.

Penrod, S.D. and Heuer, L. (1997). Tweaking commonsense — assessing aids to jury decision making. *Psychology Public Policy and Law*, 3, 259–84.

Pritchard, M.E. and Keenan, J.M. (1999). Memory monitoring in mock jurors. *Journal of Experimental Psychology-Applied*, 5, 152–68.

Ramaekers, J.G. and Kuypers, K.P.C. (2006). Acute effects of 3,4-methylenedioxymetham-phetamine (MDMA) on behavioral measures of impulsivity: Alone and in combination with alcohol. *Neuropsychopharmacology*, **31**, 1048–55.

Rezvani, A.H. and Levin, E.D. (2001). Cognitive effects of nicotine. *Biological Psychiatry*, **49**, 258–67.

Riby, L.M., McLaughlin, J. Riby, D.M., *et al.* (2008). Lifestyle, glucose regulation and the cognitive effects of glucose load in middle-aged adults. *British Journal of Nutrition*, **100**, 1128–34.

Rosenhan, D.L., Eisner, S.L., and Robinson, R. J. (1994). Note taking can aid juror recall. *Law and Human Behavior*, **18**, 53–61.

Sahakian, B. and Morein-Zamir, S. (2007). Professor's little helper. *Nature*, **450**, 1157–9.

Slomka, J. (1992). Playing with Propranolol. *Hastings Center Report*, **22**, 13–17.

Smith, A. (2002). Effects of caffeine on human behavior. *Food and Chemical Toxicology*, **40**, 1243–55.

Stewart, S.A. (2005). The effects of benzodiazepines on cognition. *Journal of Clinical Psychiatry*, **66**, 9–13.

Sunstein, C.R. (2006). *Infotopia: How Many Minds Produce Knowledge*. Oxford: Oxford University Press.

The National Center for State Courts (2002). *Through the Eyes of the Juror: A Manual for Addressing Juror Stress*. Williamsburg, VA: NCSC.

Turner, D.C., Robbins, T.W., Clark, L., *et al.* (2003). Cognitive enhancing effects of modafinil in healthy volunteers. *Psychopharmacology*, **165**, 260–9.

von Restorff, H. (1933). Über die Wirkung von Bereichsbildungen im Spurenfeld. *Psychologie Forschung*, **18**, 299–34.

Weissenborn, R. and Duka, T. (2003). Acute alcohol effects on cognitive function in social drinkers: their relationship to drinking habits. *Psychopharmacology*, **165**, 306–12.

Wesensten, N.J., Killgore, W.D., and Balkin TJ. (2005). Performance and alertness effects of caffeine, dextroamphetamine, and modafinil during sleep deprivation. *Journal of Sleep Research*, **14**, 255–66.

CHAPTER 18

....

NEUROETHICS AND THE EXTENDED MIND

....

NEIL LEVY

NEUROETHICS AND THE EXTENDED MIND

....

NEUROETHICS offers unprecedented opportunities as well as challenges. The challenges are obvious enough, and stem from the range of difficult ethical issues which confront us as neuroethicists. The opportunities arise from the fact that as we come to understand our targets, we also come to a better understanding of our tools: in coming to the kind of understanding of the mind we need to make progress on ethical problems, we also come to better understand the strengths and limitations of the ways in which we think about these problems. Because the target and the tools of ethical investigation are, for the neuroethicist, broadly the same, neuroethics is alone among the branches of applied ethics in giving us the opportunity for a profound exploration of the nature of ethical thought itself.

Because neuroethics is as much a theoretical endeavor as a practical undertaking—a practical undertaking which requires and leads to theoretical advances—progress on its subject matter requires reflection not only on issues in ethics, but also on much more abstract and apparently abstruse questions. Questions concerning the nature of consciousness, of personal identity, free will, and so on, are all grist for the neuroethical mill. One such apparently esoteric question concerns the *location* of the mind. In this chapter, I will argue that this debate bears centrally on neuroethics. Moreover, I will argue that this debate is significant for neuroethics no matter how it turns out. Whether the best interpretation of the facts to which proponents of the extended mind appeal is that the mind is genuinely extended, or merely embedded, reflection on these facts, which are not themselves in dispute, will show that the domain of neuroethics extends to all the processes and mechanisms subserving cognition, rather than just those processes and mechanisms internal to the skull. Once this fact is recognized, I claim, both the scope of neuroethics and some of its characteristic concerns will be transformed.

WHAT IS THE EXTENDED MIND HYPOTHESIS?

One of the perennial concerns of philosophers of mind is the relationship between minds and brains. Descartes famously argued that minds and matter (and hence brains) are composed of different kinds of substance. According to Cartesian dualism, the mind is categorically different to the brain. Substance dualism is no longer considered a respectable philosophical position today. Almost all philosophers are monists, believing there is only kind of substance in the universe. If there is only one kind of substance, then everything substantial is composed of it; it follows that mind and brain are made of the same kind of stuff (it must be stressed, however, that it does not follow from the claim that mind and brain are composed of the same stuff that they have the same kinds of properties). This makes the *identity* thesis attractive. On the identity thesis, minds just *are* (appropriately functioning) brains.

To the question "where is the mind?" the identity thesis answers by pointing to the brain. In all but the most unusual cases (science fiction cases involving brains in vats, for instance), the mind is to be found inside the skull of the person whose mind it is. The extended mind hypothesis holds that the mind is not to be found exclusively within the skull, though proponents concede that (again, in all but the most unusual cases) the brain is a necessary and especially significant core part of the mind. Instead, it holds that minds extend beyond the skull, and even beyond the skin, of the person whose mind it is, out into the world.

This is sometimes put in terms of a distinction between the *contents* and the *vehicles* of minds (Hurley 1998). Mental states have content, where the content of a mental state can be expressed by "that" statements. Mental states include beliefs, such as my belief *that I am typing*, desires, such as my desire *that I write well*, intentions, such as my intention *that I go home at 5 o'clock*, and so on (these mental states need not be conscious, of course). Mental states need vehicles. On the identity thesis, the vehicles of mental states are neural states. On the extended mind hypothesis, the vehicles of mental states include many things beside neural states.

The extended mind hypothesis was first explicitly defended in a short but influential article written by Andy Clark and David Chalmers (1998). In this paper, they introduced a pair of agents, Inga and Otto, who live in New York City. Inga and Otto both wish to go to see a new exhibition at the Museum of Modern Art. Inga recalls that the museum is situated on 53rd street and sets out to visit it. Otto, however, suffers from Alzheimer's disease and cannot recall the location of the museum in just the way that Inga can. However, Otto carries a handy notebook which he consults regularly. He pulls out his notebook and looks up the location of the museum. Having retrieved the information from his notebook, he sets out for the exhibition.

Clark and Chalmers claim that there is (or at least need not be) any relevant difference between the way in which Otto and Inga retrieve the information *that the Museum of Modern Art is on 53rd Street*. Prior to recall, both had a dispositional belief—that is, a mental state with the functional role of belief, but which was not currently active—with that content. There are many differences between the ways in which this belief was stored and retrieved in each person, of course, but these differences should not lead neuroethicists to say that only one of these beliefs was genuinely a mental state. Instead, we should say that both agents had a belief with the same content; only the vehicle of the content differed.

On the basis of this imaginary case, Clark and Chalmers advance the *Parity Principle*, which is an explicitly functionalist principle. If something functions in the way in which a mental state functions for an agent, then it *is* a mental state. One could, indeed, argue that the Parity Principle is an entailment of functionalism. Functionalists believe that what makes something a mental state of a particular type depends not on what its realizer or vehicle is, but on the role it plays; on its causal relations to inputs from the environment, to other mental states, and to behavior. Functionalism is motivated, among other things, by the thought that aliens or robots or the advanced computers of the far-future might have mental states, yet obviously these mental states will not be realized by neural networks in precisely the same way human mental states are realized. Instead, functionalists claim, mental states can be *multiply realized*: the same *type* of mental state (a pain, the belief *that aspirin helps headaches*, the desire *that I take aspirin*) can be realized by a variety of different vehicles, some of them made of flesh, some of silicon or what have you. If functionalism is true, there seems to be little motivation for regarding what is within the head as especially privileged. *If something outside the head plays much the same role in cognition as something within, then—given the truth of functionalism—it should be ascribed the same status as it would were it in the head.*

The Parity Principle attempts to capture the conditions which an extra-neural process or mechanism has to satisfy in order for it to count as mental. Obviously, it is not sufficient that some mechanism contribute causally to my thinking for that mechanism to count as part of my mind. In addition, Clark and Chalmers claim, the resource must be constantly and easily accessible; its contents must be automatically endorsed and must have been consciously endorsed in the past. These conditions are met by the information contained in Otto's notebook, but they are not met, for instance, by Wikipedia (in relation to me). Though I *often* consult Wikipedia, accessing it is relatively slow and effortful for me (I do not always have an internet connection available) and I often wonder whether the entry is correct. In this case, it seems that the conditions Clark and Chalmers set down give the right result, because it is clearly false that I believe everything that is written in Wikipedia (right now, before I look).

Though the conditions Clark and Chalmers set out might be sufficient for a mental state to count as mental, there are reasons to doubt that they are necessary. Take ease of access: in both normal and pathological cases (ranging from ordinary lapses through to dementia), dispositional beliefs may not be readily retrievable. Yet they are clearly mental states. In any case, it seems that if the proponent of the extended mind can show that some extended states satisfy these conditions, given that they are sufficient conditions, they will have adequately demonstrated the thesis.

The extended mind hypothesis is driven by two independent phenomena: new developments in technology, on the one hand, and new discoveries in cognitive science on the other. The new developments in technology include many which fall within the purview of neuroethics, broadly construed: cognitive enhancement technologies which do not simply target the brain and its capacities but which instead work to enhance cognition by interfacing the brain with extra-neural and extra-somatic mechanisms. For instance, brain–computer interfaces which expand their users' cognitive powers by reducing the differences between Otto's notebook and Wikipedia blur the boundaries between internal and external informational states, or reduce it to irrelevance (from the functionalist perspective). At the limit, it might be true that I (dispositionally) believe the contents of Wikipedia, if I effortlessly and automatically retrieve its contents via such an interface. Of course, it may be that the kinds of technologies envisaged here prove to be beyond the capabilities of science for the foreseeable future. But the extended mind hypothesis is not only driven by such developments. It is also motivated by work in cognitive science and evolutionary theory.

One motivation is a perspective driven by a lively respect for the parsimony of evolution. Evolution is very conservative and very frugal; in general, it will find the cheapest and simplest means for organisms to achieve their goals. Now, it seems that for those goals which involve cognition, the cheapest and simplest means often involve the organism relying upon external resources to cut down on effort and processing costs. Brain-based cognitive processes are energetically demanding, and evolution is sensitive to even small increments in such costs. Moreover, there are opportunity costs as well; cognitive resources expended on one task are not available for other tasks. If it possible to outsource cognitive tasks and such outsourcing reduces these costs (without, of course, raising other costs excessively) than evolution can be expected to hit upon ways of outsourcing.

The most obvious ways in which organisms outsource cognitive costs involve memory. When the environment is stable (enough) it makes sense to use it as (in a phrase Clark uses many times, owed originally to Rodney Brooks) "its own best model." The organism uses the world as its own best model when, rather than constructing a detailed inner representation of the environment, with all the associated costs involved in creating and storing such a representation, the organism relies upon the stability of the world and its perceptual access to it in order to retrieve information when it needs it. Studies of the visual saccades of human beings engaged in various tasks such as copying a model indicate that human beings proceed in just this way under certain circumstances, thereby reducing the burden on the brain (Clark 2008). Now if human beings *had* constructed a detailed inner representation and guided their behavior by reference to it, philosophers would have no hesitation in treating the representation as part of the mind; since the external representation—the world itself—plays precisely the same role in human behavior, including mental behavior, it ought to be counted as mental by the Parity Principle.

Using the world as an external memory store reduces the burden on the human brain, but it is far from the most spectacular (alleged) extension of the mind. It is relatively unspectacular for the following reason: it allows agents to accomplish more cheaply and efficiently a goal—representing certain states of affairs—which we could, in principle, have accomplished in a brain-based manner. But extending the mind is not just something which makes agents better at achieving goals they might have achieved in other ways; it also allows them to do things they could not otherwise have done at all.

One thing we accomplish by externalizing memory is to make it publicly accessible and resistant to decay. It then becomes available for learning and transmission, with far greater fidelity than could otherwise be achieved (with *perfect* fidelity, insofar as the externalized object is its own model). Human cultures have thus externalized information for thousands of years: material artefacts have many uses, one of which is representational (Sterelny 2004). Of course, with the advent of written language, the range of facts than can be publicly represented expands to include anything that can be thought. As a consequence, ways of *accumulating* knowledge become possible which would not be available were agents thrown back on brain-based resources. In turn, this makes far greater specialization possible. One person can specialize in using a technology (say, computers) without needing to know how that technology works, secure in the knowledge that other specialists can build and repair the technology (that specialist, in turn, can perform the task because she has specialist knowledge about how to *retrieve* information from the public store, as well as how to operate on that knowledge when it is retrieved).

External representations expand cognition in an even more direct way. There are cognitive tasks that we can perform only because we are able to operate on tokens that represent states of affairs, rather than having to work with iconic representations. This is clearest in the case of number. Human beings have two innate—brain-based—number senses. We have an innate sense of small exact numbers; we come equipped to understand the differences between quantities like "one" and "two" and "three." We also have an innate sense of large differences between approximate quantities; we intuitively grasp the difference between about seventy and about ninety-five. But we have no intuitive grasp of large or even medium-sized exact numbers, and therefore no intuitive grasp of the difference between "seventy" and "seventy-one." When agents become capable of representing exact quantities using number words, these differences for the first time become available to them for calculation. Dehaene *et al.* (1999) showed that subjects engaged in exact number tasks showed significant activation in speech-related areas, while engagement in approximate number tasks does not give rise to such activation. The ability to engage in such number tasks is dependent on the availability of extra-neural linguistic representations, representations that are, of course, available to the learner in virtue of cultural transmission. The professional mathematician can think about mathematical tasks orders more complex still, because she has available to her many more representations upon which to operate. Thus, she can think of multidimensional spaces, even though her brain is unable to represent such spaces except by using tokens.

THE DEBATE OVER THE EXTENDED MIND

The extended mind hypothesis has met with a mixed reception from philosophers. Some have embraced it as an obvious extension of functionalism; others have rejected it out of hand. Resistance to the thesis has been motivated by two major concerns: a denial that external resources have the right kinds of contents to count as mental, and the claim that only internal mental states are psychological kinds.

Mental states, recall, have contents. To that extent, my internal representational states and Otto's notebook are analogous: they both are repositories of a great deal of information including all kinds of information expressible in propositional form. According to Adams and Aizawa (2008), however, there is a dramatic difference between the kinds of content they contain. Otto's notebook contains only *derived* content; that is, its content is meaningful only in virtue of conventions and the intentions of agents. Signs, for instance, have merely derived contents: they carry information only in virtue of various conventions such as the conventions of natural languages. Minds, Adams and Aizawa claim, are different: they and they alone have content that is intrinsically referential. They must have such content, because the alternative is an infinite regress; derived content must derive from somewhere.

One obvious response to this line of argument is to claim out that ordinary minds contain derived content as well (arguably) as non-derived. Humans think in natural languages, but natural languages are only derivatively meaningful. However, the defender of intrinsic content might maintain that human minds do not contain derived content in any important sense. Some philosophers and cognitive scientists, following Fodor (1975), maintain that we think in a "language of thought," not in natural languages, where the language of thought is non-derivatively referential. On this view, propositions in natural languages must be trans-formed into equivalents in the language of thought before they can become the contents of minds. But it seems false that *all* human thinking is carried out in a language of thought: at least some thinking does seem to be carried out in natural languages (as well as by way of the manipulation of other conventional symbols). Indeed, the work of Dehaene *et al.* (1999) mentioned earlier seems to show just that. Bilinguals trained in exact mathematical tasks in one of their native tongues perform better at that task if the instructions are given in the same tongue: if they have previously translated their number words and concepts into a more basic language of thought, they should perform equally well in both their native tongues.

In any case, no matter how internal processes are implemented, insofar as thinkers are genuinely concerned with what enables human beings to perform the spectacular intellec-tual feats exhibited in science and other areas of systematic enquiry, as well as in the arts, they need to understand the extent to which the mind is reliant upon external scaffolding. Clark (2008: xxv) quotes a revealing exchange between Richard Feynman, the great physi-cist, and Charles Weiner. Weiner described a collection of Feynman's notes as "a record of the day-to-day work." Feynman rejected the description, claiming it wasn't a record of the work, it *was* the work:

> "I actually did the work on the paper," he said. "Well," Weiner said, "the work as done in your head, but the record of it is still here." "No, it's not a record, not really. It's working. You have to work on paper and this is the paper. Okay?"

Feynman's point, I take it, is that the paper should not be thought of as simply recording what passed through his head, but instead as constituting a part of the cognitive loop involved in his thinking. By externalizing and labeling ideas, they became available for a kind of representation and extension otherwise impossible. Notes on paper, or on a com-puter screen (or mathematical models, or what have you) do not make contemporary physics or other kinds of intellectual endeavor *easier*, they make it *possible*.

The second major worry advanced by critics of the extended mind hypothesis focuses on its utility as a framework for cognitive science. Some philosophers and cognitive scientists have worried that the causal processes involved in extended systems are so diverse that there could be no science of the extended mind. A science, they argue, has as its domain a set of processes that are causally individuated. And in actual fact, they argue, the sciences of the mind qualify as proper sciences on just this basis: neuroscience, cognitive psychology, and so on, reveal a set of causal regularities that characterize (properly) mental processes. Since the causal processes involved in extended processes are so diverse (looping from brains to notebooks or to computers, or to gestures, or what have you), the prospects for a science of the extended mind are slim. By delineating a unified set of causal processes, science cuts nature at its joints; thinkers should therefore be guided by science in their ontology. If there is no science of the extended mind, because it is too causally diverse, there is no genuine extended mind: instead, the "extended mind" should be seen as constituted out of a set of processes and mechanisms each of which could be the subject of a genuine science and each of which should figure by itself in the list of the constituents of the world.

One problem with this argument is that many actual sciences fail the proposed test: The science of animal communication includes causal processes as disparate as communication by the use of pheromones, threat displays, the dance of honey bees, and territory marking by birds, as well as natural language in human beings. There are few general laws which circumscribe all and only these phenomena: instead they are unified only by their functional similarities. Perhaps proponents of the causal regularities view of science would claim that animal communication is not a proper science, or perhaps they would claim that a science ought, if possible, to have as its domain a single set of causally individuated processes. In that case, however, it seems that cognitive psychology will no longer count as a science, since the mental processes it studies are too diverse to constitute the domain of a science: controlled and automatic processes seem causally quite different.

The criticism that the extended mind thesis will impede science rests, finally, on a misconception: that advocates hold that the proper object of the science of the mind is the extended mind *rather than* the brain/central nervous system (CNS). Instead, as Clark's work argues and exemplifies, proponents urge work at many levels and by many specialists simultaneously. The extended mind thesis is not the denial that the brain is special: it is only because the brain/CNS has certain characteristics that there are extended mental systems at all. Studying the extended mind requires the study of the brain; it also requires the study of how the brain interfaces with diverse extra-neural and extra-somatic processes and mechanisms.

The extended mind hypothesis
and neuroethics

Neuroethics is concerned, inter alia, with the permissibility and the advisability of intervening in the mind. Many of the biggest controversies in neuroethics centre on this topic. Is it permissible to use cognitive enhancers to increase the abilities of those who are already functioning in the normal range? Do the use of affective enhancers—say antidepressants or "love drugs"—threaten the authenticity of individuals or relationships? Does the prolonged use of methylphenidate as a treatment for ADHD threaten to alter the identity of users? These questions need to be rethought in light of the extended mind hypothesis.

Much of the heat and the hype surrounding neuroscientific technologies stems from the perception that they offer (or threaten) opportunities genuinely unprecedented in human experience. But if the mind is not confined within the skull, psychopharmaceuticals and other interventions targeted at the brain (say transcranial magnetic stimulation) are not unprecedented inasmuch as they intervene in the mind. Instead, intervening in the mind is *ubiquitous*. It becomes difficult to defend the idea that there is a difference in principle between interventions which work by altering a person's environment and those that work directly on her brain, insofar as the effect on cognition is the same; the mere fact that an intervention targets the brain directly no longer seems relevant (ethically or even psychologically). Of course, many environmental interventions target the brain *indirectly*; better education, for instance, alters the brain just as surely as might cognitive enhancing psychopharmaceuticals. But even if the effect of the intervention is to alter the environment *only*, insofar as it affects cognitive performance it is hard to see why this fact matters. Clark (2003) recounts how some dementia sufferers remain able to live independently long after neuropsychological testing indicates that their leveling of cognitive functioning is below the threshold believed to be required for someone to be capable of taking care of themselves. The tests are accurate, but they do not take into account the ways in which some people learn to structure their environment to take the burden off their brains (taking cupboard doors off, so they can see the contents at a glance, organizing their environment spatially, so that what they need comes to hand when needed, and so on). The effect is to raise their level of cognitive performance above what they could achieve given their brain alone (in a less well organized environment).

Given these facts, neuroethicists need to be alive to the possibility—indeed, I think, the likelihood—that much of the opposition to cognitive enhancements, as well as the preference for talk therapy over psychopharmacology or deep-brain stimulation, and so on, stems from internalist prejudices: from the inchoate thought that the mind is to be found within the skull and there alone. Once it is recognized that human cognitive success and even our identities as psychological beings depends on extended processes, including processes every bit as mechanical and arational as internal interventions, neuroethicists ought to begin to assess interventions based on their *effects*, and not on their *location*. Agential resources of self-control can be strengthened by altering their environment or by drugs; which should be done depends, I claim, not on the means by which the result is achieved, but on the effects: which achieves the best balance of benefits over costs? Just because one intervention is achieved by means that directly target the brain whereas another directly targets external states isn't relevant; this kind of difference is *only* relevant when it makes a difference to the costs and benefits.

The central questions of neuroethics must be rethought in light of the extended mind thesis. Questions like "ought society use our new powers to intervene into the minds of agents?"; "does the dependence of someone on external props affect their identity or their authenticity?"; "is it wrong to alter human nature?"; "ought human beings adopt an attitude of gratitude for the unforced gifts of nature, and not interfere with them?" all seem to depend, directly or indirectly, on the idea that in principle it is possible to separate the human mind from its environmental embedding. That is, the questions seem to presuppose that human beings have a choice about whether to intervene into the minds of agents; we can either continue as we are, with unaltered minds, *or* use our new technologies to intervene. Similarly, the questions presuppose that we can choose between having our identities depend on external props or not, between remaining in a natural state or becoming deeply dependent on the artificial, and so on. If the extended mind thesis is true, these claims are untenable. Human beings have always been dependent on external props to make us who we are. If human beings are rational animals—that is, if our cognitive success is definitive of what we are, as a species and as individuals—then we have always been deeply dependent on external props to make us the kinds of being we are. New technologies and psychopharmaceuticals do not mark a difference *in principle*; they give us new means to do what we have always done. That is not to say, of course, that we ought to use these new means, just that we should not reject them on the grounds suggested.

Taking the extended mind thesis seriously does not commit neuroethicists either to accepting or to rejecting new technologies. It commits us, rather, to assessing them on grounds which are not a mere reflection of internalist prejudices. That may prove harder to do than it might seem, because internalist prejudices may be deeply buried in arguments apparently turning on other considerations. Consider the oft-heard, and eminently sensible, concern that cognitive enhancers would cause inequality. Though the concern is genuine, it is also often voiced by people in whose mouths it seems confabulatory: the bioconservatives like Francis Fukuyama (2002), for instance. It seems confabulatory because these thinker are little concerned with the massive inequalities that actually exist, both within and especially between nations. Why do they overlook one set of inequalities while insisting on another? I think that the answer is because, like many conservatives, they *naturalize* inequality (Napier and Jost 2008); they see actual inequalities as the product of nature, or as reflecting the desert of agents. They do not recognize that existing inequalities are dependent on social choices; on the ways in which nations structure their environments. Indeed, the most valuable thing about the intuitions upon which they insist is that they can be turned back upon the views of those who advance them: by demonstrating that actual inequalities are as undeserved as those they contemplate, neuroethicists can motivate the thought that the public ought to be far more concerned with existing inequalities, which are far greater than anything realistically threatened by cognitive enhancement, than with new technologies. Neuroscience has a role in this project, by showing how inequalities in cognitive function are the product, in part, of environments (Farah *et al.* 2006; Noble *et al.* 2007).

Clark and Chalmers motivated the extended mind hypothesis by appealing to the Parity Principle. The significance of the hypothesis for neuroethics is that attention to it motivates an *Ethical Parity Principle*: whether a particular means of altering cognition directly targets the brain/CNS or the external scaffolding shouldn't make a difference to the assessment of its permissibility or advisability. Causal route is a difference that makes no difference; what matters is the result.

WHY THE EXTENDED MIND THESIS MIGHT NOT MATTER AFTER ALL

Clark and other proponents of the extended mind thesis appear to me to have good responses to almost all the arguments leveled against it. There is, however, one argument against the thesis which seems to me quite forceful. Some philosophers, Rob Rupert (2004) in particular, have argued on the grounds of theoretical conservatism that the mind ought to be identified with internal goings-on alone. Rupert concedes, as he should, that environmental scaffolding is absolutely essential to human cognitive success, but he argues that recognition of this fact is compatible with the internalist view. He prefers to see mind as deeply *embedded* in extra-neural and extra-somatic processes and mechanisms, not as genuinely (though partially) *constituted* by such processes. Insofar as Rupert concedes all the facts upon which proponents of the extended mind insist about external scaffolding, there can be no (direct) empirical response to this claim. Every fact about cognition that could be cited by the proponent of the extended mind Rupert can accept, consistent with rejecting the functionalist claim that if the same kinds of goals and behaviors are subserved by external processes and mechanisms as by internal, they ought to be regarded as the same kind of thing. But just insofar as this is true, the debate seems to become *merely* terminological. In the end, it doesn't matter what the mechanisms subserving cognition get called; it is recognition of how it is done that matters.

Embedded cognition views will serve multilevel cognitive science, of the kind Clark advocates, just as well as will the extended mind thesis. It will serve just as well as a basis for neuroethics. What matters to human beings as thinkers doesn't depend on how these processes are described; what matters is their effects. If neuroethicists and philosophers wish to call only some part of human cognitive machinery our minds, and call the rest its scaffolding, so be it. It remains the case that our cognition is already, and always, deeply dependent on external scaffolding, and that our new technologies do not mark a radical break with our cognitive past. It remains the case that there is no isomorphism between causal routes to mental effects and their moral or intellectual significance. All that is lost, for neuroethics, is the rhetorical power which comes from the identification of extended mechanisms with the mind. Nevertheless, the set of facts to which I appealed in arguing for an ethical parity thesis should not be in dispute.

REFERENCES

Adams, F. and Aizawa, K. (2008). *The Bounds of Cognition*. Malden, MA: Blackwell.

Clark, A. (2003). *Natural-Born Cyborgs: Minds, Technologies, and the Future of Human Intelligence*. Oxford: Oxford University Press.

Clark, A. (2008). *Supersizing the Mind*. Oxford: Oxford University Press.

Clark, A. and Chalmers, D. (1998). The extended mind. *Analysis*, **58**, 7–19.

Dehaene, S., Spelke, E., Pinel, P., Stanescu, R., and Tsivkin, S. (1999). Sources of mathematical thinking: behavioral and brain-imaging evidence. *Science*, **284**, 970–4.

Farah, M.J., Shera, D.M., Savage, J.H., *et al.* (2006). Childhood poverty: Specific associations with neurocognitive development. *Brain Research*, **1110**, 166–74.

Fodor, J. (1975). *The Language of Thought*. Cambridge, MA: Harvard University Press.

Fukuyama, F. (2002). *Our Posthuman Future: Consequences of the Biotechnology Revolution*. New York: Farrar, Straus and Giroux.

Hurley, S. (1998). *Consciousness in Action*. Harvard, MA: Harvard University Press.

Napier, J.L., and Jost, J.T. (2008). Why are conservatives happier than liberals? *Psychological Science*, **19**, 565–72.

Noble, K.G., McCandliss, B.D., and Farah, M.J. (2007). Socioeconomic gradients predict individual differences in neurocognitive abilities. *Developmental Science*, **10**, 464–80.

Rupert, R.D. (2004). Challenges to the hypothesis of extended cognition. *Journal of Philosophy*, **101**, 389–428.

Sterelny, K. (2004). Externalism, epistemic artefacts and the extended mind. In R. Schantz (ed.) *The Externalist Challenge. New Studies on Cognition and Intentionality*, pp. 239–54. Berlin: de Gruyter.

CHAPTER 19

DOES COGNITIVE ENHANCEMENT FIT WITH THE PHYSIOLOGY OF OUR COGNITION?

HERVÉ CHNEIWEISS

INTRODUCTION

IT is a common observation that people harbor ambivalent feelings about science and technology, feeling both highly suspicious and outrageously confident in these two fields. Strangely, these highly emotional but often, at times, rational views ranging between technophobia and technophilia turn to mostly confidence when it comes to medical progress as well as body and mind enhancement. In the field of medicine, this can easily be understood as a basic human brain activity that develops behavior allowing prevention and/or a fight against suffering. Indeed, shamans and ancestors of physicians are as old as humanity. It is more difficult to understand concerning enhancement since potential benefits must be more carefully analyzed and actual risks more precisely considered, leading to a conservative attitude related to a "preservation instinct." This should be particularly true when it comes to our brain. Indeed, neurosciences not only open new avenues to alleviate neurological and psychiatric disorders—and some day to repair our nervous system—but also present targeted ways to control and enhance vegetative (being awake, sleep, appetite, sexuality) as well as mood and cognitive behaviors (memory to ideation), already triggering a strong adhesion and a huge market (Farah *et al.* 2004).

The momentum is such that one may already consider that this is not a matter of discussion since "you can't stop progress." On the one hand we may consider this as a new life style, a general trend to obtain improved memory and comprehension capacities through so-called "smart pills," rewards from technical progress. Physicians or regulatory governmental agencies should only be required to check for safety and efficiency of "treatments" which should be more and more considered as a food complement. Considered as a basic need, people should only be concerned about equal access to enhancement drugs and devices. If we take this view, cognitive enhancement is just considered as any technical element in the market field, consumer needs and satisfaction being the only goals to fulfill. On the other hand, currently available drugs will not only change some quantitative aspects of neural activities, whose improvement implies no problem, but also the global internal economy of cognition. Are available "smart-pills" controlling children's behaviors or they are increasing immediate, emotional, pre-learned skill-based and short-term rewarded strategies? The answers may be detrimental to long-term goals and social interactions, and consequently challenge our philosophy of human rights. Cognitive enhancers do not only change the amplitude of a given brain capacity, i.e. memory, but also the balance between emotional and rational networks, and will thus change our relationship to others, essential to the building of our thought and social life. Furthermore we are at risk at becoming addicted to our own brain enhancement, thus succumbing to renouncing our free-will, provided it exists. Indeed, because most of our brain activity is unconscious, some neuroscientists argue that there is no free will and that cognitive enhancement is a natural need of our brain. I shall argue, on the contrary, that recent advances in neurosciences do not deny free will and that the real risk resides in a hypertrophy of the self, losing essential feedback from the eyes of the others. These fundamental changes should encourage us to understand the driving forces of our "neurotechnological gourmandize" and wonder if cognitive enhancement is not a mystification that covers up social pressure for enhanced productivity and behavior control.

THE OUT-DATED CYBERNETIC MODEL

For some time now, our nervous system has been formalized with the cybernetic scheme that considers it essentially as a feedback adaptive system, sculpted by trials and errors, experiences, and repetitions. Indeed, scientists learned from developmental neurobiology that starting from a highly redundant and poorly interconnected cellular stock, our nervous activity at critical periods selects and stabilizes less than 50% of neurons. These survivors become highly branched and interconnected, a neuron from the cerebral cortex forming, for instance, an average of 50,000 synapses (zone of communication) with neighboring or distant cells. This architecture remains highly plastic, at least at the level of synapses, allowing for the remodeling of circuits and the acquisition of new behaviors and memories. Learning may influence functional brain morphology (Peretz et al. 2009). The initial theory of phrenology of Franz Joseph Gall comparing the brain to a muscle was rejected long ago. It considered skull deformations observable, such as bumps, as the results from underlying highly developed brain activities such as maternal instinct or criminality. The "bump of mathematics" remains a popular metaphor. But the development of brain imaging, particularly functional magnetic resonance imaging (fMRI), renewed phrenology since it is now clear that training, such as with the example of learning music and becoming a violin maestro, results in an enlargement of brain areas dedicated to the learned tasks, i.e. the motor area in the cerebral cortex dedicated to the fingers of the left hand (Zarate and Zatorre 2008).

Neural systems also possess intrinsic, self-generated activities. On the one hand we have fundamental and determined activities of a living brain such as the basic 40Hz rhythm of thalamus and constraints and thresholds to generate an action potential. On the other hand, stochastic processes introduce a probabilistic view of how the central nervous system (CNS) works, perceives, and acts. Take N-methyl-D-aspartic acid (NMDA) receptor (NMDAR) of glutamate, the main excitatory neurotransmitter of the adult brain. NMDAR is a complex of five transmembrane proteins forming a channel through the plasma membrane that may, or may not, let calcium ions enter the cell and trigger multiple intracellular events (Tai *et al.* 2008). A naïve view of the synapse should be that the action potential arrives at the presynaptic cleft, triggers the release of glutamate that binds to NMDAR on the postsynaptic membrane, and results in the opening of the channel, calcium entrance, and signaling to the postsynaptic element. But in our brain, the presence of glutamate is not enough to predict the opening probability of NMDAR. Spontaneously, NMDAR opens and closes randomly. Glutamate binding should increase the probability of the open state but in basal conditions, another ion, magnesium, occupies the pore of the channel and blocks it, and glutamate does not change the probability of the open state. Glial cells, however, particularly astrocytes that wrap the synapse and are able to release D-serine, surround the neuron. In the presence of this gliotransmitter, the magnesium block is removed and glutamate then significantly increases the probability of opening and its duration. In addition, NMDAR interacts with several other proteins that modulate its activity. An example is its interaction with the calcium-dependent enzyme CAMKII, highly enriched in the postsynaptic element, which results in the addition of a phosphate group on NMDAR, thus changing its properties. Recent mathematical models that try to integrate what neuroscientists know from NMDAR consider that it may exist under 21 different conformations, more or less possible to stabilize in an open state. This means that a similar pulse of glutamate will have a very different outcome from one NMDAR to another. This will be determined by the history of the synapse and of the circuit involved. But the stochastic opening of the channel at the precise time when the pulse arrives will introduce probability in the system. In other words, a given drug may enhance glutamate release without increasing synaptic transmission.

These advances change our view of how our brain works. In the cybernetic model, the brain was a black box activated by external stimuli such as perception, or internal needs signaled by hormones. A given stimuli was associated to a coordinated reaction, more or less like a reflex. Classical illustrations are Pavlov's experiences. Today's model considers a self-generated activity modulated by life events. Most of our brain activities are anticipations and not reactions. This was recently illustrated by the analysis and formalism of changes of mind in decision making (Resulaj *et al.* 2009). The currently admitted "drift-diffusion" model considers that a decision is made when the accumulated noisy evidence (decision variable) reaches a criterion level, the decision bound. This decision is followed by reinforcement as the subject looks over the results of an action. But this does not explain the changes of decision that one may make even in the absence of a novel clue. Indeed it appears that a decision is made 400ms or so before the physical initiation of it (latency time). During this time, the brain continues to work, to evaluate… and even can change its mind.

Latency time is close to the one originally found in Libet's famous experiment on voluntary action (Libet 1985). Using electrodes on the wrist and scalp to measure, respectively, the start of the action and the start of the readiness potential in motor cortex, Libet asked people to say when they decided to move looking at a revolving spot on a clock. The brain activity began about 500ms before the person was aware of deciding to act. Conscious decision came far too late to be the cause of the action. This experience and many confirmatory ones led some neuroscientists and moral philosophers to consider that free will is a fiction, or a brain self-generated illusion, because we should not be aware of the unconscious reasons that drive our choices (Dennet 2003; Wegner 2004; Soon *et. al.* 2008; Heisenberg 2009; Suhler and Churchland 2009). Conscious free will is a post hoc rationalization since our brain is making essentially unconscious decisions, and even the few decisions that arise in our conscious field appear a few milliseconds to seconds after the real moment of our brain's choice. Thus, it seems that conscience is a distinct brain function from decision, and that a free decision does not depend on the fact that we are conscious of it. As stated by Martin Heisenberg "Conscious awareness may help improve our behavior, but it does not necessarily do so and is not essential" (Heisenberg 2009).

Unexpectedly, this anticipatory feed-forward principle links our intentions to the conscious perception of our actions. This was recently illustrated for a simple hand movement. Taking advantage of the electrical stimulations performed in the course of brain tumor neurosurgery to prevent lesions of major active cortical areas such as the motor cortex, it was reported that if direct stimulation of the motor cortex actually triggers a movement of the contralateral hand, the subject is not always conscious of this movement (Desmurget *et al.* 2009, Desmurget and Sirigu 2009). On the contrary, the same stimulation of the parietal cortex area involved in the intention to move the hand triggers the feeling that the hand moves, even if it did not. Only prestimulation of the parietal/intentional area allows the conscious perception of the movement of the hand. We may formulate the hypothesis that future work will generalize this principle linking conscience to the anticipation of the results of actions. One is aware of what s/he does if and only if it was her/his intention to do so. On the contrary one should neglect or at least be unconscious of what s/he did with no intention to do so. In other words, the neurophysiological basis of our conscious perception may yield much more attention to internal rewards from expected results than from unexpected ones. We need an external witness to warn us from neglecting or rapidly forgetting unintended effects.

Placing intention at the genesis of conscious activities is of paramount importance since a basic function of our brain is to be an intention-of-the-other detector (Behrens *et al.* 2009). Our intentions to act make us aware of acting, and we also spend most of our time observing and guessing others' intentions. This is not only true for other humans or even our preferred pets, but also for any scene we observe. Humans spontaneously imbue the world with social meaning. The amygdala, a key node in the network of interpreting social meaning, is a collection of nuclei in the temporal lobe (Kennedy *et al.* 2009). Its role in processing emotionally and socially relevant information was demonstrated a few years ago (Heberlein and Adolphs 2004). A film of animated shapes, two triangles, a big and a small one, and one small circle, moving on the screen, sometimes colliding, sometimes disappearing on the boarders of the screen, is normally seen as full of social content. Indeed a bad big triangle tries to eat the gentle small circle and the courageous small triangle tries to protect the small circle. In one case study of a patient with bilateral amygdala damage, this film was described in entirely asocial, geometric terms, despite otherwise normal visual perception (Heberlein and Adolphs 2004). As amygdala is well known to be a major crossroad of emotion processing in our brain, this finding suggests that the human capacity for anthropomorphizing draws on some of the same neural systems as do emotional responses. It also suggests that a basic and unconscious function of our brain is to fill-up the physical world that surrounds us with human-like anticipated intentions, this being finely tuned by an emotionally driven flux.

Taken altogether, these data depict a brain that works mainly on self-generated, partly stochastic, anticipatory and unconscious activities. Intention makes us consciously aware of the results of our actions. Crossroads such as amygdala are essential to process emotions and to detect intentions of others. How can cognitive enhancers be selective with such highly integrated and overlapping activities?

From support to a need:
TECHNOLOGICAL ADDICTION

Most technologies we are using daily simultaneously satisfy our feed-forward and feedback working brain. The remote control of our television allows us to reach the channel we want, satisfying Hume's learning association proposal. How do we know and trust that pitching a violin cord will produce a sound? Because we learned that reproducibly pitching the cord was associated with hearing a sound and this built up our memory and rational networks. On the same basis, we can spontaneously guess that the sun will rise tomorrow morning as it does every day. Night after night getting the channel we want reinforces that technology can be trusted, as long as the batteries work. However, this might be not true for a new technology. Our experiences demonstrate that technology improves rapidly, and that the pace is increasingly quicker. Just take cell phones as an example. Not only do they allow us to work or reach friends any time, they now guide us with GPS (global positioning system), deliver weather reports and news, and can take pictures or small movies. For an increasing number of people, cell phones have become almost another limb of their body, and any failure is felt with a moral distress similar to a real wound. It is possible to hypothesize that we can become addicted to personal technologies because our brain anthropomorphizes these objects using the same networks as it does for emotion. And so the question arises: Are we still able to decide about how we use it? This will be one of the main questions challenging any cognitive enhancing technology.

Indeed we have to evaluate the multiple aspects of this growing addiction that include personal/individual choices as well as social constraints. To continue with our cell phone example, it is easy and rather cheap to call a friend but much more difficult to move from one service provider to another. Problems of reversibility will become major when implants will do everything from enhancing, or potentially erasing memory to accelerating ideation? Is it going to interfere or even prevent our self-generated capacity to obey moral law, to stay with the classical definition of freedom or at least autonomy (Kant)[1]?

---

[1] Autonomy as "the property of the will by which it is a law to itself (independently of any property of the objects of volition)" (**Groundwork for the Metaphysics of Morals**, 4:440). From Denis, Lara, "Kant and Hume on Morality", *The Stanford Encyclopedia of Philosophy (Summer 2009 Edition)*, Edward N. Zalta (ed.), URL = <http://plato.stanford.edu/archives/sum2009/entries/kant-hume-morality/>.

Why should we resist responsible use of cognitive enhancement?

At the end of 2008, several scientists, many of them also contributing to the present book, called for a responsible use of cognitive-enhancing drugs for healthy people (Greely *et al.* 2008). It was most likely the right time to take such a position—regardless of whether one views it correct or erroneous—considering the rapidly growing demand. But we need to examine enhancement from different views. On the one hand, from an empiric and practical basis, one may consider that enhancement is a cultural common and that the brain needs to be optimized as any mechanical machine could be. On the other hand, one may wonder what kind of cognitive enhancement society will request, and even ask ourselves if individuals really need it.

One good reason to oppose the use of cognitive enhancers is their risk of toxicity and/or their lack of efficacy. This could lead us to consider them as medical treatments with the same evaluation procedures and regulatory body approval requirements as for any medical care. However, approval as a treatment is not a guarantee for the absence of abuse, as illustrated by the over-prescription of antidepressant and anxiolytic drugs. Furthermore, approval as a medical treatment may present several perverse effects. One is to consider the approval as a certificate that validates the efficacy of the drug as a cognitive enhancer. Another one is that a medical treatment is designed for a disease. This may even create a vicious circle where new diseases are invented for the sole purpose of using new drugs. The effect of the drug is then considered as proof that the diagnosis was correct and that the disease is real. We can already observe a trend towards transforming an increasing range of conditions that were previously regarded as part of the normal human spectrum into pathologies treated by medicine.

A second reason to oppose the use of enhancers should be the fact that they are already overestimated as so-called "smart pills" because they are supposed to "boost one's intellectual creativity." A century ago, these were terms used for the devastating alcohol "absinthe," a basic "booster" for the genius of French poets such as Baudelaire, Verlaine, or Rimbaud, or painters such as Van Gogh, which in fact actually drove them insane. Since one intention is to benefit from cognitive enhancement, people will anticipate a low individual risk soon to be solved by rapid technological progress. This will be supported by marketing strategies minimizing the real and/or potential risks and promoting the benefits.

Enhancement unto itself is not a problem. Getting better is a basic root of human culture and an essential way to implement our weak nature. Enhancing our immune system through vaccination, for example, allowed for a major decrease in child mortality. So, enhancing our brain capabilities is not something to blame because it would modify some untouchable natural property of human beings. Even the Levitic book of the Bible says, "I gave you life and death, you'll choose life," on which the Talmud comments as "human destiny is to finish the world." Considering progress in our understanding of how the brain works and availability of drugs or other processes to increase some of its abilities, why not use them? Indeed, since humans have existed, education has always tried to enhance the cognitive abilities of students as well as scholars. Consequently, the question of enhancement using drugs or implants is frequently focused on fairness. The transhumanist philosopher Nick Bostrom describes it this way: "If school is to be regarded as a competition for grades, then enhancers would arguably be cheating if not everyone had access to enhancements or if they were against the official rules. If school is viewed as having primarily a social function, then enhancement might be irrelevant. But if school is seen as being significantly about the acquisition of information and learning, then cognitive enhancements may have a legitimate and useful role to play."[2]

An initial problem with such an argument is that education deals with the fruit of natural selection that took a rather long period to produce the human brain, this wonderful set of 200 billions interacting cells that we are just beginning to understand. Drugs and implants must be evaluated for more than their potential toxicity and their real efficacy. They may introduce drastic quantitative but also qualitative changes in the way our brain works. One apparent advantage, for example, to stay awake longer, may be at a cost to other cognitive impairment, sooner or later. Such a cost/benefit balance should be carefully evaluated to show evidence not only of some immediate benefits but also of short-term as well as long-term side effects. A major need should be a detailed analysis of the impact of "smart pills" on the balance between emotionally-driven and rationally-grounded circuits, and on the importance given to immediate rewards toward long-term goals.

A second problem is the confusion between some basic neurophysiological functions, being awake for example, which is easy to evaluate, and cognition, a matter much more of quality than quantity.

A third problem requires us to consider cognitive enhancement within the social context wherein it takes place. Taking "awake" drugs does not have the same meaning if you are a soldier on the battlefield, a skipper in a race, or a trader fighting for bonuses.

WHAT FUNCTION OF OUR BRAIN DO COGNITIVE ENHANCERS REALLY ENHANCE?

More is far from better when we consider cognition. A classical example is Cherechevski, the mnemonist patient of the Russian neurologist Alexander Luria, a man gifted with an impressive capacity for memory but a depressed and inhibited capacity for focusing attention. This demonstrates that memory is much more than storing capacities. Cognition is not a simple aggregation of basic functions, enough to increase one of them to improve the complete process. The success obtained by implants as substitutes for sense organs that may lead to a vision better than 10/10 or an improved audition are not a good metaphor for cognition. In examining cognitive enhancers and society, one is struck by their overly simplistic view of a precise increase in the magnitude of a given activity.

Take the example of modafinil (Provigil® in the US), an "awake" promoting agent whose therapeutic effect was first discovered in France in the early 1990s. It is used as a treatment for excessive somnolence observed in the rare genetic disease known as narcolepsy/cataplexy.

---

[2] Sandberg and Bostrom: Converging cognitive enhancements *http://www.nickbostrom.com/papers/converging.pdf*

Modafinil has consistently shown efficacy in measures of alertness in narcolepsy, as well as in shift-work sleep disorder (Czeisler *et al.* 2005). Studies in rodents indicate that modafinil can improve working memory as well as the processing of contextual cues, and that these effects may be augmented with sustained dosing regimens. In healthy humans, with or without sleep deprivation, working memory, recognition memory, and sustained attention, are enhanced with modafinil. However, results also show that the magnitude of modafinil effects in healthy adults depends on underlying cognitive abilities. The mechanism of modafinil's action is controversial. Studies employing pharmacological tools or genetic ablation of α-1B-adrenoreceptors in mice suggest that modafinil increases wakefulness by activating central noradrenergic transmission. Consensus studies recently reported that modafinil changes the coupling between the brain stem locus coeruleus nucleus and the prefrontal cortex (Minzenberg *et al.* 2008). However, pharmacological elimination of the noradrenalin transporter-bearing forebrain projections in mice does not influence the efficacy of modafinil action (Wisor and Eriksson 2005). By contrast, dopamine-dependent signaling is important for the wake-promoting action of modafinil. Indeed modafinil has a direct agonist action on the D_2 dopaminergic receptor (Korotkova *et al.* 2007). In addition, modafinil can increase serotonin release, decrease GABA release, and enhance glutamate release in various brain regions. Therefore, even if modafinil possesses only minimal potential for abuse, it will affect cognition on a much more global scale than by just increasing the level of arousal or the efficiency of working memory.

Mimicking some aspect of dopamine D_2 transmission, modafinil will affect some learning processes. Reward-based decisions are guided by reward expectations, and reward expectations are updated based on prediction errors. The processing of related errors involves dopaminergic neuromodulation in a central region of the brain, the striatum. Consequently, modafinil's effect on the striatum will affect the balance between "Go" learning to make good choices and "NoGo" learning to avoid those that are less adaptive. In the prefrontal cortex, dopamine contributes to learning on a short-term scale by actively maintaining recent reinforcement experiences in a working memory-like state. Dopamine also tunes some essential interactions between the prefrontal cortex and the striatum by processing the importance that a particular prediction error has on the expectation for updating for the next decision (Moustafa *et al.* 2008). Thus, modafinil will also affect the decision-making process in the long term. One may even hypothesize that modafinil or equivalent enhancers played a part in the 2008 financial crisis. The arguments are as followed: (1) As each individual brain, the financial industry is essentially based on anticipation. (2) The mainstream that follows agents of the financial market illustrate our brains as intention detectors since they buy or sell when they feel that the others are going to buy or sell much more than considering the real value of what they buy or sell. (3) It is notorious that there is a large portion of the population in favor of arousal enhancing drugs, including modafinil. What will happen when new molecules will become available such as oxytocin, recently demonstrated to increase trust in social relationships (Baumgartner *et al.* 2008)? Will some professionals feel that they have an obligation to use enhancers as proof of their dedication to their work? Since social relationships are based on the fact that individuals are responsible for their actions, are they still responsible for what they do if they consider cognitive enhancers as a duty?

Complicating the issues is the intrinsic heterogeneity of people. For example, studies coupling human genetic analyses and learning tasks recently showed that several independent dopaminergic mechanisms contribute to reward and avoidance learning in humans

(Frank *et al.* 2007; Krugel *et al.* 2009). Individual genetic variations may influence neurobiological mechanisms underlying the ability to rapidly and flexibly adapt decisions to changing reward contingencies. Thus, a molecule such as modafinil will have a very different effect from one individual to another, introducing to the concept of "personalized enhancement" as a parallel to personalized medicine, but also making more complex the real evaluation of what benefit a given individual can really expect from cognitive enhancers.

Another example of the difficulty to determine what "enhancement" with cognitive-targeted drugs really means may be illustrated by methylphenidate, effective in getting children to be quieter. Methylphenidate is the drug of reference for attention deficit with hyperactivity disorder (ADHD) a psychiatric syndrome that remains highly controversial, some physicians considering that it was created (or at least its diagnosis definition highly extended) to support extensive prescription of this drug. Indeed, the diagnosis does not only open the door to treatment but also to many parallel social benefits for the family. On the contrary, the long-term benefits that diagnosed children get from the treatment, for instance better scholar results, are far from being demonstrated (Gonon 2009). Thus, the treatment is effective on the treated child's behavior, effective in bringing social support for parents, effective for a quiet classroom, but is not effective as a cognitive enhancer for the treated individual. Here is another real dilemma: individual rights versus social pressure.

Autonomy or social pressure

Who makes the decision of treatment and does it remain under the treated individual's control? The Nuffield Council for Bioethics in 2006 considered that the requirement for cognitive enhancement for all might be positive in a certain way: "improving the general standards or abilities across the population might not be a problem if this was driven by the public interest."[3] Notice also that in medical ethics the so-called "public interest" is never considered to be more important than the choice of the person. It might be more and more difficult to differentiate this decision, even taken freely, from the need to fulfill standards of efficacy requested by the society, for instance to get and stay in a given school, team or company. This makes cognitive enhancement improperly compared to doping in sport because the latter is a way to obtain an advantage over competitors. At the start of enhancer availability, and eventually for quite sometime, cognitive enhancement, like doping, may be a powerful means of discrimination between a cast of "enhanced" and a mass of "regulars." However, after a while enhancement will become an obligation just to stay at the same level as competitors.

Individual addiction and social pressure will make cognitive enhancement irreversible or at a great risk of social exclusion or even worse. A recent and dramatic illustration is a case of the face transplant. People requesting such surgery do not suffer from a life-threatening disease but rather from a type of social death associated with a scarred face, and are ready to risk their lives to be relieved of this disability. Since the grafted tissue comes from a stranger, this requires permanent treatment to block the immune system and prevent transplant

---

[3] *http://www.nuffieldbioethics.org*

rejection. Treatment is expensive, sometimes painful and not fully effective. The first Chinese face transplant patient stopped his immunosuppressive therapy after a year of treatment, and rapidly died from the rejection of the graft. This might become the archetype of risking life to remain socialized.

Our post-industrial society requires more and more efficiency from each of us. Several ways could be used to reach such a goal. One could be to overcome individual limitations through improved collaborative organization and enhancement of non-competitive individual interactions. However, more and more is required from each individual, placing competition above any other success motivating factors. Furthermore, competition is mostly evaluated on short-term quantitative criteria. It seems that the fact of establishing numbers, creating ranks and classifying people within percentiles, has a kind of magic effect: it makes any evaluation credible. Hence, the development of tests that can be translated into numbers. Such tests, when applied to cognition, preferentially explore certain aspects of brain functions such as speed of reaction, memory, and pre-registered logical skills. These biases were already denounced for a century in the abusive use of IQ tests. Actually, available cognitive enhancers increase these brain processes, maybe because their efficiency was validated by these tests. In addition, this targets the concept of cognitive enhancement on individual criteria whereas no individual human brain is able to work alone and by itself only: a human brain needs to interact with another human brain from its first day to its last.

COGNITIVE ENHANCEMENT IN THE EYES OF OTHERS

This road has been paved by several recent philosophers, i.e. in France Emmanuel Levinas (*Humanisme de l'autre homme, 1972*), Jean-Paul Sartre (*L'existentialisme est un humanisme, 1946*), Paul Ricoeur (Changeux and Ricoeur 1998), Michel Foucault (*Le courage de la vérité 2009*). In the introduction of his last series of lectures, delivered at the College de France in Paris in the first months of 1984,[4] Michel Foucault considers that all his work was dedicated to studies of how one is recognized as telling the truth. For years Foucault described the social practices and forms of "telling the truth" on figures of the modern society, the mad or the delinquent for instance. During this period, he developed the concept of "Biopower" defined by a generalized constraint on our bodies but not yet on our minds. He was always studying the relationship between the subject and the truth through the discourse that tells the truth on the subject. But during the last 10 years, he turned to the discourse of truth that the subject is able to deliver on himself. He developed a long analysis of "*parrêsia*," the antique practice central to Greeks and Romans to search within one's thoughts, and practice the truth on oneself. Each time he studied a case, from Socrates to present, there was always a need for another person to allow this possibility to "tell the truth on oneself." From the last

---

[4] Michel Foucault, *Le Courage de la vérité* (1984) ; *Le gouvernement de soi et le gouvernement des autres - tome 2* Seuil 2009

words of Socrates for Criton, to Catholic confessors, and more recently the extent of medicine, psychiatry, and psychoanalysis, there is always the need of the other.

Cognitive enhancement may appear as an attempt to escape from this need for alterity, the boosted brain suddenly able to understand the truth on its own without any further external oversight. This is most likely the greatest disillusion since, as already mentioned, a basic brain activity is detecting the other's intention, particularly being in the eyes of the other. Interestingly, recognition of the other and the exploration of a face starts with the eyes. By contrast, it seems that the lack of focalization on the other's eyes is a frequent disorder found in autism. This need for the other's eyes is reminiscent of Emmanuel Levinas's views. Levinas derives the primacy of his ethics from the experience of the face-to-face encounter with the other. The last words of Foucault during his last lecture concluded with the absolute need of an external view. This is the main risk of an over-individualized society where cognitive enhancement is seen as a way to escape from the eyes of the other, a phenomenon that would result, if we follow Levinas and Foucault, in a renunciation to tell the truth.

REAPPRAISING ENHANCEMENT GOALS

During the last two centuries, the concept of progress built-up by *Enlightenment thinkers*, and initially defined by Condorcet as the road to human happiness (1973 Esquisse d'un tableau historique des Progrès de l'esprit humain), has became an autonomous social value with no other goals than its own technological development. We must reintroduce human goals and finality to evaluate enhancement.

There is clearly a convergence between the natural appetite of humans for enhancement and society's needs. This convergence has led to consider our human body, including our brain, as an object to technically improve in all its functions, including cognition among them. We can wonder what kind of human being will emerge from these technical manipulations. We must carefully evaluate the potential for modern slavery that the techniques of enhancement might create through addiction and irreversibility. We must also carefully acknowledge that biology in general, and the brain in particular, is not just a huge set of simple mechanisms that some bioengineers can easily fine tune to achieve maximum efficiency. In the realm of cognition, enhancement may mean a fundamental change in the way our brain processes information. We have mentioned earlier that modafinil may interfere with mechanisms underlying the ability to rapidly adapt one's decisions when reward contingencies change. Such modification in the way our brain operates may represent a real breakthrough and surge towards a post-human creature. What this new form of humanity might resemble is simply impossible to imagine since we still do not know what novel cognitive process these "enhanced brains" will use, nor how they will need (or not) interaction with the "other." Consequently, it will be essential to evaluate how these individual performance enhancers influence social interaction capabilities. The risk is creating isolated super-brains lost within a self-centered, self-organized, virtual world wherein the absence of the eyes of the other blurs the fundamental meaning of "telling the truth" on oneself.

ACKNOWLEDGMENTS

I am particularly grateful to Lucile Chneiweiss, Judy Illes, and Jennifer Merchant for careful reading and fruitful suggestions on this manuscript.

REFERENCES

Baumgartner, T., Heinrichs, M., Vonlanthen, A., Fischbacher, U., and Fehr, E. (2008). Oxytocin shapes the neural circuitry of trust and trust adaptation in humans. *Neuron*, **58**, 639–50.

Behrens, T.E., Hunt, L.T., and Rushworth, M.F. (2009). The computation of social behavior. *Science*, **324**, 1160–4.

Changeux, J.P. and Ricoeur, P. (1998). *Ce qui nous fait penser. La nature et la règle*. Paris: Editions Odile Jacob.

Czeisler, C.A., Walsh, J.K., Roth, T., *et al.* (2005). Modafinil for excessive sleepiness associated with shift-work sleep disorder. *New England Journal of Medicine*, **353**, 476–86.

Dennett, D.C. (2003). The self as a responding-and responsible-artifact. *Annals of the New York Academy of Sciences*, **1001**, 39–50.

Desmurget, M. and Sirigu, A. (2009). A parietal-premotor network for movement intention and motor awareness. *Trends in Cognitive Sciences*, **13**, 411–19.

Desmurget, M., Reilly, K.T., Richard, N., Szathmari, A., Mottolese, C., and Sirigu, A. (2009). Movement intention after parietal cortex stimulation in humans. *Science*, **324**, 811–13.

Farah, M.J., Illes, J., Cook-Deegan, R., *et al.* (2004). Neurocognitive enhancement: what can we do and what should we do? *Nature Reviews Neuroscience*, **5**, 421–5.

Foucault, M. (2009). *Le Courage de la vérité. Le gouvernement de soi et des autres II. Cours au Collège de France, 1984*. Paris: Éditions du Seuil, coll. "Hautes Etudes."

Frank, M.J., Moustafa, A.A., Haughey, H.M., Curran, T., and Hutchison, K.E. (2007). Genetic triple dissociation reveals multiple roles for dopamine in reinforcement learning. *Proceedings of the National Academy of Sciences of the United States of America*, **104**, 16311–16.

Gonon, F. (2009). The dopaminergic hypothesis of attention-deficit/hyperactivity disorder needs re-examining. *Trends in Neuroscience*, **32**, 2–8.

Greely, H., Sahakian, B., Harris, J., Kessler, R.C., Gazzaniga, M., Campbell, P., and Farah, M.J. (2008). Towards responsible use of cognitive-enhancing drugs by the healthy. *Nature*, **456**, 702–5.

Heberlein, A.S. and Adolphs, R. (2004). Impaired spontaneous anthropomorphizing despite intact perception and social knowledge. *Proceedings of the National Academy of Sciences of the United States of America*, **101**, 7487–91.

Heisenberg, M. (2009). Is free will an illusion? *Nature*, **459**, 164–5.

Kennedy, D.P., Glascher, J., Tyszka, J.M., and Adolphs, R. (2009). Personal space regulation by the human amygdala. *Nature Neuroscience*, **12**, 1226–7.

Korotkova, T.M., Klyuch, B.P., Ponomarenko, A.A., Lin, J.S., Haas, H.L., and Sergeeva, O.A. (2007). Modafinil inhibits rat midbrain dopaminergic neurons through D2-like receptors. *Neuropharmacology*, **52**, 626–33.

Krugel, L.K., Biele, G., Mohr, P.N., Li, S.C., and Heekeren, H.R. (2009). Genetic variation in dopaminergic neuromodulation influences the ability to rapidly and flexibly adapt decisions. *Proceedings of the National Academy of Sciences of the United States of America*, **106**, 17951–6.

Levinas, E. (1972). *Humanisme de l'autre homme*. Montpellier: Fata Morgana.

Libet, B. (1985). Subjective antedating of a sensory experience and mind–brain theories: reply to Honderich (1984). *Journal of Theoretical Biology*, **114**, 563–70.

Minzenberg, M.J., Watrous, A.J., Yoon, J.H., Ursu, S., and Carter, C.S. (2008). Modafinil shifts human locus coeruleus to low-tonic, high-phasic activity during functional MRI. *Science*, **322**, 1700–2.

Moustafa, A.A., Cohen, M.X., Sherman, S.J., and Frank, M.J. (2008). A role for dopamine in temporal decision making and reward maximization in parkinsonism. *Journal of Neuroscience*, **28**, 12294–304.

Peretz, I., Gosselin, N., Belin, P., Zatorre, R.J., Plailly, J., and Tillmann, B. (2009). Music lexical networks: the cortical organization of music recognition. *Annals of the New York Academy of Sciences*, **1169**, 2565.

Resulaj, A., Kiani, R., Wolpert, D.M., and Shadlen, M.N. (2009). Changes of mind in decision-making. *Nature*, **461**, 263–6.

Sartre, J.P. (1970). *L'existentialisme est un humanisme*. Paris: Nagel.

Soon, C.S., Brass, M., Heinze, H.J., and Haynes, J.D. (2008). Unconscious determinants of free decisions in the human brain. *Nature Neuroscience*, **11**, 543–5.

Suhler, C.L. and Churchland, P.S. (2009). Control: conscious and otherwise. *Trends in Cognitive Science*, **13**, 341–7.

Tai, C.Y., Kim, S.A., and Schuman, E.M. (2008). Cadherins and synaptic plasticity. *Current Opinion in Cell Biology*, **20**, 567–75.

Wegner, D.M. (2004). Precis of the illusion of conscious will. *Behavioral and Brain Science*, **27**, 649–59; discussion 659–92.

Wisor, J.P. and Eriksson, K.S. (2005). Dopaminergic-adrenergic interactions in the wake promoting mechanism of modafinil. *Neuroscience*, **132**, 1027–34.

Zarate, J.M. and Zatorre, R.J. (2008). Experience-dependent neural substrates involved in vocal pitch regulation during singing. *Neuroimage*, **40**, 1871–87.

CHAPTER 20

··

ATTENTION DEFICIT HYPERACTIVITY DISORDER: DEFINING A SPECTRUM DISORDER AND CONSIDERING NEUROETHICAL IMPLICATIONS

··

JAMES M. SWANSON, TIMOTHY WIGAL,
KIMBERLEY LAKES, AND NORA D. VOLKOW

INTRODUCTION

ATTENTION deficit hyperactivity disorder (ADHD) is thought to affect about 5% of children around the world, although many differences in diagnostic methods make its recognition and treatment highly variable across countries and regions (see Polanczyk *et al.* 2007). Prospective follow-up studies have shown that even though some children outgrow the disorder, a childhood diagnosis of ADHD is clearly a risk factor for a broad range of adverse outcomes, with extremes including drug abuse and juvenile delinquency (see Molina *et al.* 2008). For administrative reasons, more acceptable methods are needed for defining ADHD consistently, and for clinical reasons more precise definitions of ADHD are needed that predict adverse outcomes and can be used to focus treatments.

Traditionally, ADHD has not been conceptualized as a spectrum disorder, either by the diagnostic system developed and currently recommended by the American Psychiatric Association (APA 1994) or by the World Health Organization (WHO 1993). However, clinical heterogeneity of the manifestation of ADHD does fit into the spectrum approach used for other psychiatric disorders (see Maser and Patterson 2002; Cassano *et al.* 2004). Here we will consider the use of several spectrum concepts and some neuroethical issues that accompany each one.

What are the defining features of a spectrum disorder?

The criteria in the Diagnostic and Statistical Manual (DSM) and the International Classification of Disease (ICD) manual provide lists of criterion symptoms with a threshold set for the number of symptoms required for categorical diagnoses of disorders. The current version of DSM-IV (APA 1994) provides a few examples of spectrum disorders (e.g. related to variants of schizophrenia and depression), and dimensional adjuncts have been proposed for almost all disorders in revisions for DSM-V (see Helzer *et al.* 2008) that may be used to define more disorder-related spectra in the future. A prototype spectrum approach is presented by Maser and Patterson (2002) for depression. It provides for recognition of subthreshold cases when the presence of criterion symptoms is elevated but below the established cut-offs. They point out that in psychiatric diagnosis the fundamental difference between the categorical diagnosis and the dimensional approach is that a dimension of behavior "… associated with an illness, disease or disorder has no absolute, qualitative break between 'normal' and 'abnormal.'" They also point out that a continuum approach differs from both categorical and dimensional approaches by defining "…a statistical middle range as normal and departure away from 'normality'" (Maser and Patterson 2002, p. 868). Here we will consider how these different approaches can be used to define an ADHD spectrum based on the concepts of *categorical diagnosis* (see Maser and Patterson 2002), *dimension of symptom severity* (see Helzer *et al.* 2008), and *continuum of behavior* (see Swanson *et al.* 2009).

How are definitions of an ADHD spectrum related to neuroethics?

The Society for Neuroscience (2008) suggests that the topic of neuroethics differs from general biomedical ethics because it deals with "… brain-specific issues that touch no other area of science," including "new neuroscience technologies such as brain scanning" and "pharmaceuticals to manipulate cognition" (p. 62). This has clear relevance to the definitions of ADHD as a spectrum disorder. All three spectrum approaches are based on different underlying assumptions of neural bases of this disorder, and the neural basis for its most common treatment (with stimulant medication) is based on hypotheses about the effects of this class of drug on neurotransmitters and synaptic events as well as on neural networks of the brain. In our introduction, we will provide a brief review of some brain imaging and pharmacological treatment studies of ADHD to set the stage of consideration of brain-specific issues related to neuroethics.

What is the current consensus about cognitive and neural deficits in ADHD?

Hypotheses about specific brain processes that might underlie the symptoms of ADHD date back to era when the syndrome was labeled "minimal brain dysfunction" (Wender 1971).

In the 1970s (see Douglas 1972) and 1980s (see Sergeant and Scholten 1985), neuropsychological studies emphasized the cognitive components over the motor components. This was reflected in the modern diagnostic criteria in DSM-III (APA 1980) and the label used then, attention deficit disorder (ADD), which elevated the cognitive symptoms to be the essential features of the disorder over the motor symptoms that were used to define a subtype (ADD with Hyperactivity). In the 1990s, theories emerged that propose ADHD symptoms are manifested as a consequence of a core deficit in executive functions (Pennington and Ozonoff 1996; Barkley 1997). However, subsequently extensive neuropsychological research has shown heterogeneity of cognitive deficits within typical groups of children with ADHD (see Doyle et al. 2000). Additional scholarly reviews concluded that the preponderance of evidence did not support any "core deficit" theory but instead favors theories based on multiple cognitive deficits (e.g. Nigg 2005; Willcutt et al. 2005). In comparison to groups of children without ADHD or with other disorders, some ADHD individuals do not manifest any deficit on specific neuropsychological tests of executive function or even on a composite of a battery of tests, suggesting that executive function deficits are not necessary or unique components of ADHD.

Recent studies with neuropsychological batteries (e.g. Rhodes 2005; Rubia 2007) provide evidence of multicomponent rather than unitary deficits in children with ADHD. From the perspective of cognitive neuroscience, this heterogeneity of cognitive deficits is not unexpected, since prominent theories have proposed that the neural processes underlying the cognitive symptom domains of ADHD (impulsivity and inattention) are not unitary constructs. Tests have been developed to fractionate both impulsivity and inattention into component parts. For example, Winstanley and colleagues (2006) describe two general domains of impulsivity—impulsive choice and impulsive action—and Posner and Rothbart (2007) describe three general domains of attention—alerting, orienting, and executive control.

In the 1990s, brain imaging and molecular genetic studies of ADHD identified some abnormalities that supported modern neuroscience theories of the biological basis of the ADHD disorder as a dysfunction in neural networks of the brain and functions they serve, rather than specific brain regions or cognitive processes. The early studies provided evidence of deficits in a cortical–striatal–thalamic network modulated by the neurotransmitter dopamine (Castellanos 1997). In the National Institutes of Health (NIH) Consensus Conference on ADHD (NIH 1998), Swanson and Castellanos (1999) summarized the emerging evidence of presence of abnormal brain anatomy (reduced areas of key striatal, frontal, and callosal brain regions) and association with alleles of candidate genes, the dopamine transporter (DAT) and the dopamine receptor D4 (DRD4) genes. Over the ensuing decade, others have presented reviews to update these findings, which in general have been replicated and remained consistent with these early neural network theories of ADHD (see Castellanos and Tannock 2002; Bush 2010). There have been some advances to refine these theories of ADHD, which we have reviewed and discussed in detail elsewhere (Swanson et al. 2008a,b; submitted), so only a selected few will be discussed here.

Studies using functional magnetic resonance imaging (fMRI) revealed that in ADHD children (compared to controls) some brain regions involved in the performance of cognitive tasks were underactivated (e.g. frontal) lobes) and others overactivated (e.g. parietal), suggesting that ADHD children may compensate for cognitive deficits underlying the symptoms of inattention and impulsivity by using alternative neural processes to achieve some degree of attention and reflection (Durston et al. 2003; Schulz et al. 2004; Schweitzer et al. 2003).

Recent studies (see Volkow and Swanson 2008; Volkow *et al.* 2009) of adults with ADHD using positron emission tomography (PET) and radioligands targeting the synaptic mechanisms of dopamine transmission have uncovered abnormalities in brain networks associated with processes of motivation (with involvement of dopamine transmission in the nucleus acumens) as well as with processes of attention (with involvement of dopamine transmission in the caudate nucleus), suggesting a motivation deficit as well as an attention deficit may characterize individuals with ADHD.

Studies using reaction time (RT) tasks of cognitive control (e.g. the go/no-go task), response inhibition (e.g. the stop signal task), and conflict (e.g. the attention network task or ANT) have identified interindividual variance in task performance as one of the most prominent aspects of cognitive deficits related to ADHD (see Swanson *et al.* submitted for a review). The increased variance produced skewed distributions of RTs (see Leth-Steensen *et al.* 2000). These observations led to the speculation that long response times may be the result of lapses in attention that are cyclical with relative slow waves occurring every 20–40 seconds rather than the results of random events (see Castellanos 2005). Several studies have used Fourier analyses of RTs and have shown that the power in these low frequency bands is greater in ADHD individuals than in controls (e.g. see Di Martino *et al.* 2008). The slow oscillations in RTs may be related to brain networks (see Fox *et al.* 2006) that are considered to be task-positive (a dorsal network) and a task-negative (a ventral network). The dorsal network is activated during goal-directed task performance, and it includes the dorsal lateral and ventral prefrontal brain regions that are activated by a variety of cognitive tasks. The ventral network, described as a "default network" that includes the medial prefrontal, posterior cingulate, and lateral parietal regions, is deactivated when performing a task. At rest, the ventral default network is activated ("resting state") and the dorsal network is deactivated, and during task performance the dorsal network is activated and the ventral network is deactivated. Sonuga-Barke and Castellanos (2007) proposed the default-mode interference hypothesis of ADHD: the ventral network may be deactivated when a RT task is initiated, but gradual recovery may eventually intrude on the activity of the dorsal network, and when a threshold is crossed a lapse of attention occurs and results in a long RT.

Effects of stimulant medication

The literature on the use of stimulant medications—amphetamine (AMP) and methylphenidate (MPH)—for the treatment of hyperkinetic disorder (HKD) and ADHD is enormous. In the 1990s, the number of articles was in the thousands and there were already more than 300 reviews. Swanson *et al.* (1993) used a "review of reviews" to synthesis the literature and summarized what should be expected (temporary reduction of symptoms of ADHD and management of some associated features —social, academic, and deportment deficits) and what should not be expected (large effects on higher order processes, paradoxical responses, prediction of response, absence of side effects, or improvement in the long-term). The "review of reviews" approach was also used by Conners (2002), who added contemporary reviews from through the early 2000s and summarized the consistency across time and methods about the effects on behavior (effect size approximately 0.74) and academic performance (effect size approximately 0.46).

From 1937, when the first use of stimulants was reported (Bradley 1937) until 2000 when the first use of modern controlled-release (CR) formulations was reported (see Swanson *et al.* 2000), the state-of-the-art practice of stimulant pharmacotherapy was based on multiple daily doses of immediate-release (IR) MPH. Three-times-a-day (TID) administration of IR-MPH for 7 days per week was used in the medication algorithm of the Multimodal Treatment study of ADHD (MTA). After titration based on the full range of doses from 5–20mg TID (see Greenhill *et al.* 1996), about 90% of all of the cases (children with diagnoses of ADHD Combined Type) showed a clinically significant short-term response, as expected from the massive literature (see Swanson *et al.* 1993; Conners *et al.* 2002) on response to stimulant medication. The relative benefit of medication management (MedMgt) over the non-pharmacological treatment, behavior modification (Beh), was maintained for the duration (14 months) of the treatment-by-protocol phase of the randomized clinical trial (MTA Group 1999). However, the relative benefit dissipated during the naturalistic follow-up phase of the MTA, and by the 3-year assessment there was no documented relative benefit of the initial assigned treatment (MedMgt vs. Beh) or of the actual or current treatment with stimulant medication (Jensen *et al.* 2007; Swanson *et al.* 2007a,b).

Brain imaging studies have suggested one of the primary sites of action of stimulant medication: a typical oral clinical dose of MPH blocks about 50% of the available DAT (Volkow *et al.* 1995, 1998), and significant increases in extracellular DA occur at clinically relevant oral doses of MPH (Volkow *et al.* 1999b, 2009a) and AMP (villemagne *et al.* 1999). This biochemical effect has profound effects on brain function, as shown by Volkow *et al.* (2008a) using PET and FDG (fludeoxyglucose) to measure brain glucose metabolism in non-ADHD adults when performing a cognitive task: compared to placebo, MPH significantly reduced the task-related increase in glucose by 50%, suggesting increased focal activity that may enhance or impair performance on a task.

On some measures of response there may be cognitive enhancing effects of stimulants on non-ADHD (control of normal) individuals. Challenges to the hypothesis of a paradoxical response in children with ADHD have a long history. For example, Sahakian and Robbins (1977) developed the hypothesis that the clinical improvements in activity and attention were related to the normal action of the stimulants in producing stereotyped behavior. They also pointed out that stereotyped behavior increases with dose, and they suggested that as in animal studies this drug-response might merely reflect an increased rate of responding within a reduced number of response categories. In some cases this may be related to dose-related physical side effects that occur (e.g. tics, picking and biting, etc.) and cognitive side effects (overfocusing, anxiety, etc.), as well as loss of flexibility in cognitive tasks that is essential for good performance on some neuropsychological tasks that require reversals in cognitive strategies.

The hypothesis of a paradoxical response to stimulants was tested by Rapoport *et al.* (1978), who evaluated dose-related effects of d-amphetamine on ADHD and normal children and adults. They showed that the direction of response (e.g. decreased activity level) was the same in individuals with and without diagnoses of the clinical syndrome of hyperactivity that is now labeled ADHD. Robbins and Sahakian (1979) considered factors related to response to stimulants (dose, rate dependency, and stereotypy). They point out that effects of dose are likely to be manifested as a U-shaped curve, with low doses producing enhancement but high doses impairment. The Yerkes–Dodson law describes this relationship for tasks that are complex but not for simple tasks, which has been discussed in great detail recently by Diamond *et al.* (2007). Robbins and Sahakian (1979) also point out that rate dependency may occur, which is stated as an inverse mathematical relationship between the frequency of a behavior and the relative effects of stimulants. They reported rate-dependent analyses for many studies in the literature, and discussed several complications in the analyses of data (e.g. use of baseline vs. placebo on the abscissa, the regression to the mean effect, etc.), and showed that the manifestation of rate dependent effects in these datasets was not invariant across the methods used to estimate its presence.

The general notion of cognitive enhancement has been questioned repeatedly and regularly over the past 50 years (see the reviews presented in the scholarly books by Grinspoon and Hedblom 1975 and Rasmussen 2008). Stimulants appear to produce a sense of well-being in many individuals (see Rasmussen 2008 for a description of Gordon Alles' response to the first ever dose of the newly synthesized drug amphetamine in 1929). Similar responses have been observed in modern studies of the drug methylphenidate (e.g. Bray *et al.* 2004 described the perception of well-being and benefit even in the absence of cognitive enhancement). Stimulants also appear to produce benefits on some tasks and in some individuals (see Mehta *et al.* 2004, who found that the enhancement was greatest in those who performed poorly on the laboratory tasks used for evaluation). However, literature on the effects of stimulants on individuals without ADHD is very sparse, and this leaves considerable uncertainty about the general effects of the non-medical use of stimulants.

The debate about cognitive enhancement and non-medical use of stimulant medication was revived recently by Sahakian and Morein-Zamir (2007), who proposed that "…scientists, doctors, and policy-makers should provide easy access to information about the advantages and dangers of using cognitive-enhancing drugs and set out clear guidelines for their future use" (p. 1157). This challenge generated discussion of important neuroethical issues in the scientific literature (see Greely *et al.* 2008; Swanson and Volkow 2008; Volkow and Swanson 2008) and in the popular press (see Stix 2009) about the non-medical use of stimulant drugs and the regulatory restrictions and laws that apply. These same issues about U-shaped dose-response curves addressed by Sahakian and Robbins (1977) and Robbins and Sahakian (1979) are still critical to consider in the current debate about the non-medical use of stimulants. In individuals with ADHD, the medical use may produce a U-shaped curve that would be the basis for titration to find the optimum dose, while in individuals without ADHD the non-medical use may produce a monotonic dose–response function (dose-related impairment) or a small enhancement followed by dose-related impairment. Here we will discuss how the consideration of ADHD as a spectrum can contribute to this debate.

DEFINING A SPECTRUM FOR ADHD: THREE APPROACHES

Categorical diagnosis in DSM-IV and ICD-10

The same set of 18 symptoms (see Table 20.1a) is used to make categorical diagnoses of ADHD by the DSM-IV criteria or HKD by the ICD-10 criteria. In both diagnostic systems, the gold standard is the clinical interview by which a fundamental categorical judgment is made about each symptom—present or absent—dependent on whether its manifestation is severe enough to contribute to functional impairment. Another categorical decision is required by both diagnostic systems based on symptom counts and cut-offs set for the DSM-IV diagnosis of ADHD and for the ICD-10 diagnosis of HKD.

Despite the same symptoms, differences in decision rules make HKD a subset of ADHD. The decision rules have been described by Santosh *et al.* (2005), who provided details about how these decision rules address pervasiveness across settings and symptom domains, as well as impairment and comorbidity:

1) *Settings* For both DSM-IV and ICD-10 approaches, pervasiveness of symptom pres-ence is required across settings, which for children are typically parent and teacher reports of behavior at home and school. For DSM-IV, the "Or" decision rule is used to define symptom presence (see Lahey *et al.* 1994): some symptoms must be mani-fested in more than one setting, but any particular symptom is counted if manifested in only one setting (e.g. at home or school). In contrast, for ICD-10 the "And" deci-sion rule is applied (see Taylor *et al.* 1998): a symptom is counted only when mani-fested in more than one setting (e.g. at home and school).

2) *Symptom domain* In both DSM-IV and ICD-10 the same three domains (Inattention, Hyperactivity, and Impulsivity) are used to organize the 18 symptoms. The same nine symptoms are listed in the Inattention domain, but in DSM-IV the symptoms of impulsivity are merged with the Hyperactivity symptoms while in ICD-10 these two domains remain separated. Cut-offs are set for the two DSM-IV domains (at least six of the nine symptoms of Inattention and at least six of the nine symptoms of Hyperactivity/Impulsivity) and partial syndromes are defined (ADHD Primarily Inattentive or Primarily Hyperactive/Impulsive Type) as well as the complete syndrome (ADHD Combined Type). For ICD-10, the cut-offs are set for the three domains (six or more Inattention, three or more Hyperactivity, and one or more Impulsivity symptoms) and only a single syndrome (HKD) is specified.

3) *Impairment* DSM-IV requires some impairment in at least two settings, but ICD-10 has an additional requirement of overall impairment.

4) *Comorbidity* In DSM-IV the diagnosis of ADHD plus comorbid disorders is encour-aged, but in ICD-10 the aim is to make a single primary diagnosis of HKD. For example, in DSM-IV diagnoses of comorbid internalizing disorders (anxiety and depression) are allowed if their criteria are met, but in ICD-10 the diagnosis of HKD is not recommend in the presence of internalizing disorders.

The DSM-IV decision rules already define an ADHD spectrum with provisions for a wide variation in the presence of the 18 criterion symptoms. At first glance (see Figure 20.1a), it may appear that the minimum symptom-count cut-off threshold for ADHD Combined Type (six from each of the two domains for a total of 12) is greater than for HKD (a total of ten from the three domains). However, this relationship may be reversed by the decision rule requiring pervasiveness across the two settings (home and school). This logically results in 36 setting-specific symptoms (see Table 20.1b and Figure 20.1b). We propose this dimen-sion as an ADHD-equivalent of the dimension of symptom presence proposed by Maser and Patterson (2002) for defining subthreshold conditions in the spectrum of depression.

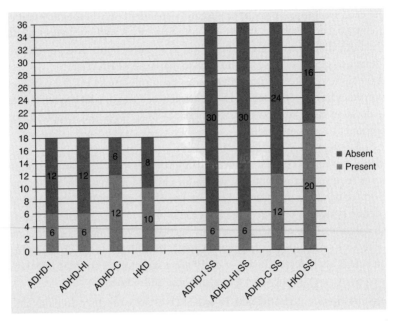

FIG. 20.1 Minimum thresholds for ADHD and HKD (a) Categorical diagnoses based on symptoms and (b) the ADHD spectrum based on setting-specific (SS) symptoms.

According to the application of the decision rules outlined earlier, the setting-specific symptoms required for a diagnosis of ADHD-Combined Type still would be six from each domain, but for the minimum this could be different items for the home and school setting for a total of 12, while for a diagnosis of HKD it still would be ten, but for the minimum this would be the same ten symptoms in both the home and school settings for a total of 20 (see Figure 20.1b).

What are the implications of the categorical (symptom count) approach in clinical application? Santosh *et al.* (2005) used the ICD-10 criteria and decision rules to evaluate the clinical sample of 579 children in the MTA (i.e. children with the categorical diagnosis of ADHD Combined Type based on a variant of the "Or" decision rule). The re-evaluation with the more stringent ICD-10 criteria resulted in diagnosis of HKD in only 25% of the MTA participants. Also, in a study of a population sample of 2452 German children, Dopfner *et al.* (2008) used DSM-IV criteria that identified about 5% of a population sample. They reported that only 25% of that group also met the ICD-10 criteria for HKD. The common finding of these two studies (i.e. a fivefold difference in the estimated prevalence) is consistent with the relative placement of ADHD and HKD on the proposed spectrum of 36 setting-specific symptoms (see Figure 20.1).

Some epidemiologic studies specifically have evaluated subthreshold manifestations of ADHD, defined operationally by the presence of three to five symptoms in one symptom domain (for subthreshold ADHD Inattentive or Hyperactive/Impulsive subtypes) or in both (for subthreshold ADHD Combined Type). In a recent example, Kim *et al.* (2009) evaluated ADHD in a random selection of ten schools in Seoul, Korea. Using the DSM-IV criteria and

Table 20.1 Eighteen symptoms and 36 setting-specific symptoms for the ADHD spectrum

Domain symptoms	a. Symptoms for categorical diagnosis	b. Setting-specific for spectrum evaluation
Inattention	1. Fails to attend to details	1. P1
		2. T1
	2. Difficult sustaining attention	3. P2
		4. T2
	3. Does not seem to listen	5. P3
		6. T3
	4. Fails to finish	7. P4
		8. T4
	5. Difficulty organizing tasks	9. P5
		10. T5
	6. Avoids sustained effort	11. P6
		12. T6
	7. Loses things	13. P7
		14. T7
	8. Distracted by extraneous	15. P8
		16. T8
	9. Forgetful	17. P9
		18. T9
Hyperactivity	10. Fidgets	19. P10
		20. T10
	11. Leaves seat in class	21. P11
		22. T11
	12. Runs about or climbs	23. P12
		24. T12
	13. Difficulty playing quietly	25. P13
		26. T13
	14. Motor excess	27. P14
		28. T14
Impulsivity	15. Talks excessively	29. P15
		30. T15
	16. Blurts out answers	31. P16
		32. T16
	17. Difficulty waiting turn	33. P17
		34. T17
	18. Interrupts or intrudes	35. P18
		36. T18

the DISC-IV interview, they found that the prevalence of the full categorical diagnosis of ADHD decreased with age, from about 7% in grades 1–3 to about 2% in grades 7–9, for an average of about 5% in school-aged children, while prevalence of subthreshold ADHD remained constant at about 9%. Thus, they also observed a substantial difference in prevalence of HKD and ADHD (see Figure 20.2), as has been observed in other countries, including Germany (Dopfner *et al.* 2008) and in the USA (Wigal *et al.* submitted).

What are some of the neuroethical implications related to such a large cross-national difference in prevalence of a condition considered to have a biological basis? Here we will discuss two neuroethical issues: first, at the population level, policy contributes to the large difference in "*administrative prevalence*" (the recognition and treatment rate) and second, at the individual level, clinical assessment contributes to *stigma and access to services*.

At the policy level, the decision rules for categorical diagnosis in DSM-IV and ICD-10 are determined by a top-down process based on clinical expertise rather than a bottom-up empirical process (see Helzer *et al.* 2008). The large cross-national difference in diagnosis may reflect differences in culture and custom that set policy rather than population differences in manifestation of the symptoms that have similar neural bases. The rate of diagnosis directly impacts rates of medication usage; in the US, where recognition and treatment rates are the highest, prescription stimulant medications (MPH and AMP) for ADHD represented two of the top five prescribed pediatric medications in terms of total expenditures (Stagnitti 2007), at a cost of more than $1 billion in 2004. When resources for healthcare are limited, the relative needs and benefits of medications across conditions must be considered (National Institute for Health and Clinical Excellence 2008). Policy decisions—such as those made for the DSM-IV and ICD-10 decision rules—have neuroethical implications since they operate to affect the allocation of scarce resources.

Sartorius (2007) discusses how stigma ("the negative attitude based on prejudice and misinformation") may be triggered by a marker of an illness, and he outlined ways to reduce stigma by reducing the visibility of markers and by increasing local and national efforts for

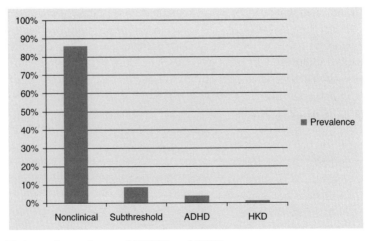

FIG. 20.2 Estimated prevalence of ADHD and HKD.

education and reduction of discrimination. In the ADHD area, over the past decade there are two good examples of successful efforts to reduce stigma. The first example is related to educational law. In the 1990s, a national effort in the US led to recognition of ADHD as a disability by Public Law 94-142, the Individuals with Disabilities Education Act (IDEA). Before the IDEA, ADHD was considered solely a medical condition and thus was not addressed in educational law, so a diagnosis did not qualify an individual for special services in the school setting where symptoms are manifested and may predominate. Some background on the prior educational law, the Education of the Handicapped Act (EHA), and details of the IDEA are summarized by Swanson (1992). ADHD was not considered a handicapping condition in the EHA, but when it was revised to become the IDEA, ADHD was considered a disability under the category of "Other Health Impaired." This was important, because this change meant that a diagnosis of ADHD could qualify a student for accommodations in the regular classroom or in some cases for special education programs "solely on the basis of the disorder." Also, it was interpreted as directing public schools to establish "procedures for locating, identifying and evaluating" children with ADHD "regardless of the severity of their disability" and to offer a "full continuum of placement alternatives." This changing perception of ADHD and recognition in educational law was accelerated by the rise of national advocacy groups such as Children and Adults with ADD (CHADD), which mounted media campaigns specifically designed to reduce stigma associated with the ADHD diagnosis and label and to increase access to services by individuals and families affected by ADHD, as recommended by Sartorius (2007) for all mental health disorders. The second example is related to the application of new technology for drug administration. In 2000, another advance in the treatment of ADHD resulted in a reduction of stigma: the development of effective long-acting formulations of stimulants dramatically reduced a visible marker of ADHD (i.e. public administration of stimulant medication in the school setting).

We have suggested that the development of effective CR formulations of the stimulant drugs was one of the most clinically significant developments of the past decade (see Swanson and Volkow 2009). In the 1990s, the use of medication increased dramatically (see Swanson, Lerner and Williams 1995) and the use of IR formulations of the short-acting stimulants (MPH and AMP) required dosing at school. Since these are Schedule II drugs and self-administration is against the law, administration by school staff was required and anecdotal reports indicated that line-ups at noon resulted in some children being embarrassed and teased. The development of effective once-a-day formulations was based on the concept of acute tolerance to MPH, which had been documented in PET studies of intravenous administration to adults (Volkow *et al.* 1995) and in proof-of-principle studies using clinical pharmacokinetic/pharmacodynamic methods to evaluate oral clinical doses of MPH (see Swanson *et al.* 1999) and AMP (see Greenhill *et al.* 2003). These studies suggested that a new first-order (ascending) drug delivery profile would be superior to the usual zero-order (flat) profile that had been assumed to be optimal, and the Osmotic Release Oral System (OROS® technology and the polymer-coated bead technology was applied to achieve a controlled drug delivery from the gastrointestinal tract after a morning dose of medication. Proof-of-product (efficacy) studies were designed to test this application of technology, and the predicted long-duration of actions was documented in laboratory school studies of Concerta® (Pelham *et al.* 2001; Swanson *et al.* 2003) and for Adderall XR® (McCracken *et al.* 2003). These efficacy trials were followed by standard clinical effectiveness trials that led to the regulatory approval of Concerta® and Adderall XR® by the US Federal Drug Administration

(FDA). The duration of effectiveness for 8 hours or more was sufficient for once-a-day dosing, and this avoided the need for a mid-day dose at school. The availability of these CR formulations of stimulant medications led to a rapid shift in prescribing practices. As documented by prescription records (see Swanson and Volkow 2009), after several decades of standard clinical practice of administration of multiple daily doses of IR formulations (typically with a noon dose at school under supervision of school personnel), the standard became administration of a morning dose of CR formulations of the stimulant medication. This acceptance in clinical practice provides an example of how findings from the neurosciences can be translated successfully into clinical applications (see Volkow and Swanson 2008 for a summary).

Dimensions of symptom severity

In preparation for the revision process for DSM-V, the APA, WHO, and the National Institute of Mental Health (NIMH) formed a "study group" to consider dimensional approaches for possible use in revision of DSM-IV criteria for future categorical diagnoses. A report of the deliberations has been published (see Helzer et al. 2008). Kraemer (2007) described the implications of a general approach that moves from a binary categorical diagnoses in DSM-IV (i.e. positive when a patient is thought to have a disorder and negative otherwise) to an ordinal diagnosis (i.e. by specifying three or more ordered values based on available and clinically relevant information —e.g. symptom counts, symptom duration, or symptom severity; certainty of diagnosis; degree of impairment). Andrews and colleagues (2008) described an epidemiological study of non-psychotic psychiatric symptoms (i.e. mixed anxiety and depression) documented by clinical interview, which created a dimension based on symptom count that is radically skewed in the population since most respondents report no current symptoms and thus have a symptom count of zero. Rather than using a symptom count, Helzer et al. (2008) proposed starting dimensionalization at the item level by using a 3-point scale for the assessment of symptom severity based on presence (0 = none, 1 = mild, or 2 = severe) or frequency (0 = never, 1= sometimes, or 2 = frequent). Hudziak et al. (2008) proposed the use of the Child Behavior Checklist (CBCL) to take advantage of norms based on age, sex, and source of rating (informant).

There are many examples in the ADHD literature of using symptom severity measures as dimensional adjuncts to categorical diagnosis. Conners et al. (1969) developed the Hyperactivity Index before the modern era of symptom lists initiated by DSM-III (APA 1980). Swanson et al. (1983) used the DSM-III items to develop the Swanson, Nolan, and Pelham (SNAP III) rating scale. Soon after the DSM-IV revisions, several ADHD symptom rating scales were developed, including the SNAP IV (Swanson 1992), the Vanderbilt Rating Scale (Wolraich et al. 1996), the DuPaul Rating Scale (DuPaul et al. 1998), and the Disruptive Behavior Disorders Rating Scale (Molina et al. 1998). All of these scales use a 4-point scale for symptom severity (e.g. not at all or never = 0; just a little or infrequently = 1; quite a bit or often = 2; very much or very often = 3). Collett and colleagues (2003) provided a thorough review of the psychometric properties of these "narrow band" approaches. They all show rather low correlations for parent and teacher ratings (about 0.3), but other psychometric properties of rating scales (test-retest reliability, validity, etc.) are adequate and about the same for all of these instruments. However, other psychometric properties may impose a serious threat to the use of these norms.

For both parent and teacher completed rating scales, the age and sex norms are typically based on the T-score (i.e. a transformation of the z-score with a mean of 50 and a standard deviation of 10), which assumes a normal distribution. Deriving T-scores from data based on a skewed distribution violates one of the basic assumptions for calculating a standard score, and the use of a T-score cut-off is not recommended by some (see Powers *et al.* 1998 for the DuPaul ADHD rating scale, and Swanson *et al.* 2000 for the SNAP). Others recommend the use of T-scores, but with torturous provisions made in an attempt to adjust for skewness (see Achenbach and Rescorla 2001). The skewed distributions for the CBCL and SNAP IV are shown in Figure 20.3.

There are many neuroethical issues related to the approach of using a dimension of symptom severity, and we will consider two here: *statistical appropriateness of norms* and *arbitrary setting of cut-offs*.

Using an ADHD dimension of symptom severity may result in overestimation of statistically extreme cases due to the skewness of the distribution of scores in the population norms. For example, in a population sample of 875 school-aged children, the z-score cut-off of 1.65 SD units (expected to identify 5% as extreme) actually identify 8.4%, representing overestimation by a factor of 1.7 (see Swanson *et al.* 2000; Wigal *et al.* submitted; and http://www.ADHD.net). The neuroethics of using a procedure known to have a serious flaw has not been discussed in the literature but should be.

Another neuroethical issue is where to place the cut-offs for the specification of threshold and subthreshold cases. Some have suggested that impairment be used to set the cut-off on the dimension of symptom severity (see Haslam *et al.* 2006). Helzer *et al.* (2008) recommended the use of a statistical approach to determine the threshold that matches the percentage of cases identified by the categorical diagnosis. For this purpose, some ADHD

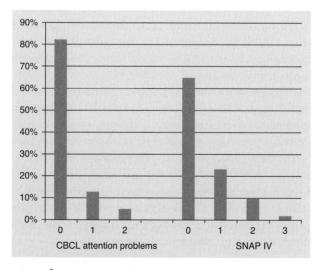

FIG. 20.3 Dimension of symptom severity.

studies have suggested that teacher ratings are superior to the parent ratings when evaluated relative to the gold standard of categorical diagnosis (see Power *et al.* 1998; Tripp *et al.* 2006). However, if the main purpose of the dimensional approach is to offer an alternative to the categorical approach, then all of these procedures may minimize the added value of the dimensional approach.

Continuum of behavior

Instead of using all negative items describing symptoms of a disorder (as in the SNAP) or problem behaviors (as in the CBCL), some items on the rating scales have been worded to be positive in order to represent the opposite of symptoms. A prime example of this approach is provided by the Strengths and Difficulties Questionnaire (SDQ) (Goodman 1997). The SDQ has 25 items, and some are worded to reflect strengths and others to reflect difficulties (but no item has both extremes). The Difficulties are rated on a 3-point scale (0 = "not true;" 1 = "somewhat true"; or 2 = "certainly true") and the Strengths are rated on a reversed 3-point scale (2 = "not true"; 1 = "somewhat true"; and 0 = "certainly true").

In the SDQ, there are five subscales each with five items, and the number of items worded to reflect strengths and difficulties varies across the subscales. The SDQ Hyperactivity–Inattention subscale lists three Difficulties ("restless, overactive, cannot stay still for long"; "constantly fidgeting or squirming"; "easily distracted, concentration wanders") and two Strengths ("thinks things out before acting" and "sees tasks through to the end, good attention span"). The scoring of Strengths is reversed compared to Weaknesses (see earlier), so the scores of all items vary from 0 (Strengths) to 2 (Weaknesses). The range of the Hyperactivity–Inattention subscale is 0 to 10, with a score of 0 indicating extreme lack of difficulties (i.e. good attention) and a 10 indicating and extreme presence of difficulties (i.e. poor attention or "attention deficit"). Unidirectional wording (i.e. either as a Strength or a Weakness, but not both) and "reversed scoring" of items reflecting Strengths (2 to 0) compared to Weaknesses (0 to 2) are used. The distribution of the SDQ Hyperactivity–Inattention subscale is highly skewed (see Figure 20.4). However, the SDQ Total Score serves as a dimensional measure of risk for psychiatric diagnosis across the range of behavior (Goodman and Goodman 2009).

Swanson *et al.* (2000, 2002) developed the Strengths and Weaknesses of ADHD-symptoms and Normal-behavior (SWAN) rating scale. The dimensionalization of the SWAN starts at the item level, but instead of considering each DSM-IV item as a symptom (as suggested by Helzer *et al.* 2008), each item was considered to cover the manifestation of behavior across the full range in the population. The DSM-IV top-down approach was taken to maintain correspondence to clinical observation, so the content remained the same, but each item was re-stated to be neutral, with an average (0) serving as an anchor that would be subjectively defined by the respondent. The same severity scale as the SNAP was used for the range of weaknesses (i.e. problem behavior that may reach the criteria for symptom presence: +1, +2, and +3), but the opposite was used for the range of strengths (i.e. −1, −2, and −3). The distribution of the SWAN is near normal in population samples (Swanson *et al.* 2002; Hay *et al.* 2005; Poderman *et al.* 2008). Figure 20.4 contrasts the behavioral continuum for the SWAN ratings of behaviors with those of the SDQ. The SDQ has a skewed distribution in the population norms, but the full range of scores at the item level on the SWAN produces a near-normal distribution in the population.

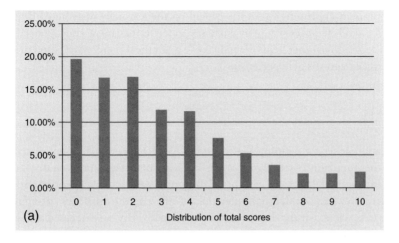

(a)   Distribution of total scores

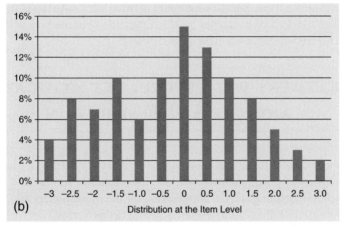

(b)   Distribution at the Item Level

FIG. 20.4 a) Distribution of SDQ hyperactivity/inattention scale in the population. b) Distribution of the SWAN in the population.

What are the ethical issues about establishing cut-offs for the SDQ and SWAN? We will discuss two here. First, the norms provided in the SDQ manual (http://www.SDQ.com) are not based on discrete cut-off values, but instead specify a band of scores to designate abnormal behavior. However, the distribution of the Hyperactivity –-Inattention subscale is highly skewed, so any cut-off based on the distribution would suffer from the same statistical flaw that affects a z-score or T-score cut-off. Several large population studies have verified that the distribution of summary ratings on the SWAN is a near-normal distribution (e.g. see Swanson *et al.* 2002; Poderman *et al.* 2007). Second, Jablensky (2005) suggested that the critical issue is the separation of psychiatric disorder from normality, and the categorical approach is based on this at both the item level (presence or absence of symptom) and the symptom count level (exceeding a threshold set by policy). Even though subjective, these decisions provide information regarding psychopathology based on clinical wisdom expressed as policy by the DSM-IV and ICD-10 criteria. This clinical wisdom is not utilized by the continuum approach. To set the cut-off on the normally distributed dimension of behavior, it would be necessary to evaluate separately impairment and the need for treatment, as is common in other fields of medicine (e.g. for the dimension of blood pressure and the categorical diagnosis of hypertension)

Summary

The three approaches for defining a spectrum of ADHD generate different distributions of scores in the population (see Figure 20.5). We have discussed some neuroethical issues related to each approach. For the categorical diagnosis, we discussed the profound impact of a top-down policy that sets decision rules and cut-offs, and the impact of cut-offs on stigma and access to services. For the dimension of symptom severity, we discussed a flaw in norms based on population distributions that are non-normal, and the statistical deceptiveness of cut-offs established on them. For the continuum of behavior, we discussed the arbitrariness of cut-off values, the lack of an anchor for the distinction between normal and abnormal, and the need for concurrent assessment of impairment.

TREATMENT WITH STIMULANT MEDICATION AND THE ADHD SPECTRUM

In clinical practice, both the categorical diagnosis of ADHD and HKD are taken as indications for treatment with stimulant medication. The implications related to the use of the three approaches of defining an ADHD spectrum for the measurement and interpretation of response to stimulant medication will be addressed in this section.

Categorical diagnosis and response to stimulant medication

It is clear that the large difference in administrative prevalence of the ADHD and HKD categorical diagnoses (see Figure 20.2) has a major impact on treatment. In North America, the first-line treatment for the multiple subtypes of ADHD diagnosed by DSM-IV is with stimulant medication (see NIH Consensus Conference on ADHD 1998), while in European and other countries stimulant medication is recommended as the first-line treatment of only severe ADHD or HKD, which is described earlier and in the literature on clinical practice, such as by the National Institute of Health and Clinical Excellence (NICE) in its recent guidelines on ADHD (NICE 2008).

The historical and cultural differences associated with the acceptance and use of different diagnostic systems (i.e. DSM-IV and ICD-10) creates very large cross-national differences in the use of stimulant medication, which is documented by records of national consumption of stimulants (see United Nations Office on Drugs and Crime 2008) and by databases of prescription records and clinical practices (see Zito *et al.* 2003). These differences in rates of use of stimulants are primarily due to high rates in North American (especially the US)

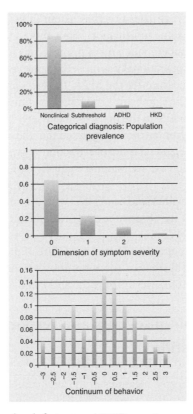

FIG. 20.5 Three approaches for defining an ADHD spectrum.

compared to other geographic regions. For example, the most recent 2008 United Nations (UN) report on national consumption of the most commonly used stimulant medication, methylphenidate (MPH), states that in the past 3 years "... the United States has accounted for 77 percent of the calculated worldwide use of the substance" (UN 2008). This dramatic difference appears to be a direct consequence of policies for making categorical diagnoses.

These cross-national differences have been noted for decades. For example, Taylor (1979) observed that despite the similarities in epidemiologic prevalence of ADHD in different counties, stimulant medications "... are used with frighteningly different frequency in different places." For example, Swanson and Volkow (2009) concluded that, despite recent increases in both the US and UK, the cross-national difference is still substantial. They used the UN estimates of national consumption (expressed as defined daily dose per 1000 inhabitants per day) to compare the use of stimulants in the US and UK from 1996–2005. In 2005, the defined daily dose was 1.33 in the UK versus 17.83 in the US—a 13.4-fold difference. Jick and colleagues (2004) provided similar national estimates based on the UK General Practice Research Database for the UK (where less than 1% of children are recognized and treated) and HMO databases in the US (where about 10% of children are recognized and treated with stimulants).

When used at a relatively high rate, as is the custom in the US, what is the evidence of benefit? The MTA provides some information about short-term response based of initial titration (see Greenhill *et al.* 1996), but a main purpose was to provide information about long-term response, defined operationally as more than one year. When categorical diagnosis is used as an outcome measure for the MTA, the assessments reveal that 22% of the MedMgt group and 18% for the Comb group no longer met the DSM-IV criteria for ADHD Combined type compared to 41% in the Beh group and 42% in the CC group. Latent class analysis of the 3-year and 8-year outcomes suggested that the relative benefit of medication was superimposed on a large general trend of reduction of symptoms in most cases, which was independent of medication use and was maintained over time in some but not in others (see Swanson *et al.* 2007).

The treatment of children with ADHD and HKD with stimulant medication is not usually evaluated by re-evaluation of the criteria for categorical diagnosis. For example, the overall goal of this treatment in the MTA was not just to reduce symptom presence to below threshold for diagnosis. Instead, an upward adjustment of dose of medication was initiated if the treating clinician considered there was "room for improvement," which was quantified by dimensional ratings of symptom severity using the SNAP and other rating scales.

Dimension of symptom severity and response to stimulant medication

In the MTA, the primary outcome measures of the large assessment battery were ratings of symptom severity on the SNAP rating scale completed by parents and teachers (see MTA Group 1999). Relative benefits of stimulant medication on the subscale scores of Inattention and Hyperactivity/Impulsivity were documented at the end of the 14-month treatment-by-protocol phase by comparison of the MedMgt and Comb groups (whose assigned treatment included the MTA medication algorithm) to the Beh and CC groups (whose assigned treatment did not).

Santosh *et al.* (2005) provided an empirical basis for the selective treatment of children with diagnosis of HKD using the symptom severity ratings on the SNAP. In their re-analysis of the MTA, the subgroup of ADHD-Combined cases that met the ICD-10 criteria for a diagnosis of HKD (145 out of the 579 participants) showed a larger beneficial effect of the MedMgt condition compared to the Beh condition (effect size approximately 1.0) than the remaining subgroup that did not meet the HKD criteria (effect size approximately 0.5). However, the benefit to the latter group was also significant and large, providing an empirical basis for treatment of the less severe as well as the severe ADHD cases.

Swanson *et al.* (2001) proposed the use of a summary measure of the dimension of symptom severity established by averaging the SNAP ratings across domains (symptoms ratings of Inattention and Hyperactivity/Impulsivity) and sources (parents and teachers). This reduced the group variances as expected by the Spearmen–Brown principles and increased effect size (see Swanson *et al.* 2001). The use of this dimensional measure of response to treatment allows for evaluation of improvement beyond the symptom count criteria of categorical diagnosis. In the MTA, the groups treated with the medication algorithm (MedMgt and Comb) showed a larger reduction in symptom severity, with individual cases moving from a high level of symptom presence (a rating of "pretty much" = 2 or "very much" = 3) to a low level of symptom presence not considered to represent psychopathology ("just a little" = 1) or symptom absence ("not at all" = 0). Rather than using a symptom count of categorical diagnosis, the measure of "remission" was a dimensional measure—the summary score on the SNAP ≤ 1.0. For this dimensional measure, 68% of the Comb, 56% of the MedMgt, and 34% of the Beh individuals showed an "excellent response."

The neuroethics of measures and characterizing response to stimulant medication is complex. This has been addressed in a summary of findings of the MTA (see Swanson *et al.* 2008). There is no clear consensus about the meaning of the measure of long-term response based on the symptom severity dimension, which was large at the 14-month assessment but dissipated and disappeared by the 3-year assessment. The confusion about the MTA outcomes has been controversial, and public reports may have been misinterpreted (see *Kids on Pills* 2010). Without an untreated control group, the lack of relative superiority of the MedMgt or Comb conditions over the positive control groups (Beh and CC) does not necessarily imply a lack of effectiveness, since all groups improved over time and the treatments converged after the treatment-by-protocol phase of the randomized control trial (RCT).

Continuum of behavior and response to stimulant medication

Recently, the SWAN was used as a measure of response to stimulant medication by Acosta *et al.* (2009) and by Arcos-Burgos *et al.* (2010). Based on latent class analysis, they used the extended range of the SWAN to form subgroups with and without high levels of hyperactive/impulsive behavior, and then they contrasted the subgroups when rated on the SWAN both on and off medication. The SWAN extended the range of measurable response, which for the dimension of symptom severity (i.e. SNAP ratings) has a minimum of 0 but for the continuum of behavior (i.e. SWAN ratings) has a minimum of −3.0.

The neuroethics of measuring response beyond the presence of psychopathology is related to the fundamental clinical rationale for the clinical use of stimulant medication—to reduce distress and impairment associated with the presence of symptoms of ADHD and HKD (i.e. the diagnostic criteria of DSM-IV and ICD-10). Response to stimulant medication can go beyond the reduction of symptoms and may produce enhancement of nonsymptom behavior. If, normal behavior (and individuals) as well as abnormal behavior (and individuals) is responsive to stimulants then, this may question the implicit clinical requirement that treatment "corrects a deficit." This requirement operates to restrict the use of stimulants to medical use for the treatment of ADHD, but this may need to be questioned in the face of frequent use for enhancement that is illegal based on this policy (see Sahakian and Morein-Zamir 2007).

TREATMENT ISSUES AND NEUROETHICS

Some neuroethical issues transcend the three spectrum approaches discussed previously. We will discuss five here: the prevalence of medication use for the treatment of ADHD that has continued to increase linearly for decades; the use of favorable response to medication to confirm the diagnoses of ADHD and HKD; the non-medical use of stimulants with the expectation of cognitive enhancement that is becoming common in some settings, such as college; the lack of evidence of long-term relative benefits of stimulant treatment over other treatments; the risk for non-medical use to escalate into abuse in vulnerable individuals in the population.

Prevalence of use of stimulant medication

The changing diagnostic criteria for ADHD may be contributing to a persistent trend in the US for the regular increase in prescription of stimulant medications for ADHD (see Safer and Krager 1985; Safer et al. 1996; Zito et al. 2003). An acceleration of this was We noticed two decades ago (Swanson et al. 1995), and it was suggested that this trend was due to correction of under-recognition and undertreatment of children compared to the estimated prevalence of ADHD according to the DSM-IV criteria and decision rules just adopted and being implemented at the time. It was predicted that at some point it would asymptote, but by 2005 the treatment rate was so high it exceeded the traditional 5% estimate of population prevalence (i.e. 9.3% of 12 year old boys and 3.7% of 11 year old girls; see Bloom and Cohen 2007). But, so far this linear increase has continued and an asymptote has not been reached. Swanson and Volkow (2008) suggested that recent increases in supply may be increasing more rapidly than the prescriptions for stimulants.

The proposed DSM-V revisions, including the increase of age of onset from 7 to 12 years of age, the addition of symptoms of impulsivity, and the reduction of cut-off for adult diagnoses (see www.apa.org), are likely to increase the recognition rate and thus the treatment rate in the future. Theoretically, if the diagnosis of ADHD is restricted to a minority of the population and the use of medication is restricted to clinical cases, then at some point an asymptote for the recognition and treatment rates should occur.

Use of response to medication to confirm diagnosis

The fundamental rationale for the clinical use of stimulant medication is to reduce distress and impairment associated with the presence of symptoms of ADHD and HKD (i.e. the diagnostic criteria of DSM-IV and ICD-10). One strategy to confirm a diagnosis has been response to treatment. This may be problematic if, as discussed above, the direction of response (improvement) is used alone to define benefit, since many individuals who do not meet the strict criteria for a diagnosis of ADHD also may show the same direction of response (see Rapoport et al. 1978). In addition to direction of response, the correction of a deficit may be used to limit those considered to benefit from treatment with medication. However, the responses to medication based on these dual criteria—improvement and correction of deficit—are dependent on setting an appropriate cut-off for defining the deficit. If the diagnostic cut-off is set low so that impairment is not present, then response to medication may not move an individual from an impaired to a non-impaired state. The extreme would exist when an individual is unimpaired (normal) and medication is used to enhance a non-impaired state.

The correction of a deficit may be conceptualized in different ways for the three diagnostic approaches. For the categorical diagnosis approach, the individual may fall well below the threshold for criterion symptoms, but may include non-criterion symptoms that create distress or dysfunction. For the dimension of symptom severity, an individual may fall below the cut-off for presence of psychopathology, but may seek enhancement to a superior level of functioning. If the dimension does not measure beyond the absence of psychopathology, then movement on the dimension beyond zero would not be evaluated. However, if the continuum approach is used for the same individuals, then, movement across the full range can be measured (see Arcos-Burgos *et al.* 2010).

Non-medical use of stimulants for cognitive enhancement

It is clear that the non-medical use of stimulant drugs has been increasing (McCabe 2006, 2007a), and that the primary reason for this use is the expectation of enhancement in educational and workplace settings (see McCabe *et al.* 2007b). Apparently, non-medical use may occur in 30% of college students (see Wilens *et al.* 2008 for a review), and if so it may even exceed the medical use for the treatment of ADHD (see Swanson and Volkow 2008).

The non-medical use of stimulant medication has been revived as a topic of debate (see Sahakian and Morein-Zamir 2007), and this has generated controversy and discussion of important neuroethical issues in the scientific literature (see Volkow and Swanson 2008) and in the popular press (see Stix 2009). In the context of modern society, the widespread non-medical use of highly regulated stimulant drugs (i.e. Schedule II in the US) is occurring, especially by high school and college students who expect that this will improve academic productivity and performance (see McCabe *et al.* 2007b). The legal issues surrounding the use of a controlled substance are serious; the use of a Schedule II drug without a prescription is technically or legally a felony. Therefore, this is an important neuroethical issue that needs to be addressed.

Greely *et al.* (2008) defined an agenda for the discussion of neuroethical concerns in three areas: safety and risk of unintended side effects; freedom from coercion to enhance by legal or other means; fairness of use in competitive situations and unequal access to cognitive enhancers. They also proposed four mechanisms to shape evidence-based policy in this controversial area: accelerated research on the effects of stimulant drugs on individuals without ADHD to clearly answer questions about potential benefits and associated risks; participation of professional organizations to set guidelines for physicians, educators, and others who interact with individuals who are using stimulants with the expectation of cognitive enhancement; education to disseminate public-health information about the non-medical use of stimulants; and legislative action to bring existing laws into line with norms of modern society.

Specific use for cognitive enhancement has been addressed in a special issue of the journal, *Psychopharmacology* (see Robbins 2009). The use of stimulants in sport practice, either for training or in competition, is banned in the name of fairness and safety (Avois 2006). Their use in the military is sometimes required in some settings when endurance and wakefulness are necessary. The use by professionals, who keep long hours, such as medical residents, has been addressed by Bray *et al.* (2004). One approach to the understanding of the effects of arousal on different tasks and across types of individuals and settings is the

Yerkes–Dodson law (see Arnsten 1998), which historically has been misapplied and even discredited (see Diamond *et al.* 2008). Recently, findings from PET imaging studies (e.g. see Volkow *et al.* 2008a) have suggested that the measurement of local brain activation may offer a way to revive this once discredited approach. We documented that compared to placebo: MPH significantly reduced the task-related increase in glucose by 50%. The stimulant-related focusing of regional brain activation during task performance may be beneficial when neuronal resources are diverted away from the task, perhaps by default mode interference that results in mind-wandering or lapse in attention (see Volkow *et al.* 2006). However, these medication effects could be detrimental when brain activity is already optimally focused. This could explain why stimulants have beneficial effects in some individuals and contexts and detrimental effects in others, generating U-shaped relationships between cognitive performance and dose of medication (Arnsten, 2008).

Long-term outcomes

The MTA was designed to evaluate long-term benefits of treatment with stimulants, either as residual effects after cessation of childhood treatment or chronic effects of continued treatment into adolescence and adulthood. The gold standard for evaluation is the RCT, in which individuals are randomly assigned to treatments with or without medication as a component, to avoid selection bias that might distort long-term medication effects. MTA treatment-by-protocol in the assigned groups was maintained in most cases through the 14-month follow-up. The initial findings at the end of the treatment-by-protocol phase (MTA Cooperative Group 1999a,b) clearly show the relative superiority of assignment to the MTA medication algorithm, and thus confirmed the initial short-term benefits of stimulant treatment documented in the titration trial and extended the evidence of superiority into the long term (defined operationally as more than one year). The findings from the first follow-up, 10 months after the end of treatment-by-protocol, revealed partial loss of the superiority of assignment to the MTA medication algorithm (MTA Group 2004), and the second follow-up revealed the complete loss of the relative superiority (Jensen *et al.* 2007; Swanson *et al.* 2007b; Molina *et al.* 2008) at the assessment 36 months after baseline and 2 years after the end of the treatment-by-protocol phase. This suggests that the superiority of assignment to intensive, carefully monitored medication management (i.e. to the MTA medication algorithm) eventually dissipates completely when the children are returned to community treatment. The relative benefits were not apparent even when compared to children who are never treated with stimulant medication.

This creates a potential neuroethical question: if stimulant medication provides short-term but not long-term benefits, should it be prescribed on the basis of short-term effects? The degree of risk associated with stimulant treatment must be weighed against what is known about potential benefits (including how long they will last),

Risks of abuse

One controversial neuroethical issue is whether treatment with stimulant medications in childhood protects against or increases risk for substance use in adolescence or adulthood.

Initial studies that showed large protective effects (see Wilens *et al.* 2003) have been contradicted by longer follow-up (Biederman *et al.* 2008). This has been discussed by us elsewhere (Volkow and Swanson 2009). These issues were addressed in the follow-up of the MTA study (Molina *et al.* 2007 and 2008), which suggested that childhood treatment does not affect risk—either by increasing or decreasing it.

However, the risk for escalation of stimulants from use to misuse or abuse (see Volkow and Swanson 2003) may be different for the non-medical use of stimulants than for medical use (see Rasmussen 2008). About 20% of the general (non-ADHD) users of stimulants, for example in the non-medical use by the military (in World War II) or in eras of lax regulatory control (in the 1960s and 1970s), escalated to dependence and abuse (see Rasmussen 2008). These questions about risk are still unresolved and require more careful evaluation.

Summary

We present here three approaches for defining a spectrum of ADHD: categorical diagnosis based on symptom counts with subtypes and comorbidities; dimensions of symptom severity based on rating scales with content defined by official manuals; and continuum of behavior based on the full range of behavior that underlies the symptoms.

For categorical diagnoses, there is a profound impact of a top-down policy that sets decision rules and cut-offs, which produces dramatic cross-national differences in recognition and treatment (e.g. of ADHD in the US and HKD in the UK). We discussed the two sides to this issue, with stigma increasing with the use of lax categorical criteria and widespread labeling of children versus access to services decreasing with the use of strict categorical criteria that limit the diagnosis to the most severe cases. Since categorical diagnosis varies so much in different counties, cross-national studies of stigma and services would be an important topic to address to understand further the neuroethics of this difference. For the dimension of symptom severity, the population distributions of ADHD ratings are non-normal, as are symptom severity ratings for other disorders if they occur rarely in the population. We discussed a possible fatal flaw in norms based some statistical properties of cut-offs based on these distributions. The use of these methods may be inappropriate and possibly deceptive (with respect to a statistical prevalence higher than assumed at any cut-off chosen), which may be a neuroethical issues to be addressed by professions that use rating scales for clinical purposes (e.g. by psychologists who are involved in the assessment of ADHD). For the continuum of behavior, the distribution of ratings is near-normal for the population. We discussed the arbitrariness of cut-off values for a continuum without any natural breakpoints, as well as without a build-in subjective anchor for the distinction between normal and abnormal. For the use of the continuum approach, there may be an increased need for concurrent assessment of impairment.

In summary, consideration of a multiple ways to consider ADHD as a spectrum disorder can contribute to discussions of the neuroethics of this controversial treatment by defining issues about stigma and services, by identifying possible unrecognized problems with the use of statistical norms that may encourage overdiagnosis, and by recommending the assessment of psychopathology based on evaluation of impairment along with evaluation of the underlying behavior that has no well-defined cut-off.

Perhaps the most obvious neuroethical issue we addressed here is about the expectation of cognitive enhancement and the resulting widespread non-medical use of stimulant medication (see Sahakian and Morein-Zamir 2007). We considered the opposing sides taken in the debate about the non-medical use of stimulant drugs and a variety of neuroethical issues in this debate (see Greely *et al.* 2008; Swanson and Volkow 2008; Volkow and Swanson 2008; Stix 2009), but the clearest conclusion might be that current scientific knowledge is inadequate to claim the presence or absence (or degree) of cognitive enhancement in non-medical use of stimulant medications.

The evaluation of long-term benefits of childhood treatment has been addressed the MTA study, which shows that the initial relative benefits of treatments that include stimulants (compared to those that do not) dissipate by 3 years after initiation of treatment (see Swanson *et al.* 2009). The claims of long-term benefits by reducing substance use and abuse have not been supported as the follow-up sample entered adulthood (see Biederman *et al.* 2008). These issues were addressed in the follow-up of the MTA (Molina *et al.* 2007 and 2008), which suggested that childhood treatment does not affect risk for substance use or abuse—either by increasing or decreasing it.

However, the risk for escalation of stimulants from use to misuse or abuse (see Volkow and Swanson 2003) may be different for the non-medical use of stimulants than for medical use (see Rasmussen 2008). About 20% of the general (non-ADHD) users of stimulants, for example, in the non-medical use by the military (in World War II) or in eras of lax regulatory control (in the 1960s and 1970s), escalated to dependence and abuse (see Rasmussen 2008). These questions about the non-medical use of stimulants and the risk of addiction to drugs are still unresolved and require more careful evaluation.

REFERENCES

Achenbach, T.M. and Rescorla, L.A. (2001). *Manual for ASEBA School-Age Forms and Profiles.* Burlington, VT: University of Vermont Press.

American Psychiatric Association. (1980). *Diagnostic and Statistical Manual of Mental Disorder, third edition.* Washington, DC: American Psychiatric Association.

American Psychiatric Association. (1994). *Diagnostic and Statistical Manual of Mental Disorder, fourth edition.* Washington, DC: American Psychiatric Association.

Andrews, G., Brugha, T. and Thase, M.E. (2008). Dimensionality and the category of major depressive episodes. *International Journal of Methods Psychiatric Research*, 16, 41–51.

Arcos-Burgos, M., Jain, M., Acosta, M.T., *et al.* (2010). A common variant of the latrophilin 3 gene, *LPHN3*, confers susceptibility to ADHD and predicts effectiveness of stimulant medication. *Molecular Psychiatry*, e1038.

Arnsten, A.F.T. (1998). Catecholamine modulation of prefrontal cortical function. *Trends in Cognitive Science*, 2, 436–47.

Avois L., Robinson N., Saudan C., Baume N., Mangin P., and Saugy M. (2006). Central nervous system stimulants and sport practice. *British Journal of Sports Medicine*, 40, 16–20.

Barkley, R.A. (1997). Behavioral inhibition, sustained attention, and executive functions: constructing a unifying theory of ADHD. *Psychological Bulletin*, 121, 65–94.

Biederman, J., Monuteaux, M.C., Spencer, T., Wilens, T.E., MacPherson, H.A., and Faraone, S.V. (2008). Stimulant therapy and risk for subsequent substance use disorders in male adults with ADHD: a naturalistic controlled 10-year follow-up study. *American Journal of Psychiatry*, **165**, 597–603.

Bloom, B. and Cohen, R.A. (2007). Summary health statistics for US children: National Health Interview Survey, 2006. *Vital Health Statistics*, **234**, 1–79.

Bradley, C. (1937). The behavior of children receiving benzedrine. *American Journal of Psychiatry*, **94**, 577–85.

Bray C.L., Cahill K.S., Oshier J.T., *et al.* (2004). Methylphenidate does not improve cognitive function in healthy sleep-deprived young adults. *Journal of Investigative Medicine*, **52**, 192–201.

Bush, G. (2010). Attention deficit hyperactivity disorder and attention networks. *Neuropsychopharmacology*, **35**, 278–300.

Cassano, G.B., Rucci, P., Frank, E., *et al.* (2004). The mood spectrum in unipolar and bipolar disorder: arguments for a unitary approach. *American Journal of Psychiatry*, **161**, 1264–9.

Castellanos, F.X. (1997). Toward a pathophysiology of attention-deficit/hyperactivity disorder. *Clinical Pediatrics*, **36**, 381–93.

Castellanos, F.X. (1999). Biological underpinnings of ADHD. In J. Swanson and. S. Sandberg (eds.) *Hyperactivity and attention disorders of children*, pp. 145–55. Cambridge: Cambridge University Press.

Castellanos, F.X. and Tannock, R. (2002). Neuroscience of attention deficit hyperactivity disorder: the search for endophenotypes. *Nature Review of Neuroscience*, **3**, 617–28.

Castellanos, F.X, Sonua-Barke, E.J. Scheres, A., Di Martino, A., Hyde, C., and Walters, J.R. (2005). Varieties of attention deficit hyperactivity disorder- related intra-individual variability. *Biological Psychiatry*, **63**, 332–7.

Castellanos F.X., Kelly C., and Milham M.P. (2009). The restless brain: attention-deficit hyperactivity disorder, resting-state functional connectivity, and intrasubject variability. *Canadian Journal of Psychiatry*, **54**, 665–72.

Collett, B.R., Ohan, J.L., and Myers, K.M. (2003). Ten-year review of rating scales. v: scales assessing attention-deficit/hyperactivity disorder. *Journal of the American Academy of Child and Adolescent Psychiatry*, **42**, 1015–37.

Conners, C.K. (1969). A teacher rating scale for use in drug studies with children. *American Journal of Psychiatry*, **126**, 884–8.

Conners, C.K. (1997). *Conners' Rating Scales -Revised: Technical manual*. North Tonawanda, NY: Multi-health Systems.

Conners, C.K. (2002). Forty years of methylphenidate treatment in attention-deficit/ hyperactivity disorder. *Journal of Attention Disorders*, **6**, S17–S30.

Diamond, D.M., Campbell, A.M., Park, C.R., Halonen, J., and Zoladz, P.R. (2007). The temporal dynamics model of emotional memory processing: a synthesis on the neurobiological basis of stress-induced amnesia, flashbulb and traumatic memories, and the Yerkes-Dodson law. *Neuroplasticity*, **7**, 1–33.

Di Martino A., Ghaffari M., Curchack J., *et al.* (2008). Decomposing intra-subject variability in children with attention-deficit/hyperactivity disorder. *Biological Psychiatry*, **64**, 607–14.

Dopfner M., Breuer D., Wille N., Erhart M., Ravens-Sieberer U., and the BELLA study group. (2008). How often do children meet ICD-10/DSM-IV criteria of attention deficit-/ hyperactivity disorder and hyperkinetic disorder? Parent-based prevalence rates in a national sample – results of the BELLA study. *European Child and Adolescent Psychiatry*, **17**, 59–70.

Doyle A.E., Biederman J., Seidman L.J., Weber W., and Faraone S.V. (2000). Diagnostic efficiency of neuropsychological test scores for discriminating boys with and without attention deficit-hyperactivity disorder. *Journal of Consulting and Clinical Psychology*, **68**, 477–88.

Douglas, V.I. (1972). Stop, look and listen: the problem of sustained attention and impulse control in hyperactive and normal children. *Canadian Journal of Behavioral Science,* **4**, 259–82.

DuPaul, G.J., Power, T.J., Anastopoulos, A.D., and Reid, R. (1998). *ADHD Rating Scale IV: Checklists, norms and interpretation.* New York: Guilford Press.

Durston S., Tottenham N.T., Thomas K.M., *et al.* (2003). Differential patterns of striatal activation in young children with and without ADHD. *Biological Psychiatry,* **53**, 871–8.

Fowler, J.S., Volkow, N.D., Ding, Y.S., *et al.* (1999). Positron emission tomography studies of dopamine-enhancing drugs. *Journal of Clinical Pharmacology,* **39**, 13S–16S.

Fox, D.J., Tharp, D.F. and Fox, L.C. (2005). Neurofeedback: an alternative and efficacious treatment for Attention Deficit Hyperactivity Disorder. *Applied Psychophysiology Biofeedback,* **30**, 365–73.

Fox, M.D., Corbetta, M., Snyder, A.Z., Vincent, J.L. and Raichle, M.E. (2006). Spontaneous neuronal activity distinguishes human dorsal and ventral attention systems. *Proceedings of the National Academy of Sciences U S A,* **103**, 10046–51.

Goodman, A. and Goodman, R. (2009). Strengths and Difficulties Questionnaire as a dimensional measure of child mental health. *Journal of the American Academy of Child and Adolescent Psychiatry,* **48**, 400–3.

Goodman, R (1997). The Strengths and Difficulties Questionnaire: a research note. *Child Psychology and Psychiatry,* **48**, 581–6.

Greely, H., Sahakian, B., Harris, J., *et al.* (2008). Toward responsible use of cognitive-enhancing drugs by the healthy. *Nature,* **456**, 702–5.

Greenhill, L.L., Abikoff, H.B., Arnold, L.E., *et al.* (1996). Medication treatment strategies in the MTA Study: Relevance to clinicians and researchers. *Journal of the American Academy of Child and Adolescemt Psychiatry,* **35**, 1304–13.

Greenhill, L.L., Findling, R.L. and Swanson, J.M. (2002). A double-blind, placebo-controlled study of modified-release methylphenidate in children with attention-deficit/hyperactivity disorder. *Pediatrics,* **109**, E39.

Greenhill, L.L., Swanson, J.M., Steinhoff, K., *et al.* (2003). A pharmacokinetic/pharmacodynamic study comparing a single morning dose of adderall to twice-daily dosing in children with ADHD. *Journal of the American Academy of Child and Adolescent Psychiatry,* **42**, 1234–41.

Grinspoon, L. and Hedblom, P. (1975). *The speed culture: Amphetamine use and abuse in America.* Boston, MA: Harvard University Press.

Haslam, N., Williams, B., Prior, M. *et al.* (2006). The latent structure of attention-deficit/hyperactivity disorder: a taxometric analysis, *Australian and New Zealand Journal of Psychiatry,* **40**, 639–47.

Hay, D., Bennett, K., Levy, F., Sergeant, J. and Swanson, J. (2006). A twin study of attention-deficit/ hyperactive disorder dimensions rated by the strengths and weaknesses of ADHD-symptoms and normal-behavior (SWAN) scale. *Biological Psychiatry,* **61**, 700–5.

Helzer, J., Kraemer, H., Krueger, R.F, *et al.* (2008). Dimensional approaches in diagnostic classification: Refining the research agenda for DSM-V. Arlington, VA: American Psychiatric Association.

Hudziak, J.J., Achenbach, T.M., Althoff, R.R., and Pine, D.S. (2007). *A dimensional approach to developmental psychopathology. International Journal of Methods Psychiatric Research,* **16**, 65–73.

IDEA (P.L. 105-17) (Education of All Handicapped Children Act) http://idea.ed.gov/

Jablensky, A. (2005). Categories, dimensions and prototypes: critical issues for psychiatric classification. *Psychopathology*, **38**, 201–5.

Jensen, P.S., Arnold, L.E., Swanson, J., *et al.* (2007). Follow-up of the NIMH MTA study at 36 months after randomization. *Journal of the American Academy of Child and Adolescent Psychiatry*, **46**, 988–1000.

Jick, H., Kaye, J.A. and Black, C. (2004). Incidence and prevalence of drug-treated attention deficit disorder among boys in the UK *British Journal of General Practice*, **54**, 345–7.

Judd, L., Hagop, A., Akiskal, S., *et al.* (2002). The long-term natural history of the weekly symptomatic status of bipolar I disorder. *Archives of General Psychiatry*, **59**, 530–7.

Kids on Pills. Panorama. British Broadcasting Corporation, United Kingdom, 10 April, 2000 [television program].

Kim, H.Y., Cho, S.C., Kim, B.N., Shin, M.S. and Kim, Y. (2009). Perinatal and familial risk factors are associated with full syndrome and subthreshold attention-deficit hyperactivity disorder in a Korean community sample. *Psychiatry Investigation*, **6**, 278–85.

Kraemer, H.C. (2007). DSM categories and dimensions in clinical and research contexts. *International Journal of Methods in Psychiatric Research*, **16**, 8–15.

Leth-Steensen, C., Elbaz, Z.K. and Douglas, V.I. (2000). Mean response times, variability, and skew in the responding of ADHD children: a response time distributional approach. *Acta Psychologica (Amsterdam)*, **104**, 167–90.

Lahey, B.B., Applegate, B., McBurnett, K., *et al.* (1994). DSM-IV field trials for attention deficit hyperactivity disorder in children and adolescents. *American Journal of Psychiatry*, **151**, 1673–85.

Maser, J.D. and Patterson, T. (2002). Spectrum and nosology: implications for DSM-V. *Psychiatric Clinics of North America*, **25**, 855–5.

McCabe, S.E., Teter, C.J., and Boyd, C.J. (2006). Medical use, illicit use and diversion of prescription stimulant medication. *Journal of Psychoactive Drugs*, **38**, 43–56.

McCabe, S.E., Cranford, J.A., Boyd, C.J. and Teter, C.J. (2007a). Motives, diversion and routes of administration associated with nonmedical use of prescription opioids. *Addictive Behaviors*, **32**, 562–75.

McCabe, S.E., West, B.T. and Wechsler, H. (2007b). Trends and college-level characteristics associated with the non-medical use of prescription drugs among US college students from 1993 to 2001. *Addiction*, **102**, 455–65.

McCracken, J.T., Biederman, J., Greenhill, L.L., *et al.* (2003). Analog classroom assessment of a once-daily mixed amphetamine formulation, SLI381 (Adderall XR), in children with ADHD. *Journal of American Academy of Child and Adolescent Psychiatry*, **42**, 673–83.

Mehta, M.A., Goodyer, I.M., and Sahakian, B.J. (2004). Methylphenidate improves working memory and set-shifting in AD/HD: Relationships to baseline memory capacity. *Journal of Child Psychology and Psychiatry*, **45**, 293–305.

Molina, B.S., Pelham, W.E., Blumenthal, J., and Galiszewski, E. (1998). Agreement among teachers' behavior ratings of adolescents with a childhood history of attention deficit hyperactivity disorder. *Journal of Clinical Child and Adolescent Psychology*, **27**, 330–9.

Molina, B.S., Hinshaw, S.P., Swanson, J.M., *et al.* (2008). The MTA at 8 Years: prospective follow-up of children treated for combined type ADHD in a multisite study. *Journal of American Academy of Child and Adolescent Psychology*, **48**, 484–500.

MTA Cooperative Group. (1999). 14-Month randomized clinical trial of treatment strategies for attention deficit hyperactivity disorder. *Archives of General Psychiatry*, **56**, 1073–86.

MTA Cooperative Group. (2004). National Institute of Mental Health Multimodal Treatment Study of ADHD follow-up: changes in effectiveness and growth after the end of treatment. *Pediatrics*, **113**, 762–9.

National Institute for Health and Clinical Excellence (2008). *The NICE Guidelines on Diagnosis and Management of ADHD in children, young people and adults.* National collaborating centre for mental health. London: NICE.

Nigg, J.T. (2005). Neuropsychologic theory and findings in attention-deficit/hyperactivity disorder: the state of the field and salient challenges for the coming decade. *Biological Psychiatry*, **57**, 1424–35.

NIH Consensus Statement (1998). Diagnosis and treatment of attention deficit hyperactivity disorder (ADHD). *NIH Consensus Statement*, **16**, 1–37.

Pelham, W.E., Gnagy, E.M., Burrows-Maclean, L., *et al.* (2001). Once-a-day Concerta methylphenidate versusthree-times-daily methylphenidate in laboratory and natural settings. *Pediatrics*, **107**, E105.

Pennington, B.F. and Ozonoff, S. (1996). Executive functions and developmental psychopathology. *Journal of Child Psychology and Psychiatry*, **37**, 51–87.

Poderman, T.J.C., Derks, E.M., Hudziak, J.J., *et al.* (2007). Across the continuum of attention skills: a twin study of the SWAN ADHD rating scale. *Journal of Child Psychology and Psychiatry*, **48**, 1080–7.

Polanczyk, G., Lima, M.S., Horat, B.L. *et al.* (2007). The worldwide prevalence of attention-deficit/hyperactivity disorder: a systematic review and meta-regression Analyses. *American Journal of Psychiatry*, **164**, 942–8.

Posner, M.I. and Rothbart, M.K. (2007). Research on attention networks as a model for the integration of psychological science. *Annual Review of Psychology*, **58**, 1–23.

Power, T.J., Doherty, B.J., Panichelli-Mindel, S.M., *et al.* (1998). The predictive validity of parent and teacher reports of ADHD symptoms. *Journal of Psychopathology and Behavioral Assessment*, **20**, 57–81.

Prendergast, M., Taylor, E., Rapoport, J.L., *et al.* (1988). The diagnosis of childhood hyperactivity. A U.S.-U.K. cross-national study of DSM-III and ICD-9. *Journal of Child Psychology and Psychiatry*, **29**, 289–300.

Rapoport, J.L., Buchsbaum, M.S., Zahn, T.P., Weingartner, H., Ludlow, C., and Mikkelsen, E.J. (1978). Dextroamphetamine: cognitive and behavioral effects in normal prepubertal boys, *Science*, **199**, 560–63.

Rasmussen, N. (2008). *On Speed: The Many Lives of Amphetamine.* New York: NYU Press.

Rhode, I.A. (2008). Is there a need to reformulate attention deficit hyperactivity disorder in future nosologic classification? *Child and Adolescent Clinics of North America*, **17**, 405–20.

Rhodes, S.M., Coghill, D.R., and Matthews, K. (2005). Neuropsychological functioning in stimulant-naive boys with hyperkinetic disorder. *Psychological Medicine*, **35**, 1109–20.

Robbins, T.W. and Sahakian, B.J. (1979). 'Paradoxical' effects of psychomotor stimulant drugs in hyperactive children from the standpoint of behavioural pharmacology. *Neuropharmacology*, **18**, 931–50.

Robbins, T.W. (2009). Special issue on cognitive enhancers. *Psychopharmacology*, **202**, 1–2.

Rubia, K., Smith, A. and Taylor, E. (2007). Performance of children with attention deficit hyperactivity disorder (ADHD) on a test battery of impulsiveness. *Child Neuropsychology*, **13**, 276–304.

Safer, D.J. and Krager, J.M. (1985). Prevalence of medication treatment for hyperactive adolescents. *Psychopharmacological Bulletin*, **21**, 212–15.

Safer, D.J., Zito, J.M. and Fine, E.M. (1996). Increased methylphenidate usage for attention deficit disorder in the 1990s. *Pediatrics,* **98,** 1084–8.

Sahakian, A. and Morein-Zamir, S. (2007). Professor's little helper. *Nature,* **450,** 1157–9.

Sahakian, B.J. and Robbins, T.W. (1977). Are the effects of psychomotor stimulant drugs on hyperactive children paradoxical? *Medical Hypotheses,* **3,** 154–8.

Santosh, P.J., Taylor, E., Swanson, J.M., *et al.* (2005). Refining the diagnosis of inattention and overactivity syndromes: a reanalysis of the multimodal treatment study of attention-deficit/hyperactivity disorder (ADHD) based on ICD-10 criteria for hyperkinetic disorder. *Clinical Neuroscience Research,* **5,** 307–14.

Sartorius, N. (2007). Stigma and Mental Health. *Lancet,* **370,** 810–11.

Schulz, K.P., Fan, J., Tang, C.Y., *et al.* (2004). Response inhibition in adolescents diagnosed with attention deficit hyperactivity disorder during childhood: an event-related FMRI study. *American Journal of Psychiatry,* **161,** 1650–7.

Schweitzer, J.B., Lee, D.O., Hanford, R.B., *et al.* (2004). Effect of methylphenidate on executive functioning in adults with attention-deficit/hyperactivity disorder: normalization of behavior but not related brain activity. *Biological Psychiatry,* **56,** 597–606.

Sergeant, J.A. and Scholten, C.A. (1985). On resource strategy limitations in hyperactivity: cognitive impulsivity reconsidered. *Journal of Child Psychology and Psychiatry Research,* **26,** 97–108.

Society for Neuroscience. (2008). Neuroethics. In *Brain Facts,* pp. 62–3. http://www.sfn.org/skins/main/pdf/brainfacts/2008/neuroethics.pdf

Sonuga-Barke, E.J. and Castellanos, F.X. (2007). Spontaneous attentional fluctuations in impaired states and pathological conditions: a neurobiological hypothesis. *Neuroscience and Biobehavioral Reviews,* **31,** 977–86.

Stagnitti, M.N. (2007). The top five outpatient prescription drugs ranked by total expense for children, adults, and the elderly. Statistical Brief #180. Rockville, MD: Agency for Healthcare Research and Quality. Available at: http://www.meps.ahrq.gov/mepsweb/data_files/ publications/st180/stat180.pdf (accessed August 2010).

Stix, G. (2009) Turbocharging the brain: pills to make you smarter. *Scientific American,* **October,** 38–43.

Swanson, J.M. (1992). *School-based Assessments and Interventions for ADD students.* Irvine, CA: K.C. Publishing.

Swanson, J.M. and Castellanos, F.X. (1998). Biological bases of attention deficit hyperactivity disorder: neuroanatomy, genetics, and pathophysiology. NIH Consensus Development Conference: *Diagnosis and Treatment of Attention Deficit Hyperactivity Disorder,* 37–42.

Swanson, J.M. and Volkow, N.D. (2008). Increasing use of stimulants warns of potential abuse. *Nature,* **453,** 586.

Swanson, J.M. and Volkow, N.D. (2009). Psychopharmacology: concepts and opinions about the use of stimulant medications. *Journal of Child Psychology and Psychiatry,* **50,** 180–93.

Swanson, J.M., Sandman, C.A., Deutsch, C., and Baren, M. (1983). Methylphenidate hydrochloride given with or before breakfast: I. Behavioral, cognitive, and electrophysiologic effects. *Pediatrics,* **72,** 49–55.

Swanson, J.M., McBurnett, K., Wigal, T., *et al.* (1993). Effect of stimulant medication on children with attention deficit disorder: a "review of reviews." *Exceptional Children,* **60,** 154–62.

Swanson, J., Lerner, M., Williams, L. (1995). Letter to the Editor. More frequent diagnosis of attention deficit-hyperactivity disorder. *New England Journal of Medicine,* **333,** 944.

Swanson, J., Gupta, S., Guinta, D., *et al.* (1999). Acute tolerance to methylphenidate in the treatment of attention deficit hyperactivity disorder in children. *Clinical Pharmacological Therapy*, **66**, 295–305.

Swanson, J., Greenhill, L., Pelham, W., *et al.* (2000). Initiating Concerta (OROS methyphenidate HC1) qd in children with attention-deficit hyperactivity disorder. *Journal of Clinical Research*, **3**, 9–76.

Swanson, J.M., Kraemer, H.C., Hinshaw, S.P., *et al.* (2001). Clinical relevance of the primary findings of the MTA: success rates based on severity of ADHD and ODD symptoms at the end of treatment. *Journal of the American Academy of Child and Adolescent Psychiatry*, **40**, 168–79.

Swanson, J., Gupta, S., Lam, A., *et al.* (2003). Development of a new once-a-day formulation of methylphenidate for the treatment of ADHD: Proof-of-concept and proof-of-product studies. *Archives of General Psychology*, **60**, 204–11.

Swanson, J.M., Hinshaw, S.P., Arnold, L.E., *et al.* (2007a). Secondary evaluations of MTA 36-month outcomes: propensity score and growth mixture model analyses. *Journal of American Academy of Child and Adolescent Psychiatry*, **46**, 1003–14.

Swanson, J.M., Elliott, G.R., Greenhill, L.L., *et al.* (2007b). Effects of stimulant medication on growth rates across 3 years in the MTA follow-up) *Journal of the American Academy of Child and Adolescent Psychiatry*, **46**, 1015–27.

Swanson, J.M., Arnold, L.E., Hechtman, L., *et al.* (2008a). Evidence, interpretation, and qualification from multiple reports of long-term outcomes in the Multimodal Treatment Study of Children with ADHD (MTA): Part I: executive summary. *Journal of Attention Disorders*, **12**, 4–14.

Swanson, J.M., Arnold, L.E., Kraemer, H., *et al.* (2008b). Evidence, interpretation, and qualification from multiple reports of long-term outcomes in the Multimodal Treatment Study of Children with ADHD (MTA): Part II: supporting details. *Journal of Attention Disorders*, **12**, 15–43.

Swanson, J.M., Wigal, T., and Lakes, K. (2009). *DSM-V* and the future diagnosis of attention-deficit/hyperactivity disorder. *Current Psychiatry Reports*, **11**, 399–406.

Swanson, J.M., Baler, R.D., and Volkow, N.D. (2010). Understanding effects of medications on cognition in ADHD individuals: a decade of progress. *Neuropsychopharmacology*, [EPUB September 29, 2010].

Taylor, E. (1979). The use of drugs in hyperkinetic states: Clinical issue. *Neuropharmacology*, **18**, 951–8.

Taylor, E., Sergeant, J., Doepfner, M., *et al.* (1998). Clinical guidelines for hyperkinetic disorder. *European Child and Adolescent Psychiatry*, **7**, 184–200.

Tripp, G., Schaughency, E.A., and Clarke, B. (2006). Parent and teacher rating scales in the evaluation of attention deficit hyperactivity disorder: contribution to diagnosis and differential diagnosis in clinically referred children. *Journal of Developmental and Behavioral Pediatrics*, **27**, 209–18.

United Nations Office on Drugs and Crime (UNODC). (2008). World Drug Report for 2007. Geneva: United Nations Publications.

US Department of Education (1990). *To Assure a Free Appropriate Public Education of All Children with Disabilities: Twenty-first Annual Report to Congress on the Implementation of the Individuals with Disabilities Education Act.* Washington, DC: US Department of Education.

Villemagne, V.L., Wong, D.F., Yokoi, F., *et al.* (1999). GBR12909 attenuates amphetamine-induced striatal dopamine release as measured by [(11)C]raclopride continuous infusion PET scans. *Synapse*, **33**, 268–73.

Volkow, N.D., Wang, G.J., Fowler, J.S., *et al.* (1998). Dopamine transporter occupancies in the human brain induced by therapeutic doses of oral methylphenidate. *American Journal of Psychiatry*, **155**, 1325–31.

Volkow, N.D., Ding, Y.S., Fowler, J.S., *et al.* (1995). Is methylphenidate like cocaine? Studies on their pharmacokinetics and distribution in the human brain. *Archives of General Psychiatry*, **52**, 456–63.

Volkow, N.D., Wang, G.J., Fowler, J.S., *et al.* (1997). Effects of methylphenidate on regional brain glucose metabolism in humans: relationship to dopamine D2 receptors. *American Journal of Psychiatry*, **154**, 50–5.

Volkow, N.D., Wang, G.J., Fowler, J.S., *et al.* (1999a). Blockade of striatal dopamine transporters by intravenous methylphenidate is not sufficient to induce self-reports of "high". *Journal of Pharmacological Experimental Therapy*, **288**, 14–20.

Volkow, N.D., Wang, G.J., Fowler, J.S., *et al.* (1999b). Reinforcing effects of psychostimulants in humans are associated with increases in brain dopamine and occupancy of D(2) receptors. *Journal of Pharmacological Experimental Therapy*, **291**, 409–15.

Volkow, N.D., Wang, G., Fowler, J.S., *et al.* (2001). Therapeutic doses of oral methylphenidate significantly increase extracellular dopamine in the human brain. *Journal of Neuroscience*, **21**, RC121.

Volkow, N.D., Wang, G.J., Fowler, J.S., *et al.* (2002). Relationship between blockade of dopamine transporters by oral methylphenidate and the increases in extracellular dopamine: therapeutic implications. *Synapse*, **43**, 181–7.

Volkow, N.D. and Swanson, J.M. (2003). Variables that affect the clinical use and abuse of methylphenidate in the treatment of ADHD. *American Journal of Psychiatry*, **160**, 1909–18.

Volkow, N.D., Wang, G.J., Ma, Y., *et al.* (2006). Effects of expectation on the brain metabolic responses to methyphenidate and to its placebo in non-drug abusing subjects. *Neuroimage*, **32**, 1782–92.

Volkow, N.D., Wang, G.J., Newcorn, J., *et al.* (2007). Depressed dopamine activity in caudate and preliminary evidence of limbic involvement in adults with attention-deficit/ hyperactivity disorder. *Archives of General Psychiatry*, **64**, 932–40.

Volkow, N.D. and Swanson, J.M. (2008). The action of enhancers can lead to addiction. [comment in Sahakian and Morein-Zamir, *Nature*, **451**, 520.

Volkow, N.D., Fowler, J.S, Wang, G.J., *et al.* (2008a). Methylphenidate decreased the amount of glucose needed by the brain to perform a cognitive task. *PLoS ONE*, **3**, epub2017.

Volkow, N.D., Fowler, J.S., Logan, J., *et al.* (2009a). Effects of modafinil on dopamine and dopamine transporters in the male human brain: clinical implications. *Journal of the American Medical Association*, **301**, 1148–54.

Volkow, N.D., Wang, G.J., Kollins, S.H., *et al.* (2009b). Evaluating dopamine reward pathway in ADHD: clinical implications. *Journal of the American Medical Association*, **302**, 1084–91.

Wender, P.H. (1971). *Minimal Brain Dysfunction in Children*. New York: Wiley-Interscience.

Wigal, T., Swanson J.M, Stelhi, A., Lee C. and Rayes, N. (submitted). ADHD diagnostic status after 14 months of treatment in randomized clinical trial: MTA outcome.

Wilens, T.E., Faraone, S.V., Biederman, J. and Gunawardene, S. (2003). Protection from drug abuse by childhood treatment with stimulants; does stimulant therapy of attention-deficit/hyperactivity disorder beget later substance abuse? A meta-analytic review of the literature. *Pediatrics*, **111**, 179–85.

Wilens, T., Adler, L.A., Adams, J., *et al.* (2008). Misuse and diversion of stimulants prescribed for ADHD: a systematic review of the literature. *Journal of the Academy of Child and Adolescent Psychiatry*, **47**, 21–31.

Willcutt, E.G., Doyle, A.E., Nigg, J.T., Faraone, S.V. and Pennington, B.F. (2005). Validity of the executive function theory of attention-deficit/hyperactivity disorder: a meta-analytic review. *Biological Psychiatry,* **57**, 1336–46.

Winstanley, C.A., Eagle, D.M. and Robbins, T.W. (2006). Behavioral models of impulsivity in relation to ADHD: translation between clinical and preclinical studies. *Clinical Psychology Review,* **26**, 379–95.

Wolraich, M.L., Hannah, J.N., Pinnock, T.Y., Baumgaertel, A. and Brown, J. (1996). Comparison of diagnostic criteria for attention-deficit hyperactivity disorder in a country-wide sample. *Journal of Academic Child and Adolescent Psychiatry,* **35**, 319–24.

World Health Organization. (1993). *The ICD-10 Classification of Mental and Behavioural Disorders: Diagnostic Criteria for Research.* WHO, Geneva.

Zito, J.M., Safer, D.J., DosReis, S., *et al.* (2003). Psychotropic practice patterns for youth: a 10-year perspective. *Archives of Pediatric Adolescent Medicine,* **157**, 17–25.

PART IV

··

NEURO-
TECHNOLOGY

··

CHAPTER 21

··

WHY NEUROETHICISTS
ARE NEEDED

··

RUTH FISCHBACH AND JANET MINDES

For all that scientists have studied it, the brain remains the most complex and
mysterious human organ.

(Carey 2009a)

INTRODUCTION

··

The Court Will Now Call Its Expert Witness: The Brain	(Chen 2009)
Poor Children Likelier to Get Antipsychotics	(Wilson 2009)
Brain Researchers Open Door to Editing Memory	(Carey 2009a)
Surgery for Mental Ills Offers both Hope and Risk	(Carey 2009b)

DISCOVERIES about the brain emerge almost daily, therefore it is hardly surprising that the
relatively new field of neuroethics is burgeoning. Headlines like those above make us pause,
and immediately bring to mind many issues that will need definition and resolution. In this
context, who will be best suited to integrate knowledge from brain science and ethics? We
contend that well-prepared neuroethicists are needed.

Medical ethics developed in the 18th century. In the mid-20th century, research ethics rose
from the ashes of the Holocaust and with the recognition of many highly problematic medical and social science research protocols (e.g. Tuskegee Syphilis Study (Jones 1981); Milgram's
Obedience to Authority Experiment (Milgram 1974)). Bioethics has had a rapid rise in the
20th century in response to dramatic advances in the life sciences, public health, engineering,
environmental sciences, and other developments. The subdisciplines of classical ethics continue to evolve in parallel, and remain robust. Their collective expertise enriches and

protects society and patients, science and scientists. Recently, neuroethics has emerged as a subspecialty of both bioethics and neuroscience. There is no reason to believe that this new subdiscipline will be any less successful, needed, or enduring than its disciplinary ancestors.

Technological and biomedical advances relevant to the brain—brain surgery, brain imaging, brain stimulation technology, neuroengineering, nanotechnology, robotics, neurogenetics, and others—will continue to spawn many significant questions. Because the brain is both symbolically and biologically such a crucial organ, and persons with brain disorders are often particularly vulnerable individuals, neuroethical questions become exquisitely compelling.

However one views the mandate of neuroethics, overarching questions about defining the field and how broad and diverse should be its scope must be addressed. In addition to monitoring brain sciences for ethical problems, and educating the public to be more neuro-literate, neuroethicists can work to constructively use the knowledge from neuroscience to benefit other disciplines. They also should speak out "against gee-whiz science that is merely fashionable, as well as against experimentation that exceeds the risk-benefit calculus" (Fischbach and Fischbach 2008).

In this chapter we will first review some of the definitions in circulation that reveal the varied perspectives and goals of the field of neuroethics. We follow this with our informal brief taxonomy of neuroethical questions. We will discuss in depth two specific contentious issues, one clinical and one from social sciences (psychosurgery and brain privacy) and show how neuroethicists can serve to inform and to protect. As neuroethicists will need education that will encompass many domains, we describe the academic grounding and qualifications that should be required. We also consider the pivotal roles neuroethicists should play. We contribute views that may help define the field of neuroethics and give structure and relevance to its activities. In conclusion, we contend that neuroethicists are needed, now more than ever.

DEFINITIONS AND SCOPE OF THE FIELD

Multiple definitions of neuroethics and calls to action have been offered. In a seminal conference, *Mapping the Field*, in 2002 in San Francisco, William Safire, late writer and journalist, is credited with bringing the term "neuroethics" to wider attention although it had been used earlier (see Cranford 1989; Pontius 1973, 1993). According to Safire:

> Neuroethics is the examination of what is right and wrong, good and bad about the treatment of, perfection of, and unwelcome invasion of or worrisome manipulation of the human brain. (Safire 2002).

Another oft-quoted view is that of Gazzaniga who wrote:

> "Neuroethics is more than just bioethics for the brain"…it is "the examination of how we want to deal with the social issues of disease, normality, mortality, lifestyle, and the philosophy of living informed by our understanding of underlying brain mechanisms" (Gazzaniga 2005).

Illes adapted a more general definition from Van Rensselaer Potter's definition of bioethics as, "a discipline that aligns the exploration and discovery of neurobiological knowledge with human value systems" (Illes 2006).

The goals of a 2005 conference, *Hard Science, Hard Choices*, held at the Library of Congress in Washington, DC could be taken as a definition. Neuroethics promotes:

exploration of new and emerging technologies, exploration of ethical, social, economic, and legal implications of new technologies, implications for public policy, and facilitates scholarly networking, a key element in any emerging field (Fischbach 2006, p. xi).

In the book produced from that conference (Ackerman 2006), a call to action is tempered with a caveat of caution:

> Our growing understanding of how the brain works and how we may manipulate, inquire into, or change it (both to treat its disorders and for nonmedical purposes) must now call forth our best efforts to seek ethical consensus while issues are taking shape – not after they have emerged as moral crises or controversies in the public arena. (Fischbach 2006, p. ix)

In 2002 Roskies described the scope of neuroethics in two divisions: the ethics of neuroscience and the neuroscience of ethics. The former addresses the ethics of the practice of neuroscience and:

> the implications of our mechanistic understanding of brain function for society... integrating neuroscientific knowledge with ethical and social thought. The latter, the neuroscience of ethics, borrows from the field of neurophilosophy and examines the neurological foundations of moral cognition. (Roskies 2002, p. 21)

Federico, Lombera, and Illes (Chapter 22, this volume) argue that this two-division view of neuroethics is overly simplistic; the neuroscience of ethics should not be placed apart or at a higher standard than neuroscience studies of other domains such as addiction or neurodegenerative diseases.

Racine asserted that:

> the single most important integrative goal underlying neuroethics is a practical one: the need to improve patient care for specific patient populations. Hence, technological advances should always be discussed in the light of their potential contribution to the good of the patients and the public. (Racine 2008, p. 3)

He points out that one of the first times the term neuroethics was used was to urge clinicians to pay more attention to the needs of neurological and psychiatric patients, especially in order to protect them from possibly harmful new interventions (see Cranford 1989; Pontius 1973, 1993).

According to cognitive neuroscientists and neuroethics scholars at the University of Pennsylvania (2009a), attempts to define the scope of the field may be premature. Nonetheless they offer two new categories of neuroethical issues: those emerging from what we can do, and those emerging from what we know:

- *The "what we can do" problems*: ethical problems raised by advances in functional neuroimaging, pharmaceutical enhancement of mood and related functions, cognitive enhancement, brain implants, and brain–machine interfaces.
- *The "what we know" problems*: ethical problems raised by our growing understanding of the neural bases of behavior, concepts of personal responsibility, personality, consciousness, and states of spiritual transcendence.

Neuroethicists will consistently confront the technological imperative: if the technology exists, use it. But they will need to recall the bioethics mantra: it is not what you can do, it is what you should do.

These definitions and field-framing statements also indicate how diverse are the issues and questions the field will address are. William Safire's definition is pithy and quotable. It was offered as an alert to the most crucial and salient concerns in early 2000. Some neuroethical questions surely will not be explored so neatly within this framework.

The present authors agree with Joseph Fins that not all neuroethical questions will be of the "sound the alarm" variety. He does caution against neuroethics having "the unintended consequence of squelching clinical progress for historically marginalized patients who might be helped by advances in neuroscience" (Fins 2003a; 2005).

Where Gazzaniga suggests a "philosophy of living *informed by our understanding of underlying brain mechanisms*"...i.e. "a brain-based philosophy of life" (Gazzaniga 2005), Fins finds this expansive stance "worrisome." Advocacy for a brain-based "universal ethics" he finds is reminiscent of a theological construct and could be seen as prescriptive, not unlike Delgado's wish decades ago to use brain implants to "psychocivilize society" (Fins 2008, p. 38; see Delgado and Anshen 1969; Fins 2003b).

Others offer practical lists of neuroethical questions and concerns that may emerge in diverse arenas. At the 2005 *Hard Science, Hard Choices* Conference one of the present authors (R.F.) suggested that we "call forth our best efforts to seek ethical consensus while issues are taking shape; we can't afford to wait." Yet it is a given that reaching consensus takes time, that new discoveries and issues are a moving target, and that controversies will inevitably erupt in the public arena.

Schiavo as a cautionary tale

While having their unproductive aspects, controversies often do bring a needed and urgent focus to important issues. A case in point is the wrenching Terri Schiavo tragedy and specifically how the neurological meaning of severe brain injury and the persistent vegetative state, "became central to the decade's most convulsive bioethics debate" (Fins 2008) that occupied national attention in 2005 (see Annas 2005; Cassell 2005; Dresser 2005) (Figure 21.1). Despite the terrible emotional and monetary cost to the extended Schiavo family, the country as a whole learned much—lay people, healthcare providers, policy makers, the media, even the President of the USA and Governor of Florida.

In the end, new neurological standards and methodologies that can help distinguish the persistent vegetative state (PVS) from the minimally conscious state (MCS) emerged "to avoid the diagnostic shortfalls that stem from clinical ignorance or ideological intent" (Fins 2008, p. 19; Hirsch 2005). In addition, the prognosis for brain injury leading to MCS, once considered untreatable, now is seen as having a variable prognosis that may respond to deep brain stimulation (Fins 2008; Schiff *et al.* 2007).

Heterogeneity of neuroethics today

While neuroscientists, neurologists, psychiatrists, and psychologists will publish about neuro-issues in their professional domains, neuroethicists can have an important role to play in synthesizing the range of neuroethical scholarly production. Neurologists will not likely read most publications in psychiatric epidemiology, nor will psychiatrists often read a paper in an experimental psychology journal. Neuroethicists are likely to explore a wide variety of professional publications, and contribute to many. They now have opportunities

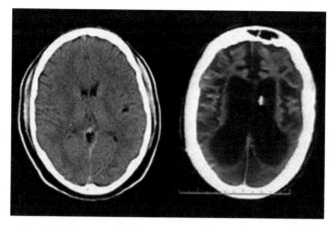

FIG. 21.1 Terri Schiavo's brain. Left: CT scan of normal brain. Right: Schiavo's 2002 CT scan provided by Ronald Cranford, showing loss of brain tissue. The black area is liquid; the small white mark in the right image is the thalamic stimulator implanted in her brain. http://en.wikipedia.org/wiki/Terri_Schiavo_case (accessed 22 December 2009).

to publish empirical research, reviews, and commentaries in their own professional periodical, the *American Journal of Bioethics Neuroscience* (*AJOB Neuroscience*). We also expect that neuroethicists will raise many new questions, prompting experts in diverse disciplines to comment further from their perspectives. Finally, in addition to monitoring brain sciences for possible ethical issues, neuroethicists can work constructively with other experts to benefit other disciplines (see Wolf 2008).

To give the reader an appreciation of the heterogeneity of neuroethics today, which is not likely to abate, one has only to refer to a recent promotional brochure (fall 2009) for *AJOB Neuroscience*. The variety and scope of "Recent topics" that appeared in the journal is as impressive as it is exciting (Table 21.1).

Neuroethics as a field is rapidly becoming international (Lombera and Illes 2009). It has garnered significant public and political attention in the US, Japan, various European nations, and others, where work groups exist to study ethical issues of translating neuroscience technologies into clinical use. The more international neuroethics becomes, the more neuroethical issues may converge within the international scientific community, and yet, new cross-cultural neuroethical issues may emerge from the very different cultures and faiths. Neuroethicists will be needed as valuable worldwide colleagues, who together contribute to improved clinical care and scientific advancement beyond what could be achieved by countries working independently.

"Neurologisms"

With the advent of interest in the brain sciences, a new vocabulary of words and concepts has developed, consisting of the prefix "neuro-" (meaning neuroscience-based or neuroscience-informed). Appended to other fields of study or practice, this has given us terms such

Table 21.1 "Recent topics," promotional brochure (Fall 2009) for *AJOB Neuroscience*

Neuroimaging and Consciousness	Memory Detection
Treating Post-Traumatic Stress	The Brain and Identity
Placebo Effects and the Brain	Neuroimaging and the Law
Animal Law and Ethics	Women's Neuroethics
Primate Stroke Research	Translational Research
Memory Suppression	Brain Privacy
Cell-based Interventions for Neurological Conditions	Pediatric fMRI
History of Neuroethics	Global Norms for Bioethics
Body Integrity Identity Disorder	Mirror Neurons
Objective and Subjective Brains	

as neurotechnology, neuromarketing, neuroengineering, neuroeconomics, and neurolaw. Judy Illes coined the term "neurologisms" to describe these hybrids (Illes 2009).

The prefix "neuro-" has become so ubiquitous that some, for example philosopher Roger Scruton, see intellectual imperialism of "neuro-thugs" claiming chunks of new intellectual territory as though those fields had no history, analytical traditions, or tools of their own (Scruton 2009). Conversely, some find anything "neuro-" sexy and thus contribute to the proliferating literature. As neuroethics as a field evolves, it will be necessary to learn when the use of "neuro" is appropriate and productive, and when merely clever and fashionable. Nonetheless, using tools of neuroscience, questions from other fields stimulate novel opportunities that may yield important new insights, justifying the faith many have in science that at times may be overhyped. Ideally these new neuro-hybrids will indeed become areas of legitimate and rigorous scientific discovery.

A related issue concerns the growing miscellaneousness of neuroethical publication. Susan Wolf cautions that her field, neurolaw, "seems increasingly about everything." As with health law, "it becomes difficult to see what is distinctive about the field, what core challenges it poses, and how to systematize our thinking about the field to make progress" (Wolf 2008, p.21). Similarly, burgeoning diversity lacking sufficient structure may be cause for concern if there is to be a recognized field of neuroethics that can develop meaningful content. Yet, valid neuroethical questions will arise in varied and unexpected places, and should be welcomed. Over time, organizing principles will emerge. Neuroethicists will be needed to serve as guides to this ever-growing literature and to give it form and definition.

D. Gareth Jones (2008) points out that there are good reasons to keep neuroethics very connected to its clinical roots. Neuroethical questions, however, do not always have primary clinical origins. Neuroethicists and others have been defining new questions at the intersection of brain sciences and many other fields. To develop optimally, neuroethics will need to respect, understand, and integrate the knowledge of other disciplines with an open mind.

Again, neuroethicists will contribute to the integration that will be needed. They also will be the ones to help determine when a course of action is "neuroethical."

Taxonomy of neuroethical questions

We offer here(see Table 21.2) a modest taxonomy for neuroethics that, for the authors of this chapter, helped create order, given the myriad vexing questions with which neuroethicists grapple, now and in the future. Complex and diverse neuroethical issues may migrate across categorical boundaries, and many topics could be examined under more than one category according to the specific question(s) posed. Our illustrative examples reflect our interests and scholarly work, and help us address the question, "Is it neuroethical?"

Below we expand on the categories in Table 21.2 and offer salient questions.

A Technologically-driven questions with wide implications for society relating primarily to bioethics

Brain stimulation

Brain stimulation modalities hold considerable promise in psychiatric treatment (see Pascual-Leone *et al.*, Chapter 25, this volume). They range from some long-used mainstream psychiatric therapies such as electroconvulsive therapy (ECT) to sophisticated devices used more widely clinically only in the last decade, such as deep brain stimulation (DBS) and transcranial magnetic stimulation (TMS). These and other modalities are more and less focal and/or invasive; they have shown varying efficacy for different indications. Some still are experimental and/or Food and Drug Administration-approved for limited indications. Brain stimulators often are viewed as complementary to brain imaging concerning the kind of neural information they can provide, and are teaching us much about brain circuitry. As therapies, however, their use occasions larger questions about our changing relationship to technologies affecting the brain.

- *Electroconvulsive therapy* for decades has been an effective, even life-saving treatment for patients with severe depression and chronic medication resistance (Figure 21.2). ECT continues to be modified to improve efficacy and safety as well as to reduce distressing aspects of its administration (Prudic 2008; Sackeim *et al.* 2008). ECT is invasive because it involves global stimulation of the brain (cortical and subcortical) with high frequency alternating current, which must cause a seizure to have any chance of therapeutic efficacy.
  - Despite its advantages, frightening images from older media continue to influence public perceptions of ECT's invasiveness causing many patients to reject ECT who could benefit (Morrison 2009; Payne and Prudic 2009a,b; Walter *et al.* 2002).
  - There are valid fears concerning post-ECT memory loss (Payne and Prudic 2009a,b). People who justly fear memory loss from ECT should concomitantly fear remaining depressed, as chronic depression exacerbates memory problems.
  - ECT is disproportionately prescribed for the elderly depressed for many reasons: it is safer than antidepressants as there are minimal cardiovascular side effects; ECT

Table 21.2 Taxonomy of neuroethical questions

Category/level	Definition, with examples
A. Technologically-driven questions with wide implications for society relating primarily to bioethics	Questions focused on the nature of brain-related technologies and their use and impact on society, in research, and clinical contexts. Examples: all types of brain imaging, brain stimulation, surgical technologies, brain-machine interfaces, central and peripheral prostheses; also technological manipulation via genetics and pharmaceuticals. Questions pertaining to bioethical implications of neuroscience and neuropsychiatric applications, and involving frequent intersection with law, public policy, media, and public perceptions. *Example:* 1. Brain stimulation (ECT, DBS, TMS)
B. Clinically-driven questions relating primarily to medical ethics	Questions focused primarily on specific neurotherapeutic interventions and contexts; concerns about safety, efficacy, appropriateness of therapeutic choices, informed choice of treatment, related issues. Questions pertaining to issues of medical ethics confronting healthcare providers in direct contact with patients and their families. *Example:* 1. Autism genetics
C. Applied philosophical, definitional, legal, cross-cultural, and psychosocial questions relating primarily to the meaning of personhood and symptomatology	Questions springing from history of psychiatry and psychology, philosophy of psychiatry, epistemology, and history of science, focused primarily on conceptual origins, historical and philosophical definitions regarding neural and mental phenomena such as individual identity, personal responsibility, cross-cultural definitions of mental ills, etc. *Examples:* 1. Revision of DSM-IV to DSM-V 2. Neuroenhancement
D. Ethically-driven questions relating primarily to protection of humans and animals in research	Questions focused primarily on ethical conduct of research with humans and animals: conduct of clinical trials concerning psychological impact, protection of brain and mind; ethical use and protection of animals used in research, particularly with relevance to their consciousness, mental capacities, and ability to feel pain. *Examples:* 1. Human: Disclosure of incidental brain research findings 2. Animal: Neuroethical care of research animals; Creating chimeras in higher primates
E. Ethically-driven "new frameworks" questions concerning the unity of mind, brain, and body relating primarily to progressive and integrative medicine	Questions pertaining to improved understanding of inherent biological systems of mind, brain, and body; consciousness; and morality, with the aims of greater scientific understanding, improved medicine and healthcare, and optimal health. *Examples:* 1. Stress and health 2. Curbing medicalization creep

a)

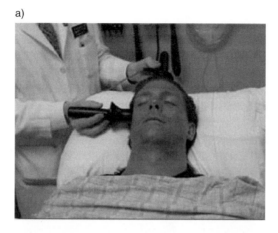

b)

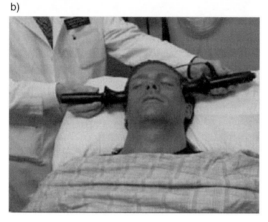

FIG. 21.2 Administration of electroconvulsive therapy (ECT). a) Right unilateral place-ment: to generate a seizure with right unilateral treatment, one electrode is placed on the crown of the head, the other on the right temple. Right unilateral treatment is typically associated with reduced memory side effects. b) Bilateral placement: bilateral treatment involves placing electrodes on both temples. This treatment may be associated with more acute memory side effects. Bilateral ECT is indicated for severe mental illnesses including depression with psychosis, manic episodes of bipolar disorder, psychosis related to schizo-phrenia and catatonia.

will not contribute to polypharmacy; chronic treatment resistance is common in this population; and very importantly, ECT is most likely to rapidly improve disabling deep depression and suicidality (Rosenberg *et al.* 2009; Sherman 2009; Sackeim *et al.* 2007).

Q: How can neuroethicists help the public better understand ECT and mitigate fears, so patients and families can make more informed therapeutic choices, while also understanding that therapies seldom are perfect?

• *Deep brain stimulation* involves implanting an electrode in the brain to stimulate subcortical areas (Figure 21.3). Current indications include treatment of movement

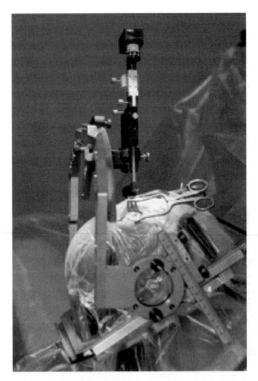

FIG. 21.3 Implantation of deep brain stimulation (DBS) electrode, to treat Parkinson's disease (PD). http://commons.wikimedia.org/wiki/File:Parkinson_surgery.jpg (accessed 22 December 2009).

disorders such as Parkinson's disease (PD) (target: subthalamic nucleus of basal ganglia); and treatment of refractory depression (target: experimental only—subgenual cingulate cortex). The electrodes cannot be explanted easily but can be turned off. Surgery usually is successful, but surgical complications and serious side effects can occur (Carey 2009a).

- DBS for PD can lead to significant cognitive and emotional impulsivity, even as it ameliorates the primary movement disorder (Halbig *et al.* 2009; Hardesty and Sackeim 2007; Witt *et al.* 2008). Given the complexity and plasticity of brain networks, the safety and efficacy of all approaches to brain stimulation must be evaluated carefully.

  Q: As we only partially understand current brain stimulating modalities to treat neuropsychiatric conditions, a necessary question is whether the cost/benefit ratio is good enough compared to other therapies?

  Q: How can neuroethicists promote advancing this promising science while cautioning about the "technological imperative" and the reality that brain stimulating modalities may result in serious complications?

Transcranial magnetic stimulation (Figure 21.4) for depression requires extensive clinician involvement and is very expensive (cost at one major center is approximately $12,000 for a 6–8 week course of 5 days/week treatment). It is only affordable to the affluent, apart from participating in clinical trials. Yet if its usefulness and safety hold up, TMS may become a treatment of choice for treatment-resistant patients (i.e. patients for whom multiple drugs and ECT have failed to lessen symptoms).

Q: If insurance companies or Medicare begin to cover TMS, can the expense be justified, compared to much less expensive pharmaceuticals or other therapies for depression?

Q: How will society manage questions of equitable treatment for promising but expensive therapy?

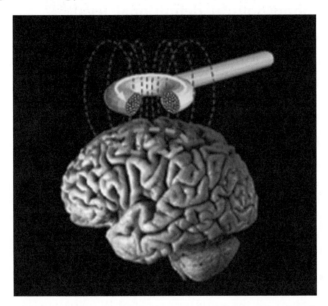

FIG. 21.4 (Also see Plate 8). Transcranial magnetic stimulation (TMS). Schematic image of electromagnetic action. TMS is a safe and non-invasive means of getting electrical energy across the insulating tissues of the head and into the brain. http://intra.ninds.nih.gov/Research.asp?People_ID=196 (accessed 1 January 2010).

B Clinically-driven questions relating primarily to medical ethics

Autism genetics

A deletion of a segment that includes 29 genes on the short arm of chromosome 16 occurs in approximately 1% of the autism population. This structural variant is highly penetrant: chances are high (between 30–50%) a person with this deletion will fall somewhere on the autism spectrum. Others with the same deletion may exhibit mental retardation or a different developmental disorder.

- A husband over 40 and his 38-year-old wife may choose *in vitro* fertilization and pre-implantation genetic screening to eliminate embryos with the 16p deletion.

  Q: How can neuroethicists, working with a clinical team, assist couples making these extremely difficult choices?

C Applied philosophical, definitional, legal, cross-cultural, and psychosocial questions relating primarily to the meaning of personhood and symptomatology

Revision of the Diagnostic and Statistical Manual of Mental Disorders (DSM-IV)

In revising DSM-IV to produce DSM-V, a particularly contentious issue is the proposal to abandon the diagnosis of Asperger's syndrome. Asperger's advocates see many negatives if they are identified as autistic individuals rather than as a distinct category. Those diagnosed with Asperger's often have a more favorable societal profile, are more likely to be able to work or function independently, and often possess unusual or creative abilities. They may not wish to be "cured" of these qualities and most oppose research seeking the genetic risk factors that might lead to genetic screening or elimination of their special status.

  Q: In what ways will the restructuring of DSM-IV (1994) into DSM-V (2013) affect diagnosis and treatment of autism spectrum disorders and many other mental health conditions? Will all changes be for the better?

Neuroenhancement

Neuroenhancement has been defined as "a pharmacological attempt to increase cognitive performance in healthy humans" (Normann and Berger 2008).

  Q: Is non-medical neuroenhancement ever ethical and possibly appropriate? If yes, at what ages, and for what specific purposes? (Sahakian and Morein-Zamir 2010; Chneiweiss, Chapter 19 this volume)

  Q: Legally and philosophically, how authentic are enhanced personality traits, and how legally autonomous, in various contexts, are people using such enhancements (Bublitz and Merkel 2009)?

D Ethically-driven questions relating primarily to protection of humans and animals in research

Human research: disclosure of incidental brain research findings

What should be done when an incidental finding of possible clinical relevance is revealed in a research study involving brain technology? Incidental findings that have not been validated generally are not disclosed; currently there is no consensus for appropriate action in response to medically significant findings (Illes 2008; Illes and Chin 2008; Wolf *et al.* 2008).

> Q: How can research volunteers' right to know or be reassured be balanced with other issues?

> Q: How should neuroethicists contribute to re-framing research protocols and informed consent forms concerning disclosure of incidental findings, and how can they help educate participants?

Animal research: neuroethical care of research animals; creating chimeras in higher primates

Use of animals in research and questions of animal rights and welfare have become high profile concerns in recent years.

- Research into comparative human and animal brain function, consciousness, and physiological function reveals that mammals possess more advanced awareness and sensation than historically recognized.

  > Q: What are the most neuroethical, affordable standards for housing, care, pain mitigation, and legal protections that research animals are owed by science and society?

- While common in a human to rodent model, creation of chimeras (physically mixing cells from two different species) in a human to primate model is only recently being explored.

  > Q: Is it neuroethical to create a chimera in higher primates by implanting human brain cells into their brains (see University of Minnesota, Center for Bioethics document on chimeras)?

E Ethically-driven and future-oriented questions concerning the unity of mind, brain, and body relating primarily to progressive and integrative medicine

Stress and health

Neuroscientists and proponents of complementary and alternative medicine have been documenting how mind, brain, and body are inextricably intertwined with respect to health and illness. This effort has provided new insights into how people respond to stress. Stress can be useful for creativity and even survival, but chronic, excessive stress, especially if present from an early age, can cause systemic over-activation of the hypothalamic/pituitary/adrenal axis (HPA axis) (McEwen 2009) and of key areas of the "social brain" (Urry *et al.* 2006). These patterns contribute to stress-related physical and psychological illness.

> Q: How can neuroethicists contribute to more rapid integration of discoveries about stress reduction and emotional functioning from psychology as well as cognitive, affective and social neuroscience, to diversify primary and neuropsychiatric care for post-traumatic stress disorder (PTSD) and other ills?

Curbing medicalization creep

Our rapidly advancing biomedical science yields a constant outpouring of ever deepening and broad knowledge of psychiatric and neural phenomena, but are our psychiatric concepts overly "medicalized?" Medicalization redefines normal psychological (and other) life occurrences such as grief or normal cognitive aging as predominantly medical in nature. Medicalization has been called "disease-mongering," and is linked as well to the excessive influence of pharmaceutical and other commercial medical interests (Conrad 2007; Horwitz and Wakefield 2007).

> Q: How can neuroethicists help integrate new perspectives on the nature of the brain and behavior to redefine the role of pharmaceuticals in mental health and neurological care, i.e. optimizing their biological benefits while expanding and redefining the nature of the illnesses and of neural wellness, meanwhile reducing the negatives of medicalization?

Neuroethicists, working in diverse settings, can be influential in addressing these and a myriad of other questions generated by all the branches of neuroscience, neurology, and psychiatry. We would now like to concentrate on two major examples that we feel illustrate the roles neuroethicists will need to play, working with other experts.

NEUROETHICISTS WILL PLAY A VITAL ROLE IN RESOLVING COMPLEX ISSUES

We present perspectives on two ethically complex issues: psychosurgery and brain privacy. We find these topics particularly compelling. They underscore why neuroethicists will play a vital role in exploring the ethical, legal, economic, social, and other medical and scientific implications of these advances.

The new psychosurgeries

A recent front-page headline in the *New York Times* read "Surgery for Mental Ills Offers Both Hope and Risk" (Carey 2009a). The article, one of a series on insights from the latest research, featured several surgical procedures that have been conducted in approximately the last 10 years on more than 500 people. While most procedures were performed as part of experimental studies, they were designed to treat a variety of problems including depression, anxiety, Tourette's syndrome, and even obesity. "The great promise of neuroscience at the end of the last century was that it would revolutionize the treatment of psychiatric problems. But the first real application of advanced brain science is not novel at all. It is a precise, sophisticated version of an old and controversial approach: psychosurgery, in which doctors operate directly on the brain" (Carey 2009a).

Concerning the high-risk experimental procedures that patients are being put through, Paul Root Wolpe opined: "We have this idea — it's almost a fetish — that progress is its own justification, that if something is promising, then how can we not rush to relieve suffering?" Wolpe went on to note that not so long ago, doctors considered the frontal lobotomy a major advance. But given the evidence of the thousands of patients left with irreversible brain damage, Wolpe concluded, "that's why we have to move very cautiously" (Carey 2009b).

Historical background

Neurosurgical procedures often follow in the tradition of Dr. Wilder Penfield (Figure 21.5) who had a passionate desire to unlock the mysteries of the human brain (Lipsman and Bernstein, Chapter 24, this volume). During the 1930s, he operated in a careful and cautious manner, probing the exposed brain tissue of patients with severe epilepsy, which was felt to be incurable. With his patients awake and reporting their sensations, his search for the scarred tissue that caused the seizures also revealed many functions performed by unmapped regions of the brain. Perfecting his "Montréal Procedure," Penfield is said to have "discovered the source of memory, tapped the reservoir of long forgotten sensations and emotions, and located the storehouse of dreams" (Penfield 1975). These findings revolutionized the study of higher brain function.

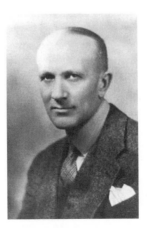

FIG. 21.5 Dr. Wilder Graves Penfield (1891–1976), 1934. http://en.wikipedia.org/wiki/Wilder_Penfield (accessed 22 December 2009)

Brain surgery continued to evolve but on a dark trajectory with the development of leucotomy and prefrontal lobotomy to treat severe behavior problems. Portuguese neuropsychia-
trist Antonio Egas Moniz, who subsequently won the Nobel Prize in 1949 for his innovative
work in neurosurgery, pioneered the procedure that was felt to be beneficial for people with
otherwise untreatable psychoses. In this crude psychosurgical procedure, connections in
the prefrontal cortex and underlying structures were severed, or the frontal cortical tissue
was destroyed, the theory being that this led to the uncoupling of the brain's emotional
center and the seat of intellect (Lerner 2005).

Walter Freeman introduced the lobotomy to the US and became its greatest advocate.
As he was a neurologist, he collaborated with neurosurgeon James Watts, to refine Moniz's
technique (Figure 21.6). Together, they developing a quick method, the so-called "ice-pick"
lobotomy, performed for the first time in 1945. At this time, prior to the availability of
Thorazine and other psychoactive drugs, lobotomy was used to reduce agitation and aggressive behaviors and to make patients easier to handle. Freeman performed ice-pick lobotomies on anyone referred to him and, during his career that lasted into the mid 1950s, he
performed almost 3500 operations (he once lobotomized 25 women in a single day
(McManamy 2009)).

The concern that troubles neuroethicists and others who currently grapple with issues
raised by psychiatric neurosurgery is that they pose high risks for patients, with only very
minimal evidence of success to date. These procedures—cingulotomy, capsulotomy, DBS,
and gamma knife surgery (targeted radiation)—are performed at only a limited number of
medical centers and generally only as a last resort (Figure 21.7). While they bring relief to
some, there remains much we need to learn about how exactly they work, specifically about
the brain's cellular and functional interconnections.

Many recognize the desperation of patients afflicted with disabling conditions that impact
almost every aspect of their lives. Neuroethicists can educate the public, work with

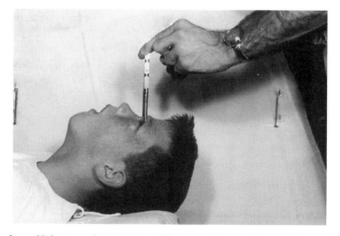

FIG. 21.6 Pre-frontal lobotomy. http://scienceblogs.com/neurophilosophy/2007/07/inventing_
the_lobotomy.php (accessed 1 December 2009).

neurosurgeons to help patients assess the major benefits, risks, adverse events, and side effects, and remind patients that anecdotal reports of the same surgery for others supposedly suffering from the same disorder may not be successful for them.

The Holy Grail in psychiatry, broadly speaking, would be to know so much more about the true, multifaceted causes of every psychiatric illness, and therefore also to know the good predictors of response for specific interventions. Ideally, treatment could be individually tailored. Many months if not years of treatment failures, frustration, loss of quality of life if not tragedy, and emergence of treatment resistance could thus be averted. However, we are far from there. Latest reports on the new psychosurgeries demonstrate once again how little we know (Carey 2009a). Desperate patients will continue to consent to surgeries that may well be too risky in their current form. Yet it seems we have no alternative but to continue to gather more data as we seek the next advance. How can we reconcile this technological imperative with the bioethical mantra to promote the responsible treatment of patients?

Treatment advancement must be balanced with honest, open, and professionally accepted, even embraced discussions of risk and failure, more publication of negative results, more transparency in the dissemination of results of clinical trials, and recognition of the limitations of current knowledge. Such discussions should also promote more curiosity about what other models of mental ills, and other medical traditions or perspectives, might have to teach us.

Most of our knowledge about possible efficacy of treatments comes from clinical trials. In the case of surgical intervention in the brain, novel study designs are needed (e.g. on/off design) to determine the impact and safety of a given therapy for the individual patient. An ablation to treat obsessive–compulsive disorder (OCD) in some patients, or DBS, as in Helen Mayberg's pioneering work with severely depressed patients (Lozano *et al.* 2008), may resolve psychiatric symptomatology, but also may lead to adverse sequelae.

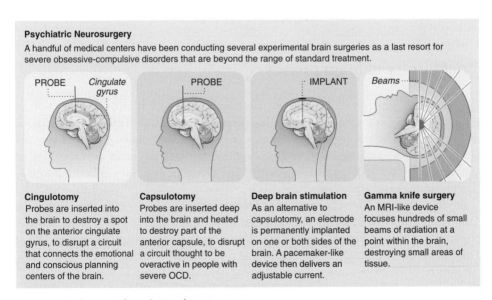

Psychiatric Neurosurgery
A handful of medical centers have been conducting several experimental brain surgeries as a last resort for severe obsessive-compulsive disorders that are beyond the range of standard treatment.

Cingulotomy
Probes are inserted into the brain to destroy a spot on the anterior cingulate gyrus, to disrupt a circuit that connects the emotional and conscious planning centers of the brain.

Capsulotomy
Probes are inserted deep into the brain and heated to destroy part of the anterior capsule, to disrupt a circuit thought to be overactive in people with severe OCD.

Deep brain stimulation
As an alternative to capsulotomy, an electrode is permanently implanted on one or both sides of the brain. A pacemaker-like device then delivers an adjustable current.

Gamma knife surgery
An MRI-like device focuses hundreds of small beams of radiation at a point within the brain, destroying small areas of tissue.

FIG. 21.7 (Also see Plate 9). Psychiatric neurosurgery.

Patients may be driven by unrealistic expectations (Kravitz, *et al.* 1996). Clinician scientists may be overwhelmingly idealistic and dedicated, but may be driven by a zeal to discover and succeed (El-Hai 2005). Companies with huge resources committed to clinical trials may be driven by the profit motive, hoping for a breakthrough drug, device, or procedure. Together these produce a perfect storm of competing interests. Neuroethicists will be needed to help resolve the dilemmas posed by the principle to respect the autonomy of the desperate patient, anxious to access innovative therapies, and the principles of beneficence and non-maleficence to protect that patient from harm caused by a high risk, unproven procedure. Neuroethicists must elaborate strong and persuasive arguments concerning the merits and drawbacks of experimental procedures, so that any participation in clinical trials can be optimized to serve the greatest good for neurological and psychiatric patients. Neuroethicists must remain unbiased, and promote clinical equipoise. They must not be seen as barriers to advancing the frontiers of brain therapy. With appropriate safeguards in place, they even can be advocates for high risks potential high gain procedures.

Medical tourism is growing more popular as many desperate people consider American medicine at times too conservative and unwilling to take risks when they, the patients, seemingly have almost nothing to lose. In addition, excellent medicine at greatly reduced cost is available in countries such as India and Thailand. The same minimally invasive neurosurgical techniques used in the US, for example, gamma-knife irradiation and DBS, are offered in India at a fraction of the US cost (PR Log 2009). On the other hand, if the irrational hope for a cure turns into a disabling disaster of its own, this only adds to the tragedy of such patients. It is often unclear if anyone can, and should, be held responsible.

The complexity of addressing such situations as those with the new psychosurgeries, rife as they are with inherently conflicting hopes and motives, and of working to make the public at large, and patient populations and advocacy groups in particular, sufficiently neuroliterate, suggests once more that neuroethicists are very needed, now more than ever.

Brain privacy

Brief history of brain privacy

Historically, the inner thoughts and personality traits of the vast majority of people were of little consequence in the wider sphere, unless persons were accused of crimes or sedition, or as an inspiration to novelists. Yet, awareness of personal and familial privacy is very old (Aries and Duby 1987). Recently, we have begun to think about "brain" privacy, whether concerning privacy of perceptions, memories, and thoughts, or privacy of health information pertaining to the status of the brain.

Aspects of personal privacy extended to privacy about health very early. *The Hippocratic Oath* reminds us that in Western culture, matters of health are not only private, between physician and patient, but considered distasteful to discuss beyond that relationship. "*What I may see or hear in the course of the treatment or even outside of the treatment in regard to the life of men, which on no account one must spread abroad, I will keep to myself, holding such things shameful to be spoken about.*" This standard clearly has been changing since the later

20th century, for mostly positive reasons, e.g. reduced shame about most health conditions, and increased discussion of health issues in all media. Concerns about privacy of electronic health records remain. Yet if worry about loss of some aspects of privacy has diminished, the ability to breach privacy of the brain and thoughts technologically has increased worries considerably.

Neuromarketing is one new concern. With the rise of mass production and then modern advertising in the later 19th century in the West, for the first time many people became major consumers of goods (Hudson 2008). Only then did the incentive to plumb material desires and buying habits arise. In the 21st century, commercial interests wish to find the means not only to influence but also to identify individuals' thoughts, choices, attitudes, and preferences, for example by accessing their online behavior, or using brain imaging. Neuroeconomics investigations have been systematizing more of our knowledge of the brain basis of choice and reward (Astolfi *et al.* 2008; Walter *et al.* 2005). So-called neuromarketers (e.g. SalesBrain) now assert they know best how to market, based on the nature of the brain. Some say neural activation patterns from imaging can reliably indicate interest in a type or brand of product, or political preference (see Caldwell 2007; Iacoboni *et al.* 2007; Lee *et al.* 2007). While neuromarketing is not yet widespread, it is troubling. It could lead to "invasion of brain privacy," and it involves distortion and potentially inappropriate commercialization of science.

Humans have always tried both to infer the thoughts of normal individuals from non-verbal cues, verbal content, and behavior, and to understand the abnormal thoughts of the psychologically ill. Yet until only recently, one's inner life remained fundamentally private and largely inaccessible, often even to oneself. The rise of experimental and psychoanalytic psychology in the later 19th century brought about fundamental changes, and led to many historically new approaches to plumbing mental contents. These included everything from psychophysical (e.g. Wundt, Fechner) and reaction time (e.g. Donders) experiments to characterize structure and function of basic perceptual and cognitive processes (see Snodgrass *et al.* 1985), to structured methods of introspection (James 1890), and the rise of early modern psychiatric and psychoanalytic methods (e.g. Charcot, Freud).

The invention of projective psychological testing (Rorschach, Thematic Apperception Test (TAT), and others) in the early to mid-20th century, also gave examiners the possibility of investigating the mind, identifying pathologies, and typing personalities. Leading clinicians refined these techniques, which still are in use (Rapaport, Gill and Shafer 1945/1978). In the popular imagination, projective tests often were seen as a means of spying into minds (Lemov 2009). Clinical psychological assessment began as a high-priority activity of the Office of Strategic Services (OSS; forerunner of the CIA) during World War II, to profile and recruit agents for intelligence work, and accomplish other wartime goals. Harvard psychologist Henry A. Murray, inventor of the TAT, guided many of these efforts, including profiling Adolf Hitler. Students in Murray's Harvard classes also were psychologically profiled, as an academic requirement. It was only understood later that psychological self-revelation can have its costs. One student in particular was alleged to have been damaged by the experience—the young Theodore Kaczynski, who became the Unabomber (Chase 2000).

The business world now often uses projective tests (Wimmer and Dominick 2006). Clinicians still do, but these tests have been criticized as relying too heavily on examiners' clinical judgment, and may lack reliability and validity (Cordón 2005). Yet despite the rise of biological psychiatry and brain imaging, the information these clinical tools can provide is strikingly different, and therefore not redundant.

Psychological and occupational assessment tools long used by potential employers (e.g. Meyers-Briggs Type Indicator (MBTI)) likely still can yield more useful information about a job candidate than a brain scan, at a much lower cost, for the vast majority of applicants and positions. We also are far from linking patterns of brain response to most job-relevant traits and behaviors. Canli (2006), however, showed that neuroimages can predict some kinds of behavior better than either self-reported measures or reaction time data. He believes that in the future, brain imaging data, combined with life history and genetic information, may predict aspects of behavior and personality very precisely. But can these predictors become inexpensive enough to use for such non-medical purposes, and will they have true practical value? SAT tests, a widely used and precisely calibrated measure of aspects of intelligence and academic performance, can be mass administered, as can some personality inventories. While SATs give college admissions offices useful data, they still can fail to predict who will be successful in college and life. Too many other factors can influence those outcomes.

We are judged primarily by what we do, not what we may privately think. People learn to restrain most harmful impulses, and can seek change through spiritual, psychotherapeutic, and other efforts. What, therefore, would be the utility of most hypothetical efforts to use brain technologies to spy on people's inner life? This is likely to be unaffordable, impractical, and unproductive in most cases, except perhaps critical forensic ones where the legal right to examine a suspect or defendant might appropriately be obtained. An identified terrorist is one such example. Attempts to "spy" on mental or behavioral patterns using brain imaging in most contexts would be considered unethical, invasive, undemocratic, and in violation of constitutional rights to privacy as well as protection from unreasonable search and seizure.

The era of documentable intrusion into experienced perceptions if not thoughts, however, may have begun. Striking recent studies using sophisticated computer vision algorithms have shown that it is possible to reconstruct or "see" what a research subject has just seen (but not "thought"). This technology, thus far used to reconstruct visual cortex content of innocuous experimental scenes, could not be used to probe the brain for older visual memory content, or probe for abstract thought or silent language (Kay *et al.* 2008; Makni *et al.* 2008; Miyawaki *et al.* 2008; Naselaris *et al.* 2009). With advancing technology, however, hypothetically more personal or meaningful mental contents from a person's past could be reconstructed and accessed.

Neuroethicists have begun and are needed to lead in establishing ethical guidelines in all these situations.

Brain privacy in psychiatry

Brain privacy is a significant issue in psychiatry. Erick Cheung (2009) asserts that "neuroscience and technology also have important ethical consequences for the practice of psychiatry that have yet to be fully considered." We would agree. Neuroethicists will be needed to help psychiatry frame many neuroethical questions it may not always consider from its disciplinary point of view. Psychiatrists obtain a wide range of information and data about individuals to optimize treatment for often grave neuropsychiatric or psychological conditions. Electronic medical records gradually are becoming the norm: electronically stored brain scans, EEG (electroencephalogram) data, results of treatment with brain stimulation modalities (e.g. TMS, ECT, DBS), and other psychological tests and measures of brain functioning, will be information potentially available to be misused. Being labeled with a psychiatric diagnosis has always had major implications including stigma.

Employment security and interpersonal bias are constant concerns for persons diagnosed with a psychiatric condition. Recall the leak concerning the depression and ECT of Senator Thomas Eagleton, running as vice-presidential candidate with George McGovern in 1972. The revelation ended his candidacy (Editorial, TIME Magazine 1972). Neuroethicists will be needed to work with psychiatrists, neurologists, and others to insure that in seeking needed treatment, patients are not subjected to a less stringent standard of personal privacy than non-patients. If the use of brain scans becomes more common in employment screening, people with a history of psychiatric illness might well show atypical or clinically suggestive scan patterns, even if they are well and able to work.

A brain scan of a person with schizophrenia or severe depression typically will show hypofrontality (abnormally low activation in key areas of frontal cortex) (Figure 21.8). If a person in a research study shows hypofrontality on a scan as an incidental finding, but has not been diagnosed with an illness, what does this mean? What action if any should be taken, concerning the participant, and the data?

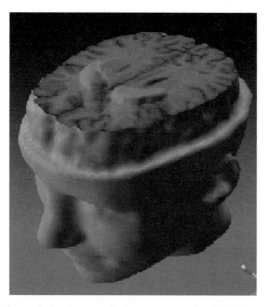

FIG. 21.8 (Also see Plate 10). Positron emission tomography (PET) image. Scan of a patient with schizophrenia. (Source: Andreas Meyer-Lindenberg, M.D., Ph.D., NIMH Clinical Brain Disorders Branch). http://www.nih.gov/news/pr/jan2002/nimh-28.htm (accessed 22 December 2009).

Scans could become a tool of discrimination and thwarted potential. Too little is known about the relationship of brain scans taken at a point in time to overt symptomatology and prognoses (Boyce 2009; Cheung 2009).

Consideration of ethical guidelines and possibly even laws to ensure brain privacy in research, clinical healthcare, and other contexts should start now. Twentieth- and 21st-century psychology and psychiatry have brought us much closer to reliably accessing and analyzing aspects of thought and personality, and yet what we still do not understand is vast.

Lie detection

The cost of brain imaging inevitably will fall in the years to come. Use of functional brain imaging (functional magnetic resonance imaging, fMRI) may become more commonplace, and could possibly be used beyond approved medical and research contexts. The visual format of imaging is powerful and can become too concretely/simplistically interpreted even among professionals ("new phrenology"); it can so more easily be misunderstood by the public or in commercial contexts. Even today, amid much concern (Fischbach and Fischbach 2005; Greely and Illes 2007; see also Murphy and Greely, Chapter 38, this volume), some companies are marketing use of brain scans for lie detection and personnel evaluation (e.g. Cephos, No Lie MRI, Inc.). These companies, aggressively marketing their services to private companies and government agencies, in some cases involve brain scientists as scientific advisors or active partners. But does the science support this use? While the techniques of some companies extrapolate from current science, the current authors believe they can mislead the public and potential clients, exaggerating the valid information that can be extracted from individual as opposed to averaged brain scans. It seems likely that regulations regarding this application of brain imaging are needed; some authors have argued vehemently in favor of such action (Greely and Illes 2007). Who will monitor regulatory compliance by these companies? Neuroethicists are needed to address these issues.

In dystopian futuristic movie scenarios such as *The Matrix* series, an agent is able to coercively access the brain to manipulate consciousness, know what people are thinking, and probe memories of past events. This fictional scenario is not entirely beyond imagining. It is possible to further imagine a time when a legal instrument such as a "brain search warrant" might exist. Courtroom use of brain scans for lie detection is being hotly debated, as is the EEG result known as the P300 component of a brain wave that can be used to probe aspects of memory (e.g. Fox 2008; Iacono 2008; Meegan 2008).

Physiological measures such as fMRI scans, P300 EEG responses, galvanic skin response, analysis of minute details of facial expression (Ekman 2003, 2009), and others, all now tell us much about emotion and cognition, in specific contexts. All these kinds of evidence, however, still are deemed inadmissible in a court of law, as they cannot reliably document "the truth."

Concern about brain privacy is warranted

Does neurotechnology encroach dangerously on the privacy of brain processes and the self today? Certainly entities such as health insurance companies, life insurance companies, and prospective employers might have the wish to use psychiatric or electronic health records to reveal the status of an individual's brain, or how that brain would function in certain circumstances (Ackerman 2006, p. 29). Illes argues that brain data should certainly have as much, if not more, protection than genetic data, which is certainly another new area involving major privacy concerns (see the Genetic Information Non-Discrimination Act of 2007; Illes and Racine 2005). It is unclear if this protection will eventually extend to neuroimaging as well, given how much less is known about the results and interpretation of brain imaging data.

Concern *is* warranted about the validity of human thought content extrapolated from brain imaging and other technologies, and the uses to which this content may be put that could be deemed invasive, harmful, and ethically inappropriate.

As neurotechnology advances, and as research results accumulate, it may seem we can make conclusions about very specific thoughts or brain states; however, mostly this assumption would be wrong. Compelling images of the brain at work have enormous appeal in these uncertain times, yet several major technical problems must be overcome before neuroscience can help resolve the contentious and challenging problem of brain privacy (Fischbach and Fischbach 2005; Glenn 2005; Wolpe *et al.* 2005).

NEUROETHICISTS AND THEIR CONTRIBUTIONS

Neuroethicists are needed now more than ever to become professionals qualified in bioethics, neuroscience, and allied areas. They will invest career time in analyzing neuroethical problems in depth, and educating about neuroethical questions by integrating diverse expertise from many domains. Clinically, they will help find more neuroethical solutions to research issues and clinical questions relevant to brain function and health. Vitally important, they will help the public and policy makers resolve neuroethical conundrums, and provide advocacy and safeguards. Neuroethicists also will play a critical role in guiding the media to avoid hype and hyperbole in their effort to report promising research.

To date, neurologists, neuroscientists, psychiatrists, psychologists (clinical and research), philosophers, historians of science, legal ethicists, bioethicists, sociomedical scientists, epidemiologists, and others have been contributing to the field of neuroethics. To the extent that we now have "professional" neuroethicists, likely they are coming from these diverse ranks.

Some argue that neuroethics should stay close to its clinical roots (e.g. Jones 2008), or be a branch of bioethics dedicated to protecting our brains and minds (Safire 2002). Some ask for a broader approach, beyond "bioethics for the brain" (Gazzaniga 2005). The clinical perspective is absolutely necessary, but we argue it is not sufficient. While many neuroethical questions will remain close to clinical medicine and neuroscience research, some neuroethical issues—and doubtless many yet to be defined—extend well beyond narrow clinical ones. Many will have ethical, legal, economic, and social implications for every citizen. It is only appropriate that knowledge and experience from other disciplines, as relevant, be weighed along with medical knowledge.

We do not argue for a neuroethics cottage industry within every academic discipline. We must not forget, however, that many recommendations that may improve our healthcare system are derived from beyond medicine—from law, public policy, and public advocacy. The public increasingly needs guidance, and needs to be educated about clinical and research issues concerning the brain, in a phrase, the public needs neuroliteracy (Illes *et al.* 2009). An informed voting public that can understand issues is a necessity in a complex society, one in which many funding and strategic priorities compete, and in which often deliberate misinformation is disseminated for political, economic, or other advantage. In addition, while a subset of society—those in medicine, neuroscience, and allied academic and clinical disciplines—develop and extend knowledge of brain sciences, they could easily leave the nonspecialist and lay public far behind. Given the likelihood that many neuroethical questions will be relevant to the wider society, in personal (medical) and general (policy, political) contexts, an ill-informed public will leave us lacking in sufficient, considered, and informed societal participation when we will need it.

Educating neuroethicists

With emerging complex issues in the brain sciences, few would doubt that neuroscientists need at least some neuroethics training (Morein-Zamir and Sahakian 2009; Sahakian and Morein-Zamir 2009; Lombera *et al.* 2010). Non-neuroscientists whose work will comment on brain sciences concomitantly need basic grounding in neuroscience. The idea of a "neuroscience bootcamp" (University of Pennsylvania 2009b) seemed timely. Academic and professional trainees need grounding in neuroethics when relevant to their work. Neuroethics curricula and increased educational efforts and outreach are needed. Neuroethicists will be needed to develop these curricula, collaboratively. The central importance to so many clinical and research activities of understanding the brain mandates that much wider, deeper, more accurate, and accessible knowledge about the brain and nervous system becomes available to learners at every stage. In this task, Web-based distance learning programs can play a large role. Some programs currently are available, such as *Neuroethics: Implications of Advances in Neuroscience,* the Columbia University Center for Bioethics online course (2008) funded by the Dana Foundation; and the Neuroethics module available on Health Sciences Online (Lombera *et al.* 2010), a portal where health professionals in training and practice can access free, comprehensive, high quality, current courses, references, and other learning resources to improve global health.

Given the need to educate neuroethicists, some universities have created Masters programs in neuroethics. Interdisciplinary 1-year certificate programs in neuroethics also could be created, tailored for well-prepared professionals or academics who are non-specialists. These programs could provide modular course offerings that would meet the learners' needs—in bioethics, neurohistory, neuroscience, law, public policy, and so on.

Neuroethicists will be needed to serve in diverse settings and capacities

In scholarly and professional contexts, neuroethics rightly has emerged as an interdisciplinary field. We feel that neuroethics, even while becoming an academic subspecialty, should not become overly self-referential. Questions neuroethicists ask should remain diverse and inherently linked to other relevant disciplinary knowledge. How exactly this will work in practice will unfold as the field continues to evolve.

In addition to scholarly work, we see a need for the neuroethicist to function in clinical settings in neurology, psychiatry, and allied clinical areas, to educate and to discuss difficult decisions with patients and family members, much as genetic counselors do. Families are likely to request the most current information and the chance to explore in depth the risks and benefits of cutting-edge options. It may reassure patients and families to know that they could consult the neuroethicist as well as the brain specialist. In the same way, Howard Gardner and others proposed that parents could consult neuroeducators, specialists in both education and neuroscience (Sheridan *et al.* 2007).

Neurological and psychiatric consultations at times may require that cross-cultural gaps and gaps of understanding about brain-related procedures and treatments be bridged. Physicians and physician/scientists are likely to have limited time for this; they could work with a consulting neuroethicist on their clinical team. In clinical settings, neuroethicists also could educate other professional personnel such as medical students, residents, nurses, social workers, clergy, and others about clinical neuroethical issues.

To educate varied disciplines in neuroethics, multiple options are available or should be created, such as specialty conferences or sections in neuroscience and ethics, continuing medical education (CME), lecture series, and tailored educational services for psychiatry, neurology, and other medical divisions.

Neuroethicists should be found not only by the hospital bedside but squarely in the university classroom. They will be needed to create graduate and undergraduate courses so that students at any level, as they advance in their understanding of brain sciences, could benefit from perspectives of neuroethicists. Fortified by their historical knowledge, neuroethicists could forestall risky or unethical academic endeavors.

Some of the most notorious behavioral science experiments of the 20th century that stretched the limits of ethical conduct of research took place in university settings.

At Yale, Stanley Milgram' 1963 obedience to authority experiments (1974) (Figure 21.9) and Philip Zimbardo's Stansford simulated prison experiments (Figure 21.10) conducted in 1971 (2007) are now seen as unacceptable.

Nonetheless they did obtain findings that revealed great insights about human behavior. These controversial and indeed infamous studies help us today to understand the tragedies of the My Lai massacre as well as the torture and prisoner abuses of Abu Ghraib and Guantanamo Bay.

We strongly urge institutional review boards (IRBs) to routinely have a neuroethicist serving as a member. With experimental protocols that offer potential promise in the face of anticipated risk, a neuroethicist can be indispensable to assess the risk–benefit calculus and guide a robust informed consent process. Faced with protocols involving dual use, controversial brain surgery and imaging procedures, neurogenetic studies, and even issues suggesting threats to brain privacy or manipulation of public attitudes, a well-prepared neuroethicist can play a pivotal role in protecting research subjects. Many terminally ill patients will state they have nothing to lose so they should be allowed to participate in extreme brain or nervous system experiments. It will fall to the neuroethicist to point out the pain and suffering that may be a consequence of the protocol, which could seem worse than death itself. Neuroethicists can serve to protect the rights and promote the welfare of those who volunteer to advance the frontiers of clinical neuroscience.

In legal contexts, neuroethicists might offer an addition or alternative to psychiatrists or neurologists having no specialty education in ethics who are asked to testify in legal proceedings. Neuroethicists might be seen as more neutral, and well rounded on points of ethics and relevant precedents.

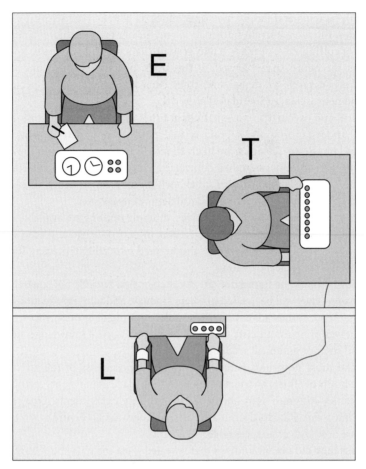

FIG. 21.9 Obedience to authority experiment of Stanley Milgram. The experimenter (E) orders the teacher (T), the subject of the experiment, to give what the latter believes are painful electric shocks to a learner (L), who is actually an actor and confederate. The subject believes that for each wrong answer, the learner was receiving actual electric shocks, though in reality there were no such punishments. Being separated from the subject, the confederate set up a tape recorder integrated with the electroshock generator, which played prerecorded sounds for each shock level.

Public and professional contributions of neuroethicists

Neuroethicists can serve as activists, contributing their knowledge as private and/or public citizens. Their unique knowledge is needed for policy and advocacy discussions in many contexts that involve complex and contentious neuroethical issues. Educating the media is an imperative to ensure public dissemination of bona fide neuroethical information rather than high-class hype.

Neuroethics expertise also will be needed in government and the private sector at many levels, e.g. federal research study sections at the National Institutes of Health (NIH), Centers for Disease Control and Prevention (CDC), and National Science Foundation (NSF); federal, state, and local policy commissions; in industry at pharmaceutical and device

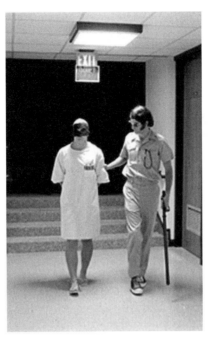

FIG. 21.10 Stanford Prisoner's Experiment of Philip Zimbardo.

companies; and in private think tanks, foundations, and policy institutes (e.g. The Hastings Center, Dana Foundation, Alzheimer's Disease Foundation, etc.).

Government and private funders will need guidance concerning neuroethical issues that will arise in the science they are evaluating for support. Having a consulting neuroethicist review proposals in advance can help avert potential ethical pitfalls in the research; neuroethically poor proposals would be flagged for revisions or rejected, and better ones strengthened.

Professional outreach and networking will be needed to obtain wider input, as new issues continue to arise that will need careful analysis from multiple perspectives. Who will mount and coordinate efforts to do so? Neuroethicists whose multidisciplinary education allows them to combine key types of expertise at a high level, and who can collaboratively tackle the epistemological and scientific challenges of today.

CONCLUSION

When we deal with brain science, we are dealing with the organ that makes us unique individuals, that gives us our personality, memories, emotions, dreams, creative abilities, and at times, our sinister selves. (Fischbach 2005, p. xiii)

In the age of neuro-everything, as we enter novel and daring new territories, neuroethicists will be needed to formulate many essential questions, and provide much-needed guidance in addressing difficult and ethically challenging problems. Neuroethics can serve as the common ground for stakeholders, and neuroethicists can bring their broad body of knowledge and critical thinking skills to the table. Neuroethicists are needed as part of a large-scale effort to speed up the integration of diverse knowledge, much as translational medicine is working to speed up valid and safe use of bench discoveries of clinical relevance, bench to bedside. We contend that neuroethicists can guide the equivalent process, and help mitigate or resolve ethical problems in research and clinical treatment. Well-prepared neuroethicists, working within a very interdisciplinary context, are needed now more than ever.

References

Ackerman, S.J. (2006). *Hard Science, Hard Choices: Facts, Ethics, and Policies Guiding Brain Science Today*. New York: Dana Press.

Annas, G.J. (2005). "Culture of life" politics at the bedside—The case of Terri Schiavo. *New England Journal of Medicine*, **352**, 1710–15.

Aries, P. and Duby, G. (1987). *A History of Private Life*. Cambridge, MA: The Belknap Press of Harvard University Press.

Astolfi, L., De Vico Fallani, F., Cincotti F., *et al.* (2008). Neural basis for brain responses to TV commercials: a high-resolution EEG study. *IEEE Trans Neural Systems Rehabilitation Engineering*, **16**, 522–31.

Boyce, A.C. (2009). Neuroimaging in psychiatry: evaluating the ethical consequences for patient care. Bioethics, **23**, 349–59.

Bublitz, J.C. and Merkel, R. (2009). Autonomy and authenticity of enhanced personality traits. *Bioethics*, **23**, 360–74.

Caldwell, M. (2007). Careers in behavioral science. Neuromarketing careers. *Science*, **316**, 1060–1.

Canli, T. (2006). When genes and brains unite: ethical implications of genomic neuroimaging. In J. Illes (ed.) *Neuroethics: Defining the Issues in Theory, Practice, and Policy*, p. 175. New York: Oxford University Press.

Carey, B. (2009a). Surgery for mental ills offers both hope and risk. *New York Times*, 26 November. Available at: http://www.nytimes.com/2009/11/27/health/research/27brain.html (accessed 16 December 2009).

Carey, B. (2009b). Brain researchers open door to editing memory. *New York Times*, 5 April. Available at: http://www.nytimes.com/2009/04/06/health/research/06brain.html (accessed 16 December 2009).

Cassell, E.J. (2005). The Schiavo case: A medical perspective. *The Hastings Center Report*, **35**, 20–3.

Center for Bioethics, Columbia University. *Neuroethics: Implications of Advances in Neuroscience*. Available at: http://ccnmtl.columbia.edu/projects/neuroethics/index.html (accessed 16 December 2009).

Chase, A. (2000). Harvard and the making of the Unabomber. *The Atlantic Monthly*, **285**, 41–65.

Chen, I. (2009). The court will now call its expert witness: the brain. The Stanford Report Online, 19 November. Available at: http://news.stanford.edu/news/2009/november16/greely-neurolaw-issues-111909.html (accessed 16 December 2009)

Cheung, E.H. (2009). A new ethics of psychiatry: neuroethics, neuroscience, and technology. *Journal of Psychiatric Practice*, **15**, 391–401.

Chneiweiss, H. (2011). Does cognitive enhancement fit with the physiology of our cognition? In J. Illes and B.J. Sahakian (eds.) *Oxford Handbook of Neuroethics*, pp.00–00. Oxford: Oxford University Press.

Columbia University, Center for Bioethics. *Neuroethics: Implications of Advances in Neuroscience*. Available at: http://ccnmtl.columbia.edu/projects/neuroethics/index.html (accessed 16 December, 2009)

Conrad, P. (2007). *The Medicalization of Society: On the Transformation of Human Conditions into Medical Disorders*. Baltimore, MD: John Hopkins University Press.

Cordón, L.A. (2005). *Popular psychology: an encyclopedia*, pp. 201–4. Westport, CT: Greenwood Press.

Cranford, R.E. (1989). The neurologist as ethics consultant and as a member of the institutional ethics committee. The neuroethicist. *Neurological Clinics*, 7, 697–713.

Delgado, J.M. and Anshen, R.N. (1969). *Physical Control of the Mind: Toward a Psychocivilized Society*. New York: Harper and Row.

Dimidjian, S. and Davis, K.J. (2009). Newer variations of cognitive-behavioral therapy: behavioral activation and mindfulness-based cognitive therapy. *Current Psychiatry Reports*, **11**, 453–8.

Dresser, R. (2005). Schiavo's legacy: The need for an objective standard. *The Hastings Center Report*, **35**, 20–2.

Editorial (1972). The Campaign: McGovern's First Crisis: The Eagleton Affair. *TIME Magazine*, 7 August. http://www.time.com/time/magazine/article/0,9171,879139,00.html (accessed 10 January, 2010).

Ekman, P. (2003). *Emotions Revealed: Recognizing Faces and Feelings to Improve Communication and Emotional Life*. New York: Times Books.

Ekman, P. (2009). *Telling Lies: Clues to Deceit in the Marketplace, Politics, and Marriage*. New York: W.W. Norton & Co.

El-Hai, J. (2005). *The Lobotomist: A Maverick Medical Genius and His Tragic Quest to Rid the World of Mental Illness*. Hoboken, NJ: John Wiley and Sons, Inc.

Federico, C.A., Lombera, S., and Illes, J. (2011). Intersecting complexities in neuroimaging and neuroethics. In J. Illes and B.J. Sahakian (eds.) *Oxford Handbook of Neuroethics*, pp.00–00. Oxford: Oxford University Press.

Fins, J.J. (2003a). Constructing an ethical stereotaxy for severe brain injury: balancing risks, benefits and access. *Nature Reviews Neuroscience*, **4**, 323–7.

Fins, J.J. (2003b). From psychosurgery to neuromodulation and palliation: history's lessons for the ethical conduct and regulation of neuropsychiatric research. *Neurosurgical Clinics of North America*, **2**, 303–19, ix–x.

Fins, J.J. (2005). The Orwellian threat to emerging neurodiagnostic technologies. *American Journal of Bioethics*, **5**, 56–8.

Fins, J.J. (2008). Brain injury: The vegetative and minimally conscious states. In M. Crowley (ed.) *From Birth to Death and Bench to Clinic: The Hastings Center Bioethics Briefing Book for Journalists, Policymakers, and Campaigns*, pp. 15–20. Garrison, NY: The Hastings Center.

Fins, J.J. and Schiff, N.D. (2005). The afterlife of Terri Schiavo (in brief). *The Hastings Center Report*, **35**, 8.

Fischbach, R.L. (2006). Foreword. In S.J. Ackerman (ed.) *Hard Science, Hard Choices: Facts, Ethics, and Policies Guiding Brain Science Today*, p. xi. New York: Dana Press.

Fischbach, R.L. and Fischbach, G.D. (2005). The brain doesn't lie. *American Journal of Bioethics*, **5**, 54–5.

Fischbach, R.L. and Fischbach, G.D. (2008). Neuroethicists needed now more than ever. *American Journal of Bioethics Neuroscience*, **8**, 47–8.

Fox, D. (2008). Brain imaging and the Bill of Rights: Memory detection technologies and American criminal justice. *American Journal of Bioethics Neuroscience*, **8**, 34–6.

Gazzaniga, M. (2005). *The Ethical Brain*. New York: The Dana Press.

Glenn, L.M. (2005). Keeping an open mind: What legal safeguards are needed? *American Journal of Bioethics*, **5**, 60–1.

Greely, H.T. and Illes, J. (2007). Neuroscience-based lie detection: the urgent need for regulation. *American Journal of Law and Medicine*, **33**, 377–431.

Halbig, T.D., Tse, W., Frisina, P.G., *et al.* (2009). Subthalamic deep brain stimulation and impulse control in Parkinson's disease. *European Journal of Neurology*, **16**, 493–7.

Hardesty D.E. and Sackeim H.A. (2007). Deep brain stimulation in movement and psychiatric disorders. *Biological Psychiatry*, **61**, 831–5.

Hirsch, J. (2005). Functional neuroimaging during altered states of consciousness: how and what do we measure? *Progress in Brain Research*, **150**, 25–43.

Horwitz, A. and Wakefield, J. (2007). *The Loss of Sadness: How Psychiatry has Transformed Normal Sadness into Depressive Disorder*. New York: Oxford University Press.

Hudson, R. (2008). Cultural political economy meets global production networks: a productive meeting? *Journal of Economic Geography*, **8**, 421–40.

Iacoboni, M., Freedman, J., Kaplan, J., *et al.* (2007). This is your brain on politics. *New York Times*, 11 November. Available at: http://www.nytimes.com/2007/11/11/opinion/11freedman. html?scp=1&sq=This%20is%20your%20brain%20on%20politics&st=cse (accessed 30 December 2009).

Iacono, W.G. (2008). The forensic application of "brain fingerprinting": Why scientists should encourage the use of P300 memory detection methods. *American Journal of Bioethics Neuroscience*, **8**, 30–2.

Illes, J. (2006). *Neuroethics, neurochallenges: A needs-based research agenda*. Stanford Center for Biomedical Ethics. Available at: http://neuroethics.stanford.edu/documents/Illes. NeuroethicsSFN2006.pdf (accessed 30 December 2009).

Illes, J. (2008). Brain screening and incidental findings: flocking to folly? *Lancet Neurology*, **7**, 23–4.

Illes, J. (2009). Neurologisms. *American Journal of Bioethics*, **9**, 1.

Illes, J. and Chin, V.N. (2008). Bridging philosophical and practical implications of incidental findings in brain research. *Journal of Law and Medical Ethics*, **36**, 298–304, 212.

Illes, J., and Racine, E. (2005). Imaging or imagining? A neuroethics challenge informed by genetics. *American Journal of Bioethics*, **5**, 5–18.

Illes, J., Moser, M.A., McCormick, J.B., *et al.* (2010). Neurotalk: improving the communication of neuroscience research. *National Review of Neuroscience*, **11**, 61–9.

James, W. (1890). *The Principles of Psychology*. Available at http://psychclassics.yorku.ca/ James/Principles/index.htm. (accessed 6 January, 2010).

Jones, D.G. (2008). Neuroethics: adrift from a clinical base. *American Journal of Bioethics*, 8, 49–50.

Jones, J.H. (1981). *Bad Blood: The Tuskegee Syphilis Experiment*. New York: Free Press .

Kay, K.N., Naselaris, T., Prenger, R.J., and Gallant, J.L. (2008). Identifying natural images from human brain activity. *Nature*, 452, 352–5.

Kravitz, R.L., Callahan, E.J., Paterniti, D., *et al.* (1996). Prevalence and sources of patients' unmet expectations for care. *Annals Internal Medicine*, 125, 730–7.

Lee, N., Broderick, A.J., and Chamberlain, L. (2007). What is "neuromarketing"? A discussion and agenda for future research. *International Journal of Psychophysiology*, 63, 199–204.

Lemov, R. (2009). Towards a data base of dreams: assembling an archive of elusive materials, c. 1947–61. *History Workshop Journal*, 67, 44–68.

Lerner, B.H. (2005). Last-ditch medical therapy — revisiting lobotomy. *New England Journal of Medicine*, 353, 119–21.

Lipsman, N. and Bernstein, M. (2011). Ethical issues in functional neurosurgery: Emerging applications and controversies. In J. Illes and B.J. Sahakian (eds.) *Oxford Handbook of Neuroethics*, pp.00–00. Oxford: Oxford University Press.

Lisanby, S.H., Husain, M.M., Rosenquist, P.B., *et al.* (2009). Daily left prefrontal repetitive transcranial magnetic stimulation in the acute treatment of major depression: clinical predictors of outcome in a multisite, randomized controlled clinical trial. *Neuropsychopharmacology*, 34, 522–34.

Lombera, S. and Illes, J. (2009). The international dimensions of neuroethics. *Developing World Bioethics*, 9, 57–64.

Lombera S. and Illes J. Health Sciences Online Neuroethics Resources and References. http://neuroethicscanada.ca/National_Core_for_Neuroethics/Initiatives_files/Neuroethics References%26Resources.pdf (accessed 14 January 2010).

Lombera S., Fine, A., Grunau, R.E. *et al.* (2010). Ethics in neuroscience graduate training programs: views and models from Canada. *Mind, Brain and Education*. March 4(1): 20–27.

Lozano, A.M, Mayberg, H.S, Giacobbe, P., Hamani, C., Craddock, R.C., and Kennedy, S.H. (2008). Subcallosal cingulate gyrus deep brain stimulation for treatment-resistant depression. *Biological Psychiatry*, 64, 461–7.

Makni, S., Idier, J., Vincent, T., Thirion, B., Dehaene-Lambertz, G., and Ciuciu, P. (2008). A fully Bayesian approach to the parcel-based detection-estimation of brain activity in fMRI. *Neuroimage*, 41, 941–69.

McEwen, B.S. (2009). The brain is the central organ of stress and adaptation. *NeuroImage*, 47, 911–13.

McManamy, J. (2009). Father of the lobotomy. Thinking of giving someone a piece of your mind? Stay clear of Walter Freeman. *McMan's Depression and Bipolar Web*, http://www.mcmanweb.com/lobotomy.html Updated Nov 1, 2009 (accessed 11 January 2010).

Meegan, D.V. (2008). Neuroimaging techniques for memory detection: Scientific, ethical, and legal issues. *American Journal of Bioethics Neuroscience*, 8, 9–20.

Milgram, S. (1974). *Obedience to Authority; An Experimental View*. New York: Harper Collins.

Miyawaki, Y., Uchida, H., Yamashita, O., *et al.* (2008). Visual image reconstruction from human brain activity using a combination of multiscale local image decoders. *Neuron*, 60, 915–29.

Morein-Zamir, S. and Sahakian, B.J. (2010). Neuroethics and public engagement training needed for neuroscientists. *Trends in Cognitive Science*, 16 November [Epub ahead of print]

Morein-Zamir, S. and Sahakian, B.J. (2011). Pharmaceutical cognitive enhancement. In J. Illes and B.J. Sahakian (eds.) *Oxford Handbook of Neuroethics*, pp.00–00. Oxford: Oxford University Press.

Morrison, L. (2009). ECT: shocked beyond belief. *Australas Psychiatry*, 17, 164–7.

Murphy, E.R. and Greely, H.T. (2011). What will be the limits of neuroscience-based mind-reading in the law? In J. Illes and B.J. Sahakian (eds.) *Oxford Handbook of Neuroethics*, pp.00–00. Oxford: Oxford University Press.

Naselaris, T., Prenger, R.J., Kay K.N., Oliver, M., and Gallant, J.L. (2009). Bayesian reconstruction of natural images from human brain activity. *Neuron*, 63, 902–15.

National Human Genome Research Institute. Genetic Information Nondiscrimination Act of 2007. Available at: http://www.genome.gov/24519851 (accessed 16 December 2009).

Normann, C. and Berger, M. (2008). Neuroenhancement: status quo and perspectives. *European Archives of Psychiatry and Clinical Neuroscience*, 258, 110–14.

Pascual-Leone, A., Fregni, F., Steven, M.S., and Forrow, L. (2011). Noninvasive brain stimulation as a therapeutic and investigative tool: An ethical appraisal. In J. Illes and B.J. Sahakian (eds.) *Oxford Handbook of Neuroethics*, pp.00–00. Oxford: Oxford University Press.

Payne, N.A., and Prudic, J. (2009a). Electroconvulsive therapy: part I: A perspective on the evolution and current practice of ECT. *Journal of Psychiatric Practice*, 15, 346–68.

Payne, N.A., and Prudic, J. (2009b). Electroconvulsive therapy: part II: A biopsychosocial perspective. *Journal of Psychiatric Practice*, 15, 369–90.

Penfield, W. (1975). *The Mystery of the Mind: A Critical Study of Consciousness and the Human Brain*. Princeton, NJ: Princeton University Press.

Pieri, E., and Levitt, M. (2008). Risky individuals and the politics of genetic research into aggressiveness and violence. *Bioethics*, 22, 509–18.

Pontius, A.A. (1973). Neuro-ethics of "walking" in the newborn. *Perceptual and Motor Skills*, 37, 235–45.

Pontius, A.A. (1993). Neuroethics vs. neurophysiologically and neuropsychologically uninformed influences in child-rearing, education, emerging hunter-gatherers, and artificial intelligence models of the brain. *Psychological Reports*, 72, 451–8.

PR Log (Press Release). (2009). Psychosurgery in India, now at a lower price. 18 August. http://www.prlog.org/10312883-psychosurgery-in-india-now-at-lower-price.html (accessed 1/14/2010)

Prudic, J. (2008). Strategies to minimize cognitive side effects with ECT: aspects of ECT technique. *The Journal of ECT*, 24, 46–51.

Racine, E. (2008). Comment on "Does it make sense to speak of neuroethics?" *European Molecular Biology Organization Reports*, 9, 2–4.

Rosenberg, O., Shoenfeld, N., Kotler, M., and Dannon, P.N. (2009). Mood disorders in elderly population: neurostimulative treatment possibilities. *Recent Patent CNS Drug Discovery*, 4, 149–59.

Roskies, A. (2002). Neuroethics for the new millennium. *Neuron*, 35, 21–3.

Rossi, S., Haslett, M., Rossini, P.M., and Pascual-Leone, A. (2009). Safety of TMS Consensus Group. Safety, ethical considerations, and application guidelines for the use of transcranial magnetic stimulation in clinical practice and research. *Clinical Neurophysiology*, 120, 2008–39.

Sackeim, H.A., Prudic, J., Fuller, R., *et al.* (2007). The cognitive effects of electroconvulsive therapy in community settings. *Neuropsychopharmacology*, 32, 244–54.

Sackeim, H.A., Prudic, J., Nobler, M.S., *et al.* (2008). Effects of pulse width and electrode placement on the efficacy and cognitive effects of electroconvulsive therapy. *Brain Stimulation*, 1, 71–83.

Safire, W. (2002). *Neuroethics: Mapping the Field*. Dana Foundation. Available at: http://www.dana.org/news/cerebrum/detail.aspx?id=2872 (accessed 30 December 2009).

Sahakian, B.J. and Morein-Zamir, S. (2009). Neuroscientists need neuroethics teaching. *Science*, 325, 147.

Schiff N.D., Giacino J.T., Kalmar K., *et al.* (2007). Behavioral improvements with thalamic stimulation after severe traumatic brain injury. *Nature*, 448, 600–3.

Scruton, R. (2009). Statement made at open session of Technology, Neuroscience and the Nature of Being: Toward a Common Morality Conference. United Nations.

Sheridan, K., Zinchenko, E., and Gardner, H. (2007). Neuroethics in education. In J. Illes (ed.) *Neuroethics: Defining the Issues in Theory, Practice and Policy*, pp. 266–75. Oxford: Oxford University Press.

Sherman, F.T. (2009). Life-saving treatment for depression in elderly. Always think of electroconvulsive therapy (ECT). *Geriatrics*, 64, 8, 12.

Snodgrass, J.G., Levy-Berger, G., and Haydon, M. (1985). Human experimental psychology. New York: Oxford University Press.

Urry, H.L., van Reekum, C.M., Johnstone, T., *et al.* (2006). Amygdala and ventromedial prefrontal cortex are inversely coupled during regulation of negative affect and predict the diurnal pattern of cortisol secretion among older adults. *Journal of Neuroscience*, 26, 4415–25.

University of Pennsylvania, Center for Neuroscience & Society. *Overview of Neuroethics*. Available at: http://neuroethics.upenn.edu/index.php/penn-neuroethics-briefing/overview-of-neuroethics (accessed 16 December 2009)

University of Pennsylvania, Center for Neuroscience & Society. *NeuroscienceBootcamp*. Available at: http://www.neuroethics.upenn.edu/index.php/events/neuroscience-bootcamp (accessed 16 December 2009).

University of Minnesota, Center for Bioethics. *Chimeras*. http://www.ahc.umn.edu/img/assets/25857/chimeras.pdf (accessed 14 January 2010).

Walter, G., Fisher, K., and Harte, A. (2002). ECT in poetry. *Journal of ECT*, 18, 47–53.

Walter, H., Abler, B., Ciaramidaro, A., and Erk, S. (2005). Motivating forces of human actions. Neuroimaging reward and social interaction. *Brain Research Bulletin*, 67, 368–81.

Wilson, D. (2009). Poor children likelier to get antipsychotics. *New York Times*, 11 December. Available at: http://www.nytimes.com/2009/12/12/health/12medicaid.html?_r=2&tntemail0=y&emc=tnt&pagewanted=print (accessed 17 December 2009).

Wimmer, R.D. and Dominick, J.R. (2006). *Mass media research: an introduction*. Belmont, CA: Thomson Wadsworth.

Witt, K., Daniels, C., Reiff, J., *et al.* (2008). Neuropsychological and psychiatric changes after deep brain stimulation for Parkinson's disease: a randomized, multicentre study, *Lancet Neurology*, 7, 605–14.

Wolf, S.W. (2008). Neurolaw: The big question. *American Journal of Bioethics Neuroscience*, 8, 21–2.

Wolf, S.W., Lawrenz, F.P., Nelson, C.A., *et al.* (2008). Managing incidental findings in human subjects research: analysis and recommendations. *Journal of Law and Medical Ethics*, 36, 219–48, 211.

Wolpe, P.R., Foster, K.R., Langleben, D.G. (2005). Emerging neurotechnologies for lie-detection: Promises and perils. *American Journal of Bioethics*, 5, 39–49.

Zimbardo, P. (2007). *The Lucifer Effect: Understanding How Good People Turn Evil*. New York: Random House.

CHAPTER 22

INTERSECTING COMPLEXITIES IN NEUROIMAGING AND NEUROETHICS

CAROLE A. FEDERICO, SOFIA LOMBERA, AND JUDY ILLES

... [T]he evaluation of health-care activities is an ethical minefield, strewn with explosive material not easily detected by the naked eye... it is our duty to rush in where others fear to tread, even if in the process we find ourselves being maligned as insensitive troublemakers...

(Williams 1992).

INTRODUCTION

NEUROIMAGING has been to neuroethics what free will and determinism have been, albeit for much longer, to philosophy: pillars for scholarly inquiry and curiosity, and entries to dialogue, debate, and discovery. Early in the days of functional neuroimaging using magnetic resonance imaging (MRI) technology, Illes and colleagues (Illes *et al.* 2003) explored studies at the juncture of this exciting new way of interrogating signals from the brain using probes for behavioral response drawn from philosophy. With interest piqued by reproducible measures of regional blood flow in the human brain under well-defined conditions such as existential problem-solving, decision making, and trust, we meticulously documented emerging trends involving functional MRI (fMRI) studies among the several thousand papers published at the time. In this short chapter here, we build on that work and examine the hypothesis that almost 20 years after the first wave of such studies, the focus on neuroimaging and its application to complex and profoundly personal human behaviors has not abated. Infact, while many topics have captivated scholars interested in neuroethics, as the chapters in this volume show, we assert that neuroimaging studies remain an unwavering source of energy for the field. Toward this goal, we review some of the reasons that they have provoked so much attention in neuroethics and elsewhere, present a 2002–2008 update to the trends we documented for 1991–2001, compare this second generation of data to the first, and share our observations.

Synchronizing ethics and science

Consideration of the ethical, legal, and social implications of emerging technologies in science and medicine has historically lagged behind the discovery of the technological capabilities themselves. Delays in contemplating the acceptability and potential applications of biomedical advances have posed significant problems for the scientific community and the public alike. Consider for example, the impact on science when significant advances preceded thorough consideration of the potential ethical and social impact of genetic screening (Rothenberg and Terry 2002), the cloning of humans (Cho et al. 1999), and even genetically modified foods (Thompson and Hannah 2008). Advanced capabilities for understanding human thought and behavior enabled by modern neurotechnologies have brought their own substantial challenges to the forefront of scientific and public scrutiny. Unlike the past, however, scientists and scholars with interests at the intersection of neuroscience and ethics have been proactively anticipating ethical, legal and social issues in this domain of scientific pursuit, raising pointed questions about the brain and human nature, whether the information is what people in fact want or ought to know, and how best to communicate it.

The understanding of why people behave as they do is closely tied to aspects of everyday life including society's laws and religious beliefs. Neuroimaging is producing increasingly comprehensive explanations of human behavior in biological terms. To this end, neuroethicists have been asking: How does the biological basis of phenomena directly related to human motivation, reasoning and social attitudes affect how people think of others and themselves? Shall any knowledge be forbidden or left untapped and is the lament of some concerned scholars and citizens that we ought to leave some human phenomena unexplored legitimate? Innovations in neurotechnology bring to the foreground the need for an appraisal of the place and the limits of technology in the relationship between mind and brain and, ultimately, between values, people, and society.

Underlying many of the claims concerning the power of modern neuroimaging is the belief that functional imaging offers a direct picture of the human brain at work (Illes 2007). Such belief brings both promise and apprehension, and in this regard there has been a historical interest in ethics in neuroimaging. The widespread use of accessible, noninvasive neuroimaging techniques, such as fMRI, raises social and legal issues including privacy of thought, prediction of violence or disease, truthfulness, and personal responsibility for behavior (Illes and Racine 2005; Aggarwal 2009; Fenton et al. 2009). Will advances in neuroimaging give the criminal justice system revolutionary or troubling new tools (Meegan 2008)? Will data on how people process information influence how they are treated by society (Farah 2005)? Do they raise the potential for unjustified discrimination (Glannon 2006)?

The increasing attention to ethics in neuroscience is not surprising, therefore, given unique concerns surrounding apparent new capabilities to monitor and translate motivation into action.

WHERE WAS FUNCTIONAL MRI 15 YEARS AGO?

In Illes *et al.* (2003), we reported on peer-reviewed journal articles of studies using fMRI, alone or in combination with other imaging techniques, published between 1991 and 2001. We analyzed and coded each article by publication type—original research or review—and into one or more classifications for study type: motor, primary sensory, integrative sensory, basic cognition, higher-order cognition, emotion, clinical, methods development, non-human primate. The journals in which all coded papers were published were also tracked.

The initial search for relevant articles yielded 3426 unique returns published across 498 different journals. Regression analyses showed a significant increase for the original research and review papers, numbers of journals, and studies reporting clinical results and methods development. More importantly for our purposes, studies classified as higher-order cognition and emotion—i.e. non-clinical studies considered to have direct translation for everyday behaviors such as human motivation, reasoning and social attitudes—also increased significantly, at a rate of 0.8% per year. Given those results, Illes *et al.* called for more ethics input than before to the increasing application of neuroscience research to complex human phenomena. In addition, we appealed for a wider perspective on the construction of scientific knowledge in general in the context of such studies, and its meaning in the context of brain and mind, identity and personhood (Illes and Racine 2005).

WHERE IS FUNCTIONAL MRI NOW?

Has the landscape changed over the past 10 years of fMRI research? Here we sought to understand whether the increasing application of fMRI technology to non-clinical studies considered to have direct meaning for everyday behavior was a transient phenomenon due, for example, to the new opportunity for noninvasive, repeatable imaging with high spatial resolution, or a continuing one with enduring characteristics. To this end, we updated the taxonomy developed by Illes *et al.* (2003) for application to studies over the next decade (Table 22.1).

Our search for new studies began in 2002, the endpoint for the original study, and the year coincident with the Dana Foundation meeting that "[brought] together scientists, ethicists, humanists, and those concerned with social policy to reflect on the broad implications of current and ongoing research on the human brain" (Marcus 2002). The formal search for the updated database closed at the end of 2008. For consistency and comparability to the previous study, the comprehensive database of all articles using functional neuroimaging techniques was compiled using PubMed and OVID search engines. As before, the search included all permutations and acronyms of the term "functional magnetic resonance imaging," although we only considered original research studies this time. The database was manually

Table 22.1 Examples of major categories with "real-world implications": higher order cognition; self and mental states

Higher order cognition	Self and mental states
Decision making	Faces/facial expressions
Impulsivity	Humor
Problem-solving	Sexual behavior
Judgment	Race
Moral behavior	Arousal
Intelligence	Fear/phobia
Anticipation (self-monitoring)	Religion
Motivation (reward)	Sex differences (with high-order processing)
Craving (as in drug craving)	Empathy
Reasoning	Self/mind
Intention	Social behavior
	Personality traits

cleaned for duplications, as well as for irrelevant returns such as fMRI investigations of non-cerebral activity (e.g. renal or cardiac function).

After establishing intercoder reliability (Cohen's Kappa = 0.95), two of us (C.F. and S.L.) blind to journal, year, and author each coded half of the articles based on paper titles and, as necessary, abstracts, as having 'implications for real-world contexts' (Table 22.1) or not. Review articles and investigations using non-human animals were excluded from further categorization.

After a first round of independent review, we further categorized all relevant articles having "real-world implications" into one of the two categories as primary, and added a code for the secondary category if appropriate (Table 22.2). For example, a study such as "fMRI

Table 22.2 Examples of article codes

Code	Examples of representative papers
Higher order cognition	fMRI evidence for a three-stage model of deductive reasoning (Knauff *et al.* 2006) Neural substrates underlying impulsivity (King *et al.* 2003)
Self and mental states	Amygdalar activation associated with positive and negative facial expressions (Yang *et al.* 2002) Neural correlates of first-person perspective as one constituent of human self-consciousness (Vogeley *et al.* 2004) The role of "shared representations" in social perception and empathy: an fMRI study (Lawrence *et al.* 2006)
Higher order cognition and self and mental states	Minds, persons, and space: an fMRI investigation into the relational complexity of higher-order intentionality (Abraham *et al.* 2008) The self as a moral agent: linking the neural bases of social agency and moral sensitivity (Moll *et al.* 2007) Reward, motivation, and emotion systems associated with early-stage intense romantic love (Aron *et al.* 2005)

evidence for a three-stage model of deductive reasoning" (Knauff *et al.* 2006) was coded as higher order cognition, and the study, "The self as a moral agent: linking the neural bases of social agency and moral sensitivity" (Moll *et al.* 2007)was coded as both (Table 22.2). In all cases, discrepancies between reviewers' codes were decided by consensus upon joint review or in consultation with the third author.

The searches returned a total of 12,967 articles across 1378 unique journals. Of these, 1198 (9%) met the criterion for real-world implications as we defined it. The number of journal articles and journals publishing these articles increased steadily from 2002–2008 at an average rate of 186 new articles ($t_7 = 4.745$, p <0.01) and 38 journals ($t_7 = 2.739$, p <0.05), annually (Figure 22.1, primary axis).

In 2007 and 2008, reports of such studies exceeded 10% of the total number of functional neuroimaging articles per year. There were more than twice as many articles pertaining to self and mental states (67%, n = 797) than those of higher order cognition (27%, n = 326), and tenfold more than pertaining to both (6%, n = 75). This pattern did not change significantly over time (p >0.7; Figure 22.2).

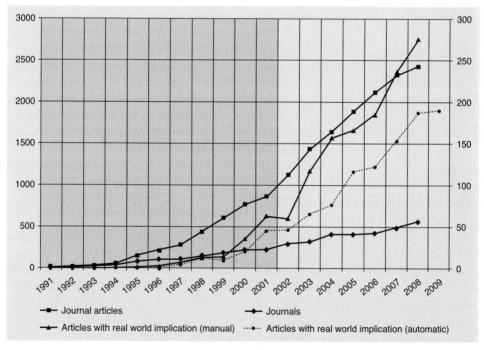

FIG. 22.1 Solid lines: number of journal articles, journals (primary y-axis) and articles with implications for real-world contexts (secondary y-axis) from 1991–2008. Data from Illes *et al.*, 2003 are shown in the shaded area. Dashed line: results of an automated query for fMRI studies with real-world implications (Garnett *et al.* 2010), also yielding up to date data. The automatic returns are predictably more conservative than the manual coding from which they are derived. 2009 data are likely low yields given still incomplete PubMed indexing for that year at the time of this writing (February 2010).

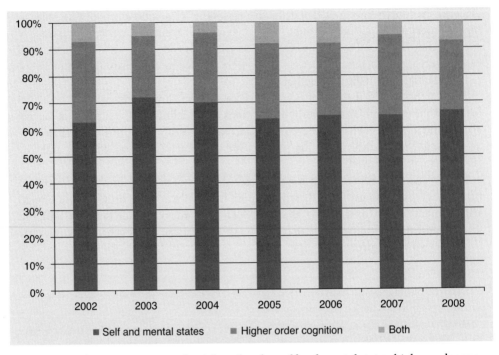

FIG. 22.2 Relative percentages of articles related to self and mental states, higher order cognition, both self and mental states and higher-order cognition from papers coded as having real-world validity between 2002–2008.

Discussion

The latest generation of fMRI

The data suggest that the power of fMRI, alone and combined with other imaging technologies such as EEG and PET, continues to be harnessed to pursue the neurobiology of complex, human phenomena. There was early momentum in the 1990s in this direction, and it was far from fleeting. Besides a sheer increase in numbers of studies, post-2002 fMRI research has revealed neural correlates and ever more intriguing results, for example, about the pain of losing a loved one and romantic love. For the former, Eisenberger et al. (2003) demonstrated that signals of social exclusion are similar to those of physical pain, and that related activity in the anterior cingulate cortex (ACC) acts as a neural alarm system during social exclusion. For the latter, Fisher et al. (2005) used stimuli invoking romantic love to produce activation in the right ventral tegmental area and right caudate nucleus, dopamine-rich areas associated with mammalian reward and motivation. Yet other studies have delved into biases and belief systems, suggesting that psychological dimensions of religion are mediated by brain networks that process intention and emotion and that engage abstract semantic processing (Harris et al. 2009; Kapogiannis et al. 2009).

The neuroscience of ethics and the neuroscience of everything else

In 2002, Adina Roskies provided thinkers in neuroethics with a clever way to conceptualize fMRI studies embodying a real-world component: she called them studies of the *neuroscience of ethics*. Besides heavily quoted definitions of neuroethics from the late William Safire and from Michael Gazzaniga, probably the next most cited is the two-part taxonomy of neuroethics provided by Roskies distinguishing these types of studies from those that focus on the conduct of research, *the ethics of neuroscience*. While the taxonomy appropriately characterizes the former classification of studies that we consider to have real-world relevance, and there are plenty of them as our data suggest, like all other fMRI research involving human subjects, these studies also contain fundamental research ethics issues captured by the *"ethics of…"* side of the taxonomy. Like studies of addiction (e.g. Volkow *et al.* 2004; Hall *et al.* 2008), minimally conscious states (e.g. Fins *et al.* 2008; Laureys *et al.* 2009), and aging (Greicius *et al.* 2004), fMRI of mental states has all the human subjects challenges of informed consent, capacity to consent, privacy, and confidentiality. Therefore, the simple dualism of the taxonomy inadvertently affords a special status to the studies having real-world implications where it does not necessarily belong.

While we are as guilty as others in perpetuating this oversimplification in now two studies (Illes *et al.* 2003; and by virtue of the data we have presented here), we wish to encourage a departure from it. We propose that *ethics of neuroscience* becomes the superordinate category for thinking about neuroimaging and ethics, and that new categories such as addiction neuroethics, and neuroethics of enhancement, of deep brain stimulation and of vegetative states, perhaps mirroring the formation of new interest groups within the professional Neuroethics Society (http://www.neuroethicssociety.org) be explicated as subcategories. This more fine-grain definition will unpackage the "other" studies according to the unique characteristics and scholarly focus they rightly possess and the new ethics challenges in neuroscience they bring forward. In parallel with this proposal, the chapter by Fishbach and Mindes (Chapter 21) and Fins (Epilogue) in this volume provide other illuminating strategies for meeting similar goals.

Forbidden knowledge?

Early studies falling into the (old) category of the *neuroscience of ethics* were quickly criticized as intruding on the very nature of humanness and, with the potential to biologize beliefs, spirituality, and human dignity, placing them at risk (Farah and Wolpe 2004). Some commentators expressed a keen need to preserve and keep them out of the hands of scientists (President's Council on Bioethics 2004). Yet others worried that such studies would lead neuroscience out of the science fiction of mind reading and into a reality that would give new meaning to what might be considered to be *truth unto its innermost parts* (the motto of the Massachusetts-based university named after Louis Dembitz Brandeis (1856–1941), Justice of the United States Supreme Court).

We reflect on these early writings and observe, first, that little has really changed about how people view themselves as moral beings, individuals and social actors as a result of relevant neuroimaging studies. In fact, after more than 15 years, there have been no shifts in religious or legal practice as a direct result of what has been learned from fMRI research, to our knowledge. Neuroscience is clearly informing policy (e.g. Greely and Illes 2007) and legal proceedings, and fMRI has now been admitted as evidence in the sentencing phase of a murder trial (Miller 2009), but to date have fundamentally changed neither policy nor the law.

Second, we observe that the publication of even some of the most remarkable studies of predictive phenomena, such as those of Haynes (Chapter 1, this volume) and Soon *et al.* (2008), or retrospective imaging evaluations of the truthfulness of past behaviors, have yet to find their place in the routine or daily life of the average person. There are anecdotes for attempts at the latter (Murphy and Greely, Chapter 38, this volume; McCormick and Brown, Chapter 40, this volume), and commercial endeavors around these applications, for lie detection in particular. They are enjoying considerable visibility but their readiness for prime time is dubious at best. Nevertheless, such studies are context-dependent, value-laden, and can be culturally sensitive. They create, therefore, a continued imperative for thoughtfulness and care at all points along the research to application trajectory, especially in the context of public understanding of neuroscience. While responsible science communication and accurate dissemination of findings are critical to ensure public support of and trust in neuroscience research (Illes *et al.* 2009), if the past predicts the future, early fears about the consequences of imaging research for our innermost sense of individuality can be calmed.

FUTURE CONSIDERATIONS AND CONCLUSIONS

Combined technologies

Where does the partnership between neuroimaging and neuroethics go from here? We predict that the coupling of technologies, such as neuroimaging with genetics-imaging genetics-is likely to propel neuroscience and medicine forward in the years to come, and the neuroethics discourse with it. Imaging genetics has emerged as a powerful and sensitive approach to the study of brain-relevant genetic polymorphisms with the potential to understand their impact on behavior (Bigos and Weinberger 2010). The combined technology has been applied, for example, to Alzheimer's and Huntington's disease with the goal of early prediction, improved disease tracking and advanced prevention strategies. It has been applied to improve the understanding of attention deficit hyperactivity disorder, depression, obsessive–compulsive disorder, anxiety, and schizophrenia, and to study emotional behavior (anxiety, response to fear) in healthy volunteers with different genotypes (Reiman 2007; Esslinger *et al.* 2009).

While imaging genetics remains a purely laboratory technique today, its potential integration into society requires careful reflection on how the knowledge may be constructed and interpreted by scientists, clinicians, patients, ethicists, and the lay public. The ethics challenges for genetics and neuroimaging have been explored at length separately, but the ethical space in which they overlap is just beginning to be explored. Tairyan and Illes (2009) suggested that the ethics issues at this juncture parallel the heightened discriminative power (the capacity to differentiate phenomena and distinguish them based on objective criteria) and cumulative power (the ability to gain greater information about the discriminated phenomena and by extension, associated ethics challenges) afforded by the powerful combination of technologies. In the new space, features of discriminative power concern better differentiation of disease, sometimes by ethnicity, and incidental findings. Features of clinical utility, prediction and intervention, and stigma and labeling share a common ground between discriminative and cumulative power. Privacy, autonomy, response sensitivity and attitudes, resource allocation for research and for health care, and commercialization, are features of cumulative power. The combined space also yields unique neuroethics considerations for science and society. These are characterized by new knowledge and new implications for health care, justice, and policy.

Implications for persons and personalized medicine

Ever-improving neurotechnologies and tools such as imaging, genetics, their combination or others to identify diseases and disease variants of the brain will bring the promise of personalized medicine to reality. Ethical issues related to the cost of health care and resource allocation notwithstanding, lives have already been changed through new knowledge about brain function, improved diagnosis of pathology, and movement toward tailored therapeutic interventions (Matthews *et al.* 2006; Monti *et al.* 2009).

The hope and promise has been and will be complicated, however, by direct-to-consumer marketing strategies adopted by an eager for profit sector both for clinical and non-clinical applications. The practical challenges of evidence for effectiveness, complexity of information, oversight and regulation, and tensions with traditional approaches to clinical practice described both for genetics (Conti 2010) and imaging (Illes *et al.* 2007; Lau and Illes 2009) will surely come into play. We are confident, however, that the type of forethought promulgated by neuroethics will pave the path by which benefits can reach people and patients, and will inform policy that sensibly and effectively mitigates risks.

Acknowledgements

The authors' work is generously supported by CIHR/INMHA CNE #85177, the British Columbia Knowledge Development Fund, NIH/NIMH #9R01MH84282-04A1, Vancouver Coastal Research Institute. Sofia Lombera is currently at the London School of Economics. We thank Emily Borgelt for her input to this manuscript and the team and the National Core for Neuroethics for ongoing and insightful discussions about neuroimaging and neuroethics.

References

Abraham, A., Werning, M., Rakoczy, H., von Cramon, D.Y. , and Schubotz, R.I. (2008). Minds, persons, and space: an fMRI investigation into the relational complexity of higher-order intentionality. *Consciousness and Cognition*, 17, 438–50.

Aggarwal, N.K. (2009). Neuroimaging, culture and forensic psychiatry. *Journal of the American Academy of Psychiatry and the Law*, 37, 239–44.

Aron, A., Fisher, H., Mashek, D.J., Strong, G., Li, H., and Brown, L.L (2005). Reward, motivation, and emotion systems associated with early-stage intense romantic love. *Journal of Neurophysiology*, **94**, 327–37.

Bigos, K.L. and Weinberger, D.R. (2010). Imaging genetics – days of future past. *Neuroimage* [Epub 18 January 2010].

Cho, M.K., Magnus, D., Caplan, A.L., McGee, D., and the Ethics of Genomics Group. (1999). Ethical considerations in synthesizing a minimal genome. *Science*, **286**, 208–90.

Conti, R., Veenstra, D.L., Armstrong, K., Lesko, L.J., and Grosse, S.D. (2010). Personalized medicine and genomics: challenges and opportunities in assessing effectiveness, cost-effectiveness, and future research priorities. *Medical Decision Making*, **30**, 328–40.

Eisenberger, N.I., Lieberman, M.D., and Williams, K.D. (2003). Does rejection hurt? An fMRI study of social exclusion. *Science*, **302**, 290–2.

Esslinger, C., Walter, H., Kirsch, P., *et al.* (2009). Neural mechanisms of a genome-wide supported psychosis variant. *Science*, **324**, 605.

Farah, M.J. (2005). Neuroethics: the practical and the philosophical. *Trends in Cognitive Sciences*, **9**, 34–40.

Farah, M.J. and Wolpe, P.R. (2004). Monitoring and manipulating brain function: new neuroscience technologies and their ethical implications. *Hastings Center Report*, **34**, 35–45.

Fenton, A., Meynell, L., and Baylis, F. (2009). Ethical challenges and interpretive difficulties with non-clinical applications of pediatric fMRI. *The American Journal of Bioethics*, **9**, 3–13.

Fins, J.J., Illes, J., Bernat, J.L., Hirsch, J., Laureys, S., and Murphy, E. (2008). Neuroimaging and disorders of consciousness: envisioning an ethical research agenda. *American Journal of Bioethics*, **8**, 3–12.

Fisher, H., Aron, A., and Brown, L.L. (2005). Romantic love: An fMRI study of a neural mechanism for mate choice. *The Journal of Comparative Neurology*, **493**, 58–62.

Garnett, A., Piwowar, H.A., Rasmussen, E.M., and Illes, J. (2010). Formulating MEDLINE queries for article retrieval based on PubMed exemplars. *Nature Precedings* [Online]. 10 March. Available from: http://precedings.nature.com/documents/4270/version/1. [Accessed: 10 March 2010]

Glannon, W. (2006). Neuroethics. *Bioethics*, **20**, 37–52.

Greely, H.T. and Illes, J. (2007). Neuroscience-based lie detection: The urgent need for regulation. *American Journal of Law and Medicine*, **33**, 377–431.

Greicius, M.D., Srivastava, G., Reiss, A.L., and Menon, V. (2004). Default-mode network activity distinguishes Alzheimer's disease from healthy aging: evidence from functional MRI. *Proceedings of the National Academy of Sciences U S A*, **101**, 4637–42.

Hall, W., Capps, B., and Carter, A. (2008). The use of depot naltroxone under legal coercion: the case for caution. *Addiction*, **103**, 1922–4.

Harris, S., Kaplan, J.T., Curiel, A., Bookheimer, S.Y., Iacoboni, M., and Cohen, M.S. (2009). The neural correlates of religious and nonreligious belief. *PLoS ONE*, **4**, e0007272.

Illes, J., Kirschen, M.P., and Gabrieli, J.D. (2003). From neuroimaging to neuroethics. *Nature Neuroscience*, **5**, 205.

Illes, J. (2007). Empirical neuroethics. Can brain imaging visualize human thought? Why is neuroethics interested in such a possibility? *EMBO Reports*, **8**, S57–60.

Illes, J. and Racine, E. (2005). Imaging or imagining? A neuroethics challenge informed by genetics. *American Journal of Bioethics*, **5**, 5–18.

Illes, J., Moser, M.A., McCormick, J.B., *et al.* (2009). Neurotalk: improving the communication of neuroscience research. *Nature Reviews Neuroscience*, **11**, 61–9.

Kapogiannis, D., Barbey, A.K., Su, M., Zamboni, G., Krueger, F., and Grafman, J. (2009). Cognitive and neural foundations of religious belief. *Proceedings of the National Academy of Science*, **106**, 4876–81.

King, J.A., Tenney, J., Rossi, V., Colamussi, L., and Burdick, S (2003). Neural substrates underlying impulsivity. *Annals of the New York Academy of Science*, **1008**, 160–69.

Knauff, M., Famgmeier, T., Ruff, C.C. , and Sloutsky, V. (2006). FMRI evidence for a three-stage model of deductive reasoning. *Journal of Cognitive Neuroscience*, **18**, 320–34.

Lau, P.W. and Illes, J. (2009). The gray zones of privatized imaging. *American Journal of Bioethics*, **9**, 21–2.

Laureys, S., Owen, A., and Schiff, N. (2009). Coma science: clinical and ethical implications. Preface. *Progress in Brain Research*, **277**, xiii–xiv.

Lawrence, E.J., Shaw, P., Giampietro, V.P, Surguladze, S., Brammer, M.J, and David, A.S. (2006). The role of 'shared representations' in social perception and empathy: an fMRI study. *Neuroimage*, **29**, 1173–84.

Marcus, S. (2002). *Neuroethics: Mapping the Field*. New York: The Dana Foundation Press.

Matthews, P.M., Honey, G.D., and Bullmore, E.T. (2006). Applications of fMRI in translational medicine and clinical practice. *Nature Reviews Neuroscience*, **7**, 732–44.

Meegan, D.V. (2008). Neuroimaging techniques for memory detection: scientific, ethical and legal issues. *American Journal of Bioethics*, **8**, 9–20.

Miller, G. (2009). fMRI evidence used in murder sentencing. *Science Insider*, *[Internet]* 23 November. Available at: http://news.sciencemag.org/scienceinsider/2009/11/fmri-evidence-u.html) [Accessed 9 March 2010]

Moll, J., de Oliveira-Souza, R., Garrido, G.J., *et al.* (2009). The self as a moral agent: linking the neural bases of social agency and moral sensitivity. *A Social Neuroscience*, **2**, 336–52.

Monti, M.M., Coleman, M.R., and Owen, A.M. (2009). Neuroimaging and the vegetative state: Resolving the behavioral assessment dilemma. *Annals of the New York Academy of Science*, **1157**, 81–9.

President's Council on Bioethics (2004). *Reproduction and responsibility: the regulation of new biotechnologies*. Washington, DC: National Academies Press.

Reiman, E.M. (2007). Linking brain imaging and genomics in the study of Alzheimer's disease and aging. *Annals of the New York Academy of Sciences*, **1097**, 94–113.

Roskies A. (2002). Neuroethics for the new millennium. *Neuron*, **34**, 21–3.

Rothenberg, K. and Terry, S.F. (2002). Human genetics. Before it's too late – addressing fear of genetic discrimination. *Science*, **297**, 196–7.

Soon, C.S., Brass, M., Heinze, H.J., and Haynes, J.D. (2008). Unconscious determinants of free decisions in the human brain. *Nature Neuroscience*, **11**, 543–5.

Tairyan, K. and Illes, J. (2009). Imaging genetics and the power of combined technologies: a perspective from neuroethics. *Neuroscience*, **164**, 7–15.

Thompson, P.B. and Hannah, W. (2008). Food and agricultural biotechnology: a summary and analysis of ethical concerns. *Advances in Biochemical Engineering Biotechnology*, **111**, 229–64.

Vogeley, K., May, M., Ritzl, A., Falkai, P., Zilles, K., and Fink, G.R. (2004). Neural correlates of first-person perspective as one constituent of human self-consciousness. *Journal of Cognitive Neuroscience*, **16**, 327–37.

Volkow, N.D., Fowler, J.S., and Wang, G.J. (2004). The addicted human brain viewed in the light of imaging studies: brain circuits and treatment strategies. *Neuropharmacology*, **47**, 3–13.

Williams, A. (1992). Cost-effectiveness analysis: is it ethical? *Journal of Medical Ethics*, **18**, 7–11.

Yang, T.T., Menon, V., Eliez, S., *et al.* (2002). Amygdalar activation associated with positive and negative facial expressions. *Neuroreport*, **13**, 1737–41.

CHAPTER 23

....

PEDIATRIC NEUROIMAGING RESEARCH

....

MICHAEL R. HADSKIS AND MATTHIAS H. SCHMIDT

INTRODUCTION

....

RECENT decades have borne witness to raised optimism about the possibility of solving the many seemingly intractable mysteries that surround the developing human brain. The mechanisms underlying normal growth and development, intellect and personality, neurobehavioral disorders, and brain plasticity are just a few entries on the long list of unsolved mysteries. Scientific optimism is fueled, in the main, by accelerated advancements in the increasingly hi-tech world of bioimaging. A wide variety of extremely sophisticated imaging modalities are now at our disposal, including computed tomography (CT), single-photon emission computed tomography (SPECT), positron emission tomography (PET), magnetic resonance imaging (MRI), and magnetoencephalography (MEG). These methodologies make possible such things as direct imaging of brain structure, chemistry, and function (Downie *et al.* 2007). They also permit direct imaging of the effects of disease and treatment (Tempany *et al.* 2001).

Progress in our ability to combat pediatric neurological disease and in our understanding of the development of human cognition is of unchallengeable importance. How this progress is achieved through the use of neuroimaging tools in the pediatric research context does, however, require thoughtful reflection on serious legal and ethical questions. Neuroimaging acutely vulnerable populations such as minors, especially those with developmental abnormalities, arguably brings to the fore the most complex, pressing, and substantial issues in neuroethics. Pediatric neuroimaging research implicates many research ethics principles, including respect for autonomy, respect for vulnerable persons, distributive justice, respect for privacy and confidentiality, harm minimization, and benefit maximization.

This chapter will discuss relevant legal and ethical research frameworks in the United States, Canada, and the United Kingdom. Although many legal and ethical norms potentially apply to pediatric neuroimaging research in these jurisdictions, we will concentrate on

Title 45, Part 46 of the *Code of Federal Regulations* (CFR) in the United States, the *Tri-Council Policy Statement: Ethical Conduct for Research Involving Humans* (TCPS) in Canada, and the *Medical Research Council Ethics Guide: Medical Research Involving Children* (MRC Guide) in the United Kingdom. These norms play a prominent role in establishing standards for the conduct of pediatric research projects in their respective jurisdictions. In view of our multi-jurisdictional focus, the generic label Research Ethics Committee (REC) will be used to refer to the bodies in these jurisdictions (each one uses a different name for its relevant body) that are charged with determining whether proposed human research is ethically acceptable.

We begin this chapter by furnishing a brief overview of pediatric neuroimaging research risks since much of the legal and ethical analysis draws upon this information. This is followed by an examination of the importance of decisional-capacity determinations for prospective minor participants. The next several sections of the chapter deal with consider-ations applicable to the involvement of incompetent minors in neuroimaging research (i.e. limitations on surrogate consent, establishing the need for the inclusion of incompetent minor participants, restrictions on risk exposure, and the roles of assent and dissent). A discussion of incidental findings (IFs), respect for minors' privacy, and interpretation of research images rounds out the subjects that are covered in the chapter.

Pediatric neuroimaging risks

A major appeal of MRI in pediatric neuroimaging research is its lack of dependence on ionizing radiation, unlike other neuroimaging modalities, such as CT, SPECT, and PET (Schmidt and Downie 2009). Instead, the signal used to create images in MRI is derived from the nuclear "spin" of protons found in water, fat, and other biological molecules distributed throughout the body. This spin is manipulated by altering the magnetic environ-ment of protons. The returning signal can provide very precise information about the distribution of protons throughout the body, the biochemical composition of tissues, the movement of water molecules in tissues, the direction and velocity of blood flow, and the oxygenation state of blood. The combination of safety, high spatial and temporal resolution, and ability to characterize a wide variety of biological parameters make MRI the most widely used modality for neuroimaging research (Desmond *et al.* 2002; Marshall and Hadskis 2009). MRI use in the clinic and the research domain enjoys an 'enviable reputation for safety' (Goldberg 2007). However, MRI is not risk-free (Kulynych 2002; Schmidt and Downie 2009).

Since the generation of images relies on the use of a powerful magnet, a risk of physical injury to participants exists if unfastened ferromagnetic objects are brought near the scanner—the so-called "missile effect." As well, the strong pull of the magnetic field can cause any ferromagnetic material embedded in a participant's body (e.g. latent metal filings in a person's eye) to move and/or heat up, possibly leading to serious tissue damage. Magnetic forces may also cause medical devices, such as pacemakers, to fail. The prospect of such adverse events requires rigorous screening of persons and the nearby MRI environ-ment for potentially problematic ferromagnetic material (Kanal *et al.* 2007). Concerns have been raised that proper screening might not always be conducted in the MRI research realm, particularly where trained MRI technicians are not involved in the research scanning and in situations where safety procedures are less standardized. On this score, one author observes: "[I]t is sometimes the case that no member of an MRI research team will have clinical experience or technical certification, and that permission to enter the MRI suite or even to operate the MRI scanner will be granted to graduate students and research fellows solely at the discretion of the principal investigator" (Kulynych 2007, p. 311).

Screening of research participants and controlling access to the MRI scanner can be a particular challenge in the pediatric environment. Here, researchers need to consider the sometimes unpredictable behavior of children and the need for "crowd control" when siblings, parents, and/or other caregivers accompany research participants (Schmidt and Downie 2009). There are additional safety concerns unique to pediatric MRI. For example, infants do not tolerate the noise generated by the MRI scanner as well as older children and adults, necessitating particular attention to noise attenuation strategies (Schmidt and Downie 2009). Also, infants reach regulatory limits for radiofrequency energy deposition in tissues more quickly due to their smaller size, requiring careful prospective consideration of the radiofrequency energy that is deposited by each imaging sequence to be used in this population (Schmidt and Downie 2009).

To produce MRI scans, researchers place participants in a supine position within the long, narrow bore of the scanner. For some individuals, confinement in the scanner can provoke anxiety and claustrophobia. Young children, both with and without mental disabilities, may experience considerable anxiety and discomfort during MRI procedures and, anxious or not, may have difficulty remaining motionless during MRI scans. This is a significant issue, because even slight movement can render MRI images uninterpretable. For this reason, in the clinical context, children frequently are sedated for MRI scans. While the benefit of sedation to achieve appropriate images is clear, the risks also must be considered, particularly when its use is being contemplated in a research project. Relatively minor complications like gastrointestinal upset, agitation, and motor imbalance are not uncommon, while potentially fatal complications like cardiorespiratory arrest, though rare, can occur (Hinton 2002; Kulynych 2002, 2007; Schmidt and Downie 2009).

Similar to the debate about the use of sedative and hypnotic drugs—although not unique to pediatric MRI—there are ethical concerns regarding the use of intravenous contrast material for the enhancement of images or for the study of blood flow and tissue perfusion in the research setting. While the incidence of contrast-related serious adverse events is very low, life-threatening reactions have been reported (Jordan and Mintz 1995; Dillman *et al.* 2007). Moreover, individuals with pre-existing kidney failure are at risk of nephrogenic systemic fibrosis, a painful, disabling, potentially fatal and—to date—incurable condition caused by the toxic gadolinium ion contained in MRI contrast materials (Marshall *et al.* 2007; Marshall and Hadskis 2009).

Finally, an area of risk that has recently attracted considerable attention and debate in the research ethics literature concerns IFs, which have been aptly defined as "observations of potential clinical significance unexpectedly discovered in healthy subjects or in patients recruited to… imaging research studies and unrelated to the purpose or variables of the study" (Illes *et al.* 2006, p. 783). The subject of IFs is discussed more fully below (see "Incidental findings" section). Suffice it to say here that psychological distress, exposure to confirmatory diagnostic tests or invasive procedures, and negative effects on the participants' insurability can flow from such discoveries, particularly if imaging researchers have not developed thoughtful plans to deal with them effectively.

DETERMINING WHETHER A MINOR CAN
CONSENT TO PARTICIPATION

Respectful engagement with minors in the neuroimaging research context requires that they participate in the decision whether to be involved in such research to the fullest extent possible. If a prospective minor participant is legally competent to provide a valid consent to study participation, then the neuroimaging researcher must seek the minor's consent (Hadskis 2007; MRC Guide Section 1.3; 46 CFR 116; TCPS Art. 2.1). Should a minor lack the capacity to consent, then the minor still may be able to participate in the decision-making process, as discussed later.

Neuroimaging researchers must exercise great care when determining whether a prospective minor participant is competent. An erroneous finding that a minor is incompetent may infringe their right to self-determination; on the other hand, a mistaken determination that the minor is competent may foreclose the engagement of safeguards for persons who are vulnerable due to their diminished capacity (Hadskis 2007). Minors may be considered competent if they are able to understand the relevant information about the specific study and are able to appreciate the potential consequences of agreeing or refusing to participate in the project (Wendler and Shah 2003; TCPS Section 2(E); MRC Guide Section 5.1.4)—competent minors are often referred to as "mature minors." The information relevant to a given neuroimaging study will include, among other things, the purpose of the research, the procedures to be followed, and any reasonably foreseeable risks or benefits to the participant. A particular minor's decisional capacity may vary according to the complexity of the decision concerning study participation; in this sense competence is not global or static. The extent to which a minor's maturity is scrutinized increases in accordance with the severity of the potential consequences of participating or not participating in the neuroimaging study. For instance, a healthy 14-year-old prospective participant for an MRI study that will use a novel contrast agent may well not meet the applicable competency definition. The complex issues surrounding the prospect of an IF being made add to the demanding nature of a minor's deliberations.

Neuroimaging researchers must inform themselves of the competency laws that are applicable in the jurisdiction(s) in which the research will be conducted. These may not always offer researchers clear guidance. For instance, in Canada, there is a lack of clarity in the law on whether the mature minor doctrine applies to research participation, although some believe that it likely does (Baylis *et al.* 2000; Nelson 2005; Hadskis 2007). Even if the doctrine applies, it is unclear whether a mature minor would always be able to make the decision to participate in research. This is due to a 2009 Supreme Court of Canada decision, A.C. v. Manitoba (Director of Child and Family Services), which dealt with the issue of minors' capacity to consent to medical treatment. According to the Court, even if a person is a mature minor, he or she may not be able under the common law (the law made by judges as opposed to the law established by the government in the form of legislation) to make a treatment decision if abiding the decision would not accord with his or her best interests. In its decision, the Supreme Court of Canada noted that United Kingdom, United States, and Australian courts have also not given mature minors the automatic ability to make any treatment decisions.

While the A.C. case involved the issue of mature minors' decision-making authority in the treatment context, the Court's reasoning is of potential application to their ability to make decisions regarding research participation. As a result, a neuroimaging researcher in Canada may not only need to be satisfied that a prospective participant is a mature minor, but may also need to be satisfied that the minor's decision regarding study participation is in this person's best interests. Outside of situations where participation in a neuroimaging study may medically benefit a minor (e.g. research on the use of preoperative fMRI to achieve safer resection of brain tumors), it may not always be clear whether a minor's involvement in a study is in his or her best interests (e.g. participation of a healthy minor in an imaging study of a normal psychological process, like learning or memory).

INVOLVEMENT OF INCOMPETENT MINORS

Neuroimaging projects that will involve incompetent minors, whether their incompetency is due to their young age and/or a mental disability, raise a number of difficult ethical issues. Perhaps the paramount challenge is grappling with the tension that can exist between the ethical principles of respect for vulnerable persons and distributive justice. Persons with diminished or no decision-making capacity are considered vulnerable to abuse, exploitation, and discrimination in research; thus, adequate protective measures must be in place to address this vulnerability. At the same time, care should be taken to ensure that the desire for protection does not lead to over-protection in the form of exclusion of incompetent minors from neuroimaging research, contrary to the tenets of distributive justice which caution against unfairly preventing vulnerable segments of the population from reaping the ultimate fruits of this research—for to do so may make them therapeutic orphans (MRC Guide Section 2.1). Hinton (2002) speaks to this issue when she notes, "In pediatric neuroimaging, an ethical tautology exists – because children are more vulnerable, working with them is more problematic, so less work has been done, limiting interpretation." Thus, "the protective impulse to shield children entirely from harms of research participation has the potential to cause them significant harm" (Miller and Kenny 2002, p. 218). The next several sections discuss the implications for pediatric neuroimaging research that flow from research ethics precepts that have been developed to respond to these considerations.

Surrogate consent

Consent must be sought from an incompetent person's legally-authorized representative (TCPS Art. 2.5(b); 46 CFR 116; MRC Guide Section 5.1.4.a). Where incompetent minors are involved, the appropriate substitute decision-makers are typically the minors' parents or legal guardians (Nelson 2005). When parents/guardians are approached about enrolling their child in a research project, their paramount responsibility is to make this decision on the basis of what they believe to be in their child's best interests. This involves weighing the risks and benefits of consenting to study participation. Survey evidence confirms that most parents keenly feel their responsibility to act in their children's best interests when enrolling them in research (Shilling and Young 2009). Nonetheless, pediatric neuroimaging researchers ought to remain alert to any signs that parental decision making is being unduly influenced by interests held solely by the parents. For example, authorization for research participation which is motivated by parental intrigue generated by media accounts of high-tech neuroimaging research tools, despite their child's unflagging anxiety about interacting with this technology, is of doubtful ethical validity (Hinton 2002).

In some jurisdictions, a lack of clarity exists respecting when parents can, in view of the obligation to make decisions that reflect their child's best interests, consent to the participation of their child in non-therapeutic research. For instance, one American state's (Maryland) highest court held that a parent cannot consent to the participation of a child "in nontherapeutic research or studies in which there is any risk of injury or damage to the health of the subject" (Grimes v. Kennedy Krieger Institute, Inc., p. 49). In an effort to subsequently clarify the use of the words "any risk" in its judgment, the Court stated: "…by 'any risk,' we meant any articulable risk beyond the minimal kind of risk that is inherent in any endeavor. The context of the statement was a nontherapeutic study that promise[d] no medical benefit to the child whatsoever, so that any balance between risk and benefit [was] necessarily negative" (Grimes v. Kennedy Krieger Institute, Inc., p. 53). Regarding this attempt at clarification, one legal commentator has opined: "It is difficult to reconcile the first sentence of this statement, which seems to permit some minimal risk, with the second sentence, which seems to mean that *any* risk is too great in the context of nontherapeutic research" (Glantz 2002). No greater clarity on this issue has since emanated from the United States courts.

Canadian researchers are plagued by a similar lack of clarity (Hadskis 2007). In 1986, the Supreme Court of Canada decided in *Eve v. E. (Mrs.)* that a non-therapeutic sterilization procedure could not be lawfully performed on an incompetent person because this procedure was not in accord with her best interests. While this decision did not discuss the limits of proxy consent in the biomedical research sphere, it has nonetheless been interpreted by a number of legal academics as potentially impeding parents from being able to lawfully consent to the inclusion of incompetent minors in research that poses any risks to their child if there is no immediate medical benefit to him or her (Dickens 1998; Grover 2003; Nelson 2005). It has been contended that this would mean that parents cannot even consent to interventions such as heel or finger-prick blood testing of their children that is being conducted for research purposes alone, and that the possibility of the research benefiting other children is immaterial (Dickens 1998). Taking a less restrictive slant on the Supreme Court of Canada's decision, other commentators have argued that the decision can be read as indicating that parents can authorize research with no direct medical benefit, provided there is potential for other forms of benefits including psychological, social, and religious benefit (Baylis *et al.* 2000). It has been speculated that the uncertainty around how future courts may interpret this case "has probably had a chilling effect on research involving children in Canada" (Baylis *et al.* 2000, p. 8).

The measure of restrictiveness the law places on parental decision making has profound implications for pediatric neuroimaging research. Many of these protocols rely on incompetent minors—whether their incompetence is due to their young age or is attributable to a mental disorder—who will not derive any direct medical benefit through their participation. Yet, as outlined earlier, their participation will involve at least some risk exposure (the degree of risk presented by neuroimaging study participation is canvassed later). Pediatric neuroimaging researchers, indeed pediatric researchers of all stripes, would greatly benefit from judicial clarity on this fundamental point.

Even if the application of the best interest principle does not bar a parent from enrolling their child in a given neuroimaging study, in order for parental substitute decision making to be ethically and legally valid, parents' consent will have to be given voluntarily after they have been properly informed about the research, including the project's reasonably foreseeable potential harms and benefits to their child (Hadskis 2007). Concerns have been raised that "therapeutic misconception"—the misapprehension that therapeutic benefits may accrue to individual research participants (Appelbaum *et al.* 1982)—can reside in pediatric neuroimaging research (Hadskis *et al.* 2008). Parents may not have accurate information about the risks and benefits of neuroimaging research for a variety of reasons, including: aggressive marketing of this research (Racine *et al.* 2006); the tendency by some members of the media to present findings of fMRI in an uncritical and sensationalist fashion (Racine *et al.* 2006); misinformation from some health advocacy groups (Racine *et al.* 2005); the possible influence of contemporary Western society's belief in the power of technology (Hadskis *et al.* 2008); and overstatements by the scientific community about the explicative power of fMRI (Racine and Illes 2006).

As well, some parents of children with profound developmental disability, degenerative neurological conditions, and serious psychiatric disorders may be particularly susceptible to therapeutic misconception. Their need for relief from the burden of care for their child and/or their deep desire to improve their child's mental health may cause them to exaggerate potential benefits and deemphasize research risks. In the end, if parents possess an inflated sense of potential benefit to their child, their best interest determinations will be impaired. Therefore, neuroimaging researchers and REC members must remain alert to the possibility that parents may labor under a therapeutic misconception and, with this in mind, they should ensure that parents receive full and clear information on the risks and benefits, if any, of study participation (Hadskis *et al.* 2008).

Recognizing that parents may make decisions contrary to the best interests of their child, research ethics frameworks make parental consent a necessary but insufficient condition for research participation. Some of the additional conditions that are imposed and their implications for pediatric neuroimaging research are considered next.

Demonstrable need for incompetent minor participants

A common condition found in research ethics frameworks for the enrolment of incompetent minor participants is that the research question can only be addressed using such minors (TCPS Art. 2.5(a); MRC Guide Section 4.1). If the question can be adequately answered by enrolling competent persons, then researchers must only recruit them. Many neuroimaging studies will satisfy this condition. Since the "developing brain is quite distinct from the developed brain" (Downie *et al.* 2007, p. 86), adult neuroimaging research cannot merely be extrapolated to minors. In order to realize the full benefits of research into brain structure and function, large numbers of healthy minor participants are needed to establish normative images. Neurologically compromised minor participants will also be required to answer many of the scientific questions being posed. In view of this, the condition requiring a demonstrable need for minor participants, both with and without neurological disorders, is unlikely to act as an impediment for many proposed pediatric neuroimaging studies.

Limitations on risk exposure

Research ethics frameworks require that measures be taken to minimize research risks to minor participants and that the risks, even when duly minimized, be reasonable in relation to the anticipated benefits of the study. These considerations can present significant ethical challenges for pediatric neuroimaging research.

Risk minimization

Ethics norms oblige researchers to not expose participants to unnecessary risk (46 CFR 111(a)(1); TCPS Introduction; MRC Guide Section 4.3) and, whenever possible, procedures already being performed on participants for diagnostic or treatment purposes should be used (46 CFR 111(a)(1); MRC Guide Section 4.3.2). To minimize the chance of physical injury to participants, pediatric neuroimaging studies should use persons properly credentialed to perform scans and, where MRI is involved, that procedures appropriate for screening children are employed. Also critically important is the need for rigorous plans for monitoring the safety of minor participants and for responding to emergencies. Professionals with the appropriate expertise in pediatrics ought to be included in such plans (MRC Guide Section 4.3.2; Schmidt and Downie 2009). As well, to the extent the research design will allow, studies should recruit minors who are already undergoing a neuroimaging procedure for clinical purposes. However, this will often not be possible because studies of normal brain structure and function should not be performed on children with known or suspected neurological issues, lest these issues confound the interpretation of the data. If children with non-neurological issues (e.g. musculoskeletal problems) are recruited instead, combined clinical and research imaging may become cumbersome, as subjects may need to be repositioned in the scanner and imaging coils may need to be exchanged (e.g. an extremity coil for a head coil). More importantly, even if there is no need for repositioning or coil exchange, combined clinical and research scans may become so long that subjects are unable to tolerate them.

The use of sedation for the conduct of neuroimaging research should never be considered acceptable if alternative methods can be effectively employed to both reduce the anxiety and fear commonly experienced by minor participants and to train them to remain sufficiently still during image acquisition. Some tools have been developed. For example, the use of an audio-visual system consisting of video goggles and earphones has been shown effective in reducing the number of individuals requiring sedation for some pediatric age groups, MRI procedure time, and financial costs (Harned et al. 2001; Hinton 2002). A behavior management program drawing upon feedback and success approximation techniques to desensitize children to the MRI setting has been proven helpful (Slifer et al. 1993; Bookheimer 2000). Age-relevant visual/written material has been used to ease apprehension and create an understanding of participation in MRI scanning (Hinton 2002).

Acceptable risk thresholds

Uniformly, research ethics frameworks establish limitations respecting the degree of risk to which incompetent minor participants can be exposed for research purposes. Determining whether a research project will involve greater than "minimal risk" to participants is often of pivotal importance under these frameworks. According to United States norms, minimal risk exists if the probability and magnitude of harm or discomfort anticipated in the research is not greater than those ordinarily encountered in daily life or during the performance of routine physical or psychological examinations or tests (45 CFR 46.102(i)). Canada has adopted a similar definition, although it does not specifically reference risks associated with routine examinations or tests (TCPS Section 1(C1)). The United Kingdom's MRC Guide states that it "is expected that research of minimal risk would not result in more than a very slight and temporary negative impact on the health of the person concerned," such as "obtaining bodily fluids without invasive intervention" (Section 4.3).

Neuroimaging research involving no greater than minimal risk to incompetent minor participants is permitted under research ethics frameworks (although, as noted earlier, the legality of surrogate consent to minimal risk research is not entirely clear). However, if the proposed research project exceeds the minimal risk threshold and study participation carries no prospect of direct benefit for the participants, the study may not receive REC approval. In some jurisdictions, such as Canada, research ethics standards prohibit such research (TCPS Art. 2.5(c)). Under UK norms, in the absence of a potential benefit to the minor, 'parents/guardians can still consent provided the risks are sufficiently small to mean that research can be reasonably said not to go against the child's interests' (MRC Guide Section 5.1.4.a). In the US, these projects are permitted, but only if certain narrow conditions are met (46 CFR 406 and 407). Thus, whether a neuroimaging study involving incompetent minors falls within the definition of minimal risk is a critical question. Studies that make use of imaging modalities that expose participants to radiation—PET and CT scans for instance—are generally regarded as exceeding the minimal risk standard (Hinton 2002).

Minimal risk classification is less clear for MRI research projects. Although MRI scans do not expose participants to radiation, participation is not devoid of risks, as discussed earlier. Some commentators have observed that pediatric MRI studies have generally been considered by RECs as entailing minimal risk to the health of minor participants (Hinton 2002; Kumra et al. 2006; Kulynych 2007). Yet, others have queried whether MRI research involving healthy controls exceeds the minimal risk threshold (Kulynych 2002; Wolf et al. 2008). Clearly, the level of risk is elevated by sedation, which as noted above may be necessary to achieve immobility of very young minors or developmentally delayed older minors. Although some authors assert that sedation can be performed safely in the research context with appropriate participant selection, supplemental oxygen delivery, and supervision by an experienced pediatric anesthesiologist (Amundsen et al. 2005), consensus appears to have emerged that if the study procedures call for the use of sedation, the study's risk level is elevated beyond minimal (Kulynych 2002, 2007; Schmidt and Downie 2009). The same holds true for study procedures that employ intravenous contrast media, which can have unpleasant side effects and may—though rarely—induce serious allergic reactions (Kulynych 2007; Schmidt and Downie 2009).

In the US, there is some disagreement among RECs on whether the use of sedation or contrast enhancement represents a "minor increase" or "more than a minor increase" over the minimal risk threshold. This is of importance for pediatric neuroimaging researchers who wish to enroll minors with a disorder or condition that is the subject of their research, where the participants will not directly benefit from their participation, but the research is likely to yield generalizable knowledge that is of vital importance for understanding or ameliorating the disorder or condition (e.g. infants with hypoxic/ischemic brain injury, who may require sedation for adequate research scans and, in the context of a particular research protocol, may require contrast enhancement to study cerebral perfusion). If the risk represents a minor increase over minimal risk then it can proceed in the US in some circumstances (46 CFR 406) "absent the extensive review and approval at the federal agency level" (Kulynych 2007, p. 313) that would be needed if the risk represented more than a minor increase (46 CFR 407).

Role of assent and dissent

Research ethics frameworks encourage respect for incompetent minors by requiring researchers to involve them in the decision-making process by seeking their assent, to the extent that their maturity and intellectual development makes such engagement possible. A minor's dissent is binding if the research is non-therapeutic (TCPS Art. 2.7; 46 CFR 408; MRC Guide Section 5.1.4.a), but their objection may not have to be heeded if there is a prospect of direct benefit that is important to the health and well-being of the minor and is only available in the context of research (46 CFR 408) (e.g. participation of a pediatric cancer patient in a trial of an imaging sequence touted to improve detection of metastases, and hence allow for more accurate tumor staging). Overriding their dissent in such circumstances is considered ethically appropriate to advance the minor's long-term medical interests (Ross 2004) over his or her short-term interest in, for example, not being put in the MRI bore due to fear of enclosed spaces.

Treating minor participants respectfully requires that all of the neuroimaging procedures must be communicated to the minor in an effective, age-appropriate manner (MRC Guide Section 5.1.5). Neuroimaging researchers can adopt a number of strategies to enhance the meaningfulness of the assent process. Child life specialists can be asked to evaluate researchers' communication tools or to take part in the actual assent process. Creative ways of gently introducing minors to the research environment can be developed, such as coloring books depicting various aspects of participation (e.g. children inside a magnet), pamphlets containing pictures of the environment together with straightforward written explanations of what the participant can expect, and videotapes of minors taking part in the research procedures. Mock MRI scanners can also be used to allow participants to safely interact with these machines on their own terms (Hinton 2002).

Care must be taken to ensure that a minor participant continues to assent to participation after the study procedures are initiated. This can be challenging when minors are in the MRI bore, since some common signals respecting willingness to continue (e.g. facial expressions) are not observable. Thus, it is recommended that a clear signal for distress be established in advance. As well, it may be prudent to allow for breaks and inquire through the intercom or headphones, at regular intervals, whether the minor is content remaining in the study (Rosen and Gur 2002).

INCIDENTAL FINDINGS

IFs are becoming an increasingly pressing ethical issue, as they are more common than one might suppose, and as they can potentially cause serious harm to research participants

(Downie *et al.* 2007). In a recent meta-analysis of occupational, commercial and clinical screening MRI studies predominantly involving adults, neoplastic IFs occurred with an overall frequency of 0.7% and non-neoplastic IFs (excluding white matter hyper-intensities, silent infarcts, and microhemorrhages) occurred with an overall frequency of 2.0% (Morris *et al.* 2009). The frequency of IFs was noted to increase with participant age and use of high resolution protocols (Morris *et al.* 2009). Specific data on the spectrum and frequency of IFs in children are still scant, but when common anatomical variants and benign conditions such as paranasal sinus inflammation are included, the frequency of IFs in children ranges from 13–25.7% (Kim *et al.* 2002; Kumra *et al.* 2006; Gupta and Belay 2008).

On the one hand, identification of IFs is important so that participants do not miss the opportunity to benefit by seeking timely medical advice. Indeed, researchers may find themselves liable if they fail to alert participants promptly to the presence of a potentially harmful condition (Kulynych 2002). On the other hand, serious consideration must be given to the negative impact of such findings on children. This is particularly true for artifacts, normal variants, abnormalities of uncertain significance, and serious abnormalities for which there is no good treatment. Any potential abnormality can lead to unpleasant and potentially risky further medical investigations. It can engender anxiety in child participants and/or their families. A perceived brain abnormality, even if it does not require medical intervention, could affect a child's self-perception and lead to stigmatization within the child's family or community. In a child, the impact of an IF may be more far-reaching than it would be in an adult. A perceived threat to normal intellectual development could potentially become a self-fulfilling prophecy. Moreover, it may affect future insurability, employability or career choices.

For these reasons, it is imperative that best management strategies for IFs be developed. This includes, but is not limited to, such issues as: how IFs should be addressed in the informed consent process; who should disclose IFs to research participants and determine whether or not medical referral is warranted; whether research scans should include diagnostic quality sequences in anticipation of IFs; and whether or not research scans should be reviewed systematically for IFs by qualified neuroradiologists. Consensus and policy on this issue are still lacking, but there is a move toward the development of collaborative guidelines (Illes *et al.* 2006, 2008; Wolf *et al.* 2008).

RESPECT FOR MINORS' PRIVACY

Privacy and confidentiality concerns are common to all human participant research. However, there are a few issues that arise specifically with respect to pediatric neuroimaging research. In order to perform MRI safely, it is important to screen all subjects for contraindications before they enter into the scanner. Since contraindications to study participation necessarily include contraindications to MRI, the consent discussion and safety screening often occur together. Depending on the age of participants and local standards, parents or guardians of potential research participants may well be part of the consent process. They may therefore also be present during the administration of a safety screening questionnaire. Typical questionnaires include questions about tattoos (metal-based dyes may heat up in the scanner and cause skin burns), skin piercings (metallic jewelry may move in the magnetic field), and pregnancy (the safety of MRI in the first trimester has not been established conclusively, and pregnancy therefore remains a relative contraindication to MRI). Teenage participants may have tattoos or piercings, and they may be pregnant. However, they may not wish to reveal such information to their parents or guardians at that time, and therefore might be placed in a very awkward position by the consent and safety screening processes (Downie *et al.* 2007). It is therefore imperative that safety screens occur in a private setting, and that participants be given an opportunity to withdraw their consent in a way that does not reveal their specific motivation for withdrawal.

An additional issue somewhat unique to MR neuroimaging research is the fact that the data themselves may allow identification of participants. Identifying demographic information is typically embedded in the headers of image files, and care must be taken to "de-identify" images prior to archiving (Kulynych 2002, 2007). Interestingly, concern has been raised about three-dimensional surface renderings from the high-resolution anatomical images that accompany fMRI studies. Since archives are being created to allow sharing of image databases, there is the potential for life-like images of participants' faces to become public (Kulynych 2002, 2007). This concern may be particularly relevant to MR neuroimaging research involving children with rare congenital malformations and metabolic syndromes. The rarity of these conditions, together with any characteristic facial features, may particularly predispose to the identification of participants.

INTERPRETATION OF RESEARCH IMAGES

Incidentally discovered anatomical abnormalities can be evaluated in light of what is already known about neuroanatomical variability and the manifestations of neurological illness on imaging studies. However, anomalous research results from an individual participant in a functional neuroimaging study should never lead to the participant being labelled "abnormal." First, given the complexity of data acquisition and processing, it is quite possible that an apparently anomalous result is artefactual. Second, it is important to remember that cutting edge functional neuroimaging research is being done precisely because we do not know how the brain gives rise to our thoughts and feelings, much less how it shapes our attitudes and character. Researchers seek generalizable knowledge about the relationship between mind and brain by studying brain activation patterns in groups of research participants. These activation patterns are no more than epiphenomena of the mental processes under examination, and should not be equated to these processes. Therefore, until we truly understand the neural basis of processes like cognition and emotion, whatever we observe in an individual research participant only informs us about the range of possible brain activation patterns that may be observed (Hadskis *et al.* 2008). This range may be quite large, particularly in children who develop at different rates.

Shifting attention from research participants to society at large, it should be noted that concern has been expressed about the potential for the invasion of fMRI into the most private recesses of our brains by virtue of such "mindreading" applications as lie detection and character assessment (Greely and Illes 2007). However, there is a more urgent ethical concern about the erroneous belief that fMRI can actually already do this. This fallacy is illustrated by the ill-advised introduction of fMRI as evidence in legal proceedings. As suggested above, too little is known about the cognitive processes that underlie fMRI activations, and about the normal range of activation patterns that might be observed in a large population, to support consequential judgments about the fMRI activations seen in any individual. The sporadic use of fMRI in the judicial arena might well raise concern about other potential non-scientific and non-medical applications of fMRI, such as aptitude testing. The very suggestion of using fMRI in children for educational or vocational streaming purposes should be resisted on scientific grounds, as well as ethical grounds (Fenton *et al.* 2009). However, the limited availability, high cost and complexity of fMRI should render any concern about its imminent use in mass screening exercises moot.

In order to assuage concerns about the potential for anomalous activation patterns to become another form of IF that might adversely impact research participants, and to dispel dystopian visions of the use of fMRI in the public arena, researchers must advertise the limits to fMRI interpretation with respect to individuals as vigorously as they advertise the things that are learned from the study of groups of research participants. Ethicists can help in this process by demanding a critical appraisal of the limitations of fMRI that make its use as a "mindreading" tool not only ethically objectionable, but also scientifically untenable.

Conclusion

In pediatric neuroimaging research, the ethical challenges of working with vulnerable child participants are convolved with the challenges of dealing with sophisticated, rapidly evolving technology that probes into the mechanisms of perception, cognition, and emotion— the very essence of human experience. In this field, there are special ethical considerations that require a very good understanding of children as well as MRI. Some of the issues touched on in the foregoing discussion are different in the clinical setting, compared to the research context. For example, assent is not required from incompetent minors who are patients requiring MRI for their clinical care. Other issues are similar. For example, unforeseen grief may come in the form of IFs from diagnostic imaging examinations as readily as it may come from research studies, cautioning against the use of sophisticated imaging tests for weak clinical indications.

Clinical need often drives neuroimaging research, as for example the need for more sensitive and specific diagnostic tools, as well as the need to understand how growth and development affect the imaging appearances of normal neuroanatomy and neurological illnesses. Pediatric neuroimaging research is an important source of normative data for clinical imaging, and it serves as a proving ground for advanced technologies that eventually find their way into the clinic. Progress in pediatric neuroimaging research is of vital importance to the health of children. At the same time, ethical debate dedicated to this field is vital to ensure that research proceeds with due regard for the rights, safety and well-being of participants, and that the information gained from this research is communicated and used responsibly.

Acknowledgements

This project was supported by a Neuroethics New Emerging Team Grant from the Institute of Neurosciences, Mental Health, and Addiction of the Canadian Institutes of Health

Research. The authors hasten to warmly thank Laura Dowling for her superb and timely research assistance.

References

A.C. v. Manitoba (Director of Child and Family Services), 2009 SCC 30.

Amundsen, L., Artru, A., Dager, S., *et al.* (2005). Propofol sedation for longitudinal pediatric neuroimaging research. *Journal of Neurosurgical Anesthesiology*, **17**, 180–92.

Appelbaum, P., Roth, L. and Lidz, C. (1982). The therapeutic misconception – Informed consent in psychiatric research. *International Journal of Law and Psychiatry*, **5**, 319–29.

Baylis, F., Downie, J. and Kenny, N. (1999). Children and decision-making in health research. *Health Law Review*, **8**, 3–10.

Bookheimer, S. (2000). Methodological issues in pediatric neuroimaging. *Mental Retardation and Developmental Disabilities Research Reviews*, **6**, 161–5.

Desmond, J. and Chen, S. (2002). Ethical issues in the clinical application of fMRI: Factors affecting the validity and interpretation of activations. *Brain and Cognition*, **50**, 482–97.

Dickens, B. (1998). The legal challenge of health research involving children. *Health Law Journal*, **131**, 135.

Dillman, J.R., Ellis, J.H., Cohan, R.H., Strouse, P.J. and Jan, S.C. (2007). Frequency and severity of acute allergic-like reactions to gadolinium-containing IV contrast media in children and adults. *American Journal of Roentgenology*, **189**, 1533–8.

Downie, J., Schmidt, M., Kenny, N., D'Arcy, R., Hadskis, M. and Marshall, J. (2007). Paediatric MRI research ethics: The priority issues. *Bioethical Inquiry*, **4**, 85–91.

E. (Mrs.) v. Eve, [1986] 2S.C.R. 388.

Fenton, A., Meynell, L. and Baylis, F. (2009). Ethical challenges and interpretive difficulties with non-clinical applications in pediatric fMRI. *American Journal of Bioethics (AJOB Neuroscience*, **9**, 3–13.

Glantz, L. (2002). Nontherapeutic research with children: Grimes v. Kennedy Krieger Institute. *American Journal of Public Health*, **92**, 1070–3.

Goldberg, S. (2007). MRIs and the perception of risk. *American Journal of Law and Medicine*, **33**, 229–37.

Greely, H. and Illes, J. (2007). Neuroscience-based lie detection: The urgent need for regulation. *American Journal of Law and Medicine*, **33**, 377–431.

Grimes v Kennedy Krieger Institute Inc (KKI) 366 Md 29. 366 Md 29; 782 A2d 807; 2001 Md LEXIS 496 (2001). Also available at: http://www.courts.state.md.us/opinions/coa/2001/128a00.pdf (PDF file) (accessed October 29, 2009).

Grover, S. (2003). On the limits of parental proxy consent: Children's right to non-participation in non-therapeutic research. *Journal of Academic Ethics*, **1**, 349–83.

Gupta, S. and Belay, B. (2008). Intracranial incidental findings on brain MR images in a pediatric neurology practice: A retrospective study. *Journal of the Neurological Sciences*, **264**, 34–7.

Hadskis, M. (2007). The regulation of biomedical research in Canada. In J. Downie, T. Caulfield, and C. Flood, (eds.) *Canadian Health Law and Policy*, 3rd ed. pp. 257–310, Toronto: Butterworths.

Hadskis, M., Kenny, N., Downie, J., Schmidt, M., and D'Arcy, R. (2008). The therapeutic misconception: A threat to valid parental consent for pediatric neuroimaging research. *Accountability in Research*, **15**, 133–51.

Harned, R. and Strain, J. (2001). MRI-compatible audio/visual system: impact on pediatric sedation. *Pediatric Radiology*, **31**, 247–50.

Hinton, V. (2002). Ethics of neuroimaging in pediatric development. *Brain and Cognition*, **50**, 455–68.

Illes, J., Kirschen, M., Edwards, E., *et al.* (2006). Incidental findings in brain imaging research. *Science*, **311**, 783–4.

Illes, J., Kirschen, M., Edwards, E., *et al.* (2008). Practical approaches to incidental findings in brain imaging research. *Neurology*, **70**, 384–90.

Jordan, R. and Mintz, R. (1995). Fatal reaction to gadopentetate dimeglumine. *American Journal of Roentgenology*, **164**, 743–4.

Kim, B., Illes, J., Kaplan, R., Reiss, A. and Atlas, S. (2002). Incidental findings in pediatirc MR images of the brain. *American Journal of Neuroradiology*, **23**, 1674–7.

Kulynych, J. (2002). Legal and ethical issues in neuroimaging research: human subjects protection, medical privacy, and the public communication of research results. *Brain and Cognition*, **50**, 345–57.

Kulynych, J. (2007). The regulation of MR neuroimaging research: Disentangling the Gordian knot. *American Journal of Law & Medicine*, **33**, 295–317.

Kumra, S., Ashtari, M., Anderson, B., Cervellione, K. and Kan, L. (2006). Ethical and practical considerations in the management of incidental findings in pediatric MRI studies. *Journal of the American Academy of Child and Adolescent Psychiatry*, **45**, 1000–6.

Marshall, J. and Hadskis, M. (2009). Canadian research ethics boards, MRI research risks, and MRI risk classification. *IRB: Ethics & Human Research*, **31**, 9–15.

Marshall, J., Martin, T., Downie, J. and Malisza, K. (2007). A comprehensive analysis of MRI research risks: In support of full disclosure. *The Canadian Journal of Neurological Sciences*, **34**, 11–17.

Medical Research Council (2004). *MRC Ethics Guide: Medical Research Involving Children*. Available at: http://www.mrc.ac.uk/Utilities/Documentrecord/index.htm?d=MRC002430 (accessed October 30, 2009).

Medical Research Council of Canada, Natural Sciences and Engineering Research Council of Canada, Social Sciences and Humanities Research Council of Canada (1998). *Tri-Council Policy Statement: Ethical Conduct for Research Involving Humans* Ottawa: Public Works and Government Services Canada.

Miller, P. and Kenny, N. (2002). Walking the moral tightrope: Respecting and protecting children in health-related research. *Cambridge Quarterly of Healthcare Ethics*, **11**, 217–29.

Morris, Z., Whiteley, W., Longstreth, *et al.* (2009). Incidental findings on brain magnetic resonance imaging: Systematic review and meta-analysis. *British Medial Journal*, **339**, b3016.

Nelson, E. (2005). Legal and ethical issues in ART 'Outcomes Research.' *Health Law Journal*, **165**, 182.

Racine E. and Illes, J. (2006). Neuroethical responsibilities. *Canadian Journal of Neurological Sciences*, **33**, 269–77.

Racine, E., Bar-Ilan, O. and Illes, J. (2005). FMRI in the public eye. *Nature Reviews Neuroscience*, **6**, 159–64.

Racine, E., Bar-Ilan, O. and Illes, J. (2006). Brain imaging – A decade of coverage in the print media. *Science Communication*, **28**, 122–43.

Rosen A. and Gur R. (2002). Ethical considerations for neuropsychologists as functional magnetic imagers. *Brain and Cognition*, **50**, 469–81.

Ross, L. (2004). Informed consent in pediatric research. *Cambridge Quarterly of Healthcare Ethics*, **13**, 346–58.

Schmidt, M. and Downie J. (2009). Safety first: Recognizing and managing the risks to child participants in magnetic resonance imaging research. *Accountability in Research*, **16**, 153–73.

Shilling, V. and Young, B. (2009). How do parents experience being asked to enter a child in a randomized controlled trial? *BMC Medical Ethics*, **10**, 1.

Slifer, K., Cataldo, M.F., Cataldo M.D., *et al.* (1993). Behavior analysis of motion control for pediatric neuroimaging. *Journal of Applied behavior analysis*, **26**, 469–70.

Tempany, C. and McNeil, B. (2001). Advances in biomedical imaging. *Journal of the American Medical Association*, **285**, 562–7.

Title 45. *Code of Federal Regulations*, Part 46.

Wendler, D. and Shah, S. (2003). Should children decide whether they are enrolled in nonbeneficial research? *The American Journal of Bioethics*, **3**, 1–7.

Wolf, S., Lawrenz, F., Nelson, C., *et al.* (2008). Managing incidental findings in human subjects research: Analysis and recommendations. *Journal of Law, Medicine and Ethics*, **36**, 219–48.

CHAPTER 24

ETHICAL ISSUES IN FUNCTIONAL NEUROSURGERY: EMERGING APPLICATIONS AND CONTROVERSIES

NIR LIPSMAN AND MARK BERNSTEIN

BACKGROUND

IN 1961, Wilder Penfield, the great Canadian neurosurgeon, was invited to speak at a neuroscience conference at the University of California (Penfield 1963). At that point, his reputation as a clinician, surgeon, and scientist had been firmly established, and he had long achieved pioneer status in the field of surgical epilepsy, as well as medical education. His talk, which he titled "The physiological basis of the mind," wasn't his first or last foray into the mind–body debate. Indeed, he would author a book, and several chapters on the topic, and was already an invited speaker and honorary member of the American Philosophical Society (Penfield 1977). Having synthesized his years of operations on awake epileptic patients, for whom he had resected epileptogenic cortex after meticulous cortical stimulation and mapping, he found himself in the ideal position to comment on the makeup of the mind, and hypothesize about its organic origins. His talk surprised many by describing a separate mind that was beyond the brain's physical mechanisms, but more importantly for Penfield, the talk did not in the least represent a digression from his neurosurgical practice. His philosophy was a direct extension of his clinical practice and was informed by concrete physical findings from his operating room, effectively his laboratory. Penfield provided his listeners with first-hand accounts of mind exploration occurring in real time, in real life, and which contextualized his hypotheses and ideas. Not only was this not unusual for him, it was perfectly natural. The recipient of a classical, and enviable, neurosurgical training under the likes of Charles Sherrington and Ramón y Cajal, Penfield learned early on the value of translational research, as well as the importance of a healthy respect and love for the human-ities, philosophy, in his case (Penfield 1977). For Penfield it required no leap of reason or imagination, for a neurosurgeon to be invited to a neuroscience conference and speak about an age-old philosophical argument. Philosophers, for the aging neurosurgeon, held no monopoly on the mind.

When thinking about the role of neurosurgery in neuroethics, one needs to first reflect, briefly, on the development of the specialty and its origins. Penfield's career, and that of his contemporaries was largely possible because of a substantial shift in the 1920s and 30s that saw the role of the neurosurgeon change from one of passive receiver of instruction and executor of risky and complex interventions to that of active prescriber and clinician (Bliss 2007). With the development of ventriculography, rudimentary radiography, and eventually angiography, neurosurgeons freed themselves from their reliance on neurologists for their localizations, and proceeded to independently diagnose, localize, and treat nervous system pathology. Neurosurgery, born a hybrid of general surgery, pathology, and neurology, matured and grew into its own, respectable profession, as clinicians also began to realize the power of their field to explore the myriad functions of the human brain. Further advances in the mid-20th century and onward, including those in anesthesia, critical and ventilatory care, and specific to neurosurgery, the development of stereotaxy, and microsurgery, solidified the neurosurgeon's role as chief navigator through the sea of complex and challenging central nervous system pathology. As with other surgical specialties, the establishment of structured academic residency programs in neurosurgery coupled to a spirit of innovation and inquiry led to a flurry of development. The difference, however, was that neurosurgeons dealt with scenarios unique to the nervous system, and found themselves then, as now, confronted with ethical dilemmas on a routine basis in their clinical practices. Issues such as brain death, withdrawal of care, autonomy of brain-damaged patients, informed consent, and the application of new and novel technology, were issues that although were not monop-olized by neurosurgery, certainly acquired a new dimension for those practitioners dealing with the organ responsible for their patients personality, memory and higher human faculties.

We can think of ethical questions in neurosurgery as falling into two categories, namely those surrounding what neurosurgeons are currently doing, i.e. their current practices, and those surrounding what neurosurgeons will, theoretically, be capable of doing in the future, i.e. their future practices. Further categorizations can be made according to whether ethical questions are related to a given technology or innovation (e.g. its use, safety and efficacy) those surrounding the disease or pathology (e.g. its classification and definition), and those surrounding the patient (e.g. including their understanding of informed consent etc.; see Table 24.1. for examples).

Neurosurgery, as mentioned, does not lack ethical challenges. Patients who are moribund, comatose, terminally ill, traumatized, or at the very least neurologically unstable make up a large portion of the clinician's challenges (Diringer et al. 2001). These patients, and their associated management challenges, are beyond the scope of this chapter, and therefore will not be addressed in great detail. Instead, we will focus on the growth of functional neurosur-gery as a discipline and scientific field, which contains not only a dramatically different patient population but an entirely new set of ethical challenges and questions. For the first time, neurosurgeons have the option to electively intervene in diseases of brain function, in morphologically normal brains, with an array of novel technologies. When they should

Table 24.1 Classifying ethical challenges in functional neurosurgery, with examples

	Current practice challenges	Future practice challenges
Technology	The rational and thoughtful use of current novel technology, and issues surrounding its access and distribution of use, e.g. DBS for mood and anxiety disorders Selecting the right technology for the right indication (DBS, Vagal nerve stimulation, GammaKnife, etc.)	Same as current, plus: The relationship between implantable technology, culture, and the dynamic between society and the individual. Future reliance and dependence on implantable technology Ensuring adequate access to, and responsible use of, enhancement technology, within and across cultures
Disease	The selection of appropriate diseases as substrates for neuromodulation, given adequate knowledge of anatomy, physiology, and circuitry Determining the threshold that must be met before a disease is deemed adequate for surgical treatment	Same as current, plus: The changing definition of disease and health and the rise of cosmetic neurosurgery for cognitive and physical enhancement Intervening prophylactically in predisposed individuals
Patient	Identifying, by a multidisciplinary panel, of appropriate patients for neuromodulation, with attention to informed consent and patient autonomy	Same as current, plus: The evolving spectrum from "patient" to "consumer" Obtaining consent in psychiatrically and otherwise neurologically compromised patients Privacy of thoughts and actions.

intervene, with what kind of technology, for which conditions and in which patients, are questions that are now under intense scrutiny.

FUNCTIONAL NEUROSURGERY

Functional neurosurgery is a subspecialty of neurosurgery that deals with restoration of function through stereotactic means. According to the World Society of Stereotactic and Functional Neurosurgery (WSSFN), the most appropriate definition for the field is:

> …a branch of neurosurgery that utilizes dedicated structural and functional neuroimaging to identify and target discrete areas of the brain and to perform specific interventions (for example ablation, neurostimulation, neuromodulation, neurotransplantation, and others) using dedicated instruments and machinery in order to relieve a variety of symptoms of neurological and other disorders and to improve function of both the structurally normal and abnormal nervous system. (WSSFN 2009)

Although many areas within neurosurgery are fraught with ethical challenges, functional neurosurgery offers practitioners a unique set of those challenges, and will continue to do so in the years to come. This is for several reasons. It is often the case that the pathology being addressed through functional means is not visible on conventional diagnostic imaging, such as computed tomography or magnetic resonance imaging scanning. For example, movement disorders, pain syndromes, and epilepsy, with some notable exceptions, frequently have no findings on neuroimaging and diagnoses are made based on the clinical picture. Surgeons are thus effectively operating on "normal" brains, and dealing macroscopically with a process most likely taking place on a microscopic, cellular level. Furthermore, functional neurosurgery makes its primary objective to alter brain function. Nervous system pathology, such as brain tumors, aneurysms, and congenital malformations, are all associated with changes in brain function, which of course can also be a consequence of their treatment. Changes in memory and personality, for example, can accompany an indolent frontal lobe tumor, but so can prolonged retraction on the frontal lobes during the clipping of an aneurysm. In both cases, brain function is altered, in the former as a direct consequence of the disease, and in the latter as an indirect, incidental consequence of treatment. With functional neurosurgery, the *primary objective* is a change in brain function, be it the perception of pain, the reduction of a tremor, or the improvement of mood.

Here we will divide our discussion into the current and emerging applications of functional neurosurgery as well as the future controversies that will stem from them. Our discussion will be limited to psychosurgery, enhancement (cognitive and physical) and brain–machine interface (BMI), in order to illustrate the pertinent ethical challenges and the role of the neurosurgeon in helping to address them. Of note, psychosurgery represents less than 10% of the current functional surgeons' clinical practice, with enhancement and brain machine interface currently under investigation only. These three applications represent natural extensions of each other, as exploration of the underlying mechanisms of psychopathology will ultimately provide insight into normal brain function. The neurosurgeon, and the neuroethicist, will by necessity need to be involved at every stage.

CURRENT AND EMERGING APPLICATIONS

In 1997 the Food and Drug Administration in the United States approved the use of deep brain stimulation (DBS) for the treatment of medically refractory essential tremor (Yu and Neimat 2008). This was followed several years later by similar approval for the treatment of Parkinson's disease and then dystonia. Its success in neurodegenerative disease and movement disorders in general, underscored the increasing utility of stimulation technology. Neuromodulation, up until then had largely been restricted to ablative procedures, which although very effective were irreversible, allowing practitioners essentially one chance to identify the correct deep brain target. DBS was not only reversible, i.e. the internalized leads can be removed or the current turned off, it allowed titration of effect, monitoring of side-effects, and facilitated double-blind, controlled trials effectively proving the utility of the technology. A detailed discussion of the proposed mechanisms of DBS is outside the scope of this chapter, but several hypotheses do exist (for review, see Dostrovsky and Lozano 2002; McIntyre et al. 2004; Montgomery and Gale 2008). Most theories center on the influence of chronic high-frequency stimulation on either inhibitory or excitatory neuronal pathways, mediated by the neurotransmitters GABA and glutamate, respectively. Whether stimulation involves a "jamming" of circuits or the promotion of specific neuronal firing rates, which facilitate physiologic functioning, is unknown. What has been recognized, however, is that stimulation in one part of the brain, for example, the globus pallidus internus, can influence the physiologic milieu in a more remote brain region, such as supplementary motor cortex (Davis *et al.* 1997). This suggests that various neuroanatomic regions can be influenced as distinct "nodes" along a physiologic circuit, and in this way potentially modulate activity along that circuit. The implications for disorders of not only movement, but of cognition and mood, are thus broad and far-reaching, and raise important questions about the possibility of modulating both normal and pathological behavior.

Psychiatric neurosurgery

It has been known for nearly 70 years that different circuits mediate different brain functions from voluntary movement to affect (Kopell *et al.* 2004; Fins *et al.* 2006; Wind and Anderson 2008). Mayberg and colleagues hypothesized that since it is known that the cingulate cortex is involved in a specific cortico-striato-thalamo-cortical circuit mediating the brain functions believed dysfunctional in depression, then modulation of the cingulate with stimulation should attenuate those maladaptive behaviors (Mayberg *et al.* 2005). Done together with a team of neurosurgeons, the first study examining DBS for depression, showed that four of six study patients achieved "...sustained clinical response or remission at the end of six months" (Mayberg *et al.* 2005). The age of modern neurosurgery for psychiatric indications had effectively been reborn, now with a stimulation twist.

The study was picked up and reported widely in the popular press. Newspapers, magazines and television news reported the successful treatment of refractory depression with brain surgery and touted its potential and promise (Canada.com 2009; Globe and Mail.com 2009). Similar attention had greeted the results of other studies with DBS in the movement disorder literature, reflecting a trend of increasing media attention to the neurosciences and to neuromodulation in particular (Racine *et al.* 2007). Clearly, the idea of "brain implants" affecting human mood and behavior, tapped into a collective public interest in the brain and its inherent mysteries; the presence of mind control, brain chips, androids, and telekinesis in the science fiction and general literature speaks to that interest as well.

The principal investigators of the Depression study, wary of the tarnished past of "psychosurgery" had selected patients carefully, with independent review by psychiatrists and involvement of family members at all stages of the study. Ethical issues and their consideration permeated the study, and were given as much attention as other methodological details in the final manuscript. Indeed, attention to the acquisition of informed consent, independent review and patient selection, as well as proper post-procedural follow-up have become staples of any manuscript attempting to present clinical evidence of stimulation effectiveness for any psychiatric indication. The tentative, early success in depression spurred researchers to explore DBS for other psychiatric indications. Although reports of DBS for refractory obsessive–compulsive disorder (OCD) had been known for at least 2 years prior to the DBS and depression study, research and trial development accelerated after 2005. Several high quality trials, including at least one randomized double blind study (Mallet *et al.* 2008), have been done and are in progress evaluating DBS for depression, OCD, Tourette's syndrome and alcoholism (Kuhn *et al.* 2007; Zabek *et al.* 2008; Mink 2009). In parallel with the seemingly exponential growth, and interest, in surgical psychiatry, the bioethics literature has grown correspondingly, and neuroethics emerged as a result of the growing advances in the neuromodulation field (Glannon 2006).

Despite the early successes, it appears that the specter of surgery for psychiatric indications is still unnerving to some in the healthcare community, as well as in the media and general public. Most likely, this is due to a perceptual error, that generates a natural resistance to and fear of an external agent, be it another individual, a chip or an implanted electrode, taking ownership over one's own mind. The thought of an external force applied to change one's thoughts and behaviors, in general, is unappealing, and has been the source of many a Hollywood horror film. Whether it is a positive change, defined as a change resulting in some alternate action not in keeping with the individuals' interests (e.g. aliens or government agents controlling the mind and body) or a negative change, defined as a change resulting in the individual being stripped of their ability to act (e.g. zombies) people find the idea of mind-tampering disturbing. Precisely why this is disturbing is unclear, but most likely has something to do with the inability to conceive of oneself as being disconnected from one's own sense of self. Feelings such as deja vu, depersonalization, and even migrainous or pre-ictal auras, are all associated with similar "strangeness" and discomfort that one cannot describe but can instantly recognize. Is this the cause of the general fascination, and possible trepidation, surrounding the idea of neuromodulation?

We conducted a qualitative interview based study asking patients undergoing neurosurgery for brain tumors, who are presumably well versed in the risks of surgery, about their attitudes towards surgery for psychiatry, identity change and neuro-enhancement (Lipsman *et al.* 2009). Patients were, perhaps surprisingly, overwhelmingly in favor of surgery for psychiatric disease citing the prerequisite importance of informed consent and the proven safety and efficacy of a given intervention. Also surprising was that patients viewed the hypothetical enhancement of a negative trait, for example greed or short-temperedness, as less ethically troublesome than the enhancement of an ostensibly normal trait, such as improving one's mood from average to above average. Not only did patients not universally dismiss neuromodulation for pathological states they expressed some approval for modifying non-pathological traits as well. Could it be that societal and cultural conditions are changing, and that neuromodulation, for pathologic indications or not, is not as unpalatable as it once was?

Enhancement

Definitions of enhancement have been difficult to formulate and are perhaps made more difficult in the context of functional neurosurgery. Does improving the mood of a depressed patient count as enhancement? Does one need to exclude the presence of pathology and focus only on the improvement from a seemingly "normal" state? Most modern definitions focus on the latter, with enhancement being generally defined and understood as an "improvement in the absence of medical need" (DeGrazia 2005). According to this definition, neurosurgeons have yet to be involved in the application of true enhancement technology. However, any member of a functional neurosurgical team who has seen the results of surgery for psychiatry, pain, movement disorders, or epilepsy, knows that this is not the case. We propose that definitions of enhancement include any improvement in functional status, cognitive or physical, as measured by objective, standardized measures, that allow the subject to engage in or perform activities otherwise not possible as a direct consequence of their pre-enhancement state. With this definition, a depressed patient that resumes their occupation following DBS would have been enhanced, as would a hearing impaired child who has received a cochlear implant, and a hypothetical patient of the future who receives memory enhancement technology to achieve a better SAT score. More than simply an "improvement," enhancement needs to demonstrate objective evidence that there has been a change, beyond that possible without the aid of technology. Distinguishing medical or therapeutic enhancement, from elective or "non-medical" enhancement, implies an endorsement of one, the former, and a rejection of the other, the latter. By removing health and pathology from the definition, we are including both possibilities.

As with all medical applications, improving the lives of the healthy must not come at the expense, be it financial or otherwise, of improving the health of the ill and disabled. The role of BMI, DBS, motor cortex stimulation and gamma-knife radiosurgery as they all relate to pathology must be well enough established prior to exploring their use in healthy populations. That ethical imperative must remain unwavering, and accordingly, the involvement of neurosurgeons in enhancement technology should be focused largely on how that improvement in health will come about. However, two points need to be mentioned, both related to the enhancement definition posed above. First, as cultural definitions of disease evolve and change, the notion of patient health will change accordingly. As diagnostic criteria contract and expand with increasing knowledge and research, as well as the changing proclivities of the societies that prescribe them, one generations ill and disabled may be another generations normal variant, and vice versa. As several authors have argued, to base a definition of enhancement on what is "normal" or "healthy" will in due course prove to be inadequate (Hansson 2005). Second, although neurosurgery's involvement in enhancement and its expanding role in psychiatry is still in its infancy, neurosurgeons must be engaged now, prior to developing trials and engaging in clinical research, to ensure their research is ethically oriented. This will be of particular importance when researchers begin to tackle some of functional neurosurgery's most fascinating, and controversial, applications.

FUTURE CONTROVERSIES

The application of DBS and other implantable technology to patients in a minimally conscious state (MCS) (Schiff et al. 2007; Schiff 2009) as well as those who have suffered the devastating effects of motor-neuron disease or strokes (Birbaumer et al. 2009) has shown some promise. In the former, DBS allowed a patient in a MCS to obtain statistically significant "functional improvement" (Schiff et al. 2007). With such studies, motor volition and consciousness itself are the respective substrates, but the theoretically possible substrates are limited only by the myriad functions of the human brain. As in plastic surgery, where technology and innovation first meant to treat pathology and disfigurement was ultimately used for elective, aesthetic procedures, we have previously used the term cosmetic neurosurgery to prophesy a similar direction in functional neurosurgery (Lipsman et al. 2009).

Clearly, however, important differences exist between cosmetic plastic surgery and neurosurgery for cognitive or physical enhancement. The brain is the seat of memory, affect, and personal identity, all of which can potentially be altered with neurosurgical operations. Further, as a science we are very far from understanding the anatomy, let alone the physiology and circuitry of many of the traits and conditions that some have hypothesized will be the targets of enhancement, or modification, such as memory or creativity. Also, issues such as fair and equal access to enhancement technology are much more salient and carry much broader societal and cultural implications when discussing memory enhancement, for example, versus breast augmentation. Despite these differences, however, similarities do exist, but need to be compared on an equal footing: if the science is far enough along, and strict federal regulations are put in place, one can easily argue that a personality "defect" such as predilection to addiction, or even greed and pessimism, are more "harmful" or disruptive to one's life than a smaller than average bust size. Is enhancement with a safe and effective technology not permissible then? We are currently conducting several qualitative studies gauging the attitudes of neurosurgery patients, and neurosurgeons towards these and similar questions. Preliminary results look promising, and suggest that, as with our previous results, individuals find the correction of a negative personality trait ethically permissible, and the improvement of a "normal" trait or the use of neuromodulation in a coercive setting (e.g. with prisoners) as ethically ambiguous at best, and generally inappropriate.

MEETING THE CHALLENGES AHEAD

Neurosurgeons, and their collaborators, will need to consider these questions soon. With regards to psychosurgery, as functional imaging, tractography, tracer studies and animal models evolve and improve, questions will shift from what drives a certain behavior to how can the behavior be prevented or modified. Several centers have already reported results on DBS for alcoholism (Kuhn *et al.* 2007), obesity (Halpern *et al.* 2008), and hypothesized targets for schizophrenia (Mikell *et al.* 2009), just as some critics argue that the biology of these diseases and others for whom DBS has been considered are not close to being understood. Until then, they argue, surgical treatment should not be performed. This is only partially true. Most centers have used DBS as a last resort, and moreover as a research tool to learn more about the diseases in question. Few, if any, centers are suggesting that DBS or any neuromodulation procedure will cure psychiatric disease, but all centers judiciously report their results in an effort to identify important targets, eliminate dangerous or ineffective ones and further our knowledge about the underlying circuitry of these conditions. Importantly, as the conditions that become candidates for surgical treatment change, ethical issues, such as adequate informed consent and respect for patient autonomy, remain unchanged and indeed acquire an additional complexity. The adequacy of proxy consent, the impossibility of foretelling all known risks and the questionable voluntariness of sometimes desperate and often unstable patients, remain unaddressed and will be sources of future investigation.

The future of enhancement in a neurosurgical context will likely involve a significant overlap with BMI. Some authors have already hypothesized about the potential uses of implantable technology and how these will change the face of society and what it ultimately means to be human: "Brain–machine interfaces will put new forms of stress on privacy, autonomy, and justice, and more importantly, on what it means to be human" (McGee and Maguire 2007). Although some of their predictions sound like science fiction to us, they are right that the time to establish regulations is now. Certainly, as technology is made available that will provide paralyzed patients with greater independence and strength; similar technology will gradually begin to be adapted to less severe pathology and eventually to healthy individuals. One can easily envision a DBS device or subdural recordings that guide the thought evoked movements of a quadriplegic patient, being applied to a hemiplegic patient, and then to a victim of stroke with a mild deficit, and ultimately, to a healthy fighter pilot acquiring targets with his mind. Each step is in turn accompanied by further debate, and a shift in cultural values and definitions of "impairment."

Concerns about the future of implantable technology, and the neurosurgeon's role in installing them, need to be addressed. The issues of privacy of thoughts and actions, and even the loss of human nature and the changing dynamic between society and the individual, are not minor and reflect a general fear that enhancement and/or implantable technology will either: (1) be usurped for less than noble means; (2) represent a shift towards a paternalistic, big-brother society; or (3) either create chasms of inequality between the enhanced or unenhanced, or homogenize society so that aptitude, cognitive or physical, will be commonplace and effectively mundane. All are valid concerns, but not insurmountable, given adequate preparation and transparent discussion. The future practice of the functional neurosurgeon will involve several points of contact with a multidisciplinary team that will, by necessity, include non-medical members. Between development and implementation, the surgeon's role will be to synthesize the legal, ethical, and moral dimensions of a proposed intervention as he or she will ultimately be responsible for the pre- and postoperative care of these patients. This can start now, with clinical trials that recognize the value of oversight, supervision and transparency, as well as the active involvement of neurosurgeons in ethical debates surrounding implantable and enhancement technology.

CONCLUSION: DRAMATIS PERSONAE AND
THE ROLE OF THE NEUROSURGEON

In July of 2009, the *Journal of Neurosurgery*, the flagship publication of the American Association of Neurological Surgeons published a special issue on the development and promise BMIs. Among articles exploring the science and clinical perspectives of the technology, an official statement from the National Institute of Neurological Disorders and Stroke outlined their fervent support for BMI in improving the lives of stroke patients and those stricken by neurodegenerative disease. "[BMI] offers the promise of restoring communication, enabling control of assistive devices, and allowing volitional control of extremities in paralyzed individuals" (Pancrazio 2009). Although both the National Institute of Health and NINDS have a long history of funding research into BMI, most notably leading to cochlear implant technology, their statement in a neurosurgical journal is significant. It recognizes that neurosurgeons will be involved in many of the developmental steps in BMI, from conceptualization to implementation and that engaging them early is vital to progress in the field.

The future applications of functional neurosurgery, including psychiatry, enhancement and BMIs, are certainly exciting and hold much promise. Within the cast of characters, the neurosurgeon will play a prominent role, not only in research and implementation but also hopefully in allaying the fears that the technology may foster. One important step is recognizing that we cannot use the highly hypothetical, often fanciful scenarios quoted in the implant literature, which strike equal parts fear and excitement in the reader, to establish current regulatory guidelines. We are indeed very far off from our brains melding into machines and from being able to download our brains onto microchips. Instead, those interested in the development of the field need to work together to identify the weaknesses of current research, and to immunize protocols and designs at an early stage from the detractors who will question their merits and value (Fins *et al.* 2006; Kimmelman *et al.* 2009). Bioethicists interested in neuromodulation have all ready begun this important work, and are identifying vulnerabilities in functional research that may hamper further progress (Bell *et al.* 2009; Ford 2009).

Wilder Penfield's participation in the mind–body debate was both prescient and ahead of its time. Surely he would have been fascinated with the latest developments in the search for the cortical representation of self and consciousness that is now an intense area of investigation (David *et al.* 2008; Schwartz and Schwartz 2008; Immordino-Yang *et al.* 2009). Although his legacy in epilepsy surgery and brain mapping will continue to live on, he was also the first neurosurgeon to engage the non-surgical world in a conversation about the mind, philosophy, and ethics, and grounded his opinions in clinical research. He saw beyond the brain, and explored the mind, and recognized the chance that neurosurgeons have on a daily basis to explore the most human of human qualities: our selves. The future of functional neurosurgery will involve building on that legacy and exploring corners of the mind previously out of reach to clinicians and philosophers alike.

References

Bell, E., Mathieu, G., and Racine, E. (2009). Preparing the ethical future of deep brain stimulation. *Surgical Neurology*, 72, 577–86.

Birbaumer, N., Ramos Murguialday, A., Weber, C., and Montoya, P. (2009). Neurofeedback and brain-computer interface clinical applications. *International Review of Neurobiology*, 86, 107–17.

Bliss, M. (2007). *Harvey Cushing: A Life in Surgery*. Toronto: University of Toronto Press.

Canada.com. *A cure for depression?* Available at: http://www.canada.com/topics/bodyand-health/story.html?id=ea7ec14d-ca4d-4763-8814-be6c72f558b8 (accessed 14 August 2009).

David, N., Newen, A., and Vogeley, K. (2008). The "sense of agency" and its underlying cognitive and neural mechanisms. *Conscious Cognition*, 17, 523–34.

Davis, K.D., Taub, E., Houle, S., *et al.* (1997). Globus pallidus stimulation activates the cortical motor system during alleviation of parkinsonian symptoms. *Nature Medicine*, 3, 671–4.

DeGrazia, D. (2005). Enhancement technologies and human identity. *Journal of Medicine and Philosophy*, 30, 261–83.

Diringer, M.N., Edwards, D.F., Aiyagari, V., and Hollingsworth, H. (2001). Factors associated with withdrawal of mechanical ventilation in a neurology/neurosurgery intensive care unit. *Critical Care Medicine*, 29, 1792–7.

Dostrovsky, J.O. and Lozano, A.M. (2002). Mechanisms of deep brain stimulation. *Movement Disorders*, 17, S63–8.

Fins, J.J., Rezai, A.R., and Greenberg, B.D. (2006). Psychosurgery: avoiding an ethical redux while advancing a therapeutic future. *Neurosurgery*, 59, 713–16.

Ford, P.J. (2009). Vulnerable brains: research ethics and neurosurgical patients. *Journal of Law, Medicine and Ethics*, 37, 73–82.

Glannon, W. (2006). Neuroethics. *Bioethics*, 20, 37–52.

Globe and Mail. *Mending a broken mind*. Available at: http://v1.theglobeandmail.com/servlet/story/RTGAM .20080627.wmhdepression28/BNStory/mentalhealth/ (accessed 14 August 2009).

Halpern, C.H., Wolf, J.A., Bale, T.L., *et al.* (2008). Deep brain stimulation in the treatment of obesity. *Journal of Neurosurgery*, 109, 625–34.

Hansson, S.O. (2005). Implant ethics. *Medical Ethics*, 31, 519–25.

Immordino-Yang, M.H., McColl, A., Damasio, H., and Damasio, A. (2009). Neural correlates of admiration and compassion. *Proceedings of the National Academy of Sciences USA*, 106, 8021–6.

Kimmelman, J., London, A.J., Ravina, B., *et al.* (2009). Launching invasive, first-in-human trials against Parkinson's disease: ethical considerations. *Movement Disorders*, 24, 1893–901.

Kopell, B.H., Greenberg. B., and Rezai, A.R. (2004). Deep brain stimulation for psychiatric disorders. *Clinical Neurophysiology*, 21, 51–67.

Kuhn, J., Lenartz, D., Huff, W., *et al.* (2007). Remission of alcohol dependency following deep brain stimulation of the nucleus accumbens: valuable therapeutic implications? *Journal of Neurology, Neurosurgery and Psychiatry*, 78, 1152–3.

Lipsman, N., Zener, R., and Bernstein, M. (2009). Personal identity, enhancement and neurosurgery: a qualitative study in applied neuroethics. *Bioethics*, 23, 375–83.

Mallet, L., Polosan, M., Jaafari, N., *et al.* (2008). Subthalamic nucleus stimulation in severe obsessive-compulsive disorder. *New England Journal of Medicine*, 13, 2121–34.

Mayberg, H.S., Lozano, A.M., Voon, V., *et al.* (2005). Deep brain stimulation for treatment-resistant depression. *Neuron*, 45, 651–60.

McGee, E.M. and Maguire, G.Q. Jr. (2007). Becoming borg to become immortal: regulating brain implant technologies. *Cambridge Quarterly of Healthcare Ethics*, 16, 291–302.

McIntyre, C.C., Savasta, M., Walter, B.L., and Vitek, J.L. (2004). How does deep brain stimulation work? Present understanding and future questions. *Journal of Clinical Neurophysiology*, 21, 40–50.

Mikell, C.B., McKhann, G.M., Segal, S., McGovern, R.A., Wallenstein, M.B., and Moore, H. (2009). The hippocampus and nucleus accumbens as potential therapeutic targets for neurosurgical intervention in schizophrenia. *Stereotactic and Functional Neurosurgery*, 87, 256–65.

Mink, J.W. (2009). Clinical review of DBS for Tourette syndrome. *Frontiers in Bioscience*, 1, 72–6.

Montgomery, E.B. Jr and Gale, J.T. (2008). Mechanisms of action of deep brain stimulation (DBS). *Neuroscience & Biobehavioral Reviews*, 32, 388–407.

Pancrazio, J.J. (2009). National Institute of Neurological Disorders and Stroke support for brain-machine interface technology. *Neurosurgical Focus*, 27, E14.

Penfield, W. (1963). *The Second Career*. Toronto: Little, Brown and Company.

Penfield, W. (1977). *No Man Alone*. Toronto: Little, Brown and Company.

Racine, E., Waldman, S., Palmour, N., Risse, D., and Illes, J. (2007). "Currents of hope": neurostimulation techniques in U.S. and U.K. print media. *Cambridge Quarterly of Healthcare Ethics*, 16, 312–16.

Schiff, N.D. (2009). Central thalamic deep-brain stimulation in the severely injured brain: rationale and proposed mechanisms of action. *Annals of the NY Academy of Sciences*, 1157, 101–16.

Schiff, N.D., Giacino, J.T., Kalmar, K., *et al.* (2007). Behavioural improvements with thalamic stimulation after severe traumatic brain injury. *Nature*, 448, 600–3.

Schwartz, R. and Schwartz, M. (2008). The risks of reducing consciousness to neuroimaging. *American Journal of Bioethics*, 8, 25–6.

Wind, J.J. and Anderson, D.E. (2008). From prefrontal leukotomy to deep brain stimulation: the historical transformation of psychosurgery and the emergence of neuroethics. *Neurosurgical Focus*, 25, E10.

World Society for Stereotactic and Functional Neurosurgery (WSSFN). *Stereotactic and functional neurosurgery. A contemporary definition by members of the WSSFN and ESSFN.* Available at: http://www.wssfn.org/STEREO_FUNCT_NS_Contemporary_Definition_ Version_3_0.pdf (accessed 14 August 2009).

Yu, H. and Neimat, J.S. (2008). The treatment of movement disorders by deep brain stimulation. *Neurotherapeutics*, 5, 26–36.

Zabek, M., Sobstyl, M., Koziara, H., and Dzierzecki, S. (2008). Deep brain stimulation of the right nucleus accumbens in a patient with Tourette syndrome. Case report. *Neurologia Neurochirugia Polska*, 42, 554–9.

CHAPTER 25

NON-INVASIVE BRAIN STIMULATION AS A THERAPEUTIC AND INVESTIGATIVE TOOL: AN ETHICAL APPRAISAL

ALVARO PASCUAL-LEONE, FELIPE FREGNI, MEGAN S. STEVEN-WHEELER, AND LACHLAN FORROW

INTRODUCTION

TRANSCRANIAL magnetic stimulation (TMS) allows for the safe and non-invasive stimulation of the human brain (Hallett 2000; Pascual-Leone 1999; Wagner *et al.* 2007). TMS can be used to complement other neuroscience methods to study the pathways between the brain and the spinal cord, and between different cortical and subcortical brain structures. Furthermore, TMS can be used to validate the functional significance of neuroimaging studies in determining the causal relationship between focal brain activity and behavior. Most relevant to the present chapter, is the way in which modulation of brain activity by repetitive TMS (rTMS) can transiently change brain function and be utilized as a therapeutic tool for treatment of a variety of neurological and psychiatric illnesses.

In the past decades, the uses of and accessibility to non-invasive brain stimulation have greatly increased. The potential risks and appropriate precautions in the use of TMS are increasingly well established (Machii *et al.* 2006; Rossi *et al.* 2009). New applications of TMS are being explored in normal subjects, and clinical treatment programs for TMS in various neuropsychiatric disorders are being launched. Such expansion has been further catalyzed by the approval of certain clinical applications of TMS in several countries, and most recently the approval by the Food and Drug Administration (FDA) in the United States (US) of the Neurostar treatment for specific forms of medication-resistant depression (Janicak *et al.* 2008; O'Reardon *et al.* 2007). In addition to TMS there are other methods of non-invasive brain stimulation, such as transcranial direct current stimulation (tDCS)

(Nitsche *et al.* 2003), which are becoming increasingly established. The number of subjects studied worldwide and the number of research studies published annually has increased yearly (Rossi *et al.* 2009). Therefore, it seems important to revisit the ethical considerations upon which one should reflect when applying non-invasive brain stimulation to humans. We aim to build on and update the work published by Green *et al.* (1997) during the early stages of rTMS testing and have aimed at updating our discussion of ethical considerations in the use of TMS in the prior edition of this textbook (see Table 25.1). For example, since 1997, clinical trials have been conducted to evaluate the efficacy of rTMS treatment for major depression and over 100 papers have been published. In a meta-analysis of controlled studies, Burt and colleagues (2002) showed that there was a definite antidepressant effect of rTMS in patients with major depression and a very favorable efficacy–side-effect balance. The positive results of these trials have encouraged researchers to continue these investigations, and there are currently large, multisite studies being conducted in the US and Europe for other conditions including stroke rehabilitation and Parkinson's disease. Certainly, rTMS appears to be an attractive approach to treat medication-resistant major depression, especially given the significant side effects of the alternative, electroconvulsive therapy (ECT). ECT, while often effective, is associated with adverse effects on cognition and a substantial social burden (O'Connor *et al.* 2003; UK ECT Review Group 2003). Despite recent FDA approval of a TMS device and application protocol for medication-resistant depression, the efficacy of rTMS in the cited trial was small (Janicak *et al.* 2008; O'Reardon *et al.* 2007). Thus even for medication-resistant depression significant ethical questions regarding the use of rTMS remain. For example: (1) Should rTMS only be offered to the relatively few patients who fit the narrow FDA indication? (2) Should other patients with resistant depression be treated with rTMS, and if so, what type of depressed patients—those refractory to medication only or a broad population of depressed patients? (3) Should this new technique be studied as an add-on therapy? (4) Should patients who experience a positive response with this treatment be offered a possibility of "maintenance" treatment, even though that has not been proven safe and effective? (5) Should other patients with depression (young patients or those who have failed multiple medications or have never tried one, for instance) be offered the possibility of receiving this treatment as an off-label therapy? Of course, none of these questions are unique to rTMS—most, if not all, are relevant to any new treatment for depression, including new medications.

Although the use of rTMS to treat other neuropsychiatric disorders has been investigated to a lesser extent, there is a growing body of evidence suggesting that rTMS might be useful, for instance, for Parkinson's disease (see (Fregni *et al.* 2005a; Wu *et al.* 2008) and schizophrenia (Freitas *et al.* 2009; Hoffman *et al.* 2003). Questions similar to those posed here regarding treatment of depression also apply to the use of rTMS for patients suffering from these diseases.

Another technique of non-invasive brain stimulation, transcranial direct current stimulation (tDCS), also has a positive effect in depression amelioration (Fregni *et al.* 2006a). TDCS is inexpensive and relatively simple to administer and might prove to be a suitable alternative for the treatment of depression in areas that lack the financial and technical resources necessary for rTMS. In fact, rTMS opened the field to explore other techniques of non-invasive brain stimulation and novel method such as transcranial alternate and intermittent stimulation are being investigated (Zaghi *et al.* 2010).

Table 25.1 List of recent advances in the field of non-invasive brain stimulation that bring about new ethical challenges

Approval by the US Food and Drug Administration of repetitive TMS with the Northstar system for the treatment of certain patients with medication refractory depression

Expansion of existing and establishment of new clinical programs and clinics offering TMS for therapeutics in a variety of neuropsychiatric disorders (on- and particularly off-label)

Establishment of new TMS protocols that enable greater modulation of cortical excitability and plasticity with shorter exposure

Growing number of applications of TMS and other neuromodulation techniques in neuroscience research

Expansion of TMS protocols to other subject populations, including vulnerable patient populations (e.g. autism spectrum disorders) and children

Development of new, simpler non-invasive brain stimulation method (e.g. transcranial direct current stimulation)

The potential uses of non-invasive brain stimulation that raise important ethical issues are not limited to therapeutic applications in patients with various neuropsychiatric disorders who fail to benefit from traditional interventions. TMS has also been utilized in healthy subjects in experimental settings. The use of TMS for neuroenhancement—the "non-therapeutic" uses of TMS for enhancing cognitive or affective function—raises fundamental ethical questions about the very nature of medicine. Should medical interventions (not just TMS, but also pharmacologic or genetic modifications) be limited to "treatment" of "disease", or is enhancement of "normal" functioning a legitimate use of medical techniques?

Several authors have shown that rTMS might enhance motor function (Kobayashi *et al.* 2004), attention (Hilgetag *et al.* 2001) and working memory (Kahn *et al.* 2005) in normal subjects—(for review see Pascual-Leone 2006). The modulatory effects of rTMS could also be used, hypothetically, to control or reinforce certain behaviors such as deception, violence, trust, and altruism. In fact, several studies have already moved beyond mere hypothesis, with published results revealing that tDCS can modulate deception (Karim *et al.* 2009; Priori *et al.* 2008). Work from Delgado (1976) in primate models illustrates the possibility of guiding complex behavior by brain stimulation. Non-invasive stimulation might permit a safer and easier means of inducing similar behaviorally modifying changes in brain activity in humans. Is neuroenhancement ethically appropriate? If so, with what aims and controls?

BASIC MECHANISMS OF TMS

The principles that underlie TMS were discovered by Faraday in 1831 (Walsh and Pascual-Leone 2003). A pulse of electric current flowing through a coil of wire generates a magnetic field (Figure 25.1). The rate of change of this magnetic field determines the induction of a secondary current in a nearby conductor. In TMS, the stimulating coil is held over a subject's

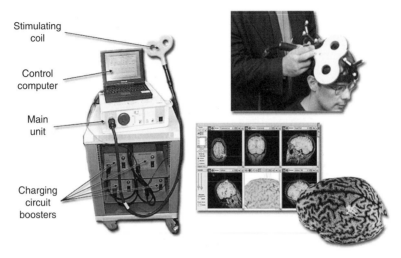

Stimulating coil

Control computer

Main unit

Charging circuit boosters

FIG. 25.1 A typical TMS module and MRI guided frameless stereotactic guidance system.

head (Figure 25.1) and, as a brief pulse of current is passed through it, a magnetic field is generated that penetrates through the subject's scalp and skull without attenuation (only decaying by the square of the distance). This time-varying magnetic field induces a current in the subject's brain that depolarizes neurons and generates effects depending on the brain area targeted. Therefore, in TMS, neural elements are not primarily affected by the exposure to a magnetic field, but rather by the current induced in the brain by electrodeless, non-invasive electric stimulation.

In the early 1980s, Barker and colleagues developed the first compact magnetic coil stimulator at the University of Sheffield. Soon thereafter, TMS devices became commercially available. The design of magnetic stimulators is relatively simple. Stimulators consist of a main unit and a stimulating coil. The main unit is composed of a charging system, one or more energy storage capacitors, a discharge switch, and circuits for pulse shaping, energy recovery, and control functions (Figure 25.2). Different charging systems are possible; the simplest design uses step-up transformers operating at line frequency of 50–60Hz. Energy storage capacitors can also be of different types. The essential factors in the effectiveness of a magnetic stimulator are the speed of the magnetic field rise time and the maximization of the peak coil energy. Therefore, large energy storage capacitors and very efficient energy transfer from the capacitor to the coil are important. Typically, energy storage capacity is around 2000 joules and 500 joules are transferred from the capacitors into the stimulating coil in less than 100μs via a thyristor, an electronic device that is capable of switching large currents in a few microseconds. The peak discharge current needs to be several thousand amperes in order to induce currents in the brain of sufficient magnitude to depolarize neural elements (approximately 10mA/cm²).

During transcranial magnetic brain stimulation only the stimulating coil needs to come in close contact with the subject (Figure 25.1). Stimulating coils consist of one or more well-insulated coils of copper wire frequently housed in a molded plastic cover and are available in a variety of shapes and sizes. The geometry of the coil determines the focality of brain stimulation. Figure-of-eight coils (also called butterfly or double coils, Figure 25.2) are constructed with two windings placed side by side and provide the most focal means of brain

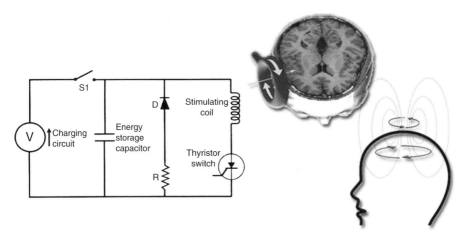

FIG. 25.2   A simple TMS pulse circuit and resultant effects.

stimulation with TMS available to date. Current knowledge, largely based on mathematical modeling, suggests that the most focal forms of TMS available today affect an area of 0.5 × 0.5cm at the level of the brain cortex (Wagner *et al.* 2007). Stimulation is restricted to rather superficial layers in the convexity of the brain (cortex or gray–white matter junction) and direct effect onto deep brain structures is not yet possible. Digitization of the subject's head and registration of the TMS stimulation sites onto the magnetic resonance image (MRI) of the subject's brain addresses the issue of anatomical specificity of the TMS effects by identifying the actual brain target in each experimental subject (Figure 25.1). The use of optical digitization and frameless stereotactic systems represents a further improvement by providing on-line information about the brain area targeted by a given coil position on the scalp.

The precise mechanisms underlying the brain effects of TMS remain largely unknown (Pascual-Leone *et al.* 1999; Robertson *et al.* 2003; Wagner *et al.* 2007). Currents induced in the brain by TMS flow primarily parallel to the plane of the stimulation coil (approximately parallel to the brain's cortical surface when the stimulation coil is held tangentially to the scalp). Therefore, in contrast to electrical cortical stimulation, TMS preferentially activates neural elements oriented horizontally to the brain surface. Exactly which neural elements are activated by TMS remains unclear and, in fact, might be variable across different brain areas and different subjects. The combination of TMS with other neuroimaging and neurophysiologic techniques provides an enhanced understanding of the mechanisms of action of TMS and a novel approach to study functional connectivity between different areas in the human brain.

ETHICS OF CLINICAL INVESTIGATION OF rTMS
TREATMENT FOR NEUROPSYCHIATRIC DISEASES

Guidelines for research on human subjects in the US are articulated in the 1979 *Belmont Report* by the US National Commission for the Protection of Human Subjects of Biomedical and Behavioral Research. This report defines three governing principles that remain the gold standard for human subject research ethics: (1) respect for persons, (2) beneficence, and (3) justice.

The first principle of respect and the third principle of justice have been addressed in the TMS literature, especially with respect to the basic ethical treatment of subjects (e.g., consent, exclusion, and inclusion criteria, e.g. see Green *et al.* (1997) and Steven and Pascual-Leone (2006). The first clause of the second principle (i.e. *risks reduced to a minimum*) is considered at length in the literature on the guidelines for safe use of single pulse TMS as well as rTMS on the normal human brain (Hallett *et al.* 1999; Rossi *et al.* 2009; Wassermann 1998). Taking these principles into account, we focus specifically on the issues of beneficence, and on finding the appropriate balance between benefit and risk of TMS.

In the clinical population, TMS has shown promise for treatment of depression (Gross *et al.* 2007), Parkinson's disease (Wu *et al.* 2008), writer's cramp (Siebner *et al.* 1999) and chronic pain (Jensen *et al.*2008), as well as for the rehabilitation for motor neglect (Hilgetag *et al.* 2001), motor stroke (Mansur *et al.* 2005), and aphasia (Martin *et al.* 2004; Naeser *et al.* 2005a,b) among others (see Table 25.2).

As is common with potential new treatments for which risks are not yet well defined, rTMS was initially studied in patients who have exhausted other, more established forms of treatment. This has meant offering rTMS to patients with relatively severe forms of neurological or psychiatric disorders refractory to conventional therapy. These patients, however, may have diminished autonomy, either as a result of their neuropsychiatric illness, or because they are "desperate" (or both), necessitating special efforts to ensure appropriate informed consent (F. G. Miller and Brody 2003; Minogue *et al.* 1995). Because studies to date have provided increasing evidence for the relatively benign profile of side-effects of rTMS (Rossi *et al.* 2009), at least for the duration (usually short term) of the studies, rTMS is now

Table 25.2 List of the clinical applications of TMS research that are currently being pursued in research laboratories worldwide

Currently investigated therapeutic applications of rTMS	
Acute mania	Obsessive compulsive disorder
Aphasia	Pain:
Auditory hallucinoses	Visceral pain
Bipolar disorder	Atypical facial pain
Depression	Phantom pain
Epilepsy:	Parkinson's disease
Myoclonic epilepsy	Post-traumatic stress disorder
Focal status epilepsy	Schizophrenia
Focal dystonia	Stuttering
Neglect	Tics

being offered to broader populations, including patients with less severe conditions and those who have not necessarily proven refractory to all available alternatives.

The nature, frequency, and severity of adverse effects of rTMS in a variety of populations are now well documented. A recent review of the experience at the Center for Non-invasive Brain Stimulation at Beth Israel Deaconess Medical Center and Harvard Medical School provides an up-to-date overview of extensive experience in patients with neuropsychiatric diseases as well as subjects recruited as normal healthy controls (Machii et al. 2006). Approximately 10 to 20% of subjects studied with TMS develop a muscle tension headache or a neck ache (23% in Machii and colleagues' review). These are generally mild discomforts that respond promptly to an aspirin, acetaminophen (Tylenol®) or other common analgesics. Because the sound of the TMS procedure is loud, repetitive TMS can also cause transient hearing loss if the subjects do not wear earplugs during the rTMS studies. Furthermore, TMS can cause very mild and transient memory problems and other cognitive deficits, as well as mood and hormone changes (these rare adverse effects are usually resolved within hours of cessation of TMS). A recent consensus conference on the safety of TMS (Rossi et al. 2009) similarly concluded that the risks of TMS were relatively minor, provided that appropriate guidelines are followed and precautions are taken.

The major risk of TMS is the risk of producing a seizure. The likelihood of inducing a seizure is small. Only 16 seizures induced by rTMS have been reported world-wide among the many thousands of patients studied resulting in a projected risk of less than 1:1000 patients and probably less than 1:10000 TMS sessions (Rossi et al. 2009). The parameters of TMS that have produced seizures during experimentation are well known and documented (Rossi et al. 2009). However even though the risk of seizures is small if safety guidelines are followed, these guidelines are primarily based on experiments in healthy subjects and the risk of seizures may be higher in patients with neuropsychiatric diseases such as stroke and major depression and in patients on certain neuropsychotropic drugs. For example, patients with infarcts or neurological disorders that cause cortical atrophy should be stimulated with great care as the presence of excess cerebrospinal fluid (CSF) can alter the electro-magnetic field properties and stimulation near CSF can cause adverse effects (Wagner et al. 2006). Finally, TMS has only been studied for approximately 25 years and the data on potential long-term effects in humans remains insufficient. Although animal studies using TMS have not indicated any risks of brain damage or long-term injury, caution remains imperative.

Since safety guidelines were generated from information on TMS in adults, relatively little is known about the appropriate safety guidelines for application of TMS in children (Frye et al. 2008). A recent study reviewed English-language published studies of TMS (single- and paired-pulse and rTMS) in persons younger than 18 years (the majority with neuropsychiatric disorders) from 1990–2005. The author of this study found 49 studies that in total applied TMS in 1036 children. No seizures were reported for any of the 1036 studied children; although the number of repetitive TMS studies (in contrast with single and paired pulse TMS studies that are safer) were low (Quintana 2005). More generally, the effects of TMS on the developing brain remain unknown. Thus, even though rTMS offers the potential for treating developmental disorders like autism, childhood depression, and obsessive–compulsive disorder among others, particular caution is needed when carrying out research on children until more is known about safety in younger populations from both studies on humans and animal models. Some authors have suggested that clinical trials on children who have medication refractory focal epilepsy represent a reasonable entry point given the current state-of- the-art (Fregni *et al.* 2005b; Thut *et al.* 2005).

RTMS treatment for major depression

The investigation for the treatment of depression using rTMS has been developing quickly and to date represents the most studied clinical application of this technique. The only FDA-approved application of TMS at this writing involves medication-resistant depression. We will discuss some ethical issues associated with this application of TMS, such as clinical trial design and its use outside of the experimental environment and outside the specific (and quite narrow) FDA indication. Furthermore, we will briefly discuss the ethical use of tDCS for the treatment of depression.

Randomized controlled clinical trials for the treatment of depression using non-invasive brain stimulation

Randomized controlled clinical trials are the gold standard for the investigation of new treatments. In neuropsychiatric populations, several variables, such as patient recruitment, trial duration, and type of control group, can be modified in order to provide the results in an ethical manner without compromising the scientific findings. For instance, in investigating treatment of depression using rTMS, which type of patients would be most appropriate— those refractory to medication or a broad spectrum of patients including, for instance, patients with newly diagnosed depression for whom medication has not yet been tried? There are advantages and disadvantages to both approaches. The investigation of patients with depression who are refractory to other medical therapies, such as antidepressants, is widely accepted—these patients do not have any other therapeutic options and, therefore, the best proven treatment will not be withheld from them in a randomized placebo-controlled trial. However this approach has an important caveat: patients with depression resistant to other antidepressant therapies might also be more likely not respond to rTMS— therefore a negative result might be hard to translate to other populations. Indeed, a recent meta-analysis showed that five out of seven studies that used this approach showed no significant depression improvement after active rTMS when compared to sham stimulation (Couturier 2005). In another investigation conducted by our own group, we pooled data from six different studies of rTMS treatment for depression and modeled these data to derive predictors of positive response. The results from the 195 aggregate patients showed that refractory patients have a less effective antidepressant response to rTMS compared with the non-refractory patients (Fregni *et al.* 2006b). Therefore, studies of refractory patients alone are inadequate to determine the possible effectiveness in broader populations of depressed patients. This conclusion and the large impact of the degree of medication refractoriness on the efficacy of rTMS in depression is further illustrated by the results of the trial that eventually led to the FDA's approval of one use of rTMS. (Janicak *et al.* 2008; O'Reardon *et al.* 2007). The initial overall results of this multisite, carefully designed and controlled trial were essentially negative and only the analysis of subpopulations of patients according to the number of medication trials failed, led to evidence of efficacy of rTMS. Indeed, the FDA approved the treatment for patients who have failed one good trial of an antidepressant, but not more than two, a strikingly narrow but understandable indication, given the poor efficacy data for patients who had failed multiple medication trials.

Another option is to investigate in a general population of depressed patients, including those that could potentially respond to the treatment of standard antidepressant medications. If there is a proven effective therapy (e.g. a certain antidepressant medication), and there is some reason to believe that a new therapy (rTMS) might work, then one could randomize to meds v. rTMS. Or one could have multiple arms: meds v. rTMS v. placebo rTMS. This method quickly becomes complicated; trials become very large and thus also quite expensive.

Another concern is that some patients will be denied an effective treatment if the trial uses a standard placebo control (e.g. placebo medication or sham rTMS). Because depression is common, and because some patients decline to take standard recommended medications, one might also recruit patients from those who have refused pharmacologic treatment. Randomizing them to rTMS or placebo (sham rTMS) would not be depriving them of known effective treatment.

But for patients for whom antidepressant medications are known to be effective, and who are willing to take them, why should non-invasive brain stimulation be investigated? There are several possible advantages to rTMS. First, rTMS has a different profile of risks compared to antidepressant medications and might be better suited to some patients that could eventually respond to either therapy. Second, efficacy of treatment with rTMS might be superior to medication for a subgroup of non-refractory patients. Finally, depending on the antidepressant drug used for comparison, rTMS can be less costly.

In order to perform a randomized, double-blind placebo-controlled clinical trial to investigate the effects of non-invasive brain stimulation in non-refractory depressive patients, the investigators would need to withhold the best proven therapy from the patients in the placebo arm. According to the declaration of Helsinki: "….in any medical study, every patient – including those of a control group, if any – should be assured of the best proven diagnostic and therapeutic methods." However, some authors defend the use of placebo, against the recommendations of the declaration of Helsinki, if patients with moderate or mild depression without suicide risk are studied on the principle that the lack of treatment for a short period of time would not expose these patients to great risk. Some authors consider this ethically permissible if these patients are adequately informed about this risk (S. M. Miller *et al.* 2000) and every attempt is made to mitigate it.

The alternative of active-controlled trials comparing new treatments only with standard drugs can lead to the use of new treatments that appear equivalent in efficacy to standard treatment but may be no more effective than placebo. This might be particularly valid if the specific population that is being tested for a new treatment has primarily a placebo response to the standard drug. In this situation, if the new treatment is found to have benefits similar to the standard drug, this new treatment might be equivalent to placebo only. Here the phenomenon of biocreep needs to be considered as well. In other words if active comparisons are made there is the risk that each new comparison treatment, even though it appears roughly similar to standard treatment, will in fact be slightly less effective. Over time it is possible that new treatments may become accepted even though they are not any more effective than placebo. For these reasons, despite the mandate of the declaration of Helsinki, the FDA continues to defend the use of placebo-controlled trials for the development of a new treatment even if effective therapy exists.

Rothman *et al.* (1994) disagree, basing their argument on the view that no patient should suffer unnecessary pain, even if the condition is not life-threatening (Rothman and Michels 1994). They argue that "active control" testing of brain stimulation—i.e. comparing it against standard antidepressant therapy—is adequate. The advantages of this approach are that: (1) patients in both groups receive active treatments for depression, and (2) results can guide the clinician regarding the choice between antidepressant treatment or brain stimulation. Still as mentioned before, a significant drawback is that the therapeutic effect of the active control might not be different than placebo in the population being investigated. One method to avoid, or at least reduce the likelihood of this problem, is to use of placebo "run-in" phase in which patients are excluded if they present a placebo response in the first weeks of the trials, "placebo-responders" (Lee *et al.* 2004).

Another drawback of this approach is the large sample size needed to perform this type of study. Because a lack of difference between two treatments is a function of the variance within datasets, a relatively large sample size is needed to decrease the risk of type II error using this study design. In contrast, the sample size needed to perform a placebo-controlled trial is much smaller, thus exposing fewer patients to unnecessary risks and discomforts. Accurate sample size calculations are imperative, therefore, to decide the best study design. Another important issue here is that future research showing patients who are likely to respond to rTMS may increase the effect sizes of a given trial, reducing therefore the number of patients who need to be part in a given research study.

Yet another alternative to placebo-control trials that has been tested is non-invasive brain stimulation as an add-on therapy. In this scenario, all patients receive the standard treatment, and half receive the experimental treatment in addition. Using this approach Rumi *et al.* (2005) showed that active rTMS and amitryptiline results in a larger antidepressant effect than amitryptiline alone. This approach however is limited in determining whether rTMS has any role in treatment of depression. For example, if there is a ceiling effect, i.e. the improvement induced by antidepressants cannot be further extended, then addition of rTMS would show no added benefit even if rTMS alone were highly effective. Indeed, several rTMS studies were conducted using this approach and some of them showed that rTMS does not add efficacy over the use of standard antidepressant medication (Garcia-Toro *et al.* 2001; Hausmann *et al.* 2004).

In summary, in exploring the effectiveness of rTMS for treatment of depression, several alternatives might be pursued: (1) inclusion only of patients that are refractory to available antidepressant medications; (2) investigation of the use of non-invasive brain stimulation as an add-on therapy (to medication); (3) comparison of the effects of non-invasive brain stimulation against an active control; and (4) comparison of rTMS versus placebo among patients who have declined pharmacologic treatment;. Given the evidence that rTMS has some effectiveness in depression, and given the scientific limitations of designs (1) and (2) reviewed earlier, approaches (3) and (4) seem most likely to provide ethically appropriate and scientifically useful information about possible roles for rTMS in depression.

OFF-LABEL TREATMENT FOR DEPRESSION

While the initial FDA approval for rTMS in depression is quite narrow, as explained earlier, it is possible that other patients might benefit. For example, what if a patient in an rTMS study appears to benefit and wants to continue rTMS beyond the study period for an indication that is not FDA-approved? Is it ethical to deny treatment after the study is terminated? One alternative is to offer it as an off-label intervention for those patients—a treatment not approved by the FDA—for which those patients might be asked to sign a consent form acknowledging that the treatment remains experimental. There is an intense debate about the use of an off-label treatment (Bickerstaffe *et al.* 2006). The practice of prescribing medicines for indications or in dosage regimens that are different than the terms of the products specification is common in medicine (Bickerstaffe *et al.* 2006). For example, a national report from a healthcare organization in Canada concludes that pediatric prescriptions in Canada are often prescribed off-label, as pharmaceutical companies do not have an incentive to obtain approval for a drug for more than one purpose (http://www.law.utoronto.ca/healthlaw/docs/student_Rabinovitch-NationalFormulary.pdf). In the case of off-label rTMS, the benign profile of side effects provides support for belief in a favorable benefit–risk ratio, since even among patients for whom efficacy is unproven the risks (at least for short-term use) are almost certainly low. (As mentioned earlier, thousands of rTMS trials on patients and healthy subjects have been conducted and data from these studies demonstrate short-term safety if technical guidelines are carefully followed (Rossi *et al.* 2009; Wassermann 1998).) Nonetheless, few data regarding long-term effects of rTMS are available, and both clinical caution and scrupulously careful informed consent are both clearly warranted.

As new data are gathered, both FDA-approved and off-label use of rTMS for patients may become more and more widespread. Depending on whether rTMS is covered by medical insurance, and on the extent of continued problems of uninsured patients, issues of distributive justice may surface. If rTMS is believed effective but is not covered by medical insurance, then equitable access to this approach to treating suffering may not be possible.

In a broader context, approval of a certain form of TMS for a given indication (major depression) has led to a further expansion of already existing clinics offering rTMS for treatment of various neuropsychiatric conditions. Such clinics often bank on the patients' hope and faith in help from a novel therapy. The efficacy data for many of the offered indications is at best limited. Such practices should thus be viewed with caution and a responsible, conservative approach by the involved physicians is critical.

USE OF tDCS FOR THE TREATMENT OF DEPRESSION: AN ALTERNATIVE TO TREAT DEPRESSION IN RESOURCE-LIMITED AREAS?

Like rTMS, tDCS is a technique of brain stimulation that can modulate brain activity, and therefore be used for depression treatment. In fact several trials have shown positive results (see review (Murphy *et al.* 2009). In tDCS, the cerebral cortex is stimulated through a weak constant electric current in a non-invasive and painless manner (Wagner *et al.* 2007). This weak current is presumed to induce focal changes in cortical excitability—increases or decreases depending on the electrode polarity—that last beyond the period of stimulation. Several studies reveal that this technique might modulate cortical excitability in the human motor cortex (Baudewig *et al.* 2001; Nitsche and Paulus 2000; Rosenkranz *et al.* 2000), and visual cortex (Antal *et al.* 2001, 2002). Although this technique has already been shown to be a promising treatment for major depression (Fregni *et al.* 2006a), continuous methodological improvements on electrode size and position and paradigms of stimulation, might yield an enhanced outcome in the future.

TDCS and rTMS have similar modulatory effects, but in the treatment of depression, tDCS might have two important advantages over both rTMS and drugs: (1) tDCS treatment is inexpensive and (2) it is easy to administer (Fregni *et al.* 2005c; Nitsche *et al.* 2003). The device used to deliver the tDCS is simple, can cost less than 100 USD, and can be manufactured locally (Fregni *et al.* 2005d). The equipment is fully reusable and utilizes one standard battery that can last several weeks. This treatment is easily administered and used after specific but relatively minimal training. Finally, tDCS has other mechanisms of action such as it is a purely neuromodulatory tool that can change the resting neuronal membrane threshold thus can modulate the neuronal spontaneous firing, being therefore an interesting technique to enhance the effect of other behavioral interventions such as cognitive behavioral therapy. Establishing efficacy in various populations requires, however, rigorous assessments, with the same issues as discussed earlier for rTMS.

The ease of application and access make tDCS potentially appealing though also raise concerns for the ease of abuse. As an approach to improve mental health in areas of the world with limited resources, tDCS might prove to be a promising solution. However, developing world issues are extremely complex and cannot be taken lightly. Naturally, the implementation of tDCS for depression treatment should be considered for any nation *only if* it is proven to be at least as efficacious as the gold standard. The standard of proof in this regard has to be as stringent for its implementation in developing countries as elsewhere. However, as antidepressants—the gold standard for depression—are often not available in poor countries, it has been argued that a treatment that is more effective than placebo but less effective than drugs (or TMS) could have value (Lenfant 2001). Again, this is a complex issue where multiple solution approaches are needed, including making antidepressants more widely available worldwide, but for the time being, the shortage of medications is a critical problem in low-income countries. Even in developed countries, people without health insurance are regularly faced with the decision of stopping antidepressant treatment because of the high cost. Poor patients often interrupt treatment for the same reason, endangering themselves through risks of worsening or relapse of their depression. Moreover, is well established that a higher prevalence of depression is found among poor, illiterate, and urban migrants (Almeida-Filho *et al.* 2004; Wohlfarth 1997). Therefore, the sickest population is the one with the greatest inability to attain or afford a regular antidepressant treatment. Given such a scenario, it can be argued that investigating low-cost approaches such as tDCS has the potential to be very beneficial.

As reasonable as these arguments may be, the history of debates regarding HIV treatments in resource-poor settings provides instructive guidance. The HIV treatment regimens in wealthy nations were not only extraordinarily expensive, but also far more complex than antidepressant medications. It was widely believed that providing access to highly-effective antiretroviral medications in developing countries was unrealistic, and many experts have discussed either settling for less effective treatment approaches or even for no treatment at all. But great progress has been made in less than a decade in reducing the price of medications, in expanding distribution systems, and in proving that compliance rates equaling or exceeding those in developed countries can be achieved even in the poorest regions of the world. The moral acceptability of any approach to HIV treatment that does not aspire to the same quality of care that is offered in developed countries is now quite properly widely questioned. Similar considerations need to be applied to the temptation of widespread implementation of certain device-based interventions in developing countries on the basis of expense.

Despite the scientific, technical, and economic potential of tDCS, further phase II trials showing efficacy of this technique are necessary. Another issue is the safety of this technique. Among the data available, Nitsche and Paulus (2001) showed that tDCS does not change serum neuron specific enolase concentration (a sensitive marker of neuronal damage), blood–brain barrier function, or cerebral vasculature (Nitsche and Paulus 2001; Nitsche et al. 2003, 2004). In another study, the safety of tDCS was tested with respect to neurocognitive and motor function (simple reaction test and Pegboard Grooved test). No significant deterioration with tDCS was found. On the contrary, the authors reported a significant improvement of verbal fluency after stimulation of the prefrontal cortex. These findings are in agreement with safety studies performed in our lab (Fregni et al. 2006c). Finally, a recent study reviewed the safety of tDCS, concluding the tDCS is associated with only a few and mild adverse effects (Nitsche et al. 2008). Although these early data and a recent review by Wasserman and Grafman (2005) suggest that the technique may prove to be intrinsically safe, more studies are clearly needed to determine full safety guidelines (Wassermann and Grafman 2005).

Use of rTMS as a placebo-inducer and placebo-blocker

Placebo and nocebo represent important concepts in medicine as they can impact neurophysiological processes and, thus, interfere in the disease pathophysiology (de la Fuente-Fernandez et al. 2001; Strafella 2006). The placebo/nocebo effect is also an important confounder in clinical trials. For instance, placebos induce an antidepressant response, on average, in 30% of patients with major depression (Laporte and Figueras 1994).

The consequence of changes in the activity of neural networks in response to plastic changes induced by organic afferents and emotional expectations from placebo or nocebo effects provides a target for neuromodulation. It is conceivable that by increasing activity in specific nodes of these networks, so as to maximize placebo, the healing powers of the patient's own body may be enhanced. At the same time, by suppressing activity in other nodes, the deleterious effects of nocebo may be reduced. To this end, rTMS could be used in clinical practice to enhance placebo and decrease nocebo effects and in randomized trials to disrupt and perhaps block the placebo effect and (thus, disentangling the effect of a new treatment from the placebo effect).

However, if placebo can help some patients that undergo placebo-controlled clinical trials, one can argue that it would be unethical to block this potential therapeutic effect of placebo in order to improve the scientific quality of a clinical trial. This assumes, however, that the "placebo effect" interferes with scientific "rigor." If the point of a clinical trial is to determine the likely effectiveness of an intervention in actual clinical practice, then since we know that for many interventions overall effectiveness includes some degree of placebo effect, research interventions that included blocking any placebo effects might not be generalizable to clinical practice in the real world. If the point of a clinical trial is to determine effects that are specifically attributable to the active pharmacologic agent under study, however, then if rTMS were able to block the placebo effect, it is possible that fewer patients would be needed in a phase III clinical trial. This would in turn mean that fewer non-placebo responders would be exposed to receive no adequate treatment. Certainly, all research subjects would have to be adequately informed about the use of a placebo-blocker method.

Ethical considerations of TMS in basic neuroscience research

Until recently, scientists relied on naturally occurring lesions in the human brain to draw conclusions about the functioning of specific neural regions. The effects of naturally-occurring lesions are, however, imprecise, often irreversible, variable from patient to patient, and do not always occur in isolation of other neurological disorders. Since TMS (at least single pulse TMS) has only a transient effect, it can be utilized to investigate the importance of a given brain area in the normal, functioning human brain by creating a temporary "virtual lesion" (Pascual-Leone 2006; Pascual-Leone *et al.* 1998; Walsh and Pascual-Leone 2003; Walsh *et al.* 2005, 2006). For this reason, TMS is used today to investigate a myriad of neuroscientific questions about the functioning of the normal human brain. Some studies have aimed at understanding early sensory processing system using single-pulse TMS at different time-points after visual stimulation (e.g. Amassian *et al.* 1991; Corthout *et al.* 1999), while others have investigated higher visual processing (e.g. Ashbridge *et al.* 1997) with the same relatively safe parameters. Motor processing is also studied extensively with single pulse TMS on normal subjects (e.g. De Gennaro *et al.* 2003; Robertson *et al.* 2003; Theoret *et al.* 2004).

RTMS studies at rates of repetition well below safety limits are also conducted on normal subjects to investigate phenomena varying from self-recognition (Keenan *et al.* 2000) to sequence learning (Robertson *et al.* 2001). Other studies utilize rTMS at parameters nearing the limit of safety guidelines, and some appear to exceed reasonable ethical criteria. For example, researchers have recently begun to investigate the induction of long-term depression (LTD) and long-term potentiation (LTP) (the mechanisms of neuroplasticity) using rTMS protocols in the normal human brain (Iyer *et al.* 2003 and Huang *et al.* 2005 respectively). These studies, while potentially producing valuable scientific knowledge, raise significant questions about the risk–benefit ratio for research subjects. The scientific value of such research is that learning how to induce LTD and LTP could provide major new understanding of brain function that might have significant implications for diagnosis and treatment of diseases like depression, epilepsy, Parkinson's and other neurological disorders. However, as described earlier, increasing the length and rate of stimulation both contribute to the higher risk of seizure. LTP induction requires only 20–190s, but stimulation must be applied at 50Hz (in the theta range) for its induction. The parameters necessary to induce LTD are not as concerning since they involve stimulation at a relatively low repetitive rate (for example 6Hz followed by 1Hz), though it might need to be applied for a long period of time (20min). Other forms of repetitive TMS, for example asynchronous trains in the theta burst pattern have also been introduced recently. All these forms of stimulation attempt to produce a potentially deleterious effect without precise knowledge of how long this effect will last, or how treatable the effect would be. That appears to violate basic standards of research on human subjects, especially when seeking maximal knowledge first through animal models has not always been done. In fact, a recent study showed that a 5-day course of rTMS is associated with structural changes in the gray matter (May *et al.* 2006) and raises a red flag for the use of repetitive sessions of rTMS in healthy subjects. Although these effects could have also been a result of changes in brain perfusion, investigators must be aware of a possible detrimental effect of consecutive sessions of rTMS in healthy subjects when planning TMS studies on healthy subjects.

RTMS to control behavior: beneficence or maleficence?

Given that rTMS can modulate brain function, an important question arises: Is it ethical to use rTMS to inhibit some behaviors such as or aggressive behavior or reinforce others such as altruistic behavior, trust, and moral behavior? Should rTMS be used to improve some aspects of cognition such as working memory? Is it ethical to use it in normal subjects to improve their performance? We will briefly discuss the aspects of using rTMS in otherwise healthy subjects.

Socially undesirable behaviors: aggression and deception

RTMS can be used to inhibit some undesirable behaviors such as aggression and deception. Deception occurs, for example, when one person attempts to deliberately make someone believe things that are not true. Because society values the ability to detect, and perhaps prevent, deception, the polygraph was developed in 1921 as a device to monitor physiological function associated with deception. More sophisticated approaches to deception detection include brain finger-printing based on scalp-recorded EEG (Dickson and McMahon 2005) and fMRI. A study using the latter technique has shown more activation in right anterior frontal cortices anterior cingulate and posterior visual cortex associated with well-rehearsed lies, i.e. the ones that fit into a coherent story, versus spontaneous lies (Ganis *et al.* 2003). Rather than recording neural correlates of such behaviors, the possibility of inhibiting them exists with rTMS: imagine a scenario of inhibiting rehearsal of lies before a criminal trial. Indeed, intellectual property protection for such notions have been filed and granted in the US. On the one hand TMS could be used to help establish one's innocence or to inhibit aggressive behaviors. On the other, even in the face of national security, the use of brain stimulation is likely to be widely (though not universally) considered unethical if coerced or against subjects' will.

Socially desirable behaviors: altruism and trust

The advance of the neuroimaging techniques has furthered the understanding of some behaviors such as altruism and trust. For instance, de Quervain (2004) has shown that people can feel rewarded from punishing norm violations and this behavior is associated with an activation of reward-related brain areas such as the dorsal striatum. Trust has been shown to be associated with an activation of the amygdala and the specific neurotransmitter oxytocin (Damasio 2005). Currently rTMS cannot stimulate such deep brain areas selectively, but this capability might become available in the future and special coil designs capable to reach deep into the brain are already available (e.g. Brainsway's H-coil). With the rapid development of neurotechnology, implantable brain stimulators are entirely within the range of possibilities and the "psycho-civilized" society envisioned by Delgado (1969) might not always be science fiction. Akin to the genetic manipulation to obtain better, more fit people, brain stimulation might create a superior, privileged society (or at least a group of individuals that, rightly or not, judge themselves "superior" and might have power to take advantage of that), a divide that would be ethically unjust.

Neurocognitive enhancement

Are non-therapeutic uses of TMS for enhancing cognitive or affective function, ethical? Does the benefit of increasing mental facility above and beyond natural levels justify an increased risk in the patient population?

The idea that targeted brain stimulation (excitatory or inhibitory) can enhance or beneficially alter cognitive function has not been lost by the Hollywood industry (see *Total Recall* 1990 or *Eternal Sunshine of the Spotless Mind* 2004) let alone the scientific community. But this is not a futuristic issue, as recent studies using TMS and other forms of non-invasive stimulation like direct current stimulation, are exploring neuroenhancing applications in the normal population (e.g. Kobayashi *et al.* 2004; Antal *et al.* 2004; Fregni *et al.* 2005d, respectively). For instance, Kobayashi *et al.* (2004) discovered that by inhibiting cortical activity in the right motor cortex (which controls the left hand), the reaction time to a sequential finger movement task can be increased in the right hand without affecting the performance in the left hand. Similarly, Hilgetag *et al.* (2001) found enhanced attention to the ipsilateral field of a person's spatial environment in normal subjects following suppression of the parietal cortex by rTMS. Others have reported facilitatory behavioral effects of rTMS on working memory, naming, abstract thinking, color perception, motor learning, and perceptual learning (Theoret *et al.* 2003).

Snyder and his colleagues (2003) reported that latent savant-like qualities could be revealed in normal control subjects following low-frequency rTMS to the left frontotemporal cortex. Subjects (11 right-handed males) performed a battery of tests before, immediately after, and 45 minutes following rTMS treatment. These tests included drawing animals from memory, drawing novel faces from images provided by the researcher and proofreading. Of 11 subjects, four showed dramatic stylistic changes in drawing immediately after rTMS as compared to the drawings produced before and 45min after stimulation (Snyder *et al.* 2003). This TMS-induced unmasking of increased artistic and language abilities was surprising to the subjects. One subject, who wrote an article about his experiences comments that he "could hardly recognize" the drawings as his own even though he had watched himself render each image. He added: "Somehow over the course of a very few minutes, and with no additional instruction, I had gone from an incompetent draftsman to a very impressive artist of the feline form" (Osborne 2003).

Whether or not savant-like capabilities can be revealed in all persons is a matter of debate. Morrell *et al.* (2000) conducted a study similar to the Snyder *et al.* (2003) study with only minimal success, suggesting that factors like sex, age, genes, and environment might play a role in determining whether or not TMS can induce savant-like responses in the normal population (just as these factors likely play a role in whether or not neurological damage leads to savant symptoms in the patient population) (Snyder *et al.* 2003). However, it remains a distinct possibility that TMS could, soon, induce reliable neurocognitive enhancement of motor, attentional, artistic or language abilities in the normal human brain.

Some believe neurostimulation is no different than enhancement by other mechanisms, as both are presumably a result of altering neuronal firing and modulating brain plasticity (see Pascual-Leone *et al.* 1998). There exist ethicists who argue both for (e.g. Caplan 2003) and against (e.g. Kass 2003; Sandel 2002—see http://www.bioethics.gov/background/ sandelpaper.html) enhancement. Michael Sandel, a member of the President's Council on Bioethics, raises the concern that non-therapeutic enhancement poses a threat to human dignity. Sandel believes that "…what is troubling about enhancement is that it represents the triumph in our time of willfulness over giftedness, of dominion over reverence, of molding over beholding." However, the capacity of being molded (plasticity) is an intrinsic property of the human brain and represents evolution's invention to enable the nervous system to escape the restrictions of its own genome and to thus adapt to environmental pressures, physiologic changes, and experiences. Dynamic shifts in the strength of pre-existing connections across distributed neural networks, changes in task-related cortico-cortical and cortico-subcortical coherence, and modifications of the mapping between behavior and neural activity take place continuously in response to any and all changes in afferent input or efferent demand. Such rapid, ongoing, changes might be followed by the establishment of new connections through dendritic growth and arborization. Plasticity is not an occasional state of the nervous system; instead, it is the normal ongoing state of the nervous system throughout the lifespan. We should therefore not conceive of the brain as a stationary object capable of activating a cascade of changes that we shall call plasticity, nor as an orderly stream of events, driven by plasticity. We might be served better by thinking of the nervous system as a continuously changing structure of which plasticity is an integral property and the obligatory consequence of each sensory input, each motor act, association, reward signal, action plan, or awareness. In this framework, notions of psychological processes as distinct from organic-based functions or dysfunctions cease to be informative. Behavior will lead to changes in brain circuitry, just as changes in brain circuitry will lead to behavioral changes. Therefore, all environmental interactions, and certainly educational approaches, represent interventions that mold the brain of the actor. Given this perspective, it is conceivable that neuromodulation with properly controlled and carefully applied neurophysiologic methods could be potentially a safer, more effective and more efficient means of guiding plasticity and thus shaping behavior. Plasticity is a double-edged sword, to be sure, and harbors dangers of evolving patterns of neural activation that might in and of themselves lead to abnormal behavior. Plasticity is the mechanism for development and learning, as much as it can be the cause of pathology.

The challenge we face as scientists, therefore, is to learn enough about the mechanisms of plasticity to be able to determine the parameters of TMS that will *optimally* modulate neuronal firing for patients, and perhaps for the non-patient population. Defining "optimal" is the accompanying immediate ethical challenge. Challenges of preventing or overcoming inequities of access to the underserved, and ethical issues of coercion will also be important (see Farah *et al.* 2004). TMS scientists and neuroethicists would do well, therefore, to jointly take the lead in pursuing these issues further and in ensuring that the utilization of rTMS as a clinical and a possibly enhancement tool become clearly defined. Otherwise, we risk in the not too distant future, being face with depressed patients using their at-home TMS machines instead of following a regimen of drug therapy or college students "zapping" their frontal or parietal lobes before taking the SATs. Ultimately such applications might prove appropriate; however, they require carefully designed, well controlled trials, based on suitable ethical considerations. Without such a cautious approach, ease of application of TMS, tDCS, and future non-invasive neuromodulatory techniques threaten to cause more harm than good.

ACKNOWLEDGEMENTS

Work on this chapter was supported in part by Grant Number UL1 RR025758 – Harvard Clinical and Translational Science Center, from the National Center for Research Resources and National Institutes of Health grant K 24 RR018875 to APL and a grant within the Harvard Medical School Scholars in Clinical Science Program (NIH K30 HL04095-03) to FF. The content of this chapter is solely the responsibility of the authors and does not necessarily represent the official views of the National Center for Research Resources or the National Institutes of Health.

The authors would like to thank Dan W. Brock, Professor of Medical Ethics in the Department of Social Medicine, Harvard Medical School, for his comments in an earlier version of this paper, and Jennifer Perez for editorial assistance.

REFERENCES

Almeida-Filho, N., Lessa, I., Magalhaes, L., *et al.* (2004). Social inequality and depressive disorders in Bahia, Brazil: interactions of gender, ethnicity, and social class. *Social Science & Medicine*, **59**, 1339–53.

Amassian, V.E., Somasundaram, M., Rothwell, J.C., *et al.* (1991). Paraesthesias are elicited by single pulse, magnetic coil stimulation of motor cortex in susceptible humans. *Brain*, **114**, 2505–20.

Antal, A., Nitsche, M.A., and Paulus, W. (2001). External modulation of visual perception in humans. *Neuroreport*, **12**, 3553–5.

Antal, A., Kincses, T.Z., Nitsche, M.A., *et al.* (2002). Pulse configuration-dependent effects of repetitive transcranial magnetic stimulation on visual perception. *Neuroreport*, **13**, 2229–33.

Antal, A., Kincses, T.Z., Nitsche, M.A., Bartfai, O., and Paulus, W. (2004). Excitability changes induced in the human primary visual cortex by transcranial direct current stimulation: direct electrophysiological evidence. *Investigational Ophthalmology & Visual Science*, **45**, 702–7.

Ashbridge, E., Walsh, V., and Cowey, A. (1997). Temporal aspects of visual search studied by transcranial magnetic stimulation. *Neuropsychologia*, **35**, 1121–31.

Baudewig, J., Nitsche, M.A., Paulus, W., and Frahm, J. (2001). Regional modulation of BOLD MRI responses to human sensorimotor activation by transcranial direct current stimulation. *Magnetic Resonance in Medicine*, **45**, 196–201.

Bickerstaffe, R., Brock, P., Husson, J.M., *et al.* (2006). Ethics and pharmaceutical medicine – the full report of the Ethical Issues Committee of the Faculty of Pharmaceutical Medicine of the Royal Colleges of Physicians of the UK. *International Journal of Clinical Practice*, **60**, 242–52.

Burt, T., Lisanby, S.H., and Sackeim, H.A. (2002). Neuropsychiatric applications of transcranial magnetic stimulation: a meta analysis. *International Journal of Neuropsychopharmacology*, **5**, 73–103.

Caplan, A.L. (2003). Is better best? A noted ethicist argues in favor of brain enhancement. *Scientific American*, **289**, 104–5.

Corthout, E., Uttl, B., Walsh, V., Hallett, M., and Cowey, A. (1999). Timing of activity in early visual cortex as revealed by transcranial magnetic stimulation. *Neuroreport*, **10**, 2631–4.

Couturier, J.L. (2005). Efficacy of rapid-rate repetitive transcranial magnetic stimulation in the treatment of depression: a systematic review and meta-analysis. *Journal of Psychiatry & Neuroscience*, **30**, 83–90.

Damasio, A. (2005). Human behaviour: brain trust. *Nature*, **435**, 571–2.

De Gennaro, L., Ferrara, M., Bertini, M., *et al.* (2003). Reproducibility of callosal effects of transcranial magnetic stimulation (TMS) with interhemispheric paired pulses. *Neuroscience Research*, **46**, 219–27.

de la Fuente-Fernandez, R., Ruth, T.J., Sossi, V., Schulzer, M., Calne, D.B., and Stoessl, A.J. (2001). Expectation and dopamine release: mechanism of the placebo effect in Parkinson's disease. *Science*, **293**, 1164–6.

Dickson, K. and McMahon, M. (2005). Will the law come running? The potential role of "brain fingerprinting" in crime investigation and adjudication in Australia. *Journal of Law and Medicine*, **13**, 204–22.

Farah, M.J., Illes, J., Cook-Deegan, R., *et al.* (2004). Neurocognitive enhancement: what can we do and what should we do? *Nature Reviews Neuroscience*, **5**, 421–5.

Fregni, F., Simon, D.K., Wu, A., and Pascual-Leone, A. (2005a). Non-invasive brain stimulation for Parkinson's disease: a systematic review and meta-analysis of the literature. *Journal of Neurology, Neurosurgery & Psychiatry*, **76**, 1614–23.

Fregni, F., Thome-Souza, S., Bermpohl, F., *et al.* (2005b). Antiepileptic effects of repetitive transcranial magnetic stimulation in patients with cortical malformations: An EEG and clinical studY. *Stereotactic and Functional Neurosurgery*, **83**, 57–62.

Fregni, F., Boggio, P.S., Nitsche, M., and Pascual-Leone, A. (2005c). Transcranial direct current stimulation. *British Journal of Psychiatry*, **186**, 446–7.

Fregni, F., Boggio, P.S., Mansur, C.G., *et al.* (2005d). Transcranial direct current stimulation of the unaffected hemisphere in stroke patients. *Neuroreport*, **16**, 1551–5.

Fregni, F., Boggio, P.S., Nitsche, M.A., Marcolin, M.A., Rigonatti, S.P., and Pascual-Leone, A. (2006a). Treatment of major depression with transcranial direct current stimulation. *Bipolar Disorders*, **8**, 203–4.

Fregni, F., Marcolin, M.A., Myczkowski, M.L., *et al.* (2006b). Predictors of antidepressant response in clinical trials of transcranial magnetic stimulation. *International Journal of Neuropsychopharmacology*, **9**, 641–54.

Fregni, F., Thome-Souza, S., Nitsche, M.A., Freedman, S.D., Valente, K.D., and Pascual-Leone, A. (2006c). A controlled clinical trial of cathodal DC polarization in patients with refractory epilepsy. *Epilepsia, 47,* 335–42.

Freitas, C., Fregni, F., and Pascual-Leone, A. (2009). Meta-analysis of the effects of repetitive transcranial magnetic stimulation (rTMS) on negative and positive symptoms in schizophrenia. *Schizophrenia Research, 108,* 11–24.

Frye, R.E., Rotenberg, A., Ousley, M., and Pascual-Leone, A. (2008). Transcranial magnetic stimulation in child neurology: current and future directions. *Journal of Child Neurology, 23,* 79–96.

Ganis, G., Kosslyn, S.M., Stose, S., Thompson, W.L., and Yurgelun-Todd, D.A. (2003). Neural correlates of different types of deception: an fMRI investigation. *Cerebral Cortex, 13,* 830–6.

Garcia-Toro, M., Mayol, A., Arnillas, H., *et al.* (2001). Modest adjunctive benefit with transcranial magnetic stimulation in medication-resistant depression. *Journal of Affective Disorders, 64,* 271–5.

Green, R.M., Pascual-Leone, A., and Wasserman, E.M. (1997). Ethical guidelines for rTMS research. *IRB, 19,* 1–7.

Gross, M., Nakamura, L., Pascual-Leone, A., and Fregni, F. (2007). Has repetitive transcranial magnetic stimulation (rTMS) treatment for depression improved? A systematic review and meta-analysis comparing the recent vs. the earlier rTMS studies. *Acta Psychiatrica Scandinavica, 116,* 165–73.

Hallett, M. (2000). Transcranial magnetic stimulation and the human brain. *Nature, 406,* 147–50.

Hallett, M., Wassermann, E.M., Pascual-Leone, A., and Valls-Sole, J. (1999). Repetitive transcranial magnetic stimulation. The International Federation of Clinical Neurophysiology. *Electroencephalography and Clinical Neurophysiology Supplement, 52,* 105–13.

Hausmann, A., Kemmler, G., Walpoth, M., *et al.* (2004). No benefit derived from repetitive transcranial magnetic stimulation in depression: a prospective, single centre, randomised, double blind, sham controlled "add on" trial. *Journal of Neurology, Neurosurgery and Psychiatry, 75,* 320–2.

Hilgetag, C.C., Theoret, H., and Pascual-Leone, A. (2001). Enhanced visual spatial attention ipsilateral to rTMS-induced 'virtual lesions' of human parietal cortex. *Nature Neuroscience, 4,* 953–7.

Hoffman, R.E., Hawkins, K.A., Gueorguieva, R., *et al.* (2003). Transcranial magnetic stimulation of left temporoparietal cortex and medication-resistant auditory hallucinations. *Archives of General Psychiatry, 60,* 49–56.

Huang, Y.Z., Edwards, M.J., Rounis, E., Bhatia, K.P., and Rothwell, J.C. (2005). Theta burst stimulation of the human motor cortex. *Neuron, 45,* 201–6.

Iyer, M.B., Schleper, N., and Wassermann, E.M. (2003). Priming stimulation enhances the depressant effect of low-frequency repetitive transcranial magnetic stimulation. *Journal of Neuroscience, 23,* 10867–72.

Janicak, P.G., O'Reardon, J.P., Sampson, S.M., *et al.* (2008). Transcranial magnetic stimulation in the treatment of major depressive disorder: a comprehensive summary of safety experience from acute exposure, extended exposure and during reintroduction treatment. *Journal of Clinical Psychiatry, 69,* 222–32.

Jensen, M.P., Hakimian, S., Sherlin, L.H., and Fregni, F. (2008). New insights into neuromodulatory approaches for the treatment of pain. *Journal of Pain, 9,* 193–9.

Kahn, I., Pascual-Leone, A., Theoret, H., Fregni, F., Clark, D., and Wagner, A.D. (2005). Transient disruption of ventrolateral prefrontal cortex during verbal encoding affects subsequent memory performance. *Journal of Neurophysiology, 94,* 688–98.

Karim, A.A., Schneider, M., Lotze, M., *et al.* (2010). The truth about lying: inhibition of the anterior prefrontal cortex improves deceptive behavior. *Cerebral Cortex,* **20,** 205–13.

Kass, L.R. (2003). Ageless bodies, happy souls: biotechnology and the pursuit of perfection. *New Atlantis,* **1,** 9–29.

Keenan, J.P., Wheeler, M.A., Gallup, G.G., Jr., and Pascual-Leone, A. (2000). Self-recognition and the right prefrontal cortex. *Trends in Cognitive Science,* **4,** 338–44.

Kobayashi, M., Hutchinson, S., Theoret, H., Schlaug, G., and Pascual-Leone, A. (2004). Repetitive TMS of the motor cortex improves ipsilateral sequential simple finger movements. *Neurology,* **62,** 91–8.

Laporte, J.R., and Figueras, A. (1994). Placebo effects in psychiatry. *Lancet,* **344,** 1206–9.

Lee, S., Walker, J.R., Jakul, L., and Sexton, K. (2004). Does elimination of placebo responders in a placebo run-in increase the treatment effect in randomized clinical trials? A meta-analytic evaluation. *Depression and Anxiety,* **19,** 10–19.

Lenfant, C. (2001). Can we prevent cardiovascular diseases in low- and middle-income countries? *Bulletin of the World Health Organization,* **79,** 980–7.

Machii, K., Cohen, D., Ramos-Estebanez, C., and Pascual-Leone, A. (2006). Safety of rTMS to non-motor cortical areas in healthy participants and patients. *Clinical Neurophysiology,* **117,** 455–71.

Mansur, C.G., Fregni, F., Boggio, P.S., *et al.* (2005). A sham stimulation-controlled trial of rTMS of the unaffected hemisphere in stroke patients. *Neurology,* **64,** 1802–4.

Martin, P.I., Naeser, M.A., Theoret, H., *et al.* (2004). Transcranial magnetic stimulation as a complementary treatment for aphasia. *Seminars in Speech and Language,* **25,** 181–91.

May, A., Hajak, G., Ganssbauer, S., *et al.* (2006). Structural brain alterations following 5 days of intervention: dynamic aspects of neuroplasticity. *Cerebral Cortex,* **17,** 205–10.

Miller, F.G. and Brody, H. (2003). A critique of clinical equipoise. Therapeutic misconception in the ethics of clinical trials. *Hastings Center Report,* **33,** 19–28.

Miller, S.M., Liu, G.B., Ngo, T.T., *et al.* (2000). Interhemispheric switching mediates perceptual rivalry. *Current Biology,* **10,** 383–92.

Murphy, D.N., Boggio, P., and Fregni, F. (2009). Transcranial direct current stimulation as a therapeutic tool for the treatment of major depression: insights from past and recent clinical studies. *Current Opinion in Psychiatry,* **22,** 306–11.

Naeser, M.A., Martin, P.I., Nicholas, M., *et al.* (2005a). Improved naming after TMS treatments in a chronic, global aphasia patient – case report. *Neurocase,* **11,** 182–93.

Naeser, M.A., Martin, P.I., Nicholas, M., *et al.* (2005b). Improved picture naming in chronic aphasia after TMS to part of right Broca's area: an open-protocol study. *Brain and Language,* **93,** 95–105.

Nitsche, M.A. and Paulus, W. (2000). Excitability changes induced in the human motor cortex by weak transcranial direct current stimulation. *Journal of Physiology,* **527,** 633–9.

Nitsche, M.A. and Paulus, W. (2001). Sustained excitability elevations induced by transcranial DC motor cortex stimulation in humans. *Neurology,* **57,** 1899–901.

Nitsche, M.A., Liebetanz, D., Antal, A., Lang, N., Tergau, F., and Paulus, W. (2003). Modulation of cortical excitability by weak direct current stimulation–technical, safety and functional aspects. *Supplements to Clinical Neurophysiology,* **56,** 255–76.

Nitsche, M.A., Niehaus, L., Hoffmann, K.T., *et al.* (2004). MRI study of human brain exposed to weak direct current stimulation of the frontal cortex. *Clinical Neurophysiology,* **115,** 2419–23.

O'Connor, M., Brenninkmeyer, C., Morgan, A., *et al.* (2003). Relative effects of repetitive transcranial magnetic stimulation and electroconvulsive therapy on mood and memory: a neurocognitive risk–benefit analysis. *Cognitive and Behavioral Neurology,* **16,** 118–27.

O'Reardon, J.P., Solvason, H.B., Janicak, P.G., *et al.* (2007). Efficacy and safety of transcranial magnetic stimulation in the acute treatment of major depression: a multisite randomized controlled trial. *Biological Psychiatry,* **62**, 1208–16.

Osborne, L. (2003). Savant for a day. *New York Times,* 22 June, pp. 38 (col 31).

Pascual-Leone, A. (2006). Disrupting the brain to guide plasticity and improve behavior. *Progress in Brain Research,* **157**, 315–29.

Pascual-Leone, A., Tormos, J.M., Keenan, J., Tarazona, F., Canete, C., and Catala, M.D. (1998). Study and modulation of human cortical excitability with transcranial magnetic stimulation. *Journal of Clinical Neurophysiology,* **15**, 333–43.

Pascual-Leone, A., Bartres-Faz, D., and Keenan, J.P. (1999). Transcranial magnetic stimulation: studying the brain-behaviour relationship by induction of 'virtual lesions'. *Philosophical Transactions of the Royal Society of London B: Biological Sciences,* **354**, 1229–38.

Priori, A., Mameli, F., Cogiamanian, F., *et al.* (2008). Lie-specific involvement of dorsolateral prefrontal cortex in deception. *Cerebral Cortex,* **18**, 451–5.

Quintana, H. (2005). Transcranial magnetic stimulation in persons younger than the age of 18. *Journal of ECT,* **21**, 88–95.

Robertson, E.M., Tormos, J.M., Maeda, F., and Pascual-Leone, A. (2001). The role of the dorsolateral prefrontal cortex during sequence learning is specific for spatial information. *Cerebral Cortex,* **11**, 628–35.

Robertson, E.M., Theoret, H., and Pascual-Leone, A. (2003). Studies in cognition: the problems solved and created by transcranial magnetic stimulation. *Journal of Cognitive Neuroscience,* **15**, 948–60.

Rosenkranz, K., Nitsche, M.A., Tergau, F., and Paulus, W. (2000). Diminution of training-induced transient motor cortex plasticity by weak transcranial direct current stimulation in the human. *Neuroscience Letters,* **296**, 61–3.

Rossi, S., Hallett, M., Rossini, P.M., and Pascual-Leone, A. (2009). Safety, ethical considerations, and application guidelines for the use of transcranial magnetic stimulation in clinical practice and research. *Clinical Neurophysiology,* **120**, 2008–39.

Rothman, K.J. and Michels, K.B. (1994). The continuing unethical use of placebo controls. *New England Journal of Medicine,* **331**, 394–8.

Rumi, D.O., Gattaz, W.F., Rigonatti, S.P., *et al.* (2005). Transcranial magnetic stimulation accelerates the antidepressant effect of amitriptyline in severe depression: a double-blind placebo-controlled study. *Biological Psychiatry,* **57**, 162–6.

Siebner, H.R., Tormos, J.M., Ceballos-Baumann, A.O., *et al.* (1999). Low-frequency repetitive transcranial magnetic stimulation of the motor cortex in writer's cramp. *Neurology,* **52**, 529–37.

Snyder, A.W., Mulcahy, E., Taylor, J.L., Mitchell, D.J., Sachdev, P., and Gandevia, S.C. (2003). Savant-like skills exposed in normal people by suppressing the left fronto-temporal lobe. *Journal of Integrated Neuroscience,* **2**, 149–58.

Steven, M.S. and Pascual-Leone, A. (2006). *Transcranial Magnetic Stimulation and the Human Brain: An Ethical Evaluation.* In J. Illes (ed.), *21st Century Neuroethics: Defining the Issues in Research, Practice and Policy.* Oxford: Oxford University Press.

Strafella, A.P., Ko, J.H., and Monchi, O. (2006). Therapeutic application of transcranial magnetic stimulation in Parkinson's disease: The contribution of expectation. *Neuroimage,* **31**, 1666–72.

Theoret, H., Kobayashi, M., Valero-Cabre, A., and Pascual-Leone, A. (2003). Exploring paradoxical functional facilitation with TMS. *Supplements to Clinical Neurophysiology,* **56**, 211–19.

Theoret, H., Halligan, E., Kobayashi, M., Merabet, L., and Pascual-Leone, A. (2004). Unconscious modulation of motor cortex excitability revealed with transcranial magnetic stimulation. *Experimental Brain Research,* **155,** 261–4.

Thut, G., Ives, J.R., Kampmann, F., Pastor, M.A., and Pascual-Leone, A. (2005). A new device and protocol for combining TMS and online recordings of EEG and evoked potentials. *Journal of Neuroscience Methods,* **141,** 207–17.

UK ECT Review Group. (2003). Efficacy and safety of electroconvulsive therapy in depressive disorders: a systematic review and meta-analysis. *Lancet,* **361,** 799–808.

Wagner, T., Fregni, F., Eden, U., *et al.* (2006). Transcranial magnetic stimulation and stroke: A computer-based human model study. *Neuroimage,* **30,** 857–70.

Wagner, T., Valero-Cabre, A., and Pascual-Leone, A. (2007). Noninvasive human brain stimulation. *Annual Review of Biomedical Engineering,* **9,** 527–65.

Walsh, V. and Pascual-Leone, A. (2003). *TMS in Cognitive Science: Neurochronometrics of Mind.* Cambridge, MA: MIT Press.

Walsh, V., Pascual-Leone, A., and Kosslyn, S.M. (2005). *Transcranial Magnetic Stimulation : A Neurochronometrics of Mind.* Cambridge, MA: MIT Press.

Walsh, V., Desmond, J.E., and Pascual-Leone, A. (2006). Manipulating brains. *Behavioral Neurology,* **17,** 131–4.

Wassermann, E.M. (1998). Risk and safety of repetitive transcranial magnetic stimulation: report and suggested guidelines from the International Workshop on the Safety of Repetitive Transcranial Magnetic Stimulation, June 5–7, 1996. *Electroencephalography and Clinical Neurophysiology,* **108,** 1–16.

Wassermann, E.M. and Grafman, J. (2005). Recharging cognition with DC brain polarization. *Trends in Cognitive Science,* **9,** 503–5.

Wohlfarth, T. (1997). Socioeconomic inequality and psychopathology: are socioeconomic status and social class interchangeable? *Social Science & Medicine,* **45,** 399–410.

Wu, A.D., Fregni, F., Simon, D.K., Deblieck, C., and Pascual-Leone, A. (2008). Noninvasive brain stimulation for Parkinson's disease and dystonia. *Neurotherapeutics,* **5,** 345–61.

Zaghi, S., Acar, M., Hultgren, B., Boggio, P., and Fregni, F. (2010). Noninvasive brain stimulation with low-intensity electrical currents:putative mechanisms of action for direct and alternating current stimulation. *Neuroscientist,* **16,** 285–307.

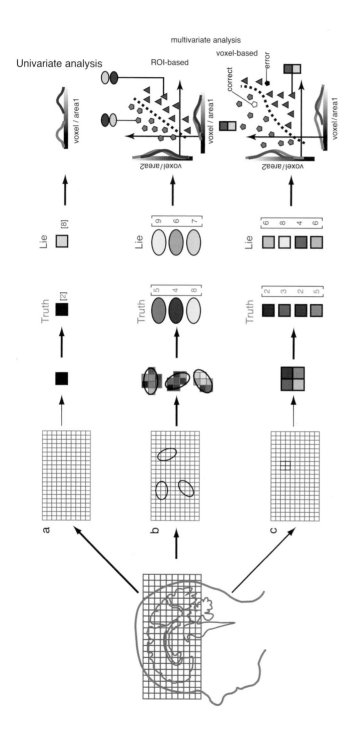

PLATE 1 (Also see Figure 1.1). Decoding mental states from brain activity using statistical pattern recognition techniques. Reproduced from Detecting concealed information using brain-imaging technology, Bles and Haynes, *Neurocase*. Reprinted with permission of the publisher (Taylor and Francis Group http://www.informaworld.com).

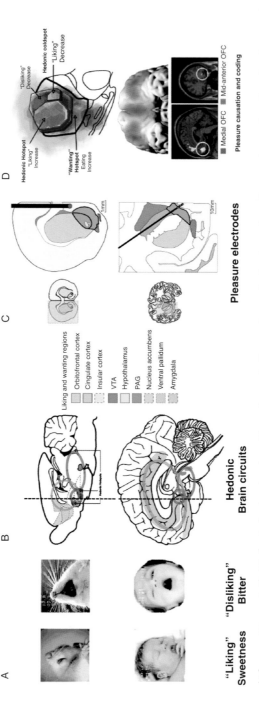

PLATE 2 (Also see Figure 2.2). Hedonic brain circuitry. The schematic figure shows the brain regions for causing and coding fundamental pleasure in rodents and humans. (a) Facial "liking" and "disliking" expressions elicited by sweet and bitter taste are similar in rodents and human infants. (b, d) Pleasure causation has been identified in rodents as arising from interlinked subcortical hedonic hotspots, such as in nucleus accumbens and ventral pallidum, where neural activation may increase "liking" expressions to sweetness. Similar pleasure coding and incentive salience networks have also been identified in humans. (c) The so-called "pleasure" electrodes in rodents and humans are unlikely to have elicited true pleasure but perhaps only incentive salience or "wanting." (d) The cortical localization of pleasure coding may reach an apex in various regions of the orbitofrontal cortex, which differentiate subjective pleasantness from valence processing of aspects the same stimulus, such as a pleasant food. PAG, periaqueductal gray; VTA, ventral tegmental area.

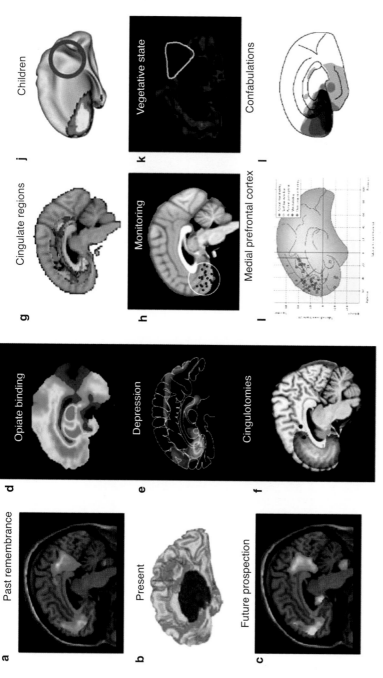

a Past remembrance

b Present

c Future prospection

d Opiate binding

e Depression

f Cingulotomies

g Cingulate regions

h Monitoring

i Medial prefrontal cortex

j Children

k Vegetative state

l Confabulations

PLATE 3 (Also see Figure 2.3). The brain's default network and eudaimonic–hedonic interaction.

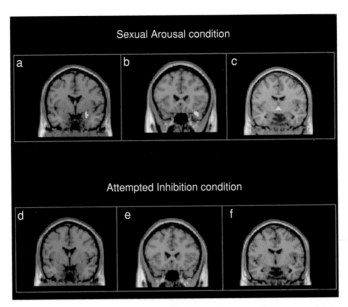

PLATE 4 (Also see Figure 5.1). Statistical activation maps showing limbic–paralimbic structures defined a priori. In the sexual arousal condition, greater activation during the viewing of erotic film excerpts relative to the viewing of emotionally neutral film excerpts was noted in the right amygdala (a), right anterior temporal pole (b), and the hypothalamus (c). In the suppression condition, no significant loci of activation were seen in the amygdalae (d), the anterior temporal polar region (e), and the hypothalamus (f). Reproduced with permission of the Society for Neuroscience from Beauregard, M. et al. (2001). Neural correlates of the conscious self-regulation of emotion. *Journal of Neuroscience*, **21**, 1–6.

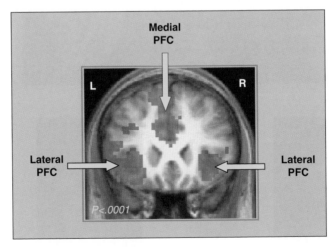

PLATE 5 (Also see Figure 6.2). Coronal section through the prefrontal cortex (y = 20) showing lateral and medial prefrontal regions in which stronger activation (*p* <0.0001, with a minimum cluster size of 15 voxels) was elicited by the subject's date of birth (probe) than by other dates not familiar to the subject (irrelevants) in a group of 14 subjects. A 3-item CIT paradigm was employed. The left side of the brain is on the left.

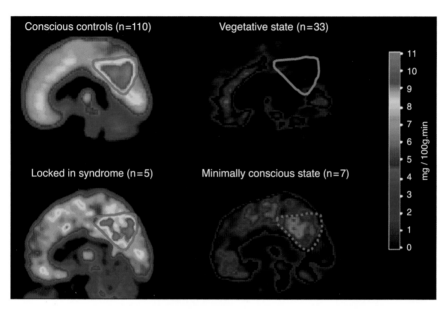

PLATE 6 (Also see Figure 7.4). Resting cerebral metabolism in healthy individuals and patients in a vegetative state, locked-in syndrome, and minimally conscious state. In healthy conscious individuals and locked-in patients the medial posterior cortex (encompassing the precuneus and adjacent posterior cingulate cortex, red line) is the most metabolically active region of the brain; in patients in vegetative state, this same area is the most dysfunctional (blue line). The precuneus and posterior cingulate cortex of patients in a minimally conscious state shows an intermediate metabolism, higher than in a vegetative state, but lower than in healthy subjects. Colors represent how much mg of glucose is consumed per mg of brain tissue per minute (adapted from Laureys S. *et al.* (2004). Brain function in coma, vegetative state and related disorders. *The Lancet Neurology*, **3**, 537–46.

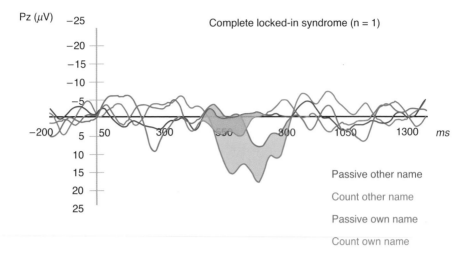

PLATE 7 (Also see Figure 7.5). Grand-averaged event-related potentials in a LIS patient at Pz. Response to the subject's own name (SON) in the passive condition (listened target SON; in green) and in the active condition (counted target SON; in pink) vs. unfamiliar names in passive (listened non-targets UN; in blue) and active condition (counted target UN, in red). Adapted from Schnakers C. *et al.* (2009). Detecting consciousness in a total locked-in syndrome. *Neurocase*, **15**, 271–7. Reprinted with permission of the publisher (Taylor and Francis Group http://www/informaworld.com).

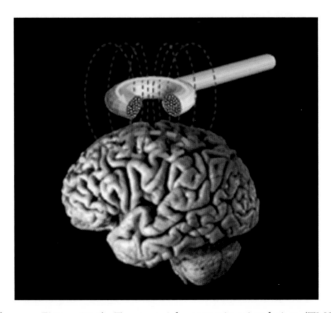

PLATE 8 (Also see Figure 21.4). Transcranial magnetic stimulation (TMS). Schematic image of electromagnetic action. TMS is a safe and non-invasive means of getting electrical energy across the insulating tissues of the head and into the brain. http://intra.ninds.nih.gov/Research.asp?People_ID=196 (accessed 1 January 2010).

Psychiatric Neurosurgery

A handful of medical centers have been conducting several experimental brain surgeries as a last resort for severe obsessive-compulsive disorders that are beyond the range of standard treatment.

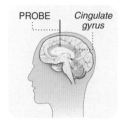 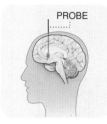 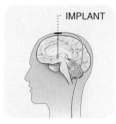 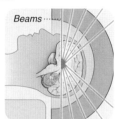

Cingulotomy
Probes are inserted into the brain to destroy a spot on the anterior cingulate gyrus, to disrupt a circuit that connects the emotional and conscious planning centers of the brain.

Capsulotomy
Probes are inserted deep into the brain and heated to destroy part of the anterior capsule, to disrupt a circuit thought to be overactive in people with severe OCD.

Deep brain stimulation
As an alternative to capsulotomy, an electrode is permanently implanted on one or both sides of the brain. A pacemaker-like device then delivers an adjustable current.

Gamma knife surgery
An MRI-like device focuses hundreds of small beams of radiation at a point within the brain, destroying small areas of tissue.

PLATE 9 (Also see Figure 21.7). Psychiatric neurosurgery.

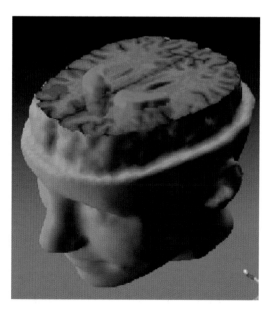

PLATE 10 (Also see Figure 21.8). Positron emission tomography (PET) image. Scan of a patient with schizophrenia. (Source: Andreas Meyer-Lindenberg, M.D., Ph.D., NIMH Clinical Brain Disorders Branch). http://www.nih.gov/news/pr/jan2002/nimh-28.htm (accessed 22 December 2009).

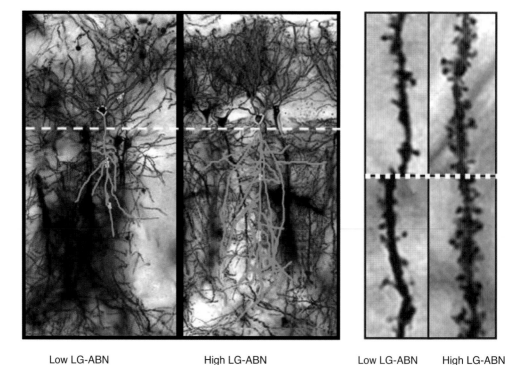

| Low LG-ABN | High LG-ABN | Low LG-ABN | High LG-ABN |

PLATE 11 (Also see Figure 44.1). Apical (blue) and basal (green) dendritic branching in adult rats who received lower (left) or higher (right) amounts of licking and grooming as infants. Stained neurons are pyramidal cells from the hippocampus. The study found significantly more branching in the rats who had received more licking and grooming. This is also visible in the photographs of branching points along the axonal spine shown on the right. (From Champagne *et al.* 2008).

....

CHAPTER 26

DEEP BRAIN STIMULATION FOR TREATMENT-RESISTANT NEUROPSYCHIATRIC DISORDERS

....

DEBRA J.H. MATHEWS, PETER V. RABINS, AND BENJAMIN D. GREENBERG

INTRODUCTION

....

IN recent decades, the treatment of Parkinson's disease and other movement disorders has been revolutionized by the advent of deep brain stimulation (DBS), a procedure in which electrodes are stereotactically implanted into specific deep brain structures and a constant electrical current is applied via a pulse generator implanted in the chest. The electrical current can be turned on and off, and "tuned" to achieve optimal symptom control. DBS has been approved by the Food and Drug Administration (FDA) for use in the treatment of Parkinson's disease, essential tremor, and dystonia. To date, DBS has been performed as a treatment for these conditions more than 60,000 times (Medtronic Inc. 2009a). However, in addition to alleviation of motor symptoms, DBS has also been found to both lessen obsessive–compulsive symptoms (Nuttin *et al.* 1999) and improve treatment resistant depression (Giacobbe *et al.* 2009), and to induce transient depression (Bejjani *et al.* 1999) and mania (Krack *et al.* 2001; Kulisevsky *et al.* 2002).

In part due to these observed effects, as well as a significant prevalence of debilitating, treatment resistant mood disorder and obsessive–compulsive disorder (OCD), DBS has been proposed as a therapy for highly treatment-resistant depression (TRD) and highly treatment-resistant OCD. Preliminary reports suggest that DBS might be effective for both diseases (Abelson *et al.* 2005; Mayberg *et al.* 2005), although these studies are of insufficient size to demonstrate statistically significant effects. However, there are several research teams exploring DBS for the treatment of TRD (Lozano and Kennedy; Mayberg *et al.*; Schlaepfer), and the efficacy of DBS for treating OCD (Agid and Mallet; Goodman). Furthermore, in response to accumulating data and a request from the device manufacturer Medtronic, in early 2009, the FDA issued a Humanitarian Device Exemption (HDE) for use of DBS in OCD (Medtronic Inc. 2009b). DBS is also currently under investigation for use in a range of other disorders (both neurologic and psychiatric) (Agid and Mallet; Goodman; Schlaepfer).

While new alternatives for chronically disabling and otherwise untreatable neuropsychiatric illness are welcome, the historical context of the treatment of psychiatric disorders (and those living with such diagnoses) suggests the need for special attention to emerging technologies in this area. In addition, the invasive nature of DBS, the resource-intensive nature of the intervention, and the possibility that continued benefit might require use over decades suggest the need for careful scrutiny of the science and ethics of the procedure. Here we review some of the ethical issues raised by the emergence and use of DBS as a treatment for neuropsychiatric disorders. Many of the same ethical considerations also apply to the continuing use of contemporary stereotactic ablation in neuropsychiatry, which has been reviewed recently (e.g. Greenberg *et al.* 2009) but will not be discussed at length here.

BACKGROUND

Many will be at least somewhat familiar with the disturbing history of psychosurgery, in particular the heyday of crude freehand procedures in the middle of the 20th century. During this time, and following a few earlier attempts to employ neurosurgical treatments for psychiatric disorders, Walter Freeman began his controversial and now infamous campaign popularizing transorbital frontal lobotomies using an instrument modeled after an ice pick. Freeman would insert the instrument through the eye socket, and sweep the probe laterally through prefrontal cortex. In his view, this procedurally simple approach would require minimal resources and training as compared to a procedure performed by a trained surgeon using standard techniques. Freeman traveled throughout the US demonstrating the technique, and his proselytizing led to widespread and indiscriminate use (more than 5000 procedures were performed in 1949, the peak year (Valenstein 1986)). In that year, the Graystone study demonstrated that the procedure did not improve the symptoms of schizophrenia, the primary disease for which it was developed (The Columbia-Greystone Associates 1949). The actions of Freeman, in concert with the development of effective pharmacological interventions in the early 1950s, lead to an abandonment of psychosurgery as a treatment for schizophrenia, though it continued to be used as a treatment for severe OCD.

The past 15 years has seen a reemergence of interest in using surgical therapies, including DBS, for severe treatment resistant cases of depression and OCD. These include anterior cingulotomy, subcaudate tractotomy, limbic leucotomy, anterior capsulotomy, and DBS (multiple targets) (for a brief review of the history of and data supporting these procedures, see Read and Greenberg 2009). Prospective research on a subset of these procedures is continuing. The most recently developed ablative procedure, gamma knife ventral capsulotomy, is now being studied in a sham-controlled trail for OCD, the first of its kind in psychiatry (Lopes *et al.* 2009). Gamma ventral capsulotomy is non-invasive (does not require craniotomy) but intentionally destroys brain tissue. DBS is the reverse: invasive but not intended to ablate more tissue than is occupied by the stimulating lead itself. Unintended hemorrhage on device insertion may occur, however.

DBS is usually performed bilaterally and the electrodes are placed using imaging (e.g. magnetic resonance imaging) and stereotactic methods. Leads, typically with a series of four electrodes evenly spaced from the lead tip, are inserted through burr holes in the skull into specific brain targets. The leads are connected to wires that are threaded subdermally to a neurostimulator (similar to a cardiac pacemaker) usually implanted in the chest. The neurostimulator allows activation of the electrodes, which can be activated individually in specified polarities. Each of the bilateral leads is programmable for electrical pulse frequency, intensity, and duration. The patient/research subject is awake but lightly sedated when the leads are tested in the operating room after implantation. Assessing acute positive and adverse effects of this intraoperative stimulation helps guide electrode placement.

While DBS was first attempted as a therapy for severe depression and anorexia in 1948 (Greenberg *et al.* 2008), its first clinical use was in medically intractable movement disorders. Use in essential tremor gained FDA approval in the US in 1997, and DBS for Parkinson's disease was approved in 2002. Approval for use in dystonia was issued in 2003, through a HDE, which requires local ethics committee (institutional review board, IRB) approval but not the full oversight of a clinical research protocol. It was not until the 1990s that clinical studies of DBS as a therapy for disorders of mood, behavior, and thought began, with the first published study in 1999 (Nuttin *et al.* 1999). Since then, interest and research in this area has blossomed (Kopell and Greenberg 2008; Larson 2008; Schlaepfer and Lieb 2005). Though the number and size of completed clinical trials remains small, two larger-scale industry-led multicenter trials of DBS for depression are underway, as is a medium-scale controlled trial of DBS for OCD supported by the National Institute of Mental Health (NIMH).

For OCD, following the Nuttin *et al.* paper, Loes Gabriëls, Paul Cosyns, and coworkers (Gabriels *et al.* 2003) published a small study, followed by a report of ten patients by Greenberg and colleagues (Greenberg *et al.* 2006). To date, approximately 100 individuals with severe and highly refractory OCD have received DBS. However, for OCD, as for other neuropsychiatric conditions, there is not yet consensus on the optimal anatomical target for stimulation. Symptom reduction has been reported after stimulation of several different targets for the same diagnoses. This is unsurprising, since it is most likely that DBS, like lesion procedures, can affect multiple nodes of brain circuitry that may help mediate therapeutic change (Greenberg *et al.* 2009). The diversity of targets, among other factors, has limited the comparability across studies and reduces the power of the total published experience. Since positive effects on symptoms have been reported using different targets, an adequately large trial directly comparing DBS sites in psychiatric conditions (the best way to establish relative efficacy and burdens) appears prohibitively expensive with current technology.

For major depression, the total published experience is yet smaller, around 70 patients (Lozano *et al.* 2008; Malone *et al.* 2009; Mayberg *et al.* 2005; Schlaepfer *et al.* 2008). For Tourette syndrome, over 30 cases have been reported (Maciunas *et al.* 2007; Mink *et al.* 2006; Servello *et al.* 2008; Temel and Visser-Vandewalle 2004).

Recently, an NIMH-funded consensus conference was held to consider key scientific and ethical issues for the use of DBS in disorders of mood, behavior, and thought (MBT), and to recommend guidelines (Rabins *et al.* 2009).

ETHICAL ISSUES TO CONSIDER

While many of the ethical issues raised by the use of DBS to treat neuropsychiatric illness are no different from those raised by its current use in movement disorders, the history of the era of "psychosurgery" in the mid-20th century remains an enduring caution. Issues include concerns about the capacity of persons with severe mental illness to give authentic informed consent, protecting vulnerable individuals from being exposed to unproven and potentially irreversible therapies, the use of DBS for psychiatric disorders in minors, the necessary organization of the interdisciplinary teams required to deliver these demanding treatments (which pose difficult ethical challenges for the teams themselves), and the degree and quality of oversight.

An additional complement of issues is raised by DBS for disorders of MBT because of the relatively early stage of the science. The challenges raised by this emerging technology include clarifying distinctions between research and clinical care; balancing the goals of advancing knowledge via data sharing, including sharing of data from "clinical" uses, which is essential to optimize patient outcomes; availability and access to clinical care; and costs and other restrictions associated very long-term follow-up and withdrawal from clinical trials.

Finally, the use of treatments that directly invade the brain raise issues related to the locus of responsibility of behavior; the meaning of personal identity and its origin; the role of, concomitant need for, and provision of psychosocial support, and questions about the extent to which patients should directly control stimulation devices. Again, these issues are also raised in uses of neurosurgery for movement disorders and other conditions, and even by conventional uses of medications with intended or unintended psychotropic effects across medicine.

Sensitive science

The paradigmatic "psychosurgical" operation was lobotomy, which even in its most careful uses in conventional operating rooms was a crude, freehand procedure. It emerged at a time when therapeutic nihilism for severe psychiatric disorders was pervasive, before the modern era of empirical psychiatry. Ethical and regulatory contexts for research and clinical treatment as we know them today did not exist. Reports of successful outcomes after lobotomy, which from the beginning included patients with severe obsessional symptoms, were highly publicized (Laurence 1937). As is well documented (Pressman 1998; Valenstein 1986), lobotomy's use, especially that of the transorbital ("ice pick") lobotomy accelerated at a tremendous rate (more than 5000 procedures performed in 1949 alone). Notably, early proponents, even Walter Freeman, who later developed an evangelist's zeal for transorbital lobotomy, emphasized careful patient selection and systematic, multidisciplinary study of outcomes when he began this work (Freeman *et al.* 1942). Despite this, the procedure was performed indiscriminately, without attention to the restraints on conventional surgeries of the day, on a stigmatized and vulnerable population (Feldman and Goodrich 2001; Valenstein 1986).

There was indeed skepticism from the beginning (Fins 2003), which later included Freeman's former colleague, the neurosurgeon James Watts, who challenged the procedure as unsafe. But voices urging caution did not carry the day until effective therapeutic alternatives appeared and lobotomy's heavy adverse effect burden was recognized (El-Hai 2005). These factors among others lead to widespread criticism of transorbital lobotomy, a decline in use of the procedure, and ultimately to the stigmatization of psychosurgery generally. It was only decades later, when wide use of lobotomy had already faded in favor of a dramatically more limited use of stereotactic procedures, that opposition rose to the attention of governments. This included a National Ethics Commission in the US, which contrary to its own expectations recommended that careful and well documented work with stereotactic psychiatric neurosurgery be allowed to continue (National Commission 1977). This is in fact the paradigm that is being followed by researchers in the field today. Media reports now, while echoing the enthusiasm of that earlier era, have a much more balanced view of burdens as well as potential benefits. And, interestingly, they sometimes highlight a new phenomenon-skepticism about the motivations of the doctors and companies involved (e.g. Carey 2009).

Despite improvements in awareness of both the prevalence and treatability of psychiatric illness, it continues to carry stigma (Henderson and Thornicroft 2009; Pinto-Foltz and Logsdon 2009). And the popular conception remains that individuals with psychiatric disorders may be vulnerable to inappropriate influence in treatment decisions. However, available research demonstrates that individuals suffering from neuropsychiatric conditions are not, as a group, less able to give informed consent than those with other chronic, debilitating disease. And even though individuals hospitalized for major depression have decreased decisional capacity, most are still scored as competent to make independent decisions about their care (Appelbaum et al. 1999; Cohen et al. 2004; Grisso and Appelbaum 1995; Lapid et al. 2003). Furthermore, depressive symptoms have not been correlated with capacity to consent. While additional research may be warranted to assess other populations of patients with psychiatric diagnosis (e.g. OCD), there is no evidence that these individuals are any more impaired than individuals with major depression or serious non-psychiatric medical diagnoses.

Nonetheless, the perception of vulnerability of the population, the possibility that concerns will be raised about exploitation, and the history of psychosurgery, suggest that special attention should be paid to the informed consent process in current studies of DBS for disorders of MBT, at least for the present stage of development of the field. For example, protocols for early phase studies of DBS for disorders of MBT should include an IRB-approved assessment of capacity (Rabins et al. 2009). While there are no data to suggest that, as a group, these individuals are less capable of providing informed consent as other groups involved in similarly novel or invasive research, it is likely that there will be individuals who do not meet criteria for capacity to consent and therefore should not be enrolled as subjects in early phase studies of DBS for disorders of MBT. Because longitudinal follow-up is required to demonstrate efficacy, the consent process should be longitudinal, spanning the duration of the protocol and providing opportunities for questions and withdrawal. Some individuals suggest a need for additional layers of protection such as the use of an independent review panel to assess patient selection and the consent process (Nuttin et al. 2003); or the inclusion of "a close third" (e.g. the patient's caregiver) in these conversations, to enable (witnessed) informed consent, as an additional safeguard against abuse, but we do not believe these are required (Rabins *et al.* 2009). Some research groups have implemented a formal process of consent monitoring, which often includes families and caregivers, in part for research and clinical reasons. Additional safeguards in use in some clinical trials (e.g. the current NIMH-funded multicenter trial of DBS of the ventral capsule/ventral striatum for intractable OCD, ClinicalTrials.gov identifier: NCT00640133) include an independent review group of expert psychiatrists and patient advocates. The group assesses potential candidates based on detailed information provided by clinical investigators, and commonly asks for more information about past treatment history, especially to determine whether prior use of evidence-based behavioral therapies was adequate.

The history of psychosurgery and the variability of psychiatric diagnoses over time also provide strong justification for rigorously defined inclusion criteria in research studies of DBS for the treatment of neuropsychiatric disorders. Table 26.1 lists recommendations that have been made regarding patient selection. Inclusion criteria should be clear, consistent, and transparent. Optimally, inclusion criteria would be consistent across studies for each neuropsychiatric condition under consideration, enabling comparison across studies, and ensuring that the research will more quickly and efficiently arrive at answers about safety and efficacy. In practice, there are likely to be differences in inclusion criteria, especially with respect to the specific treatments a patient must have tried without benefit, the level of documentation about such past treatments, and exact definitions of severity thresholds or other clinical features of prospective trial participants.

A question for the future is whether or not children or young adults should be considered as candidates for DBS for disorders of MBT. Current consensus appears to be that minors should not be included in early phase studies (Mink *et al.* 2006; Read and Greenberg 2009). As noted by Rabins *et al.* (2009), "[t]he course of disorders of MBT can be particularly

Table 26.1 Proposed inclusion criteria*

Age	The patient must be old enough to give independent informed consent and to be reasonably certain that their condition is unlikely to improve in the course of normal human development
Diagnosis	The patient must meet clinical criteria for a primary diagnosis of major affective disorder, chronic anxiety, or OCD
Severity	The patient's symptoms fall at the severe end of the relevant measure
Disability	The illness must cause significant disability both in terms of suffering or distress and psychosocial functioning
Chronicity	The patient must have suffered with their primary diagnosis for at least 5 years
Treatment refractoriness	The patient's disorder must be refractory to an exhaustive array of pharmacological; behavioral; and, where appropriate, ECT treatments
Compliance	The patient must be actively engaged in and committed to her or his own treatment

*Table compiled based on Nuttin, *et al.* 2003; Mink *et al.* 2006; Rabins *et al.* 2009; Read and Greenberg 2009.

variable in young individuals, and the effects of DBS on the developing nervous system are unknown." Some neuropsychiatric conditions can decline significantly in severity into young adulthood (e.g. Mink *et al.* 2006; Skoog and Skoog 1999), whereas DBS, while not necessarily irreversible, carries unknown and potentially long-term risks when applied to still-developing brains. These risks may not be understood or fully appreciated either by young psychiatric patients or their parents. That said, if DBS is found to be safe and effective for adults in early stage and more advanced clinical trials, then studies of its benefit for younger individuals with severe, treatment refractory neuropsychiatric disorders may be considered (Rabins *et al.* 2009). There are some data on the safety of DBS in younger individuals from clinical trials of its use to treat pediatric movement disorders (Volkmann and Benecke 2002). While these data may not be completely generalizable, they may help inform any future discussions about the study of DBS in young neuropsychiatric patients.

Finally, two additional layers of protection should be offered to patients as this area of research moves forward: first, clinical trials should involve multidisciplinary teams of clinicians and other professionals all focused on the good of the patient; second, clinical trials should be subject to thoughtfully crafted and rigorously applied oversight.

The complexity of the surgery, post-surgical stimulator adjustment, and the treatment resistant nature of the disorders being treated require a multidisciplinary team to care for and support participants in studies of DBS for neuropsychiatric disorders. Such a team also provides checks and balances that help ensure that potential research participants are adequately assessed and if enrolled in the trial, adequately and responsibly cared for. Rabins *et al.* (2009) state that this team should include, at minimum: neurosurgeons and neurologists with extensive experience in DBS; psychiatrists with expertise in diagnosing and treating the neuropsychiatric condition under investigation; and, neuropsychologists and case managers, who should participate in both pre-enrollment evaluation and post-study follow-up. Case managers or other social workers may be particularly important if a research subject is successfully treated. Years of impairment (particularly if impairment spanned childhood or early adulthood) may have left an individual with few relationships, social skills, or job prospects. The burdens of re-entry into society for such individuals must be considered and sincere efforts made on multiple fronts to assist their transition back into a more functional life.

Finally, as long as DBS for neuropsychiatric disorders is experimental (a partial exception being DBS for OCD under the HDE mechanism in OCD, which is intermediate between that of clinical research and standard-of-care clinical practice), it should be offered only in expert centers and only with appropriate oversight by an institutional review/research ethics board (Rabins *et al.* 2009). Again, this is especially important owing to the history of psychosurgery and the degree to which those performing it were unchecked and unaccountable, leading to serious abuse.

DBS as emerging technology

While DBS may be seen as the most recent on a continuum of surgical intervention for psychiatric disease, it also represents an adaptation of the first implantable brain-interfacing device (IBID) in clinical use (excluding vagal nerve stimulation, in which the interface with the brain is indirect, mediated by the nerve itself) and as such sits at the beginning of what is likely to be a rapidly expanding field of IBIDs. These emerging technologies raise additional ethical issues.

Technologies in the proof of principle stage—including all IBIDs proposed or in clinical use in neuropsychiatric conditions—should be assessed in formal and fully vetted clinical trials (which includes regulatory as well as IRB/ethics committee oversight). Patients must be made aware of the investigational nature of the intervention, the lack of data on safety and efficacy, and the lack of consensus about optimal targeting within the brain for individual diagnoses. The number of patients involved should remain relatively small until efficacy has been demonstrated, although patient samples need to be large enough to reliably assess therapeutic effects and safety in controlled designs. The efficiency and speed of this process would be maximized by the deposition of de-identified outcomes data in an independent registry by researchers, assisted by device manufacturers. Establishing such a registry was a major recommendation of the 1977 US National Commission. This has recently been reiterated and given strong support by the NIMH (Goodman and Insel 2009). Included in the registry should be data from both clinical trials and "clinical use," though this will need to be done with great care, to ensure that the privacy of the patients and subjects involved is rigorously protected.

The expense and complexity of IBID therapy also raises ethical issues. The small number of expert centers and clinical trials that offer DBS for neuropsychiatric disorders are not the only factors limiting access, of course. Emerging technologies—particularly complex, expensive ones—are inevitably available in relatively wealthy countries first, making their way to those in developing nations only much later, if at all. DBS requires highly specialized medical personnel, equipment, and settings not only during and immediately after surgery but also long-term. Over time, patients require stimulator parameter readjustment and battery or other device replacements, which typically requires minor surgery. For patients in developing nations—and many in developed nations—such medical resources are neither available nor affordable. This inequity suggests the need to reassess or develop less resource-intensive interventions (e.g. gamma knife) to maximize access to the advances in knowledge gained through studies of DBS for neuropsychiatric disorders. Furthermore, there are data to suggest that at least in some cases, DBS and ablation produce comparable results, providing scientific and ethical justification for comparative studies of safety and efficacy for at least some targets (Rabins *et al.* 2009). Ideally, refined ablative procedures (Lopes *et al.* 2009) would have risk–burden–benefit profiles comparable to those of device-based treatments, in which case they would be expected to see continuing use in the developed world (as occurs at present). Clear differences in efficacy or burdens of treatments that are available in developed and developing nations might be perceived as compounding existing inequities, in which case there will be debate about how best to develop and deploy practicable treatments without merely perpetuating injustice.

Even in developed countries, the cost and resource-intensiveness of treatment with IBIDs raise concerns. For example, the lack of a uniform national health care plan in the US might lead to a requirement that participants in a trial of DBS for neuropsychiatric disorders have health insurance that would include coverage for the evaluation, surgery, and follow-up care that IBIDs require (Read and Greenberg 2009). We believe it is unethical to use socioeconomic criteria for inclusion in research and recommend that device manufacturers, third-party payers, researchers, research institutions, and funding organizations develop and implement a system that will reduce or eliminate barriers to access to clinical trials based on access to health insurance.

Just as there should be no financial barriers to entrance to a clinical trial, there should also be no financial barriers to patients withdrawing from a study. As noted by Rabins *et al.* (2009), "There are unique consequences of withdrawal from a trial of any implanted device, for example, the subject's right to withdraw is limited if she is personally responsible for related costs (e.g. surgical removal)." Furthermore, individuals receiving DBS for neuropsychiatric disorders, in contrast to individuals receiving DBS for Parkinson's disease, may have many decades of life ahead of them, and questions arise about who should bear the responsibility of coverage of ongoing medical costs associated with the device. One solution to the absence of national coverage would be the establishment of an insurance pool to which all stakeholders (except research participants) contribute, and on which research subjects can draw when trial- or device-related costs arise (e.g. from an adverse event or for device removal), even past the end of the trial (Rabins *et al.* 2009). Since this is not currently in place, research teams should be explicit in their consent documents and processes regarding who is financially responsible for device removal in the event of withdrawal or disenrollment from the trial, device maintenance over time, and care secondary to trial-related adverse events.

Broadly speaking, these issues raise the question of when a participant in an early-phase trial of an implantable device ceases to be a research subject, and what responsibilities the participants, research teams, device manufacturers, and other stakeholders have after the trial has ended. Similar issues are raised by other implantable devices such as cardiac pacemakers, ventricular assist devices, and spinal cord stimulators for chronic pain, but the possibility that long-term behavioral or functional changes might result from brain stimulation suggest that this issues requires specific scrutiny in the case of IBIDs.

Additional issues

Two final issues that are raised by DBS and other IBIDs as an intervention for neuropsychiatric disorders are the potential to change—reversibly and reproducibly—individuals' personalities; and the issue of patient control of the devices.

Preliminary and case report data suggest that DBS can modulate mood, behavior, and thought. These constructs are elements of personal identity and "humanness," and set IBIDs apart from other implantable devices that affect functions seen as "non-mental" (e.g. cardiac pacemakers). This raises questions about the agency of decisions that individuals with IBIDs make, and whether changes in thought and mood should be considered differently than changes induced by such devices in the realms of movement or pain. Changes in mood, behavior, and thought induced by IBIDs might lead to transient or long-term concerns in recipients or society about personhood, personal identity, and agency. Similar questions have been raised about the use of pharmacologic agents and electroconvulsive therapy to treat psychiatric illnesses, but the potential reversibility of pharmacologic approaches seems to distinguish it from IBIDs, in which irreversible changes might occur even if the device is removed. Experience in psychiatric neurosurgery research, however, raises a counterpoint to these concerns. Patients with certain kinds of psychopathology commonly view mental phenomena associated with their illnesses as alien to their own conception of self and of their sense of an authentic personality. A notable example of this is the view expressed by individuals with OCD regarding the intrusive obsessions (thoughts) and compulsions (actions or behaviors) that are the hallmark of the illness. A recently published interview with an OCD patient who had undergone DBS implantation and chronic stimulation shows that what was lost after the intervention was what the patient wanted to lose, without any indication of induction of deficits that would diminish a sense of quality of life (Merkel 2007). A different kind of challenge to patients is that IBIDs require close, persistent involvement of medical professionals. Patients may view this as a substantial curtailment of their own autonomy, including for example their ability to make a decision as fundamental as where to live, since moving away from a specialized treatment team may not be a realistic option. Again, there are other examples in medicine of similar burdens imposed by specialized or intensive treatments.

Even more challenging is the possibility that changes in behavior, mood, or personality unrelated to the condition being treated might be induced by changing stimulator parameters or by turning the stimulator on and off. Such control is already considered appropriate for those taking prescription pharmacologic agents as well as agents such as alcohol, but IBIDs raise questions about direct modulation of brain function. And what if the change is perceived by the recipient as positive but by significant others as negative? Or vice versa?

Should individuals be asked to draft an advance directive or enter into legally binding contracts with a trusted potential surrogate in such a circumstance? At minimum, we suggest that patients and research subjects be informed of the risk of personality, mood, and behavior change. That said, sufficient data are not available to estimate the risk of such changes, nor the likelihood that such changes will be subtle or minor. Clinical trials should prospectively collect such data. The core challenge will be assessing the tradeoffs necessary to relieve suffering imposed by symptoms of the primary illness and any treatment-emergent burdens, and optimizing decisions about accepting or rejecting as a package all that these treatments entail. This issue is extremely important in the current, standard-of-care uses of DBS for movement disorders, where it has emerged as a recent focus of bioethics (Glannon 2009).

Finally, while there are no data demonstrating that self-control of the stimulator is beneficial, some individuals with movement disorders turn the device down at night in order to preserve battery life. Without evidence that self-control is harmful, and since self-control is already established, no ethical objection can be raised to control by patients being treated for disorders of MBT. However, if subsequent research demonstrates harm or abuse, the issue should be revisited.

Conclusions

DBS for the treatment of disorders of MBT deserves careful study. The past history of misuse of psychosurgery in persons with such disorders suggests that they might be a vulnerable group and therefore require scrutiny not given to the use of this therapy for movement disorders, but such a view can also be seen as condescending, discriminatory, and as encouraging stigma. Indeed, many psychiatric researchers currently working in the field of neurosurgery for otherwise intractable illness are strongly motivated by their belief that demonstration of effects of neurocircuit-based interventions will help lessen stigma by reinforcing the status of neuropsychiatric illnesses as brain disorders that have primarily behavioral manifestations. The potential of IBIDs to cause changes in MBT, and in more ephemeral constructs such as personhood, do suggest that ongoing, well-designed research is needed to monitor for unintended effects, but we suggest that such scrutiny be applied to the study of IBIDs for all indications, not just those considered to be "psychiatric." The potential benefit of such therapies justifies continued study. Consideration of the ethical issues raised by such therapies will protect individuals with neurologic and psychiatric diseases from the abuses of the past.

REFERENCES

Abelson, J.L., Curtis, G.C., Sagher, O., *et al.* (2005). Deep brain stimulation for refractory obsessive-compulsive disorder. *Biological Psychiatry,* **57**, 510–16.

Agid, Y. and Mallet, L. (2005). Subthalamic Nucleus (STN) Stimulation and Obsessive-Compulsive Disorder (OCD) (Clinical Trial). Available at: http://clinicaltrials.gov/show/NCT00169377 (accessed 15 November 2009).

Appelbaum, P.S., Grisso, T., Frank, E., O'Donnell, S., and Kupfer, D.J. (1999). Competence of depressed patients for consent to research. *American Journal of Psychiatry,* **156**, 1380–4.

Bejjani, B.P., Damier, P., Arnulf, I., *et al.* (1999). Transient acute depression induced by high-frequency deep-brain stimulation. *New England Journal of Medicine,* **340**, 1476–80.

Carey, B. (2009). Surgery for Mental Ills Offers Both Hope and Risk. *New York Times.* New York.

Cohen, B.J., Mcgarvey, E.L., Pinkerton, R.C., and Kryzhanivska, L. (2004). Willingness and competence of depressed and schizophrenic inpatients to consent to research. *Journal of the American Academy of Psychiatry and the Law,* **32**, 134–43.

El-Hai, J. (2005). *The lobotomist: a maverick medical genius and his tragic quest to rid the world of mental illness,* Hoboken, NJ: Wiley.

Feldman, R.P. and Goodrich, J.T. (2001). Psychosurgery: a historical overview. *Neurosurgery,* **48**, 647–57.

Fins, J.J. (2003). From psychosurgery to neuromodulation and palliation: history's lessons for the ethical conduct and regulation of neuropsychiatric research. *Neurosurgery Clinics of North America,* **14**, 303–19, ix–x.

Freeman, W.J., Watts, J.W., and Hunt, T. (1942). *Psychosurgery; intelligence, emotion and social behavior following prefrontal lobotomy for mental disorders,* Springfield, IL: C. C. Thomas.

Gabriels, L., Cosyns, P., Nuttin, B., Demeulemeester, H., and Gybels, J. (2003). Deep brain stimulation for treatment-refractory obsessive-compulsive disorder: psychopathological and neuropsychological outcome in three cases. *Acta Psychiatrica Scandinavica,* **107**, 275–82.

Giacobbe, P., Mayberg, H.S., and Lozano, A.M. (2009). Treatment resistant depression as a failure of brain homeostatic mechanisms: implications for deep brain stimulation. *Experimental Neurology,* **219**, 44–52.

Glannon, W. (2009). Stimulating brains, altering minds. *Journal of Medical Ethics,* **35**, 289–92.

Goodman, W. (2003). Deep Brain Stimulation for Treatment-Resistant Obsessive Compulsive Disorder (Clinical Trial). Available at: http://clinicaltrials.gov/show/NCT00057603 (accessed 15 November 2009).

Goodman, W.K. and Insel, T.R. (2009). Deep brain stimulation in psychiatry: concentrating on the road ahead. *Biological Psychiatry*, **65**, 263–6.

Greenberg, B.D., Malone, D.A., Friehs, G.M., *et al.* (2006). Three-year outcomes in deep brain stimulation for highly resistant obsessive-compulsive disorder. *Neuropsychopharmacology*, **31**, 2384–93.

Greenberg, B.D., Askland, K.D. and Carpenter, L.L. (2008). The evolution of deep brain stimulation for neuropsychiatric disorders. *Frontiers in Bioscience*, **13**, 4638–48.

Greenberg, B.D., Rauch, S.L. and Haber, S.N. (2009). Invasive circuitry-based neurotherapeutics: stereotactic ablation and deep brain stimulation for OCD. *Neuropsychopharmacology*, **35**, 317–36.

Grisso, T. and Appelbaum, P.S. (1995). Comparison of standards for assessing patients' capacities to make treatment decisions. *American Journal of Psychiatry*, **152**, 1033–7.

Henderson, C. and Thornicroft, G. (2009). Stigma and discrimination in mental illness: Time to Change. *Lancet*, **373**, 1928–30.

Kopell, B.H. and Greenberg, B.D. (2008). Anatomy and physiology of the basal ganglia: implications for DBS in psychiatry. *Neuroscience and Biobehavioral Reviews*, **32**, 408–22.

Krack, P., Kumar, R., Ardouin, C., *et al.* (2001). Mirthful laughter induced by subthalamic nucleus stimulation. *Movement Disorders*, **16**, 867–75.

Kulisevsky, J., Berthier, M.L., Gironell, A., Pascual-Sedano, B., Molet, J., and Pares, P. (2002). Mania following deep brain stimulation for Parkinson's disease. *Neurology*, **59**, 1421–4.

Lapid, M.I., Rummans, T.A., Poole, K.L., *et al.* (2003). Decisional capacity of severely depressed patients requiring electroconvulsive therapy. *Journal of ECT*, **19**, 67–72.

Larson, P.S. (2008). Deep brain stimulation for psychiatric disorders. *Neurotherapeutics*, **5**, 50–8.

Laurence, W.L. (1937). Surgery used on the soul-sick; relief of obsessions is reported. *New York Times*.

Lopes, A.C., Greenberg, B.D., Norén, G., *et al.* (2009). Treatment of resistant obsessive-compulsive disorder with ventral capsular/ventral striatal gamma capsulotomy: a pilot prospective study. *Journal of Neuropsychiatry and Clinical Neurosciences*, **21**, 381–92.

Lozano, A. and Kennedy, S. (2006). Deep Brain Stimulation for Refractory Major Depression (Clinical Trial). Available at: http://clinicaltrials.gov/show/NCT00296920 (accessed 15 November 2009).

Lozano, A.M., Mayberg, H.S., Giacobbe, P., Hamani, C., Craddock, R.C. and Kennedy, S.H. (2008). Subcallosal cingulate gyrus deep brain stimulation for treatment-resistant depression. *Biological Psychiatry*, **64**, 461–7.

Maciunas, R.J., Maddux, B.N., Riley, D.E., *et al.* (2007). Prospective randomized double-blind trial of bilateral thalamic deep brain stimulation in adults with Tourette syndrome. *Journal of Neurosurgery*, **107**, 1004–14.

Malone, D.A., Jr., Dougherty, D.D., Rezai, A.R., *et al.* (2009). Deep brain stimulation of the ventral capsule/ventral striatum for treatment-resistant depression. *Biological Psychiatry*, **65**, 267–75.

Mayberg, H.S., Holtzheimer, P., and Gross, R. (2006). Deep Brain Stimulation for Treatment Resistant Depression (Clinical Trial). Available at: http://clinicaltrials.gov/ct/show/NCT00367003 (accessed 15 November 2009).

Mayberg, H.S., Lozano, A.M., Voon, V., *et al.* (2005). Deep brain stimulation for treatment-resistant depression. *Neuron*, **45**, 651–60.

Medtronic Inc. (2009a). *History of Deep Brain Stimulation*. Available at: http://www.medtronic.com/physician/activa/history.html (accessed 15 November 2009).

Medtronic Inc. (2009b). *Medtronic Receives FDA HDE Approval to Commercialize the First Deep Brain Stimulation (DBS) Therapy for a Psychiatric Indication in the United States.* Available at: http://wwwp.medtronic.com/Newsroom/NewsReleaseDetails.do?itemId= 1235065362795andlang=en_US (accessed 15 November 2009).

Merkel, R. (2007). *Intervening in the brain: changing psyche and society,* Berlin: Springer-Verlag.

Mink, J.W., Walkup, J., Frey, K.A., *et al.* (2006). Patient selection and assessment recommendations for deep brain stimulation in Tourette syndrome. *Movement Disorders, 21,* 1831-38.

National Commission (1977). *Psychosurgery: report and recommendations,* Bethesda, MD: National Commission for the Protection of Human Subjects of Biomedical and Behavioral Research.

Nuttin, B., Cosyns, P., Demeulemeester, H., Gybels, J., and Meyerson, B. (1999). Electrical stimulation in anterior limbs of internal capsules in patients with obsessive-compulsive disorder. *Lancet, 354,* 1526.

Nuttin, B., Gybels, J., Cosyns, P., *et al.* (2003). Deep brain stimulation for psychiatric disorders. *Neurosurgery Clinics of North America, 14,* xv–xvi.

Pinto-Foltz, M.D. and Logsdon, M.C. (2009). Reducing stigma related to mental disorders: initiatives, interventions, and recommendations for nursing. *Archives of Psychiatric Nursing, 23,* 32–40.

Pressman, J.D. (1998). *Last Resort: Psychosurgery And The Limits Of Medicine.* Cambridge: Cambridge University Press.

Rabins, P., Appleby, B.S., Brandt, J., *et al.* (2009). Scientific and ethical issues related to deep brain stimulation for disorders of mood, behavior, and thought. *Archives of General Psychiatry, 66,* 931–7.

Read, C.N. and Greenberg, B.D. (2009). Psychiatric neurosurgery 2009: review and perspective. *Seminars in Neurology, 29,* 256–65.

Schlaepfer, T.E. (2005). Deep Brain Stimulation for Treatment-Refractory Major Depression (Clinical Trial). Available at: http://clinicaltrials.gov/show/NCT00122031 (accessed 15 November 2009).

Schlaepfer, T.E. and Lieb, K. (2005). Deep brain stimulation for treatment of refractory depression. *Lancet, 366,* 1420–2.

Schlaepfer, T.E., Cohen, M.X., Frick, C., *et al.* (2008). Deep brain stimulation to reward circuitry alleviates anhedonia in refractory major depression. *Neuropsychopharmacology, 33,* 368–77.

Servello, D., Porta, M., Sassi, M., Brambilla, A., and Robertson, M. M. (2008). Deep brain stimulation in 18 patients with severe Gilles de la Tourette syndrome refractory to treatment: the surgery and stimulation. *Journal of Neurology, Neurosurgery and Psychiatry, 79,* 136–42.

Skoog, G. and Skoog, I. (1999). A 40-year follow-up of patients with obsessive-compulsive disorder [see comments]. *Archives of General Psychiatry, 56,* 121–7.

Temel, Y. and Visser-Vandewalle, V. (2004). Surgery in Tourette syndrome. *Movement Disorders, 19,* 3–14.

The Columbia-Greystone Associates (1949). *Selective partial ablation of the frontal cortex, a correlative study of its effects on human psychotic subjects,* New York: Paul B. Hoeber.

Valenstein, E.S. (1986). *Great and Desperate Cures: The rise and decline of psychosurgery and other radical treatments for mental illness,* New York: Basic Books.

Volkmann, J. and Benecke, R. (2002). Deep brain stimulation for dystonia: patient selection and evaluation. *Movement Disorders, 17,* S112–15.

CHAPTER 27

THE ETHICAL ISSUES OF TRIALS OF NEURAL GRAFTING IN PATIENTS WITH NEURODEGENERATIVE CONDITIONS

ROGER A. BARKER AND ALASDAIR COLES

INTRODUCTION

EFFECTIVE treatments of neurodegenerative disorders are increasing in importance, as the prevalence of these conditions increases with an aging population. These disorders include Alzheimer's disease, Parkinson's disease (PD), Huntington's disease, amyotrophic lateral sclerosis (motor neuron disease), progressive multiple sclerosis and a range of other less common conditions. In all these diseases there is progressive attrition of specific population of cells within the central nervous system (CNS) which leads to gradual, but inexorable, accumulation of disability—normally in both the physical and cognitive domains. In none of these disorders is there effective disease-modifying therapies (aggressive immunotherapy may impact on the early relapsing-remitting phase of multiple sclerosis, but has no effect on the secondary progressive phase of the disease (Compston and Coles 2008)). Consequently, there is intense research activity into innovative treatments of neurodegeneration. This includes developing more effective drug therapies (e.g. rapamycin in animal models of Huntington's disease (Floto *et al.* 2007); the use of antibodies against the pathogenic protein in misfolding disorders (Holmes *et al.* 2008); the use of ion channel blockers to reduce metabolic stresses (e.g. lamotrigine in multiple sclerosis (Kapoor 2008)); and the delivery of growth factors (e.g. GDNF in PD (Gill *et al.* 2003)).

Before any of these strategies were conceived, however, was the hope that transplantation of neuronal cells could replace or repair lost cells. This approach assumes that the brain is not capable of regenerating the lost neurons itself in neurodegenerative disease. Yet that is not always the case. In multiple sclerosis, for instance, oligodendrocyte precursors are present in the lesions of the brain, but are not activated (Scolding *et al.* 1998). It is not immediately obvious cell transplantation would activate them. Tissue restoration remains a primary aim of most neural grafting programs but it is important to recognize that cell therapies could be used in other ways, such as delivering missing enzymes or neurotransmitters, locally delivering trophic and immune modulating factors to the brain, or even providing a substrate for innate axonal repair (reviewed in Barker and Dunnett 1999). In an animal model of a lethal gangliosidosis, grafts have been shown to restore function by multiple mechanisms (Lee *et al.* 2007).

The ethical issues around these different uses of neural tissue are essentially the same. So, in this chapter, we will focus on the specific example of PD where clinical transplantation trials are most advanced.

Neural grafting and Parkinson's disease

PD is a common disorder of the CNS affecting about 1 in 800 people, typically in the seventh decade of life (Foltynie *et al.* 2004). Classically, it is thought of as a disorder of movement secondary to the loss of the dopaminergic nigrostriatal pathway. Because of this apparent anatomical specificity, treatment with neural grafting is conceptually straightforward: dopaminergic neurons need to be implanted into the diseased nigrostriatal pathway.

Research on neural grafting for PD began around 30 years ago, most notably by Björklund and colleagues in Sweden. They showed that transplantating dopaminergic tissue into the adult mammalian brain was most successful when using tissue from the fetal midbrain which contained the developing dopaminergic nigrostriatal system (6–9 weeks after conception in humans). Such tissue survives in the adult host long term, makes and receives connections with the host brain, releases dopamine, and restores many behaviors back to normal (reviewed in Wijeyekoon and Barker 2008). It was on this background that the first clinical trials were started in the late 1980s and have continued into the early part of this century.

These trials were undertaken in a number of centers within Europe (e.g. Lund, Sweden; Paris, France) as well as North America (e.g. Denver and Florida). They were small open-label studies recruiting patients with advanced disease that were failing standard drug therapies, who tended to be younger than the average patient with PD. They were assessed using a recognized international protocol called CAPIT-PD and allografted with fetal ventral mesencephalic (VM) tissue. This tissue was obtained from surgical terminations of pregnancies. Various national guidelines ensured that women were consented to the use of this tissue only after they had made a firm decision to terminate the pregnancy. The VM is that part of the developing brain which contains the neurons that will form the dopaminergic nigrostriatal pathway in the adult brain and which is lost as part of the core pathology in PD. The yield of dopaminergic cells from such a source is low, so tissue from between 4–6 fetuses was needed for grafting one side of the brain. The pooled VM tissue so collected was directly implanted into the striatum where dopamine acts. In most cases, patients also received standard immunosuppressive drugs, in protocols similar to those given to kidney transplant patients.

The main conclusions from these early open-label studies were that:

- The procedure itself is safe, with very few perioperative complications.
- The use of immunotherapy in patients with advanced neurological disease did not pose safety issues additional to those seen with these drugs in other settings.
- Some patients had a clear, sustained, and dramatic improvement following the transplant, both clinically and on F-Dopa positron emission tomography demonstrating the integrity of presynaptic dopaminergic terminals.
- Postmortem studies on those few patients who died after grafting, for unrelated reasons, showed the graft had survived and produced dopamine, and had extended axons into the host striatum.

The initial enthusiasm generated by these open-label trial results was dulled by reports of the success of deep brain stimulation in advanced PD (Wider *et al.* 2008), a technique that can more easily be set up and delivered and the negative outcomes from two double blind placebo-controlled studies investigating VM transplants in patients with PD (Freed *et al.* 2001; Olanow *et al.* 2003). These latter studies, while adopting different approaches, showed after VM transplants that:

- Patients did not significantly improve clinically compared to sham/placebo treatment.
- Some patients developed involuntary movements that did not resolve after stopping their drug therapies (so-called "graft induced dyskinesias"—GIDs).

The immediate response of the media was that a "miracle cure" had turned into a "disaster" (Boseley 2001). Uncritical acceptance of this interpretation has meant that no further trials in this area have been undertaken, although open-label studies continue to show encouraging results (Mendez *et al.* 2005). More sober responses have been to try to understand the apparent divergence of the trial results with previous open-label experience. For instance, one critical issue may be patient selection; PD is more heterogeneous than often appreciated, so some subtypes of the disease may be more or less responsive to transplantation (see, e.g. William-Gray *et al.* 2009). In addition, the pathology of PD extends outside the dopaminergic nigrostriatal pathway, involving a range of other sites within and outside the CNS which may also influence the individual response to dopaminergic transplants. Further work has suggested that GIDs may relate to the distribution of dopaminergic cells across the transplanted striatum along with contamination of the graft with co-transplanted serotoninergic neurons (Ma *et al.* 2002; Carlsson *et al.* 2007). Finally the use of immunosuppression may be more important than once thought for optimizing graft survival and efficacy.

So, there remains cautious optimism that, with more refined patient selection and graft preparation along with better trial design and immunosuppression, there may be a place for better conducted cellular transplantation trials in PD.

The ethical issues generated by the transplantation of this fetal material does though remain pressing and cannot be avoided. These can be categorized as those relating to (a) the patient and physician, (b) the trial design, and (c) the tissue.

THE PATIENT AND PHYSICIAN

The recruitment of patients to clinical trials requires a great deal of care and is an iterative process as the optimal patient group is chosen. In early development, when safety rather than efficacy is the major issue, recruited patients tend to have more advanced disease and have failed standard therapies. As the safety profiles of therapies become more established, clinical trial recruitment is widened to include as broad a section of the patient group as sober risk/benefit assessments allow.

This tendency, to recruit patients with advanced disease, who have "least to lose," to trials of novel therapies seems intuitively fair. However, it may compromise the trial, especially when it is difficult to sensitively measure outcome in such advanced patients. Furthermore, this approach misses the point that the potential threat of a disease is greatest before a patient has become very handicapped.

For the individual patient considering participation in a trial, the acceptable risks of an experimental treatment are balanced against the perceived threat of the disease. It is important, therefore, that the physician not only explains the trial procedures and risks, but also ensures that the patient has a reasonable perception of his or her disease and its prognosis. Several factors confound this process. Firstly, cognitive deficits in advanced PD are common (Williams-Gray et al. 2009) and interfere with the ability to fully appreciate the risks of treatment. Dysexecutive problems in PD have been well described in early disease (Foltynie et al. 2004; Williams-Gray et al. 2009); whilst it is not clear how they affect everyday activities of daily living, they may well impede the ability to assimilate complex and competing sets of information—as would be needed to consent for any cell therapy trial. Even subtle deficits may interfere with a full understanding of the risks inherent in a trial of an experimental therapy. Secondly, even in cognitively normal patients, rational thinking may be clouded by the hope, even desperation, that the treatment might give personal benefit. Sometimes these hopes have been inflamed by histrionic media reports, internet chatroom rumors, or relatives struggling to cope with the affected person. Thirdly, a particularly difficult element of the consenting process in experimental therapies is the attitude of the patient and physician to uncertainty. In fetal cell therapies for PD there may be considerable unforeseeable risks. It is worth overtly discussing a patient's attitude to risk, much in the way an investment broker might. For someone who values safety above all else, fetal grafting may not be appropriate.

The person taking consent needs to be aware of all these dynamics, and ensure that a realistic account of the known advantages and disadvantages of the trial is understood. In our experience, the patient information sheet, which is so scrutinized by the ethics committee, cannot be relied upon. Each potential trial participant has to receive an explanation of its pros and cons in language and detail tailored for their particular situation and background. This is usually best done at several meetings. And the process of information delivery does not stop once the patient is recruited. An audit of patients in trials, of which one of us was the principal investigator, found a high level of satisfaction with the consenting process, but a surprising inability of participants to remember the aim of the trial and the chief adverse effects of the investigational drug (Cox, Association of British Neurologists, 1999). We concluded that these important points need to be regularly reiterated as the trial proceeds.

Given the highly technical and sophisticated nature of fetal grafting for PD, it is likely that it will only take place in a few centers internationally. To begin with, at least, the few physicians involved will naturally be advocates of the approach and may well have considerable career investment in a successful outcome. Whilst ensuring enthusiasm, this tendency allows the possibility that the physician consenting a patient either consciously, or more likely unconsciously, "sells" the trial to boost recruitment. In principle, a neutral third party would be better placed to advise and consent the patient. But, in early trials of complex treatments, it is hard to find physicians with sufficient understanding who are not already committed to the program.

In summary, various pressures bear on the physician and patient considering a trial of neural transplantation. The investigator needs to be aware of these, particularly the possibility of subtle cognitive impairment in many of the relevant diseases. He or she ultimately needs to ensure that trial participants understand, in their own terms, their disease, its prognosis, best standard therapy, and the possible benefits and harm of the grafting procedure. This understanding needs to be regularly checked and reinforced as the trial proceeds, which of course may be on a background of changing cognitive abilities in the affected trial patient.

THE ETHICS OF TRIAL DESIGN

Trial design is an ethical issue. The utilitarian approach is to define the ethical position of any clinical trial as the balance between management of the individual participant and the potential gains to the wider community. For those trial patients taking an active agent, the possible good of a successful treatment should outweigh the potential harmful effects of the drug or disease progression. To the wider community of disease sufferers, there is the potential good that an effective treatment will be discovered. In addition a well-conducted trial, irrespective of its result, should always advance understanding of the disease and so benefit a wide population. A definite negative trial result minimizes the potential harm to the wider community, whereas an inconclusive trial is a waste of resources, time, and participants' good will. Underpowered trials fall into this category. Concerns have been raised about the power of the two NIH PD transplantation studies, with 20 and 23 initially grafted in the two trials respectively with control arms (sham surgery) of 20 and 11 respectively, and of the GDNF trials in PD (Barker 2009). One way of improving power, without exposing more patients to transplantation, is to randomize patients to immediate or delayed grafting. This allows for a comparison between grafted and non-grafted patients during the first half of the trial and before and after grafting of the delayed group, acting as their own controls. This approach has been adopted in a large transplant study in Huntington's disease, where patients that are not grafted in the first phase of the study are transplanted 2 years later (A. Bachoud-Levi, personal communication).

Utilitarianism needs to be constrained by deontological ethics, where primacy is given neither to outcome nor utility but to motive and ethical principles. One such approach, for instance, would be the principle of non-maleficence, "first do no harm." Superficially, a strict application of this rule would disallow all clinical trials. But, appealing to the principle of autonomy, Schafer wrote that: "human dignity can be severely undermined by serious illness as well as by the human experimentation designed to eliminate such illness. There is an ethical cost attached to not doing such research as well as to proceeding with it" (Schafer 1982).

This is manifestly true of progressive neurological diseases such as PD and multiple sclerosis.

The relative weight of collective and individual ethics depends on the aims of the trial. In phase 1 studies, individual ethics should predominate, as the information derived from such a trial will not be applied directly to the wider community but will lead at most to a phase 2 study. This means that the iconic placebo-controlled double-blinded design of drug trials may not be most appropriate for phase 1 transplantation studies. For instance, the sham surgery of recent PD transplantation trials is clearly more risky than a placebo pill. Patients went to theatre to have a burr hole drilled through their skull but without penetrating the dura. In one of trials (Olanow *et al.* 2003) all patients had 6 months of immunosuppression, including those who had imitation transplant surgery. The question is not whether such controls are technically correct, as they clearly are, but whether the risks to the individual participants, which for imitation transplant surgery and 6 months of immunosuppression are appreciable, are justifiable. We believe they may not be, because the techniques for graft preparation and insertion are not yet sufficiently optimized. So the benefit to the collective is likely to be small from current trials, as different grafting regimens are explored, and the emphasis must be on reducing risk to the trial participants themselves.

Once a transplantation trial has concluded, media attention can be expected. Results may be widely and uncritically cited, and may well be given more prominence than is justified by their true clinical impact. This is particularly damaging when negative trial results are used to damn the strategy of neural grafting. A transplant may fail to help a disease, not because there is anything wrong with the cell therapy itself, but because the wrong patients have been included, or the trial design was inappropriate.

A particular problem in transplantation trials, which rarely affects drug development, is that patients can purchase cellular therapies. "Stem cells" are sold all over the world in an unregulated way. One company, for instance, took to selling stem cells in the toilets of a ferry between the UK and Ireland in order to avoid regulatory compliance (*Panorama: Stem Cells and Miracles* 2009)! Trading off the publicity generated by reputable centers doing transplantation trials, such unscrupulous businesses exploit desperate patients. They undermine the reputation of neural grafting and fail to provide any useful scientific data to advance the field. Very likely, the only beneficiaries are the businesses and its investors.

We believe that the development of neural grafting cannot be directly borrowed from the well-honed system for drug approval. At present, we believe the primary goal of clinical studies of fetal transplantation should be to consolidate the technical issues around patient selection, graft preparation, and surgical delivery. In this context, we do not think imitation transplant surgery or immunosuppression of ungrafted patients can easily be justified. Only when the technique is more consolidated can power calculations be reasonably made and controlled trials set up.

The grafted tissue

A number of different cell sources have been considered for use in patients with neurological disease (Laguna Goya *et al.* 2008). These have included:

- Fully differentiated adult tissue that can then be autografted (e.g. carotid body transplants in PD).

- Adult cells that have been simply manipulated to adopt more of a neuronal, dopaminergic phenotype (e.g. adrenal medullary transplants in PD).

- Adult cells that have been de-differentiated into more primitive neural precursor cells (e.g. induced pluripotent stem cells (iPS cells) in motor neuron disease (Ebert *et al.* 2009).

- Fetal cells derived from the developing brain, which involves collecting tissue from elective termination of pregnancies (e.g. fetal VM or striatal allografts in PD and Huntington's disease respectively).

- Cells derived from the embryo at a very early stage of development, such as the blastocyst—so-called embryonic stem or embryonic stem cell cells (e.g. dopaminergic neurons for use in PD).

- Engineered cell lines derived from a range of sources (e.g. the cell lines MHP36 used in a variety of experimental CNS disease and soon to be used in clinical trials in patients with stokes).

Each of these cells brings with them their own unique advantages and disadvantages. In the early stages of development, transplantation of adult adrenal medullary tissue was used in PD. However, whilst some initial success was claimed (Madrazo *et al.* 1987), it soon became apparent that this tissue survived poorly, if at all, and had minimal lasting clinical benefits in patients (Goetz *et al.* 1989). This has been the usual outcome whenever adult post-mitotic tissue has been used as graft. The best hope for adult tissue grafting come from improved carotid body autografts or using induced pluripotent stem cells (iPS cells).

Stem cells are an exciting potential future source of cells for transplantation programs. They are defined by their capacity to divide and self-propagate whilst also retaining the capacity to differentiate into other cell types. There are many different sources of stem cells, with unique benefits and disadvantages. Three in particular could be treatments of neurodegenerative disorders. Mesenchymal stem cells derived from the adult bone marrow are now being trialed in a range of neurological disorders including stroke, multiple system atrophy, and, more recently, multiple sclerosis (Freedman *et al.* 2010) Their mechanism of action is complex. It has not yet been shown that they can truly transdifferentiate into mature neural elements. Nevertheless they may be able to support the degenerating CNS networks through the release of trophic and immunosuppressive factors. These cells are relatively easy to obtain but we remain to be convinced that they can truly make a clinically significant long-term impact in patients with neurological disorders (e.g. Quinn *et al.* 2008).

The second stem cell source for cell therapy is the embryonic stem cell. These cells are derived from blastocysts redundant to the needs of couples undergoing *in vitro* fertilization programs. The key ethical issue is the moral status of the inner cell mass of the blastocyst, which has not yet differentiated into any recognizable fetal elements. At what point, in the long and complex process from fertilization to delivery of baby, does humanness or personhood start? This complex question cannot be adequately addressed here. Simplistically put, there are two positions. Some take a gradualist approach, where the embryo becomes more human and more deserving of protection as it develops biologically. In effect, this is the position adopted in law in most countries. The alternative position is to identify an absolute threshold at which a non-living lump of material becomes a fully-fledged person, with all human rights. Historically, different times have been suggested for the emergence of personhood or ensoulment: at fertilization, quickening (first movements), at the time beyond which twinning is no longer possible, or at birth. To our knowledge, the most helpful and comprehensive survey of these various positions, and their implications, is that of David Jones (2004).

Attempts to harvest stem cells without raising these ethical concerns have been developed. Widely publicized techniques to isolate individual cells from the developing blastocyst without destroying it (Klimanskaya *et al.* 2006) have yet to be replicated. Alternatively, and most excitingly, has been the announcement that adult cells can be reprogrammed to a more primitive pluripotent state, which resembles an embryonic stem cell. The technology to generate these iPS cells has made much progress over the last few years. IPS cells have now been made from both adult mouse and human cells from a variety of sources but most notably skin fibroblasts. These are then back-differentiated to stem cells and driven down a new differentiation pathway, initially using oncogenes and viral vectors (Takahashi *et al.* 2007), but more recently by safer technologies (Soldner *et al.* 2009). The current situation is that, in mice, neuronal elements can be generated from adult skin cells which have some functional benefits in a model of PD (Wernig *et al.* 2008). Not only does this technology avoid the ethical issues of embryo harvesting, but it provides tissue that is easily available (from the patient directly), which is uninfected and will not be immunologically rejected. However, these cells are not yet ready for clinical use. Furthermore, if the cells are derived from the patient with a neurological disease themselves, it is possible that the derived tissue may be vulnerable to the original pathology. And there are concerns, as with all embryonic stem cell treatments, over the extent to which all cells can be directed to a mature neural fate. Any residual undifferentiated cells could form a tumor; the proliferative potential of differentiated human embryonic stem cell transplants in vivo has been reported (Roy *et al.* 2006) and there is a case report of a brain tumor arising from a neural graft used to treat ataxia telangiectasia (Amariglio *et al.* 2009). The moral status of iPS cells remains largely undiscussed. A key issue is whether or not such cells can generate a human person in much the same way as an embryonic stem cell. But at least their source is not ethically contentious; as tattooing and cosmetic surgery is socially acceptable, using adult human skin to treat disease seems positively lofty!

Although there are great hopes that iPS cells could be used in transplantation, that prospect remains distant. Pragmatically, there is currently only one viable option for cell transplantation in PD: fetal tissue.

The use of human fetal tissue requires the collection of material acquired through elective terminations of pregnancy. Unfortunately, fetal material from spontaneous miscarriages cannot be used for a number of reasons: (1) it is often unclear how long the material has been dead for; (2) the tissue may have acquired an *in utero* infection; and (3) the cause of the miscarriage, which is usually unknown, may have been a problem with the developing fetus which would preclude its use as donor tissue. For this reason, the fetal material for grafting has to be collected from elective surgical termination of pregnancy, although there is a growing interest in whether tissue from medical terminations could also be used.

In some countries, the medical use of fetal material is not permitted. This does not avoid ethical difficulties though. For example, before Bill Clinton came to power in 1992 in the US, human fetal allotransplant work in patients with neurodegenerative disorders could not be federally funded, so it became the preserve of the private sector. This decision placed greater value on the ethic of the free market. It is not at all clear that rescinding to commerce promotes an ethical approach to fetal transplantation. Furthermore, medical tourism means that physicians may be asked by patients to comment on trials, which would not be permitted in his or her country, but are nevertheless accessible.

Some will argue that, in countries where termination of pregnancy is legal, there are no ethical issues involved in using the "waste products." In this line of thinking, it is better to make some good use of the material, to potentially benefit others, than let it be thrown away. This is an intuitively powerful argument and, superficially, is similar to cadaveric organ donation. One does not wish for people to die in accidents, but it will happen and it is good that their organs can be used to help others, and their use does not condone the cause of death.

However attractive this argument appears, it fails to address two key points, the first being the status of the fetus. In the cadaveric organ transplantation example, the status of the dead person is fairly universally recognized and this leads to social strictures around the treatment of the body. For instance, many would be offended by the use of a cadaver for cosmetic research. So, to define whether or not the use of fetal grafts as treatment is acceptable, it is necessary to address what the fetus is, whether person, human, animal, or none of these. As with the moral status of the blastocyst, this topic is too complex to address fully but we make some comments briefly here. Secondly, it is not possible to completely divorce the ethics of the use of the products of termination of pregnancy from the ethics of the procedure itself. To stretch the analogy: if traffic accidents were deliberately committed in order to farm organs for transplantation, the use of the material, however effective in relieving suffering, would be seen to be complicit with murder and unethical. Of course, all fetal cell transplantation programs are structured to ensure that there is no coercion of women considering termination. Nevertheless individuals involved in transplantation programs may feel involved in the source of the tissue. The relation between distance from the act of termination, and complicity in it, is finely argued by Edward Furton (2003). A more systemic issue is that if society allows fetal cell transplantation, as in the UK, this may impact on the ethical environment in which people make decisions about termination of pregnancy. It is possible that the perception that "some good will come from a bad situation" may nuance occasional decisions in favor of termination. Even if this happens very infrequently, it ties the ethics of termination with the use of fetal material.

CONCLUSION

In this chapter we have laid out the major issues with respect to the ethical problems confronting the field of neural transplantation. These issues encompass the patient themselves, the cell to be used and the trial design. Each of these areas presents major problems and in some ways the field, still early in development, is defining the issues as it moves forward. Exactly how these issues will be resolved in the future requires active debate and the involvement of those outside of the medical profession including ethicists, social scientists, and philosophers. It also will involve a wider discussion with governmental agencies that regulate much of this work and the society that they serve and protect.

REFERENCES

Amariglio, N., Hirshberg, A., Scheithauer, B.W., *et al.* (2009). Donor-derived brain tumor following neural stem cell transplantation in an ataxia telangiectasia patient. *PLoS Medicine*, **6**, e1000029.

Barker, R.A. (2009). Parkinson's disease and growth factors - are they the answer? *Parkinsonism Relat Disord* Suppl 3: S181-4.

Barker, R.A. and Dunnett, S.B. (1999). *Neural repair, transplantation and rehabilitation.* Hove: Psychology Press Ltd.

Boseley, S. (2001). Parkinson's miracle cure turns into a catastrophe. *The Guardian*, March 13, 2001.

Carlsson, T., Carta, M., Winkler, C., Björklund, A., and Kirik, D. (2007). Serotonin neuron transplants exacerbate L-DOPA-induced dyskinesias in a rat model of Parkinson's disease. *Journal of Neuroscience*, **27**, 8011–22.

Compston, A. and Coles, A. (2008). Multiple sclerosis. *Lancet*, **372**, 1502–17.

Cox, R. (1999). Association of British Neurologists relates to an oral presentation at the annual meeting of the Association of British Neurologists.

Ebert, A.D., Yu, J., Rose, F.F. Jr., *et al.* (2009). Induced pluripotent stem cells from a patient with spinal muscular atrophy. *Nature*, **457**, 277–80.

Floto, R.A., Sarkar, S., Perlstein, E.O., Kampmann, B., Schreiber, S.L., and Rubinsztein, D.C. (2007). Small molecule enhancers of rapamycin-induced TOR inhibition promote autophagy, reduce toxicity in Huntington's disease models and enhance killing of mycobacteria by macrophages. *Autophagy*, **3**, 620–2.

Foltynie, T., Robbins, T.W., Brayne, C., and Barker, R.A. (2004). Cognitive impairments are common among a population cohort of newly diagnosed PD patients – the CamPaIGN study. *Brain*, **127**, 550–60.

Freed, C.R., Greene, P.E., Breeze, R.E., *et al.* (2001). Transplantation of embryonic dopamine neurons for severe Parkinson's disease. *New England Journal of Medicine*, **344**, 710–19.

Freedman, M. S., Bar-Or, A., Atkins, H.L., *et al.* (2010). The therapeutic potential of mesenchymal stem cell transplantation as a treatment for multiple sclerosis: consensus report of the International MSCT Study Group. *Multiple Sclerosis*, **16**, 503–8.

Furton, E.J. (2003). Levels of moral complicity in the act of human embryo destruction. In N. E. Snow (ed.) *Stem cell research. New frontiers in science and ethics*, pp.100–21. Indiana, IN: University of Notre Dame Press.

Goetz, C.G., Olanow, C.W., Koller, W.C., *et al.* (1989). Multicenter study of autologous adrenal medullary transplantation to the corpus striatum in patients with advanced Parkinson's Disease. *New England Journal of Medicine*, **320**, 337–41.

Gill, S.S., Patel, N.K., Hotton, G.R., *et al.* (2003). Direct brain infusion of glial cell line-derived neurotrophic factor in Parkinson disease. *Nature Medicine*, **9**, 589–95.

Holmes, C., Boche, D., Wilkinson, D., *et al.* (2008). Long-term effects of Abeta42 immunisation in Alzheimer's disease: follow-up of a randomised, placebo-controlled phase I trial. *Lancet*, **372**, 216–23.

Jones, D. (2004). *The Soul of the Embryo*. London: Continuum.

Kapoor, R. (2008). Sodium channel blockers and neuroprotection in multiple sclerosis using lamotrigine. *Journal of the Neurological Sciences*, **274**, 54–6.

Klimanskaya, I., Chung, Y., Becker, S., Lu, S.J., and Lanza, R. (2006). Human embryonic stem cell lines derived from single blastomeres. *Nature*, **444**, 481–5.

Laguna Goya, R., Tyers, P., and Barker, R.A. (2008). Sources of cells for brain repair in Parkinson's disease. *Journal of the Neurological Sciences*, **265**, 35–42.

Lee, J. P., Jeyakumar, M., Gonzalez, R., *et al.* (2007). Stem cells act through multiple mechanisms to benefit mice with neurodegenerative metabolic disease. *Nature Medicine*, **13**, 439–47.

Ma, Y. Feigin, A., Dhawan, V., *et al.* (2002). Dyskinesia after fetal cell transplantation for parkinsonism: a PET study. *Annals of Neurology*, **52**, 628–34.

Madrazo, I., Drucker-Colin, R., Diaz, V., Martinez-Mata, J., Torres, C., and Becerril, J.J. (1987). Open microsurgical autograft of adrenal medulla to the right caudate nucleus in two patients with intractable Parkinson's disease. *New England Journal of Medicine*, **316**, 831–4.

Mendez, I., Sanchez-Pernaute, R., Cooper, O., *et al.* (2005). Cell type analysis of functional fetal dopamine cell suspension transplants in the striatum and substantia nigra of patients with Parkinson's disease. *Brain*, **128**, 1498–510.

Olanow, C.W., Goetz, C.G., Kordower, J.H., *et al.* (2003). A double-blind controlled trial of bilateral fetal nigral transplantation in Parkinson's disease. *Annals of Neurology*, **54**, 403–14.

Panorama: Stem Cells and Miracles (2009). BBC 1, UK. 18 May 2009 [television program].

Quinn, N., Barker, R.A., and Wenning, G.K. (2008). Are trials of intravascular infusions of autologous mesenchymal stem cells in patients with multiple system atrophy currently justified and are they effective? *Clinical Pharmacology and Therapeutics*, **83**, 663–5.

Roy, N.S., Cleren, C., Singh, S.K., *et al.* (2006). Functional engraftment of human ES cell-derived dopaminergic neurons enriched by coculture with telomerase-immortalized midbrain astrocytes. *Nature Medicine*, **12**, 1259–68.

Schafer, A. (1982). The ethics of the randomized clinical trial. *New England Journal of Medicine*, **307**, 719–24.

Scolding, N., Franklin, R., Stevens, S., *et al.* (1998). Oligodendrocyte progenitors are present in the normal adult human CNS and in the lesions of multiple sclerosis. *Brain*, **121**, 2221–8.

Soldner, F., Hockemeyer, D., Beard, C., *et al.* (2009). Parkinson's disease patient-derived induced pluripotent stem cells free of viral reprogramming factors. *Cell*, **136**, 964–77.

Takahashi, K., Tanabe, K., Ohnuki, M., *et al.* (2007). Induction of pluripotent stem cells from adult fibroblasts by defined factors. *Cell*, **131**, 861–72.

Wernig, M., Zhao, J.P., Pruszak, J., *et al.* (2008). Neurons derived from reprogrammed fibroblasts functionally integrate into fetal brain and improve symptoms in rats with Parkinson's Disease. *Proceedings of the National Academy of Sciences USA*, **105**, 5856–61.

Wider, C., Pollo, C., Bloch, J., Burkhard, P.R., and Vingerhoets, F.J. (2008). Long-term outcome of 50 consecutive Parkinson's disease patients treated with subthalamic deep brain stimulation. *Parkinsonism and Related Disorders*, **14**, 114–19.

Wijeyekoon, R. and Barker, R.A. (2009). Cell replacement therapy for Parkinson's Disease. *Biochimica et Biophysica Acta*, **1792**, 688–702.

Williams-Gray, C.H., Evans, J.R., Goris, A., *et al.* (2009). The distinct cognitive syndromes of Parkinson's disease: 5 year follow-up of the CamPaIGN cohort. *Brain*, **132**, 2958–69.

CHAPTER 28

....

THE ETHICS OF NANO/NEURO CONVERGENCE

....

GEORGE KHUSHF

In this chapter, I outline a few representative areas of research in nano- and neuroscience, and then consider the complex continuum of entangled research practices that results. The point of this review is to give a realistic sense of the distributed, opportunistic character of this research, and to show how such emergent practices challenge conventional assumptions about how ethics and science should be advanced. When ethicists consider nano/neuro convergence, they should not just look for some standard type—for example, of a medical, nano-enabled brain–machine interface (BMI)—and then evaluate the risk profile of research related to that type as if it designated some discrete project. Instead, there are a host of entangled types in a complex possibility space: nano/neuro interfaces range from the use of quantum dots (QDs) as sensors for understanding neuron function *in vitro* all the way to specific military enhancement-related projects. Along this continuum, engineers look for opportunities to apply their new tools. Mission-driven agencies or clinicians also look for tools to solve existing problems. In their dialogue, both the nature of the tools and the framing of the problems are altered. Here research does not fit the conventional model of a discrete, applied science where top-down political control can be established. There are a host of distributed practices and visions at multiple scales of time and space, and there are complex sets of transactions between these distributed practices. Instead of a conventional ethical assessment of some discrete interventional type, we need an ethic that is continually in process, and that arises in the interstitial spaces where these transactions occur. Such an ethic of nano/neuro convergence will be opportunistic in the same way that the practices themselves are, and it will be oriented toward dispositions, capacities, and ends, rather than just oriented toward discrete actions. Such an ethic of nano/neuro convergence will be informed by, and inform, the new models of understanding and control integral to the emerging research. The contrast between the conventional type-based ethic and the needed interstitial ethic of nano/neuro convergence will be illustrated by critically reflecting on US and EU initiatives that consider the use of nano-enabled BMIs for enhancing human performance.

ON THE NOVELTY OF NANOSCIENCE: ESTABLISHING A NEW KIND OF INTERFACE WITH THE MOLECULAR SCALE

Nanoscience involves the study and manipulation of material systems that have components 1–100 nanometers (nm) in size. On the bottom end of this scale, we approach the size of atoms; for example, a hydrogen atom is about one angstrom, which is a tenth of a nanometer. Quantum mechanical principles are needed to understand the behavior of matter at this scale—all is a weird blur, accounted for by a set of well-established formal tools, but not easily understood by standards of ordinary human experience. As we move to the upper end of the nanoscale, there is a kind of averaging effect that stabilizes phenomena, yielding bulk level material properties. While there is a general understanding of how these bulk level properties arise from the ground up, even modestly complex systems cannot be modeled in quantum mechanical terms. The nanoscale thus signifies a middle level or mesorange, where *ab initio* computational tools break down, and a complex, multiscale alignment of theoretical and experimental methods is needed. This is a frontier, where solid-state physics, supramolecular chemistry, and molecular biology converge with one another and with cutting edge applications in fields as diverse as materials science, biotechnology, and medicine.

Since nearly everything of interest to humans has nanoscale components, the scale alone cannot be used to define nanoscience. By that criterion, most chemistry, biology, and a host of other science and engineering disciplines would all be nanoscience. In order to more narrowly circumscribe the field, the US National Nanotechnology Initiative (NNI) has advanced a definition that highlights the understanding and manipulation of meso-level principles "to create materials, devices, and systems with *essentially new properties and functions because of their small structure*" (Roco and NSTC 2004, p. 890, my emphasis; NSTC 2002, p. 11). Of course, much here depends on what is meant by such essential novelty of properties and functions. A careful analysis of several representative examples would show there is considerable variability in meaning—indicating a set of family resemblances, rather than necessary and sufficient conditions.

The manner in which novelty depends on size can be illustrated by QDs, which have several uses in neuroscientific research (Pathak *et al.* 2006). QDs are nanosized semiconducting materials (approximately 5–15nm); for example, they might involve a cadmium selenide (CdSe) core in a zinc sulfide (ZnS) shell (with shell size ranging up to 120nm). When excited, they fluoresce, with the color of fluorescence related to the size and shape of the QD. The color can thus be tuned by synthesizing dots of different size. The relation between color of the light emitted and size is understood according to quantum mechanical principles (e.g. quantum confinement effect). If we consider an electron confined in a small box (less than about 20nm), the uncertainty relation tells us that as we decrease the box size we get an increase in the electron's kinetic energy. If we consider a photon (a particle of light) exciting an electron from its valence band into the conduction band (the difference between these giving a band gap), then the smaller the box size, the greater the energy needed to excite the electron, and thus the greater the energy released when the electron relaxes back to its valence band. (A full account of the phenomenon depends on multiple factors, including a complex combination of two kinds of quantization, one related to size and the other related to capacitance of the semi-conductor and amount of charge within it (Reed 1993; Vanmaekelbergh and Liljeroth 2005)) If we consider the visible spectrum, greater energy light (shorter wavelength) is on the blue side, and lower energy light (longer wavelength) is on the red side of the spectrum. Thus as dot size decreases, the wavelength of the light shifts from red to blue. Here we can see how the novelty of the properties and functions (e.g. the size tunable wavelength of QDs) depends on the characteristics of the meso-realm.

In some ways, a QD is like an artificial atom, allowing for exploration of basic quantum mechanical principles (Michler *et al.* 2000). Interest in the nanoscale, however, does not just depend on this capacity to exploit quantum principles for the creation of new products that enable fundamental scientific investigation. Additionally, there is an interest in imaging and interfacing with complex systems at this fundamental scale, and exploitation of their properties for human ends (Ratner and Ratner 2003, provides an accessible overview by a leading research group). Once synthesized, QDs can be used in areas as diverse as renewable energy (photovoltaic devices), quantum computing, and sensing. In biomedical applications, the surface of QDs can be functionalized so they bind to structures of interest; for example, to proteins, DNA, or viruses (Sutherland 2002; Zhou and Ghosh 2006). Since QDs photo-bleach at a much slower rate than traditional fluorescent markers (as much as 100 times as stable), are brighter (as much as 20 times), and they allow for tuning of wavelength according to size, they greatly expand the capacity of the biologist to track what is going on in cells (Chan and Nie 1998). QDs can be used to tag cells, track molecules across cell boundaries, or track single molecules within cells (Cai *et al.* 2007).

In these biomedical uses of the QD, the novelty of nano is more difficult to specify: it concerns the qualitative advance that arises from many quantitative, incremental developments that coalesce to provide a *new level of resolution and control* of the simplest elements of biological systems (Silva 2005, 2006). Here there is a kind of convergence of the specific, coordinated functions of elements in a hierarchically organized ensemble (associated with the logic of biological systems) and the kind of mass action integral to chemical systems. "Nano" as a general category thus connotes a *new kind of interface* with the molecular building blocks of living systems, and can thus be taken as the general science for enabling a long-awaited molecular medicine (Khushf 2008).

Many of the proposed clinical applications of QDs depend on their multi-functional character (Gomez *et al.* 2005; Azzazy *et al.* 2007). They can be used diagnostically to image pathological processes; for example, the surface of a QD can be functionalized so it binds to cancer cells, revealing their location when excited by light. But they can also be used to target specific cells; for example, when binding to or ingested by neoplastic cells, their potentially toxic effects might be exploited (Trojan horse). The same QD might thus perform both diagnostic and therapuetic functions, leading to so-called theranostics (Gao *et al.* 2004; Yezhelyev 2006).

In characterizing the development of nanoscience, Renn and Roco (2006) have identified four stages, ranging from simple particles (such as QDs) to multifunctional, hierarchically organized nanosystems. As research moves to the latter stages, QDs perform diverse clinical functions, depending on the environment or internal state of the nanosystem; for example, they might have optical properties that are modulated, have membrane-crossing equipment, and even be given an enzymatic function (Michalet *et al.* 2005). In these biomedical contexts, the meso-level considerations that account for the size dependent optical properties of

QDs are generally black-boxed, and emphasis is placed upon the diverse functions of QDs in the engineered interface. This leads to medical definitions of nanoscience that downplay the "intrinsic" novelty of nano-products (associated with meso-level quantum effects) in favor of "extrinsic" novelty associated with higher level organization of diverse nano-components. "In this functional definition of nanotechnology, it is implicit that this is not a new area of science per se, and that the interdisciplinary convergence of basic fields (such as chemistry, physics, mathematics, and biology) and applied fields (such as materials science and the various areas of engineering) contributes to the functional outcomes of the technology" (Silva 2006, p. 66). For Silva, who is a leading nano/neuro researcher, the novelty of nano-phenomena concerns the way systems components such as DNA or QDs can be adapted to new functions; for example, the way DNA that does not have the intrinsic capacity to function as a nanowire might be turned into such a wire as part of a new application (p. 65).

Finally, the novelty of nano might relate to the methods of synthesis, rather than to intrinsic or extrinsic properties of products or applications. It is common within nanoscience to distinguish between top-down and bottom-up methods of design (Ratner and Ratner 2003). These reflect general engineering strategies: Do you start with some plan—like the sculptor's vision of the end product—and then inscribe this from the top-down, for example, by lithographic techniques? Or do you discover ways of evoking the desired structures so they self-organize from the bottom-up? Often within nanoscience, a combination of the two will be used. But researchers hope that more and more can be done by bottom-up self-assembly, because this will be needed for accomplishing some of the more ambitious research goals and also for developing products and services that are commercially viable (Zhang 2003).

Both top-down and bottom-up methods have been developed for the synthesis of QDs (Murray *et al.*1995; Tersoff 1996). However, the questions of synthesis go beyond the formation of the QD itself. There are also top-down and bottom-up methods for integrating QDs among themselves and for engineering the interface between QDs and some system of interest. For example, Angela Belcher and her collaborators have re-engineered viruses (M13 bacteriophage) so they bind to ZnS at one end (Lee *et al.* 2002; Mao *et al.* 2003). For this, they generated a large phage library, and then selected for those variants that had the appropriate characteristics. M13 bacteriophage is about 880nm long, and 6.6nm in diameter. The variant that had a peptide on one end that binds to ZnS was termed A7 phage. When suspended in ZnS precursor solutions, an A7 phage-ZnS liquid nanocrystalline suspension was created. Belcher and colleagues used these methods to create highly organized thin films. They also used the A7 phage to generate nanowire arrays. In this way, "natural" systems and combinatorial/evolutionary design strategies guide a self-assembly process that is orchestrated to generate complex, highly ordered systems of QDs.

Nano/neuro convergence

There is a fuzzy boundary between nano research and several other kinds of research in areas like solid state physics, synthetic biology, information technology, and neuroscience. Among these emerging research domains, there is a pervasive cross-traffic of tools and concepts, and advancements in one field often have complex implications for the way research in other fields might be advanced (Khushf 2009). It is thus a mistake to assume that "nano" involves some discrete set of tools that are then "applied" to "neuro," as if the two domains were neatly distinguished. Instead, "nano/neuro convergence" should be taken as a designation for a broad continuum of emerging research practices where there is a complex entanglement of inter-related tools and concepts. The contrast class of interest is thus not between nano and related areas of emerging research in neuroscience, but between much of this emerging research and more conventional, disciplinary science and engineering, where it is possible to modularize the practices and products of research. Here nanoscience is of interest because of the way it is representative of these emerging technologies.

Nano/neuro research on quantum dots

In order to appreciate some of the challenges associated with characterizing nano/neuro convergence, we might ask how we could distinguish the "nano" from the "neuro" in the earlier-mentioned QD research. As a first approximation, we could assume that "nano" involves a kind of tool-oriented, applied science, and "nano/neuro convergence" involves application of those tools to neuroscience (Silva 2006). QDs have been used to track glycine receptors as they diffused into synaptic and extrasynaptic domains in cultured spinal neurons, showing that diffusion dynamics depended on whether receptors were synaptic, perisynaptic, or extrasynaptic (Dahan *et al.* 2003; general review of QD surface trafficking of neurotransmitter receptors can be found in Groc *et al.* 2007). They have been used to investigate how neuronal activity (and by implication, memory and learning) modifies diffusion properties of neurotransmitter receptors (Bannai *et al.* 2009). QDs can also control specific physiological or pharmacological responses; for example, to initiate downstream signaling of neurite growth (Vu *et al.* 2005). When combined with other methods (both within nanoscience and in more traditional areas of molecular biology/genetics), it is possible to directly control neural physiology at multiple systems levels, ranging from the constitutive electrical and molecular events up through the complex, functional organization of neural circuits (Lima and Miesenbock 2005; Deisseroth *et al.* 2006; Silva 2006; Andrews 2007; Elder *et al.* 2008;). Nano/neuro convergence would then concern this cluster of enabling capacities. But this would give just one side of the convergence.

Mihail Roco brings into view the other side when he characterizes nano/bio convergence: "Nanotechnology provides the tools and technology platforms for the investigation and transformation of biological systems, and biology offers inspiration models and bio-assembled components to nanotechnology" (Roco 2003, p. 337). When speaking of how biology "inspires" nanoscience, Roco has in mind something like the QD research of Angela Belcher and colleagues (Lee *et al.* 2002): by genetically altering viruses, establishing selection mechanisms for properties of interest, and then using the selected viruses to assemble her QD nanosystems, Belcher is both imitating and exploiting biological systems for human purposes. Neural models for designing nanoelectronics would provide another example of a biologically inspired research agenda. Thus, when QDs are used to image or manipulate neural systems, we have one kind of nano/neuro convergence: we could call this nano-enabled neuroscience. But when the meso-level properties of QDs are studied, or when they are synthesized by chemists, or when they are self-assembled by viruses into novel materials, then we have nano, but not neuro. This would make all the QD research outlined in the previous section "nano," but not "neuro" (although we would have nano/bio in the case of Belcher's self-assembled systems). However, if we use "neuro" as an "inspiration" for "nano," then we have another kind of nano/neuro convergence. According to Roco's definition, nano-enabled neuroscience and neuro-inspired nanoscience constitute two distinct domains that are encompassed under the general category of nano/neuro convergence.

Roco's account of nano/neuro convergence works as a first approximation, but it breaks down when we consider some of the more complex lines of influence, and when we view these over a longer historical time line. For example, some look to neuroscience for the new architectures that are needed for nanoelectronics. Here we have neuro-inspired nano. The QD might be taken as a model of a neuron, and systems of QDs as neural systems (Toth *et al.* 1996). By understanding how neural systems handle uncertainty and error (e.g. by redundancy and adaptivity, which uses feedback from some functional interaction organized at higher systems levels to tune lower level circuits) or by exploring the integration of top-down and bottom-up pathways integral to neural interconnections, electrical engineers can develop new design strategies for circuits (van Roermund and Hoekstra 2000). However, once the electronic circuits are biomimetically designed, they can be taken as physical models of neural systems, and insights from these models can be used to ask new questions in neuroscience (Arenkiel and Ehlers 2009). Or the solutions to the electrical interconnection and control problems can inspire new ways of developing brain/machine interfaces (Miesenbock and Kevrekidis 2005; Aravanis *et al.* 2007; Shalk 2008). Here we get nano-inspired neuro. But when the inspiration maps back in a circle, the two distinct domains become entangled. There is thus a kind of iterative adjustment and alignment of disciplines, which leads to both convergences and divergences of disciplinary tools. In this cross-traffic, it becomes impossible to isolate just one strand and consider it in isolation. This will have significant implications for ethics, since we will not be able to neatly specify "the ethics of X" and consider it in isolation from "the ethics of Y."

If we consider nanoscience as the general science for understanding and interfacing with living systems at the meso-scale where the smallest functional units are constituted, then neuroscience can be viewed as a subcategory of nanoscience. While such an over-reaching definition of nano is problematic, it does capture at least one aspect of nano/neuro convergence. In one recent review for *Science*, neuroscience was understood in exactly this way: an integration of meso-scale models of micro-circuits with the architecture of higher scale processing was seen as the key to harmonizing the currently fragmented bits of neuroscientific knowledge (Arenkiel and Ehlers 2009).

NBIC Convergence for electrophysiological brain–machine interfaces

When considering nano/neuro convergence, the distinction between pure and applied science breaks down. Establishing an interface with neural systems is a task of both. Basic science is advanced by technological means that directly interface with the neural systems, and medical interfaces serve as platforms for advancing basic science. As a result, medical and other applied neuroscientific projects at the nano/neuro intersection will have the same characteristics that we identified when describing the novelty of nanoscience: they will represent a continuum of entangled practices, and move toward multi-functional capacities. To illustrate this, I turn now to research on nano-enabled brain-machine interfaces (BMIs) that was part of a US policy initiative cosponsored by the US Department of Commerce and the National Science Foundation. The stated goal of the initiative was to facilitate the convergence of nanoscience, biomedicine, information technology, and cognitive science (NBIC Convergence) and orient this toward advancing human performance. (Roco and Bainbridge 2002a,b; Khushf 2007 provides an overview.) Fairly radical enhancements of strength, lifespan, and cognitive function were proposed. Here I consider just two of the contributions related to nano-enabled BMIs.

The title of Miguel Nicolelis' (2002) contribution to the first US Convergence conference nicely captures the goals of the initiative: "Human-machine interaction: potential impact of nanotechnology in the design of neuroprosthetic devices aimed at restoring or augmenting human performance." Note how conventional medical treatment (= restoring) and enhancement (= augmenting) are used together. This reflects the general, multifunctional, capacity-oriented character of the US convergence initiative. Nicolelis' experiments with monkeys have provided one of the most vivid demonstrations of the mid-term potential of BMIs. After implanting electrodes into their sensorimotor cortex, his team was able to develop a computer algorithm to interpret the neural signals associated with arm movement, and then use this to drive a robotic arm. Eventually, monkeys were trained to use the robotic arm without moving their own arm, indicating how the prosthetic limb was incorporated into the monkey's body schema. These kinds of experiments have been taken as proof-of-principle that fairly radical BMI-based enhancements lie on our immediate horizon. Some of the most high profile research on BMIs—including that of Nicolelis—has been funded by the US military because of this potential for enhancement (Hoag 2003; Moreno 2006; Barr 2008).

In his Convergence contribution, Nicolelis (2002) highlights non-medical, general purpose reasons for pursuing this research. He argues that the "realization of the full potential of the 'digital revolution' has been hindered by its reliance on low-bandwidth and relatively slow user-machine interfaces (e.g. keyboard, mice, etc.)." For human operators, computers are just another "external tool." However, "if such devices could be incorporated into 'neural space' as extensions of our muscles or senses, they could lead to unprecedented (and currently unattainable) augmentation in human sensory, motor, and cognitive performance." Nicolelis then considers how electrophysiological methods of the kind he studies could be used to provide that kind of "seamless" human/machine interface (see also Cauller and Penz 2002).

For Nicolelis (2002), the rate-limiting step for advanced human BMIs depends on nano-science and technology: they provide the tools for developing invasive interface with neural tissue (see also Moxon *et al.* 2004; Lebedev and Nicolelis 2006; Andrews 2007). In turn, such interfaces will enable us to further extend our understanding and control of meso-level phenomena, for example, by using them to create "a complete new generation of actuators, designed to operate in micro- and nanospaces" (Nicolelis 2002). Nicolelis presupposes the goals of systems neuroscience, and then regards research in nano as instrumental for realizing those goals. But there is also a more subtle and complex influence of nano on his research—an influence that can even been seen in the tone of his convergence contribution, with its blending of treatment and enhancement. When "nano" informs research on human/machine interfaces, researchers don't just "use" it. Beyond that, they come to understand the task of establishing an interface in new ways; for example, in the multifunctional, opportunist, capacity-oriented way exhibited in Belcher's viral QD research (Stieglitz 2007; Schalk 2009). This understanding is not *just* due to the nanoscale research. It reflects a thought-style that is found in many areas of emerging research, including neuroscience. But that thought-style is reinforced by means of the nano/neuro convergence. This more subtle influence of nano is also well exhibited in another contribution to the US Convergence conference.

At the second US Convergence conference, Rodolfo Llinas quipped that his medical colleagues do not always respond positively when they hear about BMI research like that of Nicolelis. To get around this, Llinas and his colleagues developed a new, remote control strategy for establishing a BMI (Llinas and Makarov 2002; Llinas *et al.* 2005). For this, a catheter could be threaded through the vascular system to the place where blood bathes a region of the brain where an interface is sought. Nanowires small enough to cross the blood–brain barrier could then be released. These would not interfere with blood flow exchange of gases or introduce any disruption of brain activity. A small number of electrodes with an amplifier converter could then be used to establish the interface. At the time of the second Convergence conference (2004), Llinas and colleagues had already demonstrated in vitro that the nanowire could receive and relay signals from a firing neuron and that it could be used to trigger such a firing. He also demonstrated in mice that the vascular system could be used to target brain regions of interest, and provided functional magnetic resonance images showing nanowires as they cross the blood–brain barrier and snuggle next to neurons in ways that are likely to be safe and allow for the desired interface. Since that time, he has been awarded a patent for this interface. In this patent, Llinas (2008) asserts that "the brain–machine bottleneck will ultimately be resolved through the application of nanotechnology." (The patent actually uses much of the wording from his Convergence workshop presentation, later published in the *Journal of Nanoparticle Research* (Llinas *et al.* 2005).) In prominent reviews by Lebedev and Nicolelis (2006) and Leary *et al.* (2006), Linnas' research is presented as an example of the kind of BMI that nanoscience makes possible.

Optogenetic brain–machine interfaces

Electrophysiological interfaces like those of Nicolelis and Llinas have some weaknesses. One of the most significant of these is referred to as the "specificity problem" (Miesenbock and Kevrekidis 2005). When electrodes are used, they indiscriminately activate all kinds of neurons and fibers of passage in the area. Even in the case of Llinas' nanowires, primary lines are needed that would be used with a multiplex amplifier. This would indiscriminately activate or receive signals from all nanowires within the receiving range of the primary line. Current BMIs such as those used in deep brain stimulation (DBS) for Parkinson's disease have side effects that are thought to arise from this non-specific action, which yields extensive "collateral damage" (Aravanis 2007). This problem cannot be addressed by current electrophysiological technologies, because these depend on relatively large scale, mass-activation of multiple neurons within the region of an electrode. Initially, one might expect to address the problem of specificity by means of the reduction of scale associated with nanoscience and technology. If one could use a large number of very small electrodes, then one could activate all and only those neurons that are important in some circuit of interest. However, this strategy assumes that one can move down scale to the smallest functional unit (as modular, and independent), and then independently interface with each unit that constitutes some circuit of interest. But even the simplest of functions is associated with a large number of such units, and these associated units (the ensemble that constitutes the circuit) are not themselves addressable as a single unit. Rather, they are distributed among a host of other cells. As a result of this non-local, distributed character, establishing such a fine grained interface would require a process of individually discriminating and interfacing with each of the smallest, locally addressable units. As one moves down scale, the complexity of information to be managed increases exponentially, and such a process of interface becomes practically insurmountable. This problem of managing complexity is why nanotechnology needs bottom-up methods of self-assembly.

To solve these problems of specificity and complexity, new optogenetic interfaces have been developed (Deisseroth *et al.* 2006; Henderson *et al.* 2009). These take advantage of biologically based mechanisms for interfacing with the circuits (Zemelman *et al.* 2003). Vectors are developed that introduce genes into the specific cell types of interest, and the "natural" machinery of these cells is used to make proteins that either generate light when cells are activated (sensors) or that excite (or inhibit) neurons when light is introduced (actuators). Fiber optic cables (microendoscopes) can then be inserted instead of electrodes, and light can be used to receive signals or target only those cells that have been genetically altered to interact with the light (Deisseroth *et al.* 2006). In addition to the new specificity of action, optogenetic interfaces avoid the biofouling/scaring problems that lead to degradation of electrophysiological interfaces (Moxon *et al.* 2004; Elder *et al.* 2008). In this way, "the organism itself generates the tools necessary for investigating its function; biology is revealed through biology" (Miesenbock 2009, p. 395).

In several proof-of-principle experiments, optogenetics was used to modulate behavior of flies (Lima and Miesenbock 2005), zebra fish (Arrenberg *et al.* 2009), mice (Hira *et al.* 2009; Tsai *et al.* 2009), and monkeys (Berdyyeva and Reynolds 2009). Preliminary research indicates the genetic interventions are safe, and this technology is already moving to human trials. This may be an area where some of the long awaited, more radical developments associated with gene therapy are first realized in clinical practice. These genetic interventions have the interesting characteristic of introducing new properties to cells (allowing them to optically interface with artificial mechanisms of control), rather than addressing a defect associated with some pathology (as in many gene therapy protocols).

The relation between optogenetics and nano is similar to that between electrophysiology and nano: in both cases nano/neuro convergence denotes a broad set of enabling tools and connotes a thought-style oriented to new capacities for understanding and manipulating neural systems at the most basic level. To advance this convergence, the US National Institutes of Health has recently established a major Nanomedicine Center for the Optical Control of Biological Function (NIH 2009).

QDs thus provide just one development among many in nanoscience that might be used for establishing an optical interface with neural systems. In fact, there is a convergence between all three of the strands outlined in this essay (Arenkiel and Ehlers 2009). Although electrophysiological and optogenetic BMIs are sometimes presented as competing alternatives, they too should be regarded as complementary, converging technologies (Scanziani and Hausser 2009). Such convergence is clearly demonstrated in two sets of recent studies, which bring optogenetics closer to human application. In the research of Han *et al.* (2009; see also Berdyyeva and Reynolds 2009), published in *Neuron*, an optogenetic interface was used to modulate neural circuits in a monkey, and an electrophysiological interface in the same animal was used to identify complex cascades of excitation and inhibition. Here optogenetic and electrophysiological technologies are integrated in a hybrid BMI that enables both sensing and control of neural circuits. A different kind of convergence is demonstrated by two essays in *Science* on the mechanisms of action of DBS for Parkinson's patients. In optogenetic research by a team in the lab of Karl Deisseroth (Gradinaru 2009), genes encoding light-sensitive ion pumps were inserted into the subthalamic nucleus (STN) of mice, and optical signals were used to inhibit the activity of these neurons, thus testing the hypothesis that DBS works by a kind of mini-lobotomy of STN hyperactivity generated as a result of withering dopaminergic cells in the substantia nigra. The research team was also able to selectively excite cells in the STN, testing an opposing hypothesis. In both cases, they did not find the beneficial effects associated with DBS. However, when they activated cells in the primary motor cortex whose axons extend into the STN, they were able to generate the beneficial DBS effects. They also found that different effects could be found when the same cells were driven at different frequencies, indicating the importance of temporal precision in optogenetic control. In another study published in the same issue of *Science*, Nicolelis' team (Fuentes *et al.* 2009) showed that DBS effects on Parkinsonian mice could be generated by placing electrodes on the surface of the spinal chord. This involved indirect stimulation of the cortex that compensated for degenerating effects of Parkinson's disease. Thus, in different ways, both of these investigations "point to the cortex as an important player in the therapeutic effect of DBS for Parkinson's disease" (Miller 2009, p. 1555).

On the Entanglement of Ethical and Scientific Concepts

In the previous sections I gave more detail about QDs and BMIs than might seem necessary for an encyclopedia article that looks at the *ethics* of nano/neuro convergence. But the detail is important. Too often, summary judgments are made about the ethics of nanoscience and nano/neuro convergence—that there is "nothing new" (Gordijn 2006; Allhoff 2007; Litton 2007; Alpert 2008)—but an insufficient account is provided of the research. The earlier overview exhibits a slice of this research, so such claims about ethical novelty (or its lack) can be assessed. But before I can provide this assessment, I need to take a brief detour away from the nano/neuro research. It turns out that summary judgments dismissing any ethical novelty in nanoscience depend on implicit assumptions about the nature of ethical reflection, and these, in turn, depend on assumptions about the nature of pure and applied science. By undermining the conventional assumptions about science, nano/neuro convergence undermines associated assumptions about the character of applied ethics. In order to appreciate the ramification of nano/neuro convergence, I thus need to first consider the underlying linkage between conventional science and applied ethics.

Forms of practical rationality integral to ethics mirror assumptions about the nature of science and its rationality (a detailed review is provided in Khushf 2009). In many contexts, something like a linear model of scientific research and development is still assumed (Bush 1945). Science is divided into two kinds: pure and applied. The first involves the pursuit of understanding for its own sake, and yields descriptively accurate portrayals of the world.

The second kind of science involves intervention in that world, and thus a modification of what is antecedently given. This pure/applied distinction depends on a related distinction between what is natural and artificial. The pre-interventional given is called "nature," and the task of pure science is to understand it. In contrast, applied science alters what is given; as such, it is artificial and yields "artifacts." In an applied science, ends and values from outside science orient the activity—for example, medicine seeks to promote health and eliminate disease among humans. Basic science and technology provide means that are "used" to advance the extra-scientific ends—thus the "linear" movement from the basic to the applied domains. (An outstanding account of this model of applied science and its associated technical rationality is found in Schon, 1983, part I.)

The linear model yields two kinds of ethical reflection roughly corresponding to the two kinds of science. Pure science is governed by internal norms—for example, honesty in reporting of data, fair attribution of credit, and so on. Here the free and open pursuit of truth is advanced, and ethical norms assure that claims are sifted in the appropriate way to assure they are reliable. The internal norms of science foster the flourishing of the science itself. (The classic account of these norms is provided in Merton 1979; a nuanced justification in terms of internal and external goods is found in MacIntyre 1984, ch. 14.) In applied domains, however, the ethic needs to go beyond the purely internal concerns of the practice and assure that the change brought about in the world does not disrupt the flourishing of other activities external to that practice. The intervention is thus regarded as a modular unit that is rationally organized toward the advancement of some specified end. This whole unit is then taken as a perturbation in the world, and the ripple effects of the perturbation are assessed. Applied ethics assures that the positive aspects of the perturbation outweigh the negative aspects. According to this model, applied ethics is like a meta-applied science that reasons backward: instead of moving from pre-given ends to sufficient means, ethics considers the complete applied intervention as the means and considers the ends/consequences that follow. The task of the applied ethic is then to regulate applied science so that negative consequences are blocked or mitigated, and positive consequences are optimized. (J.S. Mill provides the classic statement of this model of ethical reflection; the associated risk model is reviewed in Macnaughten *et al.* 2005; Wynne 2005)

To simplify analysis of proposed applications of science, applied ethicists often categorize new interventions or products according to pre-existing ethical types. For example, a new drug for treatment of heart disease does not call for a new ethical type. Such a drug would provide an instance of a standard type—"new pharmaceutical"—and there are well-defined ethical/policy guidelines for managing such instances. For conventional applied ethicists contemplating some emergent research domain such as nano/neuro convergence, the question is then: "Is there anything new here?" (Gordijn 2006; Allhoff 2007; Litton 2007; Alpert 2008). By this they do not mean "is there new science or technology?" That is taken for granted. Instead, they ask whether the existing taxonomic structure of ethical types is sufficient to understand and socially manage the consequences of some proposed development. They are thus asking whether there is a *novel ethical type* that requires some modification of the background taxonomy. This approach thus assumes a neat division of labor between the work of the applied scientist and that of the applied ethicist. The ethics work comes downstream of the science, and presupposes some potential or actual intervention that can be discretely regarded. The ethicist then asks whether the antecedent ethical types are sufficient for managing the consequences of that intervention.

Despite extensive criticisms of the linear model, these background assumptions about applied ethics are pervasive. They directly inform the incessant worry about whether there is "anything new" in nano or nano/neuro convergence research. But this approach to ethics misses exactly what is most significant about much of the emerging research. Namely, it misses how research does not fit the conventional pure/applied distinction; how it resists categorization according to existing taxonomies; and how it concerns enabling capacities, rather than modular interventions. In the fuzzy world of emerging research, there is even a breakdown of the conditions for a neat division of labor between the work of the scientist or engineer, on one side, and the work of the ethicist or social scientist, on the other side (Gorokhov and Lenk 2009; I provide a more detailed account of this in Khushf 2009). This, in turn, undermines the conditions for post hoc ethical analysis. Instead, ethics needs to move upstream and be integrated as part of the research and development process. But that requires a deep change in research cultures of both the ethicists, who often know little about the science, and the scientists, who know little about ethics.

The European Union Convergence
Initiative as a Type-Framed Ethic

In addressing the ethical issues integral to electrophysiological and optogenetic BMI research, we are faced with a fundamental framing problem. What exactly do we mean, when we speak of BMIs? This can be interpreted as a question about the ethical type featured in the ethical analysis. Are we referring here to specific, already developed BMIs, such as those currently used in DBS for treatment of Parkinson's patients? Do we consider the research projects of people like Deisseroth, Miesenboch, Nicolelis, and Llinas, and take what has been accomplished with animals as evidence of the human BMIs on the mid-term horizon? How is this BMI research related to the more speculative visions integral to NBIC Convergence and military funded initiatives for enhancing human performance? Should we address all these as variants on a single type—that of BMIs—or see a set of distinct types, each raising different kinds of ethical concerns? And what role does nanoscience play in addressing any of these questions?

A traditional applied ethic will begin with such type-questions (usually implicit), and then, after clarifying the type at issue, move on to consider specific problems integral to that pre-given type. Generally, the framing associated with the specification of type is viewed as external to the ethical analysis. It provides the condition for the ethic. In the rare cases when it is made explicit, such framing is seen as a matter of proper description of some emergent phenomenon that calls for the ethical analysis. When ethics researchers ask "what's new about BMIs associated with nano/neuro convergence?" they usually are asking such a type-question. They want specification of some feature or property of nano/neuro convergence that would require a different ethical analysis from the BMIs already considered as part of neuro-ethics. (Here novelty functions like "specific difference" in Aristotelian definitions and taxonomies.) Since the framing is taken as establishing the conditions for ethics, I will call such ethical analysis a "type-framed ethic."

A European Union High Level Expert Group (HLEG 2004) was commissioned to develop an EU counterpart to the US NBIC Convergence initiative. This Group was highly critical of the US workshops, and they presupposed a type-framed ethic in their analysis. Here I focus on the arguments of Alfred Nordmann, who was the *rapporteur* for the HLEG. I'll consider both the official EU report that he drafted and also some of Nordmann's individually authored essays (2007a,b, 2009) where distinctions integral to that report are defended. Even beyond the specific topic of nano-enabled BMIs, the approach of the EU High Level Expert Group can be taken as representative of how applied ethical problems are generally addressed. By critically evaluating some of Nordmann's claims, I thus show how nano/neuro convergence challenges a type-framed ethic.

The EU Group wants to make a sharp distinction between the development and use of BMIs for medical application—such as DBS for Parkinson's patients—and BMIs for human enhancement. They think ethicists should not focus on enhancement projects, because they are unrealistic, and they divert our attention from the more pressing, real world challenges. For Nordmann, this means that calls for "upstream ethics" of such enhancement projects are misguided. "[E]thical concern is a scarce resource and must not be squandered on incredible futures, especially when they distract from on-going developments that demand our attention" (2007b, p. 34). They think the US NBIC Convergence initiative inappropriately framed the task of science, ethics, and policy. Radical human–machine interfaces are assumed to be on the immediate horizon—taken as given—and we are then supposed to ask about the ethics of this soon-to-be-realized development. But for Nordmann and the HLEG, this involves an inappropriate relation to history and technology. Instead, we should start with our current needs and challenges, and then ask: what research provides a solution to these challenges? Nordmann thinks that the US Convergence workshops undermine the very possibility of genuine ethical reflection when they presuppose a speculative and problematic technological development as if it were already realized. By taking some anticipated development as if it were given, they deprive ethics of its standpoint. "Rather than adopt a believing attitude towards the future, an ethics beholden to present capabilities, needs, problems, and proposed solutions will begin with vision assessment. Envisioned technologies are viewed as incursions on the present and will be judged as to their likelihood and merit." (2007b, p. 41) When considering BMIs that might allow for thought-control of robotic arms or mind-mind communication, Nordmann thinks that there is no proof of principle. He sees nothing special about Nicolelis' experiments: the monkeys only have a robotic arm that poorly mimics the motion of an actual arm. In humans, there are only the partial lobotomies of DBS or the terribly slow manipulation by ALS patients of a cursor to spell out words. In all of this, there is nothing radical. For Nordmann, the task is thus to make clear to scientists the difference between the medical and enhancement visions, and to reorient research and debate to the real world problems and prospects (Nordmann 2007b, 2009; HLEG 2004).

Summarizing, Nordmann and the EU Group introduce a sharp distinction between two types of BMI research. They dismiss the enhancement oriented work associated with the US Convergence initiative, and want to frame ethical deliberation in terms of discrete, therapeutically oriented projects like DBS for Parkinson's disease or artificial hands for those who are disabled. For them, "ethics" must take human capacities and limits as given, and then, in a second step, consider how some technological intervention might best address needs that are already specified. This is what is already done in medical, therapeutically oriented research: researchers and clinicians respond to some pre-given need associated with some disease. Nordmann and his EU colleagues want an ethic that is therapeutic and problem-oriented in the same way: ethics becomes a kind of applied social science. They suggest that ethics of enhancement should not be discussed, and any enhancement projects should be blocked politically at the stage when they arise.

ON THE DEFICIENCIES OF A TYPE-FRAMED ETHIC

In substance, the EU High Level Expert Group wants to impose upon nano/neuro convergence the conventional view of an applied science (on this linkage, see Khushf 2007 commentary on Nordmann 2007a). What converges are technologies, not the basic sciences. The EU Group thus explicitly excludes "science" from the name: "NBIC Convergence" becomes "Converging *Technologies*" (CT). As befits the classical ideal of an applied science, they want specific, targeted projects that start with a clear delineation of the end/vision, and then, step by step organize disciplinary pursuits so that end is realized. They want to divert policy away from the kind of general, multifunctional, open-ended, capacity-oriented focus found in the US Convergence initiative. Their type-framed ethics simply presupposes this normative ideal, and then attempts to implement it. All of their recommendations could be taken as a political call to construct CT as an applied science, thus establishing a predictable order out of the otherwise chaotic ensemble of diverse technoscientific practices. But this simply amounts to a kind of nostalgia: they wish for a kind of transparent, predictable science that is no more (and probably never was). Consideration of the QD and BMI research outlined earlier makes clear why this ideal is problematic.

First, there is no clear type that captures common properties of interfaces associated with nano/neuro convergence. Instead, there are many kinds of brain–machine, human–machine, and neural–system interfaces. We should view the QD, electrophysiological, and optogenetic research as constituting a complex continuum, whose possibility space involves a range of variant, but overlapping types (this is apparent in scientific reviews like Miesenbock and Kevrekidis 2005; Deisseroth *et al.* 2006; Lebedev and Nicolelis 2006; and Arenkiel and Ehlers 2009). Some of these interfaces are developed primarily for purposes of basic research in neuroscience. Others are developed for medical or human enhancement purposes. And still others are developed for applications in electronics, cognitive science, systems management, and materials science. But most significantly, there is a blurring between all of these areas, and a kind of distributed, opportunistic adjustment of goals according to context, grant funding, and to the affordances provided by existing research capacity.

We can follow this entanglement of ideas and research projects over all scales. Consider, for example, the QD research outlined earlier. When a QD is functionalized so it binds to some neural structure of interest, then, when it is excited by light and fluoresces, an interface has been established between the human researchers and the neural system. Here we might define the interface in terms of the mediating agency of light. This would make optogenetical interfaces continuous with those established by QDs. Alternatively, we might define the interface in terms of the scale and the qualitative advance associated with the confluence of new capacities. In a central way, nanoscience is about establishing such interfaces. In all sorts of review essays, roadmaps, and grand challenges, establishing of interfaces between macro-scale and nano-scale structures has been viewed as integral to the development of both nanotechnology and neuroscience. Only by this means is understanding and control of systems at the most basic level possible. Further, most scientists agree that establishing these interfaces will require novel strategies; we cannot simply scale down current micro-level interfaces. As a result, new ways for managing failure/error will be needed; new ways of communicating; new ways of working with natural, self-organizing processes (van Roermund and Hoekstra 2000; Zhang 2003). Some of the needed novel strategies are already seen in QD and optogenetic research (Miesenbock and Kevrekidis 2005; Sjulson and Miesenbock 2008). These, in turn, challenge current models for managing risk and understanding safety: for example, when a QD or some other nanoparticle is used in a multifunctional way—perhaps as a sensor that triggers some latent capacity to destroy a cancer cell when some additional environmental condition is met—what does this do to current models for testing; e.g. to the time frame for assessing safety or to assumptions about what is needed in the preclinical stage of testing? (Kelty 2009 provides a nice account of how conventional views of the science and ethics/policy of toxicity are challenged by nanoscience.) Viewed in this way, all of the QD research was about a kind of BMI, or at least about a neural-interface. This should not just be thought of in the trivial sense that all neuroscience is about establishing an interface. The key here is to notice how, by means of nano/neuro convergence, the research interface is at the same time a kind of functional interface that could be naturally extended into practice settings. In the US Convergence initiative there is an attempt to further cultivate these kinds of opportunistic extensions. They want to cultivate those kinds of transfers in the same way Belcher's team (Lee *et al.* 2002) wants to cultivate variants on some phage type in order to generate some library on which her selection function can operate.

In the nano/neuro convergence continuum, there is no sharp line between basic and applied research, and thus no place where we can gate control to block enhancement research. Nordmann views the whole nano/neuro convergence research program as if it were a giant applied science project. For him, vision comes first, before any large scale project. "Envisioned technologies" are "incursions on the present" and are to be "judged as to their likelihood and merit" (2007b, p. 41). This assumes we can distinguish between these "envisioned technologies" and the fundamental research that would provide the basis for the technological interventions. But in practice, the basic research necessary for enhancement is the same basic research necessary for the medical BMIs. In both cases, basic research advances by establishing functional interfaces that enable both understanding *and control* of the neural systems that are studied.

Miesenbock did some of the path-breaking work establishing optogenetic interfaces. For him, the central goal was to advance neuroscience. But he seeks to advance this by breaking out of the purely descriptive, observational mode of pure science. "Mechanistic understanding requires intervention" (Miesenbock 2009, p. 398). Drawing on control theory, Miesenbock and colleagues suggest that "scientific fields shift emphasis from observation to control as they mature" (Miesenbock and Kevrekidis 2005, p. 534). Although he seeks "to do in order to understand," he advances this understanding by establishing artificial interfaces that enable novel functions and control of the systems he studies. He thus blurs the distinction between "natural" and "engineered" interfaces. By using "natural" mechanisms (e.g. of genetics), he solves the specificity problem associated with cruder kinds of interfaces.

Note again the similarity between this kind of approach and that used by Belcher when she re-engineers viral self-assembly so it becomes a tool for organizing complex structures. In the research of Miesenbock and Belcher, "natural" systems that are currently not fully understood and transparent are "used" to "solve" an engineering problem. This is not just "like" genetically modified organisms (one of the concerns raised in the early days of nanoethics). These are GMOs, but now the "genetic" component is just one element of a more elaborate design. For Miesenbock, once the optogenetic interface is established, the organism (e.g. fly) can be placed in a more "natural" setting, allowing for study of relations between neural circuits and behavior. The organism no longer needs to be immobilized in the manner necessary with earlier interfaces, and thus is brought closer to the unperturbed state. But at the same time, far more radical modulation of behavior becomes possible: "remote control of behavior through genetically targeted photostimulation of neurons" (Lima and Miesenbock 2005). In this research, the most "natural" behavior is achieved by the greatest artifice.

There is already a multifunctional character to the developing BMIs that makes them distinct from conventional medical therapies. According to the EU Convergence report, interfaces like those for ALS or Parkinson's patients are always for very specific purposes, and they compensate for some lost function. These special purposes devices are sharply contrasted with general purpose interfaces that might be used for human enhancement. But this simple either/or is inappropriate. We don't face a simple choice between fully specific, single function interfaces, on one side, and completely nonspecific, general purpose interfaces, on the other hand. Instead, BMIs initially developed for specific purposes such as treatment of Parkinson's disease are found to serve other functions, as well. This multifunctionality of the interface can arise from unplanned, opportunistic discoveries that are made after the interface was initially developed. Again, much of nano/neuro convergence is concerned with understanding and facilitating the conditions that foster such opportunistic discoveries. An ethic of nano/neuro convergence should consider the norms that might inform these processes.

The need for a third category—of multifunctional interfaces—can already be seen in the crude interfaces used for DBS. Nordmann simply takes these as a mini-lobotomy to address symptoms of late Parkinson's disease (2007b, p. 44). But it is now clear that these interfaces function in more complex ways (Gradinaru et al. 2009; Miller 2009). Once the interfaces are established, they provide a window into more complex mental states and processes, and this provides an "opportunity" to ask more general questions about things like mood (Schneider et al. 2003), pain (Smith 2007), or about dopamine altering drugs and the importance of high frequency oscillations in sustaining voluntary control (Foffani et al. 2003). This almost natural extension of interface functionality should be more carefully studied as part of an ethics of nano/neuro convergence. Such extensions seem to be inherent to functional BMIs, and may have something to do with conditions needed for establishing a functional interface of this kind in the first place. Also, the extension of function arises naturally from mechanisms used to increase specificity. In the case of DBS for Parkinson's disease, an electrode needed to be threaded into a tiny, cubic millimeter region of the brain. To provide greater control in targeting the appropriate region, several contacts were placed along the electrode, allowing the clinician to experiment with the contacts. By this means, physicians could independently target different regions along the electrode, thereby honing in upon the contact that provides the best symptom profile. When clinicians did this, they accidentally discovered that in some cases the mood of a patient could be significantly altered (Bejjani et al. 1999). This led to experimentation with mood, and immediately suggested alternate medical conditions that might be managed by DBS. This control of mood by itself raises some disturbing possibilities: patients at times seem like puppets, manipulated by strings and wires, and it is easy to imagine how this technology might be misused (Nordmann 2007b). However, it is also not too hard to imagine how patients might be given greater control over their own emotional states by such means, although the ramifications of doing this are anything but clear.

Experimental extensions of functional interfaces arise naturally for at least three reasons: (1) because things like mood and voluntary control are already implicated in the disease process that is addressed by the BMI; (2) because the neural structures (e.g. associated with the STN) addressed by the interface are themselves complex and multifunctional; and (3) because the specificity needed for the interface is partly obtained by introducing redundancy and then selection (as with the multiple contacts on the electrodes), and once that redundancy is introduced, it allows for addressing additional structures that were not originally targeted by means of the interface. Consider, for example, the way Llinas uses the vascular system to introduce nanowires within a region, or the way Miesenbock genetically targets specific kinds of neurons to introduce the novel, light-related property (sensor or actuator). In both cases, complex structures and mechanisms of the organism are "used" to solve the problems of specificity. But this only provides a kind of course grained solution. After that, additional control is gained by means of the central lines (electrical or fiber optical) used to interface with the nanowires or with the novel proteins arising from the genetic intervention. Once this hardware is introduced, all sorts of extensions are possible in relatively non-invasive ways.

The EU Convergence Group assumes that general purpose BMI enhancements would need to be advanced as separate, large-scale projects, and that these can be politically blocked when they arise (Kjolberg *et al.* 2008). They make a sharp distinction between envisioned military uses for an artificial hand and therapeutic uses (HLEG 2004). But when we recognize how therapeutically oriented BMIs can be extended, it becomes clear that the first enhancements will arise as extensions of treatments. For example, DARPA, the Air Force, and the Army have been major sponsors of BMIs (Moreno 2006), and have supported some of the most high profile research, including the above-mentioned work of Nicolelis (Hoag 2003) and Llinas (2005, Acknowledgements on p. 125). In a *Washington Post* review (Barr 2008), the director of DARPA explains how neural–machine interfaces for a prosthetic arm "hold promise that disabled soldiers can stay in the military 'and contribute as before' rather than be discharged." Obviously, DARPA's interest in such a disabled soldier arises from the "opportunity" a treatment-oriented human/machine interface would provide for extension. By dismissing these possibilities as speculative, Nordmann and the EU Group divert ethical reflection away from visions and values that inform prominent strands of BMI research. Instead of openly discussing these visions, they want to politically legislate them away. This approach only makes the issues invisible (Khushf 2006).

THE ETHICS OF NANO/NEURO CONVERGENCE: UNDERSTANDING THE TASK

Taken together, the earlier-mentioned aspects of nano/neuro convergence problematize a traditional type-framed ethic. But this does not completely undermine the standpoint of ethics, as Nordmann contends (2007b, p. 40). He and the EU High Level Expert Group work with too narrow a conception of ethics, and with too great a confidence in what might be accomplished by political means. Ethics is more than just the politics of vision/needs assessment, implementation, and regulation. To responsibly address the emergent capacities associated with nano/neuro convergence, a much richer kind of ethical reflection is required, one that is more fit for the practices integral to emerging research. I close by considering what is needed for this ethic.

1) An ethic of nano/neuro convergence needs to move upstream (Wilsdon and Willis 2004). It needs to be anticipatory and not just reactionary, and needs to work with a mid-term time horizon (Khushf 2007). But moving upstream does not mean making ethics political. Too often, the metaphor of a stream and flow is still interpreted in terms of a variant of the older linear model. It is assumed that ethics means control of some discrete intervention, and control means a capacity to specify the ends that, in turn, govern how subcomponents of a research endeavor are coordinated and integrated (HLEG 2004). Moving ethics upstream then means: use political mechanisms to control the projects that are initiated. But this kind of top-down control is neither desirable nor possible. A more realistic model of science and engineering involves the recognition that "new" research always starts in the middle, when there are a host of other diverse research pathways already underway. These jump together in complex ways. In formal initiatives like the US NBIC Convergence workshops, there are attempts to facilitate the cross-talk (Khushf 2004a). But this does not follow older models of applied science.

   When considering nano/neuro convergence, "ethicists" need to start with an appreciation of some of the diverse strands of research in nanoscience and neuroscience, and then consider how these strands come together. But this does not mean the strands are taken as fixed, fully determinate trajectories. In this essay, I considered QD and BMI work, and tried give a sense of the opportunistic ways these strands link up with one another to specify an interface with neural systems. My attempt to sketch this work presupposed that I was in dialogue with those who are developing the research, and thus that the current state of this research is accurately reflected in my overview. But this overview is not mere description. It is already a work of ethics, since it seeks to re-present that research in a way that rightly discloses what is given and what is yet open for reconstruction. This task of framing needs to be seen as a component of ethical deliberation, and it needs to be explicitly put into play as part of ethical discourse. What I offer here—and what anyone offers—can only be a first draft, open to correction and revision in the same way any other research contribution is open for revision. To move ethics upstream thus means that ethics needs to be located at the place where the research first arises, and it needs to uncover the possibilities inherent within that research. It also needs to be adaptive in the same ways any first efforts in research are adaptive.

2) In place of top-down control, ethics should be oriented toward management of processes that are already underway (Khushf 2007). Such management might initiate new eddies and currents. Here a decentralized management among distributed actors is needed (Guston and Sarewitz 2002). For this, the ethics of nano/neuro

convergence needs to be worked out in the context of genuine, collaborative dialogue with the researchers involved (Fisher *et al.* 2006). And beyond this, the very character of communication between scientists and ethics/policy researchers needs to be altered. The pure/applied science distinction works against this dialogue. Traditionally, it was assumed that scientists are masters of fact; engineers masters of artifacts; and ethics and policy researchers are masters of visions and values. The splits between research cultures reflect these presumed differences between realms of expertise, and each field guards against encroachment upon its own domain. Since there was no presumed overlap of jurisdictions, exchange between scientists and ethics/policy researchers was too often viewed in terms of a turf war. Ethics and policy researchers tend to view scientists as naïve when they reflected on visions and values. Thus, Nordmann (2009) discounts statements by scientists about the enhancement prospects of their own research, seeing such statements as evidence of a kind of "ignorance at the heart of science." He wants something like a reverse deficit model, where those in the humanities educate scientists about the naivety of their visions. On the other hand, scientists generally resent new requirements and expectations that they explicitly reflect upon the ethics of their own research. They see these as inappropriate, bureaucratic encroachment on their freedom to pursue science where it leads. In both cases, there is insufficient appreciation of the entanglement between the work of even the purest science and the work of ethics and policy. Both ethicists and scientists do not want to expend their "scarce resources" worrying about unneeded details integral to the other's domain. They do not want to expend the effort to learn what the other knows, and they do not see the value of dialogue with those who have that knowledge.

For conventional applied ethicists, the incessant worry about "what's new in nano" reflects this attempt to guard against diversion. But how can ethicists or scientists ever know if there is anything ethically novel if neither works at the intersection of both the emerging science (which by definition is scientifically novel) and the ethics/policy arenas where there is a nuanced appreciation of the scope and limits of existing ethical taxonomies. Without an active, ongoing dialogue between the "two cultures," there is no social capacity for appropriately taking stock of the realistic possibilities and challenges inherent to that emerging research. Researchers and regulators then miss opportunities for modulating such research trajectories so potential downstream disruptions are mitigated at the outset, as part of the research and development process that realizes the promise inherent in the novel science. Establishing genuine dialogue thus stands as one of the central challenges for an ethic of nano/neuro convergence, and this, in turn, requires a significant change in the cultures of research in both the scientific and the ethics/policy communities (Stieglitz 2007).

3) Instead of focusing on standard types in some pre-given taxonomy of ethical problems, an ethic of nano/neuro convergence should consider regions in a possibility space. Older taxonomies are still helpful in organizing this space, but a much freer relation is needed between background assumptions and types and the space of emerging research practices. For a type-framed ethic, there is some discrete intervention, which is taken as an instance of some problem with specific, well-defined ramifications. The goal of the ethic is to gate and control the discrete intervention, so

negative ramifications are minimized. This is how Nordmann frames the task of an ethics of nano/neuro convergence. "Ethics" reflects a kind of heightened socio-political control that arises at the nexus of specific kinds of discrete action. Instead of this act-oriented ethic, we need something closer to a virtue theory (MacIntyre 1984).

The goal of an ethic should be to cultivate responsible research practices that are proactively responsive to broader ramifications of the practices. For scientists, this means more reflective practices: they must reflect upon what they do and how this might foster or undermine the flourishing of what others are doing (Schon 1983). Here the "internal" ethic of science needs to be extended so it encompasses "external" concerns. When this arises, then scientists learn to gate their own practices. They learn to discern where social expertise is insufficient for understanding or managing potentially disruptive aspects of research that is underway, and they learn to draw into their practice settings those who might explore with them how best to configure the next stage of the research. Even beyond this, the goal is to have scientists who appreciate that others may see things in their own work that they do not recognize, and thus that a transparency and openness to critical reflection is needed. They already appreciate how such openness to their scientific peers is essential to science. Now this needs to be extended to a broader set of peers. But we will never get this, if the people in the humanities and social sciences dismiss or patronize the researchers, or if they want to come in and politically control things as soon as something seems risky. As long as ethics is viewed in terms of politics, scientists will legitimately guard their secrets. They will seek to downplay ethical novelty and forestall disclosure of more radical possibilities of disruption until later stages. But that delay undermines vital opportunities of midstream adjustments that could mitigate such problems. In place of top-down, large-scale, political control at nodes where research transitions from "basic" to "applied," we should seek to cultivate a host of partial, small-scale, distributed adjustments that permeate the possibility space of research (Guston and Sarewitz 2002). Only when this occurs will we have the general capacity for strategic political action that is carefully targeted to address a narrow subset of those ethical issues that are not best addressed in a more free, decentralized manner.

4) Like the science, the ethics of nano/neuro convergence must be more reflexive (Rabinow and Bennett 2009 provide an outstanding overview of the challenge emerging research poses for both conventional mode 1 and even mode 2 approaches to ethics). An ethic should continually explore how the very character and content of ethical deliberation and action is (and ought to be) informed by developing notions of understanding and control integral to the emerging science. In practice, this means that the science, the ethics, and the philosophical and social scientific study of these will be deeply entangled, and will co-evolve in mutual dialogue (Khushf 2009). Scientists will play a greater role in framing and addressing the ethical issues, and ethicists will play a greater role in framing and even advancing the science. Here it is important to appreciate how traditional precautionary and cost/benefit models of ethical deliberation depend upon assumptions about gated control that are not applicable to many emerging research practices. Humans do not and cannot have that kind of control, and ethics should not work with such control as an ideal. An ideal of transparent or "see-through science" (Wilsdon and Willis 2004) should thus be

abandoned. For the alternative, ethics can learn from the science. In research areas associated with embodied cognition, control theory, human factors engineering, nanoscience, complexity theory, and a host of other areas, we find strategies of understanding and control that do not involve complete transparency of the systems being manipulated. This is, of course, true for neuroscience and for all medical BMIs, as well. When Miesenbock utilizes an organism's own mechanisms to solve the specificity problem, he doesn't fully understand the system he is utilizing. In fact, the alterations precede the understanding, and become a vehicle toward stabilizing the system so it can be transparent to understanding. But the neural system that is stabilized is the one that now has the novel capacities that he introduced for controlling it. Here the capacity for control arises through an anticipation of a not-yet-realized stability that depends on the scientist's innovative practice. Similarly, for Angela Belcher's nanoscience, design of the complex array of QDs involves generation of large libraries of viral variants together with artificial selection mechanisms that isolate specific variants that have properties of interest. In both the research of Miesenbock and Belcher, there is a complex loop between a smaller scale, partially blind action and larger scale architectures that structure those small scale experiments so specific kinds of outcomes are rapidly identified. An ethic of nano/neuro convergence needs to explore how these new models might help us more appropriately manage the complex possibility space associated with emerging research.

REFERENCES

Allhoff, F. (2007). On the autonomy and justification of nanoethics. *NanoEthics*, 1, 185–210.

Alpert, S. (2008). Neuroethics and nanoethics: do we risk ethical myopia? *Neuroethics*, 1, 55–68.

Andrews, R. (2007). Neuroprotection at the nanolevel – part I, Introduction to nanoneurosurgery. *Annals of the New York Academy of Sciences*, 1122, 169–84.

Arenkiel, B. and Ehlers, M. (2009). Molecular genetics and imaging technologies for circuit-based neuroanatomy. *Nature*, 461, 900–7.

Arrenberg, A., Bene, F.D., and Baier, H. (2009). Optical control of zebrafish behavior with halorhodopsin. *PNAS*, 106, 17968–73.

Azzazy, H., Mansour, M., and Kazmierczak, S. (2007). From diagnostics to therapy: prospects of quantum dots. *Clinical Biochemistry*, 40, 917–27.

Bannai, H., Levi, S., Schweizer, C., *et al.* (2009). Activity-dependent tuning of inhibitory neurotransmission based on $BABA_AR$ diffusion dynamics. *Neuron*, 62, 670–82.

Barr, S. (2008). The idea factory that spawned the Internet turns 50. *Washington Post*, April 7, p. D01.

Bejjani, B-P., Damier, P., Arnulf, I., *et al.* (1999). Transient acute depression induced by high-frequency deep-brain stimulation. *The New England Journal of Medicine*, 340, 1476–80.

Berdyyeva, T. and Reynolds, J. (2009). The dawning of primate optogenetics. *Neuron*, 62, 159–60.

Bush, V. (1945). *Science The Endless Frontier*. Washington, DC: United States Government Printing Office. Available at http://www.nsf.gov/about/history/vbush1945.htm.

Cai, W., Hsu, A., Li Z-B., and Chen, X. (2007). Are quantum dots ready for in vivo imaging in human subjects? *Nanoscale Research Letters*, 2, 265–81.

Cauller, L. and Penz, A. (2002). Artificial intelligence and natural intelligence. *Converging Technologies for Improving Human Performance: Nanotechnology, Biotechnology, Information Technology, and Cognitive Science* (NSF/DOC-sponsored report), pp. 227–33. Arlington, VA: World Technology Evaluation Center (WTEC).

Chan, W. and Nie, S., (1998). Quantum dot bioconjugates for ultrasensitive nonisotopic detection. *Science*, **281**, 2016–18.

Dahan, M., Levi, S., Luccardini, C., Rostaing, P., Riveau, B., and Triller, A. (2003). Diffusion dynamics of glycine receptors revealed by single-qunatum dot tracking. *Science*, **302**, 442–5.

Deisseroth, K., Feng, G., Majewska, A.K., Miesenbock, G., Ting, A., and Schnitzer, M. (2006). Next-generation optical technologies for illuminating genetically targeted brain circuits. *Journal of Neuroscience*, **46**, 10380–6.

Elder, J., Liu, C., and Apuzzo, M. (2008). Neurosurgery in the Realm of 10^{-9}, Part 2: Applications of nanotechnology to neurosurgery – present to future. *Neurosurgery*, **62**, 269–84.

Fisher, E., Mahajan, R., and Mitcham, C. (2006). Midstream modulation of technology: governance from within. *Bulletin of Science, Technology, and Society*, **26**, 485–96.

Foffani, G., Priori, A., Egidi, M., *et al.* (2003). 300-Hz subthalamic oscillations in Parkinson's disease. *Brain*, **126**, 2153–63.

Fuentes, R., Petersson, P., Siesser, W., Caron, M., and Nicolelis, M. (2009). Spinal cord stimulation restores locomotion in animal models of Parkinson's disease. *Science*, **323**, 1578–82.

Gao, X., Cui, Y., Levenson, R., Chung, L., and Nie, S. (2004). In vivo cancer targeting and imaging with semiconductor quantum dots. *Nature Biotechnology*, **22**, 969–76.

Gomez, N., Winter, J., Shieh, F., Saunders, A., Korgel, B., and Schmidt, C. (2005). Challenges in quantum dot-neuron active interfacing. *Talanta*, **67**, 462–71.

Gordijn, B. (2006). Converging NBIC technologies for improving human performance: a critical assessment of the novelty and the prospects of the project. *Journal of Law, Medicine and Ethics*, **34**, 2–8.

Gorokhov, V. and Lenk, H. (2009). Nanotechnoscience as a cluster of the different natural and engineering theories and nanoethics. In M. Yuri, K. Sergey, K, and V. Ashok (eds.) *Silicon Versus Carbon: Fundamental Nanoprocesses, Nanobiotechnology and Risk Assessment*, pp. 199–222. NATO Science for Peace and Security Series B: Physics and Biophysics. Netherlands: Springer.

Gradinaru, V., Mogri, M., Thompson, K., Henderson, J., and Deisseroth, K. (2009). Optical deconstruction of Parkinsonian neural circuitry. *Science*, **324**, 354–9.

Groc, Laurent, Lafourcade, M., Heine, M., *et al.* (2007). Surface trafficking of neurotransmitter receptor: comparison between single-molecule/quantum dot strategies. *Journal of Neuroscience*, **27**, 12433–7.

Guston, D. and Sarewitz, D. (2002). Real-time technology assessment. *Technology in Society*, **24**, 93–109.

Han, X., Qian, X., Bernsetin, J.G., *et al.* (2009). Milisecond-timescale optical control of neural dynamics in a nonhuman-primate brain. *Neuron*, **62**, 191–8.

Henderson, J., Federici, T., and Boulis, N. (2009). Optogenetic neuromodulation. *Neurosurgery*, **64**, 796–804.

Hira, R., Honkura, N., Noguchi, J., *et al.* (2009). Transcranial optogenetic stimulation for functional mapping of the motor cortex. *Journal of Neuroscience Methods*, **179**, 258–63.

HLEG (High Level Expert Group). (2004). *Foresighting the new technology wave. Converging Technologies: shaping the future of European societies.* Luxemburg: Office for Official Publications of the European Communities.

Hoag, H. (2003). Remote control. *Nature,* **423,** 796–9.

Kelty, C.M. (2009). Beyond implications and applications: the story of 'safety by design.' *NanoEthics,* **3,** 79–96.

Khushf, G. (2004a). Systems theory and the ethics of human enhancement: a framework for NBIC Convergence. *Annals of the New York Academy of Sciences,* **1013,** 124–49.

Khushf, G. (2004b). The ethics of nanotechnology: vision and values for a new generation of science and engineering. In National Academy of Engineering, *Emerging Technologies and Ethical Issues in Engineering,* pp. 255–78. Washington, DC: National Academies Press.

Khushf, G. (2006). An ethic for enhancing human performance through integrative technologies. In W.S. Bainbridge and M. Roco (eds.) Managing Nano-Bio-Info-Cogno Innovations: Converging technologies in society, pp. 255–78.

Khushf, G. (2007). Importance of a midterm time horizon for addressing ethical issues integral to nanobiotechnology. *Journal of Long-term Effects of Medical Implants,* **17,** 185–91.

Khushf, G. (2008). Health as intra-systemic integrity: rethinking the foundations of systems biology and nanomedicine. *Perspectives in Biology and Medicine,* **51,** 432–49.

Khushf, G. (2009). Open evolution and human agency: the pragmatics of upstream ethics in the design of artificial life. In M. Bedau and E. Parke (eds.) *The Ethics of Protocells: Moral and Social Implications of Creating Life in the Laboratory,* pp. 223–62. Cambridge, MA: MIT Press.

Kjolberg, K., Delgado-Ramos, G.C., Wickson, F., and Strand, R. (2008). Models of governance for converging technologies. *Technology Analysis and Strategic Management,* **20,** 83–97.

Leary, S., Liu, C., and Apuzzo, M. (2006). Toward the emergence of nanoneurosurgery: Part III – Nanomedicine: targeted nanotherapy, nanosurgery, and progress toward the realization of nanoneurosurgery', *Nuerosurgery,* **58,** 1009–25.

Lebedev, M. and Nicolelis, M. (2006). Brain-machine interfaces: past, present and future. *Trends in Neurosciences,* **29,** 536–46.

Lee, S-W, Mai, C., Flynn, C., and Belcher, A. (2002). Ordering of quantum dots using genetically engineered viruses. *Science,* **296,** 892–5.

Lima, S. and Miesenbock, G. (2005). Remote control of behavior through genetically targeted photostimulation of neurons. *Cell,* **121,** 141–52.

Litton, P. (2007). Nanoethics? What's new? *Hastings Center Report,* **37,** 22–5.

Llinas, R. and Makarov, V. (2002). Brain-machine interface via a neurovascular approach. In M. Roco and W.S. Bainbridge (eds.) *Converging Technologies for Improving Human Performance: Nanotechnology, Biotechnology, Information Technology, and Cognitive Science* (NSF/DOC-sponsored report), pp. 216–22. Arlington, VA: World Technology Evaluation Center (WTEC).

Llinas, R., Walton, K., Nakao, M., Hunter, I., and Anquetil, P. (2005). Neuro-vascular central nervous recording/stimulating system: using nanotechnology probes. *Journal of Nanopartgicle Research,* **7,** 111–27.

Llinas, R. (2008). *Brain-Machine Interface Systems and Methods.* United States Patent 2008/0015459 A1.

Mao, C., Flynn, C., Hayhurst, A., *et al.* (2003). Viral assembly of oriented quantum dot nanowires. *PNAS,* **100,** 6946–51.

Macnaughten, P., Kearnes, M., and Wynne, B. (2005). Nanotechnology, governance, and public deliberation: what role for the social sciences? *Science Communication*, 27, 268–91.

Merton, R. (1979). *The Sociology of Science: Theoretical and Empirical Investigations* Chicago, IL: University of Chicago Press.

Michalet, X., Pinaud, F., Bentolila, L.A., *et al.* (2005). Quantum dots for live cells, in vivo imaging, and diagnostics. *Science*, 307, 538–44.

Michler, P., Imamoglu, A., Mason, M.D., Carson, P.J., Strouse, G.F., and Buratto, S.K. (2000). Quantum correlation among photons from a single quantum dot at room temperature. *Nature*, 406, 968–70.

Miesenbock, G. (2009). The optogenetic catechism. *Science*, 326, 395–9.

Miesenbock, G. and Kevrekidis, I. (2005). Optical imaging and control of genetically designated neurons in functioning circuits. *Annual Review of Neuroscience*, 28, 533–63.

Miller, G. (2009). Rewiring faulty circuits in the brain. *Science*, 323, 1554–6.

Moreno, J. (2006). *Mind Wars: Brain Research and the National Defense*. New York: Dana Press.

Moxon, K., Kalkhoran, N., Markert, M., *et al.* (2004). Nanostructured surface modification of ceramic-based microelectrodes to enhance biocompatibility for a direct brain-machine interface. *IEEE Transactions on Biomedical Engineering*, 51, 881–9.

Murray, C.B., Kagan, C.R., and Bawendi, M.G. (1995). Self-organization of CdSe Nanocrystallites into three-dimensional quantum dot superlattices. *Science*, 270, 1335–8.

National Institutes of Health (NIH), Division of Program Coordination, Planning, and Strategic Initiatives (DPCPSI) web page on Nanomedicine Center: *NDC for the optical control of biological function*, http://nihroadmap.nih.gov/nanomedicine/devcenters/progressreports/Isacoff_ExecSumm2009.asp (accessed December 10, 2009)

National Science and Technology Council (NSTC), Committee on Technology, Subcommittee on Nanoscale Science, Engineering and Technology (2002). *Nanotechnology Initiative: The Initiation and its Implementation Plan*. Washington, DC: Office of Science and Technology Policy.

Nicolelis, M. (2002). Human-machine interaction: potential impact of nanotechnology in the design of neuroprosthetic devices aimed at restoring or augmenting human performance. In M. Roco and W.S. Bainbridge (eds.) *Converging Technologies for Improving Human Performance: Nanotechnology, Biotechnology, Information Technology, and Cognitive Science* (NSF/DOC-sponsored report), pp. 223–6. Arlington, VA: World Technology Evaluation Center (WTEC).

Nordmann, A. (2007a). Knots and strands: an argument for productive disillusionment. *Journal of Medicine and Philosophy*, 32, 217–36.

Nordmann, A. (2007b). If and then: a critique of speculative nanoethics. *Nanoethics*, 1, 31–46.

Nordmann, A. (2009). Ignorance at the heart of science? Incredible narratives on brain-machine interfaces. In J. Ach and B. Luttenberg (eds.) *Nanobiotechnology, Nanomedicine and Human Enhancement*. Berlin: Munsteraner Bioethik-Studien.

Pancrazio, J. (2008). Neural interfaces at the nanoscale. *Nanomedicine*, 3, 823–30.

Pathak, S., Cao, E., Davidson, M., Jin, S., and Silva, G. (2006). Quantum dot applications to neuroscience: new tools for probing neurons and glia. *The Journal of Neuroscience*, 26, 1893–5.

Rabinow, P. and Bennett, G. (2009). Human practices: interfacing three modes of collaboration, in Bedau, M, Parke, E, *The ethics of protocells: moral and social implications of creating life in the laboratory*, pp .263–90. Cambridge, MA: MIT Press.

Ratner, M. and Ratner, D. (2003). *Nanotechnology: Gentle Introduction to the Next Big Idea.* Upper Saddle River, NJ: Prentice Hall.

Renn, O. and Roco, M. (2006). Nanotechnology and the need for risk governance. *Journal of Nanoparticle Research,* **8,** 153–91.

Reed, M. (1993). Quantum dots. *Scientific American,* **January,** 118–23.

Roco, M. (2003). Nanotechnology: convergence with modern biology and medicine. *Current Opinion in Biotechnology,* **14,** 337–46.

Roco, M. and Bainbridge, W.S. (2002a). Converging technologies for improving human performance: integrating from the nanoscale. *Journal of Nanoparticle Research,* **4,** 281–95.

Roco, M. and Bainbridge, W.S. (eds.) (2002b). *Converging Technologies for Improving Human Performance: Nanotechnology, Biotechnology, Information Technology, and Cognitive Science* (NSF/DOC-sponsored report). Arlington, VA: World Technology Evaluation Center (WTEC).

Roco, M., and National Science, Engineering and Technology (NSET) Subcommittee, U.S. National Science and Technology Council (NSTC) (2004). Nanoscale science and engineering: unifying and transforming tools. *American Institute of Chemical Engineers Journal,* **50,** 890–7.

Roco, M. and Montemagno, C. (eds.) (2004). Integrative technology for the twenty-first century. *Annals of the New York Academy of Sciences,* **1013.**

Scanziani, M. and Hausser, M. (2009). Electrophysiology in the age of light. *Nature,* **461,** 930–9.

Schon, D. (1983). *The Reflective Practitioner: How Professionals Think in Action.* New York: Basic Books.

Schneider, F., Habel, U., Volkmann, J., *et al.* (2003). Deep brain stimulation of the subthalamic nucleus enhances emotional processing in Parkinson disease. *Arch of General Psychiatry,* **50,** 296–302.

Scientific American Editors. (2002). *Understanding Nanotechnology.* New York: Warner Books.

Shalk, G. (2008). Brain-computer symbiosis. *Journal Neurological Engineering,* **5,** 1–15.

Silva, G. (2005). Small neuroscience: the nanostructure of the central nervous system and emerging nanotechnology applications. *Current Nanoscience,* **1,** 225–36.

Silva, G. (2006). Neuroscience nanotechnology: progress, opportunities, challenges. *Nature Reviews,* **7,** 65–74.

Smith, K. (2007). Brain waves reveal intensity of pain. *Nature,* **450,** 329.

Stieglitz, T. (2007). Restoration of neurological functions by neuroprosthetic technologies: future prospects and trends towards micro-, nano-, and biohybrid systems. *Acta Neurochir Suppl,* **97,** 435–42.

Sutherland, A. (2002). Quantum dots as luminescent probes in biological systems. *Current Opinion in Solid State and Materials Science,* **6,** 365–70.

Tersoff, J. (1996). Self-organization in growth of quantum dot superlattices. *Physical Review Letters,* **76,** 1675–8.

Toth, G., Lent, C.S., Tougaw, P.D., *et al.* (1996). Quantum cellular neural networks. *Superlattices and Microstructures,* **20,** 4.

Tsai, H-C, Zhang, F., Adamantidis, A., *et al.* (2009). Phasic firing in dopaminergic neurons is sufficient for behavioral conditioning. *Science,* **324,** 1080–4.

Van Roermund, A. and Hoekstra, J. (2000). Design philosophy for nanoelectronic systems from SETs to neural nets. *International Journal of Circuit Theory and Applications,* **28,** 563–84.

Vanmaekelbergh D. and Liljeroth P. (2005). Eletron-conducting quantum dot solids: novel materials based on colloidal semiconductor nanocrystals. *Chemical Society Reviews*, **34**, 299–312.

Vu, T., Maddipati, R., Blute, T., Nehilla, B., Nusblat, L., and Desai, T. (2005). Peptide-conjugated quantum dots activate neuronal receptors and initiate downstream signaling of neurite growth. *Nano Letters 2005*, **5**, 603–7.

Wilsdon, J. and Willis, R. (2004). *See-through Science: Why Public Engagement Needs to Move Upstream*. London: Demos.

Wynne, B. (2005). Risk as globalizing 'democratic' discourse? Framing subjects as citizens, in Leach, M, Wynne, B (ed.), *Science and Citizens: Globalization and the Challenge of Engagement*, pp. 66–82. London: Zed Books.

Zemelman, B., Nesnas, N., Lee, G., and Miesenbock, G. (2003). Photochemical gating of heterologous ion channels: remote control over genetically designated populations of neurons. *PNAS*, **100**, 1352–7.

Zhang, S. (2003). Fabrication of novel biomaterials through molecular self-assembly. *Nature Biotechnology*, **21**, 1171–8.

Zhou, M. and Ghosh, I. (2006). Quantum dots and peptides: a bright future together. *Peptide Science*, **88**, 325–9.

PART V

AGING AND DEMENTIA

CHAPTER 29

NEUROBIOLOGICAL AND NEUROETHICAL PERSPECTIVES ON THE CONTRIBUTION OF FUNCTIONAL NEUROIMAGING TO THE STUDY OF AGING IN THE BRAIN

KARIMA KAHLAOUI, MAXIMILIANO WILSON,
ANA INES ANSALDO, BERNADETTE SKA,
AND YVES JOANETTE

INTRODUCTION

ACCORDING to United Nations (UN) projections, by 2050, 20% of the world's people will be at least 60 years old (World Health Organization 2003); the proportion of older people will be higher in developed countries. In Canada, the number of people aged 65 and over will almost double by 2031, when it will represent 25% of the total population (Statistics Canada 2005). Increased life expectancy brings a higher risk not only of physical problems but also of cognitive decline (Bravo *et al.* 2005; Sachs and Cassel 1990). It is therefore crucial to improve the understanding of healthy and pathological processes of cognitive aging. This improved understanding will help both to promote healthy aging and to prevent or alleviate the negative effects of cognitive aging. Research on aging is the key to achieving this goal and, combined with neuroimaging, is the focus of this chapter.

Cognitive aging is defined as a gradual process of mental loss beginning as early as age 30. For over a century, our knowledge of the neural basis of cognitive aging came essentially from research on the cognitive neuropsychology of aging. This research focused on age-related changes in cognition, with no reference to age-related changes in the brain. But in recent decades, the development of functional neuroimaging techniques has enabled researchers to measure various indirect indices of ongoing neural activity arising from the brain "in action." This technique has had a tremendous impact on research on aging in cognitive neuropsychology and other cognitive neurosciences, because it has helped researchers to compile both structural and functional evidence about the neural basis of cognitive aging.

The evidence of age-related deterioration in the brain can be found in a variety of structural, functional, and physiological changes. Notwithstanding such changes, however, there is also growing evidence of high-level cognitive functioning in some older persons. For example, in one study, older professors at the University of California (Berkeley) were found to perform certain cognitive tasks as well as or even better than younger professors (Shimamura *et al.* 1995).

How can such successful aging be explained? Functional neuroimaging has provided some clues by enabling researchers to examine the neural substrate of cognitive aging in both healthy and pathological populations, including older people with mild cognitive impairment (MCI) and Alzheimer's disease (AD).

Like many other aspects of neuroscience research, however, research on cognitive aging has ethical, legal, and social implications and therefore faces many hurdles, in particular regulatory ones. Hence functional neuroimaging techniques and the new research topics that they have been used to investigate have given rise to a new discipline: neuroethics. Neuroethics stands at the crossroads between bioethics and neuroscience and focuses on the ethical, legal, and social implications of neuroscience and neuroscience research (Illes and Bird 2006).

This chapter has two main goals: to provide an overview of the contribution of neuroimaging to our understanding of neurocognitive aging, and to highlight the neuroethical considerations and legal implications of using neuroimaging to conduct research on aging in the brain.

NEUROCOGNITIVE AGING

Age-related changes in cognitive functions

It was long believed that the connections among brain cells remained unchanged over an individual's lifetime. Over the past few decades, however, scientific research has shown that throughout the lifespan, the brain continues to form new neural connections and thereby adjusts and reorganizes its neural networks and functions. This neuroplasticity enables the brain to adapt to environmental changes by finding new ways of learning and acquiring new skills. In some cases, this plasticity also enables the brain to compensate for damage due to injury, stroke, or disease. The mechanisms by which these changes take place, how they are affected by both healthy and pathological aging processes, and how some older people manage to maintain good cognitive functioning as they age have become a focus of intense attention for many scholars whose work spans the basic and clinical neurosciences.

Many studies apply cross-sectional designs in which younger and older adults are compared to discover the fundamental properties of neuroplasticity. Other studies have involved longitudinal designs, which are more powerful because they follow a cohort of individuals over a long period and test them in various cognitive tasks at various intervals. Taken all together, these studies have shown that, even when accounting for variability among people and tasks, some cognitive functions—such as attention, processing speed, working memory, inhibition, episodic memory, and executive function—inevitably decline with age (Hedden and Gabrieli 2004; Salthouse 1996), while others—such as vocabulary, semantic and world knowledge, and implicit and procedural memory—remain stable or even improve (Verhaeghen 2003). In addition, several studies have shown that individuals vary considerably in their performance of various cognitive tasks. Some older adults perform just about as well as younger ones, while others show a major decline in performance compared with younger adults, even in the absence of any age-related pathology.

Neuroimaging studies have contributed the most to the understanding of such cognitive variability, by documenting both structural and functional changes related to aging. Each of the main current neuroimaging techniques provides specific kinds of information about certain characteristics of the brain. Magnetic resonance imaging (MRI) gives exceptionally detailed information about the brain's anatomical structure. Diffusion tensor imaging (DTI) measures the integrity of white matter nerve fiber pathways and examines how connectivity changes in the course of aging. Functional magnetic resonance imaging (fMRI) is used to observe, in real time, how brain signals change as the result of neural activity while individuals are actually performing cognitive tasks.

Age-related changes in brain structures

Before the advent of neuroimaging techniques, age-related structural changes in the brain were observed by means of postmortem examinations. One of the most prominent findings from such studies was the age-related loss of whole-brain volume. Some studies showed that brain volume declines by at least 10% from ages 25–75 years (Skullerud 1985). Others found that it remains relatively stable from the start of adulthood to about age 45 or 50, but then starts decreasing gradually, reaching its lowest values after age 86 (Dekaban 1978). This volume loss in the aging brain is considered to be the result of a variety of factors, including reduced synapse density (Terry and Katzman 2001), deafferentation (Bertoni-Freddari *et al.* 2002), cell-body shrinkage (Haug 1985), neuropil loss (Peters *et al.* 2001), and white matter loss (Bartzokis 2004).

Over the past two decades, neuroimaging studies in general, and volumetric MRI analyses in particular, have confirmed the postmortem evidence regarding age-related loss of brain volume and added much to our understanding of many other aspects of brain aging. Neuroimaging has enabled researchers to determine which specific brain regions are more vulnerable to age-related structural changes, and when such changes begin.

Summarizing the data from two decades of neuroimaging studies is no small task, because results vary widely and are not easy to interpret. Nonetheless, numerous MRI studies have shown that reduction in gray matter volume occurs preferentially in frontal regions rather than posterior ones, and more specifically in the prefrontal cortex (Allen *et al.* 2005; Raz *et al.* 2004). Gray matter reduction has also been reported in the parietal, insular, caudate, cerebellar, and hippocampal regions (Bartzokis *et al.* 2001; Good *et al.* 2001; Raz *et al.* 2005). In contrast, minimal changes are observed in the entorhinal cortex and none occur in the primary visual cortex that retains a stable volume across the individual's lifespan.

These findings initially led to the hypothesis that cortical atrophy progresses in the opposite order from cortical maturation, that is, along an anteroposterior gradient (Raz 2000, see also Kemper 1994). More recently, Salat *et al.* (2004) investigated cortical thickness of the brain in 106 adults ranging from 18–93 years of age. Their cross-sectional study confirmed some of these previous findings but also made some interesting unexpected ones, in particular significant age-related atrophy both in the frontal cortex (near the primary motor and premotor areas) and in the calcarine cortex (near the primary visual cortex). Similarly, Ziegler *et al.* (2010) have shown greater cortical thinning in sensory and motor areas and lesser thinning in the lateral prefrontal cortex, inferior parietal cortex, and transverse temporal gyri. Discrepancies among such studies are always hard to explain, and it has been suggested that these conflicting findings may have been due to the inclusion of participants who had vascular disease resulting in frontal lobe damage (Artero *et al.* 2004). Nonetheless, these results challenge the theory that age-related gray matter loss occurs along an anteroposterior gradient; they instead suggest that atrophy is widespread across the entire cerebral cortex.

Concerning pathological aging, and particularly AD, convergent evidence shows that the entorhinal cortex and hippocampus appear to be affected in the earliest stages of the disease, with the parietal and temporal cortices involved later on. Thereafter, both frontal regions and the entire neocortex become affected (Buckner *et al.* 2004; Price and Morris 1999).

Age-related structural changes are also observed in white matter fibers. One method of assessing white matter integrity is to measure the number of age-related white matter hyperintensities (WMH): white matter signal abnormalities that are associated with cardiovascular risk factors, hypertension, and cognitive decline (Gunning-Dixon and Raz 2000). The prevalence of WMH has been found to increase with aging (Meyers *et al.* 1992), and where severe WMH were observed, cognitive performance was found to be impaired (de Groot *et al.* 2000). In healthy older persons, WMH tend to be greater in prefrontal regions (Gunning-Dixon and Raz 2000).

Recently, DTI studies have added much to current knowledge of aging. In particular, DTI studies have shown an age-related decline in regional and fractional anisotropy of white matter (a measure of coherence and orientation of diffusion), suggesting that connections from one brain region to another are compromised with age (see, for example, Head *et al.* 2004; Sullivan and Pfefferbaum 2003). These structural alterations in white matter in the course of normal aging are observed mainly in anterior brain regions, including the prefrontal cortex and the anterior corpus callosum, but also in posterior regions, and particularly in the splenium of the corpus callosum (Abe *et al.* 2002; Head *et al.* 2004). Other DTI studies have shown that the most severe age-related deterioration of the white matter is observed in association fibers, which connect brain regions in the same hemisphere (Stadlbauer *et al.* 2008). Overall, most studies have suggested an anteroposterior gradient of fractional anisotropy decline during the normal aging process (Madden *et al.* 2004; Salat *et al.* 2004). In contrast, in persons with either MCI or AD, the decline of white matter is observed in more posterior and temporal regions, suggesting that the structural changes in cases of brain pathology are different from those seen in healthy aging (Fellgiebel *et al.* 2005).

Several imaging studies have shown that volumes of gray and white matter do not change at the same rate over the human lifespan. A key question is: At what time in life do different brain tissues start "aging"? Giedd *et al.* (1999) analyzed gray matter and white matter volume in a longitudinal MRI study of a large sample of children and adolescents. The authors found that gray matter volume begins to decrease in the frontal and temporal areas after ages 12 and 16, respectively, but continues increasing in the occipital areas up to age 20. The authors also reported a linear increase in white matter density from early childhood to young adulthood. Similarly, Sowell *et al.* (2003), using high-resolution structural MRI and cortical matching algorithms to map cortical changes in 176 healthy normal individuals aged 7–87, have shown that gray matter density decreases nonlinearly from ages 7–60 on both the lateral and the interhemispheric surfaces of the frontal and parietal association cortices. In contrast, in the left posterior temporal region, gray matter density is maintained until 30 years of age, but decreases rapidly afterwards.

The relative decline of gray matter density during childhood and adolescence has been attributed both to increased myelination into the peripheral neuropil (Benes *et al.* 1994; Sowell *et al.* 2001) and to synaptic pruning, i.e. reduction in the number of synapses (Sowell *et al.* 2001). In contrast, the decline of gray matter density observed during adulthood could be attributed to late myelination and, most likely, to decreased somal size (Terry *et al.* 1987).

White matter is more vulnerable than gray matter as people age (Jernigan *et al.* 1991). Some longitudinal studies have shown that white matter density increases up to about age 20, then plateaus until age 50–60. From age 60 onward, a faster decline in white matter is observed, probably due to factors such as fiber demyelination and other pathological processes (Raz 2000). Gender-related differences have not been found in age-related changes in gray or white matter (Allen *et al.* 2005; Sowell *et al.* 2003).

In addition to the structural changes just described, brain aging results in reduced concentrations of neurotransmitters, in particular dopamine, which is associated with frontal and executive functions (Braver and Barch 2002), and acetylcholine, which contributes to learning and memory (Woodruff-Pak 1997). Age-related differences in cerebral blood flow, oxygenation, metabolic activity, and resting state, described as a default-mode, have also been reported (Davis *et al.* 2008; D'Esposito *et al.* 2003).

Age-related changes in brain function

The two hemispheres of the brain differ both structurally and functionally. In several cases, structural differences have been reported between the same areas of the brain in the two hemispheres, including the planum temporale (von Economo and Horn 1930), the sylvian fissure (Rubens *et al.* 1976), and the globus pallidus (Kooistra and Heilman 1988). Before the advent of functional neuroimaging techniques such as fMRI, the right hemi-aging model was the most prominent neuropsychological model used to explain age-related changes in cerebral lateralization (Brown and Jaffe 1978). Based mainly on behavioral data, this model proposed that the right hemisphere undergoes faster age-related decline than the left, because the right has a lower ratio of gray matter to white matter (Good *et al.* 2001). The most consistent evidence for this hypothesis comes from observations that verbal processing, supported by the left hemisphere, is preserved during aging, while spatial processing, supported by the right, is not (Goldstein and Shelly 1981).

As neuroimaging methods have improved over the past two decades, significant progress has been made in the study of neurocognitive aging. Much like past neuropsychological studies, neuroimaging studies have contrasted the performance of younger and older adults assigned the same cognitive tasks. In fMRI, for example, the blood oxygen level-dependent

(BOLD) signal provides an indirect measure of neural activation elicited during cognitive tasks. Patterns of underactivation and overactivation are often reported in the aging literature. Thus, despite the common notion that almost every cognitive function declines with age, and though these studies have, in fact, found that some changes in neural activity associated with cognitive aging do involve underactivation (i.e. lower brain activity is observed in older than younger adults), other changes involve overactivation (i.e. greater brain activity is observed in older than younger adults).

These age-related changes in brain activation are observed mainly in the frontal cortex, which also shows larger structural alterations than some other brain regions (Raz 2000). The frontal cortex, and especially the prefrontal cortex, is considered a critical structure for several higher cognitive functions, such as working memory, set shifting, problem solving, attention, and other executive functions (Stuss and Alexander 2000). In recent years, there have been a plethora of models explaining these age-related brain activation patterns. In the following paragraphs, we present only the most recent and popular models and theories on this subject.

Patterns of underactivation

Initially, the underactivation observed in older adults' frontal regions in neuroimaging studies was interpreted as an example of age-related brain changes, possibly reflecting the absence of frontal resources (Grady *et al.* 1995). But this interpretation was not shared by all, and an interesting alternative suggestion was that such underactivation (also called under-recruitment) might be context-dependent in older adults. Investigating age-related changes in memory encoding, Logan *et al.* (2002) found that older adults, using their own strategies to encode memories, had less activation in frontal regions than did younger adults. But when the older adults were given instruction on strategy, the reduced frontal activation was ameliorated and sometimes even reversed. This finding led the authors to hypothesize that older adults still have substantial frontal resources but do not recruit them effectively when self-initiated encoding is required. According to these authors, their findings might have important implications for cognitive rehabilitation, which designed the improvement of cognitive functioning and learning how to do things differently when some functions remained affected. If underactivation in frontal regions can be attributed to poor or under-utilized encoding strategies, then adults displaying such underactivation might be successfully trained to develop more effective encoding strategies.

The hemispheric asymmetry reduction in older adults (HAROLD) model

In addition to these studies on underactivation, there is a vast literature demonstrating that older adults also display overactivation, that is, in some cases they activate more brain regions than younger adults. For example, it has been shown that in encoding memory tasks that are strongly left-lateralized in the frontal cortex in younger adults, older adults show bilateral frontal activation: they activate not only the left hemisphere but also homologous regions in the right. These observations have led to the theory that aging is associated with a reduction in hemispheric asymmetry: the HAROLD model (see Cabeza 2002). This model is supported by several neuroimaging studies and behavioral data dealing with episodic memory, semantic memory, working memory, perception, and inhibitory control (Cabeza 2002).

Bilateral activation in older adults is observed not only in frontal but also in other brain regions, such as the parietal lobes (Davis *et al.* 2008), and even at the subcortical level.

For example, Maguire and Frith (2003) investigated the effect of remoteness on the neural basis of memory and showed that older adults activated both the left and the right hippocampus, while younger adults recruited only the left one. Several neuroimaging studies have also shown that age-related bilateral activation is accompanied by better performance on cognitive tasks. An elegant demonstration of this phenomenon was provided by Cabeza *et al.* (2002), who investigated brain activity in younger adults, high-performing older adults, and low-performing older adults. During a memory task, younger adults and low-performing older adults showed right prefrontal cortex activity, whereas high-performing older adults displayed bilateral prefrontal cortex activity. These results suggest that low-performing older adults activated roughly the same brain network as young adults but used it inefficiently, whereas high-performing older adults countered age-related decline through neural reorganization. Similarly, age-related bilateral activation of frontal regions has also been associated with faster response times (Reuter-Lorenz *et al.* 2000).

Since these initial findings, much more has been learned about the role of bilateral activation in aging. Typically, age-related bilateral activation has been interpreted as an advantageous compensatory brain response in which older adults maximize performance by using brain structures or networks not normally engaged in young adults. In the Cabeza *et al.* study (2002), the bilateral activation shown by high-performing older adults demonstrated the facilitative role of the additional frontal activity in cognitive task performance. The aging brain probably works "harder," and this age-related brain reorganization allows individuals to cope better with cognitive decline (Cabeza 2002; Reuter-Lorenz *et al.* 2000). This compensatory bilateral activation pattern has also been observed in studies with brain-damaged subjects. Indeed, several studies (for example, Cao *et al.* 1999) have directly linked bihemispheric activation to successful recovery of brain function following brain damage.

Another line of evidence favoring the interpretation that compensatory mechanisms underlie bilateral recruitment comes from studies of pathological aging, mainly in persons with MCI or AD. Grady *et al.* (2003) showed that, compared with healthy older adults, people with AD engaged additional prefrontal regions during both semantic and episodic memory tasks and that the degree of this engagement was positively correlated with better performance. According to these authors, the recruitment of additional brain regions, which still seems to be specific to cognitive decline, is probably "a response to the degenerative disease process that occurs early in its course, perhaps even before the onset of symptoms" (Grady *et al.* 2003, p. 992).

But the suggestion that the increase in bilateral activation with age is inherently beneficial is controversial. Divergent results from different neuroimaging studies led Persson and Nyberg (2006) to propose a tentative model to explain how bilateral activation might be related to cognitive changes attributable to pathological as well as healthy aging. This model posits three stages. First, when the aging process has not yet affected cognitive performance, older adults show little or no overactivation of brain regions. Second, as cognitive decline (whether associated with healthy or with pathological aging) begins to affect their performance, older adults display overactivation of some specific brain regions. Third, when cognitive decline has become much more advanced, underactivation is observed.

The compensation-related utilization of neural circuits hypothesis (CRUNCH)

Other interpretations of age-related bilateral activation have been proposed. For example, Reuter-Lorenz and Cappell (2008) presented the CRUNCH hypothesis, according to which, older adults require more cognitive resources than younger ones to process similar information, even at lower levels of task demands, which suggests a compensatory process. But as task demands increase, a ceiling effect is observed, resulting in insufficient processing and age-related impairment at higher levels of task demands (Reuter-Lorenz and Cappell 2008). The CRUNCH hypothesis has been confirmed by both behavioral (Reuter-Lorenz et al. 1999) and neuroimaging studies (Mattay et al. 2006; Schneider-Garces et al. 2010).

The concept of cognitive reserve (CR)

At the time of writing this chapter, explaining age-related structural and functional changes in the brain remains a challenge for cognitive neuroscientists. However, a new way of research has emerged in order to understand why some individuals maintain good cognitive functioning as they age whereas others manifest cognitive decline. Some answers are provided by the CR, defined as the ability of the brain to minimize the clinical manifestations of brain damage by recruiting brain networks differently and/or adopting alternative cognitive strategies (Stern 2002, 2009). The concept of CR has been proposed to explain the observed discrepancies between the severity of brain damage and the clinical manifestations of its symptoms in some individuals. For example, epidemiological studies have shown that about 25% of older adults who met full pathological criteria for AD upon postmortem examination had appeared cognitively intact while still alive (Ince 2001; Katzman et al. 1989). Consistent with these findings, other evidence has shown that individuals presenting with AD neuropathology, vascular damage, or both can successfully perform clinical and neuropsychological tests, thus displaying a resistance to the clinical impairment associated with the disease.

According to Stern (2002), CR enables individuals to maintain their cognitive performance despite ongoing underlying brain pathology. But CR varies from one individual to another. Hence people with less CR manifest clinical deficits sooner because they have relatively fewer resources to help them resist the cognitive decline that accompanies both healthy and pathological aging. In contrast, individuals with more CR can cope longer with clinical impairment, because their reserve of resources is greater.

An individual's level of CR before cognitive decline begins is determined not only by differences in resources at birth, but also by differences in cognitive activity as the brain matures from birth to adulthood. Recent studies have shown that across an individual's lifespan, various lifestyle factors, such as education, physical training, and social and intellectual engagement, may slow the negative effects of aging (Colcombe et al. 2003, 2006; Stern 2002), even in centenarians (Kliegel et al. 2004). For example, epidemiological evidence has shown that older adults with more education, and hence more CR, manifest clinical symptoms later than those with less education, and hence less CR (see Bennett et al. 2003); the mechanism of this protective effect remains unknown. Recently, Paradise, Cooper and Livingston (2009) found that higher levels of education can delay clinical manifestations of AD, but are not associated with earlier death after diagnosis.

The scaffolding theory of aging and cognition (STAC)

Park and Reuter-Lorenz (2009) have recently proposed a theory similar to the concept of CR: the STAC. This theory proposes that the aging brain, when confronted with age-related neural deficits with or without increased task difficulty, develops scaffolds: new circuitry that helps it to perform cognitive tasks successfully. These authors describe scaffolding as "the recruitment of additional circuitry that shores up declining structures whose functioning has become noisy, inefficient or both" (p. 183).

According to the STAC model, the age-related bilateral activation of frontal regions observed in most of the neuroimaging studies mentioned earlier reflects compensatory processes or "scaffolding" that the brain applies to respond to the challenges posed by structural and functional decline as it ages. The prefrontal cortex is regarded as the brain structure most vulnerable to aging, so it makes sense that such scaffolding would be observed mainly in this structure. The STAC model also proposes that some factors, such as cognitive training and education, increase scaffolding. Park and Reuter-Lorenz recognize strong similarities between their STAC model and the concept of CR; the crucial difference is that the STAC model describes a dynamic process that is not specific to aging adults but rather occurs across the entire lifespan. In other words, the scaffolding process may be regarded as a mechanism by which the brain responds to neurocognitive challenges throughout its lifetime.

Age-related structural and functional changes associated with cognitive performance

There is convergent evidence that environmental factors, such as special expertise and training, have an impact on brain plasticity, especially in structural terms. For example, Maguire *et al.* (2000, 2006) found that taxi drivers in London (England) had a greater volume of gray matter in the posterior hippocampus than bus drivers or ordinary adults in control groups, which suggests that personal experience determined the observed differences. Similar evidence of environmentally-driven plasticity has been found in other expert groups. For example, professional musicians have been found to have a larger volume of gray matter in both the motor and the auditory regions of the brain (Gaser and Schlaug 2003). Gray matter volume may also increase when individuals learn music or a second language. For example, Mechelli *et al.* (2004) found that individuals who are bilingual have a larger left inferior parietal cortex than individuals who are monolingual.

Aerobic physical training has also been associated with changes in brain volume during aging. Colcombe *et al.* (2006) showed that such training in older adults increases brain volume in areas usually associated with age-related decline. The authors conducted a 6-month randomized clinical trial in which they divided 59 healthy but sedentary adults ranging in age from 60–79 years into two groups, one of which then participated in an aerobic training program while the other participated in a non-aerobic one. Comparison of MRI scans before and after the trial period showed a significant increase in both gray and white matter volumes in the aerobic training group. This volume increase was observed primarily in the prefrontal and temporal areas, which often show age-related deterioration. No changes in gray or white matter volumes were found for either the non-aerobic training group or for a control group of 20 younger adults (age range 18–30). The authors concluded that brain volume loss is not an inevitable effect of aging and that regular aerobic exercise can increase brain volume in older adults, thus maintaining and enhancing brain health and cognitive functioning during aging.

Other evidence has been reported of associations between age-related changes in brain structures and cognitive performance: for example, between changes in the entorhinal cortex and memory performance (Rodrigue and Raz 2004), and between changes in the prefrontal cortex and executive functions (Gunning-Dixon and Raz 2003). As described in the preceding section, age-related changes in brain function are also associated with changes in task performance (see Grady 2008 for an interesting discussion).

RESEARCH WITH HUMAN SUBJECTS: LEGISLATION AND NEUROETHICS

Advances in neuroscience have given us a better understanding of human behavior and will ultimately contribute to improved public health. But they have also had many implications for both criminal and civil law (Tovino 2008). Under modern principles of neuroethics, neuroscience experiments must be rigorously designed to protect participants from harm and must be approved by institutional ethics committees that are well versed in the latest thinking on the moral and ethical issues involved (Miller and Fins 2006). But despite the benefits of neuroscience research and the neuroethical safeguards now surrounding it, the laws in some jurisdictions have not kept pace. These laws place such severe restrictions on recruitment of older people and people with neurodegenerative diseases as research subjects that research with these populations can be nearly impossible (Voyer and St-Jacques 2006). In this section, we seek to achieve two goals. The first is to present the neuroethical concerns and the moral and legal implications surrounding neuroscience research involving healthy older people and people with neurodegenerative diseases. The second is to critically present the limitations that current laws impose on research with these populations.

Neuroethical, moral and concerns surrounding neuroscience and aging

Much research in cognitive neuroscience involves studies with human subjects, which raises a variety of ethical concerns to begin with. Further concerns requiring especially close attention are raised when these human subjects have clinical conditions such as brain damage, AD, or other neurodegenerative conditions that might compromise their cognitive capacities and hence their ability to fully understand the nature of the research and to provide their informed consent (Jaworska 2006). Such subjects are regarded as vulnerable (Miller and Fins 2006) and are afforded special protection under the law.

Incidental findings

One ethical concern about having older persons participate in neuroimaging studies is that these studies might increase the chances of incidental findings such as unusual brain atrophy or tumors. Most of these incidental findings may not be clinically significant, but when a clinically significant finding is made, the basic neuroethical principle seems to be to consult a neuroradiologist first, to confirm the diagnosis, and then refer the participant for a clinical consultation if necessary. But there are no universal, explicit guidelines for such cases (Illes *et al.* 2007). This issue also raises questions of confidentiality and privacy. Should all images, in every study, be reviewed by a neuroradiologist? If a clinically relevant abnormal finding is made, who should inform the participant: a physician from the research team, or the participant's own previously designated physician? Illes *et al.* (2007, p. 109) suggest that the research consent form should address this issue explicitly: "[t]he investigators for this project are not trained to perform radiological diagnosis, and the scans performed in this study are not optimized to find abnormalities", and it should explain the procedure that will be followed if a significant incidental finding is made.

Informed consent

It is common practice—and a legal and moral imperative—to obtain voluntary, informed consent from individuals who are competent to give it, before they are selected as participants in research studies (Chen *et al.* 2002). This is also the case for studies of any modality, including neuroimaging. The principle comes from the *Nuremberg Code*, which was adopted after World War II in response to the abuses committed in research with human subjects. But when the *Nuremberg Code* was drafted, it did not address the issues of cognitively impaired participants or third-party consent (Bravo and Duguet 2005). These shortcomings were addressed in the World Medical Association's *Declaration of Helsinki*, which was adopted in 1964 and has been amended several times since.

In research involving aging, the question arises: Should all older persons be automatically considered incapable of providing informed consent? According to Sachs and Cassel (1990), there is no reason to assume a priori that the same guidelines and principles that are applied to other healthy populations cannot be applied to healthy seniors.

What about the many individuals who have neurodegenerative diseases but whose symptoms are relatively mild, such as people diagnosed with early stage dementia or even MCI? These people may still have some ability to make their own decisions (Bravo and Duguet 2005), and there may be no clear cut-off point beyond which such people can be categorically considered so cognitively impaired as to be unable to give informed consent. In order to address the issue of obtaining informed consent for such people to participate in research studies, a process should be established to assess their ability to understand the nature of the studies and to give their consent accordingly (Miller and Fins 2006).

That leaves the population of older people with neurodegenerative diseases that impair their intellect and emotions, which makes them a vulnerable population (Leshner 2007) with an impaired capacity to make personal decisions and, therefore, to consent to participate in research. In most such cases, a legally appointed person or a surrogate decision-maker should be able to give informed consent on behalf of the incapable potential participant (Miller and Fins 2006).

When a potential participant does not have someone who is legally empowered to give consent to research on their behalf, researchers usually try to find a responsible relative or other person who can give such consent (Sachs and Cassel 1990). In cases where individual incapacity has already been legally established, there are guidelines and codes governing their enrollment as research participants. The World Medical Association's *Declaration of Helsinki* states that where a person has been declared legally incompetent, that person's legal guardian can give informed consent for that person to participate in research, but that such individuals "must not be included in a research study that has no likelihood of benefit for them unless it is intended to promote the health of the population represented by the potential subject" (World Medical Association 2008, art. 27).

Current laws in different jurisdictions

European Union

In Europe, subject to other protective conditions prescribed by law, the Council of Europe's *Convention on Human Rights and Biomedicine* allows research with participants who are unable to consent, provided that the research has the aim of contributing to "significant improvement in the scientific understanding of the individual's condition, disease or disorder" (Council of Europe 1997, art. 17, paragraph 2, subparagraph 1). To recruit an adult for a research study who is unable to give consent, researchers must have "the authorization of his or her representative or an authority or a person or body provided for by law." (Council of Europe 1997, art. 6, paragraph 3). This international convention has been signed by most of the member states of the Council of Europe, though not ratified by all of them.

Canada

In Canada, Bravo *et al.* (2005) have made a comprehensive study of the country's current legislation governing substitute consent for research. They found that the laws on this subject are largely provincial and territorial rather than federal, and that the provinces and territories vary widely as to who may give substitute consent for incapable persons to participate in research studies and the conditions under which such consent may be given. The permissible arrangements vary from mediation by a lawyer to advance directives that an individual signs while still healthy, appointing a third party to make this decision if he or she becomes incapable of doing so. Quebec is the only Canadian province where a judge must give permission before someone who has been appointed as a substitute decision-maker by advance directives can exercise his or her authority to provide substitute consent.

Quebec

The current legislation of the province of Quebec merits special attention here, because it imposes particular constraints on research with incapable participants (Bravo and Duguet 2005; Voyer and St-Jacques 2006). Article 21 of the Civil Code of Quebec establishes that substitute consent should be given by a legally designated representative. But in Quebec, legal representation is a right and not a requirement. As a result, many incapable older people in Quebec have no legally designated substitute decision-maker; it has been estimated that only 3% of this population have such legally appointed proxies (Bravo and Duguet 2005).

Article 15 of Quebec's Civil Code recognizes the right of a spouse, close relative, or other proxy, even if not legally appointed, to give consent on behalf of an incapable elderly person, but only for healthcare, with no reference to research or experiments. In 1998, article 21 of the Civil Code was amended so that if an adult suddenly becomes incapable of consent, and an "experiment" must be "undertaken promptly after the appearance of the condition giving rise to it," meaning that there is no time to designate a legal representative, consent may be given by the person authorized to consent to any health care that this person may require. But the article goes on to state that "innovative care required by the state of health of the person concerned does not constitute an experiment." Hence there is some ambiguity as to the nature of the activities to which the new consent provision applies (Bravo and Duguet 2005; Bravo *et al.* 2005).

France

Another French-speaking jurisdiction, France, once had a law similar to Quebec's that limited participation in research. The French Civil Code (art. 488) specifies that if a person becomes incapable of taking care of his or her interests, then legal representation is necessary. In 2004, an amendment of the Huriet-Sérusclat Law (French Public Health Code, articles 1121-1 and onwards) made it possible, under certain conditions, for a proxy to give consent for an incapable person to participate in research, even if that proxy was not legally appointed as such (Bravo and Duguet 2005). The most important contribution of this amendment is that it clearly states under what circumstances consent must be obtained from the potential participant, or from a proxy previously appointed by that person, or from a family member, and that, unlike the Quebec law, it clearly defines the procedures to be followed in each case, leaving little or no room for ambiguity (Bravo and Duguet 2005).

Limitations of current laws

The preceding discussion shows that the legislation regarding older persons who are incapable of understanding the aims and potential consequences of research protocols and are therefore incapable of giving informed consent to research studies varies from one country to another and, in the case of Canada, from one province or territory to another.

Current approaches to research ethics clearly make implicit philosophical assumptions about the nature of human life (Illes and Bird 2006; Miller and Fins 2006), and these assumptions are embodied in consent laws designed to protect the human right of free will. But despite the great pains that neuroscientists have taken in recent years to address neuro-ethical issues in designing their studies (Illes and Bird 2006), the laws in some jurisdictions still impose severe constraints on the pursuit of knowledge on certain subjects, especially aging and neurodegenerative diseases. In particular, the current legislation in the Canadian province of Quebec places very tight constraints on the participation of cognitively impaired individuals in research studies, even though it is precisely these people whose participation would do so much to advance scientific knowledge of neurodegenerative diseases, of brain changes due to healthy and pathological aging, and of aging-related behavioral changes. Article 21 of Quebec's Civil Code should therefore be amended to simplify the procedures by which representatives who have not been legally appointed as such can provide consent to participate in research studies on behalf of older people who are incapable of giving consent but have not yet been legally declared so, provided that these studies pose no particular risk to the individuals concerned (Voyer and St-Jacques 2006).

CONCLUSION

The emergence of neuroimaging techniques has had a tremendous impact on the study of cognitive aging and is revolutionizing our understanding of the neural basis of both healthy and pathological aging. Thanks to neuroimaging, we can now detect neurobiological markers of pathological aging, such as AD, and track the progression of cognitive decline in older people over time. The resulting knowledge of how brain function changes with age will be crucial not only for helping people to maintain successful cognitive performance as they grow older, but also for helping to prevent, to slow, or perhaps even to reverse pathological processes.

However, ethical concerns and current laws may impede research and the development of new knowledge in these areas. In particular, the conditions and procedures for recruiting research subjects who are incapable of informed consent vary so widely from one country to another that the possibilities for international and multilingual studies are severely limited (Bravo and Duguet 2005; Bravo et al. 2005). Such studies would be highly beneficial for our understanding of optimal and impaired aging and for the development of more effective protocols for treating people who have neurodegenerative diseases. We conclude here by calling upon legal and regulatory decision-makers to work with neuroscientists and neuroethicists to effect positive change in this regard.

REFERENCES

Abe, O., Aoki, S., Hayashi, N., *et al.* (2002). Normal aging in the central nervous system: quantitative MR diffusion-tensor analysis. *Neurobiology of Aging*, **23**, 433–41.

Allen, J.S., Bruss, J., and Damasio, H. (2005). The aging brain: the cognitive reserve hypothesis and hominid evolution. *American Journal of Human Biology*, **17**, 673–89.

Amieva, H., Jacqmin-Gadda, H., Orgogozo, J.M., *et al.* (2005). The 9-year cognitive decline before dementia of the Alzheimer type: a prospective population-based study. *Brain*, **128**, 1093–101.

Artero, S., Tiemeier, H., Prins, N.D., Sabatier, R., Breteler, M.M., and Ritchie, K. (2004). Neuroanatomical localisation and clinical correlates of white matter lesions in the elderly. *Journal of Neurology, Neurosurgery and Psychiatry*, **75**, 1304–8.

Bartzokis, G. (2004). Age-related myelin breakdown: a developmental model of cognitive decline and Alzheimer's disease. *Neurobiology of Aging*, **25**, 5–18.

Bartzokis, G., Beckson, M., Lu, P.H., Nuechterlein, K.H., Edwards, N., and Mintz, J. (2001). Age-related changes in frontal and temporal lobe volumes in men: a magnetic resonance imaging study. *Archives of General Psychiatry*, **58**, 461–5.

Benes, F.M., Turtle, M., Khan, Y., and Farol, P. (1994). Myelination of a key relay zone in the hippocampal formation occurs in the human brain during childhood, adolescence, and adulthood. *Archives of General Psychiatry*, **51**, 477–84.

Bennett, D.A., Wilson, R.S., Schneider, J.A., *et al.* (2003). Education modifies the relation of AD pathology to level of cognitive function in older persons. *Neurology*, **60**, 1909–15.

Bertoni-Freddari, C., Fattoretti, P., Delfino, A., *et al.* (2002). Deafferentative synaptopathology in physiological aging and Alzheimer's disease. *Annals of the New York Academy of Sciences*, **977**, 322–6.

Braver, T.S. and Barch, D.M. (2002). A theory of cognitive control, aging cognition, and neuromodulation. *Neuroscience and Biobehavioral Review*, **26**, 809–17.

Bravo, G. and Duguet, A.M. (2005). La recherche chez les personnes âgées inaptes à consentir : présentation des cadres éthiques et juridiques en vigueur au Québec et en France. *L'Année Gérontologique*, **19**, 327–45.

Bravo, G., Gagnon, M., Wildeman, S., Marshall, D.T., Pâquet, M., and Dubois, M.F. (2005). Comparison of provincial and territorial legislation governing substitute consent for research. *Canadian Journal on Aging*, **24**, 237–50.

Brown, J.W. and Jaffe, J. (1975). Hypothesis on cerebral dominance. *Neuropsychologia*, **13**, 107–10.

Buckner, R.L., Head, D., Parker, J., *et al.* (2004). A unified approach for morphometric and functional data analysis in young, old, and demented adults using automated atlas-based head size normalization: reliability and validation against manual measurement of total intracranial volume. *Neuroimage*, **23**, 724–38.

Cabeza, R. (2002). Hemispheric asymmetry reduction in older adults: the HAROLD model. *Psychological Aging*, **17**, 85–100.

Cabeza, R., Anderson, N.D., Locantore, J.K., and McIntosh, A.R. (2002). Aging gracefully: compensatory brain activity in high-performing older adults. *Neuroimage*, **17**, 1394–402.

Cao, Y., Vikingstad, E.M., George, K.P., Johnson, A.F., and Welch, K.M. (1999). Cortical language activation in stroke patients recovering from aphasia with functional MRI. *Stroke*, **30**, 2331–40.

Chen, D.T., Miller, F.G., and Rosenstein, D.L. (2002). Enrolling decisionally impaired adults in clinical research. *Medical Care*, **40**, V-20-9.

Colcombe, S.J., Erickson, K.I., Raz, N., *et al.* (2003). Aerobic fitness reduces brain tissue loss in aging humans. *The Journal of Gerontology, Series A: Biological Sciences and Medical Sciences*, **58**, 176–80.

Colcombe, S.J., Erickson, K.I., and Scalf, P.E. (2006). Aerobic exercise training increases brain volume in aging humans. *The Journal of Gerontology, Series A: Biological Sciences and Medical Sciences*, **61**, 1166–70.

Council of Europe (1997). Convention for the Protection of Human Rights and Dignity of the Human Being with regard to the Application of Biology and Medicine: Convention on Human Rights and Biomedicine. Available at: http://conventions.coe.int/Treaty/EN/Treaties/html/164.htm

Davis, S.W., Dennis, N.A., Daselaar, S.M., Fleck, M.S., and Cabeza, R. (2008). Que PASA? The posterior-anterior shift in aging. *Cerebral Cortex*, **18**, 1201–9.

de Groot, J.C., de Leeuw, F.E., Oudkerk, M., *et al.* (2000). Cerebral white matter lesions and cognitive function: The Rotterdam scan study. *Annals of Neurology*, **47**, 145–51.

Dekaban, A.S. (1978). Changes in brain weights during the span of human life: relation of brain weights to body heights and body weights. *Annals of Neurology*, **4**, 345–56.

D'Esposito, M., Deouell, L.Y., and Gazzaley, A. (2003). Alterations in the BOLD fMRI signal with ageing and disease: a challenge for neuroimaging. *Nature Reviews Neuroscience*, **4**, 863–72.

Fellgiebel, A., Müller, M.J., Wille, P., *et al.* (2005). Color-coded diffusion-tensor-imaging of posterior cingulate fiber tracts in mild cognitive impairment. *Neurobiology of Aging*, **26**, 1193–8.

Gaser, C. and Schlaug, G. (2003). Gray matter differences between musicians and nonmusicians. *Annals of the New York Academy of Sciences*, **999**, 514–17.

Giedd, J.N., Blumenthal, J., Jeffries, N.O., *et al.* (1999). Brain development during childhood and adolescence: a longitudinal MRI study. *Nature Neuroscience*, **2**, 861–3.

Goldstein, G. and Shelly, C. (1981). Does the right hemisphere age more rapidly than the left? *Journal of Clinical Neuropsychology*, **3**, 65–78.

Good, C.D., Johnsrude, I.S., Ashburner, J., Henson, R.N., Friston, K.J., and Frackowiak, R.S. (2001). A voxel-based morphometric study of ageing in 465 normal adult human brains. *Neuroimage*, **14**, 21–36.

Grady, C.L. (2008). Cognitive neuroscience of aging. *Annals of the New York Academy of Sciences*, **1124**, 127–44.

Grady, C.L., McIntosh, A.R., Horwitz, B., *et al.* (1995). Age-related reductions in human recognition memory due to impaired encoding. *Science*, **269**, 218–21.

Grady, C.L., McIntosh, A.R., Beig, S., Keightley, M.L., Burian, H., and Black, S.E. (2003). Evidence from functional neuroimaging of a compensatory prefrontal network in Alzheimer's disease. *The Journal of Neurosciences*, **23**, 986–93.

Gunning-Dixon, F.M. and Raz, N. (2000). The cognitive correlates of white matter abnor-malities in normal aging: a quantitative review. *Neuropsychology*, 14, 224–32.

Gunning-Dixon, F.M. and Raz, N. (2003). Neuroanatomical correlates of selected executive functions in middle-aged and older adults: A prospective MRI study. *Neuropsychologia*, 41, 1929–41.

Haug, H. (1985). Are neurons of the human cerebral cortex really lost during aging? A mor-phometric evaluation. In J. Traber and W.H. Gispen (eds.) *Senile Dementia of the Alzheimer Type*, pp. 150–63. Berlin: Springer.

Head, D., Buckner, R.L., Shimony, J.S., *et al.* (2004). Differential vulnerability of anterior white matter in nondemented aging with minimal acceleration in dementia of the Alzheimer type: evidence from diffusion tensor imaging. *Cerebral Cortex*, 14, 410–23.

Hedden, T. and Gabrieli, J.D. (2004). Insights into the ageing mind: A view from cognitive neuroscience. *Nature Reviews Neuroscience*, 5, 87–96.

Illes, J. and Bird, S.J. (2006). Neuroethics: a modern context for ethics in neuroscience. *Trends in Neurosciences*, 29, 511–17.

Illes, J., Desmond J.E., Huang, L.F., Raffin, T.A., and Atlas, T.W. (2007). Ethical and practical considerations in managing incidental findings in functional magnetic resonance imaging. In W. Glannon (ed.) *Defining Right and Wrong in Brain Science. Essential Readings in Neuroethics*, pp. 104–14. New York: Dana Press.

Ince, P. (2001). Dementia with Lewy bodies. *Advances in Experimental Medicine and Biology*, 487, 135–45.

Jaworska, A. (2006). Ethical dilemmas in neurodegenerative disease: respecting patients at the twilight of agency. In J. Illes (ed.) *Neuroethics: Defining the Issues in Theory, Practice, and Policy*, pp. 87–101. New York: Oxford University Press.

Jernigan, T.L., Archibald, S.L., Berhow, M.T., Sowell, E.R., Foster, D.S., and Hesselink, J.R. (1991). Cerebral structure on MRI, Part I: Localization of age-related changes. *Biological Psychiatry*, 29, 55–67.

Katzman, R. (1989). Alzheimer's disease is a degenerative disorder. *Neurobiology of Aging*, 10, 581–2.

Kemper, T.L. (1994). Neuroanatomical and neuropathological changes during aging and dementia. In M.L. Albert, and J. Kusefel (eds.) *Clinical Neurology of Aging*, pp. 3–67. New York: Oxford University Press.

Kliegel, M., Moor, C., and Rott, C. (2004). Cognitive status and development in the oldest old: a longitudinal analysis from the Heidelberg Centenarian Study. *Archives of Gerontology and Geriatrics*, 39, 143–56.

Kooistra, C.A. and Heilman, K.M. (1988). Motor dominance and lateral asymmetry of the globus pallidus. *Neurology*, 38, 388–90.

Leshner, A.I. (2007). Ethical Issues in Taking Neuroscience Research from Bench to Bedside. In W. Glannon (ed.) *Defining Right and Wrong in Brain Science. Essential Readings in Neuroethics*, pp. 75–82. New York: Dana Press.

Logan, J.M., Sanders, A.L., Snyder, A.Z., Morris, J.C., and Buckner, R.L. (2002). Under-recruitment and nonselective recruitment: dissociable neural mechanisms associated with aging. *Neuron*, 33, 827–40.

Madden, D.J., Whiting, W.L., Huettel, S.A., White, L.E., MacFall, J.R., and Provenzale, J.M. (2004). Diffusion tensor imaging of adult age differences in cerebral white matter: relation to response time. *Neuroimage*, 21, 1174–81.

Maguire, E.A., Gadian , D.G.,Johnsrude, I.S., *et al.* (2000). Navigation-related structural change in the hippocampi of taxi drivers. *Proceedings of the National Academy of Sciences of the United States of America*, 97, 4398–403.

Maguire, E.A., and Frith, C.D. (2003). Lateral asymmetry in the hippocampal response to the remoteness of autobiographical memories. *Journal of Neuroscience*, **15**, 5302–5307.

Maguire, E.A., Woollett, K., and Spiers, H.J. (2006). London taxi drivers and bus drivers: a structural MRI and neuropsychological analysis. *Hippocampus*, **16**, 1091–101.

Mattay, V.S., Fera, F., Tessitore, A., *et al.* (2006). Neurophysiological correlates of age-related changes in working memory capacity. *Neuroscience Letters*, **392**, 32–7.

Mechelli, A., Crinion, J.T., Noppeney, U., *et al.* (2004). Neurolinguistics: structural plasticity in the bilingual brain. *Nature*, **431**, 757.

Meyer, J.S., Kawamura, J., and Terayama, Y. (1992). White matter lesions in the elderly. *Journal of the Neurological Sciences*, **110**, 1–7.

Miller, F.G. and Fins, J.J. (2006). Protecting human subjects in brain research: a pragmatic perspective. In J. Illes (ed.) *Neuroethics: Defining the Issues in Theory, Practice, and Policy*, pp. 123–40. New York: Oxford University Press.

Paradise, M., Cooper, C., and Livingston, G. (2009). Systematic review of the effect of education on survival in Alzheimer's disease. *International Psychogeriatrics*, **21**, 25–32.

Park, D.C. and Reuter-Lorenz, P. (2009). The adaptive brain: aging and neurocognitive scaffolding. *Annual Review of Psychology*, **60**, 173–96.

Persson, J. and Nyberg, L. (2006). Altered brain activity in healthy seniors: what does it mean? *Progress in Brain Research*, **157**, 45–56.

Peters, A., Moss, M.B., and Sethares, C. (2001). The effects of aging on layer 1 of primary visual cortex in the rhesus monkey. *Cerebral Cortex*, **11**, 93–103.

Price, J.L. and Morris, J.C. (1999). Tangles and plaques in nondemented aging and "preclinical" Alzheimer's disease. *Annals of Neurology*, **45**, 358–68.

Raz, N. (2000). Aging of the brain and its impact on cognitive performance: Integration of structural and functional findings. In F.I.M. Craik and T.A. Salthouse (eds.) *Handbook of Aging and Cognition – II*, pp. 1–90. Mahwah, NJ : Erlbaum.

Raz, N., Gunning-Dixon, F., Head, D., Rodrigue, K.M., Williamson, A., and Acker, J.D. (2004). Aging, sexual dimorphism, and hemispheric asymmetry of the cerebral cortex: replicability of regional differences in volume. *Neurobiology of Aging*, **25**, 377–96.

Raz, N., Lindenberger, U., Rodrigue, K.M., *et al.* (2005). Regional brain changes in aging healthy adults: general trends, individual differences and modifiers. *Cerebral Cortex*, **15**, 1676–89.

Reuter-Lorenz, P.A. and Cappell, K.A. (2008). Neurocognitive aging and the compensation hypothesis, *Current Directions in Psychological Science*, **17**, 177–82.

Reuter-Lorenz, P.A., Stanczak, L., and Miller, A.C. (1999). Neural recruitment and cognitive aging: two hemispheres are better than one, especially as you age. *Psychological Science*, **10**, 494–500.

Reuter-Lorenz, P.A., Jonides, J., Smith, E.E., *et al.* (2000). Age differences in the frontal lateralization of verbal and spatial working memory revealed by PET. *Journal Cognitive Neuroscience*, **12**, 174–87.

Rodrigue, K.M. and Raz, N. (2004). Shrinkage of the entorhinal cortex over five years predicts memory performance in healthy adults. *Journal of Neuroscience*, **24**, 956–63.

Rubens, A.B., Mahowald, M.W., and Hutton, J.T. (1976). Asymmetry of the lateral (sylvian) fissures in man. *Neurology*, **26**, 620–4.

Sachs, G.A. and Cassel, C.K. (1990). Biomedical research involving older human subjects. *Law, Medicine and Health Care*, **18**, 234–43.

Salat, D.H., Buckner, R.L., Snyder, A.Z., *et al.* (2004). Thinning of the cerebral cortex in aging. *Cerebral Cortex*, **14**, 721–30.

Salthouse, T.A. (1996). The processing-speed theory of adult age differences in cognition. *Psychological Review*, 103, 403–28.

Schneider-Garces, N.J., Gordon, B.A., Brumback-Peltz, C.R., *et al.* (2010). Span, CRUNCH, and Beyond: Working Memory Capacity and the Aging Brain. *Journal of Cognitive Neuroscience*, 22, 655–669.

Shimamura, A.P., Berry, J.M., Mangels, J.A., Rusting, C.L., and Jurica, P.J. (1995). Memory and cognitive abilities in university professors: evidence for successful aging. *Psychological Science*, 6, 271–7.

Skullerud, K. (1985). Variations in the size of the human brain. Influence of age, sex, body length, body mass index, alcoholism, Alzheimer changes, and cerebral atherosclerosis. *Acta Neurologica Scandinavica Supplementum*, 102, 1–94.

Sowell, E.R., Thompson, P.M., Tessner, K.D., and Toga, A.W. (2001). Mapping continued brain growth and gray matter density reduction in dorsal frontal cortex: Inverse relationships during postadolescent brain maturation. *Journal of Neuroscience*, 21, 8819–29.

Sowell, E.R., Peterson, B.S., Thompson, P.M., Welcome, S.E., Henkenius, A.L., and Toga, A.W. (2003). Mapping cortical change across the human life span. *Nature Neuroscience*, 6, 309–15.

Stadlbauer, A., Salomonowitz, E., Strunk, G., Hammen, T., and Ganslandt, O. (2008). Age-related degradation in the central nervous system: assessment with diffusion-tensor imaging and quantitative fiber tracking. *Radiology*, 247, 179–88.

Statistics Canada (2005). Deaths, 2003 (84F0211XIE). Available at: http://www.statcan.ca

Stern Y. (2002). What is cognitive reserve? Theory and research application of the reserve concept. *Journal of the International Neuropsychology Society*, 8, 448–60.

Stern Y. (2009). Cognitive reserve. *Neuropsychologia*, 47, 2015–28.

Stuss, D.T. and Alexander, M.P. (2000). Executive functions and the frontal lobes: a conceptual view. *Psychological Research*, 63, 289–98.

Sullivan, E.V. and Pfefferbaum, A. (2003). Diffusion tensor imaging in normal aging and neuropsychiatric disorders. *European Journal of Radiology*, 45, 244–55.

Terry, R.D. and Katzman, R. (2001). Life span and synapses: will there be a primary senile dementia? *Neurobiology of Aging*, 22, 347–8.

Terry, R.D., DeTeresa, R., and Hansen, L.A. (1987). Neocortical cell counts in normal human adult aging. *Annals of Neurology*, 21, 530–9.

Tovino, S.A. (2008). The impact of neuroscience on health law. *Neuroethics*, 1, 101–17.

Verhaeghen, P. (2003). Aging and vocabulary scores: a meta-analysis. *Psychology and Aging*, 18, 332–39.

von Economo, C. and Horn, L. (1930). Über Windungsrelief, Maße und Rindenarchitektonik der Supratemporalfläche, ihre individuellen und ihre Seitenunterschiede. *Zeitschr Ges Neurol Psychiat*, 130, 678–757.

Voyer, P. and St-Jacques, S. (2006). *L' article 21 du code civil et la recherche auprès des aînés atteints de démence dans les milieux de soins de longue durée au Québec. Une analyse, un constat et une proposition*. Québec City: Faculté des sciences infirmières.

Woodruff-Pak, D.S. (1997). *The Neuropsychology of Aging*. Malden, MA: Blackwell.

World Health Organization (2003). *Gender, Health and Ageing*. Published online at: http://www.who.int/gender/documents/en/Gender_Ageing.pdf

World Medical Association (2008). *Declaration of Helsinki – Ethical Principles for Medical Research Involving Human Subjects*. Available at: http://www.wma.net/en/30publications/10policies/b3/index.html

Ziegler, D.A, Piguet, O., Salat, D.H., Prince, K., Connally, E., and Corkin, S. (2010). Cognition in healthy aging is related to regional white matter integrity, but not cortical thicknesss. *Neurobiology of Aging*, 31, 1912–26.

....

CHAPTER 30

CLINICAL RESEARCH ON CONDITIONS AFFECTING COGNITIVE CAPACITY

....

SAMIA HURST

INTRODUCTION

....

RESEARCH is crucial to improve medicine's ability to care for the sick, and this includes research on conditions affecting cognition. At the same time, however, participation in clinical research places human subjects at risk of harm for the benefit of others, and this concern is particularly great in the case of vulnerable persons. Studies designed to address health problems specific to a vulnerable population, however, are needed to improve care for this very population and often cannot be conducted on others.

This tension—to protect participants in research while also taking into account the interests of future patients by allowing research to be conducted—is intrinsic to all clinical research, and underlies the need for protection of human subjects (The National Commission for the Protection of Human Subjects of Biomedical and Behavioral Research 1979; ICH Steering Committee 1996; CIOMS 2002; World Medical Association 2008; Department of Health and Human Services revised as of March 1983). The number and length of the relevant texts can be overwhelming to individual investigators, yet they all refer to similar basic principles, which have been synthesized thus: social value, scientific validity, fair subject selection, favorable risk:benefit ratio, independent review, informed consent, and respect for enrolled participants (Emanuel, Wendler *et al.* 2000). Finding the right balance in the inherent ethical tension of research, and respecting specific criteria for its ethical conduct are both particularly important and difficult in situations where vulnerable persons are potential research participants. In the case of persons with cognitive impairment, it is broadly recognized that special safeguards are needed (National Bioethics Advisory Commission 1998; European Parliament and the Council of the European Union 2001; CIOMS 2002; Karlawish 2003). This chapter will focus first, on whether persons suffering from diseases affecting cognition can be enrolled in research when the purpose is to investigate the condition leading to this impairment and second, on when they may be enrolled and on the precautions which are necessary if they are. Finally, it will examine, and reject, the idea that there could be circumstances in which persons suffering from diseases affecting cognition could have an obligation to participate in research addressing these disorders.

CAN PERSONS WITH COGNITIVE IMPAIRMENT BE ENROLLED IN RESEARCH?

That vulnerable persons require special protection in the conduct of research is recognized in a number of international (ICH Steering Committee 1996; CIOMS 2002; World Medical Association 2008) and national regulations, including the US federal regulations on research with human subjects (US Department of Health and Human Services 1991). When designing and conducting a research study, it is important to know which potential participants are vulnerable, which sorts of studies do or do not justify their inclusion, and what protections are necessary when they do participate in research.

"Vulnerability" in research on human subjects is usually linked either to consent (ICH Steering Committee 1996; CIOMS 2002), or to the risk of harm (Kottow 2004), or exploitation (Lott 2005): conditions which persons with cognitive impairment clearly sometimes meet. One way to synthesize these different definitions, and to make headway towards defining what protections are needed, is to consider that vulnerability as a claim to special protection is any identifiably increased likelihood of being wronged (Hurst 2008). Adequate protections require identification of the sorts of wrongs likely to occur in the conduct of research and those more likely to suffer these wrongs. Protections then need to be tailored to specific wrongs, and specific sources of vulnerability, and outlined in the research project.

Concerns for coercion and exploitation

Concerns regarding the inclusion of vulnerable persons—including persons unable to give informed consent—in research often point to risks of coercion or exploitation. What is meant by that and does it apply here (Emanuel *et al.* 2005)? The clearest explanation defines coercion as a credible and strong threat exerted by a person that limits the options in a negative way available to another person (Hawkins and Emanuel 2005). Therefore having limited options through no fault of anyone's does not constitute coercion. Rather than removing options, the possibility of enrolling in a clinical trial actually gives patients with chronic conditions an additional option. Although coercion can exist in research, and although of course care should be taken to avoid it, the mere offer to participate in an otherwise ethically justifiable study does not constitute coercion.

Exploitation is the unfair distribution of the benefits and burdens of a transaction (Hawkins and Emanuel 2005). Are patients suffering from diseases affecting cognition at greater risk, or are they less likely to benefit from research participation, than they should? This is not an easy question to answer: effects deemed sufficient by researchers—and which underlie the choice of research questions and methodology—may or may not reflect what patients would consider a clinically interesting effect (Horrobin 2003). Our evaluation of both risks and benefits can shift during chronic disease and changes in cognitive ability, and we should expect this shift to vary between individuals. At minimum, the risks incurred by patients suffering from diseases affecting cognition should never be discounted. More specifically, the risk:benefit assessment must take into account their circumstances. This does, however, means that exploitation can be avoided in studies enrolling vulnerable persons, including persons with diseases affecting cognition.

Concerns for coercion or exploitation, then, cannot be sufficient to warrant a general exclusion of patients with diseases affecting cognition from research. Moreover, it would be ethically problematic if the need for special protection meant that vulnerable persons should never be enrolled in research. Historically, scandals have involved abusive studies where vulnerable persons were included because they were less able to resist (Emanuel *et al.* 2008). This has led to concerns about involving them in research at all, and investigators are currently still often uncertain as to when they may or may not include vulnerable persons in a protocol, and under which conditions. Excluding vulnerable persons from research entirely, however, can lead to their exclusion from 1) research with potential benefit and 2) the more general benefits of the research endeavor: knowledge about conditions relevant to them, their sometimes specific needs and risks, and the possibility to generalize available data to the situations they present with. Exclusion thus carries a moral cost, which would be borne by the very people such protections would attempt to protect. Inclusion with adequate protections will often be the morally preferable alternative.

Special precautions for research on conditions affecting cognition

Protections for vulnerable persons in research have two components: fair subject selection (when to enroll), and the specific care required to minimize wrongs to vulnerable persons once they are enrolled in research (how to enroll) (Hurst and Elger, in press). Recruitment of research subjects should respect fairness in the distribution of research-related risks and benefits. It is not justifiable to conduct research on an "easily available" population—for example, the rural poor in developing countries (Tangwa 2009)—simply because the study will be easier to conduct with them than with persons living in better circumstances. Neither is it defensible to reserve access to potentially beneficial research to the socially privileged. The rationale for the planned recruitment strategy must be based on the balance of potential harms and benefits and the need to obtain generalizable results, and discussed in the protocol.

The conduct of research with vulnerable persons once enrolled should start with a good grasp of criteria for ethical research in general (Emanuel *et al.* 2000), and define protections based on which criteria are at risk of remaining unfulfilled without special protection. Under the definition provided earlier, persons suffering from disease affecting cognition are vulnerable in several ways. Although issues related to informed consent in the presence of cognitive impairment are the most obvious, they are not the only ones. Other aspects include difficulties related to fair subject selection, scientific methodology, a favorable risk/benefit ratio, as well as respect and confidentiality.

In the context of diseases affecting cognition, it is also especially important for ethics review committees (ERCs) and researchers to remember exactly whom we are trying to protect, and why. While such conditions can lead to impaired decision-making capacity, they do not by themselves signify such impairment. The relevant difference here is not the diagnosis, but whether or not a specific source of vulnerability is present. This is especially important as patients suffering from mental disorders have been—and often still are—subject to stigma (Michels 1999). There is a real risk of underestimating the cognitive ability of individuals who bear this label. Some special precautions will only apply when decision-making capacity is impaired. Attempts to substitute informed consent through proxy decision making, assent, or advance research directives are of this kind, as are the more restrictive limits on the risk:benefit ratio, which the lack of patient consent imposes. Others, such as difficulties with scientific validity or misleading expectations, will apply to all patients with diseases affecting cognition. Some, such as concerns for respect and confidentiality, will apply especially to those whose decision-making capacity is not impaired, but whose diagnosis places them at special risk of seeing their abilities underestimated.

Fair subject selection: when to enroll

In some cases, excluding vulnerable persons from participation in a research project will be an appropriate way to minimize the risk of harm or other wrongs. Sometimes, however, it won't be. A study could be designed to address health problems specific to a vulnerable population, and research on conditions affecting cognition often falls within this category. In such cases, preventing the enrollment of vulnerable persons in research would be harmful to the very individuals which regulations intend to protect (Michels 1999). It would also be harmful to them as a group: studies benefiting the same population of vulnerable persons from which subjects are recruited often cannot be conducted on non-vulnerable subjects: a condition known as the *subsidiarity principle*. This characteristic of research projects helps to outline which can include vulnerable persons, and which should not.

Fair subject selection should also take into account the timing of a protocol within the course of a research program. Limiting risks in the case of cognitively impaired individuals who are unable to consent to research can imply that interventions relevant both to persons who are, or are not, capable of decision making should first undergo testing on those able to understand the implications of research participation. The goal is to minimize unknown risks at the time when those with greater cognitive impairment will be recruited to assess questions more specific to them.

Timing within the course of the disease is also relevant. In research on degenerative disease, such as various forms of dementia, the disease stage at which potential subjects are recruited will affect research-related risks and benefits. For example, the effect size of benefits will sometimes be predictably lower in the initial stages, where patients have fewer symptoms (Vellas *et al.* 2008a). In some cases it will also be the case in late-stage disease, when impairments are too great for subjects to benefit significantly even from an intervention otherwise deemed successful. Late-stage patients are also more likely to be lost to follow-up (Vellas *et al.* 2008a). Timing within the disease course can also affect how we value risks and benefits (Kahneman *et al.* 2006; Gilbert and Wilson 2009), and this in turn can affect informed consent. In the period immediately following the diagnosis of a chronic disorder, patients' priorities can be in a state of rapid flux. Recruiting patients at this time can lead to informed consent based on priorities which are more unstable than is usually the case, and could be problematic for this reason.

Scientific validity

Although individual patients may benefit indirectly from research participation, the main intention of research is to generate valid data to inform the care of future patients. The investigator is responsible for avoiding unnecessary harm to research subjects, and therefore accountable for the clinical relevance of the research question and scientific validity of the study design. Failure to give proper attention to methodological issues can make the results of a trial difficult to interpret, and prevent comparisons. This limits usefulness in clinical practice, causing research to come short of its purported goal and fail to fulfill its commitments towards patients and society. Inasmuch as risks to human subjects are justified, in part, by the social benefit of research, any risk, however small, run within a study that cannot answer its research question is an excessive risk.

Outcome measurements in diseases affecting cognition are subject to discussion. While several large primary prevention trials in Alzheimer type dementia (AD) have used incidence as a primary endpoint (Vellas *et al.* 2008b), the transition between normal aging, very early AD, and AD, makes a threshold difficult to identify (Petersen 2006). Proposed alternatives include delegating the identification of new cases to an independent attribution committee, or replacing the threshold altogether and using changes in cognitive performance instead (Vellas *et al.* 2008b). This may have the added benefit of reducing the required sample size, thus making a greater number of studies feasible and perhaps reflecting the priorities of patients somewhat better (Horrobin 2003).

As clinical trials can continue for several years, selected outcome measures should be valid at different stages of the disease under study. This is difficult: in degenerative dementias, distinct assessment tools can be needed depending on the disease stage, for both cognitive and functional domains of impairment. In the case of AD, the cognitive subscale of the AD assessment scale (ADAS-cog) has been considered the standard primary cognitive outcome for symptomatic trials. As a greater number of studies include patients with early disease, it has, however, been pointed out that this measurement may not be appropriate for trials in very early dementia, where it may need to be complemented with other tests. In complex diseases affecting different aspects of mental and social functioning, a single type of measurement is unlikely to be the best one in every stage of progression. A task force of the European Alzheimer Disease Consortium proposed to combine changes in the slope of cognitive decline with quality of life and (instrumental) activities of daily living assessments, to establish the clinical relevance of measured differences between treatment groups in clinical trials (Vellas *et al.* 2008b). Behavioral and psychological symptoms should also be taken into account, but their diversity makes this difficult to do: for example, changes in individual items on the neuropsychiatric inventory (Cummings *et al.* 1994), may be masked if the overall result is used as the outcome. In studies of secondary prevention, the use of compound scores measuring performance on different validated tests is recommended (Vellas *et al.* 2008b).

Biomarkers—for example, cerebrospinal fluid analysis or magnetic resonance imaging—are increasingly used in dementia research. Currently, none predicts clinical decline sufficiently to serve as surrogate endpoint (Coley *et al.* 2009). Although many correlate with diagnosis, and some do correlate with decline, their use still warrants caution: in one study (Fox *et al.* 2005), greater cerebral atrophy was recorded in the active arm of the study, but without an increase in cognitive decline.

The large inherent variability of diseases affecting cognition means that the potential of multicenter trials to introduce added site-related effects can be problematic. Specific training and assessment of investigators has been proposed (Morris 1997), as have higher thresholds for the minimum number of research subjects recruited in each included center (Vellas *et al.* 2008b).

For results to be readily understandable, data must be measured and reported in a way which relates to clinical practice. Currently, no true consensus exists on the definition of the minimally clinically important difference in dementia trials (Molnar *et al.* 2009). The important variability of disease and treatment effect will sometimes mean that giving mean values does not reflect clinical reality. Graphical representation of the data showing the full range of response has been proposed in other areas of research, and may be useful here as well (Farrar *et al.* 2006).

A favorable risk: benefit ratio

When cognitively impaired patients are recruited in research, protections are required to circumscribe acceptable risks, and to compensate the lack of valid consent. The Council for International Organizations of Medical Sciences (CIOMS) guidelines specify that:

> When there is ethical and scientific justification to conduct research with individuals incapable of giving informed consent, the risk from research interventions that do not hold out the prospect of direct benefit for the individual subject should be no more likely and not greater than the risk attached to routine medical or psychological examination of such persons. Slight or minor increases above such risk may be permitted when there is an overriding scientific or medical rationale for such increases and when an ethical review committee has approved them. (CIOMS 2002, p. 49)

In the somewhat similar case of research with children, US regulations stipulate that ERCs may approve research involving children under three sets of circumstances: "prospect of direct benefit," "minimal risk," and "minor increase over minimal risk." A prospect of direct benefit is defined as a research situation where risks are "justified by the anticipated benefit to the subjects" and where "the relation of the anticipated benefit to the risk is at least as favorable" as that of alternatives available to potential subjects (US Department of Health and Human Services 1991).

Linking the acceptable risk threshold to the prospect of direct benefit has come under criticism in the case of children for conflating risks acceptable in therapy and in research (Wendler 2008). Wendler proposes an alternative based on the "net risks test" (Wendler 2006). As any assessment of risk in research, this one should focus on the *research-related risk*: risks which potential research subjects would not run outside the protocol. Patients enrolled in research will often undergo standard therapy as well as experimental interventions, and risks inherent to the standard therapy are not research-related. The assessment should further focus on the *net risk*: risks that are not balanced by the prospect of direct benefit to the research subject. Pharmacokinetic studies, for example, hold no prospect of direct benefit: their entire risk is a net risk. A phase III study of a novel therapy with promising results in phase II, however, does hold a prospect of direct benefit for subjects. Such a study can still have a net risk, however, especially if the expected benefit is modest. Finally, ERCs should assess this *net research-related risk* and accept it if it is no greater than "those associated with routine medical and psychological examination" (CIOMS 2002), or "those ordinarily encountered in daily life" (US Department of Health and Human Services 1991). US regulations combine these two thresholds.

What are risks "ordinarily encountered in daily life"? CIOMS proposes that research interventions considered to carry low or minimal risk be similar to clinical interventions that subjects may have experienced. This requirement, which would allow greater research-related risk in situations of greater therapy-related risk, is justified by CIOMS based on the likelihood that consent will then be better informed. But this may still be excessive. In the case of children, to avoid placing an excessive burden on patients suffering from diseases requiring invasive treatment or living in circumstances such as war-torn countries, whose risks in daily life far exceed what is acceptable in research (Freedman 1993), stricter definitions of low or minimal risk has been proposed. Comparison of the net research-related risks posed by a study should be with "the level of risk average children face in daily life (or during routine examinations)" (Wendler 2006), or the level "normally encountered in the daily lives of people in a stable society" (South African Research Council 2006). Although the exact degree of net risk which is acceptable in a trial including adults incapable of giving consent is a point on which there is currently no consensus, these considerations do provide some guidance.

Consent and decision-making capacity

Informed consent is particularly important in research, because it allow subjects to make an informed and voluntary choice to participate—or refuse to participate—in a project where they will take risks for the benefit of others. Adequate informed consent requires that potential subjects understand the relevant aspects of their choice, are capable of decision making, and are free to accept or refuse participation (Faden and Beauchamp 1986). Importantly, the mere presence of a disease affecting cognition does not mean that a specific person is not capable of giving valid consent. The relevant difference here is not the diagnosis, but whether or not decision making is impaired (Michels 1999). The disease may be in an early stage, or mild, and its effects on cognition limited. Moreover, the presence of cognitive impairment is itself imperfectly correlated with capacity to give consent (Warner *et al.* 2008). This is not entirely surprising: valid consent requires not just understanding, but a degree of appreciation of the situation as well. It has affective and evaluative components (Elliott 1997), all of which can be affected by disease in a manner different from cognition. Studies planning the inclusion of patients suffering from a disease affecting cognition should provide for formal assessment of decision-making capacity. They should plan to evaluate the patient's understanding of the relevant information, the patient's appreciation of the significance of this information for the circumstances, the patient's ability to reason with the relevant information and weigh options logically, and the patient's ability to express a choice

(American Psychiatric Association 1998; Grisso and Appelbaum 1998). This assessment must be described in the protocol, and the evaluation targeted specifically for the purposes of research participation. Even in persons who are capable of decision making for clinical care, consent for research requires something more: research-related risks are borne for the benefits of others, a fact potential subjects are at risk of misunderstanding even in the best of cases (Appelbaum *et al.* 2004). Decision-making capacity for research participation is thus distinct from the abilities required for capacity to consent to medical treatment or for decisions in everyday life (Karlawish 2008). For subject to understand, specifically, that they are involved in research can be demanding (Wendler and Grady 2008). Barring such an assessment, decision-making capacity in persons with conditions affecting cognition can be underestimated as well as overestimated (Stocking *et al.* 2008). When decision-making capacity is present, consent for research on conditions affecting cognitive capacity shares the same process—and the same difficulties—as any other consent for research with human subjects (Flory and Emanuel 2004).

The problem of misleading expectations

Another difficulty is that patients suffering from chronic conditions, and their proxies, have often experienced various treatments which showed less than satisfactory efficacy, and are likely to welcome the opportunity to gain access to a novel treatment. This makes the likelihood of the "therapeutic misconception" particularly high. Their hope for direct benefit to themselves or a sick loved one can also expose them to minimizing or overlooking inconveniences and risks. Furthermore, many persons suffering from diseases affecting cognition experience impaired physical, emotional, and social functioning, all of which have been associated with the therapeutic misconception (Appelbaum *et al.* 2004). Failure to address the therapeutic misconception in potential participants undermines the validity of consent, and constitutes a breach of obligations.

The therapeutic misconception is also ethically problematic because it is a case of misplaced trust, which can endanger the physician-patient relation (de Melo-Martin and Ho 2008). Participants, or their family members, may come to question the researcher's competence and blame him or her if their expectations are not fulfilled. Patients' distrust towards physician investigators can extend and impact on their relationship with their own physician. It will then affect and possibly jeopardize routine clinical care (Escher and Hurst, in press).

Assent and dissent

When persons who are not capable of decision making are recruited for research, the investigator should seek the person's agreement—officialized in some jurisdictions as "assent"—to the extent of the potential subject's capabilities, and respect his or her dissent (CIOMS 2002). Concerns underlying the requirement for assent are based on the need to continue respecting the priorities of potential subjects of research and their right to self-determination to the degree they are capable of (Jaworska 1999). Rejecting potential subjects' stated choices outright, when they are capable of voicing them even in part, can also be humiliating to them (Winick and Goodman 2006).

While the requirement to respect assent and dissent in cognitively impaired subjects is accepted, there are no widely accepted standards either for judging the extent to which persons can assent to participation, or for obtaining such assent. When agreement—or assent—is sought, a formal process should nevertheless be planned. Relying on simple indications of willingness to participate is insufficient. Difficulties in verbal and non-verbal communication are frequent in dementia, making the risk of misunderstanding high (Warner and Nomani 2008). Investigators should indicate what abilities will determine whether a potential subject can assent, and ERCs should examine these procedures (Karlawish 2003).

Dissent—disagreement or resistance—to participation in a research project should be respected regardless of ability to assent. Respect for dissent is not only required because we should respect the expression of the patient's priorities (as in assent), but also to avoid exerting abusive power, and to avoid causing harm through constraints in the conduct of research.

Advance research directives

In some cases, subjects can be recruited before a predictable loss of capacity occurs and advance informed consent then becomes an option. When this is done, research subjects should also be asked to name a person to serve as their proxy for decisions to be reached at a future date during the conduct of the study. Advance informed consent only applies to specific projects enrolling persons known to be eligible, who are capable of decision making at the outset, and who may lose this capacity during the course of the same study. Informed consent is thus close enough to present potential subjects with information likely to be relevant in their current situation. In cases where loss of decision-making capacity is predictable, but the question of research participation relates to research in general rather than to a specific protocol because it addresses participation in future research, it has been proposed that an "advance research directive" could stipulate potential subjects' preferences independently of an actual study. This would allow competent individuals who know in advance that they wish to participate in research, to prospectively state this rather than depend exclusively on surrogate decision-makers in the future (Pierce 2009). The legal status of advance research directives is, however, unclear (Lotjonen 2006; Pierce 2009). A number of difficulties with their use have also been put forward. Concerns focus on the difficulty of anticipating a future experience of research participation as an incompetent subject, and lack of ability to withdraw consent after capacity is lost. There are also questions regarding abilities required to write such directives, the degree of risk which can be consented to in advance, and the legitimacy of binding a incompetent future self (Pierce 2009). Despite this, advance research directives have been endorsed by advocacy groups as a means of fostering research designed to help persons with diseases affecting cognition. Advances in early diagnosis also make advance research directives before any loss of capacity appears a more realistic option. One study of such directives found that a significant minority of adult inpatients (9%) indicated willingness to participate in research that would not help them and posed greater than minimal risk (Muthappan *et al.* 2005). Although further research is required to define appropriate conditions for advance research directives, their implementation may thus provide such patients with a way of accepting research which may otherwise not be considered ethically acceptable.

Proxies and surrogates

In some countries including the US, patients who are incapable of giving consent can be enrolled in research following proxy consent (US Department of Health and Human Services 1991; CIOMS 2002). The possibility for proxy, or surrogate, consent is designed to delegate the decision to someone who is likely to know what the potential subject would have wanted (Buchanan and Brock 1990), and who takes their best interest to heart (Karlawish 2003). It also reflects a prevalent—though not general—attitude of willingness on the part of potential subjects to give leeway to their family members for such decisions (Chenaud *et al.* 2009; Karlawish *et al.* 2009; Kim *et al.* 2009).

Identifying the most appropriate proxy is not easy, and legally provided hierarchies among family members may be misaligned with affective proximity and knowledge of a potential subject's preferences. This has led to a proposal that investigators should identify the ethically most appropriate surrogate, and obtain consent from both proxies when the law requires them to obtain is from a legal surrogate as well (Karlawish 2003). Even when an appropriate proxy is identified, there is no clear guidance on how ERCs should oversee their involvement (Kim *et al.* 2004). Moreover, substituted judgment, attempting to decide as the patient would have done, is a difficult exercise. A fact reflected in the finding that next-of-kin as well as patient-designated proxies incorrectly predict patient preferences in approximately a third of cases (Shalowitz *et al.* 2006). Among patients, reluctance to give leeway to a surrogate was found to increase with the risk of the research scenarios (Stocking *et al.* 2006). Despite these difficulties, it is important to note that patients may remain capable of appointing a proxy even when they are no longer capable of writing an advance research directive (Kim and Kieburtz 2006).

Respect and confidentiality

Respect for research subjects as persons also includes respect of patients' more general clinical needs, concerns for their safety including at times when it becomes necessary to withdraw them from a research protocol, and protection of their private sphere. Like clinical care, research often involves the collection of intimate information, which persons would not otherwise divulge. In clinical care, respect for patient confidentiality is based on the requirement to respect a patient's private sphere and his or her control over personal information. It is also based on the need to provide patients with a private space where they can divulge to clinicians the information needed in order to treat them, without fear that others will hear it. These considerations also apply in research but, in both research and clinical care, confidentiality is more difficult to implement in the case of conditions affecting cognition. When decision-making capacity is impaired, reliance on proxies and surrogates will mean that the relevant information must be made available to them. This is not the case for patients whose decision-making capacity is intact. As outlined earlier, however, decision-making capacity in persons with conditions affecting cognition can be underestimated (Stocking *et al.* 2008). Confidentiality is thus an additional reason to assess decision-making capacity specifically. Furthermore, diseases affecting cognition are often chronic disorders, during which healthcare providers will often rely to varying degrees on support from family members in the care of the patient. This can lead them to value disclosure to family caregivers as being in the patient's best interest. Patients, however, still value a high degree of control over disclosure of personal information to family members (Tracy *et al.* 2004), and researchers should be aware that confidentiality is not less important in their case than in others.

RESEARCH TO PREVENT THE LOSS OF SELF: A SPECIAL CASE?

Much focus rests on whether, and how, we *may* enroll persons with diseases affecting cognition in research. Part of the reason why special protections are needed, however, is that impaired cognition can lead to loss of autonomy. The value we attach to self-determination thus underlies much of the special attention prescribed when such persons are enrolled in research. This can seem to lead to something of a paradox. The entire field of research on conditions affecting cognition, or most of it, can be fairly described as attempting to find interventions likely to protect, or hopefully correct the loss of, self-determination in affected patients. Yet we assume as a default position that patients with diseases affecting cognition should not be enrolled in research unless there is a good reason to do so. Would we have reason, based on the importance of protecting autonomy in such patients, to assume enrollment unless there are good reasons against it? Perhaps even to place limits on the sorts of research project patients, or their surrogates, can refuse to participate in? A similar, stronger point is sometimes made as regards end-of-life choices: that making a choice which could lead to the loss of autonomy may be considered contradictory, and thus not part of the scope of choices we should allow persons to make even for themselves (ten Have and Clark 2002). Although I will argue that this argument fails, it is worth presenting here as it focuses on a rather specific characteristic of research on conditions affecting cognition: a concern to prevent the loss of self (Dekkers and Rikkert 2007). If the worth of persons—their Kantian dignity—is based on their rational nature, why does it not follow that persons affected with a disease affecting cognition have an obligation to take all available chances of maintaining autonomy, including research participation?

There are three arguments against this conclusion. First, accepting it would require that we buy into the therapeutic misconception (Appelbaum *et al.* 2004), and presume that research interventions are effective whereas this is by definition uncertain. Nevertheless, uncertainty cannot truly counter this argument, as the mere chance of maintaining the capacity for self-determination may still be sufficient. Second, as Dekkers points out, the currently available drugs are not effective enough to truly prevent the loss of self brought about by diseases affecting cognition. Although this reason is contingent on the current state of medical progress, it does seem valid for now. Third, as McMahan argues in the context of end-of-life choices, for a person to have worth, or dignity, is for this person to matter in some way. True, one possibility is to consider that a person's "rational nature" provides us with a reason why this person should matter to us. But even under such a view, the end of a person's "rational nature" does not cause this person to cease to matter (McMahan 2002). Even if we accept that self-determination is central to that which we should protect in persons, this does not mean we should protect self-determination exclusively, or that persons have a duty to protect their own self-determination above all other considerations. Velleman put it as follows: "Respecting…people is not necessarily a matter of keeping them in existence; it is a matter of treating them in the way that is required by their personhood-whatever way that is." (Velleman 1999, pp. 616).

There is also a more general debate regarding whether there exists an obligation to participate in clinical research for all persons, and some of these arguments may apply here as well. Arguments in favor of such an obligation to participate in research include that this would form a part of a general duty of beneficence, that the failure to participate in research is a form of free-riding, and that participation in research is the condition for generating a public good: generalizable biomedical knowledge (Schaefer *et al.* 2009). John Harris, for example, argues that we have an obligation to participate in research both because we must support the institutions that sustain us, including research, and because beneficence requires us to prevent harm to others "including by supporting potentially beneficial, even life-saving- research" (Chan and Harris 2009). Schaefer and colleagues argue that the beneficence argument and the free-riding arguments ultimately fail. The first because there are many alternative manners in which people can do good, and the second because participating in research does not diminish the burden borne by others for the same goal. They do, however, convincingly defend a duty to participate in research in order to help generate a public good. To some degree, then, it does seem that a duty to participate in research could exist. Would this apply to persons with conditions affecting cognition? Although this could in theory apply to anyone, there are limit to how far it can do so as regards patients with cognitive impairment. First, as the duty to participate rests on the fact that research results benefit everyone, this would be limited to research with the potential to benefit persons with cognitive disorders. In effect, the subsidiarity principle would still largely apply. More importantly, Schaefer and colleagues as well as Chan and Harris propose what amounts to an opt-out system, rather than a binding obligation to participate in research (Chan and Harris 2009; Schaefer *et al.* 2009). Since opting out requires either decision-making capacity or a delegation of the power to opt out to a surrogate, their proposal will be sharply limited as regards persons with cognitive capacity. Harris further delimits the duty of incompetent persons to participate in research to situations where they do not resist participation, and where competent individuals cannot usefully participate (Harris 2005). In effect, applying this form of obligation to participate in research—with these limitations—to persons with cognitive impairment may not change very much to the sort of practices we would already find acceptable.

Conclusion

In conducting research on diseases affecting cognition, it is important to remember exactly whom we are trying to protect, and why. Some special precautions will only apply when decision-making capacity is impaired, while others will apply especially when it is present, or to all patients. As with any other group for which questions of vulnerability in research and its protection arise, the challenge is to find the right balance between protection from abuse and the need to grant vulnerable populations access to participation in research, and to progress in medicine's ability to help them. In the case of persons whose decision making is impaired by a disease affecting cognition, as with other vulnerable subjects of research, exclusion from a specific study will sometimes be an appropriate way to minimize patients' risk of being wronged in the conduct of research. This, however, will not always be the case. Studies designed to address health problems specific to a vulnerable population are needed to improve care for this very population, and often cannot be conducted on others. Participation in research can hold a prospect of benefit from which it is sometimes wrong to exclude vulnerable persons. In such cases, enrollment with special protections tailored to the sort of wrong to be avoided is ethically preferable to exclusion.

REFERENCES

American Psychiatric Association (1998). *Guideline for Assessing the Decision-Making Capacities of Potential Research Subjects with Cognitive Impairment*. Washington, DC: The American Psychiatric Association.

Appelbaum, P.S., Lidz, C.W., and Grisso, T. (2004). Therapeutic misconception in clinical research: frequency and risk factors. *IRB*, **26**, 1–8.

Buchanan, A.E. and Brock, D.W. (1990). *Deciding for Others; The Ethics of Surrogate Decision Making*. Cambridge: Cambridge University Press.

Chan, S. and Harris, J. (2009). Free riders and pious sons – why science research remains obligatory. *Bioethics*, **23**, 161–71.

Chenaud, C., Merlani, P., Verdon, M., and Ricou, B. (2009). Who should consent for research in adult intensive care? Preferences of patients and their relatives: a pilot study. *Journal of Medical Ethics*, **35**, 709–12.

CIOMS (2002). *International Ethical Guidelines for Biomedical Research Involving Human Subjects*. Geneva: Council for International Organizations of Medical Sciences.

CIOMS (2002). *Guideline 4: Individual Informed Consent, International Ethical Guidelines for Biomedical Research Involving Human Subjects*. Geneva: Council for International Organizations of Medical Sciences.

Coley, N., Andrieu, S., Delrieu, J., Voisin T., and Vellas, B. (2009). Biomarkers in Alzheimer's disease: not yet surrogate endpoints. *Annals of the NY Academy of Sciences*, **1180**, 119–24.

Cummings, J.L., Mega, M., Gray, K., Rosenberg-Thompson, S., Carusi, D.A., and Gornbein, J. (1994). The Neuropsychiatric Inventory: comprehensive assessment of psychopathology in dementia. *Neurology*, **44**, 2308–14.

de Melo-Martin, I. and Ho, A. (2008). Beyond informed consent: the therapeutic misconception and trust. *Journal of Medical Ethics*, **34**, 202–5.

Dekkers, W. and Rikkert, M.O. (2007). Memory enhancing drugs and Alzheimer's disease: enhancing the self or preventing the loss of it? *Medicine, Health Care and Philosophy*, **10**, 141–51.

Department of Health and Human Services (revised as of March 1983). Rules and Regulations. Title 45, part 46.

Elliott, C. (1997). Caring about risks. Are severely depressed patients competent to consent to research? *Archives of General Psychiatry*, **54**, 113–16.

Emanuel, E.J., Wendler, D., and Grady, C. (2000). What makes clinical research ethical? *JAMA*, **283**, 2701–11.

Emanuel, E.J., Currie, X.E., and Herman, A. (2005). Undue inducement in clinical research in developing countries: is it a worry? *Lancet*, **366**, 336–40.

Emanuel, E.J., Grady, C., Crouch, R.A., Lie, R., Miller F., and Wendler D. (2008). *The Oxford Textbook of Clinical Research Ethics*. Oxford: Oxford University Press.

Escher, M. and Hurst, S.A. (in press). The ethics of research on pain and other symptoms. In G. Van Norman, S. Palmer, S. Jackson, S. Rosenbaum and A. Cahana (eds.) *Clinical Ethics in Anesthesiology*. Cambridge: Cambridge University Press.

European Parliament and the Council of the European Union (2001). On the approximation of the laws, regulations and administrative provision of the Member States relating to the implementation of good clinical practice in the conduct of clinical trials on medicinal products for human use. 2001/20/EC. European Union, Official Journal of the European Communities.

Faden, R. and Beauchamp, T. (1986). *A History and Theory of Informed Consent*, Oxford: Oxford University Press.

Farrar, J.T., Dworkin, R.H., and Max, M.B. (2006). Use of the cumulative proportion of responders analysis graph to present pain data over a range of cut-off points: making clinical trial data more understandable. *Journal of Pain Symptom Management*, **31**, 369–77.

Flory, J. and Emanuel, E. (2004). Interventions to improve research participants' understanding in informed consent for research: a systematic review. *JAMA*, **292**, 1593–601.

Fox, N.C., Black, R.S., Gilman, S., *et al.* (2005). Effects of Abeta immunization (AN1792) on MRI measures of cerebral volume in Alzheimer disease. *Neurology*, **64**, 1563–72.

Gilbert, D.T. and Wilson, T.D. (2009). Why the brain talks to itself: sources of error in emotional prediction. *Philosophical Transactions of the Royal Society of London B: Biological Sciences*, **364**, 1335–41.

Grisso, T. and Appelbaum, P.S. (1998). *Assessing Competence to Consent to Treatment. A Guide for Physicians and Other Health Care Professionals*. New York: Oxford University Press.

Harris, J. (2005). Scientific research is a moral duty. *Journal of Medical Ethics*, **31**, 242–8.

Hawkins, J.S. and Emanuel, E.J. (2005). Clarifying confusions about coercion. *Hastings Center Report*, **35**, 16–19.

Horrobin, D.F. (2003). Are large clinical trials in rapidly lethal diseases usually unethical? *Lancet*, **361**, 695–7.

Hurst, S.A. (2008). Vulnerability in research and health care: describing the elephant in the room? *Bioethics*, **22**, 191–202.

Hurst, S.A. and Elger, B. (in press). Research with vulnerable persons. In G. Van Norman, S. Palmer, S. Jackson, S. Rosenbaum, and A. Cahana (eds.) *Clinical Ethics in Anesthesiology*. Cambridge: Cambridge University Press.

ICH Steering Committee. (1996, May 1 1996). *ICH Harmonized Tripartite Guideline* available at: http://www.emea.europa.eu/pdfs/human/ich/013595en.pdf (accessed 25 September 2008)

Jaworska, A. (1999). Respecting the margins of agency: Alzheimer's patients and the capacity to value. *Philosophy Public Affairs*, **28**, 105–38.

Kahneman, D., Krueger, A.B., Schkade, D., Schwarz, N., and Stone, A.A. (2006). Would you be happier if you were richer? A focusing illusion. *Science*, **312**, 1908–10.

Karlawish, J. (2008). Measuring decision-making capacity in cognitively impaired individuals. *Neurosignals*, **16**, 91–8.

Karlawish, J., Rubright, J., Casarett, D., Cary, M., Ten Have, T., and Sankar, P. (2009). Older adults' attitudes toward enrollment of non-competent subjects participating in Alzheimer's research. *American Journal of Psychiatry*, **166**, 182–8.

Karlawish, J.H. (2003). Research involving cognitively impaired adults. *New England Journal of Medicine*, 348, 1389–92.

Kim, S.Y. and Kieburtz, K. (2006). Appointing a proxy for research consent after one develops dementia: the need for further study. *Neurology*, 66, 1298–9.

Kim, S.Y., Appelbaum, P.S., Jeste, D.V., and Olin, J.T. (2004). Proxy and surrogate consent in geriatric neuropsychiatric research: update and recommendations. *American Journal of Psychiatry*, 161, 797–806.

Kim, S.Y., Kim, H.M., Langa, K.M., Karlawish, J.H., Knopman, D.S., and Appelbaum, P.S. (2009). Surrogate consent for dementia research: a national survey of older Americans. *Neurology*, 72, 149–55.

Kottow, M.H. (2004). Vulnerability: what kind of principle is it? *Medicine, Health Care and Philosophy*, 7, 281–7.

Lotjonen, S. (2006). Medical research on patients with dementia – the role of advance directives in European legal instruments. *European Journal of Health Law*, 13, 235–61.

Lott, J.P. (2005). Module three: vulnerable/special participant populations. *Developing World Bioethics*, 5, 30–54.

McMahan, J. (2002). *The Ethics of Killing; Problems at the Margins of Life*. Oxford: Oxford University Press.

Michels, R. (1999). Are research ethics bad for our mental health? *New England Journal of Medicine*, 340, 1427–30.

Molnar, F.J., Man-Son-Hing, M., and Fergusson, D. (2009). Systematic review of measures of clinical significance employed in randomized controlled trials of drugs for dementia. *Journal of the American Geriatric Society*, 57, 536–46.

Morris, J.C., Ernesto, C.Schaefer, K. *et al*., Clinical dementia rating (CDR) training and reliability protocol: The Alzheimer's Disease Cooperative Study Unit Experience. *Neurology* 1997; 48: 1508–1510.

Muthappan, P., Forster, H., and Wendler, D. (2005). Research advance directives: protection or obstacle? *American Journal of Psychiatry*, 162, 2389–91.

National Bioethics Advisory Commission (1998). Research involving persons with mental disorders that may affect decisionmaking capacity. Rockville, MD: NBAC.

Petersen, R.C. (2006). Conversion. *Neurology*, 67, S12–13.

Pierce, R. (2009). A changing landscape for advance directives in dementia research. *Social Science & Medicine*, 70, 623–30.

Schaefer, G.O., Emanuel, E.J., and Wertheimer, A. (2009). The obligation to participate in biomedical research. *JAMA*, 302, 67–72.

Shalowitz, D.I., Garrett-Mayer, E., and Wendler, D. (2006). The accuracy of surrogate decision makers: a systematic review. *Archives of Internal Medicine*, 166, 493–7.

Stocking, C.B., Hougham, G.W., Danner, D.D., Patterson, M.B., Whitehouse, P.J., and Sachs, G.A. (2006). Speaking of research advance directives: planning for future research participation. *Neurology*, 66, 1361–6.

Stocking, C.B., Hougham, G.W., Danner, D.D., Patterson, M.B., Whitehouse, P.J., and Sachs, G.A. (2008). Variable judgments of decisional capacity in cognitively impaired research subjects. *Journal of the American Geriatric Society*, 56, 1893–7.

Tangwa, G.B. (2009). Research with vulnerable human beings. *Acta Tropica*, 112S, S16–S20.

ten Have, H.A. and Clark, D. (2002). *The Ethics of Palliative Care; European Perspectives*. Buckingham: Open University Press.

The National Commission for the Protection of Human Subjects of Biomedical and Behavioral Research (1979). The Belmont Report: Ethical Principles and Guidelines for the Protection of Human Subjects of Research. Washington D.C.: Department of Health, Education, and Welfare.

Tracy, C.S., Drummond, N., Ferris, L.E., *et al.* (2004). To tell or not to tell? Professional and lay perspectives on the disclosure of personal health information in community-based dementia care. *Canadian Journal of Aging,* **23**, 203–15.

US Department of Health and Human Services (1991). 45 Code of Federal Regulations 46. *Federal Register,* **56**, 28012.

Vellas, B., Coley, N., and Andrieu, S. (2008a). Disease modifying trials in Alzheimer's disease: perspectives for the future. *Journal of Alzheimers Disease,* **15**, 289–301.

Vellas, B., Andrieu, S., Sampaio, C., Coley, N., and Wilcock, G. (2008b). Endpoints for trials in Alzheimer's disease: a European task force consensus. *Lancet Neurology,* **7**, 436–50.

Velleman, J.D. (1999). A right of self-termination. *Ethics,* **109**, 606–28.

Warner, J. and Nomani, E. (2008). Giving consent in dementia research. *Lancet,* **372**, 183–5.

Warner, J., McCarney, R., Griffin, M., Hill, K., and Fisher, P. (2008). Participation in dementia research: rates and correlates of capacity to give informed consent. *Journal of Medical Ethics,* **34**, 167–70.

Wendler, D. (2006). Three steps to protecting pediatric research participants from excessive risks. *PLoS Clinical Trials,* **1**, e25.

Wendler, D. (2008). Is it possible to protect pediatric research subjects without blocking appropriate research? *Journal of Pediatrics,* **152**, 467–70.

Wendler, D. and Grady, C. (2008). What should research participants understand to understand they are participants in research? *Bioethics,* **22**, 203–8.

Winick, B.J. and Goodman, K.W. (2006). A therapeutic jurisprudence perspective on participation in research by subjects with reduced capacity to consent: a comment on Kim and Appelbaum. *Behavioral Science & The Law,* **24**, 485–94.

World Medical Association. (2008). *Declaration of Helsinki: Ethical Principles for Medical Research Involving Human Subjects* available at: http://www.wma.net/e/policy/b3.htm (accessed 24 February 2009).

CHAPTER 31

ETHICAL CONCERNS AND PITFALLS IN NEUROGENETIC TESTING

GING-YUEK ROBIN HSIUNG

INTRODUCTION

OVER the last two decades, there has been an explosion of new scientific knowledge on the genetic and molecular pathogenesis of diseases of the central nervous system. While the familial aggregation of diseases has been observed and suggested for thousands of years, the era of genetic and biochemical explanations of human hereditary diseases actually began about a century ago in 1909, with the initial publication on *Inborn Errors of Metabolism* by Garrod, the well-recognized father of biochemical genetics. Since then, over 2000 genetic disorders have been defined (GeneTests 2009). The rapid progress in recent years is largely fuelled by the Human Genome Project, an international collaborative effort which began in the 1990s to map and identify the approximately 30,000 genes encoded in the 23 pairs of human chromosomes. The progress on the Human Genome Project was swift as fierce competition between the public and private sector grew when Celera Genomics Corporation made headlines publicly declaring its intention to patent genes that the company sequenced first. In June 2000, 5 years ahead of schedule, the directors of the Human Genome Project and Celera jointly announced the completion of the first working draft of the human genome (McPherson *et al.* 2001). As the exponential growth of genetic information became difficult to keep up with in traditional printed media, McKusick and colleagues had the foresight to move to the Internet as a more effective medium to categorize and distribute new genetic knowledge. They created *Online Mendelian Inheritance in Man* (OMIM), a free public resource available through the internet by the National Library of Medicine (McKusick 2009).

This growth of genetic knowledge and technology is especially relevant in the field of neurology, as it has been estimated from tissue-specific expression experiments that nearly half of all human genes are expressed in the brain (Walton 1998; Sempere *et al.* 2004; Yeo *et al.* 2004; Parkhomchuk *et al.* 2009). In fact, some scholars have argued that no other medical specialty has benefited more from molecular genetic technology than neurology. A partial list of neurological conditions for which genetic testing is currently available is shown in Table 31.1. New conditions are added to the list almost daily, and an up-to-date resource on the clinical and laboratory aspect of genetic testing can be found at the GeneTests website (GeneTests 2009). This novel technology has also introduced a burden of ethical dilemmas for clinical neuroscience that we have not had to face in the past: (1) the information on genetic tests has implications on not just the individual tested, but also blood-relatives, and (2) genetic information can predict future disease development in asymptomatic individuals who are currently healthy, including Alzheimer's disease (AD) for which a cure remains elusive. This raises a number of concerns. For example, who should be tested when a new neurogenetic diagnostic test becomes available? What other knowledge is needed to make the test meaningful? Who should have access to this information? Who should provide the testing? Should children be tested? For the still incurable neurodegenerative diseases with an age of onset that is late in life, the questions of when to test, and whether to test, are acute: with the current rising cost of healthcare globally, is the cost of performing these relatively expensive tests justified, especially when definitive treatment for these conditions lags the ability to diagnose it?

The answers to these questions are complex. The pursuit of them is enabled by the Human Genome Project that has devoted about 3% of its total funding to specifically address these ethical, legal, and social issues (ELSI). Similar initiatives have also been launched in Europe and Japan with the goal to derive practical recommendations on policies including provision of genetic tests, banking of genetic data for research, storage of genetic information and testing for insurance and employment, and population screening (Godard *et al.* 2003a,b,c,d; Fukushima 2005a,b).

In this chapter, I explore some of the issues that arise in the post-human genome era and use various cases to illustrate some of the scenarios that a clinician may encounter in decision making. The overarching goal is to improve awareness and encourage discussion among the scientific and social academics, clinicians, patients, and stakeholders, as well as society at large.

EVOLUTION OF GENETIC TESTS

In the broadest sense, any test that can identify and diagnose a genetic brain disease could be regarded as a "neurogenetic test." Historically, the recognition of the role of inheritance in the cause of diseases began with Garrod's (1909) concept of "inborn error of metabolism," after suggestions by Bateson (Bearn 1993). The first of these disorders he investigated was alkaptonuria, a metabolic disease associated with joint cartilage damage and valvular heart problems, which he recognized as a probable Mendelian recessive condition because of the observed cluster of cases in male and female children of apparently normal parents who were often consanguineous. Garrod's prediction of the biochemical defect was later confirmed by the demonstration of the enzyme deficiency in homogentisic acid oxidase in human (La Du and Zannoni 1956). The gene responsible for alkaptonuria was eventually identified in homogentisate 1,2 dioxygenase, an enzyme involved in the catabolism of the amino acids phenylalanine and tyrosine (Fernandez-Canon *et al.* 1996). Large-scale biochemical screening for a number of autosomal recessive metabolic diseases have been

Table 31.1 Some of the neurological conditions in which genetic testing is currently available

Neurological systems	Specific conditions
Neurometabolic syndromes	Wilson's disease, Gaucher's disease, Canavan's disease, Lesch–Nyhan disease, phenoketouria, ornithine-transcarbamylase deficiency, mitochondrial encephalopathy with lactic acidosis and stroke-like epidsodes (MELAS), mitochondrial encephalomyopathy with ragged red fibres (MERRF), Leber's optic neuropathy, Kearns–Sayre syndrome, progressive external ophthalmoplegia, Leigh Syndrome, X-linked albinism-deafness syndrome, adrenoleukodystrophy, metachromatic leukodystrophy, Krabbe disease, Canavan disease, Cockayne syndrome, creatine deficiency syndromes, Menkes disease, Refsum disease, gangliosidoses, glycogen storage disease (some types), mucorlipidosis, mucopolysaccharidosis
Childhood developmental neurogenetic disorders	Angelman's syndrome, Prader–Willi syndrome, fragile X syndrome and FMR1-related disorders, Down syndrome, Lujan syndrome, MASA syndrome, fragile X mental retardation 2, Miller–Dieker syndrome, Rett syndrome, X-linked and 17-linked lissencephaly
Hereditary movement disorders	Friedreich's ataxia, Huntington's disease, spinocerebellar ataxias (types 1, 2, 3, 6, 7, 8), dentatorubral-pallidoluysian atrophy, episodic ataxias (type 1 and 2), early-onset primary dystonia (DYT1), chorea and dementia
Dementias	Familial early onset Alzheimer disease due to presenilin mutations and APP mutations, familial frontotemporal dementia due to tau and progranulin mutations, familial Creutzfeldt–Jakob disease, fatal familial insomnia
Disorders of muscles and nerves	Myotonic dystrophy, Duchenne and Becker muscular dystrophy, Emery–Dreifuss muscular dystrophy, facioscapulohumeral muscular dystrophy, sarcoglycanopathies, spinomuscular atrophy types 1-3, Charcot-Marie-Tooth disease (type 1, 2, 4, and X-linked, as well as subtypes), hereditary neuropathy with liability to pressure palsy, familial transthyretin amyloidosis, familial dysautonmia
Headache	Familial hemiplegic migraine (type 1, 2 & 3)
Epilepsy	Benign familial neonatal epilepsy, juvenile myoclonic epilepsy related to CACNB4, CLCN2, EFHC1, GABRA1, GABRD, autosomal dominant nocturnal frontal lobe epilepsy
Strokes	Cerebral autosomal dominant arteriopathy with small vessels ischemic leukoencephalopathy (CADASIL), Fabry disease
Neurocutaneous syndromes	Neurofibromatosis, types 1, 2, tuberous sclerosis complex, Von Hippel–Lindau syndrome

developed and implemented. These include neonatal screening of phenylketouria and hypothyroidism, in which early diagnosis and treatment has help reduced the incidence of mental retardation in children significantly over the last several decades.

Advances in cytogenetics characterize another important era in the history of human genetic testing. Since the depiction of the human chromosome by Flemming in 1882, a number of attempts were made to determine the correct number of chromosomes in the human. In the 1950s, improvements in cytogenetics technology allowed visualization of chromosomes as the "organ of interest" for medical geneticists, analogous to the heart for cardiologists, and the brain for neurologists. This "golden age" of cytogenetics from the 1950s to 60s came with the identification of a number of genetic disorders based on an abnormal number of chromosomes or chromosomal rearrangements (Allen *et al.* 1961). With more recent refinement of fluorescent markers in cytogenetics technology, very fine and specific abnormalities on the chromosomes can now be visualized using fluorescent *in situ* hybridization (FISH) methods. Neurodevelopmental conditions that can now be tested using FISH technology include Prader–Willi syndrome, Angelman syndrome, and some forms of Down syndrome related to chromosomal translocation.

Contemporary human molecular neurogenetics began with the identification of molecular markers linking families with Huntington's disease (HD) to chromosome 4. Even before the actual gene responsible for HD was identified, genetic predictive testing was made possible by the use of these polymorphic genetic markers surrounding the Huntington locus and tracing the inheritance pattern of affected individuals through the family tree (genetic linkage analysis). After a decade-long effort, the disease causing the trinucleotide repeat in the Huntington gene was finally identified (Gusella *et al.* 1993). Most of the current molecular genetic tests require direct sequencing of DNA fragments to identify the mutations. While these tests are highly specific, they are laborious and expensive to conduct, and in some situations, the results can be indeterminate (see section on limitations of genetic tests later in this chapter). This gives rise to another set of challenges related to test availability and provisioning, and the value of genetic testing to people and society.

APPLICATIONS OF GENETIC TESTS

The United States Task Force for Genetic Testing defines a genetic test as "the analysis of human DNA, RNA, chromosomes, proteins, and metabolites in order to detect heritable disease related to genotypes, mutations, phenotypes, or karyotypes for clinical purposes" (Task Force on Genetic Testing 2003). Genetic tests can be used in healthcare to detect gene variants associated with a specific diseases or conditions, and in non-clinical applications such for forensics, paternity testing and anthropological research. Clinical genetic testing is generally utilized in one of the five following situations:

1) Diagnostic testing of a symptomatic patient.

2) Pre-natal testing of a pregnant symptomatic or at-risk individual or carrier couple.

3) Carrier testing in a parent, sibling, or other relative of an individual with a autosomal or X-linked recessive disorder, or screening of high-risk ethnic groups or population isolates.

4) Predictive testing of an asymptomatic individual at-risk for a specific disorder.

5) Risk factor assessment of asymptomatic individuals with (or without) a family history of a particular condition.

Most clinicians are accustomed to using genetic tests to confirm a clinical diagnosis of a particular neurogenetic disease. However, once a genetic diagnosis is made in a symptomatic patient, there are immediate implications for the family as certain blood relatives will be at risk. Therefore, it is imperative for the clinician ordering the genetic test to be cognizant of the diagnostic and predictive power of the test, and the connotations of positive and negative results with respect to how they affect the probabilities that a patient, family member, or potential child has or will develop a particular disease.

In non-medical settings, one of the most common applications is in forensics. Since the number of DNA variations in human is in the order of 10^9, it is extremely unlikely that the molecular DNA profile of a person (DNA-fingerprint) would randomly match that of another person in the population (National Research Council (USA) 1996). In Canada, the Royal Canadian Mounted Police uses three multiplex systems which is said to have excellent discrimination potential of any biological sample obtain from a victim or suspect at a crime scene. The estimated frequency of the average genetic profile in the Canadian population across 10 single tandem repeat loci (the molecular DNA variation used in the system) is one in 94 billion (Curran 1997). DNA-fingerprinting for paternity testing has also become common in civil use. Because of its high specificity, a matching result would practically confirms with certainty that the child is an offspring of the individual in question. The only exception in these cases of identity testing would be the existence of an identical twin, who would have the same genetic make up of the person of interest, and cannot be simply differentiated using a DNA sample. Molecular DNA genotyping also enabled significant advances in human anthropological and genealogical research. Since Y chromosomes are passed on exclusively from fathers to sons while mitochondrial DNA are passed on exclusively from mothers to children, molecular variations in these structures can be examined to determine the origin of paternal and maternal lineage. This proved to be a powerful tool in the study of genetic history of an individual or a whole population (Cavalli-Sforza and Feldman 2003; Pakendorf and Stoneking 2005).

Confirmation of diagnosis

The most common scenario in which a genetic test is ordered is for confirmation of a diagnosis. For example, if a patient presents with symptoms of abnormal movements of chorea suspicious of HD, a genetic test can help the physician to expeditiously confirm the specific diagnosis and exclude other conditions. Similarly, a patient with progressive peripheral neuropathy with an autosomal dominant family history can be tested for Charcot–Marie–Tooth disease, eliminating the exhaustive screen for other causes of neuropathy. Using genetic tests in this situation usually has little ethical concern because the results enable clinicians to establish an accurate and specific diagnosis in symptomatic patients that expedite further treatment and minimize other unnecessary investigations. Even if there is no treatment available for the condition, a clear and specific diagnosis will help clarify the natural history, progression, and prognosis of the disease, and allow the patient and family to make informed decisions on long-term life plans. The psychological benefits of simply putting a name to the previously unknown sets of mysterious symptoms cannot be ignored either (Wiggins *et al.* 1992; Meiser *et al.* 2000; Butow *et al.* 2003). However, good counseling is particularly essential if a test is not completely diagnostic and the full implications of the results unknown (Rantanen *et al.* 2008).

PRENATAL TESTING

Prenatal genetic testing is sometimes an option for parents-to-be who are at risk for carry-ing a fetus with a neurogenetic condition. Unlike other medical screening tests to detect a treatable condition such as diabetes or high cholesterol, prenatal genetic testing is centered on reproductive decisions rather than management of a disease. Furthermore, many of the current prenatal tests are intended for screening only, and further invasive testing such as amniocentesis or chorionic villus biopsy may be required for confirmation of a diagnosis. When no treatment is available, the women and couples may be faced with the decision of termination of pregnancy. An obvious contentious issue is the use of selective abortion as a form of treatment. The sequence of tests and decision-making options must be openly dis-cussed in advance during genetic counseling sessions and prior to testing so that the patient is fully aware of the potential options they may encounter.

CARRIER TESTING

Like pre-natal testing, carrier testing is also used for making reproductive choice rather than diagnostic or treatment choices. Carrier testing is most pertinent to recessively inherited conditions in which a carrier of a single abnormal disease gene will not be affected by the disease, but can pass the gene on to offspring. It is also relevant to X-linked disorders, such as Duchenne muscular dystrophy (DMD) and fragile X mental retardation, in which a woman carrying one copy of an abnormal X-linked gene may not develop disease symptoms because of the presence of a second normal copy on her other X chromosome, but can have affected sons whose only X chromosome contains the abnormal gene (Jarvinen *et al.* 1999). For adults, the rationale for carrier testing is simply to provide the reproductive risk assess-ment; however, there are legitimate concerns about carrier testing in minors due to differing levels of maturity and ability of children to understand such health-related information (Wertz and Reilly 1997; Davis 1998).

PREDICTIVE TESTING

Predictive (or presymptomatic) testing is the use of genetic test for the sole purpose of deter-mining the presence or absence of a disease-causing gene in an asymptomatic individual. Unlike traditional medical transactions, predictive genetic testing is a medical procedure performed on healthy individuals often with no therapeutic decisions to make, other than the patient's perceived psychosocial benefits, as most neurogenetic conditions do not have any effective preventive or disease-modifying treatment available to date. In addition, unlike a simple blood test which is usually a reflection of the health status of the individual only at the time of the test, a genetic test predicts future disease development which remains for the rest of his or her life. Once the knowledge is known, it cannot be unlearned. Moreover, a genetic test can intrude family and personal relationships (Sobel and Cowan 2000;

Williams *et al.* 2000; Decruyenaere *et al.* 2004). Potential harm of discovering an eventual death from an incurable disease includes exacerbation of anxiety, a sense of fatalism, depression, and even suicide (Wiggins *et al.* 1992; Almqvist *et al.* 1999). On the other hand, potential benefits of predictive testing include relief of anxiety in those found to be free of the disease gene, and perhaps relief of uncertainty in those found to carry it. Family, career, financial, and personal planning might be quite different for a particular individual if his or her genetic condition were known. The pros and cons of predictive testing were central to a number debates over the past decade, and different arguments have been put forth using medical, empirical, philosophical, religious, and ethical viewpoint (Bird 1989; Bloch and Hayden 1990; Jaki 1994; Jonsen *et al.* 1996; Tibben *et al.* 1997; Heinrichs 2005; Duncan and Delatycki 2006; Richards 2006). It is expected that the future driving force for predictive testing will be dictated by the discovery of effective preventive treatments and early interventions. For now, the choice to test or not remains in the hands of the individual, and an informed consent after adequate genetic counseling is a minimal prerequisite.

RISK FACTOR ASSESSMENT

Genetic risk factor analysis is expected to play an increasingly important role in healthcare for many common disorders, including many in the neurological realm (Paulson 2002). It is expected that most diseases are genetically complex; that is, the genes do not directly cause disease in the classical Mendelian manner, but alter the risk of development of a disease. In other words, the risk genes increase an individual susceptibility to develop the disease rather than directly causing the disease. The best-known example of a neurogenetic risk factor is apolipoprotein E (ApoE). There are three common polymorphisms of APOE: e2, e3, and e4. These are "polymorphisms" rather than "mutations" because they exist in more than 1% of the population, and are present in normal individuals. It is well-documented that the APOE e4 allele increases risk of developing AD, but it is neither necessary nor sufficient to cause the disease (Corder *et al.* 1993; Strittmatter *et al.* 1993). Not everyone with the Apo E4 allele will develop AD, and many people without the Apo E4 allele can still develop AD. Due to the relatively low predictive value of APOE, it is not currently recommended for diagnostic use in AD, or for screening of AD in the population (Hsiung and Sadovnick 2007). However, it may have some utility in assessing patients with cognitive impairment who are at risk of progression to AD (Petersen *et al.* 1995; Farrer *et al.* 1997; Hsiung *et al.* 2004). The benefits of genetic risk factor analysis may include relief of anxiety for those who are found to have a low-risk gene, and relief of uncertainty for those who do. Like predictive genetic testing, risk factor analysis will be much more valuable if the risk of developing the disease can be modified, either through medication or modification of risk factors in some way.

LIMITATIONS OF CURRENT GENETIC TESTS

When used properly, genetic information can enhance patients' ability to learn important facts about their own health and childbearing risks, thereby empowering them to make rational choices about life decisions based on accurate information. In the ideal situation, a clinical test should be 100% sensitive and 100% specific; that is, the test should exclude the presence of the disease when the test result is negative, and identify all cases of the disease when the test result is positive. While most genetic tests have been investigated in large samples of populations and therefore the actual predictive value is known, none of them are actually 100% sensitive and specific. This gives rise to the risk of providing incorrect diagnosis or interpretation of the results to the patients and their family. There are situations when a negative test result does not necessarily ensure that the tested person does not have a genetic disease. It simply implies that the person tested does not have the abnormality detected in using the particular laboratory technique (Laing 1993; Hoffman *et al.* 1996). For example, screening for DMD and a related but less severe phenotype Becker muscular dystrophy using serum creatine kinase, is only positive in about 70% of maternal carriers or patients in the early stages of disease patient. Even with more specific molecular genetic testing with polymerase chain reaction or Southern blot techniques, there are still up to 40% of DMD cases with undetectable mutations, requiring a muscle biopsy for definitive diagnosis. Furthermore, some genetic mutations can occur *de novo*, making genetic counseling and carrier detection for DMD more complicated than other genetic diseases with less frequent new mutations (Mukherjee *et al.* 2003; Helderman-van den Enden *et al.* 2009).

The current test for HD also exemplifies the complexities of genetic testing and interpretation. The screen targets an abnormal expansion of the trinucleotide CAG repeat sequence (Gusella *et al.* 1993). The correct interpretation of the test requires knowledge of the CAG repeat length and its relationship to disease expression. If a patient has an expansion of the CAG repeat in the HD gene with 40 or greater, there is 100% certainty that if the person lives long enough the disease will manifest. If the test result shows 26 or fewer CAG repeats, then the patient does not have HD. However, if the repeat length is 37–39, the individual is at risk for developing HD, but may not always develop symptoms (Rubinsztein *et al.* 1996). Finally, for individuals with intermediate CAG repeats in the 27–35 range, the genetic instability of the CAG trinucleotide sequence places them at risk of passing an expansion of this sequence. In this case, the offspring may inherit a fragment of the DNA in the disease-causing range (Potter *et al.* 2004; Semaka *et al.* 2006).

Diseases are also known to mimic each other with one disease presenting similarly to another—a phenocopy—but not from the same mutation. Such genetic heterogeneity is demonstrated, for example, by families with autosomal dominant inheritance presenting with a progressive choreiform movement disorder very similar to HD, but who do not have the HD gene mutation (Meenakshi-Sundaram *et al.* 2004; Wild and Tabrizi 2007). Recently, a new gene, JPH3 which codes for the protein junctophilin-3, has been associated with the "Huntington disease-like syndrome" type 2 (Margolis *et al.* 2001). In addition to HD and HD-like syndromes, there are a number of genetic conditions in which different genes can cause clinically indistinguishable phenotypes, as in the spinocerebellar ataxias, hereditary neuropathies, spinal muscular atrophies, and spastic paraplegias. For added complexity, there is also phenotypic heterogeneity of the same genetic mutation even within the same family. For example, mutations in the MAPT (tau) gene can lead to frontotemporal dementia, but some patients present with mostly with a parkinsonian type movement disorder rather than dementia, and the age of onset can be quite variable, even within the same pedigree (Grover *et al.* 1999; Reed *et al.* 2001; Baba *et al.* 2005).

ETHICAL CONCERNS AND DILEMMAS

Like most other situations in medical decision making, the ethical principles of autonomy, beneficence, non-maleficence, confidentiality, and justice should be applied to genetic testing. The duty to respect autonomy of others is paramount in the practice of medicine, and performing a genetic test is no exception. The principles of beneficence and non-maleficence should similarly be observed when assessing the risk and benefits of genetic testing. These principles are best applied through the informed consent process in which the purposes, potential benefits, risks, and limitations of a specific genetic test are openly discussed and explained to the potential subject. Confidentiality is also an important aspect of medical practice and is no different in genetic testing, but it is a fine line to tread as genetic records are often multigenerational and kindred based, and therefore requires extra care in ensuring privacy and data protection. A list of considerations when deciding on the potential benefits and harms of testing is shown in Table 31.2.

Justice is the assurance that all people receive fair and equal opportunity to treatment. While justice is a highly valued ethical principle, it is limited by the variation in medical provision in different parts of the world. In a universal healthcare system as in Canada, providing one type of medical service may necessitate the elimination of another procedure because of cost limitations. Furthermore, as some genetic tests are quite expensive to perform and are only available in certain academic medical centers, it may not be available to all geographic and socioeconomic groups. In addition, some genetic diseases are more common in certain ethnic groups and may be applied to specific populations at risk. For instance, Tay–Sachs disease is more common in Ashkenazi Jews with a carrier frequency of 1 in 30, whereas it is much lower in other ancestries. Therefore, it may not be practical to provide the genetic tests to other populations unless the family is specifically known to be at risk (i.e. having an affected child). By contrast, in a private user-payer healthcare system, many genetic tests are simply not covered by insurance. In these situations, the well-heeled will likely have much better access to these new technologies than others. Concerns have also been raised regarding disproportionate acquisition of genetic knowledge on Caucasians, as almost all large-scale genome-wide association studies to date have been focused on individuals of European ancestry while other racial and ethnic groups are only sparsely represented (Need and Goldstein 2009). Whilst there is clearly scientific basis and advantage to limit genomic studies to a specific population, for instance, minimizing the statistical bias of population stratification, any clinically informative research findings from these studies would have been applicable more to Europeans and less to other racial groups. The complexities of applying the principles of justice in genomic medicine in the context of public health have been explored by others and require close scrutiny to achieve maximum benefits for the whole society without leaving others behind (Jonsen *et al.* 1996; Clayton 2003).

PATIENT CONFIDENTIALITY AND THE FAMILY UNIT

As genetic test may reveal information pertains not only to the individual tested but to other family members, conflicts may arise when family members have opposite wishes, as exemplified in the situation described in Box 31.1.

Table 31.2 Issues to consider when deciding for or against genetic testing

	Potential benefits	Potential harm
Cost of the test	Free (test covered by medical insurance, or research funding)	Expense (test not covered by medical insurance or research funding, and patients have to pay out of pocket)
Treatment of underlying condition	Potential for earlier treatment, stabilization of disease	Current treatment not very effective or not available; Potential side effects of treatment
Planning for future	Family/reproductive planning Financial and employment planning	Negative impact on career choice Limitations in employment, genetic discrimination
Relationships	Positive: support from family and friends	Negative: altered relationships, isolation from family and friends
Research	Understanding of the research—promise of future advances Potential to contribute to society to understand of the condition/diagnosis	Understanding of the research—limitations of current knowledge Perception of being used as "guinea pigs"
Psychological impact	Comfort of knowing not being affected, and ability to make long-term plans if affected	Anxiety and/or depression after learning about disease status Hypervigilance to symptoms Fear of loss of confidence, autonomy, independence Fear of inadvertent disclosure to others Survivor guilt if not affected
Social impact	Legal or social uses of genetic information—e.g. application for disability Availability and access to treatment or care	Social isolation Stigmatization, labeling, Higher insurance premium Healthcare disparities
Religious influence	Spiritual support from friends and family	Against some religions to "interfere with the will of God"

When the test result reveals the genetic status of another family member, the conflict of autonomy may arise because testing one individual (who wishes to know his/her genetic status) may affect another's autonomy (who does not wish to know). A more blatant, albeit rare, example would be the situation for identical twins who possess the same genetic make-up. What if one twin wishes to receive the genetic test, but the other does not? Could genetic testing and counseling be provided to the sibling who consented and the result kept confidential without ever inadvertently disclosing it to the other non-consenting sibling? While possible, it would be highly impractical; and clearly, such disagreements should ideally be openly discussed and resolved prior to testing to minimize untoward feelings among involved members afterwards.

Box 31.1 The case of the family feud

Mrs A, age 45, is at risk for developing HD because her mother, who is now 65, has recently been diagnosed with the disorder. Mrs A has been told by genetic counselors that she has a 50% chance of inheriting the disease gene from her mother, and has been advised to discuss this with the rest of her family. Mrs A has decided not to receive predictive testing herself, as she would not want to live with the burden and anxiety of knowing if she turns out to be a carrier of the disease gene, she will be destined to the same fate as her mother in the future. However, her daughter Mrs B, age 22, has recently married, and after learning about her own risk, she and her husband both feel that it would be beneficial for her to receive predictive testing so that they can make proper family planning decisions. The problem is that if Mrs B is indeed tested positive, then Mrs A, being her biological mother, must also be a carrier of the disease gene. Testing Mrs B, who is fully informed and consenting, would indirectly test Mrs A against her wish.

Another situation where conflict may arise is when a patient does not want to disclose genetic information that may be beneficial for other family members to know. The protection of privacy of a genetic test result for one family member may mean other family members who are at risk of the disease remain unaware of this risk (see Box 31.2).

In the situation described in Box 31.2, identifying Mrs C as a carrier for the fragile X gene mutation means that other maternal family members, including her mother and sister, may also be carriers of this gene mutation. This raises the issue about whether the clinician has a duty to warn other family members of their risk against the patient's wish to keep the genetic results private. Depending on the jurisdiction, disclosure of health information is governed by local privacy legislations, which usually identifies genetic test results the same as confidential medical information and is protected by the privacy rule (Burgess *et al.* 1998; Godard *et al.* 2003a). Some have argued that when the health of others are jeopardized, the clinician

---

Box 31.2 The case of the untold secret

Mrs C is in her first trimester of her first pregnancy. She has a younger sister who is also married but who does not yet have children. She also has a brother who has developmental delay, but the cause is unknown. Her mother believed it was due to birth trauma, but no genetic tests have ever been done on her brother. However, Mrs C is concerned about her own risk of carrying a child with developmental delay. She asks her obstetrician to determine "her own chance of having a child with mental retardation." Genetic testing performed on her revealed that she is indeed a carrier of a fragile X mutation, an X-linked disorder that always cause developmental delay and mental disability in male carriers. The phenotype is heterogeneous in females because they carry two copies of the X chromosome, with one copy variably inactivated. Mrs C decided to pursue further prenatal testing on her fetus, and it is determined that she has a boy who has not inherited the fragile X gene mutation. She is relieved by this news, but she also realizes that her mother is probably a carrier, and her sister is also at risk for being a carrier. However, she does not want anyone else in the family to know about her own test, because her mother may become very upset upon learning this news. On the other hand, her sister is at risk of carrying the disease mutation and passing on to her children.

should have an affirmative obligation to raise this issue during counseling and to go beyond the traditional non-directive model of genetic counseling in leading the proband to optimal health values with regard to disclosure (Minkoff and Ecker 2008). Of course, such measures should not be taken lightly, but how serious a disease must be before such action is required is open for debate. In Canada and the US, a clinician must not disclose any genetic information without the signed consent from the patient (McMahon and Lee-Huber 2001). However, this notion is being challenged as some genetic diseases are now treatable and preventable, as in the case of certain familial cancer syndromes such as BRCA1 for familial breast cancer, or APC gene-associated familial polyposis. In these situations, early screening and treatment may be life-saving, and the harm of not warning others at risk may be much greater than the benefit of protecting the privacy of a few.

As demonstrated in the boxed scenarios, ethical conflicts between family members are not uncommon in genetics, often occurring in situations where the care, needs, or desires of one family member conflict with those of another family member. It must be recognized that the basic unit of care in genetics is really the family rather than a single patient, so conflicts such as these may be inevitable. Valuable lessons learned from predictive testing in HD have led the way for defining a safe and reasonable clinical approach (IHA and WFN 1994). Emphasis is placed on the process of genetic counseling, during which accurate information about the patient's disease risk, as well as the nature, limitations, uncertainties, and medical implications of the test, are provided to the patient. An ongoing supportive rapport is established with the patient to help minimize the risk of psychosocial harm during or after the test.

Balancing risk and harm

When a genetic test is used for confirmation of a diagnosis, there is usually little ethical concern because finding out the exact diagnosis is often in the interest of the already symptomatic patient. However, the situation is less clear for predictive testing, as the benefits of knowing the future disease occurrence must be weighted against the psychological and social risk. It has been argued that it is morally wrong to use predictive genetic testing for HD because of the severe psychological burden a patient must face, as it would be "kinder to ask those at risk of the illness, but lucky enough not to have inherited it to forego such a test and live with their uncertainty, in order to provide the other 50% who carry the lethal gene with some hope during their remaining years." (Marsden 1981). This potential psychosocial burden has in fact been investigated in various studies. While severe psychiatric distress after predictive testing for HD has been shown to be quite low, milder degrees of depression and anxiety are common and can occur even in individuals found to be free of the disease gene (Meiser and Dunn 2000). The Canadian Collaborative Study of Predictive Testing for Huntington's Disease explored the psychological impact of test results on at-risk subjects, and sure enough found that psychological distress scores were lower in those who tested negatively as opposed to those who tested positively. Interestingly, it is also found that the psychological distress scores were lowered in those who tested positively compared to those who remained untested (Wiggins et al. 1992). This suggests that just knowing for certain, even when tested positive, relieves much of the anxiety of at-risk patients and diminishes their psychological suffering. The psychological benefits to the patient and partner persist at 3-year follow-up (Tibben *et al.* 1997). In a more recent randomized controlled trial comparing the psychological and emotional outcomes of revealing the APOE genotype to children of parents with AD, there were no significant differences between those who received their APOE genotyping results vs. those who did not in measures of anxiety, depression, or test-related stress. Not surprisingly, the APOE e4-positive subgroup (with increased risk of developing AD) had significantly higher level of test-related distress than did the APOE e4-negative subgroup (Green *et al.* 2009). However, these feelings were transient and were not associated with clinically significant psychological distress.

GENETIC TESTING IN MINORS

Genetic testing in children remains a controversial topic. When a child becomes symptomatic from a genetic disease, it is generally justified to obtain genetic testing for the purpose of confirmation of a diagnosis. However, testing of asymptomatic children at-risk for a genetic disease is generally not recommended or even allowed (Clarke 1994; IHA and WFN 1994; ASHG 1995; ESHG 2009).

In the scenario in Box 31.3, testing the children would have violated their right to decide for themselves for genetic testing when they become an adult, and worse, the results might have led to discrimination against the siblings who tested positive. Many arguments have been developed opposing the use of predictive genetic tests in children (Duncan 2004). First, they would lose the opportunity to make an autonomous decision about testing as an adult. This is supported by the fact that many adults at risk for HD choose not to undergo predictive testing (Bloch and Hayden 1990). Second, there is concern about confidentiality since test results are given to their parents, whereas in an adult, he or she may choose not to disclose this information to anyone else. Third, there is always a concern for potential psychological harm, as children may misunderstand the complex information related to the genetic test, or perceive a positive result as a punishment. Others have shown the risk of developing a sense of unworthiness or even clinical depression. On the contrary, some have argued that many young people are indeed competent enough to make a decision about

---

Box 31.3 The case of unconsented testing

Mrs D has developed HD in her 40s. She is a single mother with 4 children, Adam, Bella, Charlie, and David, ages 5 to 12. Her husband has passed away from a tragic accident. Because of the decline in her health, Mrs D is not able to care for her children any longer, and they are placed through the local social service agency for adoption. There is a couple interested in adopting one her children, but would not want to adopt a child carrying the HD gene because it would be a traumatic event to go through, and would "bring the disease" into their family. None of the children have any symptoms of HD. The neurologist of Mrs D performed genetic testing in her four children and found that Charlie and David are normal, but Adam and Bella are carriers of the HD mutation.

testing themselves and cope very well with learning their gene status (Clayton 1997; Dickenson 1999; Clayton 2008). The knowledge of the genetic result may even help them to better prepare for the future (Malpas 2008). In any case, further empirical evidence to guide future policy development on this issue is needed (Duncan and Delatycki 2006; Borry *et al.* 2008).

DILEMMAS IN PRENATAL TESTING

Prenatal testing is generally acceptable for severe diseases that begin in childhood. For example, childhood Tay–Sachs disease is particularly stressful for parents since an affected new-born baby appears perfectly healthy in the first few months of life, but developmental milestones are delayed by the first year of life. This is followed by progressive blindness, mental regression, seizures, and invariably death by age 3–4 years. Few would argue against the benefits of relieving parents from the years of stress and trauma caring for their dying child versus the harm of aborting a fetus that would have no hope of growing up. However, the line is less clear for adult onset of disorders such as AD and HD that occur much later in life. Should one deny the right of a fetus to live 30–40 good years before he or she develops disability and dementia (Squitieri *et al.* 2001; Godbolt *et al.* 2004)? For a child with developmental disability such as Down syndrome, early diagnosis can optimize disease management. By contrast, for an adult onset neurological disease such as AD, what if a parent decided to screen the fetus but later decided not to abort after the fetus was tested positive? This child would then be growing up with the burden of knowledge that he or she will develop AD later in life. This clearly violates the principle of autonomy and informed consent of the child to decide when and whether to know about his or her genetic status as an adult. Further issues on prenatal testing and selective abortion include the debate about the ethics of sterilizing disabled children in the context of the eugenics movement (Raz 2005; Landeweerd 2009), which will not be elaborated here. In general, prenatal testing of adult-onset diseases is not recommended, although in some specific situations, it may be offered in a case-by-case basis after discussion with the local institutional ethics review board (Hsiung and Sadovnick 2007).

INAPPROPRIATE USE OF GENETIC INFORMATION

One of the greatest concerns of genetic testing is the possibility of workplace or insurance discrimination for those who tested positive for genetic condition. This remains the subject of ongoing investigation, discussion, and legislation. Some have cited fear of losing insurance as a major reason to avoid genetic testing (Lapham *et al.* 1996). Citing an example provided in an article by Clayton on the ELSI of genomic medicine (Clayton 2003), a US railroad company started obtaining blood for DNA testing from employees who were seeking disability compensation for carpal tunnel syndrome when testing for the genetic condition of hereditary neuropathy with liability to pressure palsy (HNPP) became available. This recommendation allegedly came from its company physician, who in turn had apparently relied on the representations of a genetic diagnostic company which offered the test, but the employees were not told of the purpose of the test. Although not stated explicitly, it was suspected that the company intention was to deny disability to any employee who possessed this mutation, arguing the mutation rather than injury from work, caused the carpel tunnel syndrome. When this was uncovered, the federal Equal Employment Opportunity Commission immediately stopped this practice, and the company settled claims brought by its employees for an undisclosed sum of money. This made no sense medically because HNPP is rare, affecting only 3–10 persons per 100,000 (Chance and Lupski 1994). Therefore, most carpal tunnel syndrome sufferers are not carriers of this mutation. Nonetheless, this case illustrated the potential for genetic information misuse in employment and insurance situations. Needless to say, this led to widespread criticism and immediate calls to ban genetic discrimination in the workplace. The Health Insurance Portability and Accountability Act (HIPAA) now prohibits group health insurers from excluding presymptomatic persons from coverage based on genetic test results (McMahon and Lee-Huber 2001; U.S. Department of Health and Human Services 2009). In the US, many states have enacted genetic non-discrimination legislation, with provisions that, in some cases, exceed those of HIPAA. The Genetic Information Nondiscrimination Act has recently been passed in the U.S. which prohibits employers "from hiring, firing, or determining promotions based on genetic make up". It also prohibits discrimination on the basis of genetic background in group and individual health insurance plans (A Ban on Genetic Discrimination, *New York Times* 2009). However, no limits were placed on rate setting of the insurance policy. On the other hand, certain genetic conditions may affect a person's ability to perform on certain jobs that could not be reasonably accommodated. For example, persons with uncontrolled genetic epilepsy or untreatable cardiac arrhythmia ought not be truck drivers or commercial pilots due to the risk to third parties. Debates on optimal solutions are still ongoing, and the challenge with clinicians and stakeholders will be to determine the most appropriate use of genetic information in an equitable society.

DIRECT-TO-CONSUMER MARKETING OF GENETICS

With new technologies making genetic testing much more affordable, direct-to-consumer genetic testing is now available by a number of private companies, with regulation lagging behind (Shirts and Parker 2008; Goddard *et al.* 2009). Test kits can now be ordered through the Internet, and all people have to do is to spit into tubes, send in the samples by mail for DNA analysis, and out comes a detailed genetic report including their ancestry, plus their possible susceptibility to disorders that have been linked, but often unconfirmed, to particular genes. Companies that offer these tests often promote the privacy of their results, bypassing the clinician. However, consumers are not reminded that failure to indicate results of genetic testing in life insurance or disability application could be considered as fraud. Furthermore, many companies do not indicate on their policies what is done with the DNA sample after the analysis; hence, the perceived privacy and confidentiality may actually be jeopardized. In addition, most of these companies do not offer any assistance for the consumer regarding the proper interpretation of the genetic results, and there is no support to handle the emotional effects of learning about risks of any diseases. A few companies do offer some counseling, but concerns have been raised regarding potential conflict of interest because the company employing the counselor receives no compensation unless the consumer orders the test. The US Food and Drug Administration have issued a public statement advising consumers to be skeptical of the claims that the tests offered. Similarly, the UK Human Genetics Commission recently developed a set of principles to help guide consumers and to promote high standards and consistency among personal-genomics providers. Some argue that these guidelines are not enough, and government regulators may need to interfere when self-policing by the industry does not offer consumers adequate protection (Putting DNA to the test, *Nature* 2009).

Genetic counseling is now considered an essential step when advising a patient with a neurogenetic disorder. Sometimes counseling can be relatively uncomplicated and can be provided by qualified healthcare professionals. For complex cases, referral to a genetic counselor or medical geneticist is advised. Appropriate pre-test and post-test counseling must be provided, including a discussion of the correct diagnosis, recurrent risk, expression and penetrance of the disease, natural history, need for further testing (i.e. confirmatory tests), genetic options such as prenatal testing, adoption, artificial insemination, pre-implantation, treatment options, and plan for follow-up, including referral to relevant specialists and support groups. Unless all of these considerations are addressed, direct and home genetic testing should be discouraged because the potential harm of a misinterpreted or inaccurate result far outweighs the benefits of convenience of home testing (American College of Obstetricians and Gynecologists 2008).

EMERGING CONFLICTS: MOLECULAR GENETICS MEETS BEHAVIORAL NEUROSCIENCE

As genetic research moves from the search for disease genes to those of behavior, the provision of genetic testing in such situations becomes even more contentious (Newson 2004). Genes responsible for certain behavioral traits such as aggression, violence, anxiety, and even "novelty seeking" have been reported (Hill *et al.* 1999; Caspi *et al.* 2002; Luciano *et al.* 2004; Lesch 2005; Nelson and Trainor 2007; Wray *et al.* 2007). While scientists may perceive many potential benefits of such discoveries to society, such as improving our understand of these troubled behaviors and developing new therapies based on these findings, there are two obvious dilemmas arising from these new discoveries. First, if genes can be proven to be largely responsible for a person's behavior, then at what point is one person truly accountable for his or her own action? I can foresee a crisis happening in the criminal justice system. Analogous to the insanity argument that can overturn an alleged charge of criminal action in a schizophrenic, a defendant might use a similar hereditary argument to claim that the violent behavior that led to a criminal action is a result of his/her genetic make up rather than his/her own free will (Levitt and Manson 2007; Pieri and Levitt 2008). Second, if selective abortion is allowed for certain genetic disorders, could prenatal testing also be applied to choose a child with a preferred behavioral trait (i.e. one that is calm and attentive) against another (i.e. one who is violent and has attention deficit) (Birch 2005; Savulescu *et al.* 2006)? One could not help but conjure up memories of the eugenic movements from the late

19th century to after the Second World War (Smith and Nelson 1989; Gejman and Weilbaecher 2002; Schulze *et al.* 2004). Perhaps society must draw a line to distinguish a behavioral trait from a disease trait, and determine how this knowledge can be applied when making reproductive choices. Fortunately, our technology has not reached such a level of sophistication yet, but anticipating these problems and trying to resolve them with public input and open debate prior to mayhem seems prudent.

CONCLUSION

Genetic tests have proven to be extremely valuable in many clinical neurological situations. The availability of genetic tests for diseases such as the hereditary neuropathies, muscular dystrophies, HD, progressive ataxias, and other neurodegenerative disorders, has greatly simplified the diagnostic process for these conditions. However, the ability to provide an accurate and specific diagnosis of a neurogenetic disorder moves us beyond the realm of one-to-one care and extends our responsibility of care to other family members. After giving a genetic diagnosis, one must also be prepared to address questions about risks to other family members, including the children of the tested individual. As more gene tests become available for a wider range of disease-causing genes and disease-predisposing genetic variants, clinicians will be called upon to explain complex genetic concepts to their patients. It is also important to be aware of the potential ethical conflicts inherent in genetic testing, so that one can maximize the benefits of these tests to patients and minimize their harm.

ACKNOWLEDGMENTS

Dr. Hsiung is supported by a Canadian Institute of Health Research Clinical Genetics Investigatorship award, as well as funds from the Alzheimer Society of British Columbia and the Fisher Professorship. The author would also like to thank Dr Lynn Beattie for her helpful comments on the initial draft.

REFERENCES

A Ban on Genetic Discrimination (2009). [editorial] *New York Times*, 21 November 2009.

Allen, G., Benda, C.E., Book, J.A., *et al.* (1961). Mongolism. *American Journal of Human Genetics*, 13, 426.

Almqvist, E.W., Bloch, M., Brinkman, R., Craufurd, D., and Hayden, M.R. (1999). A worldwide assessment of the frequency of suicide, suicide attempts, or psychiatric hospitalization after predictive testing for Huntington disease. *American Journal of Human Genetics*, 64, 1293–304.

American College of Obstetricians and Gynecologists (2008). ACOG Committee Opinion No. 409: Direct-to-consumer marketing of genetic testing. *Obstetrics and Gynecology*, **111**, 1493–4.

ASHG (1995). Points to consider: ethical, legal, and psychosocial implications of genetic testing in children and adolescents. American Society of Human Genetics Board of Directors, American College of Medical Genetics Board of Directors. *American Journal of Human Genetics*, **57**, 1233–41.

Baba, Y., Tsuboi, Y., and Baker, M.C., *et al.* (2005). The effect of tau genotype on clinical features in FTDP-17. *Parkinsonism & Related Disorders*, **11**, 205–8.

Bearn, A.G. (1993). *Archibald Garrod and the Individuality of Man*. Oxford: Clarendon Press.

Birch, K. (2005). Beneficence, determinism and justice: an engagement with the argument for the genetic selection of intelligence. *Bioethics*, **19**, 12–28.

Bird, S.J. (1989). Genetic testing for neurologic diseases. A rose with thorns. *Neurologic Clinics*, **7**, 859–70.

Bloch, M. and Hayden, M.R. (1990). Opinion: predictive testing for Huntington disease in childhood: challenges and implications. *American Journal of Human Genetics*, **46**, 1–4.

Borry, P., Goffin, T., Nys, H., and Dierickx, K. (2008). Predictive genetic testing in minors for adult-onset genetic diseases. *Mount Sinai Journal of Medicine*, **75**, 287–96.

Burgess, M.M., Laberge, C.M., Knoppers, B.M. (1998). Bioethics for clinicians: 14. Ethics and genetics in medicine. *Canadian Medical Association Journal*, **158**, 1309–13.

Butow, P.N., Lobb, E.A., Meiser, B., Barratt, A., and Tucker, K.M. (2003). Psychological outcomes and risk perception after genetic testing and counselling in breast cancer: a systematic review. *The Medical Journal of Australia*, **178**, 77–81.

Caspi, A., McClay J., Moffitt. T.E., *et al.* (2002). Role of genotype in the cycle of violence in maltreated children. *Science*, **297**, 851–4.

Cavalli-Sforza, L.L. and Feldman, M.W. (2003). The application of molecular genetic approaches to the study of human evolution. *Nature Genetics*, **33**, 266–75.

Chance, P.F. and Lupski, J.R. (1994). Inherited neuropathies: Charcot–Marie–Tooth disease and related disorders. *Baillieres Clinical Neurology*, **3**, 373–85.

Clarke, A. (1994). The genetic testing of children. Working Party of the Clinical Genetics Society (UK). *Journal of Medical Genetics*, **31**, 785–97.

Clayton, E.W. (1997). Genetic testing in children. *Journal of Medicine and Philosophy*, **22**, 233–51.

Clayton, E.W. (2003). Ethical, legal, and social implications of genomic medicine. *New England Journal of Medicine*, **349**, 562–9.

Clayton, E.W. (2008). Testing teens: a commentary. *Journal of Genetic Counseling*, **17**, 526–7.

Corder, E.H., Saunders, A.M., Strittmatter, W.J., *et al.* (1993). Gene dose of apolipoprotein E type 4 allele and the risk of Alzheimer's disease in late onset families. *Science*, **261**, 921–3.

Curran, T. (1997). *Forensic DNA Analysis: Technology and Application*. Ottawa, ON: Parliametary Research Branch (PRB), Library of Parliament, Canada.

Davis, D.S. (1998). Discovery of children's carrier status for recessive genetic disease: some ethical issues. *Genetic Testing*, **2**, 323–7.

Decruyenaere, M., Evers-Kiebooms, G., Cloostermans, T., *et al.* (2004). Predictive testing for Huntington's disease: relationship with partners after testing. *Clinical Genetics*, **65**, 24–31.

Dickenson, D.L. (1999). Can children and young people consent to be tested for adult onset genetic disorders? *British Medical Journal*, **318**, 1063–5.

Duncan, R.E. (2004). Predictive genetic testing in young people: when is it appropriate? *Journal of Paediatrics and Child Health*, **40**, 593–5.

Duncan, R.E. and Delatycki, M.B. (2006). Predictive genetic testing in young people for adult-onset conditions: where is the empirical evidence? *Clinical Genetics*, **69**, 8–20.

European Society of Human Genetics. (2009). Provision of genetic services in Europe: current practices and issues. Available at: https://www.eshg.org/fileadmin/eshg/documents/20090519DraftRecommendationsGeneticTestingandCommonDisorder.pdf

Farrer, L.A., Cupples, L.A., and Haines, J.L. (1997). Effects of age, sex, and ethnicity on the association between apolipoprotein E genotype and Alzheimer disease. A meta-analysis. APOE and Alzheimer Disease Meta Analysis Consortium. *Journal of the American Medical Association*, **278**, 1349–56.

Fernandez-Canon, J.M., Granadino, B., and Beltran-Valero de Bernabe, D. (1996). The molecular basis of alkaptonuria. *Nature Genetics*, **14**, 19–24.

Fukushima, Y. (2005a). [Ethical guidelines on genetic testing and gene therapy]. *Nippon Rinsho*, **63**, 389–93.

Fukushima, Y. (2005b). [Guidelines on genetic research and genetic testing]. *Nippon Rinsho*, **63**, 9–15.

Gejman, P.V. and Weilbaecher, A. (2002). History of the eugenic movement. *The Israeli Journal of Psychiatry and Related Sciences*, **39**, 217–31.

GeneTests (2009). GeneTests website. Available at: http://www.ncbi.nlm.nih.gov/sites/GeneTests/?db=GeneTests

Godard, B., Kaariainen, H., Kristoffersson, U., Tranebjaerg, L., Coviello, D., and Ayme, S. (2003a). Provision of genetic services in Europe: current practices and issues. *European Journal of Human Genetics*, **11**, S13–48.

Godard, B., Raeburn, S., Pembrey, M., Bobrow, M., Farndon, P., and Ayme, S. (2003b). Genetic information and testing in insurance and employment: technical, social and ethical issues. *European Journal of Human Genetics*, **11**, S123–42.

Godard, B., Schmidtke, J., Cassiman, J.J., and Ayme, S. (2003c). Data storage and DNA banking for biomedical research: informed consent, confidentiality, quality issues, ownership, return of benefits. A professional perspective. *European Journal of Human Genetics*, **11**, S88–122.

Godard, B., ten Kate, L., Evers-Kiebooms, G., and Ayme, S. (2003d). Population genetic screening programmes: principles, techniques, practices, and policies. *European Journal of Human Genetics*, **11**, S49–87.

Godbolt, A.K., Cipolotti, L., Watt, H., Fox, N.C., Janssen, J.C., and Rossor, M.N. (2004). The natural history of Alzheimer disease: a longitudinal presymptomatic and symptomatic study of a familial cohort. *Archives of Neurology*, **61**, 1743–8.

Goddard, K.A., Duquette, D., Zlot, A., *et al.* (2009). Public awareness and use of direct-to-consumer genetic tests: results from 3 state population-based surveys, 2006. *American Journal of Public Health*, **99**, 442–5.

Green, R.C., Roberts, J.S., Cupples, L.A., *et al.* (2009). Disclosure of APOE genotype for risk of Alzheimer's disease. *New England Journal of Medicine*, **361**, 245–54.

Grover, A., Houlden, H., Baker, M., *et al.* (1999). 5′ splice site mutations in tau associated with the inherited dementia FTDP-17 affect a stem-loop structure that regulates alternative splicing of exon 10. *Journal of Biological Chemistry*, **274**, 15134–43.

Gusella, J.F., MacDonald, M.E., Ambrose, C.M., and Duyao, M.P. (1993). Molecular genetics of Huntington's disease. *Archives of Neurology*, **50**, 1157–63.

Heinrichs, B. (2005). What should we want to know about our future? A Kantian view on predictive genetic testing. *Medicine, Health Care and Philosophy*, **8**, 29–37.

Helderman-van den Enden, A.T., de Jong, R., den Dunnen, J.T., *et al.* (2009). Recurrence risk due to germ line mosaicism: Duchenne and Becker muscular dystrophy. *Clinical Genetics*, **75**, 465–72.

Hill, S.Y., Zezza, N., Wipprecht, G., Locke, J., and Neiswanger, K. (1999). Personality traits and dopamine receptors (D2 and D4): linkage studies in families of alcoholics. *American Journal of Medical Genetics*, **88**, 634–41.

Hoffman, E.P., Pegoraro, E., Scacheri, P., *et al.* (1996). Genetic counseling of isolated carriers of Duchenne muscular dystrophy. *American Journal of Medical Genetics*, **63**, 573–80.

Hsiung, G.Y. and Sadovnick, A.D. (2007). Genetics and dementia: Risk factors, diagnosis, and management. *Alzheimers & Dementia*, **3**, 418–27.

Hsiung, G.Y., Sadovnick, A.D., and Feldman, H. (2004). Apolipoprotein E e4 genotype as a risk factor for cognitive decline and dementia: data from the Canadian Study of Health and Aging. *Canadian Medical Association Journal*, **171**, 863–7.

IHA and WFN (1994). Guidelines for the molecular genetics predictive test in Huntington's disease. International Huntington Association (IHA) and the World Federation of Neurology (WFN) Research Group on Huntington's Chorea. *Neurology*, **44**, 1533–6.

Jaki, S.L. (1994). Consistent bioethics and Christian consistency. *Linacre Quarterly*, **61**, 87–92.

Jarvinen, O., Lehesjoki, A.E., Lindlof, M., Uutela, A., and Kaariainen, H. (1999). Carrier testing of children for two X-linked diseases: a retrospective evaluation of experience and satisfaction of subjects and their mothers. *Genetic Testing*, **3**, 347–55.

Jonsen, A.R., Durfy, S.J., Burke, W., and Motulsky, A.G. (1996). The advent of the 'unpatients'. *Nature Medicine*, **2**, 622–4.

La Du, B.N. and Zannoni, V.G. (1956). A requirement for catalase in tyrosine metabolism: the oxidation of p-hydroxyphenylpyruvic acid to homogentisic acid. *Nature*, **177**, 574–5.

Laing, N.G. (1993). Molecular genetics and genetic counselling for Duchenne/Becker muscular dystrophy. *Molecular and Cell Biology of Human Diseases Series*, **3**, 37–84.

Landeweerd, L. (2009). Prenatal diagnosis and the trouble with eugenics. *Law and the Human Genome Review*, **30**, 35–61.

Lapham, E.V., Kozma, C., and Weiss, J.O. (1996). Genetic discrimination: perspectives of consumers. *Science*, **274**, 621–4.

Lesch, K.P. (2005). Serotonergic gene inactivation in mice: models for anxiety and aggression? *Novartis Foundation Symposium*, **268**, 111–70.

Levitt, M. and Manson, N. (2007). My genes made me do it? The implications of behavioural genetics for responsibility and blame. *Health Care Analysis*, **15**, 33–40.

Luciano, M., Zhu, G., Kirk, K.M., *et al.* (2004). Effects of dopamine receptor D4 variation on alcohol and tobacco use and on novelty seeking: multivariate linkage and association analysis. *American Journal of Medical Genetics, B Neuropsychiatric Genetics*, **124B**, 113–23.

Malpas, P.J. (2008). Predictive genetic testing of children for adult-onset diseases and psychological harm. *Journal of Medical Ethics*, **34**, 275–8.

Margolis, R.L., O'Hearn, E., Rosenblatt, A., *et al.* (2001). A disorder similar to Huntington's disease is associated with a novel CAG repeat expansion. *Annals of Neurology*, **50**, 373–80.

Marsden, C. (1981). Prediction of Huntington's disease. *Annals of Neurology*, **10**, 202–3.

McKusick, V. (2009). Online Mendelian Inheritance in Man (OMIM). Available at: http://www.ncbi.nlm.nih.gov/sites/entrez?db=OMIM

McMahon, E.B. and Lee-Huber, T. (2001). HIPPA privacy regulations: practical information for physicians. *Pain Physician*, **4**, 280–4.

McPherson, J.D., Marra, M., Hillier, L., *et al.* (2001). A physical map of the human genome. *Nature*, **409**, 934–41.

Meenakshi-Sundaram, S., Arun Kumar, M.J., Sridhar, R., Rani, U., and Sundar, B. (2004). Neuroacanthocytosis misdiagnosed as Huntington's disease: a case report. *Journal of the Neurological Sciences*, **219**, 163–6.

Meiser, B. and Dunn, S. (2000). Psychological impact of genetic testing for Huntington's disease: an update of the literature. *Journal of Neurology, Neurosurgery & Psychiatry*, **69**, 574–8.

Meiser, B., Gleeson, M.A., and Tucker, K.M. (2000). Psychological impact of genetic testing for adult-onset disorders. An update for clinicians. *The Medical Journal of Australia*, **172**, 126–9.

Minkoff, H. and Ecker, J. (2008). Genetic testing and breach of patient confidentiality: law, ethics, and pragmatics. *American Journal of Obstetrics and Gynecology*, **198**, 498 e1–4.

Mukherjee, M., Chaturvedi, L.S., Srivastava, S., Mittal, R.D., and Mittal, B. (2003). De novo mutations in sporadic deletional Duchenne muscular dystrophy (DMD) cases. *Experimental and Molecular Medicine*, **35**, 113–17.

National Research Council (USA) (1996). *The Evaluation of DNA Evidence*. Washington, DC: National Academy Press.

Need, A.C. and Goldstein, D.B. (2009). Next generation disparities in human genomics: concerns and remedies. *Trends in Genetics*, **25**, 489–94.

Nelson, R.J. and Trainor, B.C. (2007). Neural mechanisms of aggression. *Nature Reviews Neuroscience*, **8**, 536–46.

Newson, A. (2004). The nature and significance of behavioural genetic information. *Theoretical Medicine and Bioethics*, **25**, 89–111.

Pakendorf, B. and Stoneking, M. (2005). Mitochondrial DNA and human evolution. *Annual Review of Genomics and Human Genetics*, **6**, 165–83.

Parkhomchuk, D., Borodina, T., Amstislavskiy, V., *et al.* (2009). Transcriptome analysis by strand-specific sequencing of complementary DNA. *Nucleic Acids Research*, **37**, e123.

Paulson, H.L. (2002). Diagnostic testing in neurogenetics. Principles, limitations, and ethical considerations. *Neurologic Clinics*, **20**, 627–43.

Petersen, R.C., Smith, G.E., Ivnik, R.J., *et al.* (1995). Apolipoprotein E status as a predictor of the development of Alzheimer's disease in memory-impaired individuals. *Journal of the American Medical Association*, **273**, 1274–8.

Pieri, E. and Levitt, M. (2008). Risky individuals and the politics of genetic research into aggressiveness and violence. *Bioethics*, **22**, 509–18.

Potter, N.T., Spector, E.B., and Prior, T.W. (2004). Technical standards and guidelines for Huntington disease testing. *Genetics in Medicine*, **6**, 61–5.

Putting DNA to the test (2009). [editorial] *Nature*, **461**, 697–98.

Rantanen, E., Hietala, M., Kristoffersson, U., *et al.* (2008). What is ideal genetic counselling? A survey of current international guidelines. *European Journal of Human Genetics*, **16**, 445–52.

Raz, A.E. (2005). Disability rights, prenatal diagnosis and eugenics: a cross-cultural view. *Journal of Genetic Counseling*, **14**, 183–7.

Reed, L.A., Wszolek, Z.K., and Hutton, M. (2001). Phenotypic correlations in FTDP-17. *Neurobiology of Aging*, **22**, 89–107.

Richards, F. (2006). Letter to the Editor in response to Duncan RE and Delatycki MB. Predictive genetic testing in young people for adult-onset conditions: where is the empirical evidence? *Clinical Genetics*, **69**, 450–4.

Rubinsztein, D.C., Leggo, J., Coles, R., *et al.* (1996). Phenotypic characterization of individuals with 30-40 CAG repeats in the Huntington disease (HD) gene reveals HD cases with 36 repeats and apparently normal elderly individuals with 36-39 repeats. *American Journal of Human Genetics*, **59**, 16–22.

Savulescu, J., Hemsley, M., Newson, A., and Foddy, B. (2006). Behavioural genetics: why eugenic selection is preferable to enhancement. *Journal of Applied Philosophy*, **23**, 157–71.

Schulze, T.G., Fangerau, H., and Propping, P. (2004). From degeneration to genetic susceptibility, from eugenics to genethics, from Bezugsziffer to LOD score: the history of psychiatric genetics. *International Review of Psychiatry*, **16**, 246–59.

Semaka, A., Creighton, S., Warby, S., and Hayden, M.R. (2006). Predictive testing for Huntington disease: interpretation and significance of intermediate alleles. *Clinical Genetics*, **70**, 283–94.

Sempere, L.F., Freemantle, S., Pitha-Rowe, I., Moss, E., Dmitrovsky, E., and Ambros, V. (2004). Expression profiling of mammalian microRNAs uncovers a subset of brain-expressed microRNAs with possible roles in murine and human neuronal differentiation. *Genome Biology*, **5**, R13.

Shirts, B.H. and Parker, L.S. (2008). Changing interpretations, stable genes: responsibilities of patients, professionals, and policy makers in the clinical interpretation of complex genetic information. *Genetics in Medicine*, **10**, 778–83.

Smith, J.D. and Nelson, K.R. (1989). *The Sterilization of Carrie Buck*. Far Hills, NJ: New Horizon Press.

Sobel, S.K. and Cowan, D.B. (2000). Impact of genetic testing for Huntington disease on the family system. *American Journal of Medical Genetics*, **90**, 49–59.

Squitieri, F., Cannella, M., Giallonardo, P., Maglione, V., Mariotti, C., and Hayden, M.R. (2001). Onset and pre-onset studies to define the Huntington's disease natural history. *Brain Research Bulletin*, **56**, 233–8.

Strittmatter, W.J., Saunders, A.M., and Schmechel, D., *et al.* (1993). Apolipoprotein E: high-avidity binding to beta-amyloid and increased frequency of type 4 allele in late-onset familial Alzheimer disease. *Proceedings of the National Academy of Sciences USA*, **90**, 1977–81.

Task Force on Genetic Testing. (2003). Promoting safe and effective genetic testing in the United States. Available at: http://www.genome.gov/10002335

Tibben, A., Timman, R., Bannink, E.C., and Duivenvoorden, H.J. (1997). Three-year follow-up after presymptomatic testing for Huntington's disease in tested individuals and partners. *Health Psychology*, **16**, 20–35.

U.S. Department of Health and Human Services (2009). HIPAA. Available at: http://www.hhs.gov/ocr/privacy/

Walton. (1998). Decade of the brain: neurological advances. *Journal of the Neurological Sciences*, **158**, 5–14.

Wertz, D.C. and Reilly, P.R. (1997). Laboratory policies and practices for the genetic testing of children: a survey of the Helix network. *American Journal of Human Genetics*, **61**, 1163–8.

Wiggins, S., Whyte, P., Huggins, M., *et al.* (1992). The psychological consequences of predictive testing for Huntington's disease. Canadian Collaborative Study of Predictive Testing. *New England Journal of Medicine*, **327**, 1401–5.

Wild, E.J. and Tabrizi, S.J. (2007). The differential diagnosis of chorea. *Practical Neurology*, 7, 360–73.

Williams, J.K., Schutte, D.L., Holkup, P.A., Evers, C., and Muilenburg, A. (2000). Psychosocial impact of predictive testing for Huntington disease on support persons. *American Journal of Medical Genetics,* **96**, 353–9.

Wray, N.R., James, M.R., Mah, S.P., *et al.* (2007). Anxiety and comorbid measures associated with PLXNA2. *Archives General Psychiatry*, **64**, 318–26.

Yeo, G., Holste, D., Kreiman, G., and Burge, C.B. (2004). Variation in alternative splicing across human tissues. *Genome Biology*, **5**, R74.

CHAPTER 32

NEUROETHICAL ISSUES IN EARLY DETECTION OF ALZHEIMER'S DISEASE

MARILYN S. ALBERT AND GUY M. MCKHANN

INTRODUCTION

ALZHEIMER'S disease (AD) was first identified as a brain disorder in 1907 (Alzheimer 1907). It was not until almost 70 years later that it became recognized as a major public health problem (Katzman 1976), initiating an international effort to understand the neurobiology of the disease and develop disease-modifying therapies.

Initial research efforts were focused on examining patients with established disease. This was facilitated by the development of widely accepted clinical criteria for use in both research and clinical settings (McKhann *et al.* 1984; American Psychiatric Association Diagnostic and Statistical Manual 1994), in parallel with pathological criteria permitting a definitive diagnosis (Mirra *et al.* 1993). This consensus regarding diagnostic standards greatly facilitated the conduct of clinical trials for AD, leading to the approval of five medications (four cholinesterase inhibitors and one NMDA (N-methyl-D-aspartic acid) antagonist). Although these medications offer only symptomatic relief, their development has increased the optimism that agents will be developed that alter the rate at which patients decline over time (i.e. the requirement for a claim of disease modification).

At the same time that such drugs have been under development, it has become increasingly clear that AD has a long prodromal phase, during which symptoms are evolving but the individual does not yet meet criteria for dementia. The application of disease-modifying therapies during this prodromal phase would clearly be preferable, since it would delay the time to full-blown dementia. It has been hypothesized that treatment during the prodromal phase of AD might be more efficacious than treatment at a later stage of the disorder.

Moreover, recent evidence indicates that a substantial portion of individuals who are cognitively normal have the pathological hallmarks of AD in their brains (i.e. neuritic plaques and neurofibrillary tangles). These individuals do not, however, have evidence of neuronal loss. Thus, intervention at this very early stage of disease would be ideal.

The importance of early diagnosis and treatment for AD therefore cannot be overemphasized. It is, nevertheless, currently faced with a number of practical and ethical challenges, which are the topic of this chapter.

TRANSITION PHASE BETWEEN NORMAL FUNCTION AND DEMENTIA

There is considerable evidence to support the argument that there is a transitional phase between normal function and the dementia of AD, as noted earlier. Various terms have been used to describe this prodromal phase, but the term mild cognitive impairment (MCI) has gained the widest recognition (Flicker *et al.* 1991; Petersen *et al.* 1999).

Neuropsychological studies of individuals defined as neither normal nor demented, demonstrate progressive declines in cognition over time. Declines in cognition are particularly striking in the area of episodic memory, but other domains appear to be affected as well (Albert *et al.* 2001; Storandt *et al.* 2001; Bennett *et al.* 2002).

Likewise, studies of imaging and other biomarkers of AD pathology demonstrate alterations in non-demented cognitively impaired individuals that are intermediate between normal individuals and those with mild AD. This is true for structural magnetic resonance imaging (MRI) measures of the medial temporal lobe structures targeted by the pathology of AD (e.g. the hippocampus and entorhinal cortex), as well as for measures of whole brain atrophy (Fox *et al.* 1999; Jack *et al.* 2000; Killiany *et al.* 2000). Functional imaging measures, such as 18-FDG (fludeoxyglucose) photon emission tomography (PET) show similar findings (e.g. Jagust 2006). Cerebrospinal fluid (CSF) measures of the amyloid beta protein (Abeta), tau, and phosphylated tau (ptau), the primary constituents of the plaques and tangles, are altered in cognitively impaired non-demented individuals, though to a lesser degree than that seen in established AD cases (Blennow 2004; Andreason and Blennow 2005; Shaw *et al.* 2009). Perhaps most importantly, each of these measures is a significant predictor of progression from mild impairment to AD. That is, individuals who are cognitively impaired but not demented *and* have these intermediate levels of risk factors are at significantly elevated risk of being diagnosed with AD within a few years (Atiya *et al.* 2003; Blennow and Hampel 2003; Kantarci and Jack 2003; Jagust 2006; Vemuri *et al.* 2009).

Pathological findings in non-demented cognitively impaired individuals are particularly important in this context, though the number of studies is small, given the difficulty of obtaining brain tissue at a time that individuals are not demented. These studies have found that a substantial number of individuals who died when they were mildly impaired had evidence of AD pathology (i.e. a "high likelihood" of AD, based on NIA-Reagan criteria (NIA-Reagan Institute Working Group 1997)). The absolute percentage of such cases has varied (Morris *et al.* 2001; Bennett *et al.* 2005; Petersen *et al.* 2006) depending on the age of the subjects.

CHALLENGES FOR THE CLINICAL DIAGNOSIS OF MILD COGNITIVE IMPAIRMENT

Despite the wealth of evidence, and widespread agreement, that there is a transitional phase between normal function and dementia, there has, nevertheless, been debate about the utility of the clinical diagnosis of MCI. Some of the concern has been based on the heterogeneity of the subjects who met criteria for MCI, based on the original criteria published by Petersen and colleagues (Petersen *et al.* 1999). Although many subjects progressed from MCI to AD dementia within a few years, there were alternative outcomes: some progressed to other forms of dementia, some remained stable and, particularly in epidemiological settings, some were diagnosed as normal at subsequent follow-up (Ritchie *et al.* 2001; Lopez *et al.* 2003; Manly *et al.* 2008; Palmer *et al.* 2008).

In response to these reports, Petersen modified the criteria to permit clinical subtypes with variable outcomes, based on the presumed etiology underlying the disorder (Petersen 2004). Two primary subtypes were delineated, based on whether a predominant memory disorder was present ("amnestic MCI") or absent ("non-amnestic MCI"). The revised criteria also acknowledged the possibility that more than one cognitive domain may be impaired within each of these subtypes (e.g. single or multiple domain impaired). Thus, amnestic MCI (single and multiple domains impaired), is hypothesized to represent the majority of individuals who will progress to a diagnosis of AD over time. Those with non-amnestic MCI (single and multiple domains impaired) were hypothesized to pertain to the transitional phase of other dementias (e.g. vascular dementia, frontotemporal dementia) as well as psychiatric disorders (e.g. depression). In practice, however, there is evidence that some individuals who meet criteria for non-amnestic MCI are also at increased risk for a diagnosis of AD over time (Boyle *et al.* 2006).

In retrospect it seems clear that the original clinical criteria for MCI were targeted at amnestic MCI, as Petersen and colleagues were attempting to focus on individuals likely to be in the prodromal phase of AD. Nevertheless, some of the current concern about the term MCI stems from the belief that it has been used to describe a syndrome of MCI that is not sufficiently tied to the underlying neurobiology of AD. The argument of these investigators is that we should be focused on the disease entity of AD, and develop criteria for identifying it as early as possible, as opposed to using terminology that mixes individuals with multiple underlying diseases into the same overall category (i.e. MCI). They argue that research studies over the last decade permit the identification of a subgroup of individuals at highest risk for AD, and that this relatively homogeneous group should be the one that is targeted for treatment with potential disease-modifying therapies, regardless of whether or not they meet criteria for dementia (e.g. Dubois *et al.* 2007).

Those who believe that the term MCI continues to be useful believe that it is important from both a clinical and a research perspective to recognize and study individuals who are neither normal nor demented in order to learn as much as possible about them. From this perspective, it should be possible to identify a subgroup with MCI who should be included in clinical trials for AD (based on very targeted criteria, including assessments of imaging and CSF), but at the same time enable other clinical researchers (including epidemiologists), as well as primary care physicians, to identify individuals in this intermediate stage, but without requirements for potentially invasive procedures (such as CSF sampling, which may not be feasible). They therefore recommend a common set of basic diagnostic criteria for "MCI of the AD type," with differing degrees of intensity (or invasiveness), depending on the setting in which the criteria are applied.

This ongoing debate has clear ethical implications. The first pertains to the fact that the term MCI has become widely used in some medical circumstances, even though researchers recognize that those who meet the broad criteria represent a heterogeneous group for whom effective treatment is unclear.

For example, a recent survey about the attitudes and practices of neurologists in the US (J. Roberts, personal communication) indicates that these physicians find the term useful because they see many patients in their practice who fit the general criteria (90% of the survey respondents). They report that the diagnosis of MCI is beneficial because it enables them to discuss dementia risk (63%), it motivates them to engage in risk reduction activities, such as physical and mental exercise (85%), and it involves them in planning for the future (86%). Moreover, the majority of the respondents in this survey (70%) sometimes prescribed cholinesterase inhibitors for patients they diagnose with MCI. This survey clearly indicates that, despite the fact that the criteria for MCI were enunciated to facilitate research in the field, they have been adopted by many practicing clinicians, perhaps prematurely, while there is continuing debate among researchers about how best to refine the criteria and in which circumstances.

It is unclear that the physicians who responded to this survey understand that the outcome of a diagnosis of MCI can vary greatly, based on a variety of factors. Recent evidence suggests that the severity of the cognitive and/or functional impairment of the subjects, as well as their genetic status, greatly influence the likelihood that subjects will progress from amnestic MCI to dementia within a few years. For example, subjects whose episodic memory performance is unusually poor (i.e. 1.5 standard deviations below the mean of their age and education adjusted peers on specific memory tests), or who carry at least one copy of the ApoE-4 allele are at greater risk for progression from MCI to dementia within 2–3 years than are MCI subjects whose memory performance is less impaired or whose ApoE-4 status is negative (Blacker et al. 2007). The presence of these characteristics likely identifies individuals who are at the severe end of the spectrum of MCI and thus, closer to the point where dementia will be diagnosed. This variability in outcome, even among individuals with amnestic MCI, is completely consistent with a disorder that is gradually progressive, with no fixed line demarcating the "onset" of dementia. However, it presents substantial practical and ethical challenges when community physicians employ this diagnostic framework.

It also appears that physicians in the community are making recommendations about lifestyle changes and medication use that is not well substantiated by results from clinical trials. While it is true that recent evidence suggests that increased levels of mental and physical activity are associated with a lower risk of cognitive decline, the most convincing data is from individuals who are cognitively normal (not those with memory problems), and the majority of the data are from observational studies, as opposed to randomized clinical trials (see Hendrie et al. 2006 for a review). Likewise, the clinical trials that have been done in subjects with MCI have not demonstrated that cholinesterase inhibitors are beneficial in reducing cognitive decline over time (Petersen *et al.* 2005; Thal *et al.* 2005; Feldman *et al.* 2007; Winblad *et al.* 2008; Doody *et al.* 2009). It should be noted that interpretation of these trials is hindered by the fact that some of the trials were not successful in identifying MCI subjects likely to progress to AD over a 2-3-year period, and thus there were insufficient outcomes with which to judge whether or not the drugs were efficacious. Furthermore, cholinesterase inhibitors are effective in treating cognitive symptoms in people with mild and moderate AD.

The overarching ethical concern is that the term MCI is being applied to patients in clinical settings, when the majority of the data pertains to risk for groups of subjects, as opposed to individuals. Moreover, this is happening when no effective treatments are available. It is therefore not the same as telling someone that they have elevated blood pressure and cholesterol, which puts them at increased risk for stroke, because there are effective ways to lower blood pressure and cholesterol levels. In the latter case, even if we cannot be certain that this specific individual will have a stroke, we can recommend lifestyle changes or medications that have demonstrated efficacy. The increased anxiety and worry which may be caused by telling some individuals that they are in the prodromal phase of AD, when, in fact, the diagnosis is currently probabilistic, is also of ethical concern.

CHALLENGES FOR THE CLINICAL DIAGNOSIS OF "NORMAL"

These same challenges regarding the boundary between normal and abnormal, and the probabilistic nature of predicting progression apply to individuals with normal cognition. There is increasing evidence that it may be possible to identify a subset of individuals with normal cognition who are at risk for developing AD over time.

This is based on studies demonstrating that some individuals who are cognitively normal show the hallmark pathological features of AD in their brain (i.e. neuritic plaques and neurofibrillary tangles). The percentage of individuals with evidence of substantial AD pathology varies among studies, largely based on the age of subjects examined (Hulette *et al.* 1998; Price and Morris 1999; Schmitt *et al.* 2000; Knopman *et al.* 2003; Bennett *et al.* 2006). Despite abundant pathology, most investigators have, however, *not* reported that these individuals have significant neuronal loss. In fact, there is evidence of changes that suggest neurobiological compensation among cognitively normal individuals with abundant AD pathology (e.g. increases in neuronal and nuclear volume, and enhancement of presynaptic markers) (Bell *et al.* 2007; Riudavets *et al.* 2007; Head *et al.* 2009). It therefore seems likely that the evolution of AD is a multiphase process; the first involving the accumulation of AD pathology, which may be contained in the early stages of disease. However, as compensatory systems begin to fail, progressive pathology and clinical symptoms evolve.

These findings suggest that there may be a "window of opportunity" to prevent AD, if treatments can be initiated when individuals are cognitively normal despite evidence of some AD pathology in their brain. The scientific challenge is, therefore, to identify biomarkers that can be used to predict which cognitively normal individuals will subsequently develop cognitive decline and dementia.

However, some investigators in the field argue that AD should be diagnosed on the basis of pathology, rather than symptoms, in much the same way that we diagnose cancer on the basis of a biopsy, even if someone is asymptomatic. That is, we should say that someone has AD if there is substantial biomarker evidence of AD pathology, even if someone is cognitively normal. The ethical challenges raised by this position are even more striking than they are when one discusses MCI.

Since studies of risk for AD among cognitively normal individuals are relatively recent, we know much less about the outcome of individuals who carry various risk factors (e.g. decreased CSF Abeta-42, increased amyloid imaging, etc.). Moreover, the time course over which cognitively normal individuals may become symptomatic is particularly unclear. Thus, the risks of saying that someone who is asymptomatic has AD, on the basis of our current knowledge about these risk factors, are substantial. The benefits, given the absence of effective treatments, are unclear.

This balance between risks and benefits would, of course, change, when disease-modifying therapies are identified. Then potentially beneficial treatments could be instituted even when someone is cognitively normal.

Conclusions

Neuroethical issues in the early detection of AD are likely characteristic of any disorder where the boundary conditions between being impaired and unimpaired are unclear. In this case, the absence of clearly demarcated boundaries is particularly problematic because they are at both ends of the cognitive spectrum, i.e. between normal cognition and mild impairment and between mild impairment and dementia. No one doubts that the scientific imperative is to identify those individuals at greatest risk for progression to dementia as early as possible. The rationale is that this will permit early intervention, when disease-modifying therapies are identified.

Differences of opinion arise, however, regarding how to define "prodromal disease" and the risks and benefits of transmitting this information to individual patients. Ethical concerns are raised when researchers and clinicians act without recognizing the underlying risks and benefits of their decisions. The important thing would seem to be to enunciate these risks and benefits as clearly as possible so that ethically-informed action is possible.

References

Albert, M., Moss, M., Tanzi, R., and Jones, K. (2001). Preclinical predictions of AD using neuropsychological tests. *Journal of the International Neuropsychology Society*, 7, 631–9.

Alzheimer, A. (1907). Uber eine eigenartige Erkrankung der Hirnrinde. *Allgemeine Zeitschrift für Psychiatrie und Psychisch-gerichtliche Medzin*, 64, 146–8.

American Psychiatric Association. (1994). *Diagnostic and Statistical Manual*, 4th edn. Washington, DC: American Psychiatric Association.

Andreason, N. and Blennow, K. (2005). CSF biomarkers for mild cognitive impairment and early Alzheimer's disease. *Clinical Neurology and Neursurgery*, 107, 165–73.

Atiya, M., Hyman, B., Albert, M., and Killiany, R. (2003). Structural magnetic resonance imaging in established and prodromal Alzheimer's disease: A review. *Alzheimer Disease & Associated Disorders*, 17, 177–95.

Bell, K.F., Bennett, D., and Cuello, A. (2007). Paradoxical upregulation of glutamatergic pre-synaptic boutons during mild cognitive impairment. *Journal of Neuroscience*, 27, 10810–17.

Bennett, D., Wilson, R., Schneider, J., *et al.* (2002). Natural history of mild cognitive impairment in older persons. *Neurology*, 59, 198–205.

Bennett, D., Schneider, J., Bienias, J., *et al.* (2005). Mild cognitive impairment is related to Alzheimer pathology and cerebral infarctions. *Neurology*, 64, 834–41.

Bennett, D., Schneider, J., Arvanitakis, Z., *et al.* (2006). Neuropathology of older persons without cognitive impairment from two community-based studies. *Neurology*, 66, 1801–2.

Blacker, D., Lee, H., Muzikansky, A., *et al.* (2007). Neuropsychological measures in normal individuals that predict subsequent cognitive decline. *Archives of Neurology*, 64, 862–71.

Blennow, K. (2004). CSF biomarkers for mild cognitive impairment. *Journal of Internal Medicine*, 256, 224–34.

Blennow, K. and Hampel, H. (2003). Cerebrospinal fluid markers for incipient Alzheimer's disease. *Lancet Neurology*, 2, 605–13.

Boyle, P., Wilson, R., Aggarwal, N., Tang, Y., and Bennett, D. (2006). Mild cognitive impairment: risk of Alzheimer's disease and rate of cognitive decline. *Neurology*, 67, 441–5.

Doody, R., Ferris, S., Salloway, S., *et al.* (2009). Donepezil treatment of patients with MCI : a 48-week randomized, placebo-controlled trial. *Neurology*, 72, 1555–61.

Dubois, B., Feldman, H., Jacova, C., *et al.* (2007). Research criteria for diagnosis of Alzheimer's disease: Revising the NINCDS-ADRDA criteria. *Lancet Neurology*, 6, 734–46.

Feldman, H., Ferris, S., Winblad, B., *et al.* (2007). Effect of rivastigmine on delay to diagnosis of Alzheimer's disease from mild cognitive impairment: the InDDEx study. *Lancet Neurology*, 6, 501–12.

Flicker, C., Ferris, S., and Reisberg, B. (1991). Mild cognitive impairment in the elderly: predictors of dementia. *Neurology*, 41, 1006–9.

Fox, N.C., Warrington, E.K., and Rossor, M.N. (1999). Serial magnetic resonance imaging of cerebral atrophy in preclinical Alzheimer's disease. *Lancet*, 353, 2125.

Head, E., Corrada, M., Kahle-Wroblenski, K., *et al.* (2009). Synaptic protein, neuropathology and cognitive status in the oldest-old. *Neurobiology of Aging*, 30, 1125–34.

Hendrie, H., Albert, M., Butters, M., *et al.* (2006). The NIH cognitive and emotional health project: report of the critical evaluation study committee. *Alzheimer's & Dementia*, 2, 12–32.

Hulette, C., Welsh-Bohmer, K., Murray, M., Saunders, A., Mash, D., and McIntyre, L. (1998). Neuropathological and neuropsychological changes in "normal" aging: Evidence for preclinical Alzheimer disease in cognitively normal individuals. *Journal of Neuropathology & Experimental Neurology*, 57, 1168–74.

Jack, C.R., Petersen, R.C., Xu, Y., *et al.* (2000). Rates of hippocampal atrophy correlate with change in clinical status in aging and AD. *Neurology*, 55, 484–90.

Jagust, W. (2006). Positron emission tomography and magnetic resonance imaging in the diagnosis and prediction of dementia. *Alzheimers and Dementia*, 2, 36–42.

Kantarci, K. and Jack, C. (2003). Neuroimaging in Alzheimer's disease: an evidenced-based review. *Neuroimaging Clinics of North America*, 13, 197–209.

Katzman, R. (1976). The prevalence and malignancy of Alzheimer disease. A major killer. *Archives of Neurology*, 33, 217–18.

Killiany, R., Gomez-Isla, T., Moss, M., *et al.* (2000). Use of structural magnetic resonance imaging to predict who will get Alzheimer's disease. *Annals of Neurology*, 47, 430–9.

Knopman, D., Parisi, J., Salvati, A., *et al.* (2003). Neuropathology of cognitively normal elderly. *Journal of Neuropathology & Experimental Neurology,* **62,** 1087–95.

Lopez, O., Jagust, W. and DeKosky, S., *et al.* (2003). Prevalence and classification of mild cognitive impairment in the Cardiovascular Health Study Cognition Study: Part 1. *Archives of Neurology,* **60,** 1385–9.

Manly, J., Tang, M., Schupf, N., Stern, Y., Vonsattel, J.P., and Mayeux, R. (2008). Frequency and course of mild cognitive impairment in a multiethnic community. *Annals of Neurology,* **63,** 494–506.

McKhann, G., Drachman, D., Folstein, M.F., Katzman, R., Price, D., and Stadlan, E. (1984). Clinical diagnosis of Alzheimer's disease: Report of the NINCDS-ADRDA Work group under the auspices of Department of Health and Human Services Task Force. *Neurology,* **34,** 939–44.

Mirra, S., Hart, M., and Terry, R. (1993). Making the diagnosis of Alzheimer's disease. A primer for practicing pathologists. *Archives of Pathology & Laboratory Medicine,* **117,** 132–44.

Morris, J., Storandt, M., Miller, J., *et al.* (2001). Mild cognitive impairment represents early-stage Alzheimer's disease. *Archives of Neurology,* **58,** 397–405.

National Institute on Aging/Reagan Institute Working Group. (1997). Consensus recommendations for the postmortem diagnosis of Alzheimer's disease. The National Institute on Aging, and Reagan Institute Working Group on Diagnostic Criteria for the Neuropathological Assessment of Alzheimer's disease. *Neurobiology of Aging,* **18,** S1–S2.

Palmer, K., Backman, L., Winblad, B., and Fratiglioni, L. (2008). Mild cognitive impairment in the general population: occurrence and progression to Alzheimer's disease. *American Journal of Geriatric Psychiatry,* **16,** 603–11.

Petersen, R. (2004). Mild cognitive impairment. *Journal of Internal Medicine,* **256,** 183–94.

Petersen, R., Smith, G., Waring, S., Ivnik, R., Tangalos, E., and Kokmen, E. (1999). Mild cognitive impairment: clinical characterization and outcome. *Archives of Neurology,* **56,** 303–8.

Petersen, R., Dickson, D., Parisi, J., Johnson, R., Ivnik, R., and Smith, G. (2000). Neuropathologic substrate of mild cognitive impairment. *Neurobiology of Aging,* **21,** S198.

Petersen, R., Thomas, R., Grundman, M., *et al.* (2005). Vitamin E and donepezil for the treatment of mild cognitive impairment. *New England Journal of Medicine,* **352,** 2379–88.

Petersen, R., Parisi, J., Dickson, D., *et al.* (2006). Neuropathologic features of amnestic mild cognitive impairment. *Archives of Neurology,* **63,** 655–72.

Price, J.L. and Morris, J.C. (1999). Tangles and plaques in nondemented aging and "preclinical" Alzheimer's disease. *Annals of Neurology,* **45,** 358–68.

Ritchie, K., Artero, S., and Touchon, J. (2001). Classification criteria for mild cognitive impairment: a population-based validation study. *Neurology,* **56,** 37–42.

Riudavets, M.A., Iacono, D., Resnick, S.N., *et al.* (2007). Resistance to Alzheimer pathology is associated with hypertrophy in neurons. *Neurobiology of Aging,* **28,** 1484–92.

Roberts, J., Karlawish, J., Petersen, R., Uhlmann, W., and Green, R. Mild cognitive impairment in clinical care: A survey of neurologists attitudes and practice, personal communication.

Schmitt, F., Davis, D., Wekstein, D., Smith, C., Ashford, J., and Markesbery, W. (2000). "Preclinical" AD revisited: Neuropathology of cognitively normal older adults. *Neurology,* **55,** 370–6.

Shaw, L., Vanderstichele, H., Knapik-Czajka, M., *et al.* (2009). Cerebrospinal fluid biomarker signature in Alzheimer's disease neuroimaging initiative subjects. *Annals of Neurology*, **65**, 403–13.

Storandt, M., Albert, M., Moss, M., Tanzi, R., and Jones, K. (2001). Preclinical predictions of AD using neuropsychological tests. *Journal of the International Neuropsychological Society*, 7, 631–9.

Thal, L., Ferris, S., Kirby, L., *et al.* (2005). Rofecoxib Protocol 078 study group. A randomized, double-blind study of rofecoxib in patients with mild cognitive impairment. *Neuropsychoparmacology*, **30**, 1204–15.

Vemuri, P., Wiste, H., Weingand, S., *et al.* (2009). MRI and CSF biomarkers in normal, MCI and AD subjects: predicting future clinical change. *Neurology*, **73**, 294–301.

Winblad, B., Gauthier, S., Scinto, L. *et al.* (2008). GAL-INT-11/18 Study Group. Safety and efficacy of galantamine in subjects with mild cognitive impairment. *Neurology*, **70**, 2204–35.

CHAPTER 33

THE NEUROETHICS OF COGNITIVE RESERVE

JERRY SAMET AND YAAKOV STERN

THE idea of reserve against brain damage stems from the repeated observation that there does not appear to be a direct relationship between the degree of brain pathology or brain damage and the clinical manifestation of that damage. For example, Katzman *et al.* (1989) described 10 cases of cognitively normal elderly women who were discovered to have advanced Alzheimer's disease (AD) pathology in their brains at death. They speculated that these women did not express the clinical features of AD because their brains were larger than average, providing them with "brain reserve." Parallel findings have shown that individuals with enriched lifestyles, such as higher educational or occupational attainment, also have a reduced risk of expressing AD pathology clinically. These observations have led to the concept of "cognitive reserve." The literature suggests that both brain reserve and cognitive reserve (CR) are not entirely determined at birth but are influenced by experiences and environmental factors throughout the lifespan. These most likely include not only education and occupation, but also social relationships, leisure activities, exercise, and factors influencing postnatal development. Recently, investigators have been looking at the possibility of imparting reserve via lifestyle enrichment, cognitive training, exercise, and other interventions. In this chapter we review the concept of CR. We then discuss the potential ethical implications connected with this concept.

DEFINING RESERVE

Brain reserve (Katzman 1993) is an example of what might be called passive models of reserve, where reserve derives from brain size or neuronal count. The models are passive because reserve is defined in terms of the amount of brain damage that can be sustained before reaching a threshold for clinical expression. The threshold model (Satz 1993), one of the best articulated passive models, revolves around the construct of "brain reserve capacity." While brain reserve capacity is a hypothetical construct, concrete examples might include brain size or synapse count. The model recognizes that there are individual differences in brain reserve capacity. It also presupposes that there is a critical threshold, and once brain reserve capacity is depleted past this threshold specific clinical or functional deficits emerge.

In contrast, the CR model suggests that the brain actively attempts to cope with brain damage by using pre-existing cognitive processing approaches or by enlisting compensatory approaches (Stern 2002, 2009). Individuals with more CR would be more successful at coping with the same amount of brain damage. Thus, the same amount of brain damage or pathology will have different effects on different people, even if brain reserve capacity (e.g. brain size) is held constant. The concept of CR provides a ready explanation for why many studies have demonstrated that higher levels of intelligence and of educational and occupational attainment are good predictors of which individuals can sustain greater brain damage before demonstrating functional deficit. Rather than positing that these individuals' brains are grossly anatomically different than those with less reserve (e.g. they have more synapses), the cognitive reserve hypothesis posits that they process tasks in a manner that allows them to cope better with the brain damage.

The simplest explanation for how CR forestalls the clinical effects of AD pathology does not posit that experiences associated with more CR directly affect brain reserve or the development of AD pathology. Rather, CR allows some people to better cope with the pathology and remain clinically more intact for longer periods of time. This has been the working assumption underlying the design and interpretation of many studies. However, as mentioned earlier, many of the factors associated with CR may also have direct impact on the brain itself. There is a demonstrated relationship between intelligence quotient (IQ) and brain volume (Willerman et al. 1991). Thus, the child development literature suggests that intracranial brain volume and aspects of lifetime exposure are predictive of differential susceptibility to the effects of traumatic brain injury (Kesler et al. 2003). Also, it is now clear that stimulating environments and exercise promote neurogenesis in the dentate of animals (Brown et al. 2003; van Praag et al. 2005). In addition, there is evidence to suggest that environmental enrichment might act directly to prevent or slow the accumulation of AD pathology (Lazarov et al. 2005). Thus, a more complete accounting of CR would have to integrate these complex interactions between genetics, the environmental influences on brain reserve and pathology, and the ability to actively compensate for the effects of pathology.

Epidemiologic evidence for cognitive reserve

The concept of reserve is relevant to any situation where the brain sustains injury. In addition, the concept of reserve might be extended to encompass variation in healthy individuals' performance, particularly when they must perform at their maximum capacity. The reviewed studies will address cognitive reserve in the context of AD. The key conceptual point is that there is a disconnection between the underlying AD pathology and the clinical expression of that pathology. AD pathology affects cortical circuitry that subserves a wide range of cognitive functions, and is also inexorably progressive. This provides an effective research setting for exploring the severity of brain insult that is required before cognitive networks change. While this is comparable to many other conditions that affect the brain and result in clinical changes, it differs from other situations such as traumatic brain injury where recovery of function is a greater interest.

A host of studies have examined the relation between CR proxy variables and incident dementia. Parallel studies have often examined the relation between these variables and cognitive decline in normal aging. Several studies reported no association between education and incident dementia (Paykel *et al.* 1994; Cobb *et al.* 1995; Graves *et al.* 1996; Hall *et al.* 2000; Chandra *et al.* 2001). However, lower incidence of dementia in subjects with higher education has been reported by at least eight cohorts, in France (Letenneur *et al.* 1994), Sweden (Qiu *et al.* 2001), Finland (Anttila *et al.* 2002), China (Zhang *et al.* 1990), and the US (Evans *et al.* 1993, 1997; Stern *et al.* 1994; White *et al.* 1994). Similar associations emerged in a pooled analysis of four European population-based prospective studies of individuals aged 65 years and older (Launer *et al.* 1999).

There is also evidence for the role of education in age-related cognitive decline, with several studies of normal aging reporting slower cognitive and functional decline in individuals with higher educational attainment (Snowdon *et al.* 1989; Colsher and Wallace 1991; Albert 1995; Farmer *et al.* 1995; Butler *et al.* 1996; Christensen *et al.* 1997; Lyketsos *et al.* 1999; Chodosh *et al.* 2002). These studies suggest that the same education-related factors that delay the onset of dementia also allow individuals to cope more effectively with brain changes encountered in normal aging. In an ethnically diverse cohort of non-demented elders in New York City, increased literacy was also associated with slower decline in memory, executive function, and language skills (Manly *et al.* 2005).

No or equivocal association between occupation and incident AD was found in several population-based longitudinal studies (Jorm *et al.* 1998; Helmer *et al.* 2001; Anttila *et al.* 2002). In two other prospective studies, occupational position did not predict incident dementia (Paykel *et al.* 1994), or its predictive value might have been mediated by educational status (Evans *et al.* 1997). Nevertheless, many studies have noted a relationship between occupational attainment and incident dementia (Bickel and Cooper 1994; Stern *et al.* 1994; White *et al.* 1994; Schmand *et al.* 1997; Zhang *et al.* 1999; Qiu *et al.* 2003). As mentioned earlier, occupational attainment was often noted to have independent effects or interact with educational attainment.

Studies have also explored the relationship between leisure activities and incident dementia. A study from France reported that traveling, doing odd jobs, and knitting were associated with lower risk of incident dementia (Fabrigoule *et al.* 1995; Helmer *et al.* 1999). Community activities and gardening were also protective for incident dementia in China (Zhang *et al.* 1999). A longitudinal study in Sweden reported that having an extensive social network was protective for development of incident dementia (Fratiglioni *et al.* 2000). The same group later reported that engagement in mental, social, and productive activities was associated with decreased risk for incident dementia (Wang *et al.* 2002). Participation in a variety of leisure activities characterized as intellectual (e.g. reading, playing games, going to classes) or social (e.g. visiting with friends or relatives etc.) was assessed in another population study of non-demented elderly in New York (Scarmeas *et al.* 2001). During follow-up, subjects with high leisure activity had 38% less risk of developing dementia. In another prospective study, frequency of participation in common cognitive activities (i.e. reading a newspaper, magazine, books) was assessed at baseline for 801 elderly Catholic nuns, priests, and brothers without dementia (Wilson *et al.* 2002). Additionally, engagement in cognitive activities was also associated with slower rates of cognitive decline. Finally, in another prospective cohort from New York, participation in leisure activities, particularly reading, playing board games or musical instruments, and dancing, was associated with a reduced risk for incident dementia (Verghese *et al.* 2003). Increased participation in cognitive activities was also associated with reduced rates of memory decline in this study.

A meta-analysis examined cohort studies of the effects of education, occupation, premorbid IQ, and mental activities on dementia risk (Valenzuela and Sachdev 2005). A summary analysis was based on an integrated total of 29,279 individuals from 22 studies. The median follow-up was 7.1 years. The summary OR of incident dementia for individuals with high brain reserve compared to low was 0.54 (95% confidence interval 0.49–0.59, $p < 0.0001$)—a decreased risk of 46%. Eight out of 33 datasets showed no significant effect, while 25 out of 33 demonstrated a significant protective effect. The authors found a significant negative association between incident dementia risk (based on differential education) and the overall dementia rate for each cohort ($r = -0.57$, $p = 0.04$), indicating that in negative studies there was a lower overall risk of incident dementia in the cohort.

In contrast to these studies, in which greater reserve was associated with better outcomes, a series of studies of patients with AD have suggested that those with higher reserve have poorer outcomes. In prospective studies of AD patients matched for clinical severity at baseline (Stern *et al.* 1995b; Geerlings *et al.* 1999), patients with greater education or occupational attainment died sooner than those with less attainment. Although at first these findings appear contra-intuitive, they are consistent with the CR hypothesis. The hypothesis predicts that at any level of assessed clinical severity, the underlying pathology of AD is more advanced in patients with CR than in those with CR. This would result in the clinical disease emerging when pathology is more advanced, as suggested by the incidence studies reviewed earlier. This disparity in degree of pathology would be present at more advanced clinical stages of the disease as well. At some point the greater degree of pathology in the high reserve patients would result in more rapid death. Higher educational attainment, and greater engagement in leisure activities has also been associated with more rapid cognitive decline in patients with AD (Stern *et al.* 1999; Scarmeas *et al.* 2006; Hall *et al.* 2007; Helzner *et al.* 2007). Explanation of this finding is along similar lines. At some point AD pathology must become too severe to support the processes that mediate CR. This point should arrive at an earlier stage of clinical severity in patients with higher CR because the underlying AD pathology is more severe.

Evidence for cognitive reserve from studies of regional cerebral blood flow

Our first imaging studies of CR were designed to test the hypothesis that at any given level of clinical AD severity an individual with a higher level of CR should have greater AD pathology. In these studies, we used resting regional cerebral blood flow (rCBF) as a surrogate for AD pathology. In AD patients matched for clinical severity (as assessed with measures of cognition and function), we found negative correlations between resting rCBF and years of education (Stern *et al.* 1992), such that higher education was associated with more depleted flow specifically in parietotemporal areas that are affected in AD. These findings imply that patients with higher education can tolerate more AD pathology than those with lower education and still appear clinically similar. This finding has been replicated many times (Alexander *et al.* 1997; Scarmeas *et al.* 2003; Perneczky *et al.* 2006).

In a subsequent analysis of the same subjects we found a similar inverse relationship between rCBF and occupational attainment, even after controlling for educational attainment, suggesting that some aspects of occupational experiences imparted reserve over and above that obtained from education (Stern *et al.* 1995a). We used data from the Dictionary of Occupational Titles to characterize occupational demands and found that two features of occupation were protective in this model. The first was interpersonal skills, which reflects the degree to which a job requires interaction with people vs. machines. The second was physical demands, which is consistent with the subsequent observations that physical exercise is beneficial for cognition. In a later O15 PET study, we re-extended the findings to leisure activities (Scarmeas *et al.* 2003): we found an inverse relationship between rCBF and increased engagement in leisure activities, even after controlling for educational and occupational attainment.

The implications of these imaging findings were confirmed in a prospective clinical study with subsequent neuropathological analysis. Education was found to modify the association between AD pathology assessed postmortem and levels of cognitive function proximate to death: for the same degree of brain pathology there was better cognitive function with each year of education (Bennett *et al.* 2003).

Neural mechanisms underlying
cognitive reserve

Stern and colleagues have suggested that the neural implementation of CR might take two forms: neural reserve and neural compensation (Stern *et al.* 2005; Stern 2009). The idea behind neural reserve is that there is interindividual variability in the brain networks or cognitive paradigms that underlie the performance of any task. This variability stems from innate factors as well as life exposures. It could be in the form of differing efficiency or capacity of these networks, or in greater flexibility in the networks that can be invoked to perform a task. While healthy individuals may invoke these networks when coping with increased task demands, the networks could also help an individual cope with brain pathology. An individual whose networks are more efficient, have greater capacity, or are more flexible might be more capable of coping with the disruption imposed by brain pathology.

Neural compensation refers to the process by which individuals suffering from brain pathology use brain structures or networks (and thus cognitive strategies) not normally used by individuals with intact brains in order to compensate for brain damage. Again, individuals with higher CR might be more able to invoke these compensatory strategies.

CR might also be mediated by brain networks that are not directly associated with performance of the task at hand. That is, there may be some general cognitive functions that could be useful to the performance of many tasks. Two candidate domains would be executive control and attentional allocation. Both of these cognitive functions would play a role in diverse activities, and therefore may be candidates for the cognitive substrate of CR. In one study, we sought to identify a generic cognitive reserve brain network that was expressed across two different tasks. In both tasks, task difficulty was systematically varied. We reasoned that a "CR network" would increase in expression as task difficulty increased. We also reason that individuals with higher measured CR (e.g. higher IQ) would be more able to express this network. Finally, we reasoned that this network would be separate from those cognitive networks that were directly involved in the performance of the two different tasks. Our analysis did identify a network that was expressed by younger subjects in both tasks as a function of CR. This network included areas of the frontal lobe that have been implicated executive control processes. While this study supports the idea that CR networks may exist, much more work will be needed to identify such networks.

NEUROETHICAL IMPLICATIONS OF
COGNITIVE RESERVE

As our summary makes clear, CR is a theory. At this point, we don't know enough about the brain, about AD, and about cognition to understand why some people can sustain severe brain pathology and suffer only mild functional effects. We are making progress in figuring out the features that are positively correlated with reserve, and we are developing hypotheses about the mechanisms at work in the brain that enable it to deal with the severe pathology. The CR hypothesis is that the "reserve" of these relatively spared people can be best understood in terms of cognitive processes—what their brains are doing—as opposed to anatomical properties of the brain.

The situation we are in is somewhat akin to responses to pain. We know that the same stimuli, and the same activation in the brain's pain centers in response to those stimuli, can result in different levels of felt pain. Some people seem to have higher pain thresholds—pain reserve, if you will. Here too we are still in the dark: there is much that we don't understand about pain and consciousness.

CR represents a gap in our understanding, and as such does not give rise to specific ethical quandaries or have any specific ethical implications of its own. There is no "downside" to worry about here, and it is hard to think of issues of patient safety or consent that are especially pertinent. Nor do we see any profound philosophical issues—having to do with the autonomy, the nature of the self, personal responsibility, and so on—that are especially connected to it. These issues are certainly relevant to dementia in general, but not to CR in particular. Nevertheless, what we have learned so far about CR—specifically which groups may be expected to have it—reinforces other recent findings about the determinants of cognitive and neural well-being, and this body of work does have important policy implications.

What we are learning is that the determinants of reserve are to a very significant extent environmental (as opposed to genetic), and that these environmental factors are largely under our control. Reserve is obviously good. If we could give everyone greater reserve we would all be better off, both cognitively and in terms of the social costs of care for those with severe dementia. It is fortunate that the "enriched lifestyles" that are correlated with reserve—educational levels, occupational attainment, socioeconomic status, social relationships, regular exercise, etc.—do more than offer protection against the possible ravages of AD. They are not like painful deposits into a retirement scheme that will benefit us only when we get older. They are goods that enhance the quality of a whole life. Findings about reserve give us all the more reason to support policies that promote these goods, and suggest that they might also be promoted as health issues.

Consider education. Those in economically-advanced societies tend to value educational opportunity and achievement as instrumental goods that contribute to economic advancement. On a global scale, societies prosper to the extent that they can capitalize on their resources. Fifty years ago, "resources" meant tin and oil. But we've come to understand that resources include, usually first and foremost, the cognitive resources of the members of the society. Education is a key to prosperity because it maximizes the productivity and the quality of life. But the CR literature takes this line of thought a step further. It suggests that education pays unexpected dividends beyond productivity and economic success. Education functions as an early treatment—like a childhood vaccination, perhaps—that can extend the time that people can stay cognitively healthy. Failing to educate our citizens deprives them of a health benefit. There is also evidence that CR is not fixed, and that further exposure to educational opportunities can be effective throughout the lifespan (like booster shots). Life-long education should also be recognized as a health benefit.

What are the policy implications of thinking of education in terms of health? At a concrete level, we may consider whether our health insurance system ought to provide coverage for educational "interventions"—e.g. reading materials, cognitive interventions (video games?), etc.—in the way many plans cover gym membership. But thinking of education as a component of health opens the door for bigger changes in the way we think about the availability of education and learning. We might be better off getting away from the idea that to advance (beyond compulsory levels) one needs to excel. Excellence and advanced training aside, we might be better off including a component of education as cognitive exercise. Educational content here would aim less at economic productivity, and more to creating interests that can be pursued through the lifespan.

Along the same lines, we may need to rethink the widely-held dichotomy between schooling as serious and challenging, and adult education as a form of entertainment and leisure. Adult learning can be promoted as an important way of staying healthy, not only as a diversion for those who happen to enjoy a particular subject on offer. Current programs that make college and university resources available to adult learners might in the long run make a significant contribution to CR and overall cognitive well-being. The key lesson of CR is not a design for a repurposed or multipurposed educational system, but rather the acknowledgment of the education–health connection.

Similar rethinking might apply to the other factors that have been identified as positively correlated with reserve. Consider the quality of work. Work is almost exclusively designed in terms of economic function and productivity. There is a growing realization that one cannot retain the best employees unless one also provides certain lifestyle advantages, and some well-situated employers provide flexible work hours, on-site child care, and so on as perks that "make economic sense." Indeed, employers sometimes provide or subsidize access to gyms in an effort to maintain employee health. CR research suggests that we may need to go further, and consider aspects of work itself in terms of what makes health sense. So, for instance, that patterns of specialization that sharply distinguish manual labor from desk jobs, white from blue collar jobs, and so on, might be reparsed so that more cognitively-stimulating challenges are integrated with physical work and more physical demands are integrated into the typical desk job. The point, again, would be to recognize, as CR research does, that occupations have an intrinsic health dimension, and that the design of work needs to include more than economic efficiency and competitiveness. The "Eat Healthy" campaign might be paired with a "Work Healthy" ethic.

The findings about CR are also relevant to the ongoing rethinking of the importance of social relationships throughout the lifespan. We intuitively know that social isolation is unhealthy, especially for the elderly. Group living for elders—in the form of assisted living facilities and group homes—is on the rise. Current CR research suggests that these arrangements may have powerful health benefits, and would provide further support for promoting such arrangements.

Finally, we consider a more speculative matter about the cultural barriers that may need to be overcome as we move to promote cognitive exercise as a health priority. We are in the middle of a physical fitness and exercise boom (we think so, anyway). The psychology of physical fitness is no doubt complicated, but the basic appeal of physical activity and exercise—even for those who may not enjoy it for its own sake—is not. We all have bodies, it makes sense that we ought to take care of our bodies to keep them in shape. Of course, many are weak-willed and are less physically active than they know they ought to be, but even those who fail in practice recognize the ideal. We change the oil in our cars to take care of the engine, and we realize that the body needs to be kept up as well.

We suspect that these patterns of thought do not carry over easily to the case of cognitive fitness, and that it may be a challenge to convince people who may not enjoy cognitive activity for its own sake, to recognize such an activity as an ideal. Part of the reason probably has to do with the fact that our bodies live in a public space and are almost inevitably part of our public image. But there may be more to it than that. There is good empirical reason to believe that, to some degree, we remain in the grip of an inborn dualistic presumption about our own natures. On this prescientific view, our bodies are physical mechanisms, and as such, it makes perfectly good sense that we ought to do what is necessary to keep them in good operating order. But even though we learn more and more about the brain as the organ of mentality, the naïve conception, which sees the mind as non-physical, is difficult to dislodge. Despite what science tells us, the mind does not seem to be the kind of thing that needs exercise. Its capabilities and strengths and weaknesses seem inherent features of its makeup. We can realize its potential or let it languish, but the idea that we can "keep it up" in the way we do a machine—although it makes sense and may be well-supported by research—may meet intuitive resistance.

ACKNOWLEDGMENTS

This work was supported by a grant from the National Institutes on Aging (RO1 AG26158).

REFERENCES

Albert, M.S. (1995). How does education affect cognitive function? [editorial; comment]. *Annals of Epidemiology*, **5**, 76–8.

Alexander, G.E., Furey, M.L., Grady, C.L., Pietrini, P., Mentis, M.J., and Schapiro, M.B. (1997). Association of premorbid function with cerebral metabolism in Alzheimer's disease: Implications for the reserve hypothesis. *American Journal of Psychiatry*, **154**, 165–72.

Anttila, T., Helkala, E.L., Kivipelto, M., *et al.* (2002). Midlife income, occupation, APOE status, and dementia: a population-based study. *Neurology*, **59**, 887–93.

Bennett, D.A., Wilson, R.S., Schneider, J.A., *et al.* (2003). Education modifies the relation of AD pathology to level of cognitive function in older persons. *Neurology*, **60**, 1909–15.

Bickel, H. and Cooper, B. (1994). Incidence and relative risk of dementia in an urban elderly population: findings of a prospective field study. *Psychological Medicine*, **24**, 179–92.

Brown, J., Cooper-Kuhn, C.M., Kemperman, G., Van Praag, H., Winkler, J., and Gage, F.H. (2003). Enriched environment and physical activity stimulate hippocampal but not olfactory bulb neurogenesis. *European Journal of Neuroscience*, **17**, 2042–6.

Butler, S.M., Ashford, J.W., and Snowdon, D.A. (1996). Age, education, and changes in the Mini-Mental State Exam scores of older women: findings from the Nun Study. *Journal of the American Geriatrics Society*, **44**, 675–81.

Chandra, V., Pandav, R., Dodge, H.H., *et al.* (2001). Incidence of Alzheimer's disease in a rural community in India: the Indo-US study. *Neurology*, **57**, 985–9.

Chodosh, J., Reuben, D.B., Albert, M.S., and Seeman, T.E. (2002). Predicting cognitive impairment in high-functioning community-dwelling older persons: MacArthur Studies of Successful Aging. *Journal of the American Geriatrics Society*, **50**, 1051–60.

Christensen, H., Korten, A.E., Jorm, A.F., *et al.* (1997). Education and decline in cognitive performance: compensatory but not protective. *International Journal of Geriatric Psychiatry*, **12**, 323–30.

Cobb, J.L., Wolf, P.A., Au, R., White, R., and D'agostino, R.B. (1995). The effect of education on the incidence of dementia and Alzheimer's disease in the Framingham Study. *Neurology*, **45**, 1707–12.

Colsher, P.L. and Wallace, R.B. (1991). Longitudinal application of cognitive function measures in a defined population of community-dwelling elders. *Annals of Epidemiology*, **1**, 215–30.

Evans, D.A., Beckett, L.A., Albert, M.S., *et al.* (1993). Level of education and change in cognitive function in a community population of older persons. *Annals of Epidemiology*, **3**, 71–7.

Evans, D.A., Hebert, L.E., Beckett, L.A., *et al.* (1997). Education and other measures of socioeconomic status and risk of incident Alzheimer disease in a defined population of older persons. *Archives of Neurology*, **54**, 1399–45.

Fabrigoule, C., Letenneur, L., Dartigues, J.F., Zarrouk, M., Commenges, D., and Barberger-Gateau, P. (1995). Social and leisure activities and risk of dementia: a prospective longitudinal study. *Journal of American Geriatrics Society*, **43**, 485–90.

Farmer, M.E., Kittner, S.J., Rae, D.S., Bartko, J.J., and Regier, D.A. (1995). Education and change in cognitive function: The epidemiologic catchment area study. *Annals of Epidemiology*, **5**, 1–7.

Fratiglioni, L., Wang, H.X., Ericsson, K., Maytan, M., and Winblad, B. (2000). Influence of social network on occurrence of dementia: a community-based longitudinal study. *Lancet*, **355**, 1315–19.

Geerlings, M.I., Deeg, D.J., Penninx, B.W., *et al.* (1999). Cognitive reserve and mortality in dementia: the role of cognition, functional ability and depression. *Psychological Medicine*, **29**, 1219–26.

Graves, A.B., Mortimer, J.A., Larson, E.B., Wenzlow, A., Bowen, J.D., and Mccormick, W.C. (1996). Head circumference as a measure of cognitive reserve. Association with severity of impairment in Alzheimer's disease. *British Journal of Psychiatry*, **169**, 86–92.

Hall, C.B., Derby, C., Levalley, A., Katz, M. J., Verghese, J., and Lipton, R.B. (2007). Education delays accelerated decline on a memory test in persons who develop dementia. *Neurology*, **69**, 1657–64.

Hall, K.S., Gao, S., Unverzagt, F.W., and Hendrie, H.C. (2000). Low education and childhood rural residence: risk for Alzheimer's disease in African Americans. *Neurology*, **54**, 95–9.

Helmer, C., Damon, D., Letenneur, L., *et al.* (1999). Marital status and risk of Alzheimer's disease: a French population-based cohort study. *Neurology*, **53**, 1953–8.

Helmer, C., Letenneur, L., Rouch, I., *et al.* (2001). Occupation during life and risk of dementia in French elderly community residents. *Journal of Neurology, Neurosurgery and Psychiatry*, **71**, 303–9.

Helzner, E.P., Scarmeas, N., Cosentino, S., Portet, F., and Stern, Y. (2007). Leisure activity and cognitive decline in incident Alzheimer disease. *Archives of Neurology*, **64**, 1749–54.

Jorm, A.F., Rodgers, B., Henderson, A.S., *et al.* (1998). Occupation type as a predictor of cognitive decline and dementia in old age. *Age and Ageing*, **27**, 477–83.

Katzman, R. (1993). Education and the prevalence of dementia and Alzheimer's disease. *Neurology*, **43**, 13–20.

Katzman, R., Aronson, M., Fuld, P., *et al.* (1989). Development of dementing illnesses in an 80-year-old volunteer cohort. *Annals of Neurology*, **25**, 317–24.

Kesler, S.R., Adams, H.F., Blasey, C.M., and Bigler, E.D. (2003). Premorbid intellectual functioning, education, and brain size in traumatic brain injury: An investigation of the cognitive reserve hypothesis. *Applied Neuropsychology*, **10**, 153–62.

Launer, L.J., Andersen, K., Dewey, M.E., *et al.* (1999). Rates and risk factors for dementia and Alzheimer's disease: results from EURODEM pooled analyses. EURODEM Incidence Research Group and Work Groups. European Studies of Dementia. *Neurology*, **52**, 78–84.

Lazarov, O., Robinson, J., Tang, Y.P., *et al.* (2005). Environmental enrichment reduces Abeta levels and amyloid deposition in transgenic mice. *Cell*, **120**, 701–13.

Letenneur, L., Commenges, D., Dartigues, J.F., and Barberger-Gateau, P. (1994). Incidence of dementia and Alzheimer's disease in elderly community residents of south-western France. *International Journal of Epidemiology*, **23**, 1256–61.

Lyketsos, C.G., Chen, L.-S., and Anthony, J.C. (1999). Cognitive decline in adulthood: an 11.5-year follow-up of the Baltimore Epidemiologic Catchment Area Study. *American Jounal of Psychiatry*, **156**, 58–65.

Manly, J.J., Schupf, N., Tang, M.X., and Stern, Y. (2005). Cognitive decline and literacy among ethnically diverse elders. *Journal of Geriatic Psychiatry and Neurology*, **18**, 213–17.

Paykel, E.S., Brayne, C., Huppert, F.A., *et al.* (1994). Incidence of dementia in a population older than 75 years in the United Kingdom. *Archives of General Psychiatry*, **54**, 325–32.

Perneczky, R., Drzezga, A., Ehl-Schmid, J., *et al.* (2006). Schooling mediates brain reserve in Alzheimer's disease: findings of fluoro-deoxy-glucose-positron emission tomography. *Journal of Neurology, Neurosurgery and Psychiatry*, **77**, 1060–3.

Qiu, C., Backman, L., Winblad, B., Aguero-Torres, H., and Fratiglioni, L. (2001). The influence of education on clinically diagnosed dementia incidence and mortality data from the Kungsholmen Project. *Archives of Neurology*, **58**, 2034–9.

Qiu, C., Karp, A., Von Strauss, E., Winblad, B., Fratiglioni, L., and Bellander, T. (2003). Lifetime principal occupation and risk of Alzheimer's disease in the Kungsholmen project. *American Journal of Industrial Medicine*, **43**, 204–11.

Satz, P. (1993). Brain reserve capacity on symptom onset after brain injury: A formulation and review of evidence for threshold theory. *Neuropsychology*, 7, 273–95.

Scarmeas, N., Levy, G., Tang, M.X., Manly, J., and Stern, Y. (2001). Influence of leisure activity on the incidence of Alzheimer's disease. *Neurology*, 57, 2236–42.

Scarmeas, N., Zarahn, E., Anderson, K.E., *et al.* (2003). Association of life activities with cerebral blood flow in Alzheimer disease: implications for the cognitive reserve hypothesis. *Archives of Neurology*, 60, 359–65.

Scarmeas, N., Albert, S.M., Manly, J.J., and Stern, Y. (2006). Education and rates of cognitive decline in incident Alzheimer's disease. *Journal of Neurology, Neurosurgery and Psychiatry*, 77, 308–16.

Schmand, B., Smit, J.H., Geerlings, M.I., and Lindeboom, J. (1997). The effects of intelligence and education on the development of dementia. A test of the brain reserve hypothesis. *Psychological Medicine*, 27, 1337–44.

Snowdon, D.A., Ostwald, S.K., and Kane, R.L. (1989). Education, survival and independence in elderly Catholic sisters, 1936–1988. *American Journal of Epidemiology*, 130, 999–1012.

Stern, Y. (2002). What is cognitive reserve? Theory and research application of the reserve concept. *Journal of the International Neuropsychological Society*, 8, 448–60.

Stern, Y. (2009). Cognitive reserve. *Neuropsychologia*, 47, 2015–18.

Stern, Y., Alexander, G.E., Prohovnik, I., and Mayeux, R. (1992). Inverse relationship between education and parietotemporal perfusion deficit in Alzheimer's disease. *Annals of Neurology*, 32, 371–5.

Stern, Y., Gurland, B., Tatemichi, T.K., Tang, M.X., Wilder, D., and Mayeux, R. (1994). Influence of education and occupation on the incidence of Alzheimer's disease. *Journal of the American Medical Association*, 271, 1004–10.

Stern, Y., Alexander, G.E., Prohovnik, I., *et al.* (1995a). Relationship between lifetime occupation and parietal flow: Implications for a reserve against Alzheimer's disease pathology. *Neurology*, 45, 55–60.

Stern, Y., Tang, M.X., Denaro, J., and Mayeux, R. (1995b). Increased risk of mortality in Alzheimer's disease patients with more advanced educational and occupational attainment. *Annals of Neurology*, 37, 590–5.

Stern, Y., Albert, S., Tang, M.X., and Tsai, W.Y. (1999). Rate of memory decline in AD is related to education and occupation: Cognitive reserve? *Neurology*, 53, 1942–57.

Stern, Y., Habeck, C., Moeller, J., *et al.* (2005). Brain networks associated with cognitive reserve in healthy young and old adults. *Cerebral Cortex*, 15, 394–402.

Valenzuela, M.J. and Sachdev, P. (2005). Brain reserve and dementia: a systematic review. *Psychological Medicine*, 25, 1–14.

Van Praag, H., Shubert, T., Zhao, C., and Gage, F.H. (2005). Exercise enhances learning and hippocampal neurogenesis in aged mice. *Journal of Neuroscience*, 25, 8680–5.

Verghese, J., Lipton, R.B., Katz, M.J., *et al.* (2003). Leisure Activities and the Risk of Dementia in the Elderly. *New England Journal of Medicine*, 348, 2508–16.

Wang, H.X., Karp, A., Winblad, B., and Fratiglioni, L. (2002). Late-life engagement in social and leisure activities is associated with a decreased risk of dementia: a longitudinal study from the Kungsholmen project. *American Journal of Epidemiology*, 155, 1081–7.

White, L., Katzman, R., Losonczy, K., *et al.* (1994). Association of education with incidence of cognitive impairment in three established populations for epidemiologic studies of the elderly. *Journal of Clinical Epidemiology*, 47, 363–74.

Willerman, L., Schultz, R., Rutledge, J.N., and Bigler.E.D (1991). In vivo brain size and intelligence. *Intelligence,* **15,** 223–8.

Wilson, R.S., Mendes De Leon, C.F., Barnes, L.L., *et al.* (2002). Participation in cognitively stimulating activities and risk of incident Alzheimer disease. *Journal of the American Medical Association,* **287,** 742–8.

Zhang, M., Katzman, R., Salmon, D., *et al.* (1990). The prevalence of dementia and Alzheimer's disease in Shanghai,China: Impact of age, gender and education. *Annals of Neurology,* **27,** 428–37.

Zhang, X., Li, C., and Zhang, M. (1999). [Psychosocial risk factors of Alzheimer's disease]. *Zhonghua Yi Xue Za Zhi,* **79,** 335–8.

CHAPTER 34

....

ETHICAL ISSUES IN THE MANAGEMENT OF PARKINSON'S DISEASE

....

SILKE APPEL-CRESSWELL AND A. JON STOESSL

INTRODUCTION

PARKINSON'S disease (PD) is a neurodegenerative condition affecting most prominently the neurons of the substantia nigra pars compacta in the midbrain with their dopaminergic projections to the striatum, thereby leading to the well-known motor symptoms of tremor, rigidity, and slowness (bradykinesia) of movement with difficulties initiating and sustaining movements. In addition, the illness causes patients to suffer from increasingly severe and widespread dysfunction of the central nervous system leading to disturbances of sleep, sense of smell, autonomic function, cognition, motivation, and mood, as well as decision making and personality. The clinical symptoms have a profound impact on the patient's and caregiver's quality of life and the diagnosis and treatment of PD, as well as research into the disease, raise wide-ranging ethical questions. In this chapter, we concentrate on the genetics of PD, functional imaging including imaging of pre-symptomatic subjects, and treatment of Parkinsonian diseases including novel treatments, side effects, the placebo effect, potential biases in the evaluation and promotion of therapies, and access to resources as examples of the numerous and varied ethical challenges associated with this neurodegenerative disorder.

GENETICS

Inherited forms of PD account for approximately 10% of the disease. The identification of subjects at high risk for developing PD represents an enormous opportunity for scientific study, but also raises particular challenges from an ethical perspective.

Challenges for research in patients with autosomal dominant disease

There are at least two genes in which either mutations or altered expression can lead to dominantly inherited PD. The first to be identified was α-synuclein, in which a G209A mutation was found to be responsible for parkinsonism in families of Sicilian or Greek origin (Polymeropoulos *et al.* 1997). Shortly after this mutation was identified, a much less common mutation (A30P) was found to be associated with PD in another kindred of German origin (Kruger *et al.* 1998). More recently, it has been found that increased dose of the normal synuclein gene can also induce disease (Chartier-Harlin *et al.* 2004; Fuchs *et al.* 2007; Singleton *et al.* 2003). Despite the undeniable importance of the discovery of these mutations, all together these account for a very small minority of even inherited PD.

In contrast to α-synuclein, mutations in the gene encoding leucine-rich repeat kinase 2 (LRRK2) appear to be responsible for a substantial proportion of inherited PD (Paisan-Ruiz *et al.* 2004; Zimprich *et al.* 2004), as well as approximately 1.5% of apparently "sporadic" PD worldwide (Gilks *et al.* 2005) and up to 40% in some populations (Lesage *et al.* 2005). LRRK2 is interesting from many perspectives, including pathological heterogeneity (Wszolek *et al.* 2004; Zimprich *et al.* 2004), gain of function (Smith *et al.* 2006), and variable expressivity, with some subjects remaining disease-free into advanced age (Goldwurm *et al.* 2007; Healy *et al.* 2008; Latourelle *et al.* 2008). Thus, even if an unaffected individual from an at-risk pedigree were to desire genetic testing and this confirmed the presence of the mutation, one would have difficulty advising him/her with respect to when they would develop disease, if they were to do so at all.

Challenges for research in patients with autosomal recessive disease

The first described autosomal recessive form of PD was due to mutations in the gene encoding parkin (Kitada *et al.* 1998), an ubiquitin E3 ligase (Shimura *et al.* 2000). Parkin mutations, originally thought to account for young onset parkinsonism, predominantly in the Japanese, are now known to contribute to PD in all ages, worldwide. Disease may arise from point mutations or gene deletions and many affected individuals are compound heterozygotes with 2 different abnormalities. The estimated prevalence of parkin mutations is approximately 3% (Lincoln *et al.* 2003). Less common mutations resulting in recessively inherited PD include PINK1 (PARK6) and DJ-1 (PARK7).

Available evidence to date suggests that recessively inherited forms of PD are more likely to onset at a younger than average age and that disease progression is slower compared to later onset (or dominantly inherited) PD. Apart from the very different challenges facing patients and their families when PD onsets at a younger age, such individuals may still be planning families and it may therefore be appropriate to routinely offer genetic testing to young-onset PD patients (bearing in mind that a finding of a recessively inherited mutation would only be meaningful if the partner is tested as well). The situation is made more complex by the possibility that inheritance of even a single mutant allele may be associated with subclinical dopamine dysfunction (see following section on imaging) or may act as a risk factor for sporadic PD (Satake *et al.* 2009; Simon-Sanchez *et al.* 2009).

Ethical implications of preclinical diagnosis

In families with dominantly inherited disease, it may be possible to perform DNA analysis in at risk individuals. This must be conducted within the context of an environment that provides adequate screening for emotional state, genetic counseling, and counseling for possible psychological fallout from the results of disclosing whether or not the individual has been affected. These issues are discussed in greater depth elsewhere in this volume (see Chapter 31) but it should be remembered that "good news" may not always be interpreted as such for a variety of reasons, including survivor guilt and an unexpected void in a life that had hitherto revolved around the deemed inevitability of developing serious disease (Lawson *et al.* 1996). As some mutations may not be associated with the development of disease even at quite advanced age (Goldwurm *et al.* 2007; Healy *et al.* 2008; Latourelle *et al.* 2008) in certain individuals, considerable caution is required in the interpretation of genetic results. Taking together the problems of multiple genes, reduced penetrance, variable expressivity, and the uncertain role of heterozygous mutations (in recessively inherited forms of parkinsonism) and susceptibility genes, genetic testing for PD is generally regarded as a research rather than a clinical tool, except in select circumstances (Klein and Schlossmacher 2007).

IMAGING

The complex process of producing persuasive pictures

Functional imaging studies in PD are carried out for research purposes mainly using positron emission tomography (PET) and functional magnetic resonance imaging (fMRI). Both techniques rely on sophisticated data processing and advanced statistics.

FMRI like PET depends on numerous steps in the generation and analysis of data: The image obtained is based on the blood oxygenation level-dependent (BOLD) contrast which is influenced by oxygen consumption and cerebral blood flow and which is thought to be closely related to neuronal activity. Neuronal activity, though, can change within milliseconds whereas cerebral blood flow (the "hemodynamic response") occurs with a delay of 1–2s and thus limits the temporal resolution of fMRI. Blood flow itself is dependent not only on increased demand generated by neuronal activity, but can also be influenced by many other physiological factors including age, cardiovascular function, red blood cell state, medication, and others (Illes *et al.* 2006a). The differences in BOLD contrast are very small and repetition of the task/measurement is required to obtain statistically significantly differences. Signal strength is proportional to the size of the chosen region of interest and thus small areas of neuronal activity are difficult to detect, whereas larger areas of interest are susceptible to partial volume effects. Spatial resolution is further compromised by the numerous statistical operations required: MRI image generation uses probabilistic covariances, often warping brain images into a common template and averaging scans from several subjects to derive the relative statistical intensity values for each brain region, the basis for the final color coded images. Thus the results are probabilistic associations in nature rather than causal relationships (Fuchs 2006; Illes 2007).

The condition under which a scan is obtained, and, if a task is used, the specific details of the task and the control condition which in fMRI is "subtracted" from the images obtained during the task, are crucial to the conclusions that can be drawn from the results. Ideally, the brain function under investigation is the only difference between the task and the control condition. Usually, tasks used for imaging experiments are relatively simple and caution about their generalizations to explain complex social behaviors is warranted (Fuchs 2006). Activation of a brain region during a task might not be causally related to the task and the processes employed by different individuals for a certain task can differ and thus lead to variations in activation patterns (Illes *et al.* 2006a). Multiple other factors influence a task, including word frequency, word familiarity in verbal tasks or visual frequency leading to significant variations in activation patterns (Van Orden and Paap 1997). Ideally, the studied subjects should be as uniform as possible in education, sex, age, primary language etc., on the other hand, this limits the generalizability of findings. In studies with PD patients, for example, problems can arise due to diminished color discrimination in PD or due to the effect of attentional and other, even subtle cognitive changes potentially influencing a wide range of tasks. It is also worth remembering that the fMRI signal does not differentiate between the activation of inhibitory and excitatory neurons which complicates the interpretation of findings further.

PET imaging allows the study of function rather than structure. It requires the injection of a biological substance such as glucose, or a drug such as levodopa or raclopride linked to a radiotracer. The combined molecule is taken up by different tissues and in the case of PD by different brain regions, depending on the tracer selected. The radiotracer releases a positron which soon collides with an electron in the tissue. This reaction leads to the emission of two photons which travel in exactly opposite directions and which can be detected by the tomograph allowing the spatial reconstruction of their point of origin and thus indirectly the localization of the radiotracer. The spatial resolution of currently leading PET scanners reaches 2–3mm but is more often in the realm of 5–10mm which can become worse when images are reconstructed. Compared to structural imaging techniques such as MRI the spatial resolution is poor, rendering PET vulnerable to partial volume effects, particularly when looking at small regions of interest. The problem is somewhat more complex than in structural imaging, as one may be contrasting areas of high and low function, even in the absence of significant structural abnormalities. The measured radioactivity reflects the tracer input function, non-specific uptake/binding, conversion of the biological substance in the tissue and specific binding (for receptor ligands), amongst other processes. The temporal resolution is limited and image acquisition which requires the subject to lie still takes relatively long, exact times depending on the radiotracer and biological substance used. In subjects with PD, the ability to lie still can be reduced due to motor, cognitive, urinary urge, or pain and discomfort related factors and thus degrading both PET and fMRI images. The risk related to the small dose of radioactivity used in PET is thought to be low but multiple studies in younger subjects require a particularly careful weighing of risks versus potential benefit (Appel-Cresswell *et al.* 2010).

As detailed earlier for fMRI, the choice of the control condition is crucial: In the PD literature, one recent example of potential pitfalls when choosing and interpreting a control paradigm is a PET study measuring dopamine release where PD patients with pathological gambling were compared to non-gambling PD patients during a gambling task involving cards. The control task used the same cards but only involved sorting the cards rather than the gambling aspect which included winning and losing. The authors describe differential findings between PD controls and PD gamblers during the task but also during the control condition which they interpret as evidence for an underlying, not task dependent abnormality in the dopamine system representing a marker of vulnerability to addiction (Steeves *et al.* 2009). An alternative explanation for the finding could be, though, that the cards themselves served as a gambling cue for the patients. Drug-associated cues themselves have very recently been shown to lead to dopamine release in PD patients with impulse control disorders including pathological gambling (Piccini and Brooks 2010). Drug-related stimuli are known to lead to craving and dopamine release in most addictions and exposure to drug-related stimuli is associated with an increased risk for relapse after abstinence (Volkow *et al.* 2004).

A task carried out in the scanner, even if it is well designed, will usually only address a particular aspect of the complex interplay of factors determining a behavior: For example, a study on changes in the reward system in PD visualized as dopamine release in the ventral striatum (Evans *et al.* 2006) provides valuable information on one aspect of the dopamine dysregulation syndrome but it does not assess the role of important other factors such as the influence of the prefrontal lobes or environmental factors in modulating actual behaviors.

The limitations of functional imaging techniques need to be communicated clearly to prevent simplified misleading conclusions especially if imaging techniques should be employed to predict behavior or as detailed in the next section to predict disease. This is of particular relevance when techniques or images are used outside the medical research setting for which the technique was developed, e.g. the justice system or potentially by insurance companies, educational institutions, and employers. In a world dominated by fast visual impressions a picture "of the brain in action" might appear more attractive and convincing than a detailed written and statistical discussion explaining how the images were derived.

Imaging of asymptomatic subjects at high-risk for Parkinson's disease

Imaging studies may also provide evidence of subclinical disease in high-risk populations. The symptoms of PD do not develop until people have lost approximately 50% of their nigral dopamine (DA) neurons, or up to 80% of striatal DA content. Functional imaging using PET or single photon emission computed tomography (SPECT) may detect subclinical abnormalities of nigrostriatal DA function in people exposed to dopaminergic toxins (Calne *et al.* 1985) or in subjects with increased genetic risk (Adams *et al.* 2005; Piccini *et al.* 1999). Here again, considerable caution is required in interpretation, as only limited data are available on progression from subclinical DA dysfunction to clinical disease (Nandhagopal *et al.* 2008). In the absence of more information on the progression of DA dysfunction, it is for instance possible that mutation carriers could have lifelong abnormalities of DA function but still not go on to develop PD. In the case of recessively inherited mutations, the situation is even more complex, because PET evidence of subclinical DA dysfunction has been described in single mutation heterozygous mutation carriers for both parkin and PINK1 (Khan *et al.* 2002, 2005). Whether this represents increased susceptibility to sporadic PD in single mutation carriers, haploinsufficiency or a dominant negative effect of the mutation is unclear. It is, however, worth noting that structural MRI abnormalities have also been observed in heterozygous parkin mutation carriers (Binkofski *et al.* 2007).

Ultimately, the information provided to asymptomatic subjects participating in PET studies will depend upon (i) the purpose of their involvement (in the case of PET, most subjects will be participating for research rather than diagnostic purposes—see later); (ii) how (if) this possibility was addressed in the consent form; (iii) with what degree of certainty one can interpret the results and (iv) whether one can act on them (i.e. would advance knowledge of a likely incipient diagnosis of PD result in different (neuroprotective) treatment?). As already outlined, current knowledge probably does not permit accurate prognostication, particularly not based on a single radiotracer study performed at a single point in time. Studies using multiple tracers (which may be differentially affected) and in a longitudinal fashion may provide greater insight, but this is still an area of investigation and may well differ from one genetic mutation to another. The uncertainty associated with such studies highlights the importance of careful attention to the wording of the consent form and as a corollary to ensuring that one has explored participants' motivation for participating in the study and that they are well informed in advance about possible outcomes and how information will be handled. In view of the uncertainty of interpretation of the results from imaging studies and the current lack of established neuroprotective therapies, it is our view that functional imaging studies in individuals at increased risk of developing PD should be performed for research purposes only and that attempts to perform diagnostic imaging are ethically tenuous. This view could of course be drastically modified as our knowledge of the relationship between imaging abnormalities and disease grows, or if a suitable neuroprotective therapy is discovered.

Incidental abnormalities

It is likely that in attempting to study a healthy control population an unanticipated subclinical abnormality of DA function may be detected in some individuals, which will inevitably raise questions as to the significance of the finding and whether/how this information should be disclosed to the participant. While there is an emerging literature on incidental imaging findings in other scenarios, this possibility has received relatively scant attention in the PD literature. Assuming that abnormal DA imaging is highly specific for presynaptic abnormalities of DA function (most of which could be attributed to PD, as opposed to other disorders of DA neurons), the prevalence of significant abnormalities in a healthy elderly control population could approach 10% or even higher (the generally accepted figure for incidental Lewy body disease above the age of 65 (Dickson *et al.* 2008)). It is again important to examine the original purpose of the study and the participant's motivation to participate. People with a family history of PD may be more motivated than most to participate in research, in part for altruistic reasons, and in part because they may hope to learn whether they themselves are likely to be affected. Such individuals should really not be regarded as healthy controls, as they have a known increased risk, and such information should hopefully be gleaned during the screening process. As mentioned earlier, the subject's expectations and the wording of the consent form are critical—most healthy research subjects expect that any meaningful abnormality detected will be disclosed to them (Kirschen et al. 2006). Subjects could be told that the study is being conducted entirely for research purposes and that abnormalities will not be disclosed to them. This would be deemed a relatively extreme approach as in some cases (more likely with structural MRI than for PET), an incidental abnormality that could have serious implications for the subject's health may be detected. Thus, a common compromise is to indicate to the subject in advance that in the event of an abnormality deemed "significant," the result will (with the subject's consent) be disclosed to his/her family physician. Given the uncertainty associated with the interpretation of functional imaging studies (as described earlier, it is not necessarily true that an asymptomatic individual with abnormal PET will necessarily go on to develop PD), however, this may not be a particularly helpful approach. One might indicate (again with consent) that an abnormality of uncertain significance has been detected and that periodic neurological evaluation is recommended.

This topic has received considerable attention in the last few years. However, the relevant literature deals predominantly with the problem of how to deal with structural abnormalities detected when structural MRI is conducted as part of a research protocol, often one using functional MRI. There are some overarching principles arising from this literature that may apply in general (Illes 2006; Illes et al. 2006b; 2008). However, there are also several important differences about the specific situation for functional imaging in PD. First, PET (or SPECT) images are purely functional. Especially when conducted with dopaminergic tracers, it is unlikely that any diagnostic information other than that related to the specific question of dopamine innervation can be derived. This is in sharp contrast to MRI, where a study conducted to look at cognitive activation patterns might potentially uncover a hitherto unsuspected brain tumor or aneurysm. Secondly, whereas diagnostic (as opposed to research) MRI scans are typically interpreted by neuroradiologists, this is not necessarily the case for PET. A related issue is that in contrast to MRI, where the diagnosis is predominantly based on appearance, analysis of PET data is usually dependent upon the application of a quantitative tracer model to measures of radioactivity taken from predetermined regions of interest. The interpretation requires a knowledge of various assumptions and technical limitations as detailed above and may just as readily come from a physicist looking at a printout of numbers as from a medically trained imager. As discussed earlier, there may be genuine uncertainty about the biological significance of impaired dopaminergic function as detected by PET, as opposed to the finding of a tumor, which will presumably require a plan for further investigation and/or management, even if the tissue diagnosis is not clear. A finding of impaired dopaminergic function, while potentially highly suggestive depending on the pattern, may not be specific for Parkinson's and the prognosis may therefore be unclear. Finally, even if one could be certain that the subject might be in the incipient stages of PD, it is not clear how one would use this information, as currently available treatments are for symptomatic control and there are no established neuroprotective or preventative therapies.

Use of research imaging for diagnostic purposes

Although practices vary from one center to another, functional imaging techniques are highly specialized and require major infrastructure support as well as considerable expertise in interpretation. As such, they are frequently although not invariably, conducted for research purposes, funded by research grants. From time to time, such studies may become of interest to other parties for reasons unrelated to the research. Examples would include insurance companies or a legal action, where scan information could potentially be used to confirm diagnosis, determine whether the pattern of abnormality is typical of sporadic PD or more suggestive of an alternate form of parkinsonism (this might for instance potentially be used to support or refute a diagnosis of post-traumatic parkinsonism (Turjanski *et al.* 1997)), or to try and assess level of disease at a particular point in time. An example of questionable use of PET for medicolegal purposes comes from the recent suggestion that PD in welders may reflect exposure to manganese (Racette *et al.* 2001). While prior literature suggested that parkinsonism due to manganese toxicity was associated with intact pre- and postsynaptic function (Shinotoh *et al.* 1997), more recent papers have suggested that the appearance may be similar to that seen in idiopathic sporadic PD (Racette *et al.* 2005). Regardless of the truth, it is clear that studies originally performed for purely academic purposes can potentially be used (or abused) by either side in a legal battle surrounding causation of disease. Apart from the possibility of mistaken or uncertain interpretation, it should be remembered that the original purpose of the patient's involvement and the only one for which consent was obtained, was in order to acquire data for research studies. In the authors' view, any other use of the data, even with post-hoc consent, is ethically questionable. Other potential (and more serious) misuses of imaging data are discussed in the following sections.

Imaging and personality traits, personal preferences, and deception

In 1913 Carl Camp wrote that PD affects individuals whose "lives had been devoted to hard work…and who never come under the inhibiting influences of tobacco or alcohol. In this respect, the disease may be almost regarded as a badge of respectable endeavor" (Camp 1913). PD patients have been described as "honest" and more recently, Abe and colleagues tested PD patients' perceived difficulties to lie; in their study they correlated difficulties with lying in PD patients with hypometabolism in specific areas of the prefrontal cortex, particularly the dorsolateral prefrontal cortex, compared to controls (Abe *et al.* 2009). Functional imaging in PD has further been employed to investigate decision making, cognitive function, impulse control disorders, and reward processing (Abe *et al.* 2009; Abler *et al.* 2009; Bodi *et al.* 2009; Canli 2006; Evans *et al.* 2005, 2006; Kaasinen *et al.* 2001; Pagonabarraga *et al.* 2007; Steeves *et al.* 2009) as discussed in the following section on therapy. The ethical issues related to studies of personality, preferences, and deception are relevant beyond the study of PD and the literature most poignantly discusses these questions in non-PD subjects, particularly when studies are carried out for reasons other than medical research or management. For a detailed discussion of these questions, the reader is thus referred to the dedicated section "Conciousness and intention: decoding mental states and decision making" in this volume.

THERAPY

There are several issues encountered in the management of patients with PD in which ethical considerations may be important. These include the strength of evidence used to support a decision to use newer rather than more established therapies, the potential to alter personality and behavior, the role of the placebo effect, and access to resources.

Novel versus established therapies

A full discussion of the advantages and disadvantages of the many therapeutic options available for PD is beyond the scope of this chapter. Our purpose is rather to highlight the ethical implications of scientific and non-scientific issues that may direct treatment for a given individual with PD. The potential advantage of other medications and indeed other therapeutic approaches notwithstanding, the best established and most effective therapy for PD is replacement of missing dopamine with its precursor levodopa. Because of some potential problems with levodopa therapy, including reduction in efficacy, shortened duration of action and involuntary movements or dyskinesias, numerous other approaches have been developed either as adjuncts to levodopa, or as alternatives for initial therapy. While the strength of evidence used to support these treatments may seem more appropriate for a textbook on therapy than a handbook of ethics, we argue that there are indeed serious ethical implications. First, in an age of global communication, patients often are and should be well informed about novel therapies and may demand them, or fail to understand that they are either still very much in development or, even if approved, that the advantages compared to more traditional approaches are limited. Examples of the former would include invasive treatments such as fetal tissue transplantation, stem cell therapy, or gene therapy. In all cases, evidence supporting their use is either limited or lacking and the potential risks are substantial. However, the well-intentioned enthusiasm of the scientific community may lead patients to feel that a potentially useful treatment is being withheld and they may in some cases choose to travel to other countries in order to obtain access. This of course raises additional ethical concerns, including the practice of providing unproven therapies as if they were established, as well as the obligation of the scientific and medical communities to balance optimism with realism. The ethical considerations surrounding the initiation of trials of invasive therapy for PD have recently been reviewed by Kimmelman and colleagues (Kimmelman et al. 2009). Special considerations include the relatively high potential risk associated with such procedures—on a background where the underlying disease, while potentially debilitating, is nonetheless amenable to several helpful symptomatic therapies and is not immediately life threatening (in contrast to cancer, where similar degrees of risk may be deemed more acceptable, given the lack of suitable alternatives). The problem is compounded by the limited ability of preclinical models to determine likely risk. The authors therefore conclude that such trials can be ethically justified only when the quantity and quality of preclinical evidence meets a high standard, when this evidence suggests that there is a reasonably high likelihood of clinical benefit and/or a prospect of deriving significant generalizable knowledge. In order to meet these objectives, the authors emphasize the need for statement of a priori hypotheses and associated power calculations, randomization, blinded treatment allocation and assessment in preclinical studies, as well as attention to treatment of missing data. Selection of better animal models that more closely mimic the human condition is also needed prior to embarking upon first in human use and the preclinical studies should correspond to the methodology anticipated for clinical trials. Finally, the authors point to the need to control optimism and publication bias—essentially holding preclinical studies to the more stringent standards that are set for pivotal clinical trials. While these recommendations seem to reflect common sense and the application of best scientific practice, the standards have not always been met and this may have led to undue optimism with respect to "high-tech" therapies.

A more subtle difficulty arises when one looks at the strength of evidence for certain therapies. For instance, based on neuroimaging studies, claims have been made that early dopamine agonist monotherapy is associated with a slower rate of progression of PD compared to initial therapy with levodopa (Marek *et al.* 2002; Whone *et al.* 2003), yet the clinical significance of these findings is unclear (Ahlskog 2003; Albin and Frey 2003). Furthermore, any potential benefits of early agonist therapy must be balanced against the potential disadvantages of excessive daytime sleepiness and impulse control disorders.

In assessing the numerous factors that may drive patients' demands and physicians' prescribing practices, one cannot ignore the potential role of marketing by the pharmaceutical industry. Many of the relevant studies, even though conducted by true experts and published in high quality journals, are nevertheless funded by industry and there may be commercial advantages to certain interpretations or secondary analyses. The issue is compounded by the recruitment of "Key Opinion Leaders", who may sometimes unwittingly be subject to non-scientific influences (Moynihan 2008).

MEDICATION EFFECTS

Personality

Personality factors are thought of as stable over time—they aim to describe the enduring characteristics of a person. Yet, both PD as well as the medication used to treat the disease can have profound influences on a patient's personality: dopaminergic medication influences the personality factors novelty seeking and to a lesser extent harm avoidance (Bodi *et al.* 2009; Menza 2000) which can play a key factor when a previously industrious person becomes a pathological gambler on dopaminergic medication. Thus the possibility of altering core aspects of a patient's personality, the self, with potentially devastating consequences (e.g. pathological gambling as described later) requires very careful weighing of risks and potential benefits of a medication. On the other hand, one study described increased impulsivity and reward seeking behavior in nearly 20% of PD patients treated with a dopamine agonist, but this was perceived as a negative change by less than 20% of such affected subjects, perhaps as it seemed to result in more spontaneity and rewarding experiences, usually perceived as lacking in PD patients (Kunig *et al.* 2000; Ondo and Lai 2008). Is there a risk of taking away a source of joy from the majority of patients in order to prevent harm in a few?

The perceived positive change in behavior, though, might make the slope into detrimental behavior patterns even more slippery.

Decision making

PD patients on dopaminergic therapy are impaired in learning from negative outcomes, and PD patients off dopaminergic therapy are impaired in learning from positive outcomes (Bodi *et al.* 2009; Frank *et al.* 2004; Van Eimeren *et al.* 2009). The likely reason for this phenomenon is that a positive outcome, a reward, triggers dopamine release in the ventral striatum, a structure crucial for the processing of reward, while a negative outcome is associated with a dip in dopamine release in controls (Schultz 2002). PD patients *on* medication have constant externally derived dopaminergic stimulation so the dip necessary to register a negative outcome is restricted; when *off* medication, they are not able to generate a spike in dopaminergic transmission. The assumption thus is that this mechanism contributes to the development of impulse control disorders described in the next section, as PD patients cannot learn from the negative consequences of their behavior and are more likely to continue detrimental patterns of behavior. The deficit in learning and decision making potentially has another implication as well: depending on whether an individual with PD is on or off when consenting to participation in a study, choosing a treatment or making other risk-associated decisions in their personal or private life, there might well be a bias depending on the status of their medication and researchers and physicians might have to inform patients about this potential bias in important decisions and need to keep this potential limitation in mind when consenting patients to procedures, treatments or studies.

Impulsive and compulsive symptoms

The dopaminergic medications used to treat PD can lead to impulsive and compulsive symptoms: about 6–14% of patients treated with dopaminergic medication are affected by these potentially devastating side effects (Giladi *et al.* 2007; Voon *et al.* 2006) which consist of complex often repetitive disinhibitory, addiction-like behaviors and include impulse control disorders (ICDs), punding, and the so-called "dopamine dysregulation syndrome" (Bodi *et al.* 2009; Evans *et al.* 2009). Associated with them are changes in reward-related behavior (Evans *et al.* 2006; Steeves *et al.* 2009), personality traits (Bodi *et al.* 2009), decision making (van Eimeren *et al.* 2009), and cognition (Brand *et al.* 2004; Pagonabarraga *et al.* 2007; Rossi *et al.* 2009; Santangelo *et al.* 2009; Siri *et al.* 2009). These neuropsychiatric side effects in PD are thus raising questions related to the self, autonomy, determinism, and moral agency.

The DSM-IV describes ICDs as "the failure to resist an impulse, drive, or temptation to perform an act that is harmful to the person or to others" (American Psychiatric Association 2000). It refers to repetitive, excessive behaviors that have detrimental effects on other areas of life, e.g. in the professional, financial, personal/social realm. ICDs are thought of as "behavioral addictions" and share some features with substance related addictions. The ICDs encountered in PD prominently include pathological gambling, hypersexuality, compulsive shopping, and compulsive eating (Lim *et al.* 2008; Voon *et al.* 2006). Risk factors for the development of ICDs and/or dopamine dysregulation syndrome include younger age, a previous personal or family history of substance abuse, certain personality traits such as novelty seeking and high impulsivity, male sex for most ICDs and particularly hypersexuality and pathological gambling, as well as dyskinesias (Lim *et al.* 2008).

Pathological gambling refers to recurrent gambling behavior with spending of increasing amounts, a preoccupation with gambling, unsuccessful attempts to control the spending, and chasing losses. Patients often become irritable when trying to cut down on the behavior, they might even be lying and stealing money and thus endangering relationships, jobs, and pensions. Voon *et al.* found an average loss of $129,000 in a series of PD patients with pathological gambling. Slot machine gambling, which is viewed to be particularly addictive, has been found to be the most prevalent in PD gamblers, followed by gambling in casinos and on the internet as well as lottery, betting, and bingo (Gallagher *et al.* 2007), gambling on the internet is expected to become a growing problem, though, given its nearly ubiquitous availability and frequent pop-up windows inviting users to gambling activities (Wong *et al.* 2007). Pathological gambling is the most common ICD in Parkinson's disease and like the other ICDs described here most often occurs in PD patients who before starting on dopamine agonist medication did not have a gambling problem. Patients often try to hide their behavior from their partners and families, and only when substantial amounts of money are lost, do the problems come to light. Patients and occasionally caregivers can be reluctant to share information about an impulse control disorder fearing potential stigmatization or being afraid of relapses being viewed as failures.

Hypersexuality in PD patients is marked by a preoccupation with sexual thoughts, increased sexual demands on the partner or outside the relationship, and seeking of sexual contacts on the Internet, or with sex workers. Cases of new onset exhibitionism or paraphilias such as cross-dressing as well as pedophilia have been described (Berger *et al.* 2003b; Munhoz *et al.* 2009; Quinn *et al.* 1983; Riley 2002). It has led to the break-up of families, legal consequences including incarceration in cases of pedophilia (Berger *et al.* 2003a), and serious sexual assault (Cannas *et al.* 2007).

Compulsive shopping is defined as a behavior which is driven by an intense urge to shop and leads to significant distress, particularly financially, and often includes the urge to buy items which the person does not actually need and which might be stored unopened and unused (Lim *et al.* 2008). Compulsive eating can take the shape of binge eating, particularly at night or intense cravings for certain kinds of foods and usually leads to weight gain.

Punding was first described in psychostimulant addicts (Rylander 1972) and refers to ritualistic, stereotyped behaviors usually influenced by culture and personal background; in PD patients these can be seen as sorting of items for hours, hoarding, dismantling technical objects, excessive gardening, Internet or computer use, or walkabouts amongst a multitude of similar behaviors leading to a loss of social interactions, meals, and/or sleep. "Hobbyism" lies along the same continuum of prolonged, stereotyped, and essentially unproductive behaviors (Evans *et al.* 2009). In contrast to obsessive compulsive symptoms, punding PD patients do not experience obsessions, that is intrusive thoughts driving their behavior. Some patients describe the engagement in the activity as soothing, and they might become irritable when asked to stop.

Dopamine dysregulation syndrome describes the compulsive use of increasingly high doses of dopaminergic medication, beyond what is needed to achieve optimal control of motor symptoms, despite significant physical, behavioral, and psychiatric side effects as well as negative social consequences (Giovannoni *et al.* 2000). The securing of dopaminergic drugs, including with force and deception, can become a major focus in the life of these patients. Criteria for addiction are fulfilled, yet the patients are addicted to a medication they need—albeit in lower dosages—to control parkinsonian symptoms and which is prescribed by their physician. Withdrawal is associated with intense negative emotions as well as physical symptoms usually related to drug withdrawal such as pain, sweating or palpitations. Relapses after a reduction in the dopaminergic medication dose are frequent. During episodes of particular high doses of dopaminergic drugs, self-injurious thoughts and behavior or hypomania can occur (Evans *et al.* 2009).

The occurrence of both behavioral and drug-related addictions in relation to the dopaminergic medication adds to the existing evidence of biological mechanisms underlying both patterns of addiction that are at least partially shared. Both dopamine dysregulation syndrome and pathological gambling in PD patients have been shown to be associated with sensitization processes in the ventral striatum, which is crucial in processing reward (Evans *et al.* 2006; Steeves *et al.* 2009). Pathological gambling was also found to be associated with altered orbitofrontal cortex activity in an fMRI task, the findings correlated with increased risk-taking in a task outside the scanner (van Eimeren *et al.* 2009) and thus provide evidence for an alteration in decision-making abilities in patients affected by PD pathological gambling.

Management of impulse control disorders in Parkinson's disease

The insight of patients into the abnormality of their behavior is often limited and only information from caregivers or family members might reveal the true nature and impact of a given behavior. Disagreements between family members and patients in this regard need to be handled with great care. The physician's role is to advocate for the benefit of the patient, yet also considering issues of confidentiality as related to the question of capacity of the patient, or the protection of minors from sexual offences.

Following best clinical practice principles, physicians need to ensure that the potential benefits of the medication outweigh the risks in a given patient. Possible side effects must be discussed with the patient and his/her family before starting the medication. Several risk factors for the development of impulse control disorders are known and need to be screened for before starting dopamine agonist medications or increasing L-dopa to comparatively high levels (Evans *et al.* 2009). After starting a medication, vigilant screening for signs of a developing ICD is paramount, especially since patients—as described earlier—are unlikely to connect their behavioral problems with their anti-parkinsonian medication or are reluctant to admit to socially undesirable behaviors. Reducing the dopaminergic medication dose is currently still the most effective treatment strategy and in the majority of cases ICD behaviors such as pathological gambling, hypersexuality, or compulsive shopping seem to disappear completely once dopamine agonists are discontinued. The treatment of dopamine dysregulation disorders, though, is laden with difficulties as the patients usually resist the proposed changes. Perceived suffering on the part of the patient on a lower dose needs to be weighed against the risk of serious medical, psychiatric, or social sequelae on a continuously high dose. Occasionally, family and partners of patients are asked by the medical team to act as "gatekeepers" of the dopaminergic medication: they then keep the medication in a safe place, hand out only what is required for a specific dose, and thus control the patient's medication intake. Family members taking on the role of gatekeepers of medication are at risk of becoming the target of the patient's aggression, verbally or physically, or at least having to endure constant conflict with the patient. Can we ask the family and partners to take on the role of the gatekeeper? Alternatively, a multidisciplinary approach can be employed: only one physician should prescribe the medication and medication can be collected by the patient from the pharmacy for a day or a week at a time only, reliable communication between the different professionals involved is paramount. A further consideration is whether harm reduction is important enough a goal to force patients against their will to reduce the dosage of their dopaminergic medication, essentially to cut the patient's autonomy in one sphere in order to ultimately increase it by reducing the influence of the drug on behavior, craving, and thinking? This challenging situation again touches on the issue of difficult, even hateful patients, and in this case the physician's relationship with these patients. How can equally high standards of care be ensured for these patients? Is this possible? When is it justified to refuse treatment?

The problems posed by ICDs and dopamine dysregulation syndrome are similar to those in addictions, yet the situation is more complex: The patients require treatment of motor symptoms due to PD, and are being prescribed medications by their physicians. To what extent is behavior displayed only whilst on dopaminergic medication the fault of the drug, perhaps even the drug company, the physician, and to what extent the fault of the patient? Not all patients on dopaminergic medications develop pathological behaviors – what factors predispose patients to do so or not? Are these factors within the control of the patient? What roles do casinos and proprietors of slot machines and other industries earning from pathological gambling play? Should business standards include banning of pathological gamblers from casinos? How free are patients on dopaminergic medication in their decisions given the earlier mentioned imaging findings with alterations of reward and decision-making/risk taking processes? Genetic variations within the dopamine-driven reward system are associated with a higher likelihood to develop addictions and impulse control disorders (Le Foll *et al.* 2009; Silva Lobo *et al.* 2007). Likewise, if there is a spectrum of underlying biological factors, e.g. genetic variations of the dopamine-driven reward system, reduced function of prefrontal cortices needed for behavioral regulation, what degree of responsibility should an affected individual assume for negative consequences of their behavior? Growing insight into the biological functions underlying human behavior might alter the understanding of responsibility with implications for the legal system (Goodenough and Prehn 2004), yet not all authors agree with this, arguing that imaging or other biological evidence is not a measure of (diminished) responsibility before the law (Buller 2006; Morse 2006).

The placebo effect

There is a prominent placebo effect in Parkinson's disease (Goetz *et al.* 2008), thought to be mediated by release of endogenous dopamine into the striatum (de la Fuente-Fernandez *et al.* 2001) and associated with the anticipated electrophysiological changes downstream (Benedetti *et al.* 2004). As improvement in clinical symptoms can be seen as a form of reward, we predicted that placebo-related improvements may depend upon activation of dopaminergic reward signals in mesolimbic projections both in PD as well as in other conditions such as depression and pain (de la Fuente-Fernandez *et al.* 2004; Lidstone *et al.* 2005) and this appears to be supported by functional imaging studies in those disorders (Benedetti *et al.* 2005; Scott *et al.* 2007). The importance of understanding the potential power of the placebo effect in PD is that the anticipation of benefit may substantially color not only patients' subjective responses to therapy (especially when the therapy is novel, highly publicized, and/or invasive) but the physiological basis for placebo response may result in improvement in objective measures conducted by a blinded observer. Thus, in the case of fetal transplantation, both subjective and objective measures of improvement were dictated more by the perceived treatment assignment than by the actual treatment (active vs. sham transplant) (McRae *et al.* 2004; Stoessl and Fuente-Fernandez 2004). There are numerous other examples of initial benefits described in pilot studies failing to be sustained once submitted to a double blind trial (Lang *et al.* 2006; Watts *et al.* 2001, 2009).

The ethical implications of this are many. First, as outlined earlier, patients with PD and their families are often very well informed about new scientific advances and particularly about novel therapies. Given the potentially devastating effects of the illness, they are understandably frustrated if they are not offered immediate access to such treatments. However, the potential risks of these treatments are far from trivial, yet the benefits may be entirely unproven. For instance, in the case of fetal transplants, there was a high incidence of severe dyskinesias that persisted despite withdrawal of all dopaminergic medication. In the case of stem cell transplantation, gene or trophic factor therapy, there are potentially much more serious risks. In the case of glial cell line derived neurotrophic factor (GDNF) treatment, some patients and their families (in some cases, with the support of their physicians) sued the company that was developing this treatment when a double blind trial failed to demonstrate efficacy. Such issues also raise significant questions about the ethical responsibility of the scientific community in presenting potentially promising findings in a realistic and appropriately cautious fashion. The scientific and medical communities have a particular responsibility to respect the potential power of the placebo effect and take its potential influence on preliminary findings into consideration. Some authors have argued that it may not be ethical to conduce placebo-controlled trials of surgical therapies (Clark 2002; Weijer 2002). However, given the tradeoffs between risk and benefit, others have argued the opposite (Freeman *et al.* 1999) and it should be noted that PD patients understand the need for placebo controls and are in general well disposed towards participation in placebo-controlled trials.

Surgical interventions in Parkinson's disease: focus on deep brain stimulation

Established surgical interventions in PD include lesional approaches such as thalamotomy and pallidotomy and deep brain stimulation (DBS) of the same sites as well as the subthalamic nucleus (STN). Deep brain stimulation compared to lesional approaches has the advantage of being reversible (unless permanent side effects such as hemorrhage occur), and adjustable and has favorable morbidity, mortality, and quality of life outcomes compared to thalamotomy and pallidotomy (Marconi *et al.* 2008). DBS involves the stereotactic unilateral or bilateral implantation of a stimulating electrode into specific sites of the brain, in PD usually the STN, the globus pallidus internus (GPi), or the ventral intermediate nucleus (VIM) of the thalamus. The leads are subcutaneously connected to the stimulator including battery which is implanted into a subcutaneous pouch below the clavicula in the upper thorax. VIM DBS is used to control tremor, DBS of STN or GPi can control levodopa responsive symptoms such as slowness of movement (bradykinesia), and rigidity but fails to reliably and significantly alter symptoms such as postural imbalance and falls which also do not respond well to levodopa.

As a rule of thumb, the potential benefit of DBS of the STN, the now most frequently chosen stimulation site, is comparable to the maximal benefit an individual patient experiences on levodopa. The advantage of DBS over drug therapy alone lies in the improvement of motor complications such as dyskinesias and motor fluctuations associated with dopaminergic therapy. The indication for DBS thus is PD with marked motor complications or severe tremor not controlled with medication (Marconi et al. 2008). Appropriate patient selection on medical grounds including physical, cognitive, and emotional/psychiatric suitability is crucial for the success of an intervention which realistically can only be offered to a minority of patients (Bell et al. 2009). Morgante and colleagues assessed 641 patients for their suitability for DBS, and found only 1.6% to be suitable candidates following strict criteria and 4.5% with more flexible criteria (Morgante et al. 2007); thus a realistic presentation regarding the promise of DBS for the individual patient is important. Similarly, suitability for DBS in already implanted patients is likely to change over time: Most PD patients will eventually develop dementia, yet dementia is a contraindication for implantation of DBS: An explicit agreement before the implantation of the DBS system should be in place stating under which circumstances the device will be removed again.

Side effects of deep brain stimulation

Potential side effects of DBS include those related to the surgical intervention: hemorrhage, infection at the implantation site of the electrodes and more frequently at the site of the stimulator, as well as equipment failure, particularly lead fracture. In a large series short-term study, adverse events resulting in death or permanent disability occurred in 0.4–1% of patients (Voges et al. 2007). Reports about long-term cognitive and psychiatric symptoms after DBS, particularly depression, anxiety, mania, and impulse control disorders vary considerably in the literature and a comprehensive discussion is beyond the scope of this chapter. Methodological questions with a lack of standardized assessments across studies are one reason for the discrepancy; another is that PD itself is associated with cognitive decline, depression, and anxiety. Dopaminergic medication is usually decreased after DBS implantation which can in itself have either positive or negative influences on cognition, mood and motivation. Potential cognitive deficits attributed to DBS in PD include changes in verbal fluency, working memory, executive function, and attention as well as increased impulsivity (Voon et al. 2006b). To fully evaluate the risk/benefit ratio of the intervention in the short and long-term and to aid patient selection, a more standardized approach, e.g. by using a central, anonymized, publicly accessible register for DBS outcome database as suggested for DBS in psychiatric conditions (Rabins et al. 2009b) might be helpful. The literature is somewhat more uniform when it comes to suicidal ideation/suicide attempts after DBS: Rates vary from 0.16–4.3% in different studies (Burkhard et al. 2004). The reported suicide rate for the US is estimated to be quite stable at a considerably lower rate of around 0.02% per annum, and the suicide rate in PD is thought to be only one tenth of this. Thus there seems to be an increase in suicide risk after DBS, although absolute numbers are comparatively small. Causes for increased suicide rates are likely to be multifactorial including depression, poor impulse control due to DBS (Soulas *et al.* 2008), and potentially psychological adjustment difficulties. Pre-surgical screening for risk factors and post-surgical comprehensive assessments are important measures to prevent this catastrophic outcome (Soulas *et al.* 2008). Potential candidates for DBS should also be informed before their decision to undergo surgery that as long as the stimulator is implanted, the patient's ability to have an MRI or pacemaker is limited.

Treatment efficacy, cost effectiveness, and resource allocation

The largest trial to date comparing DBS with best medical treatment for the treatment of advanced PD is a recent multicenter randomized controlled trial in the US of 225 advanced PD patients which compared DBS to best medical treatment over a period of 6 months following DBS implantation for either the STN of the GPi (Weaver *et al.* 2009). It is important to note that although the neurological raters were blinded, the subjects were not; also, follow-up was relatively short and thus the possibility of a considerable placebo effect in the DBS group must be kept in mind as detailed earlier. The authors report an increase of 4.6hours/day of dyskinesia free on-time in the DBS group compared to no change in the best medical treatment group as the primary outcome measure. They also found a significant improvement of motor function as measured by an improvement of at least 5 points in the Unified Parkinson's disease rating scale (UPDRS) in 71% of DBS versus 32% of best medical treatment subjects, as well as significant improvements in quality of life scores in the DBS group compared to the best medical treatment group. Cognitive changes in the DBS group were minor compared to the non-surgical group. Serious adverse events including one death due to hemorrhage occurred in 49/121 DBS subjects compared to 15/134 best medical treatment group subjects (Weaver *et al.* 2009). A previous large scale prospective study (n=156) from Germany comparing DBS of the STN to best medical treatment had comparably positive findings regarding improvement of motor function and quality of life; serious adverse events including one fatality due to cerebral hemorrhage occurred in 13% of DBS and only 4% of the non-surgical group subjects while the overall rate of adverse events was higher in the best medical treatment group (64% versus 50%).

In order for a treatment to be cost-effective, both efficacy of the treatment, that is improvement of clinical symptoms (in this case particularly motor symptoms) and quality of life without overriding side effects and associated costs need to be considered. Several European studies looked at the relative cost effectiveness of DBS versus best medical treatment: Overall, initial costs are high but it seems that these are more than recovered over the next few years considering both direct and indirect costs: A German multicenter study assessed costs for the 1 year before DBS surgery and the 2 years following the procedure and found that although costs were increased in the first year (total mean 21082 Euros per patient per year) due to the initial set-up costs of DBS, they then declined from year 2 (7223 Euros/patient/year) onwards compared to the presurgical year (mean 15991 Euros/patient/year). Motor improvement after DBS was significant and the authors conclude that DBS for advanced PD is a cost effective treatment (Meissner *et al.* 2005). A prospective Spanish study compared best medical treatment to DBS in patients with advanced PD and also found DBS to be associated with significantly better motor outcomes, and improved quality of life. They rated DBS as a cost effective therapy for advanced PD, mainly related to decreased medication costs (best medical treatment: 13208Euros/patient/year versus 3799 Euros/patient/year in the DBS subjects) (Valldeoriola *et al.* 2007). A French multicenter study compared direct and indirect costs including for medication, hospitalization, DBS surgery, follow-up visits, and auxiliary care in the 6 months before and after DBS implantation and found a reduction of costs from 10,087 Euros to 1673 Euros and significant improvements in motor scores and quality of life. The reduction in costs was mainly attributable to a reduction in medication. The authors estimated that the costs for the DBS surgery of nearly 37,000 Euros would be recovered after 2.2 years (Bell *et al.* 2009). Given already overstretched healthcare systems it might be difficult to convince healthcare providers to agree to the initial expenditure required for DBS despite evidence of benefit in the long run. To optimize the use and outcomes of DBS, longer-term follow-up of efficacy and cost-effectiveness is needed, the best point in time in the course of an individual's disease course for DBS needs to be determined and the influence of age on DBS outcomes needs to be addressed in more studies (Deuschl 2009).

Patient and public education

Public education and especially education of the patients and caregiver are crucial early in the process of evaluating a patient for DBS: realistic expectations are important to avoid considering all non-perfect outcomes as failures (Okun and Foote 2004). Ideally, specific target symptoms that are aimed to be improved by DBS should be identified together with the patient. Likewise, education of the public with balanced information is important as widely publicized miracle stories contribute to unrealistic expectations in patients and their families. Physicians should supply reliable internet resources for information as many patients and their families nowadays will seek to find answers to their questions on the Internet. For a more detailed discussion on public education and the internet see Bell *et al.* (2009) and Racine *et al.* (2007). Similar to the issues related to genetic testing discussed previously, the challenges of a positive change in function after DBS implantation should be discussed with the patient and his/her family before a deep brain stimulator is implanted as even a beneficial outcome can lead to adjustment issues both in the patient as well as the caregiver. These can occur in relation to the long-standing patient role with its expectations and consequences for the understanding of the self and social functioning in and outside the home similar to the discussion above about pre-symptomatic genetic diagnosis.

Research related questions

DBS is frequently used when other treatments have failed to control symptoms for a considerable length of time, patients and their families are often desperate and thus vulnerable. Medical professionals and researchers need to be aware of this vulnerability during the consenting process which can potentially compromise the objective weighing of the risks and benefits of a procedure by the patient (Lopes *et al.* 2003; Miller and Fins 2006; Racine *et al.* 2007).

Controlled trials in the assessment of DBS effects are vital given the prominent placebo effect in such an invasive procedure (de la Fuente-Fernandez 2004). Considering the practical and ethical difficulties of awake patients undergoing an invasive procedure, one possible approach is a cross-over design of studies: The control condition consists of placing the stimulator *in situ* but not turning it on. As pointed out by Rabins and colleagues, potential ethical difficulties can arise when a control subject becomes aware of his/her status and wishes to drop out of the study to have the stimulator turned on (Rabins *et al.* 2009). Another issue related to a subject's withdrawal from a study is that—as with all medical research—subjects need to be able to do so at any point and without having to bear the costs associated with withdrawal (Rabins *et al.* 2009), be this for the removal of the stimulator or further clinical follow-up with the stimulator in place. This is particularly relevant if the subject's healthcare provider would not usually financially support DBS treatment and the individual would be prevented from freely making such a decision depending on their financial means.

Infrastructure and neurodegenerative disease: access to services and outlook

The projected proportion of persons over the age of 65 in 2030 is around 25% for the European countries, around 20% for the US, and over 30% for Japan (Lutz *et al.* 2008). After Alzheimer's disease, PD is the second most common neurodegenerative disease, affecting about 1.6% of the population over 65 (de Rijk *et al.* 1997; Lutz *et al.* 2008). Aging populations will lead to a dramatic increase in the prevalence of neurodegenerative diseases—health systems of the developed world have moved beyond catering for the bare basics and, along with social advances, have contributed to prolonged survival of patients with degenerative disorders. There is a price to be paid, though: Who will be responsible for the exponentially growing need for medical care at the end of a long life and particularly during the advanced stages of neurodegenerative diseases? How are we going to allocate limited resources generated by a workforce that is shrinking relative to the percentage of the older retired part of the population?

The National Institute for Health and Clinical Excellence (NICE) has published guidelines for the management of PD in the National Health System (NHS) in the UK (National Collaborating Centre for Chronic Conditions 2006). These focus on the importance of multidisciplinary care through the implementation of the following steps as key priorities: quick (within a maximum of 6 weeks) access to an expert in PD, access to specialist nursing care, physiotherapy, speech and language therapy, occupational therapy, and palliative care. Research from the UK Parkinson's Disease Society showed that at that time only 4% of referrals to a neurologist met that criterion and 20% of PD patients never saw a specialist (Beckford-Ball 2006). In 2006 when the report was written, the net costs to implement these steps in the NHS, was estimated at £3,776,000 (ca. US$ 6,240,000) per annum.

Medical advances with longer survival of patients with PD also lead to more patients developing challenging non-motor, especially cognitive and neuropsychiatric symptoms, as their disease advances. These patients frequently require both neurological as well as (neuro)psychiatric care and services which can provide both. In one audit PD patients had longer neuropsychiatric admissions than patients with any other neurological disease with psychiatric symptoms (Appel-Cresswell *et al.* 2009). The treatment of one domain often affects another: dopaminergic medication needed for improved motor function may lead to psychotic symptoms that medical units are often ill-equipped to deal with. Waiting lists for neuropsychiatrists, who are usually only found in academic centers, are already long in most Western countries and certainly in the UK and Canada.

Canadian fee structures for neurologists do not contain an augmented fee for complex cases such as Parkinson's patients with neuropsychiatric complications therefore providing little financial incentive for physicians to provide comprehensive care. Yet, in addition to care facilities, training programs for physicians and allied medical professions will need to respond to this increasing demand of knowledge in both fields with an ever growing number of neurodegenerative disorders including PD and treating teams including long-term care facilities will need to be increasingly interdisciplinary. Societal consensus will need to be reached on how to address the growing demand for complex resources.

Acknowledgments

The authors' work is supported by the Canadian Institutes of Health Research, the Michael Smith Foundation for Health Research, the Pacific Alzheimer Research Foundation, and the Pacific Parkinson's Research Institute. AJS holds the Canada Research Chair in Parkinson's Disease.

References

Abe, N., Fujii, T., Hirayama, K., *et al.* (2009). Do parkinsonian patients have trouble telling lies? The neurobiological basis of deceptive behaviour. *Brain*, **132**, 1386–95.

Abler, B., Hahlbrock, R., Unrath, A., Gron, G., and Kassubek, J. (2009). At-risk for pathological gambling: imaging neural reward processing under chronic dopamine agonists. *Brain*, **132**, 2396–402.

Adams, J.R., van Netten, H., Schulzer, *et al.* (2005). PET in LRRK2 mutations: comparison to sporadic Parkinson's disease and evidence for presymptomatic compensation. *Brain*, **128**, 2777–85.

Ahlskog, J.E. (2003). Slowing Parkinson's disease progression: recent dopamine agonist trials. *Neurology*, **60**, 381–9.

Albin, R.L. and Frey, K.A. (2003). Initial agonist treatment of Parkinson disease: a critique. *Neurology*, **60**, 390–4.

American Psychiatric Association (2000). *Diagnostic and statistical manual of mental disorders*, 4th edition. Washington DC: American Psychiatric Press.

Appel-Cresswell, S., Morton, L., Foong, J., and Ron, M.A. (2009). Parkinsonian diseases neurological diseases associated with longest neuropsychiatric inpatient admissions. *Parkinsonism and Related Disorders*, **15**/Suppl 2, S75.

Appel-Cresswell, S., Nandhagopal, R., Adams, J.R., and Stoessl, A.J. (2010). Positron emission tomography. Submitted to R.F. Pfeiffer (ed.) *Parkinson's Disease*, 2nd edition. Boca Raton, FL: CRC Press.

Beckford-Ball, J. (2006). Implications of the latest NICE Parkinson's disease guidance. *Nursing Times*, 102, 25–6.

Bell, E., Mathieu, G., and Racine, E. (2009). Preparing the ethical future of deep brain stimulation. *Surgical Neurology*, 72, 577–86.

Benedetti, F., Colloca, L., Torre, E., *et al.* (2004). Placebo-responsive Parkinson patients show decreased activity in single neurons of subthalamic nucleus. *Nature Neuroscience*, 7, 587–8.

Benedetti, F., Mayberg, H.S., Wager, T.D., Stohler, C.S., and Zubieta, J.K. (2005). Neurobiological mechanisms of the placebo effect. *Journal of Neuroscience*, 25, 10390–402.

Berger, C., Mehrhoff, F.W., Beier, K.M., and Meinck, H.M. (2003). Sexual delinquency and Parkinson's disease. *Der Nervenarzt*, 74, 370–5.

Binkofski, F., Reetz, K., Gaser, C., *et al.* (2007). Morphometric fingerprint of asymptomatic Parkin and PINK1 mutation carriers in the basal ganglia. *Neurology*, 69, 842–50.

Bodi, N., Keri, S., Nagy, H., *et al.* (2009). Reward-learning and the novelty-seeking personality: a between- and within-subjects study of the effects of dopamine agonists on young Parkinson's patients. *Brain*, 132, 2385–95.

Brand, M., Labudda, K., Kalbe, E., *et al.* (2004). Decision-making impairments in patients with Parkinson's disease. *Behavioral Neurology*, 15, 77–85.

Buller, T. (2006). Brain, lies, and psychological explanations. In J. Illes (ed.) *Neuroethics: Defining the Issues in Theory, Practice, and Policy*, pp. 51–60. New York: Oxford University Press.

Burkhard, P.R., Vingerhoets, F.J., Berney, A., Bogousslavsky, J., Villemure, J.G., and Ghika, J. (2004). Suicide after successful deep brain stimulation for movement disorders. *Neurology*, 63, 2170–2.

Calne, D.B., Langston, J.W., Martin, W.R., *et al.* (1985). Positron emission tomography after MPTP: observations relating to the cause of Parkinson's disease. *Nature*, 317, 246–8.

Camp, C. (1913). Paralysis agitans, multiple sclerosis and their treatment. In W.A. White and S.E. Jelliffe (ed.) *Modern Treatment of Nervous and Mental Disease*, pp. 651–7. Philadelphia, PA: Lea and Febiger.

Canli, T. (2006). When genes and brains unite: ethical implications of genomic neuroimaging. In J. Illes (ed.) *Neuroethics: Defining the Issues in Theory, Practice, and Policy*, pp. 169–83. Oxford: Oxford University Press.

Cannas, A., Solla, P., Floris, G.L., Serra, G., Tacconi, P., and Marrosu, M.G. (2007). Aberrant sexual behaviours in Parkinson's disease during dopaminergic treatment. *Journal of Neurology*, 254, 110–12.

Chartier-Harlin, M.C., Kachergus, J., Roumier, C., *et al.* (2004). Alpha-synuclein locus duplication as a cause of familial Parkinson's disease. *Lancet*, 364, 1167–9.

Clark, P.A. (2002). Placebo surgery for Parkinson's disease: do the benefits outweigh the risks? *Journal of Law and Medical Ethics*, 30, 58–68.

de la Fuente-Fernandez, R., Ruth, T.J., Sossi, V., Schulzer, M., Calne, D.B., and Stoessl, A.J. (2001). Expectation and dopamine release: mechanism of the placebo effect in parkinson's disease. *Science*, 293, 1164–6.

de la Fuente-Fernandez, R. (2004). Uncovering the hidden placebo effect in deep-brain stimulation for Parkinson's disease. *Parkinsonism and Related Disorders*, 10, 125–7.

de la Fuente-Fernandez, R., Schulzer, M., and Stoessl, A.J. (2004). Placebo mechanisms and reward circuitry: clues from Parkinson's disease. *Biological Psychiatry*, 56, 67–71.

de Rijk, M.C., Tzourio, C., Breteler, M.M., *et al.* (1997). Prevalence of parkinsonism and Parkinson's disease in Europe: the EUROPARKINSON Collaborative Study. European

Community Concerted Action on the Epidemiology of Parkinson's disease. *Journal of Neurology, Neurosurgery and Psychiatry*, 62, 10–15.

Deuschl, G. (2009). Neurostimulation for Parkinson Disease. *Journal of the American Medical Association*, 301, 104–5.

Dickson, D.W., Fujishiro, H., DelleDonne, A., *et al*. (2008). Evidence that incidental Lewy body disease is pre-symptomatic Parkinson's disease. *Acta Neuropathologica*, 115, 437–44.

Evans, A.H., Lawrence, A.D., Potts, J., Appel, S., and Lees, A.J. (2005). Factors influencing susceptibility to compulsive dopaminergic drug use in Parkinson disease. *Neurology*, 65, 1570–4.

Evans, A.H., Pavese, N., Lawrence, A.D., *et al*. (2006). Compulsive drug use linked to sensitized ventral striatal dopamine transmission. *Annals of Neurology*, 59, 852–8.

Evans, A.H., Strafella, A.P., Weintraub, D., and Stacy, M. (2009). Impulsive and compulsive behaviors in Parkinson's disease. *Movement Disorders*, 24, 1561–70.

Frank, M.J., Seeberger, L.C., and O'Reilly, R.C. (2004). By carrot or by stick: cognitive reinforcement learning in parkinsonism. *Science*, 306, 1940–3.

Freeman, T.B., Vawter, D.E., Leaverton, P.E., *et al*. (1999). Use of placebo surgery in controlled trials of a cellular-based therapy for Parkinson's disease. *New England Journal of Medicine*, 341, 988–92.

Fuchs, J., Nilsson, C., Kachergus, J., *et al*. (2007). Phenotypic variation in a large Swedish pedigree due to SNCA duplication and triplication. *Neurology*, 68, 916–22.

Fuchs, T. (2006). Ethical issues in neuroscience. *Current Opinion in Psychiatry*, 19, 600–7.

Gallagher, D.A., O'Sullivan, S.S., Evans, A.H., Lees, A.J., and Schrag, A. (2007). Pathological gambling in Parkinson's disease: risk factors and differences from dopamine dysregulation. An analysis of published case series. *Movement Disorders*, 22, 1757–63.

Giladi, N., Weitzman, N., Schreiber, S., Shabtai, H., and Peretz, C. (2007). New onset heightened interest or drive for gambling, shopping, eating or sexual activity in patients with Parkinson's disease: the role of dopamine agonist treatment and age at motor symptoms onset. *Journal of Psychopharmacology*, 21, 501–6.

Gilks, W.P., Abou-Sleiman, P.M., Gandhi, S., *et al*. (2005). A common LRRK2 mutation in idiopathic Parkinson's disease. *Lancet*, 365, 415–16.

Giovannoni, G., O'Sullivan, J.D., Turner, K., Manson, A.J., and Lees, A.J. (2000). Hedonistic homeostatic dysregulation in patients with Parkinson's disease on dopamine replacement therapies. *Journal of Neurology, Neurosurgery and Psychiatry*, 68, 423–8.

Goetz, C.G., Wuu, J., McDermott, M.P., *et al*. (2008). Placebo response in Parkinson's disease: comparisons among 11 trials covering medical and surgical interventions. *Movement Disorders*, 23, 690–9.

Goldwurm, S., Zini, M., Mariani, L., *et al*. (2007). Evaluation of LRRK2 G2019S penetrance: relevance for genetic counseling in Parkinson disease. *Neurology*, 68, 1141–3.

Goodenough, O.R. and Prehn, K. (2004). A neuroscientific approach to normative judgment in law and justice. *Philosophical Transactions of the Royal Society of London B: Biological Science*, 359, 1709–26.

Healy, D.G., Falchi, M., O'Sullivan, S.S., *et al*. (2008). Phenotype, genotype, and worldwide genetic penetrance of LRRK2-associated Parkinson's disease: a case-control study. *Lancet Neurology*, 7, 583–90.

Illes, J. (2006). 'Pandora's box' of incidental findings in brain imaging research. *Nature Clinical Practice Neurology*, 2, 60–1.

Illes, J. (2007). Empirical neuroethics. Can brain imaging visualize human thought? Why is neuroethics interested in such a possibility? *EMBO Reports*, 8, S57–S60.

Illes, J., Racine, E., and Kirschen, M.P. (2006a). A picture is worth a thousand words, but which 1000?, In J. Illes (ed.) *Neuroethics: Defining the Issues in Theory, Practice, and Policy*, pp. 149–68. Oxford: Oxford University Press.

Illes, J., Kirschen, M.P., Edwards, E., *et al.* (2006b). Ethics. Incidental findings in brain imaging research. *Science*, 311, 783–84.

Illes, J., Kirschen, M.P., Edwards, E., *et al.* (2008). Practical approaches to incidental findings in brain imaging research. *Neurology*, 70, 384–90.

Kaasinen, V., Nurmi, E., Bergman, J., *et al.* (2001). Personality traits and brain dopaminergic function in Parkinson's disease. *Proceedings of the National Academy of Sciences of the United States of America*, 98, 13272–7.

Khan, N.L., Scherfler, C., Graham, E., *et al.* (2005). Dopaminergic dysfunction in unrelated, asymptomatic carriers of a single parkin mutation. *Neurology*, 64, 134–6.

Khan, N.L., Valente, E.M., Bentivoglio, A.R., *et al.* (2002). Clinical and subclinical dopaminergic dysfunction in PARK6-linked parkinsonism: an 18F-dopa PET study. *Annals of Neurology*, 52, 849–53.

Kimmelman, J., London, A.J., Ravina, B., *et al.* (2009). Launching invasive, first-in-human trials against Parkinson's disease: Ethical considerations. *Movement Disorders*, 24, 1893–901.

Kirschen, M.P., Jaworska, A., and Illes, J. (2006). Subjects' expectations in neuroimaging research. *Journal of Magnetic Resonance Imaging*, 23, 205–9.

Kitada, T., Asakawa, S., Hattori, N., *et al.* (1998). Mutations in the *parkin* gene cause autosomal recessive juvenile parkinsonism. *Nature*, 392, 605–8.

Klein, C. and Schlossmacher, M.G. (2007). Parkinson disease, 10 years after its genetic revolution: multiple clues to a complex disorder. *Neurology*, 69, 2093–104.

Kruger, R., Kuhn, W., Muller, T., *et al.* (1998). Ala30Pro mutation in the gene encoding alpha-synuclein in Parkinson's disease. *Nature Genetics*, 18, 106–8.

Kunig, G., Leenders, K.L., Martin-Solch, C., Missimer, J., Magyar, S., and Schultz, W. (2000). Reduced reward processing in the brains of Parkinsonian patients. *Neuroreport*, 11, 3681–7.

Lang, A.E., Gill, S., Patel, *et al.* (2006). Randomized controlled trial of intraputamenal glial cell line-derived neurotrophic factor infusion in Parkinson disease. *Annals of Neurology*, 59, 459–66.

Latourelle, J.C., Sun, M., Lew, M.F., *et al.* (2008). The Gly2019Ser mutation in LRRK2 is not fully penetrant in familial Parkinson's disease: the GenePD study. *BMC Medicine*, 6, 32.

Lawson, K., Wiggins, S., Green, T., Adam, S., Bloch, M., and Hayden, M.R. (1996). Adverse psychological events occurring in the first year after predictive testing for Huntington's disease. The Canadian Collaborative Study Predictive Testing. *Journal of Medical Genetics*, 33, 856–62.

Le Foll, B., Gallo, A., Le Strat, Y., Lu, L., and Gorwood, P. (2009). Genetics of dopamine receptors and drug addiction: a comprehensive review. *Behavioral Pharmacology*, 20, 1–17.

Lesage, S., Ibanez, P., Lohmann, E., *et al.* (2005). G2019S LRRK2 mutation in French and North African families with Parkinson's disease. *Annals of Neurology*, 58, 784–7.

Lidstone, S.C., de la Fuente-Fernandez, R., and Stoessl, A.J. (2005). The placebo response as a reward mechanism. *Seminars in Pain Medicine*, 3, 37–42.

Lim, S.Y., Evans, A.H., and Miyasaki, J.M. (2008). Impulse control and related disorders in Parkinson's disease: review. *Annals of the New York Academy of Sciences*, 1142, 85–107.

Lincoln, S.J., Maraganore, D.M., Lesnick, T.G., *et al.* (2003). Parkin variants in North American Parkinson's disease: cases and controls. *Movement Disorders*, 18, 1306–11.

Lopes, M., Meningaud, J.P., Behin, A., and Herve, C. (2003). Consent: a Cartesian ideal? Human neural transplantation in Parkinson's disease. *Medicine and Law*, **22**, 63–71.

Lutz, W., Marmolo, M., Potancokova, M., Scherbov, S., and Sobotka, T. (2008). *European Demographic data sheet 2008*. Vienna, Austria; Washington, DC: Vienna Institute of Demography; Population Reference Bureau.

Marconi, R., Landi, A., and Valzania, F. (2008b). Subthalamic nucleus stimulation in Parkinson's disease. *Neurological Sciences*, **29**, S389–91.

Marek, K., Seibyl, J., Shoulson, I., *et al.* (2002). Dopamine transporter brain imaging to assess the effects of pramipexole vs levodopa on Parkinson disease progression. *Journal of The American Medical Association*, **287**, 1653–61.

McRae, C., Cherin, E., Yamazaki, T. G., *et al.* (2004). Effects of perceived treatment on quality of life and medical outcomes in a double-blind placebo surgery trial. *Archives of General Psychiatry*, **61**, 412–20.

Meissner, W., Schreiter, D., Volkmann, J., *et al.* (2005). Deep brain stimulation in late stage Parkinson's disease: a retrospective cost analysis in Germany. *Journal of Neurology*, **252**, 218–23.

Menza, M. (2000). The personality associated with Parkinson's disease. *Current Psychiatry Reports*, **2**, 421–6.

Miller, F.G. and Fins, J.J. (2006). Protecting human subjects in brain research: a pragmatic perspective. In J. Illes (ed.) *Neuroethics: Defining the Issues in Theory, Practice, and Policy*, pp. 123–40. New York: Oxford University Press.

Morgante, L., Morgante, F., Moro, E., *et al.* (2007). How many parkinsonian patients are suitable candidates for deep brain stimulation of subthalamic nucleus? Results of a questionnaire. *Parkinsonism and Related Disorders*, **13**, 528–31.

Morse, S.J. (2006). Moral and legal responsibility and the new neuroscience. In J. Illes (ed.) *Neuroethics: Defining the Issues in Theory, Practice, and Policy*, pp. 33–50. New York: Oxford University Press.

Moynihan, R. (2008). Key opinion leaders: independent experts or drug representatives in disguise? *BMJ*, **336**, 1402–3.

Munhoz, R.P., Fabiani, G., Becker, N., and Teive, H.A. (2009). Increased frequency and range of sexual behavior in a patient with Parkinson's disease after use of pramipexole: a case report. *Journal of Sexual Medicine*, **6**, 1177–80.

Nandhagopal, R., Mak, E., Schulzer, M., *et al.* (2008). Progression of dopaminergic dysfunction in a LRRK2 kindred: a multitracer PET study. *Neurology*, **71**, 1790–5.

National Collaborating Centre for Chronic Conditions (2006). *Parkinson's Disease: National Clinical Guidelines for Management in Primary and Secondary Care*. London: Royal College of Physicians.

Okun, M.S. and Foote, K.D. (2004). A mnemonic for Parkinson disease patients considering DBS: a tool to improve perceived outcome of surgery. *Neurologist*, **10**, 290.

Ondo, W.G. and Lai, D. (2008). Predictors of impulsivity and reward seeking behavior with dopamine agonist. *Parkinsonism and Related Disorders*, **14**, 28–32.

Pagonabarraga, J., Garcia-Sanchez, C., Llebaria, G., Pascual-Sedano, B., Gironell, A., and Kulisevsky, J. (2007a). Controlled study of decision-making and cognitive impairment in Parkinson's disease. *Movement Disorders*, **22**, 1430–5.

Paisan-Ruiz, C., Jain, S., Evans, E.W., *et al.* (2004). Cloning of the gene containing mutations that cause PARK8-linked Parkinson's disease. *Neuron*, **44**, 595–600.

Piccini, P. and Brooks, D. presented at the WFN XVIII World Congress on Parkinson's Disease and Related disorders, Miami, December 2009. 2010.

Piccini, P., Burn, D.J., Ceravolo, R., Maraganore, D.M., and Brooks, D.J. (1999). The role of inheritance in sporadic Parkinson's disease: evidence from a longitudinal study of dopaminergic function in twins. *Annals of Neurology*, **45**, 577–82.

Polymeropoulos, M.H., Lavedan, C., Leroy, E., *et al.* (1997). Mutation in the a-synuclein gene identified in families with Parkinson's disease. *Science*, **276**, 2045–7.

Quinn, N.P., Toone, B., Lang, A.E., Marsden, C.D., and Parkes, J.D. (1983). Dopa dose-dependent sexual deviation. *British Journal of Psychiatry*, **142**, 296–8.

Rabins, P., Appleby, B.S., Brandt, J., *et al.* (2009). Scientific and ethical issues related to deep brain stimulation for disorders of mood, behavior, and thought. *Archives of General Psychiatry*, **66**, 931–7.

Racette, B.A., Antenor, J.A., McGee-Minnich, L., *et al.* S. (2005). [18F]FDOPA PET and clinical features in parkinsonism due to manganism. *Movement Disorders*, **20**, 492–6.

Racette, B.A., McGee-Minnich, L., Moerlein, S.M., Mink, J.W., Videen, T.O., and Perlmutter, J.S. (2001). Welding-related parkinsonism: clinical features, treatment, and pathophysiology. *Neurology*, **56**, 8–13.

Racine, E., van der Loos, H.Z., and Illes, J. (2007). Internet marketing of neuroproducts: new practices and healthcare policy challenges. *Cambridge Quarterly of Healthcare Ethics*, **16**, 181–94.

Riley, D.E. (2002). Reversible transvestic fetishism in a man with Parkinson's disease treated with selegiline. *Clinical Neuropharmacology*, **25**, 234–7.

Rossi, M., Gerschcovich, E.R., de Achaval, D., *et al.* (2009). Decision-making in Parkinson's disease patients with and without pathological gambling. *European Journal of Neurology*, **17**, 97–102.

Rylander, G. (1972). Psychoses and the punding and choreiform syndromes in addiction to central stimulant drugs. *Psychiatr Neurol Neurochir*, **75**, 203–12.

Santangelo, G., Vitale, C., Trojano, L., Verde, F., Grossi, D., and Barone, P. (2009). Cognitive dysfunctions and pathological gambling in patients with Parkinson's disease. *Movement Disorders*, **24**, 899–905.

Satake, W., Nakabayashi, Y., Mizuta, I., *et al.* (2009). Genome-wide association study identifies common variants at four loci as genetic risk factors for Parkinson's disease. *Nature Genetics*, **41**, 1303–7.

Schultz, W. (2002). Getting formal with dopamine and reward. *Neuron*, **36**, 241–63.

Scott, D.J., Stohler, C.S., Egnatuk, C.M., Wang, H., Koeppe, R.A., and Zubieta, J.K. (2007). Individual differences in reward responding explain placebo-induced expectations and effects. *Neuron*, **55**, 325–36.

Shimura, H., Hattori, N., Kubo, S.I., *et al.* (2000). Familial Parkinson disease gene product, parkin, is a ubiquitin-protein ligase. *Nature Genetics*, **25**, 302–5.

Shinotoh, H., Snow, B.J., Chu, N.S., *et al.* (1997). Presynaptic and postsynaptic striatal dopaminergic function in patients with manganes intoxication: a positron emission tomography study. *Neurology*, **48**, 1053–6.

Silva Lobo, D.S., Vallada, H.P., Knight, J., *et al.* (2007). Dopamine genes and pathological gambling in discordant sib-pairs. *Journal of Gambling Studies*, **23**, 421–33.

Simon-Sanchez, J., Schulte, C., Bras, J.M., *et al.* (2009). Genome-wide association study reveals genetic risk underlying Parkinson's disease. *Nature Genetics*, **41**, 1308–12.

Singleton, A.B., Farrer, M., Johnson, J., *et al.* (2003). alpha-Synuclein locus triplication causes Parkinson's disease. *Science*, **302**, 841.

Siri, C., Cilia, R., De Gaspari, D., *et al.* (2009). Cognitive status of patients with Parkinson's disease and pathological gambling. *Journal of Neurology*, **257**, 247–52.

Smith, W.W., Pei, Z., Jiang, H., Dawson, V.L., Dawson, T.M., and Ross, C.A. (2006). Kinase activity of mutant LRRK2 mediates neuronal toxicity. *Nature Neuroscience*, **9**, 1231–33.

Soulas, T., Gurruchaga, J.M., Palfi, S., Cesaro, P., Nguyen, J.P., and Fenelon, G. (2008). Attempted and completed suicides after subthalamic nucleus stimulation for Parkinson's disease *Journal of Neurology. Neurosurgery and Psychiatry*, **79**, 952–4.

Steeves, T.D., Miyasaki, J., Zurowski, M., *et al.* (2009). Increased striatal dopamine release in Parkinsonian patients with pathological gambling: a [11C] raclopride PET study. *Brain*, **132**, 1376–85.

Stoessl, A.J. and Fuente-Fernandez, R. (2004). Willing oneself better on placebo–effective in its own right. *Lancet*, **364**, 227–8.

Turjanski, N., Lees, A.J., and Brooks, D.J. (1997). Dopaminergic function in patients with posttraumatic parkinsonism: an 18F-dopa PET study. *Neurology*, **49**, 183–9.

Valldeoriola, F., Morsi, O., Tolosa, E., Rumia, J., Marti, M.J., and Martinez-Martin, P. (2007). Prospective comparative study on cost-effectiveness of subthalamic stimulation and best medical treatment in advanced Parkinson's disease. *Movement Disorders*, **22**, 2183–91.

Van Eimeren, T., Ballanger, B., Pellecchia, G., Miyasaki, J.M., Lang, A.E., and Strafella, A.P. (2009). Dopamine agonists diminish value sensitivity of the orbitofrontal cortex: a trigger for pathological gambling in Parkinson's disease? *Neuropsychopharmacology*, **34**, 2758–66.

Van Orden, G.C. and Paap, K.R. (1997). Functional neuroimages fail to discover pieces of mind in the parts of the brain. *Philosophy of Science*, **64**, 85–94.

Voges, J., Hilker, R., Botzel, K., *et al.* (2007). Thirty days complication rate following surgery performed for deep-brain-stimulation. *Movement Disorders*, **22**, 1486–9.

Volkow, N.D., Fowler, J.S., Wang, G.J., and Swanson, J.M. (2004). Dopamine in drug abuse and addiction: results from imaging studies and treatment implications. *Molecular Psychiatry*, **9**, 557–69.

Voon, V., Hassan, K., Zurowski, M., *et al.* (2006). Prevalence of repetitive and reward-seeking behaviors in Parkinson disease. *Neurology*, **67**, 1254–7.

Voon, V., Kubu, C., Krack, P., Houeto, J.L., and Troster, A.I. (2006). Deep brain stimulation: neuropsychological and neuropsychiatric issues. *Movement Disorders*, **21**, S305–27.

Watts, R.L., Freeman, T.B., Hauser, R.A., *et al.* (2001). A double-blind, randomized, controlled, multicenter clinical trial of the safety and efficacy of sterotaxic intrastriatal implantation of fetal procine ventral mesencephalic tissue (Neurocell™-PD) vs. imitation surgery in patients with Parkinson's disease (PD). *Parkinsonism and Related Disorders*, **7**, S87.

Watts, R.L., Gross, R.E., Hauser, R.A., *et al.* (2009). The STEPS Trial: A Phase 2b Study Evaluating Spheramine® in Patients with Advanced Parkinson's Disease. *Movement Disorders*, LB18.

Weaver, F.M., Follett, K., Stern, M., *et al.* (2009). Bilateral deep brain stimulation vs best medical therapy for patients with advanced Parkinson disease: a randomized controlled trial. *Journal of the American Medical Association*, **301**, 63–73.

Weijer, C. (2002). I need a placebo like I need a hole in the head. *Journal of Law, Medicine and Ethics*, **30**, 69–72.

Whone, A.L., Watts, R.L., Stoessl, A.J., *et al.* (2003). Slower progression of Parkinson's disease with ropinirole versus levodopa: The REAL-PET study. *Annals of Neurology*, **54**, 93–101.

Wong, S.H., Cowen, Z., Allen, E.A., and Newman, P.K. (2007). Internet gambling and other pathological gambling in Parkinson's disease: a case series. *Movement Disorders*, **22**, 591–3.

Wszolek, Z.K., Pfeiffer, R.F., Tsuboi, Y., *et al.* (2004). Autosomal dominant parkinsonism associated with variable synuclein and tau pathology. *Neurology*, **62**, 1619–22.

Zimprich, A., Biskup, S., Leitner, P., *et al.* (2004). Mutations in LRRK2 cause autosomal-dominant parkinsonism with pleomorphic pathology. *Neuron*, **44**, 601–7.

CHAPTER 35

THE OTHER ETHICAL CHALLENGE OF NEURODEGENERATIVE DISEASES

ADRIAN J. IVINSON

INTRODUCTION

ALL biomedical researchers owe it to the communities they serve to pause once in a while and consider the ethical dimensions of our research including the environment in which we work, the consequences of our research, and how to make it more relevant and valuable to society. As the chapters of this volume show, the special nature of the central nervous system and emerging technologies that allow us to investigate and manipulate it, make the relatively young field of neuroethics a particularly rich and vibrant field of enquiry. However, as we consider such weighty issues as determinism, enhancement, truth, equity, and access we should also give some thought to an equally compelling challenge that receives less attention from the neuroethics community. Alzheimer's and other neurodegenerative diseases take a very significant emotional and financial toll. Globally, the number of patients suffering from one or other of these diseases is set to double or triple over the next few decades, yet no effective treatments exist. In light of our collective failure to develop drugs to treat or prevent neurodegeneration, we must rethink the traditional division of labor between the academic research community and the pharmaceutical industry.

A ROLE FOR ACADEMIA IN DRUG DISCOVERY?

Much of the neuroethics debate around neurological diseases focuses on the potential to repurpose potent neurological drugs for non-medical needs, or what Anjan Chatterjee calls "cosmetic neurology" (Chatterjee 2006). This will be true particularly of drugs developed to treat Alzheimer's disease (AD), Parkinson's disease, ALS (amyotrophic lateral sclerosis or motor neuron disease), Huntington's and other neurodegenerative diseases. Put very simply, as we learn about the pathogenesis of neurodegeneration, we will uncover approaches for avoiding, delaying, and reversing the processes. Reversing neurodegeneration presumably involves neuroregeneration which, when applied to the cognitively normal, represents neuroenhancement.

The use of drugs to build upon and improve cognition in the cognitively normal raises many challenging questions, from the relatively trivial to the profound: Just as we require our athletes to avoid certain performance enhancing drugs, should chess masters and game show quiz contestants be required to remain neuroenhancement-free? Will limited access to cognitive enhancement further divide the world's haves and have-nots? Given the central place for the brain in determining human nature and behavior, will the widespread use of such technology fundamentally change what it means to be human? Important as these issues are, we must not allow them to distract us from a more immediate concern: the near-complete absence of drugs to control neurodegeneration and an emerging role for academic research institutions to contribute to the solution.

Until quite recently, the idea of drug discovery within academia was anathema to some. Popular criticism included a concern that it does not represent the sort of hypothesis-driven, fundamental science that academia is best at, that it is too close to the commercial world that the "pure as the driven snow" crowd seem so scared of, and that even if safeguards to protect the integrity of our work were in place, academia simply doesn't have the track record, resources, or skills to do it well. Although there is a seam of common sense running through each of these criticisms, they fail as arguments against university-based drug discovery initiatives.

Academia is indeed a terrific environment in which to pursue basic research—the engine that drives subsequent translational research. However, an interest in drug discovery and other forms of translational research need not diminish in any way our commitment to basic research. Rather, additional resources should be brought to bear and used to expand and strengthen our translational research capacity such that we are better prepared to pick up and apply the discoveries emerging from our basic research activities. The argument is occasionally made that biomedical research funding is a zero sum game such that every dollar committed to translation is one less available to the basic research enterprise (Marks 2006). The near doubling of the budget of the National Institutes of Health during the US Clinton administration suggest otherwise, as does the willingness of some philanthropists to commit significant sums toward the most translation aspects of our work when they would not have considered funding more basic research. There is no reason that we cannot strengthen both basic and more applied research.

We do need to be aware of the potential for commercial sector influence on our desire to be always objective and true to our aims (which, in academia, do not generally mention share holders and profits). That said, we must not throw the baby out with the bath water. Realistically, almost all ideas for drugs, devices, and services that are destined to have a positive impact on large numbers of patients will at some point transition to the commercial sector where promising ideas are converted into valuable products and services. Rather than shy away from industry, academia should be pointing out the commercial relevance of our work and looking for ways to make our discoveries more attractive to industry. This is neither an argument for or against monetizing the products of academia. Rather it recognizes the need to engage with industry in order to see our discoveries through the development, testing, and licensing phases.

Finally, and most obviously, whereas it is true that drug discovery within academia is uncommon and that as a community we are, relatively speaking, dwarfed by the capacity and skills of our industry colleagues, just because we do not currently invest much in drug discovery, does not mean that we shouldn't do more.

But there has to be a reason to expand our involvement in drug discovery. In fact, when it comes to neurodegenerative disease there are two, closely connected reasons why drug discovery in academia is a moral imperative: there is a desperate need to improve the pipeline of potential new drugs, and the culture and environment of academia brings some real benefit to the enterprise.

THE INCREASING THREAT OF NEURODEGENERATIVE DISEASES

There is something of a perfect storm forming around neurodegeneration. The number of elderly people is growing, fast. This is due to both an increase in longevity—globally, life expectancy has increased from around 48 years of age in 1950 to 68 years today—and to the overall increase in the size of the human population—just shy of 3 billion in 1950, and 6.9 billion today. Because both these trends are forecast to continue over at least the next half century (with a global population of 9 billion and a life expectation of 75, by 2050) the United Nations has estimated that the elderly population (those over the age of 60) will increase from 737 million today to 2 billion by 2050 (http://www.un.org/esa/population/unpop.htm). This population shift presents a major financial challenge and economists will doubtless be arguing about the repercussions of a larger elderly population for many years to come. Easier to predict is the effect this change will have on neurodegenerative diseases, predominantly diseases of the middle aged and elderly.

AD is the most common of the neurodegenerative diseases. In more developed countries (for which accurate numbers exist), we know that approximately 10% of those over the age of 70 suffer from AD (Plassman *et al.* 2007). This grows to around 40% of the over 90 population.

Looking at the US, a reasonable model of many developed countries when it comes to the age-related demographic changes and the consequences for neurodegenerative diseases, the number of Americans over the age of 65 will increase from approximately 40 million today to 80 million by 2050 (US Census Bureau). As a consequence it is predicted that in the absence of effective prevention the US Alzheimer's patient population will increase three-fold over the same period, from around 4.5 million today to over 13 million by 2050 (Hebert *et al.* 2003). Others have predicted an increase in the global prevalence from 26.5 million in 2006 to 106 million in 2050 (Brookmeyer *et al.* 2007).

This increase, linked to the fact that neurodegenerative diseases exact a heavy emotional and financial price, is driving an ever more urgent need for more effective treatments. It may therefore be surprising to learn that despite this pressure to step up the rate at which we produce drugs to treat these diseases, the opposite is true. The number of approved drugs for treating neurodegenerative diseases is very low. And the rate at which they are being approved is actually falling (Figure 35.1). Exactly why this picture is so bleak is hard to determine with certainty (Special Section, *Science* 2005) but characteristics of the diseases likely play a part.

THE WEAK DRUG DISCOVERY PIPELINE

Neurodegeneration is biologically complex. Despite years of research and investigation we are still unable to explain the pathogenesis of these diseases. We can accurately describe the pathology of each disease and for most of them we can point to specific inherited risk factors that either put a person at increased risk or occasionally even predict with certainty if they will develop the disease. But we cannot yet fully explain at the molecular level either the initiating events or the cascade of signals that results in disease. Without such clear understanding of pathogenesis, we are to some extent forced to guess which molecular targets we need to interfere with to prevent or halt disease.

Nor do we have animal models that recapitulate what we believe to be the most important characteristics of the diseases in patients. For sure, some animal models allow us to interrogate and observe facets of disease and can be valuable research tools. But in general, the commonly employed animal models of neurodegenerative disease do not offer a reliable test bed for developing therapies. Just as observed in so many animal models of cancers, our ability to successfully treat or delay neurodegeneration in a mouse does not predict success in a human trial.

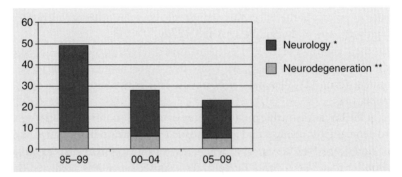

FIG. 35.1 FDA-approved neurology drugs from 1995–2009. The total number of neurology-indicated drugs approved by the FDA (including new chemical entities, new formulations and generics) has been falling over the past 15 years. Only a small subset of these drugs is aimed at treating or managing neurodegenerative diseases. *Includes drugs for treating pain, migraine, epilepsy and seizures, attention deficit hyperactivity disorder, schizophrenia, insomnia, and all neurodegenerative diseases. **Alzheimer's disease, Parkinson's disease, amyotrophic lateral sclerosis, multiple sclerosis, Huntington's disease combined. Source: Thompson CenterWatch.

Many neurodegenerative diseases have a long presymptomatic phase during which the disease is progressing silently but with ultimately devastating effects. By the time that symptoms appear, so much damage has been done that it is difficult to design therapies that can effectively and reliably reverse the damage. Although recent advances in understanding stem cell biology have provided hope that neuronal regeneration may be possible one day, that day seems a long way off. In the absence of cell therapy or other regenerative approaches we are left with just two options. We must either prevent the disease in the first place, or significantly delay (or halt) disease progression such that we can buy the patient many more years of quality life. But with, at best, an incomplete understanding of the pathogenesis, this too is a tall order.

Finally, since neurodegenerative diseases are neither acute nor short-lived phenomena, it is likely that any treatments will have to be administered chronically and probably for over decades. This creates a very restricted window of acceptable toxicity for any proposed drugs.

Combined, the listed characteristics make drug discovery aimed at neurodegenerative diseases biologically challenging in the extreme and therefore slow and expensive with a high failure rate (Adams and Brantner 2006). Layered over this biological risk is a generally unattractive market risk. Although some companies have shown that they can develop profitable drugs for treating one or more neurodegenerative diseases, the pharmaceutical industry seems more than ever focused on so-called "block buster" drugs that achieve sales over $1 billion (Cuatrecasas 2006). The sizes of the patient populations for neurodegenerative disease are therefore a disincentive to a company weighing the relative merits of multiple drug discovery opportunities. Even AD, with the highest prevalence of all the neurodegenerative disease, has an estimated US patient population of just 4–5 million. Whereas from the perspective of disease burden and personal loss this is a startling number, it pales in comparison to the US adult obesity (72 million), high cholesterol (36 million), or diabetes (24 million) populations (Centers for Disease Control, National Center Health Statistics).

A NEW PARTNERSHIP

There is a potentially critical new role for academia in making the neurodegenerative diseases more appealing to pharmaceutical and biotechnology companies as development and investment opportunities. Clearly we cannot increase the market size. Nor can we simplify the biology of the brain. However, academic researchers could "de-risk" the drug discovery proposition by undertaking the first few steps of the process and then delivering to commercial partners just those projects that look the most promising.

The process of drug discovery (Figure 35.2) typically starts with the identification of a new target upon which drugs may act, generally identified either by studying the pathology and working back to identify the molecules and pathways leading to it, or by identifying genetic abnormalities associated with the disease and working forward to determine the gene product and its role in the disease. Alternatively, targets that protect against neurodegeneration may be identified.

With a target in mind, chemical agents that can interact with and disrupt or enhance the target are sought using a biochemical or cellular assay designed to expose the target to drug-

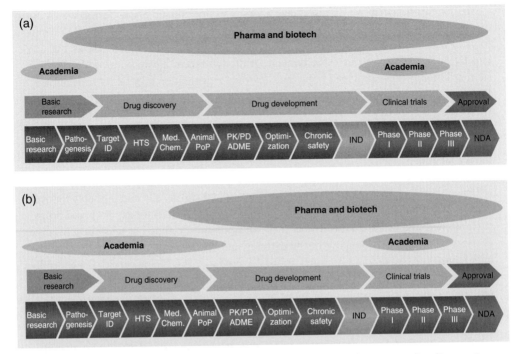

FIG. 35.2 Schematic (not to scale) showing major feature of the process for discovering, developing and testing new drugs. a) The traditional division of labor has the pharmaceutical and biotechnology sectors picking up new drug target ideas from academia and undertaking the entire process. Academia is only involved in the initial basic research, understanding pathogenesis, and in clinical trials. b) With many companies reducing their involvement in the highest risk, early-stage discovery process, particularly for neurodegenerative diseases, there is a need for academic research groups to commit more resources to early stage drug discovery and to extend their involvement. ADME, absorption, distribution, metabolism and excretion; HTS, high throughput screening; IND, investigational new drug (application); Med.Chem., medicinal chemistry; NDA, new drug application; PK/PD, pharmacokinetics/pharmacodynamics; PoP, proof of principle.

like chemicals. With the help of automation many chemicals can be tested in parallel, and the resulting high-throughput screen can test the action of many thousands of chemicals in a matter of days or weeks. The most promising hits are further investigated using an iterative process of testing, chemical modification aimed at improving the drug-like qualities of the chemical, and re-testing, before drug leads are selected and moved into an intensive phase of preclinical development. In those rare cases of drugs that have the right combination of efficacy, low toxicity, and a promising pharmacological profile, permission is sought from the appropriate regulatory authority to move the drug into the often long and expensive clinical testing phase, ultimately leading to approval to market the drug.

It is not unusual for this process to take more than a decade at a cost upward of $500 million for novel drugs, which in part explains why only 20–30 novel drugs come to market each year, for all indications (Food and Drug Administration, Center for Drug Evaluation and Research).

In light of the particularly challenging biological hurdles associated with understanding and targeting the causes of neurodegeneration, combined with the daunting commercial proposition of moving a drug candidate all the way through the discovery, development, testing, and approval process, neither is it surprising that so few new neurodegenerative diseases drugs make it to market. There are still no disease-modifying drugs approved to treat Alzheimer's, Parkinson's, ALS, or Huntington's diseases, and in the past two years just one novel symptomatic drug was approved (to treat the chorea associated with Huntington's disease). Based on the poor pipeline of new drug discovery prospects, this depressing picture seems unlikely to change in the near term.

Drug discovery has traditionally been left to biotechnology and pharmaceutical companies with the academic community generally contributing basic research and getting involved in clinical trials (Figure 35.2a). Given the dire need for novel drugs to help manage the predicted increase in neurodegenerative disease patients, it is time to reassess this arrangement.

Absent an entirely new approach to drug discovery, we must find a way of filling the early pipeline of drug discovery ideas and a means of quickly identifying the most promising. Whereas a robust and risk tolerant industry that is ready and willing to explore a larger number of early stage drug discovery projects is required for this to happen, there are also a number of steps that the academic research community can take to help fill the neurodegeneration drug pipeline. These include, for example, a significant effort to identify and validate easily measured biomarkers, the pursuit of a wide range of genetic strategies aimed at determining the inherited risk factors at work in each disease, and a continuing willingness to undertake both pilot and more formal clinical trials—all of which are traditional roles for the academic community. We should also be willing to adopt a less traditional role—that of drug discovery partner. Academic research groups are for the most part responsible for generating the basic research insight into disease pathogenesis that in turn leads to the identification of possible drug targets. These same groups must now start to put their discoveries to the test by taking the first few steps down the drug discovery path: identifying a relevant and novel target, and developing patent-protected proprietary compounds with a promising pharmacological profile and preclinical efficacy.

Most of the novel drug discovery projects that we embark upon will fail in this early stage of work—that is, unfortunately, the nature of the beast. But by investing in the appropriate laboratory infrastructure and skill set required for early-stage drug discovery we will be able to act as a filter whereby many ideas are tested and only the most successful are subsequently presented to prospective industry partners. Academic researchers are well suited to this type of work. They typically have the first and most complete understanding of emerging disease mechanisms and therefore drug targets, they regularly use a wide range of *in vitro* assays, and more often than not they have developed and characterized the animal disease models to be used for preclinical testing.

CHANGE IN CULTURE

Just as important as the technical capacity to perform this work, we must also develop the cultural expectation of university-based drug discovery and translational research in general. In some circles applied translational research such as drug discovery may still be regarded as the intellectual poor cousin to more fundamental and basic research. Increasingly this seems an outdated perspective (Ivinson 2005; Cuatrecasas 2006; Ivinson *et al.* 2008). Basic and applied research clearly represent different disciplines, the one driven more by curiosity and the other more goal oriented, and may well attract a different sort of scientist. But any inference that one is easier than the other or requires scientists of a different intellectual caliber is likely wrong. We should encourage university-based researchers to explore this relatively new opportunity by recognizing the importance of the goal and adding to and revising appropriate metrics for rewarding this activity (Crowley and Gusella 2009).

Neurodegenerative diseases represent a tidal wave of destruction bearing down on all communities. A 1994 study (Ernst and Hay 1994) estimated the annual economic cost of just AD in the US at $100 billion. Whereas more developed countries are at last waking up to the looming medical, financial and emotional burdens, the effects of Alzheimer's will be felt across the world with around half of world wide cases in the less developed and emerging economies of Asia (Brookmeyer *et al.* 2007). Given the near absence of effective drugs to treat or prevent AD and the other neurodegenerative diseases, and the startling increase in prevalence expected over the next few decades, we simply cannot afford to accept the status quo. It's time to get off the beach. One of several tangible and realistic approaches to tackling the problem is to significantly increase drug discovery interest, resources, and activity in universities and other not-for-profit settings. Universities, companies, foundations, national and international agencies, and private donors can all support this effort, which, if we are lucky, will contribute to the emergence of truly effective disease-modifying drugs for neurodegenerative disease. These will doubtless lead to challenging and important questions about access, equity, and neuroenhancement which, all things considered, would be a very good problem to have.

REFERENCES

Adams, C.P. and Brantner, V.V. (2006). Estimating the cost of new drug development: is it really 802 million dollars? *Health Affairs*, **25**, 420–8.

Brookmeyer R., Johnson E., Ziegler-Graham, K., and Arrighi, H.M. (2007). Forecasting the Global Burden of Alzheimer's Disease. *Alzheimer's and Dementia*, **3**, 186–91.

Centers for Disease Control. National Center Health Statistics. Available at http://www.cdc.gov/nchs/FASTATS/ (accessed 2 February 2010).

Chatterjee, A. (2006). The promise and predicament of cosmetic neurology. *Journal of Medical Ethics*, **32**, 110–13.

Crowley, W.F. and Gusella, J.F. (2009). Changing models of biomedical research. *Science Translational Medicine*, **1**, 1–6.

Cuatrecasas, P. (2006). Drug discovery in jeopardy. *Journal of Clinical Investigation*, **116**, 2837–42.

Ernst, R.L. and Hay, J.W. (1994). The U.S. Economic and Social Costs of Alzheimer's Disease Revisited. *American Journal of Public Health*, 84, 1261–4.

Food and Drug Administration, Center for Drug Evaluation and Research. New molecular entity approvals, 2000-2009. Data as of 1 Dec, 2009. Available at http://www.fda.gov/AboutFDA/CentersOffices/CDER (accessed 1 February 2010).

Hebert, L.E., Scherr, P.A., Bienias, J.L., Bennett, D.A., and Evans, D.A. (2003). Alzheimer disease in the US population. *Archives of Neurology*, 60, 1119–22.

Ivinson, A.J. (2005). University investment in drug discovery (letter). *Science*, 310, 777.

Ivinson, A.J., Lane, R., May, P.C., Hosford, D.A., Carrillo, M.C., and Siemers, E.R. (2008). Partnership between academia and industry for drug discovery in Alzheimer's disease. *Alzheimer's and Dementia*, 4, 230–1.

Marks, A.R. (2006). Rescuing the NIH before it is too late. *Journal of Clinical Investigation*, 116, 844.

Plassman, B.L., Langa, K.M., Fisher, G.G., *et al.* (2007). Prevalence of dementia in the United States: The Aging, Demographics, and Memory Study. *Neuroepidemiology*, 29, 125–32.

Special Section. (2005). Drug discovery; big risks, big rewards. *Science*, 309, 721–35.

United Nations, Department of Economic and Social Affairs, population Division. Available at: http://www.un.org/esa/population/unpop.htm (accessed 1 February 2010).

....

CHAPTER 36

FUTURE SCOPING: ETHICAL ISSUES IN AGING AND DEMENTIA

....

JULIAN C. HUGHES

INTRODUCTION

....

AGING and dementia are the future. Not only—whether we are from developed or developing countries—will more of us live longer, but neuroscience also provides increasing understanding of aging and dementia. Longevity, which itself will increase the prevalence of dementia, should provide a powerful impetus to governments to think seriously about the issues involved in an aging population. One tendency is to look to neuroscience to ameliorate, if not solve, the problems of aging. But is this tendency justified? Is it the case, indeed, that aging should be seen as a problem? If neuroethics is the study of the questions that arise in connection with neuroscientific advances and clinical practice, then these questions about the "problem" of aging and the tendency to look to neuroscience for solutions are pertinent, at least insofar as the aging brain as manifest by dementia is concerned.

My approach will be to start by highlighting some of the pathophysiological facts about aging and dementia. But the process of highlighting the amazing advances in terms of our neuroscientific understanding of aging and dementia will also demonstrate a conundrum. Starting with facts, we shall quickly find ourselves immersed in values. A hovering question will then be whether neuroscience can itself provide a sufficient account of such values.

With that question hanging, I shall consider potential biomedical advances and well-being. Each of these advances raises the possibility that well-being might be undermined. When, however, we raise the possibility of "curing" aging itself, we see that the argument becomes nonsensical: it is as if another language were being spoken, but not one that we could claim to understand, even in principle, because it would be embedded in a new way of life, one beyond our grasp. This is redolent of Wittgenstein (1968) saying: "If a lion could talk, we could not understand him" (p. 223). There are, thus, limits to the possibilities for human beings like us.

We arrive at these limits by considering, first, values, and secondly, the embedding context in which values are both shared and diverse. This gestures at values-based practice

(Fulford 2004), but also at the possibility of a horizon against which such values should be judged (Hughes 2009). Rather than pursue these ideas, I shall focus on mild cognitive impairment (MCI), which brings together the themes of aging and dementia. As we shall see, consideration of MCI again throws us back to the social context of aging and dementia, where values are to the fore and judgments have to be made. The point at issue in this discussion is the role of the normative in aging and dementia. And what this indicates, in my view, are the limits of the discussion. At a certain point neuroscience has little more to say; to go beyond this point is to move neuroethics into the realm of nonsense.

But the move to the social is critical. The power and importance of the move from a neuroscientific account to a more worldly account is perhaps captured best by Mary Midgley:

> People sometimes say that the human brain is the most complex item in the universe. But the whole person of whom that brain is part is necessarily a much more complex item than the brain alone. And whole people can't be understood without knowing a good deal both about their inner lives and about the other people around them. Indeed, they can't be understood without a fair grasp of the whole society that they belong to, which is presumably more complex still. (Midgley 2001, p .120)

Neuroscience, dementia, and aging

Dementia is a particular manifestation of brain aging. One way to present brain aging is to do so by disease categories. Thus, we could consider stroke as one disease of old age and Alzheimer's disease (AD) as another. Parkinson's disease (PD) might be considered as a third. We could then give a fairly accurate account of discrete pathologies that underlie these diagnostic entities. The sudden complete occlusion of a brain artery will cause anoxia, with permanent damage and death of neurons, which constitutes a stroke. AD is characterized by the accumulation of amyloid in plaques and by the phosphorylation of tau in intracellular neurofibrillary tangles. These pathological findings are associated with neuronal cell death. PD meanwhile shows evidence of Lewy bodies and degeneration in the substantia nigra of the basal ganglia. In dementia with Lewy bodies (DLB) these spherical intracellular protein deposits are found throughout the neocortex of the brain, as well as in subcortical structures (Holmes 2008; Nagy and Hubbard 2008).

Such pathological descriptions can seem clear-cut and they are supported by (or support) typical histories: the acute apoplexy of stroke; the gradual onset of memory and other cognitive impairments in AD; the characteristic movement disorders of PD—bradykinesia, rigidity, and tremor—which are also evident somewhat later in DLB. The convergence of history and neuropathology allows accurate diagnosis and rational management plans. It is the stuff of undergraduate medicine, which allows medical students to apply pattern recognition to symptoms and signs to make sense of different clinical presentations, secure in the knowledge that there is an underlying pathological reality to support the different diagnoses of stroke, AD, or PD.

Moreover, it has to be said that (at a postgraduate level) it is pretty impressive stuff. When, more than 30 years ago, a correlation was established between the deficits in cholinergic activity, plaque formation, and cognitive impairment (Perry *et al.* 1978), the implication was that a treatment that could boost acetylcholine would also improve cognitive functioning.

The cholinesterase inhibitors, which stop the breakdown of acetylcholine in the synapse between neurons, appeared in clinical use towards the end of the 1990s as the first symptomatic treatments for AD. They do, indeed, improve cognitive function, albeit modestly (Birks 2006). But occasionally, in some individuals, the results of these anti-dementia drugs have been impressive.

Meanwhile, improved neuroimaging allows us to see not only structural defects, such as atrophy in the medial temporal lobe in AD and DLB, but also functional deficits. In DLB, for instance, the deficits in dopaminergic transportation can be demonstrated—using ^{123}I-radio-labelled 2b-carbomethoxy-3b-(4-iodophenyl)-N-(3-fluoropropyl) nortropane (FP-CIT)—to a high degree of sensitivity (77.7%) and specificity (90.4%), an advance which has real clinical utility (McKeith *et al.* 2007).

Of course, as far as aging research and research into dementia go, this is just scratching the surface. The thought that there might be something about aging itself that underlies age-related diseases is an exciting one. It leads to the possibility not only of increasing longevity, but also that research into aging might decrease morbidity in the older old. This is the idea that the morbidity curve can be squared off: instead of a long period of increasing frailty and morbidity, we might lead good quality lives until roughly the time of our deaths. With this prospect in view, we can celebrate the advances in longevity and enjoy the time of our lives (Kirkwood 2000).

However, even a mere scratching of the surface reveals the deeper layers of interest. We know an immense amount about these discrete diseases. But are they discrete diseases?

> It is difficult to define the pathology of AD precisely at present. The reason for this is that the individual pathological components typical of AD brains all occur to some extent in normal ageing. (Nagy and Hubbard 2008)
> It is… increasingly clear that the spectrum of diseases that cause dementia, whilst often considered as separate disease entities clinically, have a great deal of overlap in their underlying pathogenesis. (Holmes 2008)

Not only are there significant vascular changes in AD, not only does ischemic damage coexist with AD, and not only is the pathology of AD to be found in DLB too, but also senile amyloid plaques, neurofibrillary tangles, and Lewy bodies can all be found in healthy aging brains. The lack of a clear demarcation between these conditions at the level of the brain, but also in clinical practice, means that evaluative judgments have to be made. In the clinical world this is taken for granted; but the key point is that values come into play in the concrete neuroscientific world as well.

Interestingly, this takes us back to the quote from Midgley. In deciding on a particular criterion to make a neuropathological diagnosis of definite AD, e.g. a particular number (X) of senile plaques seen in a particular region of the brain at a given age at a particular magnification, recourse has to be made to the world of persons living in a cultural and social context. Only if X senile plaques equates to such-and-such a set of behaviors will it make sense to say that X plaques is the criterion for definite AD. Normative decisions in the neuroscientific world are predicated on data derived from the real world of living people.

Leaving the point about values aside, we might take the optimistic view that the closeness of the different age-related brain diseases at the pathological level holds out the hope that research into aging will indeed provide a key to help cure all these diseases. Immediately, however, another evaluative difficulty emerges. For, we must now face not just the lack of a clear cut-off between AD and DLB, but also the absence of a clear marker to differentiate abnormal from normal aging. In many cases (or even most) we can make this differentiation quite easily: a stroke, dementia, and PD are usually identified without a problem. The point is, however, that the requisite evaluative judgments are made in the complexity of the world. What will count as normal aging must count (in a normative sense) as such in the real world, whatever the (quantitative) counts might be in the worlds of neuropathology, neurochemistry, or even of neuroimaging.

Hence, we reach the conundrum I mentioned at the start of the chapter: starting with facts, we are quickly immersed in values. The move suggested by Midgley, from neuroscience to the world, does tend to imply that neuroscience itself cannot provide a sufficient account of such values, which undermines any suggestion that neuroscience in itself will help with moral dilemmas:

> Neuroscience and neuroscientists can provide important new information about the human brain. But, while that information can feed into ethical reasoning, it cannot replace the ethical judgment needed for individual and social decision-making. (Green 2006)

I shall now leave this point hanging, but consider instead potential advances derived from biomedicine and the issues of well-being.

Biomedicine and well-being

In this section I shall consider the examples of enhancing memory, of anti-aging medicaments, and the possibility of ultimate longevity. Each can be conceived as a potential advance derived from biomedicine. The first (memory enhancement) is of direct relevance to neuroethics. Anti-aging medicaments are mainly cosmetic at present, but could (in principle) extend to medications aimed at slowing aging in the brain. The possibility of living forever remains science fiction, but it is a fiction that some people seriously hope will become a reality and for which they plan.

Another example I might have considered is the use of assistive technology to help older people and people with dementia in particular. The relevant issues are considered elsewhere (ter Meulen *et al.* 2007). One way to think of the issues is in terms of well-being: whether we are thinking of something as straightforward as electronic tagging for those at risk of getting lost, or of something much more interactive, which would in some sense anticipate cognitive deficits and act to rectify them (e.g. by providing prompts when a person was carrying out domestic chores), assistive technologies can both enhance and undermine both well-being and the person's autonomy (Nuffield Council on Bioethics 2009). The tendency for an interest in well-being to cut in different directions turns out to be common.

If tablets can now improve memory, then (given that memory loss is ubiquitous) might it not be very reasonable for drug companies to sell their cognitive enhancing drugs to everyone, since we might all benefit? Indeed, given that there is no clear biological line to be drawn between normal and abnormal, this would seem to be perfectly rational: use the drugs if they are beneficial and only avoid them if they are harmful. A similar rationale would support the use of treatments for aging itself, whether this applied to anti-wrinkle cream or the science-fiction technique of fraitching.

Tom Kirkwood (2000), one of the foremost contemporary gerontologists, concluded *Time of Our Lives* with a fictional account of the world in which people could live forever through "fraitch technology", which allows cell damage to be repaired. Given that it is—according to Kirkwood's "disposable soma theory"—the stochastic process of an accumulation of damage that accounts for aging (because the body sets greater evolutionary store on reproduction than it does on cell repair), providing a means to repair the damage that random hits cause in our somatic cells would spell the end of aging. In Kirkwood's futuristic world, however, to deal with the problem of over-population, the State allocates people a quota of children, having achieved which they are not allowed to have further fraitches. Then they become "Timed Ones" and die after a few decades.

So, we have three things that are more or less possible: creams to cope with the signs of aging, medications that might enhance normality, and futuristic technologies that might abolish death. We should treat these different possibilities differently since they raise different sorts of concern and argument. However, we can think of them all from the perspective of well-being: although the arguments are then similar, it is a line that fails when we get to the possibility of living forever.

Anti-aging creams, for instance, contribute to well-being in that they can make a person feel good. But such creams act against something, which turns out to involve the possibility of well-being too. A lined face is not something that necessarily precludes the possibility of well-being and may, indeed, reflect a life filled with smiles and vivacity.

Cognitive enhancement, inasmuch as it aims at a good (namely, improved mental powers), might be taken to enhance well-being too. But, again, the suggestion that a lack of cognitive powers is inimical to well-being does not ring true. Even if we hold that it is on the whole better to be intelligent than the reverse, we can still recognize that a simple life can be one in which there is well-being. In any case, cognitive enhancement is about improving cognitive function above a level that is not necessarily impaired, and normal cognitive function has always hitherto been compatible with well-being. Cognitive enhancement may be a means to an end—wealth or power say—but although they can produce some sense of well-being, the limits of human well-being are difficult to circumscribe (except by death). Hence, the implication is that even wealth and power do not exhaust the possibilities for human well-being. After all, whatever the material circumstances, it is not ludicrous to suggest that well-being only requires an acceptance of life. Almost any form of human life can be a life with well-being, especially where this is conceived as psychological well-being (to differentiate it from quality of life, which it could be argued implies some basic objective and materialistic minimal requirements perhaps).

In the case of ultimate longevity, however, the pattern of the argument breaks down. The sense in which getting rid of death contributes to well-being depends on a notion of well-being that is circumscribed by death. In the absence of death the notion of well-being is not the same. The acceptance of life that we know is one unto death. We do not know what well-being would be like in a world where death was absent. Everything changes, including our values, because our values reflect the temporal world of change too: artistic or scientific values have their purchase in this world where there are endings and decay, and where life itself has a certain shape that gives it meaning.

So the world of fraitching would have to incorporate significant psychological adjustments, as Kirkwood foresaw:

> In the early centuries after fraitch technology was developed, the emotional burden of a long life was poorly understood and the suicide rate grew alarmingly high. Psycho-fraitching of the mind quickly became as important as the regeneration of the cells and tissues of the body. (Kirkwood 2000, p. 245)

Bavidge made the following comment about this quote, which helps to emphasize the extent to which the adjustments to be made are normative, inter alia, as well as psychological:

> If life without end is a meaningless life then psycho-fraitching can only be a technique for obscuring that fact. Professor Kirkwood speculates that people may be psychologically impelled to conform to the old fallacious idea that there is a natural pattern to life that ends in ageing and death. (Bavidge 2006, p .45)

Later, Bavidge warns us against a form of ageism:

> The thought that human consciousness emerges, develops, and ages should remind us not to pathologize old age....there are mixed costs and benefits attending all stages of life. It is only when these become dysfunctional that we should start treating them as pathological symptoms. We should think of old age as offering alternative rather than impaired ways of experiencing life. (Bavidge 2006, p .49)

As we've seen, the suggestion that ultimate longevity might be possible runs up against our ways of understanding life. These understandings are normative, in the sense that we cannot ignore them and they impose a certain moral outlook, so that our whole notion of what might constitute a good life—a life filled with well-being—depends on the sense that life is bounded (Lesser 2006). As well as having normative properties, our understandings of life are also multifarious: life, especially one to be characterized in terms of well-being, requires emotional, aesthetic, cognitive, conative, spiritual, historical, cultural, and social aspects, amongst others. Life conceived in this way would tend, according to Bavidge, to see aging as just another aspect of life. To see life merely in terms of aging (and aging merely in terms of decline) is an aberration, which makes neither rational nor moral sense. Furthermore, such negative views of aging promote stigma and alienation of the elderly.

With these thoughts in place we can now consider some issues around the notion of MCI, which also reflect the tendency for well-being to cut in two directions.

MILD COGNITIVE IMPAIRMENT

MCI is potentially a pre-dementia state. Considerable effort has been put into delineating MCI in terms of its clinical features, including neuroimaging, as well as its genetic basis (O'Brien 2008). If this state could be found, there would be the possibility of future treatments being used in MCI to prevent full-blown dementia. There are other ways in which a diagnosis of MCI contributes to well-being. In a negative sense, to pinpoint this diagnosis is to exclude a treatable condition such as depression. More positively, a diagnosis at this stage enables the person to consider realistic advance care planning whilst still competent.

There are, however, a number of reasons to be cautious about this diagnostic "entity." First, it would seem to run the risk of being a clear case of pathologizing aging. The proponents of MCI (Peterson 2003) seek to show that (a) it has face validity and (b) it has potential utility. Even so, there would still be the concern that MCI does not contribute to well-being. One way in which this might be the case is if telling someone they have a pre-dementia syndrome is harmful. There has previously been considerable worry that telling a person he or she has dementia might cause a catastrophic reaction. This worry turns out not to have much foundation: not only do people (on the whole) wish to know their diagnoses (Bamford *et al.* 2004), but also the evidence that people contemplate suicide after the diagnosis of dementia is thin (Haw *et al.* 2009).

So MCI raises an ethical issue for neuroscience. There are strong neuroscientific reasons to wish to delineate MCI. But these reasons are driven by a variety of agendas, which reflect a variety of values (Moreira *et al.* 2008). The neuroscientific approach is not value-free. It reflects various social pressures, for example, to do with research funding and the influence of the pharmaceutical industry. These social and evaluative concerns in connection with MCI have their counterparts in other concerns about AD itself. The diagnosis of Alzheimer's has a complicated social and cultural history (Gaines and Whitehouse 2006),

Once the suggestion starts to be that "normal" life—a degree of forgetfulness in older age similar to that which many younger people also experience—is pathological, people begin to look more carefully at boundaries. What they then see is that the boundaries are constructed on the basis of particular cultural and historical norms, which can be challenged and which certainly do not add up to biologically discrete entities. Diagnoses are inherently value-laden (Sadler 2005).

So, the diagnostic category of MCI may enhance well-being, if it can enable earlier treatment of dementia or allow better future planning; but it cuts in another direction too, which poses a threat to well-being. The threat is of actual harm, but is also of a broader harm from its tendency to label human experience in a way that may be infantilizing, pathologizing, and malignant. Tom Kitwood (1997) spoke of the tendency for there to be a "malignant social psychology" surrounding dementia, as a direct consequence of the diagnosis; and, more recently, Steve Sabat has encouraged the use of the phrase "malignant positioning" to describe the way in which people (even those close to the person) can add to the burden of the brain disease and undermine the person's selfhood by their attitudes and behavior (Sabat 2006). We see, therefore, in this brief discussion of MCI, both the importance (from the perspective of well-being) of making a diagnosis of a pre-dementia state if possible, and the ways in which MCI raises questions of an evaluative and normative kind. Our understanding of MCI has to be rooted in a broader social understanding of aging, which reflects the value we ascribe to certain cognitive capacities; and the issues that are raised are normative ones, where background judgments have to be made about the kind of life we ought to live.

CONCLUSION

The facts of neuroscience with respect to aging and dementia are impressive and important; but they quickly raise values and their embedding context. In both our discussion of values and of well-being we came across a point at which neuroscience had little more to say. This is not in any sense meant to underplay the importance of neuroscience. It is simply to recognize that the neuroscientific discourse cannot in itself account for the content of the normative discussion about values and moral judgments, even if it might wish to explain—in a different discourse, as espoused by Churchland (2006)—the neurological foundations of such a discussion. For the ethical debate about aging and dementia takes place in the social realm, which (again) can be *causally explained* by neuroscience but not *understood in terms of its content.*

Data derived from neuroscience will inform normative decisions made in the social and evaluative world of people. Appeals to well-being turn out to cut in different directions depending on our views, but the horizon against which judgments must be made is set by life's boundedness. Our thoughts about aging and dementia inhabit this none the less multifaceted context. If aging can be a problem—one which neuroscience can help to solve—it also represents a broadening of possibilities. This tends to take us into other realms: of culture, of social discourse and companionship, of spiritual growth. On this view, the future can look a lot more positive than we might have expected.

REFERENCES

Bamford, C., Lamont, S., Eccles, M., Robinson, L., May, C., and Bond, J. (2004). Disclosing a diagnosis of dementia: a systematic review. *International Journal of Geriatric Psychiatry*, 19, 151–69.

Bavidge, M. (2006). Ageing and human nature. In J.C. Hughes, S.J. Louw, and S.R. Sabat (eds.) *Dementia: Mind, Meaning, and the Person*, pp. 41–53. Oxford: Oxford University Press.

Birks, J. (2006). Cholinesterase inhibitors for Alzheimer's disease. *Cochrane Database of Systematic Reviews*, 1, CD005593.

Churchland, P.S. (2006). Moral decision-making and the brain. In J. Illes (ed.) *Neuroethics: Defining the Issues in Theory, Practice, and Policy*, pp. 3–16. Oxford: Oxford University Press.

Fulford, K.W.M. (2004). Facts/values. Ten principles of values-based medicine. In J. Radden (ed.) *The Philosophy of Psychiatry: A Companion*, pp. 205–34. Oxford: Oxford University Press.

Gaines, A.D. and Whitehouse, P.J. (2006). Building a mystery: Alzheimer disease, mild cognitive impairment, and beyond. *Philosophy, Psychiatry, & Psychology*, 13, 61–74.

Green, R.M. (2006). From genome to brainome: charting the lessons learned. In J. Illes (ed.) *Neuroethics: Defining the Issues in Theory, Practice, and Policy*, pp. 105–21. Oxford: Oxford University Press.

Haw C, Harwood D, Hawton K. (2009). Dementia and suicidal behavior: a review of the literature. *International Psychogeriatrics*, 21, 440–53.

Holmes, C. (2008). The genetics and molecular biology of dementia. In R. Jacoby, C. Oppenheimer, T. Dening, and A. Thomas (eds.) *Oxford Textbook of Old Age Psychiatry*, pp. 103–17. Oxford: Oxford University Press.

Hughes, J.C. (2009). Horizons on the world. *Perspectives in Biology and Medicine*, 52, 442–7.

Kirkwood, T. (2000). *Time of Our Lives: The Science of Human Ageing*. London: Phoenix Press.

Kitwood, T. (1997). *Dementia Reconsidered: The Person Comes First*. Buckingham: Open University Press.

Lesser, A.H. (2006). Dementia and personal identity. In J.C. Hughes, S.J. Louw, and S.R. Sabat (eds.) *Dementia: Mind, Meaning, and the Person*, pp. 55–61. Oxford: Oxford University Press.

McKeith, I., O'Brien, J., Walker, Z., et al. (2007). Sensitivity and specificity of dopamine transporter imaging with ^{123}I-FP-CIT SPECT in dementia with Lewy bodies: a phase III, multicentre study. *Lancet Neurology*, 6, 305–13.

Midgley, M. (2001). *Science and Poetry*. London: Routledge.

Moreira, T., Hughes, J.C., Kirkwood, T., May, C., McKeith I., and Bond, J. (2008). What explains variations in the clinical use of mild cognitive impairment (MCI) as a diagnostic category? *International Psychogeriatrics*, **20**, 697–709.

Nagy, Z. and Hubbard, P. (2008). Neuropathology. In R. Jacoby, C. Oppenheimer, T. Dening, and A. Thomas (eds.) *Oxford Textbook of Old Age Psychiatry*, pp. 67–83. Oxford: Oxford University Press.

Nuffield Council on Bioethics (2009). *Dementia: Ethical Issues*, pp. 97–100. London: Nuffield Council on Bioethics. Available at: http://www.nuffieldbioethics.org

O'Brien, J.T. (2008). Mild cognitive impairment. In R. Jacoby, C. Oppenheimer, T. Dening, and A. Thomas (eds.) *Oxford Textbook of Old Age Psychiatry*, pp. 407–15, Oxford: Oxford University Press.

Perry, E.K., Tomlinson, B.E., Blessed, G., Bergmann, K., Gibson, P.H., and Perry, R.H. (1978). Correlation of cholinergic abnormalities with senile plaques and mental test scores in senile dementia. *British Medical Journal*, **2**, 1457–9.

Peterson, R.C. (2003). *Mild Cognitive Impairment*. Oxford: Oxford University Press.

Sabat, S.R. (2006). Mind, meaning, and personhood in dementia: the effects of positioning. In J.C. Hughes, S.J. Louw, and S.R. Sabat, (eds.) *Dementia: Mind, Meaning, and the Person*, pp. 287–302. Oxford: Oxford University Press.

Sadler, J.Z. (2005). *Values and Psychiatric Diagnosis*. Oxford: Oxford University Press.

ter Meulen, R.H.J., Nielsen, L., and Landeweerd, L. (2007). Ethical issues of enhancement technologies. In R.E. Ashcroft, A. Dawson, H. Draper, J.R. McMillan (eds.) *Principles of Health Care Ethics*, pp. 803–9. Chichester: John Wiley.

Wittgenstein, L. (1968). *Philosophical Investigations*. First published 1953, G.E.M. Anscombe and R. Rhees (trans.), G.E.M. Anscombe (eds.) Oxford: Blackwell.

PART VI

....

LAW AND
PUBLIC POLICY

....

CHAPTER 37

INCIDENTAL FINDINGS IN NEUROSCIENCE RESEARCH: A FUNDAMENTAL CHALLENGE TO THE STRUCTURE OF BIOETHICS AND HEALTH LAW

SUSAN M. WOLF

THE problem of incidental findings in human subjects research—findings of potential health importance to the research participant that the researcher stumbles upon while pursuing the aims of the research study (Wolf *et al.* 2008a)—may at first seem of minor significance. After all, the research enterprise is designed to produce something else: results of importance to a broader population concerning the variables under study. If researchers occasionally happen upon adventitious findings of potential clinical relevance to a single research participant, such as a brain tumor or aneurysm, surely this is a minor side note to the central activity of the research itself. Incidental findings seem, after all, incidental—minor, ancillary, of little consequence.

Nothing could be further from the truth: incidental findings are an unavoidable by-product of conducting research in human beings. Depending on the research method being used and the population being studied, researchers may encounter incidental findings in the majority of the participants in their research (Alphs *et al.* 2006; Johnson *et al.* 2008; Yee *et al.* 2005). Even in studies in which incidental findings are less common, they may include urgent and even life-threatening findings (Vernooij *et al.* 2007; Wolf *et al.* 2008a; Yue *et al.* 1997).

The number and potential gravity of incidental findings force researchers to face difficult questions. The most fundamental of these is whether researchers have any duty to identify, evaluate, and disclose these findings to the research participant. What makes these questions so difficult is that at root they ask whether researchers have some kind of duty to trigger or provide clinical care.

Merely asking this question is a profound challenge to the structure of bioethics and health law. Both fields approach the world of research and the world of medical care very differently. The problem of incidental findings challenges this traditional dichotomy. The problem forces attention to the question of whether the two-world vision that has been fundamental to the architecture of health law and bioethics is wrong. Neuroethics has played a central role in bringing this problem to the fore.

EMERGENCE OF THE
INCIDENTAL FINDINGS PROBLEM

Recognition of the scope and importance of the incidental findings problem has emerged over the last decade, especially in the domain of neuroscience research. However, clinicians have long known that although patients may present with one set of medical issues, others may emerge in the work-up of the initial ones. Indeed, even surgery undertaken for one indication may serendipitously uncover a second medical problem. In fact, the term "incidentaloma" is defined as an adrenal tumor unexpectedly discovered (*Stedman's Medical Dictionary* 2002). Thus, the problem of incidental findings has been well recognized in non-research clinical care.

In the clinical context, incidental findings raise far fewer issues than in the research context. The clinician is committed to caring for the patient no matter what medical problems may emerge. The discovery of an unexpected problem may call for inclusion of a new specialist on the patient's medical team, but does not disrupt the commitment of the patient's primary care physician and medical team as a whole to care for the full patient no matter what panoply of medical problems emerges. As a matter of ethics, law, and clinical custom, the primary care physician and team are responsible for addressing not only the presenting medical concern, but also other medical concerns that emerge in the course of addressing the concern initially presented.

Recognizing that incidental findings may also emerge in the very different context of human subjects research has taken more time. Most such research is undertaken in the United States under formal rules created by the federal government in the mid-1970s in the wake of the Tuskegee Syphilis Trials and other research scandals (Levine 1988; Shamoo and Resnik 2003). The National Commission for the Protection of Human Subjects of Biomedical and Behavioral Research made recommendations that ultimately resulted in enactment of federal regulations requiring local Institutional Review Board (IRB) approval of proposed research protocols before researchers could enroll human subjects. The most widely used set of regulations is the Common Rule (45 C.F.R. Part 46) and covers all research conducted or funded by the US Department of Health and Human Services (DHHS; http://www.hhs.gov) including the National Institutes of Health (NIH; http://www.nih.gov). The reach of the rule is even broader, as universities typically render a general assurance to the federal government that all of that university's research on human participants will undergo advance review under the Common Rule, whether or not the research is federally funded. Some agencies such as the US Food and Drug Administration (FDA; http://www.fda.gov) apply their own variant of the Common Rule (21 C.F.R. Parts 50, 56); all product sponsors who need FDA approval to market their product must assure that human subjects research on that product comports with the FDA regulations, even if that research is privately funded and outside the university context.

As a result of these rules and development of the IRB oversight system (with additional review mechanisms for certain kinds of research such as gene transfer research), researchers routinely submit their research protocol for approval. However, the protocol focuses on articulation of the research aims, research design, proposed study population, recruitment and enrollment plan, consent process and documents, intervention, and proposed analyses. It may say nothing about incidental findings—information beyond the research aims that may emerge at any stage of the research, from ascertaining the suitability of a prospective participant for enrollment, through data collection, data analysis, and even in secondary reanalysis of archived data in future research projects (Cho 2008; Wolf *et al.* 2008a).

Yet incidental findings in research have been impossible to avoid. Genetic research in a family manifesting a pattern of phenotypic disease whose genetic substrate is not yet understood inevitably runs the risk of revealing unexpected biological information such as misattributed paternity (Lucassen and Parker 2001). Genomic research involving chromosomal analysis may be designed to answer study questions about one set of concerns but may incidentally reveal a host of other abnormalities, including XYY syndrome or Klinefelter's syndrome (Van Ness 2008). Whenever tests or analytic methods used in research have the potential to reveal information beyond what is required to answer the specific research questions, the potential for incidental findings exists.

Indeed, any kind of research encounter has the potential to generate incidental findings. A researcher conducting a psychology experiment on university undergraduate students may detect signs of mental illness or substance abuse that have nothing to do with the research aims. Another researcher interviewing families with young children in the home may spot unsecured guns or other unsafe circumstances. Philosopher Henry Richardson (2008) has even queried the responsibility of researchers when they incidentally spot a suspicious lesion warranting investigation for melanoma. The possibilities are myriad.

Despite the wealth of research circumstances that can yield incidental findings, imaging research—and neuroimaging research in particular—has played a pivotal role in bringing the incidental findings problem to the fore. Imaging scans can present incidental findings with a visual force that demands attention. Thus, commentators write about the "unidentified bright object" or UBO that may signal a tumor or other potentially serious abnormality (Royal and Peterson 2008). Vernooij *et al.* (2007) published a series of neuroimaging research scans with incidental findings, many of which present obvious brain asymmetries even to the untrained eye.

Neuroimaging research can yield a high number of incidental findings. Reported prevalence ranges from 13–84% of scans, depending on study population, scan protocol, and definition of incidental findings (See, e.g. Alphs *et al.* 2006; Illes *et al.* 2004; Katzman *et al.* 1999; Kim *et al.* 2002; Kumra *et al.* 2006; Vernooij *et al.* 2007; Yue *et al.* 1997). The prevalence figures inch even higher in computed tomography (CT) colonography (sometimes called "virtual colonography") research, which involves scanning most of the torso. Prevalence of incidental findings ranges up to 89% of scans (Siddiki *et al.* 2008).

In both of these spheres of imaging research, a number of commentators have strongly argued against researchers simply ignoring incidental findings or dismissing them as beyond the scope of researcher duties (Ginnerup Pederson *et al.* 2003; Illes *et al.* 2006; Siddiki *et al.* 2008). While debate certainly continues on the scope of those duties and how to manage incidental findings appropriately, a substantial amount of work has been published on incidental findings in both research domains, documenting prevalence, types, appropriate management, positive and negative effects of pursuing incidental findings clinically, and costs. Authors in both research arenas have gone so far as to propose classification systems for incidental findings according to apparent seriousness and what action is warranted. Kim *et al.* (2002) suggest four categories in neuroimaging research: (1) need for immediate referral for clinical evaluation, (2) need for urgent referral, (3) need for routine referral, and (4) no need for referral. Zalis *et al.* (2005, Fig.3) suggest five categories in CT colonography research: (1) "Potentially Important Finding"—"Communicate to Referring Physician"; (2) "Likely Unimportant Finding, Incompletely Characterized"—"Work-up may be indicated"; (3) "Clinically Unimportant Finding"—"No work-up indicated"; (4) "Normal Exam or Anatomic Variant"; and (5) "Limited Exam".

Though both types of imaging research, neuroimaging and CT colonography, have led the way in catalyzing attention to the problem of incidental findings more broadly in research, neuroimaging has played a special role. This is partly because neuroimaging research raises more directly than CT colonography research the question of what clinical duties, if any, non-clinician researchers bear. Much neuroimaging research is conducted by non-clinicians, such as Ph.D. scientists in psychology or neuroscience who have no clinical role. The research may be conducted outside a medical setting and there may be no clinicians, including no neuroradiology specialists, on the study team. In contrast, CT colonography, which requires pumping air into the colon through a rectal catheter with an associated risk of colonic perforation, is performed by medical personnel, conducted in a medical setting, and yields scans that are read by a radiologist. Thus the researcher may be both a clinician, although not necessarily a particular research participant's clinician, and a researcher, and the study team is likely to include clinicians. The contrast means that although both kinds of research can raise the question of whether researchers bear clinical duties, neuroimaging research raises the question more starkly, because many researchers using neuroimaging are researchers only with no concurrent clinician role.

The other reason the neuroimaging research has acted as a powerful catalyst to work on incidental findings is that brain normality holds a special allure and abnormalities are particularly alarming. Certainly, abnormalities in the torso can be frightening and deadly (consider pancreatic cancer, for example). But for many people, the brain is considered to be seat of the self (Illes and Racine 2005; Smith Churchland 2006). Anomalies revealed on a brain scan thus may be quite alarming to the researchers viewing the scan as well as to the individual scanned. Because the brain integrates organic functioning and is crucial to cognitive functioning, pathology and disruption may be seen as, and may actually be, deeply threatening to the continued functioning of the individual in ways previously familiar. Thus, how researchers handle incidental findings in the brain—whether they decide that attention to such findings is beyond their research role or competence, or otherwise decline to evaluate and disclose them to research participants—is widely perceived to be a high-stakes question (Illes *et al.* 2006).

THE DILEMMA POSED BY INCIDENTAL FINDINGS

At first blush it may seem obvious that researchers should report incidental findings to research participants to allow clinical evaluation and care. Deeper analysis shows that researchers confronting incidental findings face a genuine dilemma. On the one hand, reporting a suspicious finding to a research participant could lead to life-saving care. There are, indeed, cases in the literature of a brain tumor found in the course of neuroimaging research in a supposedly normal participant (Anonymous 2005; Vernooij *et al.* 2007). On the other hand, neuroimaging research may not involve clinical-grade scans and a scan sequence optimized for diagnosis, and may be read by non-clinician researchers with no training in diagnostic interpretation (Illes *et al.* 2006; Wolf *et al.* 2008a). This means that suspicious findings may turn out to be false positives. Thus, disclosure to research participants may cause non-trivial anxiety and trigger testing with its own psychological burden, cost, and physical risk (Wolf *et al.* 2008a).

Researchers may fear a duty to spot incidental findings for which they and their team may not be trained, preferring to avoid this issue by asserting they are mere researchers with no clinical duties. A study of research consent forms found some saying just that (Lawrenz and Sobotka 2008). At the same time, such researchers may also fear that if they spot a threatening-looking incidental finding in the brain of a supposedly normal control and fail to disclose this, they have breached some ethical and perhaps legal duty to give warning.

Yet a decision to assume responsibility to communicate incidental findings does not provide safe refuge. Researchers may worry about missing some incidental findings they should have spotted. Conversely, they may worry about communicating some incidental findings that turn out to lack clinical importance, but only after a work-up that imposes anxiety and cost. There is also the thorny question of what incidental findings to communicate—all of them, no matter how trivial; only those with serious clinical implications; only those with such implications and options for treatment? Those are only three of the many possible decision rules under robust debate today (Wolf *et al.* 2008a).

Even while debate continues on what incidental findings to return, it is safe to say that the growing trend is to recognize that researchers have duties to anticipate incidental findings in their research, address in their proposed research protocol their plan for managing such findings, obtain IRB approval for that plan, assure adequate resources and personnel to execute the plan, and track their incidental findings experience (Illes *et al.* 2006; Wolf *et al.* 2008a). There is less consensus, however, surrounding the duties of secondary researchers accessing and reanalyzing data they did not originally collect that have been archived for reanalysis in future research projects (Cho 2008; Clayton 2008; Wolf *et al.* 2008a). Often, these data have been de-identified, making it difficult or impossible to re-contact the participant. Clayton (2008) and Wolf *et al.* (2008a) also point out that some genetic research may be conducted on DNA samples that were not collected for that research and that have no individual identifiers, so that the DNA source was not required to consent under current rules and may have no idea that their sample is being used in research. In the simpler case of incidental findings by the original researchers outside the archive context, there is wide agreement that research participants should be alerted in the informed consent process to the future possibility of incidental findings and asked whether they want to be contacted and informed of such findings (Illes *et al.* 2006; Wolf *et al.* 2008a).

THE CHALLENGE TO THE STRUCTURE OF BIOETHICS AND HEALTH LAW

This trend toward recognizing that researchers do indeed shoulder some duties to anticipate and address incidental findings in research is a profound challenge to the traditional structure of bioethics and health law. Both have contrasted the duties of researchers and clinicians. Much rests in each field on the dichotomy created between the world of research and the world of clinical care.

In ethics, the duties of treating physicians have been articulated in codes and writings on medical ethics for millennia, including those from Hippocrates and Maimonides. However, codes articulating the ethics to guide and limit researchers are much more recent, including the post-Second World War Nuremburg Code and Helsinki Declaration (Annas and Grodin 1995). This sharply contrasting history is mirrored in contrasting content. Physicians have fundamental obligations to advance the well-being of their patients. However, the fundamental duty of the researcher is to seek generalizable knowledge, while avoiding the infliction of harm and respecting the research participant's right to make a free and informed decision about whether to participate in the research. Even the skills and virtues that clinicians and non-clinician researchers bring to the table are different; many neuroscience researchers, for example, are not trained in clinical neuroscience or neuroradiology and have not undergone the attendant socialization as clinicians serving patients. Instead, they are trained and socialized as scientists.

The contrast in law is equally stark. Physicians are professionals licensed by the state, subject to state and institutional disciplinary rules. The law of malpractice holds physicians to the standard of practice of their peers in the same specialty. A patient claiming to be harmed by malpractice has the right to go to court for retrospective adjudication of whether the physician's practice fell below the applicable standard of care and that failure caused the purported harm, in order to seek monetary damages.

On the other hand, non-clinician scientists are not licensed by the state. No state or hospital disciplinary boards sit to consider infractions, although universities have grievance committees. In addition, the dominant US approach to research harm has been to try to prevent it by prospective IRB review and ongoing IRB supervision, rather than by retrospective review in court. Indeed, US courts have overwhelmingly rejected the notion that research participants have the right to sue researchers for harm in research and have refused to award money damages. Instead, the consequences of research malfeasance have predominantly been removal of or restrictions on federal research grants, with NIH and the federal Office for Human Research Protections (OHRP; http://www.hhs.gov/ohrp/) taking the lead (Wolf *et al.* 2008b).

To be sure, clinicians sometimes double as researchers. In some fields, such as oncology, clinical research is common, and a patient's own physician may even conduct research enrolling the patient as a research participant. However, the practice of combining the roles of clinician and researcher has spawned a substantial literature highlighting the complexities and confusions that can occur when both patient and clinician are wearing two hats.

Jay Katz (1993–94), in particular, has argued that this represents a profound confusion of roles; he insists that the clinician-researcher should resolve this confusion by approaching the patient-subject as a scientist, not an amalgam of scientist and clinician. The very fact that this clinician-researcher role is seen as a double-role and debated as such demonstrates the dichotomy animating both ethics and law (King 2000).

Most of the literature debating the conflation of researcher and clinician roles grows out of the world of clinical research and focuses on the physician-researcher. However, the problem of incidental findings in neuroscience research focuses on researchers who are not clinicians and may not even conduct their research in medical settings. These researchers are more likely to be psychologists, neuroscientists, and cognitive scientists.

To argue that researchers who are not clinicians at all bear some measure of clinical responsibility is a radical proposition. Richardson (2008) recognizes this in contrasting the professions of science and medicine. Indeed, in grappling with the question of whether researchers bear any duties of care beyond the conduct of their research, he and Belsky (Richardson and Belsky 2004) contrast two possible visions of the researcher—as pure scientist with no duties of ancillary care and as a professional akin to a personal physician with broad duties of ancillary care extending to all aspects of the health of a research participant. Richardson and Belsky reject both views. Instead, they argue that research participants entrust private information and aspects of their well-being to researchers. This "partial entrustment" gives rise to duties of ancillary care bounded by the scope of the entrustment. Richardson (2008) concludes that "Every incidental finding thus falls within the scope of the ancillary-care obligation." (p. 266).

Miller *et al.* (2008) grapple with this problem as well. They too come out in favor of imposing some clinical care responsibilities on researchers. Instead of using a partial-entrustment argument, however, they "derive the responsibility for addressing incidental findings in research from the investigator's consented access to private health-related information in the context of a professional relationship." (pp. 276–7). They argue that researchers do have a professional relationship with their research participants, albeit a different professional relationship than physicians have with their patients.

Thus, we see the problem of incidental findings forcing reconsideration of the dichotomy that has structured ethics and health law. Richardson and Belsky as well as Franklin *et al.* are arguing ethics, but Wolf *et al.* (2008b) and Milstein (2008) have argued the law. These legal commentators challenge the traditional gulf between clinician liability for malpractice and the absence of direct researcher accountability to individual research participants. The authors argue in favor of holding researchers responsible for handling incidental findings appropriately, though the two articles differ in legal approach. Milstein essentially treats researchers as if they were clinicians, and argues that researchers failing to recognize and disclose incidental findings are guilty of a form of malpractice. Wolf *et al.* avoid conflating researchers with clinicians, but nonetheless argue theories to undergird researcher liability for failure to handle incidental findings appropriately.

RECONSTITUTING BIOETHICS AND HEALTH LAW

Neuroethics scholarship has advocated researcher duties to plan for incidental findings, create a pathway allowing for expert consultation to assess suspicious findings on a timely basis, inform prospective research participants of the likelihood of incidental findings and ask whether participants wish to be contacted, and systematically evaluate whether individual incidental findings merit disclosure to participants (Illes *et al.* 2006; Wolf *et al.* 2008a). Such duties have been based not only on respect for participants and the language of the Common Rule, but also on emerging notions of researcher obligations of solidarity with participants, duties of reciprocity, and need to maintain participant trust (Illes and Chin 2007; Knoppers and Chadwick 2005; Wolf *et al.* 2008a, b). Increasingly, researchers and participants are seen as partners in the research enterprise, with research models emerging of researcher consultation with the participant community, including co-design of the research and explicit attention to sharing control over publication and intellectual property (Dickert and Sugarman 2005; Sharp and Foster 2007; Weijer and Emanuel 2000).

In discussion of incidental findings, this new partnership dynamic is most evident in research on what information research participants want. A number of studies indicate that research participants want and expect to receive individual research findings relating to their own health (see, e.g. Kirschen *et al.* 2006; Murphy *et al.* 2008; Wendler and Emanuel 2002). Indeed, data suggest that some research participants would refuse to participate in research that failed to return this information (Kaufman *et al.* 2008).

Kohane *et al.* (2007) consequently argue that the research practice that has emerged, which "disallows communicating pertinent results back to subjects," should be reconsidered (p. 836). They maintain that the paternalism that leaves researchers in control of all data and refusing to return individual findings to participants is no longer acceptable. They offer a host of reasons for returning incidental findings and research results, including the enormous stake that participants have in knowing health information of importance. One could argue that even when the clinical import of suspicious findings is not well understood, or no clinical intervention is currently available, it is the participant who has the greatest stake in pursuing the finding and following scientific progress over time, ideally to fuller understanding and eventual availability of treatment.

This changing vision of the utility of research-generated information for clinical surveillance and care is likely to gather even more momentum with time. More and more research is based on creating large datasets of neuroimages, genomic information, electronic medical records, and the like, and applying powerful informatics tools to identify significant relationships between these data, such as between genotype and brain function, or responsiveness to a medication and genotype. These large datasets have the potential to generate a substantial amount of information with potential clinical importance to individual research participants.

Great debate surrounds the questions of what information should be returned to participants, how, and at what cost (Wolf *et al.* 2008a). But what is fading into the distance is the old dichotomy between research and treatment that would absolve the researcher of any duties to evaluate and offer to disclose findings of potential clinical significance. Researchers are no longer free to work with their data in splendid isolation. We already know that researchers whose work is federally funded have duties to share their data with other researchers; Data Access Committees (DACs) deciding the details of that access are becoming an established part of the research landscape. But the incidental findings debate, together with the related debate over participant access to individual research results, opens the door still wider. Research could not be conducted without the generous participation of human subjects. Strong arguments support their access to individual research findings that may have health importance.

These realities are changing the conduct of human subjects research and its relationship to clinical care. Will these changes erase the distinction between research and care? We should hope not. It is still the case that clinical care must focus on the well-being of the individual patient; the fundamentally different enterprise of research strives to create generalizable knowledge. Yet it turns out that the dichotomy went too far when it absolved researchers of duties of clinical care and information sharing. Bioethics and health law must now reconstitute the traditional vision of researcher duties to bring the researcher back into relationship with the research participant.

CONCLUSION

Where will this lead? Funders are now demanding that researchers, including neuroscience researchers, build into their protocol attention to incidental findings. A vigorous debate surrounds return of individual research results and incidental findings in genomic research. Computer programs have been proposed to offer individual results to research participants, without disrupting the research design by identifying the individual results or participants (Kohane *et al.* 2007). The bioethics, neuroscience, and broader biomedical research communities are rapidly moving toward a new understanding of researcher duties toward research participants.

Neuroethics has led the way. By offering a model of research uncomplicated by clinical roles, then taking seriously the threat and challenge of the UBO and other pathology staring back from the scan, neuroethics has disrupted old views of the relationship of research and clinical care. Research on the brain has forced researchers to face unexpected and urgent— even life-threatening—findings that they simply could not ignore.

ACKNOWLEDGMENTS

Preparation of this chapter was supported in part by National Institutes of Health (NIH), National Human Genome Research Institute (NHGRI) grant #2 R01 HG003178 (S. M. Wolf, Principal Investigator). This article also benefited from the author's participation in the Project on Law & Neuroscience funded by the MacArthur Foundation (M. Gazzaniga, Principal Investigator). The contents of this chapter are solely the responsibility of the author and do not necessarily represent the views of the NIH, NHGRI, or the MacArthur Foundation Project of Law & Neuroscience. Thanks to Christian Krautkramer, M.P.H., J.D. candidate, for research assistance.

REFERENCES

Alphs, H.H., Schwartz, B.S., Stewart, W.F., and Yousem, D.M. (2006). Findings on brain MRI from research studies of occupational exposure to known neurotoxicants. *American Journal of Roentgenology*, 187, 1043–7.

Annas, G. and Grodin, M. (1995). *The Nazi Doctor and the Nuremberg Code: Human Rights in Human Experimentation*. New York: Oxford University Press.

Anonymous. (2005). How volunteering for an MRI scan changed my life. *Nature*, **434**, 17.

Cho, M. (2008). Understanding incidental findings in the context of genetics and genomics. *Journal of Law, Medicine & Ethics*, **36**, 280–5.

Clayton, E.W. (2008). Incidental findings in genetics research using archived DNA. *Journal of Law, Medicine & Ethics*, **36**, 286–91.

Dickert, N. and Sugarman, J. (2005). Ethical goals of community consultation in research. *American Journal of Public Health*, **95**, 1123–7.

Ginnerup Pederson, B., Sosenkilde, M., and Christiansen, T. (2003). Extracolonic findings at computed tomography colonography are a challenge. *Gut*, **52**, 1744–7.

Illes, J. and Chin, V.N. (2007). Trust and reciprocity: foundational principles for human subjects imaging research. *Canadian Journal of Neurological Sciences*, **34**, 3–4.

Illes, J. and Racine, E. (2005). Imaging or imagining? A neuroethics challenge informed by genetics. *American Journal of Bioethics*, **5**, 5–18.

Illes, J., Rosen, A.C., Huang, L., *et al.* (2004). Ethical consideration of incidental findings on adult brain MRI in research. *Neurology*, **62**, 888–90.

Illes, J., Kirschen, M.P., Edwards, E., *et al.* (2006). Incidental findings in brain imaging research. *Science*, **311**, 783–4.

Johnson, C.D., Chen, M.-H., Toledano, A.Y., *et al.* (2008). Accuracy of CT colonography for detection of large adenomas and cancers. *New England Journal of Medicine*, **359**, 1207–17.

Katz, J. (1993-94). Human experimentation and human rights. *St. Louis University Law Journal*, **38**, 7–54.

Katzman, G.L., Dagher, A.P., and Patronas, N.J. (1999). Incidental findings on brain magnetic resonance imaging from 1000 asymptomatic volunteers. *JAMA*, **282**, 36–9.

Kaufman, D., Murphy, J., Scott, J., and Hudson, K. (2008). Subjects matter: a survey of public opinions about a large genetic cohort study. *Genetics in Medicine*, **10**, 831–9.

Kim, B.S., Illes, J., Kaplan, R.T., Reiss, A., and Atlas, S.W. (2002). Incidental findings on pediatric MR images of the brain. *AJNR American Journal of Neuroradiology*, **23**, 1774–7.

King, N.M.P. (2000). Defining and describing benefit appropriately in clinical trials. *Journal of Law, Medicine & Ethics*, **28**, 332–43.

Kirschen, M.P., Jaworska, A., and Illes, J. (2006). Subjects' expectations in neuroimaging research. *Journal of Magnetic Resonance Imaging*, **23**, 205–9.

Knoppers, B.M. and Chadwick, R. (2005). Human genetic research: emerging trends in ethics. *Nature Reviews Genetics*, **6**, 75–9.

Kohane, I.S., Mandel, K.D., Taylor, P.L., Holm, I.A., Nigrin, D.J., and Kunkel, L.M. (2007). Reestablishing the researcher-patient compact. *Science*, **316**, 836–7.

Kumra, S., Ashtari, M., Anderson, B., Cervellione, K.L., and Kan, L. (2006). Ethical and practical considerations in the management of incidental findings in pediatric MRI studies. *Journal of the American Academy of Child & Adolescent Psychiatry*, **45**, 1000–6.

Lawrenz, F. and Sobotka, S. (2008). Empirical analysis of current approaches to incidental findings. *Journal of Law, Medicine & Ethics*, **36**, 249–55.

Levine, R.J. (1988). *Ethics and Regulation of Clinical Research*, 2nd edn. New Haven, CT: Yale University Press.

Lucassen, A. and Parker, M. (2001). Revealing false paternity: some ethical considerations. *Lancet*, **357**, 1033–5.

Miller, F.G., Mello, M.M., and Joffe, S. (2008). Incidental findings in human subjects research: what do investigators owe research participants? *Journal of Law, Medicine & Ethics*, **36**, 271–9.

Milstein, A.C. (2008). Research malpractice and the issue of incidental findings. *Journal of Law, Medicine & Ethics*, **36**, 356–60.

Murphy, J., Scott, J., Kaufman, D., Geller, G., LeRoy, L., Hudson, K. (2008). Public expectations for return of results from large-cohort genetic research. *American Journal of Bioethics*, **8**, 36–43.

Richardson, H.S. (2008). Incidental findings and ancillary-care obligations. *Journal of Law, Medicine & Ethics*, **36**, 256–70.

Richardson, H.S. and Belsky, L. (2004). The ancillary-care responsibilities of medical researchers: an ethical framework for thinking about the clinical care that researchers owe their subjects. *Hastings Center Report*, **34**, 25–33.

Royal, J.M. and Peterson, B.S. (2008). The risks and benefits of searching for incidental findings in MRI research scans. *Journal of Law, Medicine & Ethics*, **36**, 305–14.

Shamoo, A.E. and Resnik, D.B. (2003). *Responsible Conduct of Research*. New York: Oxford University Press.

Sharp, R.R. and Foster, M.W. (2007). Grappling with groups: protecting collective interests in biomedical research. *Journal of Medicine and Philosophy*, **32**, 321–37.

Siddiki, H., Fletcher, J.G., McFarland, B., *et al.* (2008). Incidental findings in CT colonography: literature review and survey of current research practice. *Journal of Law, Medicine & Ethics*, **36**, 320–31.

Smith Churchland, P. (2006). Moral decision-making and the brain. In J. Illes (ed.) *Neuroethics*, pp. 3–16. New York: Oxford University Press.

Stedman's Medical Dictionary, 27th edn. (2002). Philadelphia, PA: Lippincott Williams & Watkins.

U.S. Department of Health and Human Services, 45 C.F.R. Part 46 (Protection of Human Subjects) (2009) (also cited as the "Common Rule").

U.S. Food and Drug Administration, 21 C.F.R. Parts 50 (Protection of Human Subjects), 56 (Institutional Review Boards) (2009).

Van Ness, B. (2008). Genomic research and incidental findings. *Journal of Law, Medicine & Ethics*, **36**, 292–7.

Vernooij, M.W., Ikram, M.A., Tanghe, H.L., *et al.* (2007). Incidental findings in brain MRI in the general population. *New England Journal of Medicine*, **357**, 1821–8.

Weijer, C. and Emanuel, E.J. (2000). Protecting communities in biomedical research. *Science*, **289**, 1142–4.

Wendler, D. and Emanuel, E. (2002). The debate over research on stored biological samples: what do sources think? *Archives of Internal Medicine*, **162**, 1457–62.

Wolf, S.M., Lawrenz, F.P., Nelson, C.A., *et al.* (2008a). Managing incidental findings in human subjects research: analysis and recommendations. *Journal of Law, Medicine & Ethics*, **36**, 219–48.

Wolf, S.M., Paradise, J., and Caga-anan, C. (2008b). The law of incidental findings in human subjects research: establishing researchers' duties. *Journal of Law, Medicine & Ethics*, **36**, 361–83.

Yee, J., Kumar, N.N., Godara, S., *et al.* (2005). Extracolonic abnormalities discovered incidentally at CT colonography in a male population. *Radiology*, **236**, 519–26.

Yue, N.C., Longstreth, W.T., Elster, A.D., Jungreis, C.A., O'Leary, D.H., and Poirier, V.C. (1997). Clinically serious abnormalities found incidentally at MR imaging of the brain: data from the cardiovascular heart study. *Radiology*, **202**, 41–6.

Zalis, M.E., Barish, M.A., Choi, J.R., *et al.* (2005). CT colonography reporting and data systems: a consensus proposal. *Radiology*, **236**, 3–9.

CHAPTER 38

···

WHAT WILL BE THE
LIMITS OF
NEUROSCIENCE-BASED
MINDREADING IN
THE LAW?

···

EMILY R. MURPHY AND HENRY T. GREELY

It is always hard to predict things, particularly the future.
Attributed to Niels Bohr (Greely 2000, p. 1589)

Much of the legal and social interest in (and, sometimes, fear of) new neuroimaging techniques stems from the belief that they can deliver on the materialist understanding of the
relationship between the brain and the mind. According to this view, the mind is created by
the workings of the brain, so every mental state is produced by a physical state of the brain.
Therefore, as we can better discern the physical states of the brain, we should be able to find
a strong correlation between a particular mental state and a particular physical brain state.
Ultimately, we may be able to use neuroimaging to identify that a person's brain is in Brain
State A and use that knowledge to deduce that that person must be having Mental State A.
In short, we could use neuroimaging to "read minds."

That brain activity correlates with behavior or mental states is not a new discovery.
Neurologists in the 19th century began to associate lesions in particular brain areas with
particular mental or behavioral deficits. Adults lacking Broca's area could not speak; adults
missing Wernicke's area could not find words. Clinicians and researchers increasingly
connected other mental deficits to other specific brain areas, such as the visual cortex, the
auditory cortex, the somatosensory cortex, the motor cortex, and so on. No visual cortex, no
subjective mental state of seeing.

But lesions are crude tools, ethically impossible to create in random human subjects and
rarely discovered in neat and useful forms. Researchers using various neuroscientific

techniques, most notably functional magnetic resonance imaging (fMRI) but also tools like positron emission tomography scans, microelectrode implants, and (perhaps) transcranial magnetic stimulation, have been able to connect patterns of physical activity in the brain with mental states, either directly as with microelectrodes or indirectly through the blood oxygen level-dependent (BOLD) hypothesis and fMRI. Thus, researchers have been able to determine, with high accuracy, whether a particular subject in an MRI machine is seeing a drawing of a building or of a tool (Shinkareva *et al.* 2008), is seeing one of more than a hundred particular objects (Kay *et al.* 2008; Naselaris *et al.* 2009) or is seeing—or even just internally visualizing —a face or a place (Kanwisher 2001). Others have demonstrated an ability to predict, several seconds in advance, a person's future action (Haynes and Rees 2006; Haynes *et al.* 2007; Soon *et al.* 2008), or to discern evidence of consciousness in people in vegetative states (Owen *et al.* 2006, Monti *et al.* 2010). No machine is needed to spot the excitement these findings and others like them cause in neuroscientists, or the discomfort, and even fear, they cause in laymen.

The two of us believe in the materialist understanding of the brain and the mind. Yet we also believe that both the excitement about and the fear of the consequences of mindreading are too extreme. We see good reasons to expect neuroscience-based mindreading to hit major technical barriers before it reaches impressive levels of detail. And we see other kinds of good reasons to believe that the law would make some, but somewhat limited, use of even "pretty good" technical mindreading.

This chapter is an effort to explore some of those limits. It involves predictions about the future both of scientific advances and of social reactions to those predictions. Bohr was wrong about predictions. It is easy to make them; it is only hard to be right. We can make neither kind of prediction with any confidence. Although chastened by this reality, we believe some careful predictions, however tentative, may be useful. This chapter looks first at the likely technical limits on neuroscience-based mindreading, then at the likely limits in how the law might use such technologies.

LIKELY TECHNICAL LIMITS OF USING NEUROSCIENCE TO READ MINDS

Normal humans are, and need to be, mindreaders. We regularly read the minds of our fellow humans, in an effort to understand what they are feeling and to predict how they are going to behave, with or without various interventions we might try. As social animals, the ability to predict the behavior of our fellow humans is crucial to our happiness, our success, and our very survival. One of the deficits involved in autism is thought to be a limited ability to read the minds of fellow humans.

We read minds all the time, but not with anything approaching perfect accuracy. Neurotechnology seems to offer a tempting, and potentially threatening, tool to read minds better. We have each, separately, written about problems of getting legally relevant and powerful evidence from neuroimaging (Greely and Illes 2007; Brown and Murphy 2010), but in this section we want to look even deeper into the likely scientific limits of mindreading.

Based on work that has already been done, neuroscience techniques, particularly fMRI, can already improve our ability to read minds in some ways and at some levels of detail, but how great an improvement can we expect—or fear? Will neuroscience be able to determine whether a person is hungry—or whether that person wants a banana split, with vanilla and chocolate ice cream, hot fudge sauce, and Spanish peanuts, but no whipped cream? This section describes three kinds of technical barriers to detailed and useful mindreading: (1) the likely impossibility of making a complete and accurate model of a human brain in light of its incredible complexity, (2) the problems of interpersonal and intrapersonal plasticity, and (3) the problem of trying to read, now, someone's past mental state.

The most complicated thing in the universe

To be able to associate, with great confidence, a particular Brain State A with a particular Mental State A, we need to be able to define both states accurately and to be confident that the detection of one indicates the presence of the other. Defining Mental State A may prove difficult (what exactly *are* you thinking as you read these words?), but for present purposes assume we can come close enough by asking the subject what he is thinking. To define Brain State A in detail, though, we would need to understand the human brain and its relevant states in great detail. Such detail that may well be, even in theory, impossible to obtain, both for an idealized "human brain" and, for additional reasons, for any real, living human brain.

Imagine making a perfect working model of a human brain. Such a model may not be the only path toward reading minds, but considering it in some detail is a useful reminder of just how unmanageably complicated the brain is.

The human brain's roughly 1350g of tissue contain about one trillion brain cells. Neurons make up about 100 billion of them; glial cells, a term for several different categories of cells, make up most of the rest. Neurons pass information to other neurons, inside the brain and outside, through connections called synapses. Neurons communicate information by firing electrochemical "action potentials," which both trigger the release of neurotransmitters at the outbound side of synapses (presynaptic) and are triggered by the binding of neurotransmitters at the inbound (postsynaptic) side. Estimates of the average number of synapses for each brain neuron range from 100–1000 (the breadth of the estimates is evidence of the difficulty of these kinds of measurements). This leads to an estimate of anywhere from 5 trillion to 50 trillion synapses in an average human's brain.

The perfect model of a human brain would have to start with those 100 billion neurons and to designate which neurons are connected to which other neurons (or to themselves) through synapses. Using electron microscopy to map the neurons and synapses of an entire dead human brain, rendered in ultra-thin slices, is, perhaps, just barely conceivable. But the brain is more than a wiring diagram; each component has multiple functions and states that need to be accounted for.

Any particular action potential, or series of action potentials, proceeding towards the presynaptic region of a neuron may or may not trigger release of any particular kind of neurotransmitter, in large, medium, or small quantities. To know the probability of a neurotransmitter release we would have to understand the structure of that particular presynaptic region and the location and amount of the neurotransmitters and other electrically-charged ions in it. To know whether that synapse could release multiple times in response to a rapid series of action potentials, we would have to know how quickly the presynaptic region would be replenished with neurotransmitter. That would require a thorough understanding of the state of the DNA in each neuron's nucleus as well as the machinery for creating and transporting proteins and other molecules through its cytoplasm. Models predicting transmitter release are presently built through observation and testing of different kinds of synapses, and give us probabilistic estimates that may or may not be accurate in an actual brain.

On the other side of the synaptic cleft, the postsynaptic neuron responds to neurotransmitters through receptors. Any one postsynaptic neuron may have, at any one synapse, numerous receptors of many different types, with varying and sometimes counteracting effects. Some will act quickly, opening or closing ion channels. Others, such as G-protein coupled receptors, will act more slowly. The density of receptor expression on the postsynaptic surface is a dynamically-changing variable, directly affected by the presence of neurotransmitter and by other, longer-term factors. The cumulative effects of neurotransmitters from all a neuron's postsynaptic inputs determine whether or not one or more action potentials are generated in the postsynaptic neuron. Both sides of the synaptic cleft are also affected by what is inside and outside the cleft itself: how many neurotransmitter molecules, of what types, as well as how many molecules that degrade or destroy those neurotransmitters.

If an action potential does get started, whether it continues is affected by more variables. These include the concentrations of various ions on both the inside and outside of the length of the neuron's membrane as well as the degree to which the neuron's axon is covered with a layer of electrically insulating material called myelin.

And to add one more layer of complexity, action potentials often convey information not just by their presence, but by the number and timing of their firings. The firing frequency rate, affected by everything we have discussed so far and by other factors as yet unknown, provides another set of crucial variables.

So for an accurate picture of the state of the brain at any point in time, one needs not just the incredibly complex wiring diagram, but the state of many variables (1) at the presynaptic and postsynaptic sides of every synapse, (2) in the each synaptic cleft, (3) inside and outside the membrane along the neuron's full length, and (4) in the firing rates of neurons. At only 100 synapses per brain neuron, that requires knowing the state of all of these variables at each of 5 trillion synapses and along the cell membranes of all 100 billion neurons. Call it, conservatively, one quadrillion variables. If each of the variables had only two values (a gross underestimate), that leads to 2 to the quadrillionth different possible "Brain States." If one were to try, in a brute force way, to examine each and every brain state and see what mental state it correlated it, that number would be far beyond unapproachable.

And, of course, one would still need to understand, in detail, all the rules that governed the relationship between those variables to both the generation and strength of action potentials and the release of neurotransmitters. At this point we can be confident that we know neither all the relevant variables nor an appreciable fraction of the rules that govern their interaction.

The heavily studied roundworm, *Caenorhabditis elegans*, normally has 302 neurons and about 7000 synapses, as well as only—as far as we can tell—a small number of behaviors (and probably no mental states, at least not anything analogous to human mental states). And it can be studied cheaply and destructively without any significant ethical limitations. It is conceivable that one could create a richly detailed model of the functioning of the

C. elegans nervous system. It does not seem conceivable that one could create a similarly detailed model of a human brain, both because of its enormously greater complexity and because of the many problems with using humans as experimental animals.

Yet even if we could create such a magnificently detailed model of a human brain and its function, all that knowledge would only provide a static picture of that brain for one frozen instant in time. Many, if not all, of the variables would change over time, some on a micro-second scale, others over weeks or longer, with still others in between. One would have to know the rules that governed the changes in all of those variables.

Over time, an additional set of changes takes place. New synapses form; old synapses disappear. New neurons form and migrate; old neurons die. Brain structures grow or shrink. And each of these larger changes would have to be understood and accounted for, in detail, in a complete model of the functioning human brain. We cannot do this today, we will not be able to do this tomorrow—we may well never be able to do this. The impossibility of a perfect model does not mean that imperfect models and limited understandings cannot be useful—they, of course, can be. But it does say something about the likely limits of our understanding.

Assume, though, that someday it would be possible for us to create a complete and accurate model of the functioning of "the human brain." What does that mean for understanding any *particular* human's brain? Not necessarily very much.

Each brain will be different—not only in its wiring diagram but in its own set of the other variables, from neurotransmitter quantities in each neuron and synaptic cleft to myelination patterns. How could we ascertain that brain state in a living, changing brain?

Currently, we can use MRI to see small brain structures, with a resolution of a few millimeters, in living human brains. We can use fMRI to see blood oxygenation levels in volumes of under 10 cubic millimeters. These volumes contain hundreds of thousands of separate neurons and millions of separate synapses. Although we can use electron microscopes to see synapses in surgically extracted brain tissue, we cannot yet observe individual synapses in a living human brain. We can use nuclear magnetic resonance (NMR) spectroscopy to see the relative abundance of some different molecules in tissues, even living tissues, but with relatively poor spatial resolution. And we can use implanted microelectrodes to measure (and to influence) action potentials simultaneously in, perhaps, 50 neurons in the human brain—nearly 1 in 20 billion, albeit with an invasive and somewhat risky procedure. It is hard to believe that we would ever be able—safely and accurately—to make all the measurements in a living brain that would be needed to understand its (frozen in time) brain state completely.

Even if such measuring tools did exist, they might well run into a biological form of Heisenberg's uncertainty principle. Anything that measures such small quantities or spatial relationships is likely to be intrusive enough to change at least some of what it measures. Thus, any kind of energy imparted to the brain by this kind of measurement, energy that would, itself, change the brain it was trying to study, most likely in ways that could not, themselves, be perfectly predicted.

Problems of plasticity

The impossibility of a perfect understanding of brain functioning does not mean we cannot acquire some useful understanding of how an individual's brain works. As noted in the introduction, we already can use neuroimaging to determine, with reasonable accuracy, some mental states in individuals. We may be able to do "well enough" without having complete understanding.

Or we may not. At this point we do not know how much detail we will be able to determine from, for example, brain scans. Take the visual work cited earlier (Kay *et al.* 2008; Shinkareva *et al.* 2008; Naselaris *et al.* 2009). Researchers have been able to determine from fMRI which image out of roughly 100 their subjects were looking at in the scanner, with roughly 85% accuracy. Let's say one of those images was of "food." Using complicated statistical methods, the researchers "trained" their computerized algorithm on many trials with a particular subject looking at "food" in order to identify a pattern of BOLD response that corresponded with "food." We do not yet know whether this technology will be able to distinguish between a steak, a salad, ice cream, or dog food. We do not know whether it will be able to distinguish between a fudgesicle, a hazelnut gelato, or an ice cream sundae. Or notice the presence of a split banana, hot fudge sauce, and Spanish peanuts, as well as the absence of whipped cream. It might—or it might not.

As both the experiments become more complex and the tools (including, crucially, the statistical tools) become more advanced, we should get a sense of just how much detail an fMRI scan can "read" from the mind of someone on whom the scanner (and the statistical program) has been extensively trained. But even if the answer is "a great deal of detail," that may not be helpful in a legal setting because of (with apologies to *The Graduate*) one word—plasticity.

Different people's brains work differently. This can be true in very gross ways. Most people need to use parts of the left sides of their cerebrums to speak. An adult who loses the part of the left frontal lobe that includes Broca's area usually cannot speak fluently. But people who had their entire left cerebral hemisphere removed in childhood (usually as a treatment for otherwise untreatable epilepsy) sometimes are able to speak well. What in everyone else is localized in the left frontal lobe has moved, for them, to the right frontal lobe. Other highly localized brain functions can vary from person to person. If highly localized functions are plastic, across individuals, it seems likely that memories, particular emotional states, or "thoughts" also are located in different places or unique networks.

The research discussed above trained the statistical packages on specific individuals. How well does the pattern of activation for one image for one person predict the pattern of activation for that image for another person? And, as the level of detail increases, how rapidly will the ability to draw an inference about one person's mental state from a different person's mental state drop off? For many applications the law would like to make of these technologies, it may not be possible to train the scanner at length on a particular subject or even a general mindreading target. Limited time and money would create constraints. But so would the uncertainty about whether the subject is trustworthy when he tells you his mental state. If you want to test the mental state of a party or a witness and a successful test requires extensive training on that individual for the mental state you are testing, the possibilities for mischief seem great.

But what if one could confidently train the mindreading device in advance for the test on a willing and cooperative person? Plasticity of another kind may still be a problem. At the level of resolution that we can ascertain, there may be, for any individual, both more than one brain state that corresponds to a particular mental state and more than one mental state that corresponds to that brain state.

So, if someone is thinking of the ice cream sundae, he may usually be perceived on fMRI as having one brain state, but sometimes he will think of the same sundae and show another state and sometimes he might show that brain state and not be thinking of the sundae. (If we think of the fMRI pattern as a "test" for the mental state of "ice cream sundae," these are false negatives and false positives, respectively.) Furthermore, it is completely unclear how easy or difficult it would be for subjects to change their brain states for a given mental state, perhaps by thinking of other things at the same time. Thus, if the subject, when thinking of an ice cream sundae, intentionally thought of it in the context of the party for his 10th birthday, would that change the brain state? We do not know. And, it is unclear whether or how a concept such as "ice cream sundae" could *ever* be abstracted from other concurrent mental states relating to real-time desires; that is, does the "ice cream sundae" mental state when you're hungry look the same as the "ice cream sundae" concept when you have just eaten a huge bag of candy? Again, we do not know.

The time machine travel problem

There is one more problem. These technologies seem able, at best, to read present mental states. But the law often wants to know a person's mental state at some time in the past. Did the defendant actually fear for his life when he shot someone at his door, allegedly in self-defense? Did the defendant know the highway was icy when he drove too fast and caused an accident? Did the defendant fire an employee for reasons banned by employment discrimination laws? It is hard to imagine any direct way—days, months, or years later—to use neuroscience to answer those questions.

One might, occasionally, be able to say something about the subject's capabilities. One could say a defendant's current brain damage makes it impossible (or, at least, highly unlikely) that he *could* have premeditated a killing. One might be able, further, to say that the natural history of the brain damage is such that, at or just before the time of the killing, the brain damage was likely to have existed and to have had the same effect. This chain of inferences about mental capabilities may rule out (or rule in) certain mental states as possible, but it seems unlikely that strong evidence of specific, fine-grained constraints on mental capabilities will often be available.

There might be one other way to try to get around the time travel problem (the term was coined by Brown and Murphy, 2010). Instead of using neuroscientific methods to look for the mental state in question, one might ask the subject whether or not he had the relevant mental state at the relevant time and then use neuroscientific methods of lie detection (if reliable) to see if he were telling the truth. Similarly, one might, conceivably, be able to see whether a person had memories consistent, or inconsistent, with that mental state. (A major problem with this second approach is the necessity for such a device to also assess whether a memory is true—an accurate reflection of what really happened—or false—an inaccurate but fully experienced as a valid memory. It is far from clear that "true" or "false" memories are different in the brain. See, for example, recent work by Rissman *et al* (2010).) Whether either lie detection or memory detection can proceed that far, with high accuracy, is deeply uncertain. And whether (or how often) either the subsequent belief that one had a particular mental state, or a subsequent memory of having had a particular mental state, would, in fact, correspond well to the actual mental state at the time is also unclear.

HOW WOULD MINDREADING AFFECT THE LAW?

The law reads minds all the time, though not through technical means. If we could objectively know the subjective contents of someone's mind, when would the law be interested? The short answer: often, perhaps nearly all of the time… except when it wouldn't. Wherever the law needs to adjudicate the nature of relationship between two people or the relationship of one person to his community, a perfect mindreading device could be useful. On the other hand, the law already has proxies for interpreting the contents of someone's mind, built from the current best-available evidence as to the contents of someone's mind: other peoples' minds. While these assessments may be inaccurate, they are useful; they make the law administrable and they help those in a (potential) legal relationship organize their own conduct.

In some cases, the state of mind will itself be an important legal "fact," like the existence or extent of pain as a result of an injury. In other instances the state of mind will be useful in evaluating evidence, as in the case of lie detection. Sometimes a state of mind may be relevant to the internal workings of the legal system—is the judge or jury biased against a party or a witness? And, certainly, in many instances the law cares deeply about the state of mind of a criminal or civil defendant. Whether a killing, for example, was premeditated, purposeful, intentional, reckless, negligent, or a completely unforeseen and unforeseeable accident may determine the legal outcome. In all of these ways and others, the existing law might "care" about mindreading. We will discuss the first three situations together, before looking in more detail at the last example.

Mindreading might be useful for the workings of the legal system

The first three examples mentioned earlier might be grouped together as situations where mindreading affects the workings of the legal system. In each case reliable mindreading could have major effects on the legal system even if it did not change any of the underlying law.

Consider an example of using mindreading to establish a relevant mental fact—the existence (and possibly the extent) of pain. Pain is a major source of factual disputes in the legal system, arising often in personal injury cases (from car accidents to medical malpractice), but more often in workers' compensation cases and in disability determinations.

Pain is notoriously hard to diagnose objectively; many believe that claimants often exaggerate the extent of their pain. We know that sometimes people completely fabricate their pain. The difficulty of assessing pain breeds uncertainty about how the decision-maker (judge, jury, or administrator) will evaluate the claimed pain—and uncertainty means more litigation. Mindreading that could reliably tell us something about a claimant's level of pain could revolutionize much of the law, not so much by determining the outcomes of proceedings as by leading to earlier settlements through reducing uncertainty.

Of course, the neural signature of pain may not fit perfectly with the law's categories of compensable pain. Emotional pain, which the law compensates reluctantly because of the difficulties of proof, might be "visible" as a result of mindreading (see, for example, Eisenberger *et al.* 2003). So might "physical" pain that does not have a clear source, possibly helping people who would not win a recovery today.

Mindreading to aid in assessing evidence could be even more important. Reliable ways of determining whether a witness is lying, or whether a particular memory of a witness is high or low quality, would not totally eliminate litigation, but it could surely reduce it. There would always be a few cases where different witnesses had honestly differing recollections of the events or where the facts were clear but the issue was the interpretation or application of the law. A vast array of ordinary litigation, though, would likely disappear, replaced by settlement after (mental) discovery.

Bias might be the most interesting. Litigants are entitled to impartial jurors and judges, but, effectively, that means jurors and judges who are not demonstrably biased. Barring strong evidence of past bias, proving bias can be extremely difficult. If, however, mindreading technologies could show that a prospective juror disliked a defendant because of his race, religion, sexual orientation, or even appearance, he might be stricken for cause. Or the method might be used by attorneys to inform their decisions to use peremptory challenges to jurors (or, in some states, judges). Evidence of bias might also be useful in other ways, to assess the credibility of testimony of a witness or to provide reason to believe that a party took a particular action, such as firing an employee because of a protected characteristic, like sex or race.

These could be steps toward fairer adjudication, though they might prove that various biases are ubiquitous, so common that considering them could seriously interfere with operating the courts. We might ultimately have to reconsider our commitment to impartiality, a commitment that was easy to make when it was impossible to enforce rigorously.

Of course, before any of these consequences follow, neuroscience would have to provide sufficiently reliable mindreading methods—and the law would have to decide to allow their use. Furthermore, the technology may be as important as the science. Mindreading that required hours of expensive fMRI scanning, as well as costly expert testimony, would not be widely used. The scientific, legal, and technological uncertainties are vast, but, if it worked, mindreading could transform how the legal system functions.

Sometimes legal doctrine cares about the defendant's state of mind; sometimes it doesn't

The potential changes to the operation of the law, through the use of mindreading as evidence of pain, deception, or bias, among other things, could be extremely important. Such techniques might lead to changes in the law of evidence or of civil or criminal procedure, but they seem unlikely to change substantive legal doctrine. Legal doctrine often cares about subjective states of mind, but the difficulty of getting trustworthy evidence of subjective states of mind has often led the law to use objective means to determine subjective intent, or to set aside mental states as irrelevant in favor of administrative ease and policy considerations. The law is typically slow to change, particularly with respect to fundamental principles. And yet, if mindreading devices were able to provide good, direct evidence of such subjective mental states, the law might abandon at least some of its doctrinal "workarounds" for subjective states of mind.

It is worth discussing in some detail how substantive legal doctrine, in various parts of the law, might conceivably use, or not use, the results of mindreading in situations where the mental state of a party determines the legal consequences of actions. We will offer examples from criminal law, contract law, and tort law.

Criminal law: evil thoughts and evil deeds

Subjective knowledge of the contents of someone's mind may be most obviously applicable in criminal law, where the general formula for criminal liability is a harmful act done with the requisite "bad" intent, or "*mens rea*," minus any valid excuses or justifications. To determine whether or not a particular defendant actually possessed the requisite intent, jurors are typically instructed that they may infer intent from actions or other observations about the person's behavior.

On its face, this may seem to be straightforward. Not so. Actions are complex; motives are not per se punishable; mental states fluctuate and may not even be relevant unless liability for the action has been established. Actions may occur with more than one kind of intent and be performed for more than one reason. A simple example is pressing the accelerator in your car: you may be merging onto the highway, avoiding a collision, or trying to escape the police. Which actions to consider in assessing intent can also be unclear—when should we use a defendant's past actions as evidence of his intent even if his actions at the time of the alleged crime are equivocal as to intent?

Some relatively straightforward cases in criminal law might seem to be solved if, at the moment he commits what could be a criminal act, a person had a perfect mindreading device were attached to his head. In this case, useful "mindreading" would presumably tell us the content of someone's intent. Did you *mean* to run over your former lover with the car, or was it just an accident that happened because you did not expect anyone to be at the vacation house while you were backing out of the narrow driveway? Of course, even finding a criminal "intent" does not end the case. Did the "intending" defendant *do* the act, or attempt the act, or plan the act, or just wish really hard the act would occur? The act, as well as the intent, makes a difference.

Motives are not punishable by themselves, nor are they an essential part of a crime. However, motives are used to describe actions in criminal statutes, probably for lack of a better way of getting at subtle distinctions between harmless acts and bad ones. In situations with tricky statutory language about motive, perhaps a mindreading device could help clarify what action is punishable in addition to getting at the attached mental state. For example, the Ninth Circuit recently updated the standard of willful ignorance to comprise a) being suspicious (mental state) of something (like drugs being smuggled in your trunk) and b) not checking (the action, or lack thereof in this case) "because [you] don't want to know"—that is, being *motivated* by the desire not to discover contraband. (*United States v. Heredia* 2007). Perhaps mindreading could help prove (or disprove) those mental states.

Mental states pose hard problems in the criminal law, as they require judgments as to the normative quality of the intent and which particular statutory category it can be shoehorned into: generally speaking, one of the Model Penal Code's categories of purpose (desire for something to happen), knowledge (cognitive state of substantial certainty), recklessness (knowledge and disregard of the risk), or negligence (careless ignorance of the risk) (Model Penal Code § 2.02). Proving negligence would be especially difficult even with good mindreading; the mindreading device would need to say for certain that an absence of the measure of subjective awareness really indicated a true negative.

And, subjective intent does not matter at all in the narrow realm of strict liability crimes. For example, in cases of statutory rape in many jurisdictions, the only thing that matters is the actual age of the victim, regardless of the defendant's state of mind. Of course, if we had reliable mindreading, we might change this crime to immunize those who demonstrably had a reasonable, good faith belief that the other person was above the age of consent. On the other hand, we might choose to leave it the same to encourage the strongest possible level of care by potential offenders.

Contract law: it's not what you think, it's what you say

For a contract to exist, two parties have to agree. In the traditional common law, a contract was said to require that there have been a "meeting of the minds." This proved difficult to administer without clear proof of two "minds" shaking hands, clinking glasses, or patting each other on the back. The owner of one of the minds could later claim that he did not actually agree or mean to agree, leading to intractable disputes about what was said and what was meant. The law of contract evolved to incorporate two prongs to test whether an offeree's behavior in response to an offer forms a contract: either (1) subjectively, the parties themselves had to have intended to form the contract (whether or not a reasonable person would have so concluded), or (2) objectively, a "reasonable person" observing the scene would have to think the offer had been accepted *and* the actual offeror subjectively thought it was acceptance. The subjective intent is assessed by objective means, such as actions, writings, or spoken words. In short, the only method we have had to assess parties' intentions to enter into a contract is by looking at what they did, since we could not look into their minds.

So, what would happen to contract law if a mindreading device could determine an individual party's subjective intent? Such a device might simply slot into the list of factors that can be taken as "objective indicia" of subjective intent, putting the device's read-out into the same category as typing "Yes, I'll take delivery on Tuesday" in an email. Thus, the availability of a machine might not change contract doctrine, which has already been refined to require *some* objective indication of subjective assent.

In practice, however, the objective prong of contract formation only comes into play when the parties disagree about whether, subjectively, they had reached agreement. If we could assess, through a mindreading device, the "actual" subjective intent, we might eliminate the objective prong—if we *knew* that one party or the other truly did not intend to enter into an agreement, and had not yet been acting as if an agreement existed, we might not allow the other party to hold him to a contract based on his objective, reasonable (but mistaken) belief that an agreement had been intended. This could be especially true if both parties had "intent verification" devices available at the time of contracting.

Mindreading devices in business contexts—where it is generally quite clear that some sort of contract is the goal—may alter the negotiations if they help the parties to know exactly what the other party wants, and intends. But would this be an improvement over current practices? Presumably, both parties would have to consent to the use, either in formation or in arbitration in case of breach. The costs and benefits of this would have to be weighed against the complexity of the contract. On one hand, this may just create another layer of contract language surrounding the terms of use of the mindreading device and serve only to complicate the entire process. On the other, the additional hassle may be a small price to pay for achieving a better understanding at the time of formation of a (very expensive) contract, which may subsequently help with contract interpretation and efficient performance.

In contract law, the contents of someone's mind are important—but the law, thus far lacking mindreading devices and yet still needing to solve problems, has already developed ways of assessing the contents of someone's mind by looking at the outward expression of his behavior. In cases where what someone *does* diverges from what he really *meant*, contract law favors his outward expression. While sometimes this may be inaccurate, such as when someone is just joking (but, lacking skill in sarcasm their joking intent is not obvious to a reasonable person), it is a workable solution that allows people to predict what's next and plan their own conduct.

This is a classic example of the law striking a balance between creating bright-line rules and fuzzier, more individualized standards. Rules may be over-inclusive (lumping the jokester in with the sincere) or under-inclusive, but they are clear and tend to give more predictable results. Flexible standards may be more accurate, but they are hard to administer, especially if the relevant guidepost is set at the extreme: inside each person's private mind. A mindreading device could further individualize legal determinations, taking the application of standards to the extreme.

For example, consequential damages, under the classic rule of *Hadley v. Baxendale*, are limited to those that the defendant knew about at the time of the contract was made or those that were objectively foreseeable in those circumstances. With good mindreading, the rule could be limited to those damages that were known or *actually* foreseen. This would be a change in the law, and one that trades predictability for atomized case-by-case determinations. Such individualized justice may come at the expense of a system predictable enough that people organize their behavior to comply with the law and avoid disputes in the first place. The balance might hinge on how easy it would be for people to use the technology before contracting, in order to avoid ambiguities that often give rise to contract disputes.

Reliable mindreading clearly would not touch all parts of contract law. For example, damages for breach of contract typically are not affected by whether the breach was intentional, reckless, negligent, or completely innocent. If you do not perform your promise, you owe the other side the compensation for the harms it suffered as a result of your non-performance. But mindreading could have consequences under some existing doctrines and might lead to changes in other doctrines.

Tort law: where sometimes intentions matter not at all

The law of torts is distinct from criminal law in that tort law does not morally condemn actions. Tort law seeks to provide civil remedies for harm, whether or not a criminal remedy may also exist (such as for assault and battery).

"Intentional" torts require that the person acted with intent—but not intent to harm, just intent to have done the action. For example, trespass is an intentional tort: if you intended to be walking through the woods, and you walk onto your neighbor's property, it does not matter whether you intended to be on her property—just that you intended to be on your stroll. By contrast, if you were in publicly owned woods and a tornado picked you up and deposited you on top of your neighbor's house, you have not intentionally put yourself on her property and therefore not committed trespass. Or if you were in the woods, suddenly chased by an angry bear, and had to scale your neighbor's fence to escape, you have intentionally trespassed but have a pretty good necessity defense. In torts, such intent may be characterized as "acted consciously," even if you did not know you were intruding or intend to harm anyone or anything. Thus, a mindreading device could be tuned to determine that you knew what you were doing and were not sleep-walking may be occasionally useful, though in the vast majority of actual cases the intent prong of an intentional tort is not disputed.

"Negligent" torts are those where someone breaches a duty established by a reasonable standard of care. The subjective contents of the plaintiff's mind may be part of a defense to negligence: if the plaintiff knew or should have known of a risk and proceeded anyway, the defendant would not be liable for the resulting harm. If a mindreading device could tell us that the plaintiff was fully aware of the ice on the edge of the sidewalk, selected smooth-soled shoes, and headed for the ice at a run, her claim of the negligence of her apartment building manager may not survive—but it is not clear that we need a mindreading device to tell us what her behavior also indicates. A determination of negligence is a determination of fault, but one that again relies on objective, external standards—primarily the "what would a reasonable person have done" standard and whether or not the defendant has deviated from that.

One area of tort law, though, where intention and negligence are totally irrelevant is the realm of strict liability. In strict liability torts, something bad happened and someone is legally responsible, regardless of any degree of "intent" or "fault." Strict liability is used in situations of ultra-hazardous or abnormally dangerous activities. If a road-building contractor is blasting near your house and debris flies onto your property, he is strictly liable *even if* he took all possible precautions and did not intend or anticipate that the debris would rain down in your yard. Similarly, in product liability cases, normally if the product malfunctions and injures you, the manufacturer is liable without proof of intent or negligence. In this domain, subjective intent or willfulness of action does not matter at all: it happened, so the defendant pays. The justification for strict liability in law is one of policy: accidents happen, but sometimes someone has to pay for it even if they are in no way at fault.

The strict liability niche of tort law is an illustration that "the law," even the private law that seeks to provide remedies for wrongs, has also evolved to be administrable, and as such makes trade-offs in determining what is just and fair. This is not a principle that is unique to tort law—a parker's mental state does not affect fines for parking violations—but in the example of strict liability, trade-offs have been balanced in favor of clear, objectively determinable rules to classify conduct. In this circumstance, even the most accurate mindreading, lie-detecting, or truth-validating device would be largely irrelevant.

On the other hand, all three of these kinds of torts—intentional, negligent, and strict liability—may give rise to punitive damages above and beyond compensation for any injury the plaintiff suffered. One common formulation allows a jury to award punitive damages if a defendant acted "with malice, oppression, or fraud." In the classic case of exploding Ford Pintos, punitive damages were awarded when the court found that company executives knew of and disregarded the risk to consumer safety (*Grimshaw v. Ford Motor Co.*, 1981). Mindreading technology might be able to play a role in making these determinations, though subject to the time machine problem.

When the law does care, will the results be "good enough"?

Of course, for mindreading to affect the law at all, in its operation or in its doctrines, that mindreading should be reliable. In addition to the general scientific uncertainty about the accuracy of such mindreading discussed earlier in this chapter, the law presents two special problems—defining terms and deciding when the results are sufficiently reliable.

Defining terms

Perhaps the biggest challenge to tweaking any mindreading device to be useful to the law is to first decide what the device should look for. This means figuring out exactly what mental state we are interested in and what it would look like in the device. That task might (or might not) be fairly straightforward when we are asking the device to categorize thoughts or perceptions of concrete things, like types of houses or tools for which we have agreed-upon words, prototype images that everyone would recognize, and a common sense of various distinctions. It is probably more difficult when looking for mental states that correspond to pain, deception, or bias, but at least these mental states can probably be reliably induced and tested. We may not agree on the full spectrum of what we mean as "pain," but, like "house" or "hammer," there does seem to be some kind of core meaning that might not be controversial.

Now, try to imagine coming up with a universally agreed-upon definition or mental picture of "malicious," "deceptive," or "willful." The problem may be in part one of linguistic precision, but is not immediately solved by moving to the nouns or verbs from which those adjectives derive (malice, deceive, or willfulness). The problem is further complicated by terms that have different legal and plain-language meanings, such as "malice." In legal use, the meaning of "malice" can be that the person intentionally did something unlawful, such as libel, without any evil, spiteful, or wicked connotation. "Malice aforethought" is a part of the Massachusetts and California criminal statutes for first-degree murder, but lacks the "evil" connotation. According to the Supreme Judicial Court of Massachusetts, malice is a mental state that "includes any unexcused intent to kill, to do grievous bodily harm, or to do an act creating a plain and strong likelihood that death or grievous harm will follow" (*Commonwealth v. Huot* 1980).

Words for subjective mental states, especially as used in the law, often simultaneously describe degrees of conscious awareness and emotionally laden desires. They are terms of art in the law, defined in large part by the context in which they are used and the varying interpretations they have assumed in practice. The ambiguity inherent in the words the law uses to describe mental states reflects the difficulty of sharply categorizing the range of human experience. To program a mindreading device with such a human-like sensitive degree of perception that it could validate the presence, absence, or degree of a given legally relevant "mental state," we would have to create an almost human form of artificial intelligence.

This problem of defining the target of interest has been discussed with respect to neuroimaging technology development for lie detection and its applications in legal contexts (see, for example, Illes 2004). Judy Illes and others have articulated a primary difficulty with using lie detection technologies, and the theme is repeated here: the complexity of human behavior can only be assessed in context, rather than through simple labels that apply in any situation. Private law and criminal law are both contextual and relational: what, where, why, how, and with whom *matter* when judging human behavior.

Defining "good enough"

Even if we can define what the law is looking for, we then have to determine how accurately whatever it is can be assessed. Sensitivity, specificity, and underlying probabilities are critically important if a mindreading system is ever used like a diagnostic device, deciding presence or absence of mental states in a binary fashion. These are statistical realities that plague the current efforts to use neuroimaging-based lie detection technologies and almost certainly carry over into other forms of neuroscience-based mindreading applications.

A more technical question about applying mindreading to the law is how interested will the law be in this probabilistic evidence. After the first part of this paper, we know that any sort of "mindreading" is likely to produce probabilistic evidence, rather than clear "yes, definitely bad intent here" or "no, absolutely innocent thoughts."

The law deals with probabilistic evidence all the time, particularly in the realm of scientific evidence. However, courts have generally been reluctant to describe precise statistical thresholds of acceptability, deferring instead to expert determination and description, and allowing degrees of certainty to go to questions of weight, rather than admissibility of evidence. Where the law describes mental states in probabilistic terms, such as "substantial certainty," it generally avoids strict statistical thresholds. Some commentators have drawn rough statistical guidelines for different levels of burdens of proof, arguing that preponderance of the evidence means greater than 50%; clear and convincing evidence is more like 70%, and beyond a reasonable doubt is closer to 95–99%. Except the preponderance of the evidence, courts reject these kinds of statistical definitions of the levels of legal certainty.

The prospect of mindreading in a legal context creates at least three sequential filters of analysis where different probabilities are relevant. The threshold question, key to admissibility, is the degree of certainty or validity (what courts call "reliability") of the underlying science. If the mindreading device is not sufficiently "accurate," as assessed by its positive and negative predictive values, replicability, and other such measures, the question stops there.

In the event that the first threshold is cleared, the second filter is how certainly the reliable output determines a particular mental state, such as "substantial certainty." The analysis here will depend on how the target was probed in the first place: is the machine assessing the *degree* of the person's certainty, or whether or not the person was "substantially certain"? The challenges of operationalizing legal terms of art have already been discussed above.

Finally, the burden of proof filter varies with the legal context—in civil trials, such as contract disputes and tort claims, the standard is a proof by a preponderance of the evidence. In some kinds of civil actions, such as actions for fraud, the requirement is "clear and convincing evidence." And in criminal trials, the standard is proof beyond a reasonable doubt.

The law would probably deal with probabilistic evidence from mindreading technologies in the same way it handles other types of probabilistic evidence, via the series of filters described above. However, these are distinct analyses and should not be blurred, particularly by a machine that purports to get directly inside the mind of legal parties.

Possible legal prohibitions or limitations

Even if neuroscience-based mindreading turns out to be useful and reliable enough to be admitted as evidence for some purposes in court, we still may choose to limit its use. (A US federal district court recently excluded fMRI-based lie detection evidence on the grounds that it did not yet meet federal standards for scientific evidence admissibility, and that on balance it would be more prejudicial than probative to a fact finder (*United States v. Semrau* 2010).) We limit the use, in criminal trials, of evidence obtained as a result of unconstitutional actions by the government. We (usually) allow people to prevent a great deal of testimony from their spouses, lawyers, religious advisers, and physicians. And we allow a person to refuse to testify at all on the ground that his testimony may tend to incriminate him. The idea of mindreading is unsettling; its use in court is likely to be controversial. It is possible that we may end up limiting its use for policy reasons having nothing to do with accuracy, through constitutional decisions, new statutory provisions, common law decisions, or new court rules. These limits might, among other things, prohibit its compulsory use, discourage its "quasi-compulsory" use, or even forbid its truly voluntary use. We will discuss these possibilities in the context of the US legal system, but some similar issues will likely apply in other legal systems, particularly those with common law origins.

As a general matter, barring some privilege or incapacity, a person can be forced to testify or otherwise provide relevant evidence at trials, civil or criminal. Failure to obey a proper subpoena to testify, or to produce physical evidence, can be punished by fines or even imprisonment. Similar requirements apply to pretrial discovery. Sometimes that kind of compulsion can be applied to medical examinations, which we could view as somewhat analogous to a mindreading procedure. Outside the context of ongoing litigation, the government has the power to perform compulsory searches or seizures, limited in the US by the Fourth Amendment's restrictions on "unreasonable" searches and seizures. Is there anything that might prevent a party from demanding that someone produce or present evidence using a mindreading technology?

The Fifth Amendment's privilege against self-incrimination should provide one protection. The legal literature already contains at least three discussions of the applicability of this privilege to neuroscience-based lie detection (Pardo 2006; Stoller and Wolpe 2007; Farahany, forthcoming). A court might plausibly conclude that the results of a mindreading device would not be "testimonial" evidence and so would not be covered by the Fifth Amendment. We think it more likely that this kind of evidence will be covered by the privilege. In that case, people who can make good faith claims that the evidence may tend to incriminate them could prevent the introduction of mindreading evidence.

A possible broader claim might be made under the Due Process Clause of the Fifth and Fourteenth Amendments. In one important case the US Supreme Court held that the prosecution could not introduce evidence produced as a result of the involuntary pumping of a defendant's stomach (*Rochin v. California* 1952). That process, the Court held, "shocked the conscience." The contours of this doctrine are unclear, but it could provide a tool for a court that wished to restrict the use of mindreading evidence that had been acquired without the subject's consent.

Some have argued that the brain (or, at least, knowledge of the mind acquired by direct intervention in the brain) should be protected by a right of privacy (Wolpe 2009). The source of such a right is not entirely clear. The argument is often based on the idea of a broad right of privacy, derived from the implications of various parts of the Bill of Rights and used by the US Supreme Court primarily in cases about reproduction. Some also based that argument on the First Amendment, citing a 1969 Supreme Court decision about an adult's right to possess or read pornography, saying "Our whole constitutional heritage rebels at the thought of giving government the power to control men's minds." (*Stanley v. Georgia* 1969). It is probably more in keeping with current Supreme Court usage to talk about this as a "liberty" right, guaranteed by the Fourteenth Amendment's Due Process clause. Certainly the workings of the brain have traditionally been private; this kind of invasion may feel substantially different from other kinds of government intrusion. A sympathetic court might use some version of this theory to prohibit compulsory mindreading.

Even if compulsory mindreading were banned (or limited), people may be subject to "quasi-compulsory" mindreading. In these cases, the person may have the right to reject mindreading, but may be forced to pay a high price for doing so. For example, in civil cases (but not in criminal cases), counsel can discuss, and jurors can consider and draw negative inferences from, a party's invocation of the Fifth Amendment privilege against self-incrimination. The party can take the Fifth Amendment, but at likely cost to his civil action. In criminal cases, on the other hand, the Supreme Court has ruled that a judge cannot instruct the jury that it may infer the defendant's guilt from his invocation of the privilege—and prosecutors may not comment on the defendant's silence (*Griffin v. California* 1965). Courts might develop a similar protection, in civil or criminal cases, for mindreading.

Finally, courts or legislatures might conclude that mindreading technologies should always be banned, even when the person subjected to the device genuinely and freely wants the evidence admitted. The most prominent example of such a prohibition now is the exclusion of polygraph evidence, generally prohibited in US jurisdictions because of its lack of proven reliability. Interestingly, the Supreme Court of Canada has held that polygraph evidence may not be admitted, even if reliable, because it violates a ban on "oath helping" (*R. v. Béland* 1987). An American state court recently rejected fMRI-based lie detection evidence on a similar theory: that witness credibility was not the kind of question where the jury would be helped by expert testimony (*Wilson v. Corestaff Services* 2010). Four justices of the US Supreme Court stated in an opinion that a similar rationale would be a sufficient reason to uphold a complete ban on polygraph evidence, even in the face of a criminal defendant's Sixth Amendment rights (*United States v. Scheffer* 1998).

A ban on even truly voluntary mindreading might be justified instead on the need to protect reluctant witnesses. Such witnesses might believe that, if the other side uses mindreading, they have no realistic choice but to use it themselves. If a court (or legislature) believed that witnesses should be protected against such a dilemma, a total ban might be justified. And, of course, a legislature (or, in some jurisdictions, the voters through an initiative) could ban such testimony for any reason—such as the "yuck factor"—or for no reason at all.

Conclusion

So what are the likely scientific limits of neuroscience-based mindreading? We don't know. We are confident that we will not have a complete and accurate model of how a generic human brain, let alone any individual human's brain, works anytime in the foreseeable future. But we are equally confident that, in spite of the problems of plasticity, we will be able to use neuroscience techniques to read minds to some extent. Using fMRI, we already can. We may never be able to get all the details right about your fantasized ice cream sundae, but we will know something about it.

How will that affect the law? We don't know that, either, but we have a few guesses. The uses involved in the administration of the law—detecting pain, assessing honesty or memory, or looking for bias—are more scientifically plausible than those involved in discovering the legally relevant mental states associated with crucial actions. The earlier uses do not suffer from the time machine problem, because they are looking at current brain states to infer current mental states and probably will also suffer less from problems of definition. The second set of concepts have more potential for changing legal doctrine than the first, but are less likely to be the subjects of reliable mindreading.

But we do not yet know just how accurate any of these mindreading applications will prove to be—or how much accuracy the law will demand. Neither do we know whether nor how the law would choose to use even reliable mindreading.

What do we know? The ability of neuroscience-based methods to correlate brain states with mental states and thus to "read minds" is expanding rapidly. It has the potential, but only the potential, to change the world of the law—in small ways, in large ways, or in fundamental ways. We cannot convincingly predict what those changes will be, but, with all respect due to Niels Bohr, we do find at least one prediction not hard at all—the evolving intersection of neuroscience-based mindreading and the law will be both important and fascinating to watch.

References

Brown, T. and Murphy, E.R. (2010). Through a scanner darkly: Functional imaging as evidence of mental state. *Stanford Law Review*, **62**, 1119–208.

Commonwealth v. Huot, 380 Mass. 403, 403 N.E .2d 411 (1980).

Eisenberger, N.I., Lieberman, M.D., and Williams, K.D. (2003). Does rejection hurt? An fMRI study of social exclusion. *Science*, **302**, 237–9.

Farahany, N.A. (forthcoming). Incriminating thoughts.

Greely, H.T. (2000). Trusted systems and medical records: Lowering expectations. *Stanford Law Review*, **52**, 1585–91.

Greely, H.T. and Illes, J. (2007). Neuroscience-based lie detection: The urgent need for regulation. *American Journal of Law and Medicine*, **33**, 377–431.

Griffin v. California, 380 U.S. 609 (1965).

Grimshaw v. Ford Motor Co., 119 Cal. App. 3d 757, 174 Cal. Rptr. 348 (1981).

Hadley v. Baxendale, 9 Exch. 341, 156 Eng.Rep. 145 (1854).

Haynes. J.D. and Rees, G. (2006). Decoding mental states from brain activity in humans. *Nature Reviews Neuroscience*, **7**, 523–34.

Haynes, J.D., Sakai, K., Rees, G., Gilbert, S., Frith, C., and Passingham, R.E. (2007). Reading hidden intentions in the human brain. *Current Biology*, **17**, 323–8.

Illes, J. (2004). A fish story? Brain maps, lie detection, and personhood. *Cerebrum*, **6**, 73–80.

Kanwisher, N. (2001). Faces and places: of central (and peripheral) interest. *Nature Neuroscience*, **4**, 455–56.

Kay, K.N., Naselaris, T., Prenge, R.J., and Gallant, J.L. (2008). Identifying natural images from human brain activity. *Nature*, **452**, 352–5.

Model Penal Code § 2.02 (1962). American Law Institute.

Monti, M.M., Vanhaudenhuyse, A., Coleman, M.R., *et al.* (2010). Willful modulation of brain activity in disorders of consciousness. *New England Journal of Medicine*, **362**, 579–89.

Naselaris, T., Prenger, R.J., Kay, K.N., Oliver, M., and Gallant, J.L. (2009). Bayesian reconstruction of natural images from human brain activity. *Neuron*, **63**, 902–15.

Owen, A.M., Coleman, M.R., Boly, M., Davis, M.H., Laureys , S. and Pickard, J.D., (2006). Detecting awareness in the vegetative state. *Science*, **313**, 1402

Pardo, M.S. (2006). Neuroscience evidence, legal culture, and criminal procedure. *American Journal of Criminal Law*, **33**, 301–30.

R. v. Béland, 2S.C.R. 398 (1987).

Rissman, J., Greely, H.T., and Wagner, A.D. (2010). Detecting individual memories through the neural decoding of memory states and past experience. *Proceedings of the National Academy of Sciences*, **107**, 9849–54.

Rochin v. California, 342 U.S. 165 (1952).

Shinkareva, S.V., Mason, R.A., Malave, V.L., Wang, W., Mitchell, T.M., and Just, M.A. (2008). Using fMRI brain activation to identify cognitive states associated with perception of tools and dwellings. *PLoS One*, 3, e1394.

Soon, C.S., Brass, M., Heinze, H.J., and Haynes, J.D. (2008). Unconscious determinants of free decisions in the human brain. *Nature Neuroscience*, **11**, 543–5.

Stanley v. Georgia, 394 U.S. 557 (1969)

Stoller, S.S. and Wolpe P.R. (2007). Emerging neurotechnologies for lie detection and the fifth amendment. *American Journal of Law and Medicine*, **33**, 359–75.

United States v. Heredia, 483F.3d 913 (CA 9 2007), *cert. den.* (2007).

United States v. Scheffer, 323 U.S. 3030 (1996).

United States v. Semrau, Report and Recommendation from the U.S. District Court for the W.D. Tennessee, Eastern Division, docket number 1:07cr10074, (2010).

Wilson v. Corestaff Services, opinion published in *New York Law Journal* May 18, 2010, Page 41 column 4. Available through http://www.nylj.com.

Wolpe, P.R. (2009). Is my mind mine? Neuroethics and brain imaging. In A.L. Caplan, A. Fiester, and V. Ravistky (eds.) *The Penn Center Guide to Bioethics*, pp. 85–94. New York: Springer.

CHAPTER 39

FOR THE LAW, NEUROSCIENCE CHANGES NOTHING AND EVERYTHING

JOSHUA GREENE AND JONATHAN COHEN

INTRODUCTION

THE law takes a long-standing interest in the mind. In most criminal cases, a successful conviction requires the prosecution to establish not only that the defendant engaged in proscribed behavior, but also that the misdeed in question was the product of *mens rea*, a "guilty mind." Narrowly interpreted, *mens rea* refers to the intention to commit a criminal act, but the term has a looser interpretation by which it refers to all mental states consistent with moral and/or legal blame. (A killing motivated by insane delusional beliefs may meet the requirements for *mens rea* in the first sense, but not the second (Goldstein *et al.* 2003).) Thus, for centuries, many legal issues have turned on the question: "What was he thinking?"

To answer this question, the law has often turned to science. Today, the newest kid on this particular scientific block is cognitive neuroscience, the study of the mind through the brain, which has gained prominence in part as a result of the advent of functional neuroimaging as a widely used tool for psychological research. Given the law's aforementioned concern for mental states, along with its preference for "hard" evidence, it is no surprise that interest in the potential legal implications of cognitive neuroscience abounds. But does our emerging understanding of the mind as brain really have any deep implications for the law? This theme issue is a testament to the thought that it might. Some have argued, however, that new neuroscience contributes nothing more than new details and that existing legal principles can handle anything that neuroscience will throw our way in the foreseeable future (Morse 2004). In our view, both of these positions are, in their respective ways, correct. Existing legal principles make virtually no assumptions about the neural bases of criminal behavior, and as a result they can comfortably assimilate new neuroscience without much in the way of conceptual upheaval: new details, new sources of evidence, but nothing for which the law is fundamentally unprepared. We maintain, however, that our operative legal principles exist because they more or less adequately capture an intuitive sense of justice.

In our view, neuroscience will challenge and ultimately reshape our intuitive sense(s) of justice. New neuroscience will affect the way we view the law, not by furnishing us with new ideas or arguments about the nature of human action, but by breathing new life into old ones. Cognitive neuroscience, by identifying the specific mechanisms responsible for behavior, will vividly illustrate what until now could only be appreciated through esoteric theorizing: that there is something fishy about our ordinary conceptions of human action and responsibility, and that, as a result, the legal principles we have devised to reflect these conceptions may be flawed.

Our argument runs as follows: first, we draw a familiar distinction between the consequentialist justification for state punishment, according to which punishment is merely an instrument for promoting future social welfare, and the retributivist justification for punishment, according to which the principal aim of punishment is to give people what they deserve based on their past actions. We observe that the common-sense approach to moral and legal responsibility has consequentialist elements, but is largely retributivist. Unlike the consequentialist justification for punishment, the retributivist justification relies, either explicitly or implicitly, on a demanding—and some say overly demanding—conception of free will. We therefore consider the standard responses to the philosophical problem of free will (Watson 1982). "Libertarians" (no relation to the political philosophy) and "hard determinists" agree on "incompatibilism," the thesis that free will and determinism are incompatible, but they disagree about whether determinism is true, or near enough true to preclude free will. Libertarians believe that we have free will because determinism is false, and hard determinists believe that we lack free will because determinism is (approximately) true. "Compatibilists," in contrast to libertarians and hard determinists, argue that free will and determinism are perfectly compatible

We argue that current legal doctrine, although officially compatibilist, is ultimately grounded in intuitions that are incompatibilist and, more specifically, libertarian. In other words, the law says that it presupposes nothing more than a metaphysically modest notion of free will that is perfectly compatible with determinism. However, we argue that the law's intuitive support is ultimately grounded in a metaphysically overambitious, libertarian notion of free will that is threatened by determinism and, more pointedly, by forthcoming cognitive neuroscience. At present, the gap between what the law officially cares about and what people really care about is only revealed occasionally when vivid scientific information about the causes of criminal behavior leads people to doubt certain individuals' capacity for moral and legal responsibility, despite the fact that this information is irrelevant according to the law's stated principles. We argue that new neuroscience will continue to highlight and widen this gap. That is, new neuroscience will undermine people's common sense, libertarian conception of free will, and the retributivist thinking that depends on it, both of which have heretofore been shielded by the inaccessibility of sophisticated thinking about the mind and its neural basis.

The net effect of this influx of scientific information will be a rejection of free will as it is ordinarily conceived, with important ramifications for the law. As noted earlier, our criminal justice system is largely retributivist. We argue that retributivism, despite its unstable marriage to compatibilist philosophy in the letter of the law, ultimately depends on an intuitive, libertarian notion of free will that is undermined by science. Therefore, with the rejection of common-sense conceptions of free will comes the rejection of retributivism and an ensuing shift towards a consequentialist approach to punishment, i.e. one aimed at promoting future welfare rather than meting out just deserts. Because consequentialist approaches to punishment remain viable in the absence of common-sense free will, we need not give up on moral and legal responsibility. We argue further that the philosophical problem of free will arises out of a conflict between two cognitive subsystems that speak different "languages": the "folk psychology" system and the "folk physics" system. Because we are inherently of two minds when it comes to the problem of free will, this problem will never find an intuitively satisfying solution. We can, however, recognize that free will, as conceptualized by the folk psychology system, is an illusion and structure our society accordingly by rejecting retributivist legal principles that derive their intuitive force from this illusion.

TWO THEORIES OF PUNISHMENT: CONSEQUENTIALISM AND RETRIBUTIVISM

There are two standard justifications for legal punishment (Lacey 1988). According to the forward-looking, consequentialist theory, which emerges from the classical utilitarian tradition (Bentham 1982), punishment is justified by its future beneficial effects. Chief among them are the prevention of future crime through the deterrent effect of the law and the containment of dangerous individuals. Few would deny that the deterrence of future crime and the protection of the public are legitimate justifications for punishment. The controversy surrounding consequentialist theories concerns their serviceability as complete normative theories of punishment. Most theorists find them inadequate in this regard (e.g. Hart 1968), and many argue that consequentialism fundamentally mischaracterizes the primary justification for punishment, which, these critics argue, is retribution (Kant 2002). As a result, they claim, consequentialist theories justify intuitively unfair forms of punishment, if not in practice then in principle. One problem is that of Draconian penalties. It is possible, for example, that imposing the death penalty for parking violations would maximize aggregate welfare by reducing parking violations to near zero. But, retributivists claim, whether or not this is a good idea does not depend on the balance of costs and benefits. It is simply wrong to kill someone for double parking. A related problem is that of punishing the innocent. It is possible that, under certain circumstances, falsely convicting an innocent person would have a salutary deterrent effect, enough to justify that person's suffering, etc. Critics also note that, so far as deterrence is concerned, it is the *threat* of punishment that is justified and not the punishment itself. Thus, consequentialism might justify letting murderers and rapists off the hook so long as their punishment could be convincingly faked

The standard consequentialist response to these charges is that such concerns have no place in the real world. They say, for example, that the idea of imposing the death penalty for parking violations to make society an overall happier place is absurd. People everywhere would live in mortal fear of bureaucratic errors, and so on. Likewise, a legal system that deliberately convicted innocent people and/or secretly refrained from punishing guilty ones would require a kind of systematic deception that would lead inevitably to corruption and that could never survive in a free society. At this point critics retort that consequentialist theories, at best, get the right answers for the wrong reasons. It is wrong to punish innocent people, etc. because it is fundamentally unfair, not because it leads to bad consequences in practice. Such critics are certainly correct to point out that consequentialist theories fail to capture something central to common-sense intuitions about legitimate punishment.

The backward-looking, retributivist account does a better job of capturing these intuitions. Its fundamental principle is simple: in the absence of mitigating circumstances, people who engage in criminal behavior *deserve* to be punished, and that is why we punish them. Some would explicate this theory in terms of criminals' forfeiting rights, others in terms of the rights of the victimized, whereas others would appeal to the violation of a hypothetical social contract, and so on. Retributivist theories come in many flavors, but these distinctions need not concern us here. What is important for our purposes is that retributivism captures the intuitive idea that we legitimately punish to give people what they deserve based on their past actions— in proportion to their "internal wickedness," to use Kant's (2002) phrase—and not, primarily, to promote social welfare in the future

The retributivist perspective is widespread, both in the explicit views of legal theorists and implicitly in common sense. There are two primary motivations for questioning retributivist theory. The first, which will not concern us here, comes from a prior commitment to a broader consequentialist moral theory. The second comes from skepticism regarding the notion of desert, grounded in a broader skepticism about the possibility of free will in a deterministic or mechanistic world.

Free will and retributivism

The problem of free will is old and has many formulations (Watson 1982). Here is one, drawing on a more detailed and exacting formulation by Peter Van Inwagen (1982): determinism is true if the world is such that its current state is completely determined by (1) the laws of physics and (2) past states of the world. Intuitively, the idea is that a deterministic universe starts however it starts and then ticks along like clockwork from there. Given a set of prior conditions in the universe and a set of physical laws that completely govern the way the universe evolves, there is only one way that things can actually proceed.

Free will, it is often said, requires the ability do otherwise (an assumption that has been questioned; Frankfurt 1966). One cannot say, for example, that I have freely chosen soup over salad if forces beyond my control are sufficient to necessitate my choosing soup. But, the determinist argues, this is precisely what forces beyond your control do— always. You have no say whatsoever in the state of the universe before your birth; nor do you have any say about the laws of physics. However, if determinism is true, these two things together are sufficient to determine your choice of soup over salad. Thus, some say, if determinism is true, your sense of yourself and others as having free will is an illusion

There are three standard responses to the problem of free will. The first, known as "hard determinism," accepts the incompatibility of free will and determinism ("incompatibilism"), and asserts determinism, thus rejecting free will. The second response is libertarianism (again, no relation to the political philosophy), which accepts incompatibilism, but denies that determinism is true. This may seem like a promising approach. After all, has not modern physics shown us that the universe is *in*deterministic (Hughs 1992)? The problem here is that the sort of indeterminism afforded by modern physics is not the sort the libertarian needs or desires. If it turns out that your ordering soup is completely determined by the laws of physics, the state of the universe 10,000 years ago, *and* the outcomes of myriad subatomic coin flips, your appetizer is no more freely chosen than before. Indeed, it is *randomly* chosen, which is no help to the libertarian. What about some other kind of indeterminism? What if, somewhere deep in the brain, there are mysterious events that operate independently of the ordinary laws of physics and that are somehow tied to the will of the brain's owner? In light of the available evidence, this is highly unlikely. Say what you will about the "hard problem" of consciousness (Shear 1999), there is not a shred of scientific evidence to support the existence of *causally effective* processes in the mind or brain that violate the laws of physics. In our opinion, any scientifically respectable discussion of free will requires the rejection of what Strawson (1962) famously called the "panicky metaphysics" of libertarianism.[1]

Finally, we come to the dominant view among philosophers and legal theorists: compatibilism. Compatibilists concede that some notions of free will may require indefensible, panicky metaphysics, but maintain that the kinds of free will "worth wanting," to use Dennett's (1984) phrase, are perfectly compatible with determinism. Compatibilist theories vary, but all compatibilists agree that free will is a perfectly natural, scientifically respectable phenomenon and part of the ordinary human condition. They also agree that free will can be undermined by various kinds of psychological deficit, e.g. mental illness or "infancy." Thus, according to this view, a freely willed action is one that is made using the right sort of psychology—rational, free of delusion, etc.

Compatibilists make some compelling arguments. After all, is it not obvious that we have free will? Could science plausibly deny the obvious fact that I am free to raise my hand *at will*? For many people, such simple observations make the reality of free will non-negotiable. But at the same time, many such people concede that determinism, or something like it, is a live possibility. And if free will is obviously real, but determinism is debatable, then the reality of free will must not hinge on the rejection of determinism. That is, free will and determinism must be compatible. Many compatibilists skeptically ask what would it mean to give up on free will. Were we to give it up, wouldn't we have to immediately reinvent it? Does not every decision involve an implicit commitment to the idea of free will? And how else would we distinguish between ordinary rational adults and other individuals, such as young children and the mentally ill, whose will—or whatever you want to call it—is clearly compromised? Free will, compatibilists argue, is here to stay, and the challenge for science is to figure out how exactly it works and not to peddle silly arguments that deny the undeniable (Dennett 2003).

The forward-looking–consequentialist approach to punishment works with all three responses to the problem of free will, including hard determinism. This is because

---

[1] Of course, scientific respectability is not everyone's first priority. However, the law in most Western states is a public institution designed to function in a society that respects a wide range of religious and otherwise metaphysical beliefs. The law cannot function in this way if it presupposes controversial and unverifiable metaphysical facts about the nature of human action, or anything else. Thus, the law must restrict itself to the class of intersubjectively verifiable facts, i.e. the facts recognized by science, broadly construed. This practice need not derive from a conviction that the scientifically verifiable facts are necessarily the only facts, but merely from a recognition that verifiable or scientific facts are the only facts upon which public institutions in a pluralistic society can effectively rely.

consequentialists are not concerned with whether anyone is really innocent or guilty in some ultimate sense that might depend on people's having free will, but only with the likely effects of punishment. (Of course, one might wonder what it means for a hard determinist to justify any sort of choice. We will return to this issue later in this chapter.) The retributivist approach, by contrast, is plausibly regarded as requiring free will and the rejection of hard determinism. Retributivists want to know whether the defendant truly *deserves* to be punished. Assuming one can deserve to be punished only for actions that are freely willed, hard determinism implies that no one really deserves to be punished. Thus, hard determinism combined with retributivism requires the elimination of all punishment, which does not seem reasonable. This leaves retributivists with two options: compatibilism and libertarianism. Libertarianism, for reasons given earlier, and despite its intuitive appeal, is scientifically suspect. At the very least, the law should not depend on it. It seems, then, that retributivism requires compatibilism. Accordingly, the standard legal account of punishment is compatibilist.

NEUROSCIENCE CHANGES NOTHING

The title of a recent paper by Stephen Morse (2004), "New neuroscience, old problems," aptly summarizes many a seasoned legal thinker's response to the suggestion that brain research will revolutionize the law. The law has been dealing with issues of criminal responsibility for a long time; Morse argues that there is nothing on the neuroscientific horizon that it cannot handle.

The reason that the law is immune to such threats is that it makes no assumptions that neuroscience, or any science, is likely to challenge. The law assumes that people have a general capacity for rational choice. That is, people have beliefs and desires and are capable of producing behavior that serves their desires in light of their beliefs. The law acknowledges that our capacity for rational choice is far from perfect (Kahneman and Tversky 2000), requiring only that the people it deems legally responsible have a *general* capacity for rational behavior.

Thus, questions about who is or is not responsible in the eyes of the law have and will continue to turn on questions about rationality. This approach was first codified in the *M'Naghten* standard according to which a defense on the ground of insanity requires proof that the defendant labored under "a defect of reason, from disease of the mind" (Goldstein 1967). Not all standards developed and applied since *M'Naghten* explicitly mention the need to demonstrate the defendant's diminished rationality (e.g. the Durham standard; Goldstein 1967), but it is generally agreed that a legal excuse requires a demonstration that the defendant "lacked a general capacity for rationality" (Goldstein *et al.* 2003). Thus, the argument goes, new science can help us figure out who was or was not rational at the scene of the crime, much as it has in the past, but new science will not justify any fundamental change in the law's approach to responsibility unless it shows that people in general fail to meet the law's very minimal requirements for rationality. Science shows no sign of doing this, and thus the basic precepts of legal responsibility stand firm. As for neuroscience more specifically, this discipline seems especially unlikely to undermine our faith in general minimal rationality. If any sciences have an outside chance of demonstrating that our behavior is thoroughly irrational or arational it is the ones that study behavior directly rather than its proximate physical causes in the brain. The law, this argument continues, does not care if people have "free will" in any deep metaphysical sense that might be threatened by determinism. It only cares that people in general are minimally rational. So long as this appears to be the case, it can go on regarding people as free (compatibilism) and holding ordinary people responsible for their misdeeds while making exceptions for those who fail to meet the requirements of general rationality.

In light of this, one might wonder what all the fuss is about. If the law assumes nothing more than general minimal rationality, and neuroscience does nothing to undermine this assumption, then why would anyone even think that neuroscience poses some sort of threat to legal doctrines of criminal responsibility? It sounds like this is just a simple mistake, and that is precisely what Morse contends. He calls this mistake "the fundamental psycholegal error" which is "to believe that causation, especially abnormal causation, is *per se* an excusing condition" (Morse 2004, p. 180). In other words, if you think that neuroscientific information about the causes of human action, or some particular human's action, can, by itself, make for a legitimate legal excuse, you just do not understand the law. Every action is caused by brain events, and describing those events and affirming their causal efficacy is of no legal interest in and of itself. Morse continues, "[The psycholegal error] leads people to try to create a new excuse every time an allegedly valid new 'syndrome' is discovered that is thought to play a role in behavior. But syndromes and other causes do not have excusing force unless they sufficiently diminish rationality in the context in question" (Morse 2004, p. 180).

In our opinion, Morse and like-minded theorists are absolutely correct about the relationship between current legal doctrine and any forthcoming neuroscientific results. For the law, as written, neuroscience changes nothing. The law provides a coherent framework for the assessment of criminal responsibility that is not threatened by anything neuroscience is likely to throw at it. But, we maintain, the law nevertheless stands on shakier ground than the foregoing would suggest. The legitimacy of the law itself depends on its adequately reflecting the moral intuitions and commitments of society. If neuroscience can change those intuitions, then neuroscience can change the law.

As it happens, this is a possibility that Morse explicitly acknowledges. However, he believes that such developments would require radical new ideas that we can scarcely imagine at this time, e.g. a new solution to the mind–body problem. We disagree. The seeds of discontent are already sown in common-sense legal thought. In our opinion, the "fundamental psycholegal error" is not so much an error as a reflection of the gap between what the law officially cares about and what people really care about. In modern criminal law, there has been a long, tense marriage of convenience between compatibilist legal principles and libertarian moral intuitions. New neuroscience, we argue, will probably render this marriage unworkable.

What really matters for responsibility? Materialist theory, dualist intuitions, and "The Boys from Brazil" problem

According to the law, the central question in a case of putative diminished responsibility is whether the accused was sufficiently rational at the time of the misdeed in question.

We believe, however, that this is not what most people really care about, and that for them diminished rationality is just a presumed correlate of something deeper. It seems that what many people really want to know is: was it really *him*? This question usually comes in the form of a disjunction, depending on how the excuse is constructed: was it *him*, or was it his *upbringing*? Was it *him*, or was it his *genes*? Was it *him*, or was it his *circumstances*? Was it *him*, or was it his *brain*? But what most people do not understand, despite the fact that naturalistic philosophers and scientists have been saying it for centuries, is that there is no "him" independent of these other things. (Or, to be a bit more accommodating to the supernaturally inclined, there is no "him" independent of these things that shows any sign of affecting anything in the physical world, including his behavior.)

Most people's view of the mind is implicitly *dualist* and *libertarian* and not *materialist* and *compatibilist*. Dualism, for our purposes, is the view that mind and brain are separate, interacting, entities.[2] Dualism fits naturally with libertarianism because a mind distinct from the body is precisely the sort of non-physical source of free will that libertarianism requires. Materialism, by contrast, is the view that all events, including the operations of the mind, are ultimately operations of matter that obeys the laws of physics. It is hard to imagine a belief in free will that is materialist but not compatibilist, given that ordinary matter does not seem capable of supplying the non-physical processes that libertarianism requires.

Many people, particularly those who are religious, are explicitly dualist libertarians (again, not in the political sense). However, in our estimation, even people who do or would readily endorse a thoroughly material account of human action and its causes have dualist, libertarian intuitions. This goes not only for educated people in general, but for experts in mental health and criminal behavior. Consider, for example, the following remarks from Jonathan Pincus, an expert on criminal behavior and the brain.

> When a composer conceives a symphony, the only way he or she can present it to the public is through an orchestra....If the performance is poor, the fault could lie with the composer's conception, or the orchestra, or both....Will is expressed by the brain. Violence can be the result of volition only, but if a brain is damaged, brain failure must be at least partly to blame. (Pincus 2001, p. 128)

To our untutored intuitions, this is a perfectly sensible analogy, but it is ultimately grounded in a kind of dualism that is scientifically untenable. It is not as if there is *you*, the composer, and then *your brain*, the orchestra. You *are* your brain, and your brain is the composer and the orchestra all rolled together. There is no little man, no "homunculus," in the brain that is the real you behind the mass of neuronal instrumentation. Scientifically minded philosophers have been saying this *ad nauseum* (Dennett 1991), and we will not belabor the point. Moreover, we suspect that if you were to ask Dr Pincus whether he thinks there is a little conductor directing his brain's activity from within or beyond he would adamantly

---

[2] There are some forms of dualism according to which the mind and body, although distinct, do not interact, making it impossible for the mind to have any observable effects on the brain or anything else in the physical world. These versions of dualism do not concern us here. For the purposes of this paper, we are happy to allow the metaphysical claim that souls or aspects of minds may exist independently of the physical body. Our concern is specifically with interactionist versions of dualism according to which non-physical mental entities have observable physical effects. We believe that science has rendered such views untenable and that the law, insofar as it is a public institution designed to serve a pluralistic society, must not rely on beliefs that are scientifically suspect (see previous endnote).

deny that this is the case. At the same time, though, he is comfortable comparing a brain-damaged criminal to a healthy conductor saddled with an unhealthy orchestra. This sort of doublethink is not uncommon. As we will argue later in this chapter, when it comes to moral responsibility in a physical world, we are all of two minds.

A recent article by Laurence Steinberg and Elizabeth Scott (Steinberg and Scott 2003), experts respectively on adolescent developmental psychology and juvenile law, illustrates the same point. They argue that adolescents do not meet the law's general requirements for rationality and that therefore they should be considered less than fully responsible for their actions and, more specifically, unsuitable candidates for the death penalty. Their main argument is sound, but they cannot resist embellishing it with a bit of superfluous neuroscience.

> Most of the developmental research on cognitive and psychosocial functioning in adolescence measures behaviors, selfperceptions, or attitudes, but mounting evidence suggests that at least some of the differences between adults and adolescents have neuropsychological and neurobiological underpinnings. (Steinberg and Scott 2003, p. 5)

Some of the differences? Unless some form of dualism is correct, every mental difference and every difference in behavioral tendency is a function of some kind of difference in the brain. But here it is implicitly suggested that things like "behaviors, self-perceptions, or attitudes" may be grounded in something other than the brain. In summing up their case, Steinberg and Scott look towards the future:

> Especially needed are studies that link developmental changes in decision making to changes in brain structure and function....In our view, however, there is sufficient indirect suggestive evidence of age differences in capacities that are relevant to criminal blameworthiness to support the position that youths who commit crimes should be punished more leniently then their adult counterparts. (Steinberg and Scott 2003, p. 9)

This gets the order of evidence backwards. If what the law ultimately cares about is whether adolescents can behave rationally, then it is evidence concerning adolescent behavior that is directly relevant. Studying the adolescent brain is a highly indirect way of figuring out whether adolescents in general are rational. Indeed, the only way we neuroscientists can tell if a brain structure is important for rational judgment is to see if its activity or damage is correlated with (ir)rational *behavior*.[3]

If everyone agrees that what the law ultimately cares about is the capacity for rational behavior, then why are Steinberg and Scott so optimistic about neuroscientific evidence that is only indirectly relevant? The reason, we suggest, is that they are appealing not to a legal argument, but to a moral intuition. So far as the law is concerned, information about the physical processes that give rise to bad behavior is irrelevant. But to people who implicitly believe that real decision making takes place in the mind, not in the brain, demonstrating that there is a brain basis for adolescents' misdeeds allows us to blame adolescents' brains instead of the adolescents themselves.

---

[3] It is conceivable that rationality could someday be redefined in neurocognitive rather than behavioral terms, much as water has been redefined in terms of its chemical composition. Were that to happen, neuroscientific evidence could then be construed as more direct than behavioral evidence. But Steinberg and Scott's argument appears to make use of a conventional, behavioral definition of rationality and not a neurocognitive redefinition.

The fact that people are tempted to attach great moral or legal significance to neuroscientific information that, according to the letter of the law, should not matter, suggests that what the law cares about and what people care about do not necessarily coincide. To make this point in a more general way, we offer the following thought experiment, which we call "The *Boys from Brazil* problem." It is an extension of an argument that has made the rounds in philosophical discussions of free will and responsibility (Rosen 2002).

In the film *The Boys from Brazil*, members of the Nazi old guard have regrouped in South America after the war. Their plan is to bring their beloved führer back to life by raising children genetically identical to Hitler (courtesy of some salvaged DNA) in environments that mimic that of Hitler's upbringing. For example, Hitler's father died while young Adolph was still a boy, and so each Hitler clone's surrogate father is killed at just the right time, and so on, and so forth.

This is obviously a fantasy, but the idea that one could, in principle, produce a person with a particular personality and behavioral profile through tight genetic and environmental control is plausible. Let us suppose, then, that a group of scientists has managed to create an individual— call him "Mr Puppet"—who, by design, engages in some kind of criminal behavior: say, a murder during a drug deal gone bad. The defense calls to the stand the project's lead scientist: "Please tell us about your relationship to Mr Puppet…"

> It is very simple, really. I designed him. I carefully selected every gene in his body and carefully scripted every significant event in his life so that he would become precisely what he is today. I selected his mother knowing that she would let him cry for hours and hours before picking him up. I carefully selected each of his relatives, teachers, friends, enemies, etc. and told them exactly what to say to him and how to treat him. Things generally went as planned, but not always. For example, the angry letters written to his dead father were not supposed to appear until he was fourteen, but by the end of his thirteenth year he had already written four of them. In retrospect I think this was because of a handful of substitutions I made to his eighth chromosome. At any rate, my plans for him succeeded, as they have for 95% of the people I've designed. I assure you that the accused deserves none of the credit.

What to do with Mr Puppet? Insofar as we believe this testimony, we are inclined to think that Mr Puppet cannot be held fully responsible for his crimes, if he can be held responsible for them at all. He is, perhaps, a man to be feared, and we would not want to return him to the streets. But given the fact that forces beyond his control played a dominant role in causing him to commit these crimes, it is hard to think of him as anything more than a pawn.

But what does the law say about Mr Puppet? The law asks whether or not he was rational at the time of his misdeeds, and as far as we know he was. For all we know, he is psychologically indistinguishable from the prototypical guilty criminal, and therefore fully responsible in the eyes of the law. But, intuitively, this is not fair.

Thus, it seems that the law's exclusive interest in rationality misses something intuitively important. In our opinion, rationality is just a presumed correlate of what most people really care about. What people really want to know is if the accused, as opposed to something else, is responsible for the crime, where that "something else" could be the accused's brain, genes, or environment. The question of someone's ultimate responsibility seems to turn, intuitively, on a question of internal versus external determination. Mr Puppet ought not to be held responsible for his actions because forces beyond his control played a dominant role in the production of his behavior. Of course, the scientists did not have complete control—after all, they had a 5% failure rate—but that does not seem to be enough to restore Mr Puppet's free will, at least not entirely. Yes, he is as rational as other criminals, and, yes, it was his desires and beliefs that produced his actions. But those beliefs and desires were rigged by external forces, and that is why, intuitively, he deserves our pity more than our moral condemnation.[4]

The story of Mr. Puppet raises an important question: what is the difference between Mr Puppet and anyone else accused of a crime? After all, we have little reason to doubt that (1) the state of the universe 10,000 years ago, (2) the laws of physics, and (3) the outcomes of random quantum mechanical events are together sufficient to determine everything that happens nowadays, including our own actions. These things are all clearly beyond our control. So what is the real difference between us and Mr Puppet? One obvious difference is that Mr Puppet is the victim of a diabolical plot whereas most people, we presume, are not. But does this matter? The thought that Mr Puppet is not fully responsible depends on the idea that his actions were externally determined. Forces beyond his control constrained his personality to the point that it was "no surprise" that he would behave badly. But the fact that these forces are connected to the desires and intentions of evil scientists is really irrelevant, is it not? What matters is only that these forces are beyond Mr Puppet's control, that they're not really his. The fact that someone could deliberately harness these forces to reliably design criminals is an indication of the strength of these forces, but the fact that these forces are being guided by other minds rather than simply operating on their own seems irrelevant, so far as Mr Puppet's freedom and responsibility are concerned.

Thus, it seems that, in a very real sense, we are all puppets. The combined effects of genes and environment determine all of our actions. Mr Puppet is exceptional only in that the intentions of other humans lie behind his genes and environment. But, so long as his genes and environment are intrinsically comparable to those of ordinary people, this does not really matter. We are no more free than he is.

What all of this illustrates is that the "fundamental psycholegal error" is grounded in a powerful moral intuition that the law and allied compatibilist philosophies try to sweep under the rug. The foregoing suggests that people regard actions only as fully free when those actions are seen as robust against determination by external forces. But if determinism (or determinism plus quantum mechanics) is true, then no actions are truly free because forces beyond our control are always sufficient to determine behavior. Thus, intuitive free will is libertarian, not compatibilist. That is, it requires the rejection of determinism and an implicit commitment to some kind of magical mental causation.[5]

---

[4] This is not to say that we could not describe Mr Puppet in such a way that our intuitions about him would change. Our point is only that, when the details are laid bare, it is very hard to see him as morally responsible.

[5] Compatibilist philosophers such as Daniel Dennett (2003) might object that the story of Mr Puppet is nothing but a misleading 'intuition pump'. Indeed, this is what Dennett says about a similar case of Alfred Mele's (1995). We believe that our case is importantly different from Mele's. Dennett and Mele imagine two women who are psychologically identical: Ann is a typical, good person, whereas Beth has been brainwashed to be just like Ann. Dennett argues, against Mele, that if you take seriously the claim that these two are psychologically identical and properly imagine that Beth is as rational, openminded, etc. as Ann, you will come to see that the two are equally free. We agree with Dennett that Ann and Beth are comparable and that Mele's intuition falters when the details are fleshed out. But does the same hold for the intuition provoked by Mr Puppet's story? It seems to us that the more one knows about Mr Puppet and his life the less inclined one is to see him as truly responsible for his actions and our punishing him as a

Naturalistic philosophers and scientists have known for a long time that magical mental causation is a non-starter. But this realization is the result of philosophical reflection about the nature of the universe and its governance by physical law. Philosophical reflection, however, is not the only way to see the problems with libertarian accounts of free will. Indeed, we argue that neuroscience can help people appreciate the mechanical nature of human action in a way that bypasses complicated arguments.

Neuroscience and the transparent bottleneck

We have argued that, contrary to legal and philosophical orthodoxy, determinism really does threaten free will and responsibility as we intuitively understand them. It is just that most of us, including most philosophers and legal theorists, have yet to appreciate it. This controversial opinion amounts to an empirical prediction that may or may not hold: as more and more scientific facts come in, providing increasingly vivid illustrations of what the human mind is really like, more and more people will develop moral intuitions that are at odds with our current social practices (see Robert Wright (1994) for similar thoughts).

Neuroscience has a special role to play in this process for the following reason. As long as the mind remains a black box, there will always be a donkey on which to pin dualist and libertarian intuitions. For a long time, philosophical arguments have persuaded some people that human action has purely mechanical causes, but not everyone cares for philosophical arguments. Arguments are nice, but physical demonstrations are far more compelling. What neuroscience does, and will continue to do at an accelerated pace, is elucidate the "when," "where," and "how" of the mechanical processes that cause behavior. It is one thing to deny that human decision making is purely mechanical when your opponent offers only a general, philosophical argument. It is quite another to hold your ground when your opponent can make detailed predictions about how these mechanical processes work, complete with images of the brain structures involved and equations that describe their function.[6]

Thus, neuroscience holds the promise of turning the black box of the mind into a *transparent bottleneck*. There are many causes that impinge on behavior, but all of them—from the genes you inherited, to the pain in your lower back, to the advice your grandmother gave you when you were six—must exert their influence through the brain. Thus, your brain serves as a bottleneck for all the forces spread throughout the universe of your past that affect who you are and what you do. Moreover, this bottleneck contains the events that are,

---

worthy end in itself. We can agree with Dennett that there is a sense in which Mr Puppet is free. Our point is merely that there is a legitimate sense in which he, like all of us, is not free and that this sense matters for the law.

[6] We do not wish to imply that neuroscience will inevitably put us in a position to predict any given action based on a neurological examination. Rather, our suggestion is simply that neuroscience will eventually advance to the point at which the mechanistic nature of human decision making is sufficiently apparent to undermine the force of dualist/libertarian intuitions.

intuitively, most critical for moral and legal responsibility, and we may soon be able to observe them closely.

At some time in the future we may have extremely high-resolution scanners that can simultaneously track the neural activity and connectivity of every neuron in a human brain, along with computers and software that can analyze and organize these data. Imagine, for example, watching a film of your brain choosing between soup and salad. The analysis software highlights the neurons pushing for soup in red and the neurons pushing for salad in blue. You zoom in and slow down the film, allowing yourself to trace the cause-and-effect relationships between individual neurons— the mind's clockwork revealed in arbitrary detail. You find the tipping-point moment at which the blue neurons in your prefrontal cortex out-fire the red neurons, seizing control of your pre-motor cortex and causing you to say, "I will have the salad, please."

At some further point this sort of brainware may be very widespread, with a high-resolution brain scanner in every classroom. People may grow up completely used to the idea that every decision is a thoroughly mechanical process, the outcome of which is completely determined by the results of prior mechanical processes. What will such people think as they sit in their jury boxes? Suppose a man has killed his wife in a jealous rage. Will jurors of the future wonder whether the defendant acted in that moment *of his own free will*? Will they wonder if it was *really him* who killed his wife rather than his *uncontrollable anger*? Will they ask whether he *could have done otherwise*? Whether he really *deserves* to be punished, or if he is just a victim of unfortunate circumstances? We submit that these questions, which seem so important today, will lose their grip in an age when the mechanical nature of human decision making is fully appreciated. The law will continue to punish misdeeds, as it must for practical reasons, but the idea of distinguishing the truly, deeply guilty from those who are merely victims of neuronal circumstances will, we submit, seem pointless.

At least in our more reflective moments. Our intuitive sense of free will runs quite deep, and it is possible that we will never be able to fully talk ourselves out of it. Next we consider the psychological origins of the problem of free will.

FOLK PSYCHOLOGY AND FOLK PHYSICS COLLIDE: A COGNITIVE ACCOUNT OF THE PROBLEM OF ATTRIBUTIVE FREE WILL

Could the problem of free will just melt away? This question begs another: Why do we have the problem of free will in the first place? Why does the idea of a deterministic universe seem to contradict something important in our conception of human action? A promising answer to this question is offered by Daniel Wegner in *The Illusion of Conscious Will* (Wegner 2002). In short, Wegner argues, we feel as if we are uncaused causers, and therefore granted a degree of independence from the deterministic flow of the universe, because we are unaware of the deterministic processes that operate in our own heads. Our actions appear to be caused by our mental states, but not by physical states of our brains, and so we imagine that we are metaphysically special, that we are non-physical causes of physical events.

This belief in our specialness is likely to meet the same fate as other similarly narcissistic beliefs that we have cherished in our past: that the Earth lies at the centre of the universe, that humans are unrelated to other species, that all of our behavior is consciously determined, etc. Each of these beliefs has been replaced by a scientific and humbling understanding of our place in the physical universe, and there is no reason to believe that the case will be any different for our sense of free will. (For similar thoughts, see Wright (1994) on Darwin's clandestine views about free will and responsibility.)

We believe that Wegner's account of the problem of free will is essentially correct, although we disagree strongly with his conclusions concerning its (lack of) practical moral implications (see later). In this section we pick up on and extend one strand in Wegner's argument (Wegner 2002, pp. 15–28). Wegner's primary aim is to explain, in psychological terms, why we attribute free will to ourselves, why we feel free from the inside. Our aim in this section is to explain, in psychological terms, why we insist on attributing free will to *others*—and why scientifically minded philosophers, despite persistent efforts, have managed to talk almost no one out of this practice. The findings we review serve as examples of how psychological and neuroscientific data are beginning to characterize the mechanisms that underlie our sense of free will, how these mechanisms can lead us to assume free will is operating when it is not, and how a scientific understanding of these mechanisms can serve to dismantle our commitment to the idea of free will.

Looking out at the world, it appears to contain two fundamentally different kinds of entity. On the one hand, there are ordinary objects that appear to obey the ordinary laws of physics: things like rocks and puddles of water and blocks of wood. These things do not get up and move around on their own. They are, in a word, inanimate. On the other hand, there are things that seem to operate by some kind of magic. Humans and other animals, so long as they are alive, can move about at will, in apparent defiance of the physical laws that govern ordinary matter. Because things like rocks and puddles, on the one hand, and mice and humans, on the other, behave in such radically different ways, it makes sense, from an evolutionary perspective, that creatures would evolve separate cognitive systems for processing information about each of these classes of objects (Pinker 1997). There is a good deal of evidence to suggest that this is precisely how our minds work.

A line of research beginning with Fritz Heider illustrates this point. Heider and Simmel (1944) created a film involving three simple geometric shapes that move about in various ways. For example, a big triangle chases a little circle around the screen, bumping into it. The little circle repeatedly moves away, and a little triangle repeatedly moves in between the circle and the big triangle. When normal people watch this movie they cannot help but view it in social terms (Heberlein and Adolphs 2004). They see the big triangle as *trying* to harm the little circle, and the little triangle as trying to *protect* the little circle; and they see the little circle as *afraid* and the big triangle as *frustrated*. Some people even spontaneously report that the big triangle is a *bully*. In other words, simple patterns of movement trigger in people's minds a cascade of complex social inferences. People not only see these shapes as "alive." They see beliefs, desires, intentions, emotions, personality traits, and even moral blameworthiness. It appears that this kind of inference is automatic (Scholl and Tremoulet 2000). Of course, you, the observer, know that it is only a film, and a very simple one at that, but you nevertheless cannot help but see these events in social, even *moral*, terms.

That is, unless you have damage to your amygdala, a subcortical brain structure that is important for social cognition (Adolphs 1999). Andrea Heberlein tested a patient with rare bilateral amygdala damage using Heider's film and found that this patient, unlike normal people, described what she saw in completely asocial terms, despite that fact that her visual and verbal abilities are not compromised by her brain damage. Somehow, this patient is blind to the "human" drama that normal people cannot help but see in these events (Heberlein and Adolphs 2004).

The sort of thinking that is engaged when normal people view the Heider–Simmel film is sometimes known as "folk psychology" (Fodor 1987), "the intentional stance" (Dennett 1987), or "theory of mind" (Premack and Woodruff 1978). There is a fair amount of evidence (including the work described earlier) suggesting that humans have a set of cognitive sub-systems that are specialized for processing information about intentional agents (Saxe *et al.* 2004). At the same time, there is evidence to suggest that humans and other animals also have subsystems specialized for "folk physics," an intuitive sense of how ordinary matter behaves. One compelling piece of evidence for the claim that normal humans have subsystems specialized for folk physics comes from studies of people with autism spectrum disorder. These individuals are particularly bad at solving problems that require "folk psychology," but they do very well with problems related to how physical objects (e.g. the parts of machine) behave, i.e. "folk physics" (Baron Cohen 2000). Another piece of evidence for a "folk physics" system comes from discrepancies between people's physical intuitions and the way the world actually works. People say, for example, that a ball shot out of a curved tube resting on a flat surface will continue to follow a curved path outside the tube when in fact it will follow a straight path (McCloskey et al. 1980). The fact that people's physical intuitions are slightly, but systematically, out of step with reality suggests that the mind brings a fair amount of implicit theory to the perception of physical objects.

Thus, it is at least plausible that we possess distinguishable cognitive systems for making sense of the behavior of objects in the world. These systems seem to have two fundamentally different "ontologies." The folk physics system deals with chunks of matter that move around without purposes of their own according to the laws of intuitive physics, whereas the folk psychology system deals with unseen features of minds: beliefs, desires, intentions, etc. But what, to our minds, is a mind? We suggest that a crucial feature, if not the defining feature, of a mind (intuitively understood) is that it is an uncaused causer (Scholl and Tremoulet 2000). Minds animate material bodies, allowing them to move without any apparent physical cause and in pursuit of goals. Moreover, we reserve certain social attitudes for things that have minds. For example, we do not resent the rain for ruining our picnic, but we would resent a person who hosed our picnic (Strawson 1962), and we resent picnic-hosers considerably more when we perceive that their actions are intentional. Thus, it seems that folk psychology is the gateway to moral evaluation. To see something as morally blameworthy or praiseworthy (even if it is just a moving square), one has to first see it as "someone," that is, as having a mind.

With all of this in the background, one can see how the problem of attributive free will arises. To see something as a responsible moral agent, one must first see it as having a mind. But, intuitively, a mind is, among other things, an uncaused causer. Consequently, when something is seen as a mere physical entity operating in accordance with deterministic physical laws, it ceases to be seen, intuitively, as a mind. Consequently, it is seen as an object unworthy of moral praise or blame. (Note that we are not claiming that people automatically attribute moral agency to anything that appears to be an uncaused causer. Rather, our claim is that seeing something as an uncaused causer is a *necessary but not sufficient* condition for seeing something as a moral agent.)

After thousands of years of our thinking of one another as uncaused causers, science comes along and tells us that there is no such thing—that all causes, with the possible exception of the Big Bang, are caused causes (determinism). This creates a problem. When we look at people as physical systems, we cannot see them as any more blameworthy or praiseworthy than bricks. But when we perceive people using our intuitive, folk psychology we cannot avoid attributing moral blame and praise.

So, philosophers who would honor both our scientific knowledge and our social instincts try to reconcile these two competing outlooks, but the result is never completely satisfying, and the debate wears on. Philosophers who cannot let go of the idea of uncaused causes defend libertarianism, and thus opt for scientifically dubious, "panicky metaphysics." Hard determinists, by contrast, embrace the conclusions of modern science, and concede what others will not: that many of our dearly held social practices are based on an illusion. The remaining majority, the compatibilists, try to talk themselves into a compromise. But the compromise is fragile. When the physical details of human action are made vivid, folk psychology loses its grip, just as folk physics loses its grip when the morally significant details are emphasized. The problem of free will and determinism will never find an intuitively satisfying solution because it arises out of a conflict between two distinct cognitive subsystems that speak different cognitive "languages" and that may ultimately be incapable of negotiation.

FREE WILL, RESPONSIBILITY AND CONSEQUENTIALISM

Even if there is no intuitively satisfying solution to the problem of free will, it does not follow that there is no correct view of the matter. Ours is as follows: when it comes to the issue of free will itself, hard determinism is mostly correct. Free will, as we ordinarily understand it, is an illusion. However, it does not follow from the fact that free will is an illusion that there is no legitimate place for responsibility. Recall from earlier in this chapter that there are two general justifications for holding people legally responsible for their actions. The retributive justification, by which the goal of punishment is to give people what they really deserve, does depend on this dubious notion of free will. However, the consequentialist approach does not require a belief in free will at all. As consequentialists, we can hold people responsible for crimes simply because doing so has, on balance, beneficial effects through deterrence, containment, etc. It is sometimes said that if we do not believe in free will then we cannot legitimately punish anyone and that society must dissolve into anarchy. In a less hysterical vein, Daniel Wegner argues that free will, while illusory, is a necessary fiction for the maintenance of our social structure (Wegner 2002, ch. 9). We disagree. There are perfectly good, forward-looking justifications for punishing criminals that do not depend on metaphysical fictions. (Wegner's observations may apply best to the personal sphere: see later.)

The vindication of responsibility in the absence of free will means that there is more than a grain of truth in compatibilism. The consequentialist approach to responsibility generates a derivative notion of free will that we can embrace (Smart 1961). In the name of producing better consequences, we will want to make several distinctions among various actions and agents. To begin, we will want to distinguish the various classes of people who cannot be deterred by the law from those who can. That is, we will recognize many of the "diminished capacity" excuses that the law currently recognizes such as infancy and insanity. We will also recognize familiar justifications such those associated with crimes committed under duress (e.g. threat of death). If we like, then, we can say that the actions of rational people operating free from duress, etc. are free actions, and that such people are exercising their free will.

At this point, compatibilists such as Daniel Dennett may claim victory: "What more could one want from free will?" In a word: retributivism. We have argued that commonsense retributivism really does depend on a notion of free will that is scientifically suspect. Intuitively, we want to punish those people who truly deserve it, but whenever the causes of someone's bad behavior are made sufficiently vivid, we no longer see that person as truly deserving of punishment. This insight is expressed by the old French proverb: "to know all is to forgive all." It is also expressed in the teachings of religious figures, such as Jesus and Buddha, who preach a message of universal compassion. Neuroscience can make this message more compelling by vividly illustrating the mechanical nature of human action.

Our penal system is highly counter-productive from a consequentialist perspective, especially in the US, and yet it remains in place because retributivist principles have a powerful moral and political appeal (Lacey 1988; Tonry 2004). It is possible, however, that neuroscience will change these moral intuitions by undermining the intuitive, libertarian conceptions of free will on which retributivism depends.

As advocates of consequentialist legal reform, it behoves us to briefly respond to the three standard criticisms levied against consequentialist theories of punishment. First, it is claimed that consequentialism would justify extreme overpunishing. As noted earlier, it is possible in principle that the goal of deterrence would justify punishing parking violations with the death penalty or framing innocent people to make examples of them. Here, the standard response is adequate. The idea that such practices could, in the real world, make society happier on balance is absurd. Second, it is claimed that consequentialism justifies extreme underpunishment. In response to some versions of this objection, our response is the same as above. Deceptive practices such as a policy of faking punishment cannot survive in a free society, and a free society is required for the pursuit of most consequentialist ends. In other cases consequentialism may advocate more lenient punishments for people who, intuitively, deserve worse. Here, we maintain that a deeper understanding of human action and human nature will lead people—more of them, at any rate—to abandon these retributivist intuitions. Our response is much the same to the third and most general criticism of consequentialist punishment, which is that even when consequentialism gets the punishment policy right, it does so for the wrong reasons. These supposedly right reasons are reasons that we reject, however intuitive and natural they may feel. They are, we maintain, grounded in a metaphysical view of human action that is scientifically dubious and therefore an unfit basis for public policy in a pluralistic society.

Finally, as defenders of hard determinism and a consequentialist approach to responsibility, we should briefly address some standard concerns about the rejection of free will and conceptions of responsibility that depend on it. First, does not the fact that you can raise your hand "at will" prove that free will is real? Not in the sense that matters. As Daniel Wegner (2002) has argued, our first-person sense of ourselves as having free will may be a systematic illusion. And from a third-person perspective, we simply do not assume that anyone who exhibits voluntary control over his body is free in the relevant sense, as in the case of Mr Puppet.

A more serious challenge is the claim that our commitments to free will and retributivism are simply inescapable for all practical purposes. Regarding free will, one might wonder whether one can so much as make a decision without implicitly assuming that one is free to choose among one's apparent options. Regarding responsibility and punishment, one might wonder if it is humanly possible to deny our retributive impulses (Strawson 1962; Pettit 2002). This challenge is bolstered by recent work in the behavioral sciences suggesting that an intuitive sense of fairness runs deep in our primate lineage (Brosnan and De Waal 2003) and that an adaptive tendency towards retributive punishment may have been a crucial development in the biological and cultural evolution of human sociality (Fehr and Gachter 2002; Boyd *et al.* 2003; Bowles and Gintis 2004). Recent neuroscientific findings have added further support to this view, suggesting that the impulse to exact punishment may be driven by phylogenetically old mechanisms in the brain (Sanfey *et al.* 2003). These mechanisms may be an efficient and perhaps essential, device for maintaining social stability. If retributivism runs that deep and is that useful, one might wonder whether we have any serious hope of, or reason for, getting rid of it. Have we any real choice but to see one another as free agents who deserve to be rewarded and punished for our past behaviors?

We offer the following analogy: modern physics tells us that space is curved. Nevertheless, it may be impossible for us to see the world as anything other than flatly Euclidean in our day-to-day lives. And there are, no doubt, deep evolutionary explanations for our Euclidean tendencies. Does it then follow that we are forever bound by our innate Euclidean psychology? The answer depends on the domain of life in question. In navigating the aisles of the grocery store, an intuitive, Euclidean representation of space is not only adequate, but probably inevitable. However, when we are, for example, planning the launch of a spacecraft, we can and should make use of relativistic physical principles that are less intuitive but more accurate. In other words, a Euclidean perspective is not necessary for *all* practical purposes, and the same may be true for our implicit commitment to free will and retributivism. For most day-to-day purposes it may be pointless or impossible to view ourselves or others in this detached sort of way. But—and this is the crucial point—it may not be pointless or impossible to adopt this perspective when one is deciding what the criminal law should be or whether a given defendant should be put to death for his crimes. These may be special situations, analogous to those routinely encountered by "rocket scientists," in which the counter-intuitive truth that we legitimately ignore most of the time can and should be acknowledged.

Finally, there is the worry that to reject free will is to render all of life pointless: why would you bother with anything if it has all long since been determined? The answer is that you will bother because you are a human, and that is what humans do. Even if you decide, as part of a little intellectual exercise, that you are going to sit around and do nothing because you have concluded that you have no free will, you are eventually going to get up and make yourself a sandwich. And if you don't, you've got bigger problems than philosophy can fix.

Conclusion

Neuroscience is unlikely to tell us anything that will challenge the law's stated assumptions. However, we maintain that advances in neuroscience are likely to change the way people think about human action and criminal responsibility by vividly illustrating lessons that some people appreciated long ago. Free will as we ordinarily understand it is an illusion generated by our cognitive architecture. Retributivist notions of criminal responsibility ultimately depend on this illusion, and, if we are lucky, they will give way to consequentialist ones, thus radically transforming our approach to criminal justice. At this time, the law deals firmly but mercifully with individuals whose behavior is obviously the product of forces that are ultimately beyond their control. Some day, the law may treat all convicted criminals this way. That is, humanely.

Acknowledgments

The authors thank Stephen Morse, Andrea Heberlein, Aaron Schurger, Jennifer Kessler, and Simon Keller for their input.

References

Adolphs, R. (1999). Social cognition and the human brain. *Trends in Cognitive Sciences*, **3**, 469–79.

Baron Cohen, S. (2000). Autism: deficits in folk psychology exist alongside superiority in folk physics. In S. Baron Cohen, H. Tager Flusberg, and D. Cohen (eds.) *Understanding Other Minds: Perspectives from Autism and Developmental Cognitive Neuroscience*, pp. 78–82. New York: Oxford University Press.

Bentham, J. (1982). *An Introduction to the Principles of Morals and Legislation*. London: Methuen.

Bowles, S. and Gintis, H. (2004). The evolution of strong reciprocity: cooperation in heterogeneous populations. *Theoretical Population Biology*, **65**, 17–28.

Boyd, R., Gintis, H., Bowles, S., and Richerson, P.J. (2003). The evolution of altruistic punishment. *Proceedings of the National Academy of Sciences of the United States of America*, **100**, 3531–5.

Brosnan, S.F. and De Waal, F.B. (2003). Monkeys reject unequal pay. *Nature*, **425**, 297–9.

Dennett, D.C. (1984). *Elbow room: The Varieties of Free Will Worth Wanting*. Cambridge, MA: MIT Press.

Dennett, D.C. (1987). *The Intentional Stance*. Cambridge, MA: MIT Press.

Dennett, D.C. (1991). *Consciousness Explained*. Boston, MA: Little Brown and Co.

Dennett, D.C. (2003). *Freedom Evolves*. New York: Viking.

Fehr, E. and Gachter, S. (2002). Altruistic punishment in humans. *Nature*, **415**, 137–40.

Fodor, J.A. (1987). *Psychosemantics: The Problem of Meaning in the Philosophy of Mind*. Cambridge, MA: MIT Press.

Frankfurt, H. (1966). Alternate possibilities and moral responsibility. *Journal of Philosophy*, **66**, 829–39.

Goldstein, A.M., Morse, S.J., and Shapiro, D.L. (2003). Evaluation of criminal responsibility. In A. M. Goldstein (ed.) *Forensic Psychology*.vol. 11, pp. 381–406. New York: Wiley.

Goldstein, A.S. (1967). *The Insanity Defense*. New Haven, CT: Yale University Press.

Hart, H.L.A. (1968). *Punishment and responsibility*. Cambridge University Press.

Heberlein, A.S. and Adolphs, R. (2004). Impaired spontaneous anthropomorphizing despite intact perception and social knowledge. *Proceedings of the National Academy of Sciences of the United States of America*, **101**, 7487–91.

Heider, F. and Simmel, M. (1944). An experimental study of apparent behavior. *American Journal of Psychology*, **57**, 243–59.

Hughs, R.I.G. (1992). *The Structure and Interpretation of Quantum Mechanics*. Cambridge, MA: Harvard University Press.

Kahneman, D. and Tversky, A. (2000). *Choices, Values, and Frames*. New York: Cambridge University Press.

Kant, I. (2002). *The Philosophy of Law: An Exposition of the Fundamental Principles of Jurisprudence as the Science of Right*. Union, NJ: Lawbook Exchange.

Lacey, N. (1988). *State Punishment: Political Principles and Community Values*. London: Routledge and Kegan Paul.

McCloskey, M., Caramazza, A., and Green, B. (1980). Curvilinear motion in the absence of external forces: naïve beliefs about the motion of objects. *Science*, **210**, 1139–41.

Mele, A. (1995). *Autonomous Agents: From Self-Control to Autonomy*. New York: Oxford University Press.

Morse, S.J. (2004). New neuroscience, old problems. In B. Garland (ed.) *Neuroscience and the Law: Brain, Mind, and the Scales of Justice*, pp. 157–98. New York: Dana Press.

Pettit, P. (2002). *The Capacity to Have Done Otherwise. Rules, Reasons, and Norms: Selected Essays*. Oxford: Oxford University Press.

Pincus, J.H. (2001). *Base Instincts: What Makes Killers Kill?* New York: Norton.

Pinker, S. (1997). *How the Mind Works*. New York: Norton.

Premack, D. and Woodruff, G. (1978). Does the chimpanzee have a theory of mind? *Behavioral and Brain Science*, **4**, 515–26.

Rosen, G. (2002). The case for incompatibilism. *Philosophy and Phenomenological Research*, **64**, 699–706.

Sanfey, A.G., Rilling, J.K., Aronson, J.A., Nystrom, L.E., and Cohen, J.D. (2003). The neural basis of economic decisionmaking in the ultimatum game. *Science*, **300**, 1755–8.

Saxe, R., Carey, S., and Kanwisher, N. (2004). Understanding other minds: liking developmental psychology and functional neuroimaging. *Annual Review of Psychology*, **55**, 87–124.

Scholl, B.J. and Tremoulet, P.D. (2000). Perceptual causality and animacy. *Trends in Cognitive Science*, **4**, 299–309.

Shear, J. (1999). *Explaining Consciousness: The Hard Problem*. Cambridge, MA: MIT Press.

Smart, J.J.C. (1961). Free will, praise, and blame. *Mind*, **70**, 291–306.

Steinberg, L. and Scott, E.S. (2003). Less guilty by reason of adolescence: developmental immaturity, diminished responsibility, and the juvenile death penalty. *American Psychologist*, **58**, 1009–18.

Strawson, P.F. (1962). Freedom and resentment. *Proceedings of the British Academy*, **xlviii**, 1–25.

Tonry, M. (2004). *Thinking About Crime: Sense and Sensibility in American Penal Culture*. New York: Oxford University Press.

Van Inwagen, P. (1982). The incompatibility of free will and determinism. In G. Watson (ed.) *Free Will*, pp. 46–58. New York: Oxford University Press.

Watson, G. (1982). *Free Will*. New York: Oxford University Press.

Wegner, D.M. (2002). *The Illusion of Conscious Will*. Cambridge, MA: MIT Press.

Wright, R. (1994). *The Moral Animal: Evolutionary Psychology and Everyday Life*. New York: Pantheon.

CHAPTER 40

NEW DIRECTIONS IN NEUROSCIENCE POLICY

TENEILLE R. BROWN AND
JENNIFER B. McCORMICK

To some, scientific discovery is an engine that fuels the intellect, career, and even, when friends are gracious, social conversations. But even if one is not a person whose life is steered by science, there probably still have been occasions to marvel at the profound depth of what it means to be human: our complex emotions, memories, and thoughts; our sense of ourselves; our decision-making capacity; and our consciousness. How is this all possible? To be sure, the brain is at the center of this inquiry. And as the interdisciplinary field of neuroscience focuses on the brain, it is in a unique position to answer questions that are exceptionally interesting, not just to those passionate about the science, but also to humanity generally. The problem, however, is that human interest in the brain is so great that social institutions risk prematurely demanding too much of neuroscience.

This chapter is intended to accomplish two goals: first, to describe some of the diverse areas where neuroscience findings have overlapped with policy and the law; and second, to provide concrete questions that policymakers, which we mean to include judges and lawyers, interest groups, individual lobbyists, and legislators, should answer before relying on neuroscience research. The central thesis of this chapter is that neuroscience findings, particularly those that relate to complex human behavior, must be used with care and caution. Until they are thoroughly vetted through the scientific process, neuroscience findings must be interpreted narrowly and in context, or they risk being abused for political gain.

THE DEPTH OF NEUROETHICS

Before we branch out to the many domains where neuroscience and policy meet, let us first begin at the roots. Neuroethics examines the intersection between ethics and neuroscience, and as such it rests on a very rich intellectual base that for centuries has inquired into the ethical issues associated with mind and behavior (Illes and Bird 2006). As philosophers have been contemplating the ideas of free will, identity, and moral decision making for thousands of years, one scholar cleverly referred to neuroethics as in some ways representing old wine in a new bottle (Moreno 2003). Even if the ethics of neuroscience does not present completely new questions, the ability to localize activity in the brain and chart relative differences in brain activity and metabolism places neuroscience in a special position among the life sciences. Localization might lead to exciting hypotheses against which scientists are able to test basic presumptions about the neuropsychology and biology of human decision making.

Thus, not only is there an ethics of neuroscience research, but as researchers elucidate how the human brain makes decisions, neuroscience findings might enlighten the views generally held on agency, consciousness and social thought. This reciprocal nature of the relationship between ethics and neuroscience may yield what the prominent cognitive neuroscientist Michael Gazzaniga has referred to as a brain-based philosophy of life (Gazzaniga 2005). Even if neuroscience does not inform the entire life philosophy of individuals and social institutions, at the very least neuroscience findings will both inform and question the foundations of legal and policy decisions.

In order to capitalize on neuroscience findings in an intelligent and ethical manner, debate and deliberation about the science and its uses must respect the stage of discovery from which the data came. For example, neuroscience findings could hit news desks and judicial chambers at varying points on the trajectory from preliminary finding to fully grown and replicated population data. This is an obvious point generally, but it is one that is not fully appreciated by policymakers, and perhaps even scientists. One only needs to review headlines such as "This is your brain on politics" (Iacoboni *et al.* 2007) from *The New York Times*, in order to see how preliminary research findings can be co-opted for political purposes.

Part of the explanation for the co-opting of neuroscience by policymakers may be simply that the two disciplines are beholden to different social norms for knowledge production. Scientists stake truth claims based upon empirical data that are created in order to disprove or prove working research hypotheses. In science, there is no inherent value in protecting current belief based on data collected in the past, and in fact, entire careers may be made by successfully challenging the orthodox view. Policymakers, on the other hand, have to either dismiss the ideology, relevance, or facts of the status quo, or yield to it. In this way, precedent is a jealous mistress to policymakers that demands explicit genuflection. If policymakers decide to deviate from the path of those before them, they must explain this departure by relying on one of a handful of tools at their disposal.

One such tool is to distinguish a seemingly applicable law by arguing that the relevant details of a statute or case are not completely comparable and therefore the law should not apply in this instance. Policymakers can turn to non-binding authorities from other jurisdictions as persuasive text, or they can argue that a law is unfair or does not maximize social utility. After availing themselves of the traditional swords, policymakers may rely on empirical data, but it is often an instrument of last resort. Viewed like this, it becomes less surprising that policymakers may view science as yet another argumentative tool in their arsenal, and once something becomes a tool, it ceases to exist in its own right and has value only by being leveraged. In this way, policymakers are the principals and science is their agent. But to scientists, the pursuit of knowledge is their principal, and they are merely the agents for discovery.

Scientists also have their tools. They consist largely of methods, materials, and equipment: statistical analyses, stem cells, chemicals, mice, DNA sequencers, and mass spectrometers.

In its purest, ideal form, science discovery is internally agnostic to politics. We emphasize here that this is the ideal—and that because scientists are social beings, asking the research questions and designing the experiments, this ideal may be arguably unattainable, and this notion is a point of well-reasoned debate. Still, it is the cultural norm of respected scientists to attempt to remove personal bias in their methodology and data analysis. Precisely because of this pursuit of unbiased findings, science possesses the allure of resting objectively above politics. This view would be naïve; while the methodology of science ought to be agnostic, there are still limits on how the research question and findings can be *applied*, and whether the applications are fair or useful.

Just as it might not be obvious to scientists that lawyers have a hierarchy of sources they rely upon in making arguments, it may not be obvious to lawyers that science comes in many shapes and stages. Some data stem from pilot projects with very small sample sizes, some involve unusual experimental conditions that do not mirror the real world, some confirm or challenge previous findings, some are done in rats and squid, some extend a finding to a new population, some cannot be published because they produce a negative result, and some emerge from longitudinal studies in large populations that may take decades to be completed. Unlike in the law, there is no set hierarchy for which type of research data are best. Of course it is critical to make that initial, potentially paradigm-changing finding; however, it is also quite important to see if a result is generalizable to different groups and is capable of replication across different laboratories. Independent validation allows for extrapolation of a finding to create targeted drugs, devices, or other treatment programs.

Even though the sciences do not privilege one type of finding over the other, policy figures should still understand where the data fit on the methodological spectrum, as the social utility will depend greatly on how robust the findings are and how many times they have been replicated. Policymakers should also unpack what might appear to be banal details about sample size and base rates, statistical significance and external validity. These are concepts about which most law and policy people have virtually no training even though they present considerable roadblocks to effective social use of science. Absent some clarity on the methodological limitations, neuroscience data may be cloaked by opportunistic players for political gain.

This co-opting of neuroscience is quite likely, given the history of its older sibling behavioral genetics. Behavioral genetics arguments were also thought to carry an extraordinary amount of pedagogical and social weight, as the public craved genetic support for pre-existing theories about social behavior (Nelkin and Lindee 1995). Thus, individuals, and the public generally, readily consume stories about genes for adultery or genes for homosexuality, or genes for committing murder. Even though there might be considerable overlap in public appetite, thoughtful scholars have noted that the ethical issues raised by neuroscience are not identical to those raised by genetics and genomics, as "our genes are causally far removed from our behaviours" while our brains are not (Illes and Racine 2005; Roskies 2007, p. S54).

THE MAGNETISM OF NEUROSCIENCE FINDINGS

Neuroscience has the potential to energize arguments in ways that are not necessarily backed by data (Brown and Murphy 2010). This is true for many reasons. One reason is neuroessentialism, which captures the idea that we are our brains and our brains are us (Doucet 2007). Another is that humans identify and relate with our brains in ways that we do not with our prostate or adrenal glands. Humans also have a special affiliation with the brain because of what has been dubbed "neurorealism," a term used to explain how coverage of brain imaging studies "can make a phenomenon uncritically real, objective or effective in the eyes of the public" (Racine *et al.* 2005, p. 3). In other words, seeing a picture of the brain somehow explains a finding and places it on a pedestal of truth, the authority of which cannot be obtained by referencing the results of a genetic assay.

Perhaps because of this phenomenon many individuals may believe they have the ability to interpret a functional neuroimage, even if the image is a statistical construct of the metabolic activity of the brain and not, as many people misunderstand, a snapshot of the brain at work. Despite being poorly understood, the novel methods behind neuroimaging and other relatively new technologies such as transcranial magnetic stimulation (that uses a short pulse applied to the skull to boost or disrupt local brain activity) have begun to revolutionize our understanding of the human brain and its function. Of course, imaging methods and stimulation devices stand on the shoulders of psychological giants; without solid psychological theories and networks of behavior, cognition, and emotion, the meaning of "activated" neuronal networks would not be clear. Activated appears in quotes because of course the brain is always active, and the brain images merely take advantage of relative differences in metabolism in specific regions of interest.

By contextualizing the findings and building on the interdisciplinary strengths in physics, statistics, biochemistry, neurology, and psychology, neuroscience findings and their importance are coming into sharper focus. Some of these discoveries are allowing neuroscientists to determine the underlying mechanisms for diseases that affect everything from movement to mood. In addition to the many existing targeted treatments, there are thousands more on the horizon, providing hope for a huge segment of the population afflicted with neurological or mental illness. These same discoveries, however, are also finding uses outside of the medical realm—some of these good, some perhaps questionable, and others simply ugly.

It is with this theme of contextualizing neuroscience findings and placing them on the spectrum of social utility that we situate our discussion. Next, we suggest that neuroscientists ought to take more responsibility for how their apolitical research is ultimately used, while at the same time legal professionals and policymakers ought to resist the temptation to ask more of the science than it can currently provide. We then suggest that a funding model for neuroethics research be developed that would enable the creation of a body of empirical data that can be used to inform thoughtful, fair, and efficient public policies. What we propose includes some of the features of the Genome Institute's Ethical Legal and Social Implications (ELSI) program, but is different in some important respects. For example, funding responsibility for this type of research ought to belong to multiple governmental agencies and private foundations. Finally, we recommend a non-exhaustive list of questions that should be asked before going down the road of neuroscience-informed law or policy.

NEUROSCIENCE: THE GOOD, THE GRAY, AND THE UGLY

Given the multiple ways and contexts in which results of neuroscience can be applied, we propose that generally there are three domains in which these might be categorized: the Good, the Gray (or questionable), and the Ugly. The Good applications are those in which there is a fairly clear consensus that, on balance, the particular use of the finding has sufficient social and individual benefit when weighed against the costs to the same. The goals outlined at the onset are being met and there is general acceptance of the relative value of the outcomes. The Gray, on the other hand, represents those applications of neuroscience that might be questionable or controversial because of differences in religious values, cultural norms, or political motivations. These applications might also be questionable because, although the underlying finding was born out of sound scientific principles, the particular use might be exploiting or over-extending the science. Finally, the Ugly are those applications that are politically and socially unacceptable by most if not all, or involve some sense of government coercion or privacy violation that is not generally thought to be justified by the countervailing social benefit.

Virtually every finding in neuroscience has the prospect of being either socially destructive or socially beneficial, which is to say that the same research data could be used in ways that might be thought of as good, gray, or ugly. To some extent this echoes the US science policy discussions around dual use technologies, defense versus commercial use, and export controls (Neal *et al.* 2009, pp. 188–9, 321). The gray area is the most fertile ground for our discussion of neuroethics, as it presents the most challenging area for policymakers. If a scientific finding or technological development is generally considered good or bad, politicians know where to spend their political capital. But in the gray area, precisely because it is a gray area, stakeholders can highlight only the elements of the data that support their needs or can cover up interpretive limitations to let the seemingly objective science do the talking.

The likely outcome, then, is that when there is disagreement on values or social norms, science can be leaned on to arbitrate what is at its core a non-scientific problem.

Science in general and neuroscience in particular have often been summoned to answer moral dilemmas such as "which criminals are deserving of execution?" (Aronson 2007) and "how should teachers allocate resources between boy and girl students?" (Gurian and Stevens 2007). While these questions may be informed by neuroscientific findings related to cognitive development or effective learning strategies, data alone cannot provide authoritative answers. This is because most social policies are not driven by wholly empirical factors; they are also guided by our sense of justice, equality, and autonomy, among other values. Because policymakers can decide to ignore data if it suggests a normatively unattractive outcome or is merely inefficient, legal and policy decisions typically only rely on science when it is convenient to do so, or as a method of last resort. There are many examples of areas where the scientific data are solid, and yet for policy reasons, there is a decision to ignore what the data are saying (Loftus and Hoffman 1989; Faigman and Saks 2008). Perhaps it is simpler to defer to the wisdom of science to divine the answers, for example, determining punishment for wrongdoers and educational configurations for children, side stepping the hard psychosocial questions about equality of liberty. It is not to say that findings from neuroscience research cannot be properly applied to the particular social question. Rather the challenge is to know how to use the science, recognize when the science is premature, and not over-extend the data and blur the lines between the subjective and the objective. With neuroscience, the appearance of reductionist objectivity provides for an even greater disconnect between what the data can suggest, and what they are being promoted to say (Roskies 2008). With that, we will begin our analysis of some key neuroscience findings, and the ways in which they have been, or may be, applied in good, gray, and ugly ways.

Using preliminary data in laboratory settings and extrapolating to inferences about individuals: problems with external and internal validity in lie detection studies

Currently, jurors, parole boards, and civil commitment committees are using rough behavioral estimates to determine whether the person on the witness stand is telling the truth. These determinations can have significant consequences and can establish whether the person walks out to freedom or languishes in a prison cell for years. Typically, the parties perform this critical function in a very unscientific way—by looking to see whether the witness appears nervous, is making eye contact, is shifting in his seat, or if his story appears too rehearsed. Clearly, a cunning liar can easily manipulate the system.

In another setting, voters attempt to determine whether or not to trust a political candidate, based on her demeanor, behavior, and general comfort while speaking. Just as charismatic liars may be acquitted so too may disingenuous officials be elected into office, as the public believes them to be telling the truth in their promises that fall short of reality. These are just two examples within the realm of public policy for which it would be useful, to say the least, to have more reliable and valid forms of detecting individual lies.

A small number of researchers to date have had moderate successes predicting who is concealing information during brain imaging studies. These findings are compromised by a significant problem, however: in many the subjects were not in fact being asked to lie. Instead, they were being told by a research confederate to lie when asked by the investigator, thus measuring compliance rather than deception. A recent study sought to measure the act of lying, rather than compliance with instruction to lie. This study was conducted by Joshua Greene and Joseph Paxton using functional magnetic resonance imaging (fMRI). FMRI is a specific type of magnetic resonance imaging system that measures the flow of oxygenated blood in the brain. Blood flow and metabolism serve as an indirect proxy for neuronal activity. In regions of the brain where there is a large amount of oxygenated blood it is assumed that there is increased activity in that region. However, the premise behind fMRI is currently being investigated further and challenged, as a surplus of oxygenated blood may reflect a number of phenomena other than increased neuronal firing. In any event, in the Greene study, subjects were not told that the study was about detecting deception. Rather, they were told that the phenomenon under investigation was clairvoyance—whether the subjects could predict the flip of a coin as heads or tails more than 50% of the time. Using this method, the researchers probed whether individuals presented with an opportunity for dishonest gain (correctly guessing the 50/50 heads or tails flip of a coin) exhibited greater control or lack of conflict/temptation to lie (Greene and Paxton 2009). They demonstrated that individuals who behaved honestly exhibited no increased activation in areas associated with control when choosing to behave honestly. By comparison, individuals who behaved dishonestly showed relative increases bilaterally in the dorsolateral prefrontal cortex (DLPFC) associated with control, both when choosing to lie about their prediction and when they refrained from lying.

In spite of the fascinating work that has been done, using functional imaging of the brain to detect deception in individuals in the courtroom is not appropriate at this time. There is currently insufficient evidence demonstrating fMRI to be valid or reliable for this purpose. Even if relative increases in certain brain regions are evident, this does not mean that an individual is lying. As the mapping of structure to function is not a one-to-one relationship, the relative increase in blood flow may be suggestive of thoughts of disgust, frustration, or anger, or indicate the individual is performing a mental calculation such as how much or little to disclose. Further, reduced relative activation in a particular region might result from habituation and expertise rather than deficiency. Essentially, the data from functional imaging could suggest a host of possibilities, only one of which may be lying (Brown and Murphy 2010). Moreover, some of the studies being used to support the use of brain-based deception detection in the courtroom were designed in a manner that has no direct correspondence to how the technology would be used for forensic purposes.

The popular press tends to overlook the limitations of the methods and tends to shine more light on the possibilities of being able to predict whether someone is telling the truth (Sip *et al.* 2008). As a result, statements such as this are promulgated as fact: "areas of [the] brain associated with emotion, conflict, and cognitive control – the amygdala, rostral cingulate, caudate, and thalamus – were "hot" when I was lying but "cold" when I was telling the truth" (Silberman 2006). First, the amygdala appears to be involved in many sensory experiences including hunger, lust, and anger: identifying it as "hot" is almost absurd. The colors are chosen arbitrarily after the fact, and there is nothing to suggest that more activation means that one is lying, unless we know more about the psychological process underlying the art of deception. Perhaps greater activation in one area is related to conflict management or impulse control, as it implicates the networks involved in these processes. Or, the relative increase in activation in one area might not be capturing the inhibition of neurons. Neuronal inhibition is as important in the signal transmission in brain physiology as is neuronal activation, and the potential inability of fMRI to detect this aspect of brain function underscores further that merely saying an area is "hot" or "cold" is patently naïve. Further, the default networks of the brain are always active, and unless the entire brain is surveyed during every decision, the filters that are used to measure brain activation will sometimes focus the lens on one area at the expense of viewing another brain region. A more accurate description might be that these areas under investigation appeared to recruit more oxygenated blood than they normally would when the individual is telling the truth. Moreover, to specifically tie this increased activation with the act of lying is using the imagining data to make a correlation that is not truly validated by the data. The same blurring occurs with the cingulate cortex and thalamus—regions of the brain that are likewise leveraged in many daily tasks: "Look here, when you're telling the truth, this area is asleep. But when you're trying to deceive, the signals are loud and clear" (Silberman 2006). This remark is misleading, as there is never a time when regions of the brain are asleep; source: (silberman 2006) the brain is thankfully always active. But these statements by a respected researcher, in trying to convey lie detection results to a journalist, illustrate the deep misunderstanding about what neuroimaging findings can meaningfully demonstrate.

Two commercial companies have been providing lie detection services on the commercial market, at various points claiming that their reports would be admissible in courts regardless of the purpose for which they were being offered. The law, however, does not allow admissibility determinations to be made in a vacuum; the evidence being introduced must be relevant and probative for the purpose it is being used. Still, these companies have sought to market their products for legal applications. The methods are currently marginally better at confirming truth in compliant adults, so it appears that the chief audience is couples who are suspicious of adultery. This may be even more socially destructive than legal uses. Private individuals have no expert counsel to cross-examine the findings and challenge the weak methodology when confronted with "hard science" evidence that a spouse is not telling the truth about adulterous behavior. As such, these data have the potential to irresponsibly and permanently break up marriages and families, and shatter lives.

This entire discussion might seem like science fiction, but in fact in June of 2008 brain-based lie detection (or brain-based memory detection) was used in a criminal case in Pune, India, where 24-year-old Aditi Sharma was convicted of murdering her ex-fiancé, Udit Bharati. The state's circumstantial evidence against Sharma was weak. This may be why the opinion relied heavily on a form of brain-based lie detection called brain electrical oscillations signature (BEOS). The BEOS test relies on a brain response called the P300 wave detected by using an electoencephalograph (EEG). The P300 wave is an aggregate recording from many neurons as measured using electrodes applied to the scalp (Picton 1992). The P300 wave is useful for measuring cognitive decisions because the subject cannot consciously control whether it is triggered. While its neural substrates are still being determined, the P300 wave is often elicited in response to the subject making a novel, or odd, observation. This is the finding that has been manipulated for lie detection or "guilty knowledge" tests. The idea is that the presence of a P300 wave is meant to suggest whether the subject has or has not seen a particular item or heard a particular phrase.

The problem with using the P300 wave as evidence of whether someone committed a crime is that the signal cannot presently differentiate between experiential knowledge (i.e. knowledge of previous personal memory or activity) and content knowledge (i.e. familiarity based on exposure or non-personal experience). Examples of the latter would be if the defendant were familiar with elements of a particular crime because she has read about them in the newspaper or heard about them on the radio. In this case, the EEG results might not show that this information is novel, but it would not be because the subject personally engaged in the act that is being presented to her. In Sharma's case, forensic researchers placed 32 EEG electrodes on her head and read aloud their version of events, speaking in the first person ("I bought arsenic"; "I met Udit at McDonald's"), along with seemingly neutral statements (like "the sky is blue") to ostensibly distinguish between her personal memories and general facts. The state forensic scientist boldly asserted that the BEOS data were proof that Ms. Sharma committed the murder rather than just having heard about it. The trial judge agreed. Based on what appears in large part to be findings from unverified and unvalidated BEOS technology, Sharma and her husband, Pravin Khandelwal, were sentenced to life in prison. Subsequently, both have been granted bail by the Bombay High Court. Pravin's sentence was suspended on the grounds that there was no real evidence to tie him to the case as a conspirator. Sharma was released based on the fact that the evidence of her possessing the arsenic was not compelling, and indeed "the possibility of plantation [of arsenic] cannot not be ruled out." But as for the underlying methodological flaws in the BEOS technique, little is publicly known.

The ugly uses of brain-based lie detection are not unheard of in the US, either. In a juvenile sex-abuse and child protection case in San Diego, the guardian wanted to admit a report based on the results of functional neuroimaging done by a San Diego-based company registered as No Lie MRI. This is the first case known of where a party attempted to introduce brain-based lie detection in the US, even though the individual introducing the report agreed to withdraw his request for the evidence to be heard. Presumably the scan and resulting report were going to show that the man accused of abuse was telling the truth when he denied sexually abusing a child (Washburn 2009).

Brain-based lie detection that draws inferences based on research findings with limited external validity is an ugly use of the neuroscience, especially when the consequences could be imprisonment or freedom, life or death, or custody of a child or no custody. In other situations, however, there may be room for debate. Should employers be allowed to conduct brain-based lie detection tests prior to hiring someone, for example, for positions in which huge sums of money are handled? Would it be more appropriate to rely on brain-based lie detection as a crude and preliminary test of whether someone is lying to his parole board? Similarly an elite preparatory school may find it beneficial to screen all applicants not just through test scores and letters of recommendation, but also with lie detection tests, with the goal of identifying students with a propensity to cheat and plagiarize. While some may believe such screening to be a clear social misuse of science and technology, others may not, suggesting that ugliness of using brain-based lie detection in some social domains may not be clear-cut. Here, we suggest that the use of neuroscience falls into the gray area of our proposed spectrum of social utility.

Researchers are beginning to replicate their data and test it in more real-world like settings (Kozel et al. 2009). As the external validity of the lie detection studies improves, it moves the methodology one step closer in the direction of having a potentially valid social use (Kozel et al. 2004). Once the technology is deemed sufficiently reliable and valid for social uses, we must then engage in a normative discussion of whether each particular use is ethical, moral, and cost-justified.

The ethics of using neuroscience to prevent certain groups from being executed

In 2002, the Supreme Court of the US decided *Atkins v. Virginia*, which held that executions of mentally retarded criminals were "cruel and unusual punishments" prohibited by the Eighth Amendment of the US Constitution (*Atkins v. Virginia* 2002). Later on in *Roper v. Simmons*, the Court extended this opinion to children, holding that the execution of individuals who were under 18 years of age the time of their crimes is prohibited by the Eighth and Fourteenth Amendments (*Roper v. Simmons* 2005). The American Psychological Association (APA) submitted an amicus brief to the Court arguing, based on the neuroscience research of Jay Giedd and others (Johnson et al. 2009), that adolescents do not have the full capacity to control their impulses, as the prefrontal cortex does not fully develop until approximately 25 years of age. While the majority opinion did not specifically refer to the APA's amicus brief, it might have been the triggering point to reverse case law. The dissent, however, did reference the APA brief. Justice Antonin Scalia argued that neuroscience evidence was used by the APA in a previous case to argue the opposite: namely, that a "rich body of research" showed that juveniles were mature enough to decide whether or not to obtain an abortion without parental involvement (*Roper v. Simmons* 2005, 618). This manner of reasoning highlights how various types of neuroscience data presented as evidence may be confounded, facilitating sharp legal minds to inadvertently mistaken the mental processes under investigation (Steinberg *et al.* 2009, p. 585). It is entirely possible that juveniles might be both incapable of fully appreciating the consequences of their actions in moments of intense, and often unanticipated, emotion, while also having a brain that has developed enough to make decisions about long-term consequences that have less to do with impulse.

The Eighth Amendment's prohibition on cruel and unusual punishment is meant to respond to evolving standards of decency. As such, one might expect that new findings from neuroscience could be extended from *Atkins* to eliminate the death penalty in cases where the defendant suffers from a mental illness such as psychopathy or schizophrenia. That is, if neuroscience findings could provide a biomarker or biological basis for certain types of impulsive behavior, then arguments such as those made by the APA in *Roper* might be used in other populations that demonstrate similar deficits in cognitive and emotional control. However, such neuroscience evidence could be a double-edged sword—the direction of the cut depending on the sympathy a particular population evokes. If the argument is that both psychopaths and schizophrenics may be similar to children and the mentally retarded in their difficulty controlling their impulses, then the evolving neuroscience research could possibly be used as an aggravating factor against the argument, leading to greater punishment and civil commitment, rather than less (Snead 2007).

Retrofitting neuroscience findings for education policy

Several labs have discovered sex differences in the human brain (Shaywitz 1995; Gur 1999). Some suggest that women have better language aptitudes than men, and men have greater ability to build systems (Baron-Cohen 2003). Many of these findings have been replicated and are taken as a given in the research community. Some of the findings are more fringe. Even so, there are respected researchers who have concluded that the brains of girls and boys develop along different time courses, and they have, on average, relative differences between them in function. Even though there might be solid population data on the differences between girls' and boys' brains and their development, the neuroscience of sex differences does not direct us as to how we ought to engage with the sexes and how we ought to choreograph classroom and other learning settings. It is therefore not a question of the strength of the science that makes this use ugly, but rather the way that the science is abused or misused to make policy arguments that may be socially destructive.

Social institutions rejoiced in the findings that, on average, the brains of females differ from the brains of males in some ways. Some journalists published op-eds, that many—both women and men, would find offensive, making statements that women are the dumber sex, and this "is amply supported by neurological and standardized-testing evidence" (Allen

2008). It is quite tempting to use neuroscience findings in this manner, bending and twisting what the data actually say to make socially antiquated arguments (Weil 2008). To date there has not been any peer-reviewed study demonstrating a reliable measure of intelligence, defined broadly, that places men above women. Even so, inaccurate applications of neuroscience data find their way into the public domain to be absorbed and re-applied in ways that can be socially harmful to many and might seem to support antiquated social biases.

Some researchers, but mostly business people, have taken such findings on sex differences to argue for sweeping changes in the way we treat women and men, or boys and girls (Norfleet 2007). Specifically, two men, Leonard Sax and Michael Gurian are using these findings to advocate for sex-segregated education in public schools (Gurian *et al.* 2001). Michael Gurian is a corporate consultant and a novelist, and Leonard Sax is a psychologist. These men rely completely on the scientific findings of other labs, as neither conducts his own research. They advocate for disparate treatment of boys and girls by teachers. Notably, a junior high student in Louisiana filed a motion for an injunction to prevent her school from adopting the sex-segregated teaching policy that local officials planned to implement. The student's argument was that the sex-segregation violated Title IX and the Equal Protection Clause of the Fourteenth Amendment. From her legal arguments, we learn of a real example where policymakers in one district planned to use Sax's viewpoint from his book *Why Gender Matters* to structure its sex-segregated curriculum. Below are some of the suggestions from *Why Gender Matters* that the Louisiana high school planned to adopt that we learn about from the court filing:[1]

- Girls have more sensitive hearing than boys. Thus, teachers should not raise their voices at girls and must maintain quiet classrooms, as girls are easily distracted by noises. Conversely, teachers should yell at boys, because of their lack of hearing sensitivity.

- Because of biological differences in the brain, boys need to practice pursuing and killing prey, while girls need to practice taking care of babies. As a result, boys should be permitted to roughhouse during recess and to play contact sports, to learn the rules of aggression. Such play is more dangerous for girls, because girls do not know how to manage aggression.

- Having girls take off their shoes in class is a good way to keep stress from impairing girls' performance

- Girls need real-world applications to understand math, while boys understand and enjoy math theory. Girls understand number theory better when they can count flower petals or segments of artichokes, for instance, to make the theory concrete.

- Literature teachers should not ask boys about characters' emotions, and should only focus on what the characters actually did. But teachers should focus on characters' emotions in teaching literature to girls.

And from the teacher's guide that comes with Michael Gurian's book, *Boys and Girls Learn Differently!*, we learn that "[a]dolescent males receive surges of the hormone testosterone

---

[1] Memorandum of Law in Support of Plaitniffs' Motion for a Temporary Restraining Order in the United States District Court, Middle District of Louisiana, Michelle Selden v. Livingston Parish School Board

five to seven times a day; this can increase spatial skills, such as higher math. Increased estrogen during the menstrual cycle increases female performance in all skills, including spatials, so an adolescent girl may perform well on any test, including math, a few days per month." Gurian also argues that teachers should give boys Nerf baseball bats so that they can release tension during class. The training sessions that Gurian conducts for teachers are teeming with brain scans and the window-dressings of neuroscience data. On his institute's website, Gurian claims that "we in business tend to prefer science to art and anecdote, and many of popular culture's suggestions regarding women and men have felt more like artful opinion than fact-based, empirical knowledge. Fortunately, now, things have changed. PET scans and MRIs of men and women's brains are useful training tools. These are powerful and compelling, as well as easy to look at." (Lapidus and Martin 2008). In what is now perhaps a predictable story, entrepreneurs are leaning heavily on what appears to be incredibly objective neuroscience data to do exactly what it is they are critiquing—reinforcing popular culture's suggestions about the way we humans behave.

Sex segregation based on the current neuroscience data is an ugly use of science because it side steps an important question about education—and how our public education system *ought* to be teaching our children. Even if differences in learning style could be demonstrated, does that argue for carving up the group so they cannot learn strategies from each other? Policymakers have to start with articulating the goals of any education system and work backward from there. Is education meant to accommodate or to challenge? Should systems attempt to reach out to every child, or use crude proxies to reach most? By adopting sex-segregation policies, are policymakers acknowledging that they do not have the resources for teachers to model their approach differently for each child?

There are good data available arguing that students learn differently based on a whole host of idiosyncratic factors including the way they were raised, how often they read, how auditory they are, and how much they can sit still. Many of these variables do not sort neatly on sex lines. Sorting by sex based solely on findings from brain research appears to be an incredibly blunt tool to use for tailoring educational strategies. This sort of policy only takes into account the existing biological or physiological phenomena, that may or may not be broadly generalizable to every individual, and that certainly ignore environmental and social contexts.

There is potential for responsible and ethical applications of neuroscience research in education. In fact, in June 2009, the Society for Neuroscience sponsored a summit on this very topic and issued a report in which the participants outlined existing problematic uses of neuroscience in education, the needs to move beyond these, and how to move forward (Neuroscience Research in Education Summit 2009). The broad goal of the summit and the initiatives likely to arise from it is to determine how neuroscience research can inform educational strategies and ensure its appropriate use in teaching paradigms.

Using demonstrated findings for use in a new population

Devices and drugs that have been demonstrated to be clinically effective in one population—and actually quite beneficial to alleviating symptoms and allowing for some normality in daily activities—are also being used in unverified clinical contexts (i.e. potentially harmful) or for completely non-clinical (i.e. recreational) purposes. In some cases this is a good use of neuroscience, and in some cases it is gray. We will start with the development of deep brain stimulators in Parkinson's patients and the desire by some to use this experimentally in people who are clinically depressed. We will then discuss a different type of transition use—from clinical to recreational, or self-improvement.

Deep brain stimulators for Parkinson's disease

Treatments for Parkinson's disease have changed quite a bit in the last 20 years, with targeted ablation surgeries being replaced by therapeutic use of L-dopa in the 1960s, a drug that helps promote greater uptake of dopamine in the brain. While patients initially respond quite well to L-dopa, eventually many patients stop responding and develop other movement complications that can be worse than those caused by Parkinson's itself (Kleiner-Fishman *et al.* 2006). Because of these common complications, neurologists have returned to surgical therapies. One of the more recent treatments is deep brain stimulation, or DBS, which involves placing a medical device (called a "brain pacemaker") in the brain (Laitinen *et al.* 1992). Electrodes are implanted in targeted regions of the brain—the most common for Parkinson's being the subthalamic nuclei, and provide electrical impulses to modulate stimulation in these areas. The advantage of DBS over L-dopa is that rising and falling drug levels can lead to motor fluctuations, while the DBS pacemaker controls symptoms continuously. Several peer-reviewed studies have now found that DBS appears to be safe and effective in reducing Parkinson's symptoms (Rodriguez-Oroz *et al.* 2005). However, before these studies were done in the late 1990s, clinicians were experimenting with DBS (Kumar *et al.* 1998). Whether or not this was appropriate depends on the answers to a few questions. First, what was the likelihood and magnitude of harm to the patient? On how many patients had this safety and efficacy testing been demonstrated? Were the subjects similar to patient of the clinician considering DBS as treatment? What were the patient's other options? Had the safe and effective alternatives, like L-dopa, stopped working? How much does it cost?[2] So long as the parkinsonian patient was competent and understood the risk and cost of DBS, the use of this device to treat Parkinson's would likely be thought of as a "good" use of a neuroscience finding.

Given the success of DBS for treating parkinsonian patients, work is being done to determine whether there is a clinical application for individuals suffering from depression. Researchers have observed that DBS of the white matter tracts near the subgenual cingulated gyrus is associated with "a striking and sustained remission" of depression in four out of six individuals who received DBS as a treatment (Mayberg 2005). Given the highly experimental nature and the small sample size, what should clinically depressed patients need to demonstrate before they are appropriate candidates for DBS? Use of DBS in clinically depressed patients has yet to be made standard of care, and therefore a clinician's decision to

---

[2] According to data available online, DBS surgery costs about $80,000. If the pacemaker battery needs to be replaced, it will cost between around $15,000, in addition to the price of surgery. Insurance will often cover the full cost of a new battery.

use it, without ample population data and thorough clinical testing, should be informed by the risks, reliability, and validity of DBS, along with the efficacy of the alternatives. Sometimes clinicians do not have all of these data and thus their decision to use DBS to treat a patient with clinical depression might be questionable, or fall within the gray zone of our paradigm.

What is known is that the risks of DBS are significant, including infection in the brain, stroke, memory loss, personality and behavioral change, and even exaggerated depression. Given the breadth of medical options, it would appear that the clinical depression would have to be pretty severe, resistant to talk therapy and all of the many medical interventions, to contemplate undergoing experimental DBS for depression (Glannon 2008; Wolpe *et al.* 2008). Unlike advanced stage Parkinson's, clinical depression for some is not a long-term condition and can sometimes be treated successfully with the symptoms subsiding without further medication. Even so, clinical depression can be incredibly debilitating. The clinician/researcher would need to be very careful to ensure that the depressed individual fully appreciates the risks of DBS and the relative benefit that it might or might not afford him.

The use of therapeutics for recreational cognitive augmentation

One "good" use of neuroscience would be when research findings lead to the development of a targeted delivery drug that operates on specific faulty mechanisms, completely correcting or alleviating debilitating symptoms. There are abundant examples of this with a variety of antidepressants for the treatment of depression and a variety of antipsychotics for the treatment of schizophrenia. While not taking care of all symptoms, these classes of drugs have certainly improved the quality of life and productivity for millions of individuals. Another example of "good" uses of neuroscience would be the development of certain drugs prescribed for fatigue or severe sleepiness. Modafinil is one such drug, which has been demonstrated to be safe and effective for the treatment of narcolepsy and excessive daytime sleepiness associated with sleep apnea or shift-work (Rammohan *et al.* 2002). Being alert and able to stay awake after a long night shift promotes public safety, health, and productivity. If the night-shift population were never able to function with a clear head we might have many more road accidents as truckers fall asleep at the wheel and more mistakes made by pilots, flight crews, and air controllers unable to stay awake through overseas flights. Or we might have surgeons with sleep apnea who were drowsy in the middle of a critical emergency heart surgery. Given that today's society is dependent on a successfully operational 24/7 culture (which we recognize is a point of debate itself), these types of failures could have negative consequences for many. Until quite recently, modafinil was thought to have relatively few side effects or risks in this population (Broughton 1997). Given these factors, the use of modafinil in the approved population is probably a positive application of science.

An "ugly" use of modafinil may occur when a parent, with high expectations, gives her otherwise healthy kindergarten child modafinil (or methylphenidate or dextroamphetamine—two drugs prescribed for attention deficit disorder) without her child's knowledge, so that the child will gain a competitive edge in school. The reasons this is an ugly use are that the child cannot voice her desires, the motivations are not clearly beneficent, and the long-term effects on the healthy pediatric brain are not well known. Another potential ugly use would be where everyone in a particular city unknowingly or without consent received modafinil through their water supply for the sole purpose of enabling a fully operational 24/7 work-force. While these uses may be ethical to some outlier policymakers, given the balance of social and individual risk and benefit, many other individuals may view such uses as socially unacceptable, largely because of lack of full knowledge by, or consent of, the targeted individual or population. However, if the general public is comfortable restricting the autonomous choices of a particular group (such as sexually violent predators or criminal inmates generally) then the coerced use of the approved drug might appear less "ugly" and more subjective, and perhaps would fall into our gray zone of questionable use.

Any drug can have unintended long-term effects on the brain, but is even more likely when the drug is being used by people who do not exhibit the symptoms for which the drug has been tested and approved. This is often thought of as an off-label use, and it would include the two examples of involuntary dosing of healthy children and entire cities discussed above. Off-label use of drugs or devices refers to the provider prescribing something for a purpose for which it is not approved by the Food and Drug Administration (FDA). This use is allowed because the FDA does not interfere with a physician's independent practice of medicine and treatment choices; however, the drug or device company cannot market their product for an off-label use. There are examples in which drugs used for off-label purposes have been clinically tested for safety and effectiveness and professional organizations have recommended the practice: beta blockers for congestive heart failure and baby aspirin as a prophylaxis against cardiovascular disease in certain sub-populations (Stafford 2008; Healy 2009). There are debates as to whether it is ethical to insist that individuals wait for the long, expensive, and arduous FDA approval process before they can access a drug that might provide some benefit. It is not our place here to engage in that discussion. Instead we want to point to a type of off-label use of drugs in which the purpose is primarily to augment normal function or behavior—not to remedy a health condition.

One particularly common example of this is the use of modafinil in "normals" who seek not to treat a sleepiness disorder but to enhance their cognitive performance. Some leaders in the field of neuroethics find this practice to be ethically acceptable, so long as it is done responsibly in consenting adults and that concerns about unfair access are addressed (Greely 2008). Framed this way, the off-label use of this drug presents no new ethical hurdles, as many adults take drugs prescribed by their doctor for an off-label use. Even so, others worry about whether cognitive enhancement might stir up what it means to be an authentic version of yourself, whether individuals ought to strive for perfection (Satel 2004), whether wide-spread off-label use of modafinil redefines socially acceptable behavioral and performance standards, and whether these off-label uses are fair, safe, or socially destructive. Either way, new data suggests that modafinil does significantly enhance performance on various memory, cognition, and motor tasks in healthy normals (Turner et al. 2003).

While it might be tempting for a healthy college student to take modafinil to achieve a perfect score on a test, there are some risks, however difficult to measure. First, very little is known on how these biologics affect the non-disordered or diseased brain. A few studies have been done, and a recent one in rats suggested that despite what was previously thought, modafinil might affect the dopaminergic system and become a potential drug of abuse (Jeffrey 2009; Volkow et al. 2009). Second, once the drug becomes widely used on college campuses and students trade in their prescribed medication, two potentially damaging events occur: an individual does not receive the therapeutic she requires and a second individual takes a substance with unknown effects on his brain chemistry and physiology. Similar concerns arise with methylphenidate or dextroamphetamine, because of their potential to temporarily improve cognitive function and provide a competitive edge in a very competitive environment. Third, the source of the drug obtained may be questionable; recognizing a potential specialized niche, Internet entrepreneurs can sell the drugs on the black market. If and how the drugs have been altered by these entrepreneurs is a legitimate concern. No doubt the black market likely exists for other types of FDA approved drugs that can be used recreationally such as diazepam, sildenafil, or acetaminophen with hydrocodone, creating the same concern we articulate for off-label use of modafinil. And indeed, these examples ought not—cannot—be overlooked. Even so, we suggest that because a sense of competitiveness and remaining on par with peers largely drives the misuse of substances like modafinil and methylphenidate, the population susceptible to questionable sources of drugs expands, and thus so does the associated risk, to a group who might not otherwise take illegal or off-label drugs. Equality also seems to be more of a concern in drugs that enhance cognition: If individuals do not desire to put their health at risk by taking an off-label drug (from any source), are they placing themselves at an academic disadvantage? Is this a fair choice for adults, or one that is socially destructive?

Colleagues have presented cogent arguments for human enhancement using genetic technologies on the premise that there is equal access to the technologies (Caplan *et al.* 1999). The same could be said of pharmaceuticals that improve cognition. However, such universal equal access is an idealist's dream, given the culture of competitiveness, the growing divide between the haves and have-nots, and the current lack of ability to adequately meet basic human needs for all people. Arguments on the other side challenge this by referencing the status quo of unfairness in achievement (i.e. how is off-label use of modafinil any different from expensive SAT preparation courses?). But is it a defensible ethical argument to reference other types of inequity? If policymakers did not believe in mitigating discrimination and inequity this tenet, each new form of discrimination might be embraced, on the grounds that we could never eradicate implicit and deep-seeded biases. The larger argument for off-label use of modafinil comes from looking to whether the health and social risks are outweighed by the social and individual benefits (Farah 2005).

In a similar vein, the military are, and historically have been, very interested in neuroscience findings that might affect or improve cognitive function (Moreno 2001). Currently the Department of Defense and members of the intelligence community are interested in understanding the brain and potential biologics that allow soldiers to remain more alert and functional even after extremely long periods without sleep. Likewise they are also interested in understanding how to increase soldiers' resilience to pressures to divulge high-level security information and how to entice potential enemies to disclose information with minimal physical and psychological distress.

While beneficial in the context of considering the safety of a nation's military personnel and the defense of the country's citizens as a whole, this legitimization of enhancement could open the way for questionable uses outside the context of the military. Quite often, when a technology is developed for military use and is found to have use outside the context of defense, the technology can find its way into the civilian population—hence the use of the phrase dual use in the context of defense sponsored research (Neal *et al.* 2009).

For example, currently there is much debate in the physician education community as to the "right" number of work hours for medical residents. The long-held tradition has been that residents often work shifts that extend over a 24-hour period—usually with very little, if any sleep. It has long been part of the training—and one "test" to becoming a physician. There have been recent efforts to minimize shift hours (ACGME 2002; Ulmer *et al.* 2008) but anecdotal evidence suggests that many residents are resistant to the change—for various reasons (pride, fines imposed on departments, duty to their patients, etc). These residents are a likely population of off-label users of any alertness and cognitive enhancing drugs that the military would develop and use for national safety and security purposes. Whether such application is appropriate in either the physician training or the military domain we would argue is questionable. While in the context of physician training it is important to acknowledge the complexity of the situation and examine it closely, we would suggest perhaps focusing attention on policy issues such as the cost of medical education, fiscal structures that enable adequate hospital staffing, and culture change within the physician profession might also be in order.

Even if it is difficult to draw meaningful philosophical distinctions between drug-based cognitive enhancers and other forms of enhancement, it is important to note that drug-based enhancements do encourage the medicalization of normal behavior in addition to encouraging yet another form of health access inequality. Medicalization is worrisome because it often makes it more likely that importance of behavioral and social interventions will be overlooked or hugely under-valued in favor of a quick fix offered by a pill.

But not all off-label use is sinister. Sometimes clinicians prescribe a treatment that is so experimental that it is really better thought of as an "n of 1" study, where their patient is the only subject and their data may or may not ever be published or recorded. Using research findings or off-label uses to inform clinical decision making is fairly common. Some clinicians might be irresponsible in their prescribing habits, but many are partnering with their patients to problem-solve in creative ways when options are running out and desperation sets in. While clinicians might need guidance as to which questions to ask in determining which experimental therapies to try, they likely have some rough sense of comparative efficacy and appropriate care. A recent commentary in the *Archives of Internal Medicine* presents an ethical and professional guide framework for physicians (and patients) for a practice that is inevitable (Largent *et al.* 2009).

SHARED RESPONSIBILITY FOR IMPLEMENTING ETHICAL NEUROSCIENCE POLICIES

The examples discussed in the previous section are meant to emphasize the intersection of neuroscience research across several social domains. Indeed, hopefully the previous section also pointed out the balancing act that is required—the balancing of the good with the bad and an exploration of the questionable uses. A societal goal for science generated from scientific research is to facilitate, perhaps even maximize, the positive uses that can come while simultaneously minimizing and ideally avoiding, the negative outcomes. Of course imbedded in this notion is the necessity to have a discussion on what is positive and what is negative and how each is determined. That discussion belongs in the public domain, by and among policymakers, scientists, and private individuals. Because of the prominence of the brain as an image and the powerful effects of neuroessentialism, it is important, in fact one could argue imperative, that ethical and legal implications of the research be openly debated and policy and social considerations be integrated into the neuroscience research process and training (Sahakian and Morein-Zamir 2009). While many would probably agree with these statements, the question to be answered is who specifically has the responsibility to initiate these conversations and deliberations? Although there are individuals ideally positioned to help with the responsibility of balancing the positive and negative uses of neuroscience research, some are passing it off or "outsourcing" this responsibility. Even so, it must be mentioned that in the field of neuroethics, there appears to be much more involvement by the scientific community and interaction with lawyers than in other areas of bioethics.

Scientists are in a prime position to be contributing to the balancing we described—they understand what is possible technologically at the moment and what might be feasible in the future (and how feasible). Scientists are in a position to predict possible paths of translation of the knowledge they generate and to pose questions about the social and policy implications, should any of those translational paths be taken. What is more as citizens within society, while still motivated in part by self-interest, they have a general sensibility of what might be right or wrong in terms of social application of the knowledge, as they are closer to the precise findings, the methodological limitations of the research, and the specific research question. Of course opportunistic scientists could over-extend their own work, and this no doubt occurs. Policymakers will have to learn how to weed these individuals out and communicate with the scientists who are generally well respected as being less biased in their interpretations. Neal Lane, former Presidential Science Advisor, is known for his use of the phrase "civic scientist." When describing a civic scientist, Lane beseeches his fellow scientists to listen to the needs, expectations, hopes, and concerns of their fellow citizens and give consideration to these as they do their work, and to participate in the public debates to contribute their contemplations of the potential social and policy applications of the science.

Lane is not the first to make such pleas. Albert Einstein noted in a 1931 talk at Caltech that scientists of all disciplines should not get lost in their diagrams, equations, and models, but need to remember that "the concerns of mankind and his fate" ought to be a main impetus for their scientific endeavors. Our interpretation is that scientists have a responsibility to give consideration to how their work may eventually be used externally without internally manipulating methods to bias the scientific inquiry itself. Scientific integrity and responsible research is more than not engaging in fabrication, falsification, or plagiarism. It entails, incorporating into the scientific method consideration of possible ethical and social implications and how they may impact public policies. Yet, many seem to be agnostic about their work in this context.

Legal professionals and policymakers are also in a prime position to contribute to this necessary balancing act. In day-to-day practice policymakers may not see this as part of their charge, but in all practicality it is, given their place in our social institutions. Once informed by neuroscientists, policymakers may then have a better appreciation of how neuroscience findings applied in a broader social context could or would influence public policy, incentives, and individual and community well being. Unlike scientists, however, this group tends to fall short of recognizing that science outside the walls of the laboratory is no longer an independent and isolated domain of knowledge. They may overlook the fact that their use of scientific data clearly places the scientific findings into a social context. That is, those in the legal and policy communities can be "blinded by the science," and ignore questions of feasibility or ecological validity.

Indeed, scientific research is the pursuit of "truth"—but not Truth. Neuroscience research, as with most scientific research, happens in a controlled and regulated setting. The truth that is found is the truth for that situation and in the current moment, and it cannot be forgotten that science is dynamic, not a simple linear model as described by Vannevar Bush in *Science – The Endless Frontier* (5 July 1945). Several authors have suggested science is more than just a simple linear process (Stokes 1997; Neal *et al.* 2009 figure 1.3). The dynamic model as proposed by Neal, Smith, and McCormick suggests that regardless of what stage neuroscience is at, it can inform both the fundamental questions we ask, the potential ways in which we apply the knowledge, and the eventual public consumption. We take this yet one step further to suggest that at any point within the dynamic process of scientific discovery, questions of how the science might influence or impact social institutions and public policies can legitimately—and should be asked by scientists themselves, law- and policymakers, and the public.

PROPOSED FUNDING MODEL

Early on in the development of the National Institutes of Health (NIH) Human Genome Project, organizers realized that the new genomic discoveries might present unique questions that should be addressed simultaneously with the research (Meslin *et al.* 2007). Thus the ELSI program was born, which generated an impressive amount of scholarship on areas of research priority such as privacy, fairness, professional education, and clinical integration (Fisher 2005). While the researchers funded through the ELSI program have helped considerably to guide the conduct of ethics research and the public understanding of the genome, the project has also been criticized for lacking tangible policy deliverables. Without weighing in on that particular discussion, which ultimately depends on how one defines and measures policy success, it does seem that the model suffered from a few structural issues. First, in creating the ELSI program, and in particular the Centers for Excellence in Ethics Research (CEERS), a tight-knit group of researchers who could speak to each other and develop non-overlapping areas of expertise was formed. At the same time, this organizational structure of housing the ELSI program within the NHGRI encouraged an insular dynamic in the genetics and ethics community, ossifying the potential range of research topics and narrowing the number of different perspectives that were heard. As is the case in many domains of research, investigators need to "brand" themselves and their research agendas in order to receive large-scale grants. Once this branding takes place, what happens is, in effect, a market capture. What also happens is shoe-horning, where the researcher will see every additional discovery as necessitating the same type of questions they have asked before, even if more appropriate questions should be asked first. Having virtually one funding source encourages this type of market capture and internal politicization of research ideas. In a different way, projects that are publicly funded are limited in the policy suggestions they can make. As noted scholar Hank Greely has pointed out while suggesting both public and private funding of neuroethics research, "there are some inherent constraints on what government-funded ELSI-type programs can do. They are limited in the issues they can consider and the things they can say" (Greely 2002).

Given the lessons learned from the ground-breaking ELSI program and given the broad array of interdisciplinary and highly philosophical issues raised by neuroscience, it seems that researchers examining the intersection of neuroscience with ethics, law, policy, and society should pursue multiple avenues for funding. In addition to public funding through the NIH, partnerships with private foundations should be sought. An example of private foundation support is the MacArthur Foundation's Law and Neuroscience Project, which has already funded small workshops on law and neuroscience, white papers and research projects on brain-based lie detection, an empirical review of cases involving neuroimaging in California, demonstration projects on implicit racial bias in jurors, and imaging studies examining how individuals make decisions about punishments. If the MacArthur Law and Neuroscience Project continues on beyond the initially funded 3 years, it is intended to fund larger research projects that could not otherwise be funded through NIH or the National Science Foundation (NSF). Given the moderate amounts of funding so far, the project has produced some fantastic results. Another private option may be the Greenwall Foundation. This independent non-profit foundation has a rich history and provides grants for the arts, humanities, and bioethics (Otten 1999). Its board of directors has recently embarked on a developing a plan to strengthen scholarship in bioethics, which the Foundation sees as instrumental in the face of the coming challenges. One piece of this plan might be to make an explicit effort to fund research at the intersection of ethics, policy, and neuroscience.

Another way of injecting ethics into the basic neuroscience research is to approach journals like *Neuron, Cognitive Science, Nature Neuroscience, Journal of Neuroscience*, and others, to request that the publications implement standards requiring peer-reviewed articles to include a sentence or two on the potential ethical and societal implications of their research. This would not be very thorough, but it would be a great way of highlighting potential ethical concerns by the people who are most familiar with the methodological limitations of the data and its external validity. To be sure, the statements made would probably be fairly speculative, but this same critique was made of requiring scholars to disclose potential conflicts of interest, and it has also served as a signal to researchers that disclosure is important. While this technique will not resolve any of the social issues, at least it would require the bench scientists to think about the potential impact their science might have on society, and alert policy researchers to the perhaps otherwise unobvious potential or lack of potential. In order for this to be reliable and not self-aggrandizing, the peer review process would have to apply to this section, peer-review panels would need to include an ethical and social review, and a robust conflicts of interest disclosure would be required.

This of course raises the question as to whether neuroscientists are aware of ethical, social, and policy implications of their research. While studies indicate that some scientists think about the ethical and social implications of their research (McCormick *et al.* 2009), these same studies suggest that a significant number give little attention to such issues for various reasons including lack of perceived relevancy and simple lack of awareness (McCormick *et al.* unpublished). Others have called for increased attention to public engagement and communication in neuroscience training programs (Illes *et al.* 2009), and we extend that call to include both formal and informal training venues for discussions about potential ethical and legal implications and how to include policy and social considerations throughout the research process.

Another suggestion for how to inject ethics into neuroscience research would be for the field to create professional norms and internal reputation sanctions to discourage researchers from dismissing the social and ethical implications of their research. Much has been written on norm creation and internalization in psychology, sociology, and economics, and we do not have space to delve into that rich literature here. Suffice it to say that there are points of social intersection where the field could create norms. One such opportunity would involve hosting conferences where one day's plenary or panel sessions discuss ways of raising potential ethical and social implications of the neuroscience findings. Meetings could also make sure that the neuroethics and the science and society posters are not located in the far corners of the conference center, where only those actively seeking these posters venture. The Society for Neuroscience could incorporate more than just one panel session on social issues over the course of its 4-day annual meeting. These are just a few suggestions, but the idea is that from within the neuroscience community, institutional norms could be created to signal to researchers that the ethical implications of research are not entirely for separate "neuroethics" conferences. While not being a primary focus of the basic science researchers, they should at least have some sense of the neuroethics discussion and contribute to it in some way.

In addition to internal norm-structuring, political groups should encourage multi-institute funding of ELSI research across all NIH institutes and centers. What a lasting legacy the current NIH Director would have were he to adapt the ELSI program—that he oversaw as the Director of NHGR—across the Institutes. In this specific case, rather than boot-strapping on the ELSI program by tailoring research as being neuroscience + genetics, other institutes engaged in neuroscience-related research (NIMH, NIDA, NIAAA NINDS, etc.) should be approached politically for setting aside some amount of money for research on the ethical and legal implications of neuroscience. This budget allocation could require that some small percentage of their research budget deal with the policy and social issues arising from the laboratory science they support. Outside of the NIH, the Department of Defense and the Department of Education might also be approached for developing funding for neuroethics research, given the obvious military and education uses (and abuses) of neuroscience research. While this requires considerable political motivation and currency, it is not insurmountable.

SUGGESTING A FRAMEWORK FOR POLICYMAKERS

The aim of this article was to inject a little humility into the way neuroscience findings are used by policymakers. Hopefully, by walking through various uses of neuroscience—some good, most gray, and some ugly—the chapter demonstrates the extreme diversity of neuroscience data, and the varying levels of ripeness for specific policy uses. Because neuroscience data will have different value depending on the application, articulated below are ten related and non-exhaustive factors that policymakers should consider before injecting a normative or policy debate with neuroscience data.

Questions one should ask before infusing policy or law with neuroscience data

- What is the probability of harm to the person whose neuroscience data is being analyzed? To the community?
- What is the magnitude of that harm to the individual? To the community of which the individual is a member?
- How reliable are the data? Have they been sufficiently replicated in the correct population, or is this a novel first-time finding?
- Have the data been peer-reviewed thoroughly?
- How valid are the data? Does the research protocol model the relevant real life setting at all, or is the experimental design unrealistic for social use?
- Is there a lack of knowledge as to the differences between people on the given variable that might have no effect on their social functioning? (I.e. normal individual differences without functional deficit.)
- What is the positive predictive value of the finding as a "biomarker" for some trait? Do scientists know what the base rate is for this trait in the population? What is the risk of false-negatives and false-positives, and what is a socially justified amount of risk? (This will depend greatly on the context; there might be a higher tolerance with false positives in an employment screening policy than during the guilt phase of a capital trial, where someone stands to lose her life).
- How valid and reliable is the status quo alternative? Is the devil that is known (i.e. polygraphy) definitely worse than the devil that is not known (i.e. fMRI-based lie detection) or are we making assumptions about its predictive power because it looks so objective and fancy?
- What is the probability of social harm (i.e. considering elements of distributive justice, civil rights, equality, efficient allocation of resources, etc.)? Does this use encourage discrimination of groups, stigmatization, lack of equitable access, racism, sexism?
- What is the magnitude of social harm? Is it very likely that the harm could be mitigated in some way, or be offset by the social or individual benefit?

This list is not meant to be exhaustive. But perhaps it will serve as a starting point for those interested in using neuroscience data for policy arguments. If nothing else, we hope it highlights the fact that neuroscience data come in all shapes and sizes and levels of validity, and policymakers, individual lay public, and scientists must be careful not to retrofit a single finding to make arguments they are predisposed to want to make. Neuroscience might be able to inform analyses focused on the "what" of social policy and law. Once sufficiently robust and tailored to this purpose, the findings can help describe empirically what is happening in various social scenarios, which in turn may facilitate better policy responses to how humans behave individually and socially. But despite its allure, neuroscience cannot presently answer the questions about whether societies ought to have the social goals they have and when and how they ought to decide to flex scientific findings to support or confront those goals.

References

Accreditation Council for Graduate Medical Education (ACGME) (2002). *Report of the ACGME work group on resident duty hours,* 11 June 2002. Available at: http://www.acgme.org/acWebsite/dutyHours /dh_wkgroupreport611.pdf (accessed 22 November 2009).

Allen, C. (2008). We scream, we swoon. how dumb can we get? *The Washington Post,* 2 March 2008. Available at: http://www.washingtonpost.com/wp-dyn/content/article/2008/02/29/AR2008022902992_pf.html (accessed 22 November 2009).

Aronson, J.D. (2007). Brain imaging, culpability and the juvenile death penalty. *Psychology, Public Policy, and Law,* **13,** 115–42.

Atkins v. Virginia (2002). 536 U.S. 304

Baron-Cohen, S. (2003). *The Essential Difference: The Truth about the Male and Female Brain.* New York: Basic Books.

Broughton, R.J. (1997). Randomized, double-blind, placebo-controlled crossover trial of modafinil in the treatment of excessive daytime sleepiness in narcolepsy. *Neurology,* **49,** 444–51.

Brown, T. and Murphy, E.R. (2010). Through a scanner darkly: functional imaging as evidence of mental state. *Stanford Law Review,* **62,** 1119–208.

Bush, V. (1945). *Science – The Endless Frontier.* Washington, DC: US Government Printing Office.

Caplan, A. (2002). No brainer: can we cope with the ethical ramifications of new knowledge of the human brain? In S.J. Marcus (ed.) *Neuroethics: Mapping the Field,* pp.95–106 [conference proceedings]. New York: Dana Foundation.

Caplan, A., McGee, G., and Magnus, D. (1999). What is immoral about eugenics? *British Medical Journal,* **319,** 1284.

Doucet, H. (2007). Anthropological challenges raised by neuroscience. *Cambridge Quarterly of Healthcare Ethics,* **16,** 219–26.

Faigman, D. and Saks, M. (2008). Failed forensics: how forensic science lost its way and how it might yet find it. *Annual Review of Law and Social Science,* **4,** 149–71.

Farah, M. (2005). Neuroethics: the practical and the philosophical. *Trends in Cognitive Sciences,* **9,** 34–40.

Fisher, E. (2005). Lessons learned from the Ethical, Legal and Social Implications program (ELSI): Planning societal implications research for the National Nanotechnology Program. *Technology in Society,* **27,** 321–8.

Kleiner-Fishman, G., Herzog, J., Fisman, D.N., *et al.* (2006). Subthalamic nucleus deep brain stimulation: summary and meta-analysis of outcomes. *Movement Disorders,* **21,** S290–S304.

Gazzaniga, M. (2005). *The Ethical Brain.* New York: Harper Perennial.

Glannon, W. (2008). Deep-brain stimulation for depression. *HEC Forum,* **20,** 325–35.

Greely, H. (2002). Response. In S.J. Marcus (ed.) *Neuroethics: Mapping the Field,* pp.116–17 [conference proceedings]. New York: Dana Foundation.

Greely, H., Sahakian, B., Harris, J., *et al.* (2008). Towards responsible use of cognitive-enhancing drugs by the healthy. *Nature,* **456,** 702–5.

Greene, J. and Paxton, J. (2009). Patterns of neural activity associated with honest and dishonest moral decisions. *Proceedings of the National Academy of Sciences*, **106**, 12506–11.

Gur, R. (1999). Sex differences in brain gray and white matter in healthy young adults: correlations with cognitive performance. *The Journal of Neuroscience*, **19**, 4065–72.

Gurian, M., Henley, P., and Trueman, T. (2001). *Boys and Girls Learn Differently: A Guide for Teachers and Parents*, 1st edn. New York: Jossey-Bass.

Gurian, M. and Stevens, K. (2007). *The Minds of Boys: Saving our Sons from Falling Behind in School and Life*. New York: Jossey-Bass.

Healy, M. (2009). Prescribing drugs 'off-label': an ethical prescription. *Los Angeles Times*, 26 October 2009. Available at: http://latimesblogs.latimes.com/booster_shots/2009/10/prescribing-drugs-offlabel-an-ethical-prescription.html (accessed 21 November 2009).

Iacoboni, M., Freedman, J., Kaplan, J., *et al.* (2007). This is your brain on politics. *New York Times*, 11 November 2007. Available at: http://www.nytimes.com/2007/11/11/opinion/11freedman.html?_r=1&adxnnl=1&adxnnlx=1258902014-Fi2WBZbnXja1YPfaIlgkSA (accessed 22 November 2009).

Illes, J. and Racine, E. (2005). Imaging or imagining? A neuroethics challenge informed by genetics. *American Journal of Bioethics*, **5**, 5–18.

Illes, J. and Bird, S. (2006). Neuroethics: a modern context for ethics in neuroscience. *Trends in Neurosciences*, **29**, 511–17.

Illes J., Moser M.A., McCormick, J.B., *et al.* (2010). NeuroTalk: improving the communication of neuroscience. *Nature Reviews Neuroscience*, **11**, 61–9.

Jeffrey, S. (2009). Study flags potential for abuse and dependence with modafinil. *Medscape Medical News*, 20 March 2009. Available at: http://www.medscape.com/viewarticle/589934_print (accessed 21 November 2009)

Kozel, F.A., Padgett, T.M. and George, M.S. (2004). A replication study of the neural correlates of deception. *Behavioral Neuroscience*, **118**, 852–6.

Kozel, F.A., Johnson, K.A., Grenesko, E.L., *et al.* (2009). Functional MRI detection of deception after committing a mock sabotage crime. *Journal of Forensic Sciences*, **54**, 220–31.

Kumar, R., Lozano, A.M., Kim, Y.J., *et al.* (1998). Double-blind evaluation of subthalamic nucleus deep brain stimulation in advanced Parkinson's disease. *Neurology*, **51**, 850–5.

Laitinen, L.V., Bergenheim, A.T., and Hariz, M.I. (1992). Leksell's posteroventral pallidotomy in the treatment of Parkinson's disease. *Journal of Neurosurgery*, **76**, 53–61.

Lapidus, L. and Martin, E. Antiquated gender stereotypes underlie radical experiments in sex-segregated education. *ACLU Blog Of Rights*, 3 March 2008. Available at: http://www.aclu.org/blog/womens-rights/antiquated-gender-stereotypes-underlie-radical-experiments-sex-segregated-educati (accessed 21 November 2009).

Largent, E.A., Miller, F.G. and Pearson S.D. (2009). Going off-label without venturing off-course: evidence and ethical off-label prescribing. *Archives of Internal Medicine*, **169**, 1745–7.

Loftus, E. and Hoffman, H.G. (1989). Misinformation & memory: the creation of new memories. *Journal of Experimental Psychology*, **118**, 100–4.

Mayberg, H. (2005). Deep brain stimulation for treatment-resistant depression. *Neuron*, **45**, 651–60.

McCormick, J.B., Boyce, A.M. and Cho, M.K. (2009). Biomedical scientists' perceptions of ethical and social implications: is there a role for research ethics consultation? *PLoS ONE*, **4**, e4659.

McCormick, J.B., Boyce, A.M., Ladd, J.M., and Cho, M.K. (in preparation). Barriers to considering ethical and societal implications of research: perceptions of biomedical scientists.

Meslin, E., Thomson, E. and Boyer, J. (1997). Bioethics inside the beltway: The Ethical, Legal, and Social Implications Research Program at the National Human Genome Research Institute. *Kennedy Institute of Ethics Journal*, 7.3, 291–8.

Moreno, J. (2001). *Undue Risk: secret state experiments on humans*. New York: Routledge.

Moreno, J. (2003). Neuroethics: an agenda for neuroscience and society. *Nature Reviews Neuroscience*, 4, 149–53.

Neal, H.A., Smith, T.L. and McCormick, J.B. (2009). *Beyond Sputnik: American science policy in the 21st century*. Ann Arbor, MI: University of Michigan Press.

Nelkin, D. and Lindee, S. (1995). *The DNA Mystique: The Gene as a Cultural Icon*. New York: WH Freeman & Co.

Neuroscience Research in Education Summit: The promise of interdisciplinary partnerships between brain sciences and education, 22–24 June 2009, Society for Neuroscience

Norfleet, J.A. (2007). *Teaching the Male Brain: How Boys Think, Feel, and Learn in School*. Thousand Oaks, CA: Corwin Press.

Otten, A.L. (1999). *The Greenwall Foundation: A Story of a Work in Progress*. New York: The Greenwall Foundation.

Picton, T. (1992). The P300 wave of the human event-related potential. *Journal of Clinical Neurophysiology*, 9, 456–79.

Racine, E., Bar-Ilan, O. and Illes, J. (2005). fMRI in the public eye. *Nature Reviews Neuroscience*, 6, 159–64.

Rammohan, K.W., Rosenberg, J.H., Lynn, D.J., *et al.* (2002). Efficacy and safety of modafinil (Provigil®) for the treatment of fatigue in multiple sclerosis: a two centre phase 2 study. *Journal of Neurology, Neurosurgery, and Psychiatry* 72, 179-183. See also http://www.provigil.com/index.php?t=pat&p=home for additional information about the drug from its seller.

Rodriguez-Oroz, M.C., Obeso, J.A., Lang, A.E., *et al.* (2005). Bilateral deep brain stimulation in Parkinson's disease: a multicentre study with 4 years follow-up. *Brain*, 128, 2240–9.

Roper v. Simmons (2005). 543 U.S. 551.

Roskies, A. (2007). Neuroethics beyond genethics. *EMBO Report*, 8, S52–6.

Roskies, A. (2008). Neuroimaging and inferential distance. *Neuroethics*, 1, 19.

Sahakian, B. and Morein-Zamir S. (2009). Neuroscientists need neuroethics teaching. *Science*, 325, 147.

Satel, M.J. (2004). The case against perfection. *The Atlantic Online*, April 2004. Available at: http://www.theatlantic.com/doc/print/200404/sandel (accessed 22 November 2009).

Shaywitz, B. (1995). Sex differences in the functional organization of the brain for language. *Nature*, 373, 607–9.

Silberman, S. (2006). Don't even think about lying: how brain scans are reinventing the science of lie detection. *Wired Magazine*, January 2006. Available at: http://www.wired.com/wired/archive/14.01/lying.html (accessed 22 November 2009)

Sip, K.E., Roepstorff, A., McGregor W., and Frith, C.D. (2008). Detecting deception: the scope and Limits. *Trends in Cognitive Science*, 12, 48–53.

Snead, O.C. (2007). Neuroimaging and the complexity of capital punishment. *New York Law Review*, 82, 1265–339.

Stafford, R.S. (2008). Regulating off-label drug use — rethinking the role of the FDA. *New England Journal of Medicine*, 358, 1427–9.

Steinberg, L. (2009). Are adolescents less mature than adults? Minors' access to abortion, the juvenile death penalty, and the alleged APA "flip-flop." *American Psychologist*, **64**, 583–94.

Stokes, D.E. (1997). *Pastuer's quadrant: basic science and technological innovation*. Washington, DC: Brookings Institution.

Turner, D.C., Robbins, T.W., Clark, L., *et al.* (2003). Cognitive enhancing effects of modafinil in healthy volunteers. *Psychopharmocology*, **165**, 260–9.

Ulmer, C., Wolman, D.M. and Johns, M.M.E. (2008). *Resident Duty Hours: Enhancing Sleep, Supervision, and Safety*. Washington, DC: National Academies Press.

Volkow N.D., Fowler J.S., Logan J., *et al.* (2009). Effects of modafinil on dopamine and dopamine transporters in the male human brain: clinical implications. *Journal of the American Medical Association*, **301**, 1148–54.

Washburn, D. Can this machine prove if you're lying? *VoiceOfSanDiego.org*, 1 April 2009. Available at: http://www.voiceofsandiego.org/articles/2009/04/02/science/953mri040109.txt (accessed 21 November 2009).

Weil, E. (2008). Teaching boys and girls separately. *New York Times Magazine*, 2 March 2008.

Wolpe, P., Ford, P. and Harhay, M. (2008). Ethical issues in deep brain stimulation. *Neurological Disease and Therapy*, **91**, 323–38.

CHAPTER 41

··

WOMEN'S NEUROETHICS

··

STACEY A. TOVINO

THIS chapter seeks to examine a range of ethical, legal, and social issues that are raised by scientific studies that report neurobiological differences between and within the female and male sexes in the context of depression and psychosis, including postpartum depression and psychosis. As such, this chapter aims to add to the growing literature in "women's neuroethics," which may be preliminary defined by its focus on neuroscientific work that has as its primary categories of analysis sex or gender, including sex- or gender-specific conditions and diseases (Chalfin *et al.* 2008).

In the first part of this chapter, I reference a limited number of studies that explore between- and within-sex differences associated with the incidence, prevalence, and nature of depression and psychosis in order to illustrate a broader trend among scientists with respect to the neuroscientific investigation of sex differences. In the second part of this chapter, I identify and examine several legal implications of these studies, including implications for criminal infanticide law, health insurance policy interpretation, mental health parity law, and disability discrimination law. In the third part of this chapter, I examine the risks and benefits of scientific studies that report neurobiological differences between and within the sexes and conclude that these studies have the potential to assist women by providing them with additional criminal, civil, and administrative protections and benefits, although the ethical and social implications invite more concern. I conclude by supporting additional neuroscientific research in the context of between- and within-sex differences, although I caution against premature legal and social applications.

A note regarding the language I use in this chapter: Many of the scientific studies I reference use the words "sex" and "gender" interchangeably. In this chapter, I use the word "sex" very narrowly to refer to one of two groups of individuals with certain chromosomal arrangements; that is, individuals who have two of the same sex chromosomes (XX) and are biologically classified as females and individuals who have two different sex chromosomes (XY) and are biologically classified as males. I use the word "gender" more broadly to refer to the socially constructed roles, behaviors, activities, and attributes that a given society considers appropriate for individuals of the female and male sex (World Health Organization 2009). This chapter focuses almost entirely on the ethical, legal, and social issues raised by scientific studies that report neurobiological differences between and within the sexes. I recognize that additional and important work could and should be devoted to the ethical, legal, and social issues raised by scientific studies that report neurobiological differences between and among genders, as well as between and among individuals whose chromosomal arrangements are contrary to their phenotypic sex (including XX males and XY females), as well as between and among individuals with unique chromosomal arrangements (including XO, XXX, XXY, and XYY).

SCIENTIFIC INVESTIGATION OF DEPRESSION AND PSYCHOSIS

A number of scientists are investigating sex differences associated with the incidence, prevalence, and nature of a range of psychiatric, neurological, and other central nervous system-related illnesses and diseases (Cahill 2006). The question of why depression is more common in females than males is one common inquiry. In a recent study, Janet Shibley Hyde and colleagues (Hyde *et al.* 2008) proposed an integrated, developmental model that integrates affective, biological, and cognitive factors as vulnerabilities to depression that, in interaction with negative life events, heighten young females' rates of depression beginning in adolescence and is believed to account for differences in the rates of depression experienced by girls and boys and, later in life, women and men. A second common inquiry is whether females and males with depression have different treatment responses to particular depression medications. In a multicenter study involving 400 female and 235 male participants, Susan Kornstein and colleagues (Kornstein *et al.* 2000) investigated whether females and males with chronic depression have different treatment responses to sertraline, a selective serotonin reuptake inhibitor, and imipramine, a tricyclic antidepressant. The study authors found a statistically significant interaction effect between treatment and sex for rates of dropout and treatment response. Females taking sertraline had lower dropout rates than females taking imipramine, whereas no difference was seen between groups among males. Females had a greater response rate in the sertraline group than in the imipramine group, and males had a greater response rate in the imipramine group than in the sertraline group. The study authors concluded that in patients with chronic depression, sertraline was more effective than imipramine and led to fewer dropouts in females and that imipramine was more effective than sertraline in males.

The question of whether postpartum depression and psychosis are different than the depressive and psychotic episodes experienced by males and non-postpartum females is a third common inquiry. The current edition of the *Diagnostic and Statistical Manual of Mental Disorders* (DSM-IV) states that the symptoms of a postpartum-onset episode of depression or psychosis do not differ from the symptoms of a non-postpartum-onset episode of depression or psychosis (DSM-IV-TR 2000). However, recent neuroimaging studies are beginning to suggest both structural and functional differences in the brains of depressed postpartum women compared to depressed non-postpartum controls. In one study, Mario Lanczik and colleagues (Lanczik *et al.* 1998) used computed tomography to quantify the ventricular and cisternal cerebrospinal fluid (CSF) spaces in female participants who had cycloid psychoses with postpartum onset. The scientists found that certain CSF spaces were significantly larger in patients with postpartum psychoses when compared to age-matched female patients with non-postpartum psychoses. The scientists explained that their results "underline evidence of subtle, unspecified brain structural abnormalities in patients with post-partum cycloid, and possibly other types of postpartum psychosis," and concluded that, "Such abnormalities might constitute an unspecific vulnerability factor" (Lanczik *et al.* 1998, p. 47).

In a second study, Michael Silverman and colleagues (Silverman *et al.* 2007) used functional magnetic resonance imaging to compare the brain function of women with postpartum depression compared to asymptomatic postpartum female control subjects. The study, believed to be the first neuroimaging study specifically designed to identify neural activity changes in unmedicated postpartum depressed women, used emotionally-valenced word probes to investigate emotional processing, behavioral regulation, and their interaction in the context of fronto-limbic-striatal function. The findings suggested that the neural mechanisms related to postpartum depression are somewhat different than those of non-postpartum-related depression. Although Silverman and colleagues concluded that it would be premature to conclude that postpartum depression is a unique depression phenotype, they stated that their findings "suggest the potential to identify an empirically based neural characterization of [postpartum depression] that will provide a necessary cornerstone for developing more targeted, biologically based diagnostic and therapeutic strategies" (Silverman *et al.* 2007, p. 861).

In a third study, Eydie Moses-Kolko and colleagues (Moses-Kolko *et al.* 2008) used positron emission tomography to investigate brain serotonin-1A (5HT1A) receptor binding potential in seven healthy postpartum controls and nine postpartum depressed subjects. The study authors found that age, time since delivery, and reproductive hormones did not differ between groups, but that postsynaptic 5HT1A receptor binding in the depressed subjects was reduced 20–28% relative to controls. The scientists concluded that, "Recognition of this neurobiological deficit in [postpartum depression] may be useful in the development of treatments and prevention strategies for this disabling disorder" (Moses-Kolko *et al.* 2008, p. 685).

Taken together, these studies suggest that the neuroanatomy and neural mechanisms of postpartum depression and psychosis may be different than those of non-postpartum depressions and psychoses (Table 41.1). More broadly, these studies may be used to support the research and development of postpartum-specific diagnostic, therapeutic, and preventive interventions and strategies.

LEGAL IMPLICATIONS OF THE SCIENTIFIC INVESTIGATION OF DEPRESSION AND PSYCHOSIS

Scientific studies that report neurobiological differences between and within the sexes in the context of depression and psychosis have potential implications for criminal infanticide law, health insurance policy interpretation, mental health parity law, and disability discrimination law.

Criminal infanticide law

An ongoing question among American criminal law scholars is whether postpartum women who kill their children should be charged with the sex-neutral criminal offense of murder or

Table 41.1

Study	Major goal	Findings
Lanczik *et al.* 1998	To quantify ventricular and cisternal cerebrospinal fluid spaces in women with postpartum psychosis, age-matched female patients with non-postpartum psychoses or bipolar affective disorders, and neurological controls.	Left ventricular area, planimetric ventricle-to-brain ratio, and superior cerebellar cistern volume were significantly larger in the postpartum psychosis group.
Silverman *et al.* 2007	To probe the systems-level neuropathophysiology of postpartum depression (PPD) in the context of a specific neurobiological model of fronto-limbic-striatal function.	Attenuated activity in posterior orbitofrontal cortex for negative versus neutral stimuli with greater PPD symptomatology, increased amygdala activity in response to negative words in those without PPD symptomotology, and attenuated striatum activation to positive word conditions with greater PPD symptomotology.
Moses-Kolko *et al.* 2008	To measure brain serotonin-1A (5HT1A) receptor binding potential in healthy and depressed postpartum women	Postsynaptic 5HT1A receptor binding in women with PPD was reduced 20–28% relative to controls, with most significant reductions in anterior cingulate and mesiotemporal cortices.

whether the female-specific criminal offense of infanticide should legislatively be made available. Recognizing that some postpartum women suffer from severe mental illness that may impair their thought processes and judgment, some jurisdictions have established through criminal legislation the female-specific offense of infanticide. The Criminal Code of Canada, for example, provides for the lesser charge of infanticide when a "female person… by a wilful act or omission… causes the death of her newly-born child, if at the time of the act or omission she is not fully recovered from the effects of giving birth to the child and by reason thereof or of the effect of lactation consequent on the birth of the child her mind is then disturbed" (Criminal Code of Canada § 233). The Zimbabwe Infanticide Act similarly provided that, "Any woman who, within six months of the birth of her child, causes its death… intentionally; or….by conduct which she realises involves a real risk to the child's life; at a time when the balance of her mind is disturbed as a result of giving birth to the child, shall be guilty of infanticide and liable to imprisonment for a period not exceeding five years" (Zimbabwe Infanticide Act § 48). The Canadian and Zimbabwe provisions apply only to "female person[s]" and "women," respectively.

Unlike Canada and Zimbabwe, no state in the US has established a female-specific infanticide provision or recognized postpartum illness as an independent defense to homicide, either complete or partial, although evidence of postpartum psychosis has been used in particular cases to support the sex-neutral defenses of insanity and diminished capacity as well as the sex-neutral verdict of "guilty but mentally ill" (Tovino 2010). In the early 1990s, law professor Daniel Maier Katkin (Katkin 1992) studied 24 American child-murder cases in which the defendant mother introduced evidence of postpartum psychosis in support of her defense of insanity or diminished capacity. Of those cases, eight women were judged not guilty by reason of insanity, four were given probation, three were incarcerated for less than 5 years, and seven were incarcerated between 5 and 20 years.

The state-by-state and case-by-case approach in the US has been criticized for its lack of uniformity, consistency, and justice (Fisher 2003). A small number of US lawmakers have responded by introducing female-specific infanticide bills. In early 2009, for example, Representative Jessica Farrar (D-Houston) introduced to the Texas Legislature House Bill 3318, which would amend the Texas Penal Code to create the offense of infanticide, punishable as a state jail felony (H.B. 3318). According to the introduced legislation, a person commits the offense of infanticide if the person "willfully by an act or omission causes the death of a child to whom the person gave birth within the 12-month period preceding the child's death and if, at the time of the act or omission, the person's judgment was impaired as a result of the effects of giving birth or the effects of lactation following the birth" (H.B. 3318). Unlike its Canadian and Zimbabwean counterparts, H.B. 3318 does not by its terms apply only to "female person[s]" or "women"; however, a defendant must have given birth to the killed child in order to benefit from the lesser charge. As of this writing, the Texas Legislature has not yet enacted the infanticide bill.

In light of pending female-specific infanticide bills such as H.B. 3318, the question becomes whether scientific advances provide, or should provide, greater support for female-specific criminal infanticide laws. Legal scholarship addressing this question remains divided (Reece 1991; Fisher 2003; March 2005; Walker 2006), although it may be categorized into three broad groups. The first group of scholars argues that female-specific infanticide laws are necessary to recognize the unique characteristics and consequences of postpartum illness (Connell 2002). The second group argues for a broader insanity test that would provide greater protection for postpartum females (and other female and male defendants with mental illness), as long as such newly designed test is sex-neutral on its face (Huang 2002; Manchester 2003). The third category supports the status quo in the US; that is, the absence of female-specific infanticide laws coupled with the allowance of credible scientific evidence of postpartum illness, as appropriate, to support the existing and limited sex-neutral defenses of insanity and diminished capacity as well as the sex-neutral verdict of "guilty but mentally ill" (Gardner 1990; Stangle 2008). Feminist theorists might classify the first category of scholarship as accommodation-based, the second category of scholarship as acceptance-based, and the third category of scholarship as assimilation-based (Manchester 2003) (Table 41.2).

Health insurance policy interpretation

Scientific studies that report neurobiological differences between and within the sexes in the context of depression and psychosis—as well as more general studies that simply identify structural and functional correlates of depression and psychosis in participants with female-specific conditions—also may have implications for judicial interpretation of health insurance policies that distinguish physical illness and mental illness and provide less comprehensive coverage of mental illness (Tovino 2010).

Table 41.2

Legal position	Feminist theory	Legal examples
Female-specific infanticide laws are necessary to accommodate postpartum illnesses	Accommodation	Infanticide laws of Canada, New South Wales, and Zimbabwe; introduced (but not enacted) Texas infanticide bill.
Female-specific infanticide laws are not necessary, but the insanity test should be broadened.	Acceptance	Broad insanity test applied by some US jurisdictions, including Connecticut and Maine.
Female-specific infanticide laws are not necessary and the insanity test should not be broadened.	Assimilation	Narrow insanity test applied by some US jurisdictions, including Alabama, Arizona, and Texas.

The case of *Blake v. Unionmutual Stock Life Insurance Company* provides an example of how neuroscientific advances may impact judicial interpretations of health insurance policy provisions (*Blake v. Unionmutual Stock Life Ins. Co.* 1989, 1990). At issue in *Blake* was the proper interpretation of a provision within Pam Blake's health insurance policy that limited insurance coverage of mental illnesses (defined as "any mental, nervous or emotional diseases or disorders") to 30 days of inpatient care and US $1000 worth of outpatient treatments. Familiar with several hormone- and neurotransmitter-based theories of postpartum illness, Blake believed that her postpartum depression should be classified as a physical illness, defined in the policy as an "illness or disease… [including] pregnancy unless excluded elsewhere" (*Blake v. Unionmutual Stock Life Ins. Co.* 1990 at 1528). When Blake's insurance company classified her postpartum depression as a mental illness and refused to cover the entirety of its treatment, Blake sued to recover US $33,279.55 in unpaid medical bills.

At trial, the US District Court for the Southern District of Florida reviewed the evidence provided about Blake's postpartum depression and was asked to decide whether Blake had a physical or mental illness. Although several expert and treating psychiatrists and psychologists testified that imbalances in serotonin and norepinephrine, as well as other hormonal imbalances, may have played a role in Blake's postpartum depression, the court focused on Blake's failure to introduce into evidence any neurotransmitter measurements or hormonal tests that could literally prove to the court that Blake had a physical illness. The district court thus held that Blake had a mental illness that was subject to the less comprehensive insurance coverage. The Eleventh Circuit affirmed the district court's decision. Both courts, however, appeared open to recognizing postpartum depression and postpartum psychosis as physical illnesses in future cases if a plaintiff could provide physiological proof of her illness, such as a test result showing an imbalance, irregularity, or abnormality in serotonin or norepinephrine, or some other type of structural or functional abnormality.

The question becomes whether recent scientific findings provide (or should provide) greater support for the legal recognition of postpartum depression and psychosis as physical versus mental illnesses. The answer may depend on the studies or evidence admitted into evidence by the court. In their recent work, Janet Shibley Hyde and colleagues (Hyde *et al.* 2008) proposed an integrated, developmental model that integrates affective, biological, and cognitive factors as vulnerabilities to depression that, in interaction with negative life events, heighten young females' rates of depression beginning in adolescence and is believed to account for differences in the rates of depression experienced by girls and boys and, later in life, women and men. A court that relied on the Hyde model may view depression in females as both mental and physical. On the other hand, a court that relied solely on the work of Mario Lanczik and colleagues (Lanczik *et al.* 1998), Michael Silverman and colleagues (Silverman *et al.* 2007), and Eydie Moses-Kolko and colleagues (Moses-Kolko *et al.* 2008), described in the first part of this chapter, may view depression in postpartum females as a primarily physical illness.

Mental health parity law

Recent scientific findings also may have implications for mental health parity law, including by assisting postpartum women in securing more comprehensive health insurance benefits. In the US, mental health parity law refers to federal and state legislation that attempts to provide greater equality between the insurance benefits applicable to physical illnesses and the insurance benefits applicable to mental illnesses. At the federal level, Congress passed in 1996 the federal Mental Health Parity Act (MHPA'96), which required covered group health plans to provide parity with respect to annual and lifetime aggregate spending caps imposed on medical and surgical benefits and mental health benefits within the plan (29 U.S.C. § 1185a(a)(1)-(2)). Because MHPA'96 did not require parity with respect to financial requirements, cost-sharing requirements, and treatment limitations, mental health parity proponents continued to lobby Congress for more complete parity measures over the next 12 years. In 2008, Congress enacted the Paul Wellstone and Pete Domenici Mental Health Parity and Addiction Equity Act (MHPA'08), which requires covered group health plans that provide both medical and surgical benefits and mental health or substance use disorder benefits to ensure that: (1) the financial requirements, such as deductibles and co-payments, applicable to mental health and substance use disorder benefits are no more restrictive than the predominant financial requirements applicable to substantially all medical and surgical benefits covered by the plan; (2) no separate cost sharing requirements that are applicable only with respect to mental health or substance use disorder benefits exist; (3) the treatment limitations applicable to such mental health and substance use disorder benefits are no more restrictive than the predominant treatment limitations applicable to substantially all medical and surgical benefits covered by the plan; and (4) no separate treatment limitations that are applicable only with respect to mental health or substance use disorder benefits exist.

The question becomes whether postpartum depression and psychosis research will impact future judicial opinions interpreting federal mental health parity law as well as analogous state parity laws. The answer lies in the fact that neither MHPA'96 nor MHPA'08 defines the phrase "mental health benefits" other than to refer to "benefits with respect to services for mental health conditions, as defined under the terms of the plan and in accordance with applicable Federal and State law" (29 U.S.C. § 1185a(e)(4)). Because other federal laws do not direct a definition of the phrase "mental health benefits" as used in MHPA'96 and MHPA'08, the application of federal mental health parity law to individuals with particular mental health conditions will depend on the terms of the plan as regulated by state law. Insured persons who reside in states that narrowly define these terms may not receive as much, or the same, protection as insured persons who reside in states that broadly define these terms.

Some states define the mental illnesses that benefit from parity requirements in terms of whether they are "biologically-based." New Jersey, for example, requires certain health benefit plans to provide benefits for "biologically-based mental illnesses" under the same terms and conditions as provided for other sicknesses (New Jersey Statutes Annotated § 17B:27A-19.7, 2009). New Jersey defines a "biologically-based mental illness" in relevant part as a "mental or nervous condition that is caused by a biological disorder of the brain..." (New Jersey Statutes Annotated § 17B:27A-19.7, 2009). A female resident of New Jersey who is insured by a regulated health benefit plan and requests treatment for a postpartum illness thus can benefit from New Jersey's mental health parity provisions if she can prove that her postpartum condition is caused by a biological disorder of the brain. I anticipate that in future litigation in which a health insurance company refuses to provide equal insurance coverage for a woman's postpartum illness treatments due to the illness not being biologically-based (i.e. in the same manner as the previously examined *Blake v. Unionmutual Stock Life Insurance Company*, in which the defendant insurer argued that Pam Blake's postpartum depression was not a physical illness), the plaintiff would rely on one or more of the studies referenced in the first part of this chapter in an attempt to prove that her postpartum illness has identifiable structural, hormonal, and chemical correlates and therefore is biologically-based.

Other states expressly tie their definition of protected mental health conditions to those conditions that "current medical science affirms" is caused by an organic or physiological disorder. Nebraska, for example, defines a "serious mental illness" in relevant part as "any mental health condition that current medical science affirms is caused by a biological disorder of the brain..." (Nebraska Revised Statutes § 44-792(5)(b), 2009). As in New Jersey, I anticipate that in future litigation in Nebraska in which a defendant insurance company refuses to provide comprehensive health insurance coverage to a female resident with postpartum illness, the plaintiff may reference one or more of the studies discussed in the first part of this chapter in an attempt to prove that current medical science has affirmed that her postpartum illness is caused by a brain-based biological disorder. In summary, postpartum depression and psychosis research may assist postpartum women in securing more comprehensive health insurance benefits under federal and state mental health parity law.

Disability discrimination law

Advances in the understanding of female-specific brain conditions may also have implications in the context of disability discrimination, including by assisting certain women with postpartum depression and psychosis qualify as protected individuals with disabilities.

In the US, disability discrimination is prohibited in the context of employment, state and local government, and public accommodations by Titles I, II, and III of the federal Americans with Disabilities Act of 1990 (ADA), as amended by the ADA Amendments Act of 2008 (ADAAA). At the state level, disability discrimination is prohibited by stand-alone disability discrimination provisions as well as civil rights provisions that prohibit discrimination based on disability in addition to a number of other factors. Prior to the enactment of the ADAAA, a number of courts had found that individuals with mental illnesses such as depression were not protected individuals with disabilities either because their depressions or psychoses were temporary or episodic, or because their medications, counseling sessions, or other treatments constituted mitigating measures. In cases involving female plaintiffs with postpartum depression or psychosis, the courts tended to deny disability status on the ground that the plaintiff's illness only imposed a short-term or temporary restriction on her major life activities. In the Sixth Circuit case of *Novak v. MetroHealth Medical Center*, for example, an employee sought leave under the federal Family and Medical Leave Act (FMLA) to care for her 18-year-old daughter who allegedly had postpartum depression (*Novak v. MetroHealth Medical Center* 2007). The FMLA authorizes leave for employees to care for a child 18 years of age or older if the child is suffering from a serious health condition and is incapable of self-care because of a "physical or mental disability" (*Novak v. MetroHealth Medical Center* 2007). According to regulations adopted by the Department of Labor interpreting the FMLA, the phrase "physical or mental disability" as used in the FMLA means a "physical or mental impairment that substantially limits one or more of the major life activities of an individual," as defined in the ADA (*Novak v. MetroHealth Medical Center* 2007). Stated another way, an employee may take FMLA leave to care for an adult child only if that child has a disability under the ADA. The Sixth Circuit thus had to determine whether the daughter's claimed postpartum depression constituted a disability under the ADA in order to resolve the underlying FMLA claim.

The Sixth Circuit provided three overlapping reasons in support of its holding that the daughter's postpartum depression did not constitute a disability under the ADA. First, the mother did not provide sufficient evidence (other than her daughter's non-specific, non-expert testimony that she could not "follow the doctor's orders without some help" and that she was afraid she might "freak out and not know how to deal with a newborn") that her daughter's postpartum depression was severe (*Novak v. MetroHealth Medical Center* 2007). Second, evidence from a physician's brief certification form and the daughter's own testimony showed that the daughter's postpartum depression only lasted a week or two, and the court relied on judicial precedent for the legal principle that short-term restrictions on major life activities do not constitute disabilities. Third, the mother failed to provide any evidence showing that the daughter's postpartum depression "inflicted any permanent or long-term impact on her health" or caused the daughter to "endure[] any long-term adverse effects" (*Novak v. MetroHealth Medical Center* 2007).

In a similar case, *Shalbert v. Marcincin*, the Eastern District of Pennsylvania also was asked to determine whether the plaintiff's postpartum depression constituted a disability under the ADA (*Shalbert v. Marcincin* 2005). Like *Novak*, *Shalbert* found that the plaintiff (who began feeling better 2 months after she was prescribed the drug Paxil®) failed to produce evidence showing that her postpartum depression was long-lasting or permanent. The Shalbert court concluded that, "temporary, non-chronic impairment of short duration is not a disability covered by the ADA…" (*Shalbert v. Marcincin* 2005).

To remedy the narrow application of the ADA in these and other cases, President George W. Bush signed the ADAAA into law on 25 September 2008. The ADAAA clarifies that an impairment that is episodic or in remission remains a disability so long as it substantially limits a major life activity when active (ADAAA 2008). The ADAAA also clarifies that the determination of whether an impairment substantially limits a major life activity should be made without regard to the ameliorative effects of mitigating measures such as medication, behavior modification therapy, or adaptive neurological modifications. Finally, the ADAAA provides a new statutory definition of the "major life activities" that must be substantially limited in order for the plaintiff to qualify as an individual with a disability. The new definition includes the traditional life activities identified by the original ADA, such as "caring for oneself, performing manual tasks, walking, seeing, hearing, speaking, breathing, learning, and working," but also adds "the operation of a major bodily function, including but not limited to, functions of the immune system, normal cell growth, digestive, bowel, bladder, neurological, brain, respiratory, circulatory, endocrine, and reproductive functions" (ADAAA 2008). On 23 September 2009, the Equal Employment Opportunity Commission (EEOC) issued proposed regulations implementing the ADAAA, including regulations clarifying that individuals with episodic depressions and psychoses can qualify as protected individuals with disabilities due to the limitations posed on their neurological and brain functions (EEOC 2009).

Although female plaintiffs operating under the original ADA generally were not successful in arguing that their postpartum depressions and psychoses constituted protected disabilities, I anticipate that future ADA plaintiffs with postpartum illness may attempt to present neuroscientific studies as well as personal medical examination evidence to support their argument that they have substantially impaired neurological, brain, or endocrine functions and, therefore, that they qualify as protected individuals with disabilities. The new EEOC regulations, including the provisions that clarify that major depression can substantially limit the "functions of the brain," would support their argument (EEOC 2009). In summary, recent research findings may assist postpartum women in securing protection under federal and analogous state disability discrimination provisions.

RISKS AND BENEFITS OF THE SCIENTIFIC INVESTIGATION OF DEPRESSION AND PSYCHOSIS

In the first part of this chapter, I referenced examples of studies that explore between- and within-sex differences associated with the incidence, prevalence, and nature of depression and psychosis in order to illustrate a broader trend among scientists with respect to the neuroscientific investigation of sex differences. Studies examining between- and within- sex differences exist not only in the context of depression and psychosis, but also in the context of other neurological and developmental conditions such as autism (Baron-Cohen 2002; Baron-Cohen et al. 2005), aging (Berchtold et al. 2008), and preterm brain damage (Mayoral 2009), as well as in the context of cognition, including general intelligence (Haier et al. 2005), working memory (Speck 2000), verbal and spatial tasks (Gur et al. 2000), cognitive inhibition (Halari 2005), and math performance (Krendl et al. 2008), just to name a few.

The public's interest in the neuroscientific investigation of between- and within-sex differences dates back several decades. In a 1966 Scientific American article ("Sex Differences in the Brain"), Seymour Levine (Levine 1966) summarized then-current findings regarding mating behaviors in female and male rats, including evidence suggesting a primary role for sex hormones in the sex-differentiated behaviors. In a 1992 Scientific American article

("Sex Differences in the Brain"), Doreen Kimura (Kimura 1992) moved beyond Levine's focus on the mating behaviors of female and male rats and explained that, "Women and men differ not only in physical attributes and reproductive function but also in the way in which they solve intellectual problems". More recently, in 2005, Larry Cahill (Cahill 2005) high-lighted in his *Scientific American* article ("His Brain, Her Brain") recent findings illustrating the influence of sex on many areas of cognition and behavior, including memory, emotion, vision, hearing, the processing of faces, and the brain's response to stress hormones. Cahill recommended that neuroscientists include both females and males in future studies and take into account the sex of participants when analyzing data or risk obtaining and publishing misleading results.

Scientific American is not the only outlet for sex-based popular neuroscience. In the last 20 years, a number of scientific and popular books with eye-catching titles have presented studies finding sex differences to fellow scientists as well as the general public. Popular titles include, but are not limited to, *Brain Sex: The Real Difference between Men and Women* (Moir and Jessel 1992), *Sex on the Brain: The Biological Differences between Men and Women* (Blum 1998), *Why Men Don't Listen and Women Can't Read Maps* (Pease and Pease 2000), *Brain Gender* (Hines 2005), *Sex Differences in the Brain: From Genes to Behavior* (Becker *et al.* 2007), *The Female Brain* (Brizendine 2006), *Pink Brain, Blue Brain: How Small Differences Grow into Troublesome Gaps–And What We Can Do About It* (Eliot 2009), and *The Male Brain: A Breakthrough Understanding of How Men and Boys Think* (Brizendine 2010). Medical and science news articles also alert the general public to recent studies reporting between- and within-sex differences: *Scientists Find Sex Differences in Brain* (Onion 2005, ABC News), *Motherhood Boosts Female Brain Power: Having a Child Rewires a Woman's Brain, Improving Her Mental Agility and Health* (Leake 2009, TimesOnline), *Boys' and Girls' Brains Are Different: Gender Differences in Language Appear Biological* (ScienceDaily 2008), *Sex Differences in the Brain's Serotonin System* (ScienceDaily 2008), and *Pink Brain, Blue Brain: Claims of Sex Differences Fall Apart* (Newsweek, 2009).

In the second part of this chapter, I identified and examined several legal implications of advances in the neuroscientific understanding of between- and within-sex differences in the context of depression and psychosis, including implications for criminal infanticide law, health insurance policy interpretation, mental health parity law, and disability discrimination law. I suggested that females with depression and psychosis may benefit legally from advances in neuroscience through lesser criminal charges, more comprehensive health insurance benefits, and a greater likelihood of qualifying as protected individuals with disability. Although females with depression and psychosis may benefit legally from advances in neuroscience, the social dissemination of sex-based study findings, including the dissemination of summarized study findings through the popular books and news articles referenced above, raise additional questions and concerns (Chalfin *et al.* 2008). As suggested by Michael Silverman and colleagues (Silverman *et al.* 2007), females with postpartum depression could benefit medically from an empirically based neural characterization of postpartum depression, which may lead to the development of more targeted, biologically based diagnostic and therapeutic strategies. On the other hand, the social understanding of postpartum females who experience depressions and psychoses as neurologically impaired could recreate and perpetuate outdated stereotypes and support sex-based discrimination in social, political, employment, and other arenas.

Conclusion

Given the evidence at hand, the key question to address now is: How and where do we draw the line between encouraging neuroscientific work that may improve the diagnosis and treatment of female patients (with which many scholars and policy analysts agree), attempting to explain behavior for purposes of securing criminal, civil, and administrative protections and benefits (with which some but not all agree), and legitimizing practices that discriminate against females (with which few agree) (Huang 2002)? More broadly, how do we try to help some women without pathologizing all women (Oberman 2003)?

We can start by encouraging consumers of neuroscientific data, including lawmakers, judges, policy analysts, educators, employers, insurers, and the general public, to know and consider the source, purpose, and limitations of the data. We can further encourage study authors to more clearly state in their work the limitations of their research and data, and the purposes for which the authors intended that their data be used. Finally, we can encourage study authors, ethicists, and other commentators to identify in scholarship as well as conversations with the media and the public both the benefits of advances in neuroscience as well as the risks associated with the premature adoption and application of neuroscientific work in social and legal arenas. If we do take these actions, women may someday benefit from improved diagnostic, therapeutic, and preventive interventions and strategies without suffering from the stereotyping and discrimination that historically have accompanied findings of sex differences.

References

American Psychiatric Association. (2000). *Diagnostic and Statistical Manual of Mental Disorders*. Arlington, VA: American Psychiatric Association.

Americans with Disabilities Act. (1990). S .933, Pub. L. No. 101-336, codified at 42 U.S.C. §§ 12101-12206.

ADA Amendments Act. (2008). S .3406, Pub. L. No. 110-325, 122 Stat. 3533, 110th Cong., 2nd Sess., § 2.

Arkansas Mental Health Parity Act. (2008). Arkansas Code Annotated §§ 23-99-501 - 23-99-511.

Auger, A.P. and Olesen, K.M. (2009). Brain sex differences and the organisation of juvenile social play behaviour. *Journal of Neuroendocrinology*, 21, 519–25.

Baron-Cohen, S. (2002). The extreme male brain theory of autism. *Trends in Cognitive Science*, 6, 248–54.

Baron-Cohen, S., Knickmeyer, R.C., and Belmonte, M.K. (2005). Sex differences in the brain: Implications for explaining autism. *Science*, 310, 819–23.

Becker, J.B., Berkley, K.J., Geary, N., *et al.* (2007). *Sex Differences in the Brain: From Genes to Behavior*. New York: Oxford University Press.

Berchtold, N.C., Cribbs, D.H., Coleman, P.D., *et al.* (2008). Gene expression changes in the course of normal brain aging are sexually dimorphic. *Proceedings of the National Academy of Sciences*, 105, 15605–10.

Blake v. Unionmutual Stock Life Ins. Co. (1989). U.S. Dist. LEXIS 16331, Southern District of Florida.

Blake v. Unionmutual Stock Life Ins. Co. (1990). 906F.2d 1525, 11th Circuit.

Blum, D. (1998). *Sex on the Brain: The Biological Differences between Men and Women.* New York: Penguin Books.

Brizendine, L. (2006). *The Female Brain.* New York: Morgan Road.

Brizendine, L. (2010). *The Male Brain: A Breakthrough Understanding of How Men and Boys Think.* New York: Random House.

Cahill, L. (2005). His brain, her brain. *Scientific American*, 292, 40–7.

Cahill, L. (2006). Why sex matters for neuroscience. *Nature Reviews Neuroscience*, 7, 477–84.

Chalfin, M.C., Karkazis, K.A., and Murphy, E.R. (2008). Women's neuroethics? Why sex matters for neuroethics. *American Journal of Bioethics*, 8, 1–2.

Connell, M. (2002). The postpartum psychosis defense and feminism: More or less justice for women? *Case Western Reserve Law Review*, 53, 143–69.

Criminal Code of Canada, § 233, R.S., c. C-34, s. 216.

Equal Employment Opportunity Commission (EEOC) (2009). Regulations to implement the equal employment provisions of the Americans with Disabilities Act, as amended. *Federal Register*, 74, 48431–50.

Fisher, K. (2003). To save her children's souls: Theoretical perspectives on Andrea Yates and postpartum-related infanticide. *Thomas Jefferson Law Review*, 25, 599–634.

Gardner, C.A. (1990). Postpartum depression defense: Are mothers getting away with murder? *New England Law Review*, 24, 953–89.

Gur, R.C., Alsop, D., Glahn, D., *et al.* (2000). An fMRI study of sex differences in regional activation to a verbal and spatial task. *Brain Language*, 74, 157–70.

Hines, M. (2005). *Brain Gender.* New York: Oxford University Press.

Huang, C. (2002). It's a hormonal thing: premenstrual syndrome and postpartum psychosis as criminal defense. *Southern California Review of Law and Women's Studies*, 11, 345–67.

Hyde, J.S., Mezulis, A.H., and Abramson, L.Y. (2008). The ABCs of depression: Integrating affective, biological, and cognitive models to explain the emergence of the gender difference in depression. *Psychological Review*, 115, 291–313.

Katkin, D.M. (1992). Postpartum psychosis, infanticide, and criminal justice. In J.A. Hamilton and P.N. Harberger (eds.) *Postpartum Psychiatric Illness: A Picture Puzzle*, pp. 275–81. Philadelphia, PA: University of Pennsylvania Press.

Kimura, D. (1992). Sex differences in the brain. *Scientific American*, 267, 118–25.

Kornstein, S.G., Schatzberg, A.F., Thase, M.E. *et al.* (2000). Gender differences in treatment response to sertraline versus imipramine in chronic depression. *American Journal of Psychiatry*, 157, 1445–52.

Krendl, A.C., Richeson, J.A., Kelley, W.M., and Heatherton T.F. (2008). The negative consequences of threat: A functional magnetic resonance imaging investigation of the neural mechanisms underlying women's underperformance in math. *Psychological Science*, 19, 168–75.

Lanczik, M., Fritze, J., Hofmann E., Schulz, C., Knoche, M., and Becker T. (1998). Ventricular abnormality in patients with postpartum psychoses. *Archives of Women's Mental Health*, 1, 45–7.

Leake, J. Motherhood boosts female brain power: Having a child rewires a woman's brain, improving her mental agility and health. Available at http://www.timesonline.co.uk/tol/life_and_style/health/article4926736.ece (accessed 15 December 2009).

Levine, S. (1966). Sex differences in the brain. *Scientific American*, 214, 84–90.

Manchester, J. (2003). Beyond accommodation: Reconstructing the insanity defense to provide an adequate remedy for postpartum psychotic women. *Journal of Criminal Law and Criminology*, 93, 713–52.

March, C.L. (2005). The conflicted treatment of postpartum psychosis under criminal law. *William Mitchell Law Review*, **32**, 243–63.

Mental Health Parity Act (1996). 29 U.S.C. § 1185a(a)(1)-(2).

Moir, A. and Jessel, D. (1992). *Brain Sex: The Real Differences between Men and Women*. New York: Dell Publishing.

Moses-Kolko, E.L., Wisner, K.L., Price, J.C., *et al.* (2008). Serotonin 1A receptor reductions in postpartum depression: A PET study. *Fertility and Sterility*, **89**, 685–92.

Nebraska Revised Statutes (2009). § 44-792(5)(b).

New Jersey Statutes Annotated (2009). § 17B:27A-19.7.

Novak v. MetroHealth Medical Center (2007). 503F.3d 572, 574, 582, 6ᵗʰ Circuit.

Oberman, M. (2003). Lady Madonna, children at your feet. *William and Mary Journal of Women and Law*, **10**, 33–67.

Onion, A. (2005). Scientists find sex differences in brain: Controversial research revealing differences between men and women. *ABC News*. Available at http://abcnews.go.com/Technology/Health/story?id=424608&page=1&page=1 (accessed 30 October 2009).

Paul Wellstone and Pete Domenici Mental Health Parity and Addiction Equity Act. (2008). H.R. 1424, Pub. L. No. 110-343, 110ᵗʰ Cong., Subtitle B, §§ 511, 512.

Pease, A. and Pease, B. (2000). *Why Men Don't Listen and Women Can't Read Maps*. New York: Welcome Rain.

Reece, L. (1991). Mothers who kill: Postpartum disorders and criminal infanticide. *UCLA Law Review*, **38**, 699–757.

Roskies, A. (2006). A case study of neuroethics: The nature of moral judgment. In J. Illes (ed.) *Neuroethics: Defining the Issues in Theory, Practice, and Policy*, pp. 17–32 Oxford: Oxford University Press.

Shalbert v. Marcincin (2005). U.S. Dist. LEXIS 16564, *17, Eastern District of Pennsylvania.

Silverman, M., Loudon, H., Safier, M., *et al.* (2007). Neural dysfunction in postpartum depression: An fMRI pilot study. *CNS Spectrums*, **12**, 853–62.

Speck, O., Ernst, T., Braun, J., Koch, C. Miller, E., and Chang, L. (2000). Gender differences in the functional organization of the brain for working memory. *NeuroReport*, **11**, 2581–5.

Stangle, H.L. (2008). Murderous Madonna: Femininity, violence, and the myth of postpartum mental disorder in cases of maternal infanticide and filicide. *William and Mary Law Review*, **50**, 699–734.

Texas House Bill 3318 (2009).

Tovino, S.A. (2010). Scientific understandings of postpartum illness: Improving health law and policy? *Harvard Journal of Law and Gender*, **33**, 99–174.

Vasileiadis, G.T., Thompson, R.T., Han, V.K., and Gelman, N. (2009). Females follow a more 'compact' early human brain development model than males. *Pediatric Research*, **66**, 551–5.

Walker, A.J. (2006). Application of the insanity defense to postpartum disorder-driven infanticide in the United States: A look toward the enactment of an infanticide act. *Maryland Journal of Race, Religion, Gender and Class*, **6**, 197–221.

World Health Organization. (2009). What do we mean by 'sex' and 'gender'. Available at: http://www.who.int/gender/whatisgender/en/index.html (accessed 30 October 2009).

Zimbabwe Infanticide Act. (1990). ZWE-1990-L-57018, No. 27 of 1990, codified at Criminal Law Act, Chapter 5, Part I, § 48.

....

CHAPTER 42

PUBLIC
REPRESENTATIONS OF
NEUROGENETICS

....

AMY ZARZECZNY AND TIMOTHY CAULFIELD

INTRODUCTION

....

BIOMEDICAL research gets a lot of press in the popular media, and, if polls and academic commentary can be believed, the public is both interested in and influenced by this coverage (Weisberg 2008; Bubela *et al.* 2009). The media traditionally plays a critical role in educating and informing the public (Racine *et al.* 2006; Bubela *et al.* 2009), and thus in potentially shaping the public's views on contentious topics. While the relationship between media portrayals and public opinion is tremendously complex (Bates 2005), there seems little doubt that the media is an important source of health and science information (Marks *et al.* 2007), and that it can help to set the tone of public debate and policy reaction (Kitzinger and Williams 2005).

The field of neuroscience in particular receives considerable press coverage (Racine *et al.* 2006). Indeed, there seems to be an intense media fascination with this domain of biomedical research. Media headlines cover a wide range of topics from love—"Proof's in the brain scan: Romance can last; it doesn't always fade over time" (Jayson 2008)—to explaining different personal challenges—"Brain scans may help reveal math learning disability" (CBC 2006)—to mind reading—"Brain scan 'sees hidden thoughts'" (BBC 2005). These headlines reflect only a few of the diverse topics and issues for which neuroscience is suggested to be the answer, or, at the very least, to solve significant pieces of the puzzle. In fact, "[u]nderlying many of the claims concerning the power of modern neuroimaging is the belief, real or desired, that functional imaging offers a direct picture of the human brain at work" (Illes *et al.* 2006, p. 149). Indeed, it is functional magnetic resonance imaging (fMRI) technology that has, in many ways, emerged as the darling of the media and the "tool of choice for exploring brain functioning in cognitive neuroscience" (Van Horn and Poldrack 2009, p. 3).

This heightened attention to neuro-related topics is also reflected in the scientific literature, in a trend that has been emerging for some time. Interest seems to be particularly high with regard to research that examines aspects of personality, thought processes, and other areas not traditionally considered in purely health-focused inquiries. For example, a litera-ture search in PubMed (http://www.ncbi.nlm.nih.gov/pubmed) revealed that from 1995–2000, the number of publications with the terms "emotion" and "brain" more than doubled (Canli and Amin 2002). Research by Illes *et al.* looking at all peer-reviewed fMRI studies published between 1991 and 2001 showed an increase over time in "studies with evident social and policy implications, including studies of human cooperation and competition, brain differences in violent people and genetic influences on brain structure and function" (Illes *et al.* 2003, p.205). Of course, more typical areas of neuroscience research also continue to be popular. In fact, research indicates there were "over 2000 research articles published in the year 2007 alone concerning fMRI and its applications to understanding mental opera-tions and their disorders in diseased populations" (Van Horn and Poldrack 2009, p. 3).

These advances in neuroscience and related research are occurring in an era increasingly characterized by quick and easy access to information, including information about health, medical options, and scientific developments. In this so-called "information age," knowl-edge that was previously available to only a discrete population of experts is now more often readily accessible with the click of a mouse and a few Google searches. These trends are fur-ther shaped by the commercialization ethos that currently permeates biomedical research, and framed in the context of hype that often surrounds emerging areas of biotechnology. What impact do these forces have on the neurogenetic revolution? How do they affect public understandings and behavior? What is the potential long-term significance of these issues for the public and for the field?

In this chapter we outline what the data say about the nature of public representations of neuroimaging. Drawing on research from related domains, particularly genetics, we then consider social issues associated with media representations—with an emphasis on the con-cerns of determinism and fatalism. Finally, we go on to consider some of the key forces that are shaping the direction of the trends in this area. This analysis is particularly timely given the current prominence of neuroscience, and neuroimaging in particular, in the public eye. Ideally it will also contribute to the growing discourse surrounding emerging biomedical technologies and how they are framed in public representations.

The public face of neuroimaging

Most of us are likely familiar with these images: pictures of brains with different areas high-lighted in color, or with various dots marking certain regions. Such images are usually paired with explanations of where different thoughts, emotions or processes (e.g. anger, love, memory, lying) are located or, rather, of which parts of the brain are activated in association with them. Not only do these images tend to be aesthetically interesting and attention grab-bing, they are often presented as being persuasive evidence of the claimed connections. In fact, "both scientists and the media have suggested that using brain images to represent brain activity confers a great deal of scientific credibility to studies of cognition, and that these images are one of the primary reasons for public interest in fMRI research" (McCabe and Castel 2008, p. 344).

As is true in other domains of science (e.g. genomics), presentations of neuroimaging research results in the popular media seem to often lean towards the optimistic (Caulfield

2005; Racine *et al.* 2005) and the dramatic (for a comment on genetics and medicine in the media, see Petersen 2001), and away from engaging in debate about potential ethical and social issues. However, this trend may be shifting, as discussed further later in this chapter. While many areas of research are hyped (Caulfield 2005; Petersen 2009), the translation from speculative science to media reality seems to be happening particularly quickly in the world of neuroimaging, and sometimes seems to leave almost no subject untouched. Some recent headlines include: "Brain scans may soon read your thoughts" (Minsky 2009); "Brain scans show bullies enjoy others' pain" (U.S. News 2008); "The fMRI brain scan: A better lie detector?" (Narayan 2009); "Functional MRI of sex, when science is hot!" (Hermoye 2007). As even these few examples indicate, the range of topics addressed in popular media reports of neuroimaging is broad and diverse. Interestingly, however, it seems that certain areas of inquiry receive more attention than others.

In what appears to be the first published study examining how fMRI has been treated by the popular press, Racine and colleagues examined 132 unique print media articles published on the topic between 1994 (having found none prior) and 2004 (Racine *et al.* 2006). According to their results, press coverage is greater for studies of non-health-related phenomena, in particular higher order cognition, emotion, and social behaviors studies. However, even if such research is more frequent in number, health benefits are emphasized most. This suggests that the depiction of fMRI as a health technology is unrelenting, even if non-health-related research is the prevailing focus (Racine *et al.* 2006). However, they also noted that, in general, articles were largely uncritical of the technology, particularly where the research was framed as being health related. Conversely, more potentially controversial uses, such as "neuromarketing studies or possible truth-technology improvements received a fair deal of critical attention" in the articles studied (Racine *et al.* 2006).

Other commentators have reflected on the tendency of media representations of neuroimaging to "fail to capture the limitations of neuroimaging techniques, perhaps speaking to a need for the media to focus on sensationalized content that sells magazines as opposed to showcasing truly innovative work revealing new understanding of brain function" (Van Horn and Poldrack 2009, p. 4). Further, Racine and Illes reflect that "in the popular press, neuroimaging tends to be simplified and results over-interpreted, especially when results are portrayed as revealing our essence based on characteristics of our brain" (Racine and Illes 2007, p. 4). Our own research on the coverage of neuroscanning research has shown a media preference for stories dealing with higher-order cognition, emotion, and mind reading that is disproportionately high when compared to actual numbers of peer-reviewed research articles dealing with these topics. However, our results also point to increasing skepticism over time in both review and commentary pieces, as well as in the popular press (Caulfield *et al.*, accepted).

As Weisberg notes, there are at least three key reasons to be concerned about how neuroscience is presented to the public. First, as discussed further later in this chapter, neuroscientific images (e.g. pictures of a brain with different areas highlighted) are particularly persuasive and "gives us the feeling that we have a window into the brain and that we can actually see what the brain is doing" (Weisberg 2008, p. 52). Of course, this impression is not precisely accurate given that such images are in fact comprised of aggregate data and merely show areas of statistical significance, rather than areas of activation—contrary to how they might appear. This effect may also be termed "neuro-realism," which "describes how coverage of fMRI investigations can make a phenomenon uncritically real, objective or effective

718   AMY ZARZECZNY AND TIMOTHY CAULFIELD

in the eyes of the public. This occurs most notably when qualifications about results are not brought to the reader's attention" (Racine *et al.* 2005). Second, as will be discussed in greater detail later, research shows people find explanations of cognitive or medical phenomenon more satisfying when they are accompanied by neuroscientific references (Weisberg 2008). Finally, people tend to misunderstand the meaning of neuroscientific explanations presented in the popular press. A given study may explain where a particular processing occurs, but not how or why (Weisberg 2008). However, these limitations may not always be clear in the media representation.

Despite such concerns, the media unquestionably have an important role to play, both in informing the public about emerging science and in giving researchers the opportunity to share their work with a larger segment of society, including funders and policy makers (Caulfield 2004a; Illes *et al.* 2009; Van Horn and Poldrack 2009). The media also helps to "frame" issues in a manner that influences future policy debates (Nisbet and Mooney 2007). As such, the relevance and potential value of the media to science communication should not be minimized. Nonetheless, the competitive and commercial context in which the media currently operates likewise cannot be ignored. Reporters have limited time in which to produce stories and often insufficient resources to allow in-depth attention to be given to each one. These factors, among others, including the tendency to use provocative headlines to attract an audience and, in view of limited column space, maximizing "speculation on the meaning of the findings while minimizing the details of how they were obtained... can lead to gross misrepresentations of the underlying science and faulty impressions of what the technology can deliver" (Van Horn and Poldrack 2009, pp. 6–7).

For instance, let us consider some examples of how neuroimaging research on love is presented: "Brains in love; When you're attracted to someone, is your gray matter talking sense – or just hooked?" (Brink 2007); "Love is really a drug, say brain scan researchers" (Highfield 2007); "For women, pleasure is (nearly) all in the mind" (Henderson 2005); "Love really is blind... Neuroscience can at last explain why we can't see faults in our partners or children" (Persaud 2004). Depending on the context in which this research is presented, "studies investigating the neurofunctional correlates of human love may give rise to two misinterpretations: neuro-realism [defined above] and neuro-essentialism" (Fusar-Poli 2007, p. 285). Neuro-essentialism can be defined as "equating subjectivity and personal identity to the brain. In this sense, the brain is used implicitly as a shortcut for more global concepts such as the person, the individual or the self" (Racine *et al.* 2005, p. 160). Similarly, it can be used as a short-cut for inevitably complex and multifactoral human states, such as love, that are "properties of human beings, not brains" (Fusar-Poli 2007, p. 285).

Again, while certainly not unique to neuroimaging, such simplified presentations of research results may be particularly problematic in this context. Significantly, there is a growing debate in both the peer-reviewed science literature and the popular science press about the science of neuroimaging (Racine and Illes 2007), with some commentators suggesting that seeing activation (or non-activation) of an area of the brain using neuroimaging technology does not necessarily mean that area is involved (or is necessary for) a given activity (Van Horn and Poldrack 2009). Others are increasingly highlighting the various limitations of fMRI technology (Logothetis 2008; Sutton *et al.* 2009). Still others point out that the impression often left that fMRI provides "'visual proof' of brain activity" does not recognize "the enormous complexities of data acquisition and image processing" (Racine *et al.* 2005, p. 160). In light of these emerging critiques of the science, it is important to consider what impact current public representations of neuroimaging may have on the public and the development of the field as a whole.

THE ISSUES ASSOCIATED WITH PUBLIC REPRESENTATIONS

Given the amount and nature of media coverage of neuroimaging, is there any cause for concern from a broader policy perspective? In other words, does it matter that there may be problems with imprecision or misrepresentations in the coverage of this field? In addition to the general and broadly applicable interest in promoting accurate science communication so as to encourage an informed public, a number of other issues are engaged that merit consideration in this context. It is not within the scope of this chapter to provide a comprehensive review, but we will explore a few intriguing concerns including fears of determinism and fatalism. There are of course other important issues associated with scientific hype, such as the risk to public trust and the long-term health of public support (including investments) in the field, which may result from unmet expectations initially encouraged by media representations (Caulfield 2005), but these will not be the focus of this piece.

Fears of determinism and fatalism play a central role in the dialogue surrounding this area of research. "At its simplest, neurogenetic determinism argues that there is a directly causal relationship between gene and behaviour" (Rose 1995, p. 380). For example, according to a neurogenetic deterministic point of view, a person is aggressive because he or she has an aggressive, immutable, trait detectable in the brain. Fatalism has been described as "the subset of deterministic attitudes that project pessimistic rather than optimistic futures," and is often portrayed (perhaps unfairly) as being associated with decisions not to take personal action (e.g. cancer screening, quitting smoking, etc.) (Keeley *et al.* 2009). In general, the concern is that popular representations of genetics and neurogenetics are inappropriately simplistic and deterministic in nature—thus fostering an inaccurate "perception that genes are 'all powerful' determiners of human characteristics" (Condit *et al.* 2001, p. 380). If true, such accounts could lead to deterministic and even fatalistic behaviors where people do not attribute personal control or responsibility over a given action or state (e.g. obesity, lung cancer, violence).

Much of the work addressing concerns associated with deterministic and fatalistic responses has come from the field of genomics (Nelkin and Lindee 1995; Nelkin 2001; Petersen 2001). There are clear links between the realms of genetics and neuroscience and how they are framed in the public eye (Green 2006). Among other aspects, both involve communication of complex information that potentially incorporates multifaceted biomedical and environmental factors. Further, there are reasons to anticipate seeing even closer links between these fields in the near future. For instance, Van Horn and Poldrack suggest that "[w]ith the ability to obtain genetic information with relative ease from only a saliva sample, the next era of neuroimaging will see an increase in the number of fMRI studies examining the role of various allelic gene variants on patterns of BOLD signal" (2009, p. 7). As such, much of the work done in the context of genetics is highly relevant to neuroscience as well.

Nonetheless, while we certainly can—and will—draw on the genetics realm for its wealth of research in this area, it is important to acknowledge that thinking about deterministic concerns is hardly foreign to the world of neuroethics. In 1995, for example, Rose cautioned that the "[d]ramatic advances in neuroscience are changing and enriching our understanding of brain and behaviour. But reductionist interpretations of these advances can cause great harm" (p. 380). Several specific issues have been identified, including the concern that "simplistic understanding of such neuroimaging modalities may increase the risk for misuse and the possibility of the abuse of consumers who are lured by the high-tech profile of the technology" (Racine *et al.* 2006, p. 137). This concern only becomes more prevalent as the direct-to-consumer market, discussed further later in this chapter, continues to grow.

However, while concerns about potential effects may proliferate, what does research tell us about public representations of science and their links with determinism and/or fatatalism? In genetics, the data are somewhat equivocal, although there is some support for the claim that at times the media simplifies stories and overemphasizes the deterministic force of genes. For example, there is evidence that simplified and deterministic messaging can influence attitudes about controversial topics like race (Condit *et al.* 2004; Lynch *et al.* 2008). However, the effect is not as pronounced as some have speculated. Indeed, evidence regarding the degree to which media portrayals are deterministic remains somewhat ambiguous (Condit *et al.* 1998)—despite continuing concern to the contrary. While some studies have found deterministic portrayals, the magnitude of the phenomenon is not as significant as one might expect.

For instance, a study of media portrayals of the obesity gene found that initial stories were somewhat deterministic in tone, but that approach dissipated over the life of the story (Caulfield *et al.* 2009). Other research on the impact of news headlines on genetic determinism suggested that as long as the context of the piece is nondeterministic, "readers are able to construct less deterministic attitudes about genetics for themselves" (Condit *et al.* 2001, p. 393). Further, even where fatalistic beliefs are present, research suggests that they are not mutually exclusive with an awareness of and belief in the additional role of external or environmental factors (e.g. behavior change) (Keeley *et al.* 2009). Indeed, analysis of data from the 2004 Canadian National Health Risk Perception Survey "provides little evidence that Canadians hold overly deterministic attitudes about the role of genes in the induction of human disease" (Etchegary *et al.* 2009, p. 223). Further, other research indicates that some of the conflicting results in research in this area may stem from the fact that individual subjects may have both deterministic and non-deterministic beliefs existing in different neural networks, and that they will express one versus the other depending on the context or cueing (Condit *et al.* 2009). On the whole, given the range of forces influencing public perception of science—including not only the media but also "the creation and implementation of policy and legislation"—it is difficult to predict whether and, if so, for what reason, deterministic attitudes are shifting (Sharp 2007).

Accordingly, despite consistent concerns regarding deterministic and fatalistic responses to genetic information (and, arguably by extension, to neurogenetic information), a review of current literature on this topic does not produce evidence that this effect in fact occurs with any frequency. Of course, one significant limitation of this area of study is that the majority of the research is done using hypothetical situations where participants predict how they will react in the face of genetic information (e.g. Sanderson *et al.* 2010). Naturally, whether such predictions would in fact prove accurate in a given situation remains to be proven.

While the evidence regarding deterministic and fatalistic responses to genetic information may be equivocal at best, this area bears monitoring if for no other reason, then because of the influence neuroimaging seems to command in the general public. It has been noted that "the public often accepts research findings long before the investigators themselves feel they really understand what the results mean" (Check 2005, p. 255). Research into the allure of neuroscientific explanations has shown that irrelevant neuroscientific information caused neuro-novices to "judge explanations [of psychological phenomena] more favourably, particularly the bad explanations" (Weisberg *et al.* 2008, p. 475), and in fact served to mask "otherwise salient problems in these explanations" (Weisberg *et al.* 2008, p. 470). Others suggest that neuroimaging pictures may be particularly persuasive because "they provide a tangible physical explanation for cognitive processes that is easily interpreted as such. This physical evidence may appeal to people's intuitive reductionist approach to understanding the mind as an extension of the brain" (McCabe and Castel 2008, pp. 349–50).

In view of the increasing critiques regarding limitations of fMRI research (Poldrack 2008), the persuasive power of neuroimaging representations seems to justify continued monitoring and analysis of popular representations. While neuroimaging in general, and fMRI in particular, undoubtedly have much to offer scientific understandings, transparent presentations of the relevant limitations are key to accurate interpretations of the science. Accordingly, researchers, commentators and members of the media share a corresponding obligation to ensure this side of the neuroimaging story is appropriately prominent in media representations of emerging results (Illes *et al.* 2009).

FORCES THAT SHAPE THE MESSAGE

To be thorough, consideration of the issues discussed thus far requires acknowledgement of the significant societal forces that influence and shape these movements. The increasingly commercial nature of the research environment in general is one key factor that must be addressed. As one of us has previously speculated:

> [T]he nature and impact of media representations of science has become a major policy concern. Many of the suggested reforms understandably concentrate on ensuring that researchers learn effective communication skills and reporters understand basic scientific principles. However, there are reasons to believe that the hyping of research results might be part of a more systemic problem associated with the increasingly commercial nature of the research environment. (Caulfield 2004b, p. 337)

The forces of commercialization are relevant in a number of respects. Competition for research funds and the growth of the knowledge-based economy mean there is increasing pressure for scientific research to be justified on the basis of economic benefit—ideally benefit that can be expected in the near future. This type of environment can be conducive to encouraging positive portrayals of research results that emphasize their potential benefits and prospective clinical applications (Caulfield 2004b). In the context of neuroimaging, such representations may include, for example, promises that neuroimaging can explain complex states (e.g. love), can help treat or reveal the basis for difficult conditions (e.g. learning disorders, memory problems or violence), or provide an answer to our growing security fears (e.g. lie detection or other interrogative uses).

Another emerging commercial force relates to the growing amount of direct-to-consumer (DTC) advertising of heath products and services occurring largely via the internet. Although attention is increasingly being paid to the DTC marketing of genetic tests (FTC 2006; Caulfield 2009; McGuire *et al.* 2009), neuroproducts and neuroimaging services are also being captured in this mounting market. A simple Google search reveals various companies such as No Lie MRI which promises "unbiased methods for the detection of deception and other information stored in the brain" (No Lie MRI), Cephos Corp., which claims to be "the world-class leader in bringing this technology [fMRI to detect deception] to commercialization" (Cephos Corp), and Neurosense, which uses brain imaging techniques to provide "novel insights in to a marketing problem that are presently unobtainable from any other measures" (Neurosense).

In a more comprehensive study, Racine and colleagues performed Internet searches in 2005 to identify websites offering neuropharmaceuticals (15 websites), neuroimaging services (15 websites), and natural neuroproducts (21 websites) (Racine *et al.* 2007). Interestingly, their content analysis of these sites found that 40% of the websites had archived media stories which, for neuroimaging and natural neuroproduct sites, were stories that reflected positively on the product such as, for example, "Five tests worth paying for" from *The Wall Street Journal* (Racine *et al.* 2007). They also noted that "current gaps in the regulation of neuroimaging services and even more obviously for natural products leave the DTCA [advertising] field open to questionable practices" (Racine *et al.* 2007, p. 190), among other concerns.

Of course, commercial pressures do not solely account for science hype. However, they are increasingly recognized as a potential source of bias that must be acknowledged, and as a force that has the potential to influence the public's perception of research generally (Caulfield 2004a). Further, they contribute to the development of the "cycle of hype" that tends to surround emerging biotechnologies.

> Numerous commentators have remarked that the media, scientists, the public and other interest groups can become complicit in generating a 'cycle of hype'. The cycle is driven by enthusiastic researchers facing pressures from their research institutions, funders and industry; by the desire of institutions and journals to bolster their profiles; by a profit driven media; and by the need of individual journalists to define events as newsworthy. (Bubela *et al.* 2009, p. 516)

The cycle of hype has been evident in other areas such as genetics, stem cell research (Caulfield 2005), and nanotechnology (Williams-Jones 2004), for example, and is clearly emerging in the realm of neuroimaging (Caulfield *et al.*, submitted). Accordingly, researchers, commentators, media representatives and other key stakeholders may wish to draw on the wealth of resources available from other related domains in order to help guide the development of this field.

Conclusion

It is easy to blame the media for overly simplified, hyped, or inaccurate portrayals of science. While some degree of simplification and hype may be a somewhat inevitable part of the media communication process (Bubela *et al.* 2009), numerous studies have shown that, in fact, the media (at least the print media) often does a fairly good job reporting on science (Bubela and Caulfield 2004). Most errors are errors of omission, not commission. In fact, several studies have shown that scientists generally have a good relationship with the media (Peter Peters *et al.* 2008). Moreover, one should not forget the tremendous time pressures that journalists must contend with. They also face internal competition for space in the newspaper or for airtime on broadcasts, and external competition for audience. Simple, exciting messages are much easier to sell, no doubt. However, it is also important to recognize the important role the scientific community plays in communicating their results to the media. In some cases, the source of grand claims regarding the importance of particular findings may in fact lie with the researchers or their press office, rather than the media. Nonetheless, given the significant influence the media wields with the general public and also with key stakeholders and potentially policy makers (Van Horn and Poldrack 2009), it is important that media representations of neuroimaging be as informed and responsible as possible.

One commonly suggested way forward is to improve communication between scientists and journalists, particularly by encouraging scientists to become more active in holding journalists to account for inaccurate representations (Weisberg 2008). Members of the media are encouraged to not overly rely on press releases but rather to, as much as realistically possible, apply the principles of investigative journalism to scientific reporting. "Simply regurgitating uncritically the euphoric press releases issued by universities and leading scientific journals is not in the public interest" (Rose 2003, p. 311). Simultaneously, scientists must take greater responsibility for moderating the manner in which they, and their press release offices, speak about results. For instance, it has been "suggested that efforts be made to influence media coverage of brain imaging research to include discussion of the limitations of fMRI, in order to reduce the misrepresentation of these data" (McCabe and Castel 2008, p. 351). There are also improvements to be made in science communication and community dialogue regarding the social impact of neuroscience (Racine *et al.* 2006). Other potential recommendations include persuading media organizations to employ more reporters and researchers with science backgrounds, encouraging researchers to take media training courses to improve how they express the results and meaning of their research, and promoting "round table dialogues between science, media, and policy leaders that serve to educate each other about the limits of these exciting technologies" (Van Horn and Poldrack 2009, p. 7; see Illes *et al.* 2009 for other recommendations).

While again not unique to the field of neuroimaging, such efforts are important given that "[t]he scope of the issues raised by fMRI will be at least as far-reaching as those of genomics. We might even face them sooner. It is therefore necessary to promote global and proactive analysis of fMRI" (Racine *et al.* 2005, p. 162) (along with other neuroimaging technologies). As noted by Van Horn and Poldrack, "[c]ommunicating fMRI research findings to the public is an important aspect of this work but one that must be undertaken carefully if the field seeks sustained respectability moving forward" (2009, p. 4). An informed and critical press will play a key role in this process by keeping the public up-to-date on advancements in the science and, ideally, raising attendant issues and concerns so as to facilitate informed discussion and debate. "In the end, debate among neuroscientists, life science colleagues, the media and the public represents an exercise in critical thinking and self-reflection. It brings into focus and strengthens the pillars of science, medicine and our pluralist society" (Racine *et al.* 2005, p. 164).

ACKNOWLEDGMENTS

The authors would like to thank the Canadian Institutes of Health Research for funding as well as Ciara Toole and Lindsey Ehrman for their research assistance.

REFERENCES

Bates, B.R. (2005). Public culture and public understanding of genetics: A focus group study. *Public Understanding of Science*, **14**, 47–65.

BBC (2005). Brain scan 'sees hidden thoughts'. BBC News. 25 April 2005. Available at: http://news.bbc.co.uk/2/hi/health/4472355.stm (accessed 24 October 2009).

Brink, S. (2007). Brains in love; When you're attracted to someone, is your gray matter talking sense – or just hooked? Scientists take a rational look. *Los Angeles Times*, 30 July 2007.

Bubela, T. and Caulfield, T. (2004). Do the print media 'hype' genetic research?: A comparison of newspaper stories and peer-reviewed research papers. *Canadian Medical Association Journal*, **170**, 1399–407.

Bubela, T., Nisbet, M., Borchelt, R., *et al.* (2009). Science communication reconsidered. *Nature Biotechnology*, **27**, 514–18.

Canli, T. and Amin, Z. (2002). Neuroimaging of emotion and personality: Scientific evidence and ethical considerations. *Brain and Cognition*, **50**, 414–31.

Caulfield, T. (2004a). The commercialization of medical and scientific reporting. *PLoS Medicine*, **1**, 178–9.

Caulfield, T. (2004b). Biotechnology and the popular press: hype and the selling of science. *Trends in Biotechnology*, **22**, 337–9.

Caulfield, T. (2005). Popular media, biotechnology and the 'cycle of hype'. *Houston Journal of Health Law and Policy*, **5**, 213–33.

Caulfield, T. (2009). Direct-to-consumer genetics and health policy: A worst-case scenario? *The American Journal of Bioethics*, **9**, 48–50.

Caulfield, T., Alfonso, V. and Shelley, J. (2009). Deterministic?: Newspaper representations of obesity and genetics. *The Open Obesity Journal*, **1**, 38–40.

Caulfield, T., Rachul, C., Zarzeczny, A. and Walter, H. (2010). Sensationalizing scanning? Mapping the coverage of neuroimaging research. *SCRIPTed*, **7**. Available at: http://www.law.ed.ac.uk/ahrc/script-ed/vol7-3/editiorial.asp

CBC (2006). Brain scans may help reveal math learning disability. CBC News. 6 March 2006. Available at: http://www.cbc.ca/health/story/2006/03/06/dyscalculia-brain060306.html (accessed 24 October 2009).

Cephos Corp. Available at: http://www.cephoscorp.com/history.htm (accessed 28 October 2009).

Check, E. (2005). Ethicists urge caution over emotive power of brain scans. *Nature*, **435**, 254–5.

Condit, C.M., Ofulue, N., and Sheedy, K.M. (1998). Determinism and mass-media portrayals of genetics. *American Journal of Human Genetics*, **62**, 979–84.

Condit, C.M., Ferguson, A., Kassel, R., and Thadhani, C. (2001). An exploratory study of the impact of news headlines on genetic determinism. *Science Communication*, **22**, 379–95.

Condit, C.M., Parrott, R., Bates, B.R., Bevan, J., and Achter, P.J. (2004). Exploration of the impact of messages about genes and race on lay attitudes. *Clinical Genetics*, **66**, 402–8.

Condit, C.M., Gronnvoll, M., Landaur, J., Shen, L., Wright, L., and Harris, T. (2009). Believing in both genetic determinism and behavioural action: a materialist framework and implications. *Public Understanding of Science*, **16**, 730–46.

Etchegary, H., Lemyre, L., Wilson, B., and Krewski, D. (2009). Is genetic makeup a perceived health risk: analysis of a national survey of Canadians. *Journal of Risk Research*, **12**, 223–7.

Federal Trade Commission (FTC) (2006). At-home genetic tests: A healthy dose of skepticism may be the best prescription. Available at: http://www.ftc.gov/bcp/edu/pubs/consumer/health/hea02.pdf (accessed 28 October 2009).

Fusar-Poli, P. (2007). Love and brain: From mereological fallacy to "folk" neuroimaging. *Psychiatric Research Neuroimaging*, **154**, 285–6.

Green, R.M. (2006). From genome to brainome: charting the lessons learned. In J. Illes (ed.) *Neuroethics: Defining the Issues in Theory, Practice, and Policy*, pp. 105–21. New York: Oxford University Press.

Henderson, M. (2005). For women, pleasure is (nearly) all in the mind. *The Times*, 21 June 2005, p. 3

Hermoye, L. (2007). Functional MRI of sex, when science is hot! Imagilys. 27 February 2007. Available at: http://www.imagilys.com/functional-mri-fmri-sex/ (accessed 28 October 2009).

Highfield, R. (2007). Love really is a drug, say brain scan researchers. *The Daily Telegraph*, 14 February 2007.

Illes, J., Kirschen, M. and Gabrieli, J. (2003). From neuroimaging to neuroethics. *Nature Neuroscience*, **6**, 205.

Illes, J., Racine, E. and Kirschen, M.P. (2006). A picture is worth a 1000 words, but which 1000? In J. Illes (ed.) *Neuroethics: Defining the Issues in Theory, Practice, and Policy*, pp. 149–68. New York: Oxford University Press.

Illes, J. Moser, M.A., McCormick, J., *et al.* (2009). Neurotalk: improving the communication of neuroscience research. *Nature Reviews Neuroscience*, **11**, 61–9.

Jayson, S. (2008). Proof's in the brain scan: Romance can last; it doesn't always fade over time. *The Times*, 17 November 2008.

Jimenez, M. (2009). He's got a girl brain, she's got a boy brain. *Globe and Mail*, 31 March 2009. Available at: http://www.theglobeandmail.com/life/article977714.ece (accessed 27 October 2009).

Keeley, B., Wright, L., and Condit, C. (2009). Functions of health fatalism: fatalistic talk as face saving, uncertainty management, stress relief and sense making. *Sociology of Health & Illness*, **31**, 734–47.

Kitzinger, J. and Williams, C. (2005). Forecasting science futures: Legitimizing hope and calming fears in the embryo stem cell debate. *Social Science and Medicine*, **61**, 731–40.

Logothetis, N.K. (2008). What we can do and what we cannot do with fMRI. *Nature*, **453**, 869–78.

Lynch, J., Bevan, J., Achter, P., Harris, T., and Condit, C.M. (2008). A preliminary study of how multiple exposures to messages about genetics impact on lay attitudes towards racial and genetic discrimination. *New Genetics and Society*, **27**, 43–56.

Marks, L., Kalaitzandonakes, N., Wilkins, L., and Zakharova, L. (2007). Mass media framing of biotechnology news. *Public Understanding of Science*, **16**, 183–203.

McCabe, D. and Castel, A. (2008). Seeing is believing: the effect of brain images on judgments of scientific reasoning. *Cognition*, **107**, 343–52.

McGuire, A., Diaz, C., Wang, T., and Hilsenbeck, S. (2009). Social networkers' attitudes toward direct-to-consumer personal genome testing. *American Journal of Bioethics*, **9**, 3–10.

Minsky, A. (2009). Brain scans may soon read your thoughts. *Canwest News Service*, 13 August 2009. Available at: http://www.canada.com/health/Brain+scans+soon+read+your+thoughts/1888941/story.html (accessed 27 October 2009).

Narayan, A. (2009). The fMRI brain scan: A better lie detector?. *Time*, 20 July 2009. Available at: http://www.time.com/time/health/article/0,8599,1911546-2,00.html (accessed 28 October 2009).

Nelkin, D. (2001). Molecular metaphors: the gene in popular discourse. *Nature Reviews Genetics*, **2**, 555–9.

Nelkin, D. and Lindee, S. (1995). *The DNA Mystique: The Gene as Cultural Icon*. New York: W.H. Freeman.

Neurosense. Available at: http://www.neurosense.co.uk/services.html#Neuroimaging%20solutions (accessed 28 October 2009).

Nisbet, M. and Mooney, C. (2007). Framing science. *Science*, **316**, 56.

No Lie MRI. Available at: http://noliemri.com/ (accessed 28 October 2009).

Persaud, R. (2004). Love really is blind… Neuroscience can at last explain why we can't see faults in our partners or children. *The Daily Telegraph*, 2 June 2004.

Peter Peters, H., Brossard, D., de Cheveigné, S., et al. (2008). Interactions with the mass media. *Science*, **321**, 204–5.

Petersen, A. (2001). Biofantasies: genetics and medicine in the print news media. *Social Science & Medicine*, **52**, 1255–68.

Petersen, A. (2009). The ethics of expectations: Biobanks and the promise of personalised medicine. *Monash Bioethics Review*, **28**, 5.1–5.12.

Poldrack, R. (2008). The role of fMRI in cognitive neuroscience: where do we stand? *Current Opinion in Neurobiology*, **18**, 223–7.

Racine, E. and Illes, J. (2007). Emerging ethical challenges in advanced neuroimaging research: Review, recommendations and research agenda. *Journal of Empirical Research on Human Research Ethics*, **2**, 1–10.

Racine, E., Bar-Ilan, O. and Illes, J. (2005). fMRI in the public eye. *Nature Reviews Neuroscience*, **6**, 159–64.

Racine, E., Bar-Ilan, O. and Illes, J. (2006). Brain imaging: A decade of coverage in the print media. *Science Communication*, **28**, 122–42.

Racine, E., Van der Loos, A. and Illes, J. (2007). Internet marketing of neuroproducts: New practices and healthcare policy challenges. *Cambridge Quarterly of Healthcare Ethics*, **16**, 181–94.

Rose, S. (1995). The rise of neurogenetic determinism. *Nature*, **373**, 380–2.

Rose, S. (2003). How to (or not to) communicate science. *Biochemical Society Transactions*, **31**, 307–12.

Sanderson, S.C., Persky, S., and Michie, S. (2010). Psychological and behavioral responses to genetic test results indicating increased risk of obesity: Does the causal pathway from gene to obesity matter? *Public Health Genomics*, **13**, 34–47.

Sharp, M. (2007). The effect of genetic determinism and exceptionalism on law and policy. *Health Law Review*, **15**, 16–18.

Sutton, B.P., Ouyang, C., Karampinos, D.C., and Miller, G.A. (2009). Current trends and challenges in MRI acquisitions to investigate brain function. *International Journal of Psychophysiology*, **73**, 33–42.

U.S. News (2008). Brain scans show bullies enjoy others' pain. U.S. News & World Report. 7 November 2008. Available at: http://health.usnews.com/articles/health/healthday/2008/11/07/brain-scans-show-bullies-enjoy-others-pain.html (accessed 28 October 2009).

Van Horn, J.D. and Poldrack, R.A. (2009). Functional MRI at the crossroads. *International Journal of Psychophysiology*, 73, 3–9.

Weisberg, D. (2008). Caveat lector: The presentation of neuroscience information in the popular media. *The Scientific Review of Mental Health Practice*, 6, 51–6.

Weisberg, D., Keil, F., Goodstein, J., Rawson, E., and Gray, J. (2008). The seductive allure of neuroscience explanations. *Journal of Cognitive Neuroscience*, 20, 470–7.

Williams-Jones, B. (2004). A spoonful of trust helps the nanotech go down. *Health Law Review*, 12, 10–13.

CHAPTER 43

BRAIN TRUST: NEUROSCIENCE AND NATIONAL SECURITY IN THE 21ST CENTURY

JONATHAN D. MORENO

By any reasonable measure, including numbers of publications, academic positions, and research funding, interest in the multidisciplinary field known as neuroscience is rapidly growing. Another interdisciplinary field, bioethics, shows no signs of lessened interest or social importance. Although the bioethics literature on national security issues is surprisingly sparse (Moreno and Peroski 2009), the implications of neuroscience for national security are of increasing public and scholarly interest. Evidence for this assertion is limited but compelling; as I will elaborate, one important source of evidence can be found in reports by US government advisory committees over the past several years.

For various reasons there are no precise metrics of national security research and development (R&D). At least some of this work takes place under classified conditions, including "black" or unpublished budgets,[1] but even more pertinent is the fact that R&D is not always clearly identified according to budget lines. Therefore standard trend analysis in terms of agency mission or dollar investment is not available. There are also familiar problems in defining precisely what kind of work falls under the ambit of neuroscience. But, as I hope to demonstrate, the growing interest in neuroscience on the part of national security agencies can be discerned in part by reviewing recent reports from the US National Academies.

---

[1] I am not referring here to human experiments, which are at best difficult to conduct under classified conditions according to US human research rules; nor do there currently appear to be any classified human experiments funded or sponsored by the US government. It is, however, possible to conduct field tests and evaluation studies without bringing them under the ambit of the human research regulations.

THE ENCOUNTER BETWEEN NEUROSCIENCE
AND NATIONAL SECURITY

The relationship between national security concerns and neuroscience is complex. In my book *Mind Wars: Brain Research and National Defense* (Moreno 2006), I argued that national security needs are sure to be at the cutting edge of neuroscience, both in terms of research for warfighting and intelligence and, over the long term, the introduction of new neurotechnologies in society. In turn, the encounter between national security and neuroscience will provide much fodder for neuroethics. I also urged that these developments can most fruitfully be seen in historical context. An obvious and familiar example of unintended consequences is the Central Intelligence Agency and US Army LSD (lysergic acid diethylamide) experiments of the 1950s and 1960s. These projects were motivated by a number of concerns and goals, including interest in hallucinogens as a problem in counter-intelligence (e.g. the fear that they could be used as a "truth serum" with a kidnapped US nuclear scientist), and as a potential disruptor of combat units (Lee and Shlain 1994).

In short, interest in the brain, what it does, how to manipulate it, and how to benefit from modifying it is hardly new among defense officials, both in the US and elsewhere. The long-term cultural consequences of LSD's introduction into prestigious academic studies is an irony that does not seem to have been anticipated by government actors, but might be a useful warning in a new era of provocative, "enhancing" pharmacologics. New imaging devices, advanced neuropharmacology, implantable devices, imaging technologies, and other innovations are sure to take national security interest in neuroscience to a new level, leading as well to remarkable problems in ethics and public policy. One may expect that there will be unanticipated social consequences of the embrace of new and more powerful neuroscience by national security interests.

One of the obstacles to the participation of neuroethicists in the encounter between national security and neuroscience is a lack of familiarity with the national security establishment, which includes uniformed military services, those services' intelligence entities, as well as non-military services such as the Central Intelligence Agency, the Federal Bureau of Investigation, and the National Security Agency. Evidence of the national security establishment's growing interest in neuroscience may be inferred from the fact that national security agencies have recently reached out on several occasions to the US National Academies for guidance on the implications and applications of developments in neuroscience. Clients for the recent National Academies projects were the Defense Intelligence Agency, the Office of the Director of National Intelligence, and the US Army.

Comprised of the National Academy of Sciences, the National Academy of Engineering, the Institute of Medicine, and the National Research Council (regarded as the "executive arm" of the Academies), the National Academies are a non-governmental organization chartered by the US government to provide independent advice on science, engineering, and medicine. As such, the National Academies' role in assessing emerging technologies such as those in neuroscience is a metric of the directionality of US government policy concerns, and to some degree those of other major powers as well, at least insofar as the national security establishment is interested in seeking out high-profile advice from the academic world.

US Army interest in the National Academies' advice on performance enhancement is not new. The National Research Council's Committee on Techniques for the Enhancement of Human Performance produced a series of reports between 1988 and 1994 for the US Army. A brief overview of these reports illustrates how much the science and the potential security applications have changed. While the topics of interest are largely the same as those of concern today—e.g. enhanced training, deceiving and deception, managing stress—the modalities considered promising are vastly different from those of less than two decades later. These older modalities included various means of altering mental states such as sub-liminal self-help, neurolinguistic programming, hemispheric synchronization, hypnosis, and meditation.

According to the 1988 report *Enhancing Human Performance: Issues, Theories, and Techniques*, there was also significant interest within the Army in paranormal phenomena such as extra-sensory perception (ESP) and psychokinesis (PK). The committee undertook a careful analysis of the scant evidence for the effectiveness of such techniques, but their conclusion may be gauged from this passage: "The claimed phenomena and applications"... presented by several military officers, "range from the incredible to the outrageously incred-ible. The 'anti-missile time warp,' for example, is somehow supposed to deflect attack from nuclear warheads so that they will transcend time and explode among the ancient dino-saurs....One suggested application is a conception of the 'First Earth Battalion,' made up of 'warrior monks'...including the use of ESP, leaving their bodies at will, levitating, psychic healing and walking through walls." (Druckman and Swets 1988). Amusing as it is, this pas-sage exemplifies a persistent cultural tension between the felt need of intelligence agencies for cutting-edge technology, regardless of the source, and the scientific community's insistence on rigorous validation.

Modern neuroscience, boasting of new tools like functional magnetic resonance imaging (fMRI) and more targeted pharmacological approaches, has bred revived interest on the part of the military and intelligence communities. The National Academies have engaged in at least three projects directly related to neuroscience research policy since 2007 that were conducted under contract with national security agencies. The report *Emerging Cognitive Neuroscience and Related Technologies* was released in August 2008 for the Defense Intelligence Agency (National Research Council of the National Academies 2008). *Opportunities in Neuroscience for Future Army Applications* was published in May 2009 and conducted for the US Army (National Council of the National Academies 2009). In addi-tion, the Committee on Field Evaluation of Behavioral and Cognitive Sciences-Based Methods and Tools for Intelligence and Counter-Intelligence planned and hosted a public workshop in September 2009, at the request of the Defense Intelligence Agency and the Office of the Director of National Intelligence.[2]

In this chapter I will primarily address these questions: What can be learned from these projects about the current concerns and potential goals of the US national security estab-lishment with regard to neuroscience? And how do ethical and policy issues play into these

---

[2] The author was a member of the committee that released the first report mentioned and of the commit-tee to plan the September 2009 workshop on field testing of intelligence and counter-intelligence methods and tools. None of the matters discussed in the reports or the workshop or reviewed here are classified, and none of these remarks reflect the views of the committees or the Academies.

concerns and potential goals? The US national security establishment is the world's largest and perhaps most complex set of organizations, governmental and non-governmental. Understood as multiple interacting systems its "outputs" are no more the product of systematic, disinterested rational activities than those of any other human social endeavor. Therefore, although I have put my primary questions in the anthropomorphic terms of concerns and goals, there should be no inference to any particular sort of deliberations within these systems that lead ineluctably to a certain science policy agenda. Nonetheless, intentionally or not, black boxes do produce results.

Enhancing operatives

Perhaps the most (literally) spectacular aspect of modern neuroscience research are those technologies that provide visual evidence of neural function. Certain brain scanning techniques, especially fMRI, have stimulated an industry of research attempting to correlate neural activity with specific tasks or experiences. In one famous and controversial study, negative automatic responses to photographs of black faces by white research subjects have been correlated with activity in the amygdala, which processes emotion in the presence of stimuli (Hart *et al.* 2000). Or take the example of interpersonal game experiments in which mutual cooperation results in both subjects winning. When that happens it's been found that neural circuits mediated by the chemical dopamine are activated, "lighting up" pleasure centers in the brain. In other studies another neurotransmitter, serotonin, has been associated with feelings of well being and that it might modulate stress reactions (Wood *et al.* 2006). The role of many of these chemicals in brain activity is not yet well understood, however. Some neuroscientists claim to be able to ascertain via fMRI when an individual is thinking of a certain number (Haynes *et al.* 2007), or when they are lying (Langelben *et al.* 2002; Knight 2004), or what their sexual orientation is (Ponseti *et al.* 2006), and that the abilities to make these assessments will only become more refined and precise in the years ahead.

It's not hard to see how these kinds of technical capabilities would suggest all sorts of intriguing security implications. For instance, candidates for special operations may be assessed for their reactions to stress in various situations, including neurotransmitter secretions. Fighters in information-rich environments, like cockpits, could have their brain functions monitored for information overload and data flow modified accordingly; devices to provide complex "real-time" remote brain imaging are now being developed, as is software to support automated workstations to monitor cognitive states. Then there is an array of projects intended to replace old-fashioned lie detectors with neuroscience-based systems, perhaps obviating the need for more physically aggressive means of interrogating terror suspects and enemy operatives. "Locals" who are considered for employment in sensitive environments like embassies might also be subjects of advanced, neuroscience-based, deception screening.

If brain functions can be visualized perhaps they can be directed to certain ends. Interventions intended to enhance warfighters' capabilities could come in many forms, including new generations of neuropharmaceuticals, implants, and neural stimulation. New anti-sleep agents like modafinil, approved for the treatment of narcolepsy, are replacing old-fashioned amphetamines among fighter pilots as well as globe-trotting business executives and shift-workers (O'Connor 2004). Again, the history is telling: "poppers" (amphetamine tablets) were regarded as an advance over caffeine. The Department of Defense science agency, the Defense Advanced Research Projects Agency (DARPA) created a "peak soldier performance" program aiming to improve metabolism on demand so that an individual could operate at a high level for 3–5 days, without needing sleep or calories, perhaps using high nutrition pills.

Both non-invasive and invasive systems are up for consideration as neuroenhancers. Electrical stimulation has been used with some success as an adjunct to standard rehabilitation of stroke victims (Kim *et al.* 2006). Could healthy individuals acquire improved cognitive capacities through neurostimulation? More invasive technologies might someday increase the bandwidth of soldiers' brains. Dubbed a "brain prosthesis," an idea under study is a chip that, if it works and is safe for persons with stroke or epilepsy, might also enhance normal brains (Maguire and McGee 1999). There is, however, deep disagreement about the question whether a device that ameliorates a pathology can also improve normal functioning, a problem that may only be answerable empirically through ethically challenging experiments. Recalling the troubled history of psychosurgery, there are troubling safety issues in acting directly upon the brain, especially long-term risks and effects on other parts of the central nervous system.

Genetics may ultimately provide more efficient and stable opportunities to enhance desirable traits like learning and memory than mechanical devices. Perhaps extra copies of genes that code for certain neural receptor sites could be introduced to improve learning skills, as has been shown in mice (Gazzaniga 2005). In the highly competitive world of neuroscience there are devoted advocates of all sorts of approaches to ameliorating central nervous system disorders and perhaps functional improvement of medically normal persons.

FEAR IN THE FIELD

Intelligence and endurance are not the only elements that make for a promising combat soldier. Another is the ability to manage the fear response. In an interesting experiment, an American research team found that if they bred mice lacking the gene stathmin and put them in aversive situations, like giving them a mild shock in their cages, they didn't exhibit normal fear behavior as often as normal mice. Stathmin is expressed in the amygdala and is associated with both innate and learned fear. So the "knockout" mice froze in place less often because they had impaired learning capacity (Shumyatsky *et al.* 2005). Now it's unlikely that there's any such one-to-one correspondence between a particular gene and fear in people, but one can imagine an overly enthusiastic official proposing to screen recruits for the "fear gene."

Where there's fear can guilt be far behind? Trauma victims who had been given the beta-blocker propranolol (normally used to treat heart disease), scored lower on a post-traumatic stress disorder (PTSD) scale than a control group after a month of psychological counseling, though not significantly. However, 3 months later none of the beta-blocker recipients had elevated physiological responses when asked to recall their traumatic experiences but 40% of the control group members did (Pitman *et al.* 2002). These results give hope to PTSD sufferers, as the drug inhibits the release of brain chemicals that consolidate long-term memory with emotion. They also raise the question whether a drug could someday be given prophylactically before one enters what could be a traumatizing situation. How would we feel about preventing PTSD in young people sent into battle, preventing both a lifetime of harrowing memories as well as their capacity to connect their horrific experiences with negative emotions? Suppose that such a drug was so targeted that it did not inadvertently inhibit evolutionary mechanisms like "fight or flight" that are so crucial for individual survival. Would we have reservations about guilt-free soldiers?

The national security implications of modern neuroscience also raise specific policy questions about civil liberties, regulation, and safety, and about the responsibilities of neuroscientists for the ultimate "dual uses" of the technologies they develop. The role of atomic scientists in the control of nuclear weapons has achieved nearly iconic status as an exemplar of the inescapable nature of professional responsibility. More recently biologists have become key players in planning for defense against bioterror attacks and have been party to lively debates about problems such as the publication of potentially sensitive information. The same is not yet true of neuroscientists, partly because the very idea that neuroscience could be a national defense concern is only now becoming clear, and partly because neuroscience is still a complex interdisciplinary field whose practitioners work in separate silos. But the time is rapidly approaching when a more systematic accounting of some of these issues will be needed.

Academic assessments of neuroscience and national security needs

At the end of *Mind Wars* I suggested that one model is the National Science Advisory Board for Biosecurity that was established in 2004 by the National Institutes of Health. The NSABB advises all cabinet departments, including the Department of Defense. The non-governmental experts on the board supplement the expertise in federal agencies on the ways that new developments in important biological research could be misused to threaten public health and national security. A National Science Advisory Board for Neurosecurity, I argued, could address analogous problems and bring together the wide range of neuroscience disciplines that have not yet talked to each other about appropriate policies concerning brain research and national defense. It, too, could be organized and administered by the National Institutes of Health and provide advice to the Department of Defense, the Department of Homeland Security, and other relevant agencies. Although that board has not been created, the recent National Academies' studies appear to herald a new era in which the US national security establishment is seeking very public guidance from the premier civilian science advisory organization. Readers may consult the published materials for detailed information about each of these projects. Here I will only summarize their missions and findings, which represent some of the most up-to-date interactions between the academic and national security communities concerning research policy.

Neuroscience and the intelligence community

Emerging Cognitive Neuroscience and Related Technologies (National Research Council of the National Academies 2008) concerns itself with the intelligence community's need to integrate the rapid flow of information from modern neuroscience. The committee was asked to assess the current state of work for trends that should be tracked, to assess the rate of innovation, and to pay special attention to selected countries. The committee's Key Finding addressed itself to the need for intelligence collection and analysis to emphasize science and technology, to obtain intelligence professionals with advanced scientific training, and to increase collaboration with the academic community. Its Key Recommendation was that the intelligence community use a more centralized indication and warning system concerning non-US neuroscience potential. The report reviewed several promising areas of neuroscience research that could be of special interest to intelligence entities: detection of psychological states and intentions; neuropsychopharmacology; functional neuroimaging; computational biology applied to cognition, functional neuroimaging, genomics, and proteomics; human–machine systems. It also assessed the cultural underpinnings of neuroscience and ethical implications of evolving neurotechnologic capacity.

This report also provides an appendix that assesses neuroscience advances that might be achieved in two particular countries of interest: China and Iran. Both countries have substantial scientific capacity as compared to others in the developing world and have shown themselves able to mount sophisticated research programs in targeted fields, albeit in a very few mature research centers. But in general, tracking the uses of drugs or devices for non-medical purposes, as in enhancement or interrogation experiments, is difficult unless results are published. If they are not, then even if imports from particular manufacturers can be traced (e.g. of imaging devices), the actual uses to which a technology is applied once in the country are hard to discern without the presence of a clandestine intelligence operative. But such uses would normally be considered human experimentation, pointing up the fact that the international system of human experiment regulation is wholly voluntary.

Neuroscience and the army

Opportunities in Neuroscience for Future Army Applications (National Research Council of the National Academies 2009) suggests tailoring individual soldiers' training to recent discoveries about the brain from modern neuroscience can provide valuable advances in military training, both in terms of ameliorating deficits and enhancing performance over some baseline of normalcy. According to the report's summary:

> The committee reviewed neuroscience applications related to understanding, monitoring, and preventing or treating deficits in soldier performance. These deficits may affect performance during a single extended operation or over much longer time frames. The report considered prevention interventions relevant to acute deficits noticeable immediately within the time frame of a day or days as well as longer-term deficits such as post-traumatic stress disorder (PTSD) and other chronic effects of brain trauma on the central nervous system.

Ranking the potential payoffs of neuroscience for the Army as near, medium, and long term, the committee concluded that advances in learning, training, and performance are likely to prove to be of the most immediate benefit. Along with traditional areas of concern to the military like leadership and decision-making under stress, the report suggests that the services should also take cognitive fitness, brain–machine interfaces, and biomarkers (biological indicators of brain states) into consideration during basic training. Not only different ways of learning, but differences in orientation to risk-taking, decision making, and personal resilience might also be identifiable in more subtle ways than can be ascertained through simply observing behavior. Cellular and molecular neuroscience was judged to have more remote affects on military operations than cognitive neuroscience, and benefits from advances in systems neuroscience still less impact. Among the interesting opportunities identified was more investment in neuroergonomics, which "explores the ability of the brain to directly control systems beyond traditional human effector systems (hands and voice) by structuring the brain's output as a signal that can be transduced into a control input to an external system (a machine, electronic system, computer, semiautonomous air or ground vehicle, etc.)." (National Research Council of the National Academies 2009). More generally, the report found that the Army has no central monitoring system of potential neuroscience applications. Rather, research and development activities are scattered among various centers. It recommends the creation of a board to track military neuroscience R&D.

Field testing intelligence tools and methods

The remit of the Committee on Field Evaluation of Behavioral and Cognitive Sciences-Based Methods and Tools for Intelligence and Counter-Intelligence was to organize a workshop on field testing behavioral and social science-based methods that may be attractive for counter-intelligence purposes. A wide variety of tools and methods fall into this category but the often have doubtful validity. Examples are the Preliminary Credibility Assessment Screening System (PCASS), essentially a hand-held version of the traditional "lie detector"; technologies to measure voice stress; and APOLLO, a software application intended to help predict an individual's behavior, including political actors. These cases and a number of more general issues in validation were discussed in the public workshop in Washington, DC on September 22–23, 2009 and in several commissioned papers.

Unlike report projects assigned to committees, the National Research Council's workshop format does not involve the production of findings and recommendations, only a summary of the workshop proceedings. However, several key issues emerged, all touching on the tension between the pressing need for new intelligence tools in environments that are complex, dangerous, and often present unfamiliar cultural conditions for US personnel, and the slow, highly regulated and often uncertain pace of scientific validation. Speakers from several disciplines—organizational psychology, education, policing, and medicine—all noted that program evaluation in the field may ultimately produce data that are difficult for the practitioners themselves to integrate, both because of ambiguities that can emerge from formal testing and cultural resistance in the user community to science-based conclusions about the technology. The conditions of field evaluation are also challenging. In particular, field testing of new tools and methods that is intended to produce generalizable knowledge may be subject to both US and international conventions of human research ethics.

Neuroethics and national security

Scholars interested in the ethics of neuroscience have paid relatively little attention to the national security context. Yet there are reasons to believe that this setting will be crucial for the future of neuroscience. First, as these National Academies projects indicate, there is modest but serious and persistent interest in and concern about the security and intelligence implications of neuroscience and related technological developments. Second, there are many funding mechanisms available once national security objectives are at stake. Third, societal reticence about certain applications may be lessened in this context and therefore, fourth, national security applications could pave the way for public acceptability and adoption where there might otherwise be greater resistance.

But there is a great deal of room for misunderstanding about the potential for new knowledge about the brain to affect national security operations. Among the obvious problems are the obstacles to translating interesting laboratory findings into measures that can be applied in field conditions. Relatively few effective and efficient technologies for either civilian or military use are ever derived from basic science, and so far neuroscience has at best a thin record of achievement in this regard. A related issue is that fact that defense planners and intelligence analysts feel intense pressures to arrive at reliable conclusions at confidence levels that would not be satisfactory in the scientific community. Hence the concern expressed by scholars that certain technologies may be embraced by practitioners before they have been validated, and that some may find their way into common practice with little or no supporting evidence. The various so-called "lie detector" technologies are the paradigm case of this concern.

National Academies' reports tend to focus on science policy. Although ethical concerns may be inferred from their findings and recommendations, they are not usually rendered explicit. By contrast, on grounds of professional ethics several organizations within the scientific community have expressed their objections to the participation of their members in certain intelligence-related activities. Both the American Psychiatric Association (2008) and, in at least some official statements, the American Psychological Association (Bray 2002), have discouraged their members from participating in interrogation activities. Similarly, the American Anthropological Association has opposed anthropologists' participation in an experimental counter-insurgency project called the "human terrain system," in which anthropologists are embedded with combat units to assist in understanding local cultures (American Anthropological Association 2007).

There are familiar and deep cultural reservations about national security activities that challenge traditional notions of privacy and self-determination. Some of the ways these reservations express themselves are frankly without foundation; they are either pathological (as in paranoid delusions about authority, which are remarkably cross-cultural and recalcitrant), or based on unrealistic concerns about technological possibilities, or both. However, there are also important ethical concerns about plausible scenarios that raise problems in human research ethics, justifying the imposition of new technologies on warfighters, international relations, and just war theory, as well as acceptable limits on the participation of scientists in these activities. These are all rich targets for the neuroethicist.

Acknowledgment

The author expresses his gratitude to Hannah Zale for her assistance in the preparation of this manuscript.

References

American Anthropological Association (2007). *Executive Board Statement on the Human Terrain System Project* Washington, DC: American Anthropological Association.

American Psychiatric Association (2008). *Psychiatric participation in interrogation of detainees: position statement.* Washington, DC: American Psychiatric Association.

Bray, J.H. (2009). *Press Release: Saying it Again: Psychologists May Never Participate in Torture.* Washington, DC: American Psychological Association.

Druckman, D. and Swets, J.A. (eds.) (1988). *Enhancing Human Performance: Issues, Theories, and Techniques.* Washington, DC: The National Academies Press.

Gazzaniga, M.S. (2005). *The Ethical Brain.* Washington, DC: Dana Press.

Hart, A.J., Whalen, P.J., Shin, M.R., *et al.* (2000). Differential response in the human amygdala to racial outgroup vs ingroup face stimuli. *NeuroReport*, 11, 2351–4.

Haynes, J., Sakai, K., Rees, G., Gilbert, S., Frith, C., and Passingham, R.E. (2007). Reading hidden intentions in the human brain. *Current Biology*, 17, 323–8.

Kim, Y., You, S.H., Ko, M., *et al.* (2006). Repetitive transcranial magnetic stimulation—induced corticomotor excitability and associated motor skill acquisition in chronic stroke. *Stroke*, 37, 1471–6.

Knight, J. (2004). The truth about lying. *Nature*, 428, 692–4.

Langelben, D.D., Schroeder, L., Maldjian, J.A., *et al.* (2002). Brain activity during simulated deception: an event-related functional magnetic resonance study. *NeuroImage*, 15, 727–32.

Lee, M.A. and Shlain, B. (1994). *Acid Dreams: The Complete Social History of LSD: The CIA, the Sixties, and Beyond.* New York: Grove Press.

Maguire, G.Q. and McGee, E.M. (1999). Implantable brain chips? Time for debate. *The Hastings Center Report*, 29, 7–13.

Moreno, J.D. (2006). *Mind Wars: Brain Research and National Defense.* Washington, DC: Dana Press.

Moreno, J.D. and Peroski, M. (2009). Bioethics and national security. In V. Ravitsky, A. Fiester, and A.L. Caplan (eds.) *The Penn Center Guide to Bioethics.* New York: Springer Publishing Company.

National Research Council of the National Academies (2008). *Emerging Cognitive Neuroscience and Related Technologies.* Washington, DC: The National Academies Press.

National Research Council of the National Academies (2009). *Opportunities in Neuroscience for Future Army Applications.* Washington, DC: The National Academies Press.

O'Connor, A. (2004). Wakefulness finds a powerful ally. *The New York Times (New York Edition)*, 29 June 2004: 1F

Pitman, R.K., Sanders, K.M., Zusman, R.M., *et al.* (2002). Pilot study of secondary prevention of posttraumatic stress disorder with propranolol. *Biological Psychiatry*, 51, 189-92.

Ponseti, J., Bosinski, H.A., Wolff, S., *et al.* (2006). A functional endophenotype for sexual orientation in humans. *NeuroImage*, 33, 825–33.

Shumyatsky, G.P., Malleret, G., Shin, R., *et al.* (2005). stathmin, a gene enriched in the amygdala, controls both learned and innate fear. *Cell*, **123**, 697–709.

Wood, R.M., Rilling, J.K., Sanfey, A.G., Bhagwagar, Z., and Rogers, R.D. (2006). Effects of tryptophan depletion on the performance of an iterated Prisoner's Dilemma game in healthy adults. *Neuropsychopharmacology*, **31**, 1075–84.

PART VII

SCIENCE, SOCIETY, AND INTERNATIONAL PERSPECTIVES

CHAPTER 44

NEUROPLASTICITY, CULTURE, AND SOCIETY

BRUCE E. WEXLER

INTRODUCTION

THE most fundamental difference between the human brain and those of other mammals is the greater extent to which development of its structure and function is influenced by sensory input. This sensitivity to the environment rests on four features common to all mammals and one unique in extent to human beings. First, neurocognitive capacity increases across the phylogenetic hierarchy primarily through increases in the overall number of brain cells and their interconnections. Second, cells require sensory input from the environment to maintain their vitality and functionality. Third, cognitive functions such as perception, memory, and thinking arise from the integrated activity of multineuronal systems involving multiple brain areas and are not properties of a specific anatomical location dedicated to a specific cognitive operation. Fourth, neurons activated by sensory input develop connections with other neurons and thus constitute the multineuronal systems; environmentally induced activity thus shapes both the structure and function of the brain. Fifth, only human beings to any significant extent shape the environments that in turn shape their brains.

Neuroplasticity refers to change in neural structures and is usually the result of activity-dependent change in the interconnections among cells that constitute the structures. Enduring changes in structure result from repeated activation of some cells and pathways more than others, following the principle that neurons that fire together wire together. The neuroplastic potential of the human brain is greater than that of our nearest primate cousins due to changes in two parameter settings in pre- and postnatal neurodevelopment. One is a further increase in the number of neurons. The second is increased length of time after birth during which interconnections among neurons are easily shaped by environmental input. These two changes make it possible for environmental input to create more elaborate and powerful neural functional structures. The changes in parameter settings are the result of Darwinian biological evolution, but together with the fact that humans alter the environment that provides the formative sensory stimulation, they provide the foundation for cultural evolution.

Cultural evolution differs from Darwinian biological evolution in several important ways. Cultural evolution creates more rapid, more incremental, and more widespread population variability. Cultural and biological evolution also differ in the way information is stored so as to provide continuing influence on function. In biological evolution, information is stored in the largely stable base sequence of DNA molecules. In cultural evolution, the information is stored in the minds and behavior of adult members of society; in cultural artifacts such as books, architecture, and works of art; and in social institutions including laws, customs, and schools. In biological evolution the information is stored in identical and complete form in many individuals. In cultural evolution, the information is distributed in different and incomplete form across many individuals and artifacts.

The extent of our neuroplasticity, and our associated ability to alter the ways our minds and brains work by altering the environment that shapes them, has only recently become known to human beings. Attention to the implications of this for ethics is even more recent. Indeed, Judeo-Christian influences on contemporary Western thinking about morality and ethics have included the view that all aspects of human biology, including our minds and brains, were designed or created more or less in their adult form by the active hand of an external almighty. Both codes for ethical behavior and human characteristics and capabilities were largely given to us by a power external to us and much more powerful than we are. Debates about good and evil, and human responsibility and free will have taken place within this conceptual field. The first major challenge to this posed by biological science was Darwin's theory of evolution. It was hotly contested by church authorities when first introduced, and continues to be hotly contested by some religious communities today. The fact that human nature has arisen from single-cell organisms through random mutation and selective pressures from an environment that is itself also contingent, reframes the discussion about ethics, accountability, responsibility, good and evil. In this context, some have gone so far as to suggest that ethical behavior, and most important aspects of human thought, have evolved through these same Darwinian processes, although such views are increasingly at odds with current thinking about brain functional organization and their proponents are unable to ascertain the type of data necessary for real scientific inquiry. The new science of neuroplasticity provides the second major change in the terms of ethical considerations introduced by biological sciences.

Understanding the centrality of neuroplasticity in human brain development, and the power of cultural evolution that rests upon it, provides a new biologically based understanding of the relationship between human beings and the environment. The first phase of that relationship is the aforementioned transgenerational dialectic between human capabilities, human actions, and human-created expectations based on the influence of the human-made environment on neurocognitive development. In this phase, developing individuals have limited ability to act on the environment but are profoundly affected by it. A homology is created between the external environment and internal structures because the brain shapes itself to the recurring features of the specific environment in which it develops. By young adulthood, however, there is a fundamental shift in the relationship between the individual and the environment. The powerful neuroplastic processes in the developing brain are replaced by the less powerful ones of adulthood, and now established internal structures are self maintaining. Individuals are now able to act on the environment and do so to make the environment match established internal structures. They feel and function better when there is a match between internal and external. As a result, there is a "neurobiological antagonism to difference" (Wexler 2006, p. 212). These processes are central to what it means to be a human being rather than any other animal on earth, and they frame the discussion of human responsibility and free will in a different way than it was before and after application of Darwinian insights to considerations of ethics.

This chapter will review the neuroscience of neuroplasticity in human beings and other mammals. It will present a contemporary neural systems view of brain functional organization, review evidence on the importance of sensory input to maintain neuronal viability, and describe studies that demonstrate that the nature of that input influences brain structure and function. The centrality of socially generated stimulation will be discussed through citation of the work of Harlow and Mears with infant monkeys, more recent work in rats identifying epigenetic changes in DNA structure leading to lifelong effects of early maternal behaviors, and the work of the Russian developmental psychologist Vygotsky and early 20th-century psychoanalytic ego-psychologists on the role of interpersonal interactions in creating internal mental structures. The next section will present brain imaging studies that have demonstrated the effects of environmentally induced activity on human brain structure and function. The final section will describe some of the ways established internal structures act on the environment to make it match those structures. The overall goal is to lay the groundwork for broad ranging consideration of the issues raised and their ethics implications.

A CONTEMPORARY NEURAL SYSTEMS VIEW OF HUMAN BRAIN FUNCTION

There are 100 billion neurons in the human brain each directly connected to over 1000 other neurons. Consistent with this massive interconnectivity, learning simple associations between stimuli leads to altered responses in millions of cells distributed across wide expanses of cortical territory (John et al. 1986). When people perform simple cognitive operations, multiple brain areas in both cerebral hemispheres become more active, and others decrease their activity (e.g. D'Esposito 2007). Moreover, when even simple tasks are repeated minutes or hours later, there is a different pattern of task-related regional activation changes, with (e.g. Poldrack et al. 1999) or without (e.g. Kelly et al. 2006; Loubinoux et al. 2001) deliberate efforts to teach or learn the tasks. In real life, most of the things we do we have done before, so that the brain activations associated with them have been different at different times. As people get older, there are also common changes across individuals, so that the same tasks are done by different combinations of brain areas at different ages (e.g. Gaillard et al. 2000; Stebbins et al. 2002). Furthermore, if the same component cognitive operation is performed as part of different overall cognitive functions, the pattern of regional brain activation associated with that component operation is different (e.g. Friston et al. 1996; Wexler 2004).

These relatively recent observations are consistent with the notion of cerebral functional systems described by the early 20th century Russian neuropsychologist A.R. Luria (Luria 1973; see also Vygotsky 1978). Luria noted that localized injuries rarely affected only one cognitive operation, but usually affected multiple. He also noted that individual cognitive operations were affected by injuries in multiple different areas of the brain. He concluded that while groups of cells in a specific anatomic location might collectively have some elementary tissue function, such functions do not correspond to mental functions like perception, memory, or cognition. Mental operations are instead properties of multicomponent functional systems. Like other systems, cerebral functional systems perform constant functions through means or components that vary from instance to instance. Functions are properties of a system and not of a specific anatomic location. Most contemporary views of the functional organization of the human brain are based on such systems.

This modern view contrasts with 19th-century concepts of phrenology and related 20th-century concepts of modularity (see Wexler 2004, 2006). Phrenology and modularity posit that specific cognitive operations are performed at circumscribed, localized anatomic sites, and that the function of these sites is the specific cognitive operation. In contrast, the 21st-century systems view posits that ensembles of cells at different locations have different characteristics like different letters of an alphabet. Cognitive functions emerge from combinations of different local units just as words emerge from combinations of letters. In addition, there may be a few localized units in the systems model that are also stand alone modules for simple cognitive operations; perhaps operations that evolved prior to the primate, or even the mammalian line. Like the single letter words "a" and "I," such modules could serve both as free-standing cognitive modules and as components of larger systems.

The dynamic systems view helps explain the striking fact that when one hemisphere of the brain must be surgically removed in very young infants, their subsequent cognitive development is largely normal and all cognitive operations are performed with the remaining hemisphere (Ogden 1996; Werth 2006). Even when the left or language hemisphere is removed, near normal language function is supported by the right hemisphere. As with the other examples of developmental neuroplasticity discussed later in this chapter, these relocations and reconfigurations of brain functional architecture are more easily understood in the systems/emergent property view than in the phrenology/modularity view.

SENSORY STIMULATION AND NEURONAL VIABILITY AND GROWTH

The brain requires sensory stimulation to maintain structural integrity. Information processing structures along afferent pathways from peripheral sensory receptors to cortical processing centers atrophy without sensory input. The number of ganglion cells in the retina which carry excitation from photoreceptor cells in the eye to the first relay station in the brain, is decreased to 10% of normal in dark reared chimpanzees (Rasch et al. 1961); after dark-rearing, cats and rats have smaller than normal ganglion cells (Rasch et al. 1961); and rod and cone photoreceptor cells in the eyes of chicks are morphologically abnormal after 4 weeks with opaque coverings of the eye (Liang et al. 1995). Both the number and size of cells are reduced by as much as 30–40% in the lateral geniculate of cats and monkeys deprived of visual input during the initial weeks of life (e.g. Hubel 1988; Hubel and Wiesel 1970; Kupfer and Palmer 1964; Sherman and Sanderson 1972; Sherman et al. 1972; Tigges and Tigges 1993; Wiesel and Hubel 1963). The effects continue along the information input pathway to the visual cortex where the number, size, and density of connections among cells are decreased and the organization of cells is altered (e.g. Aghajanian and Bloom 1967; Cragg 1970; Fifková 1970; Kumar and Schliebs 1992, 1993; Rakic et al. 1991; Robner et al. 1993).

Studies of olfactory deprivation have yielded a similar picture (e.g. Benson *et al.* 1984; Najbauer and Leon 1995; Skeen *et al.* 1986). Effects of sensory deprivation on structural integrity can be decreased by injection of nerve growth factor into the cerebral spinal fluid within the brain during the period of deprivation (Berardi *et al.* 1992, 1993; Carmignoto *et al.* 1993; Domenici *et al.* 1993; Pizzorusso *et al.* 1994). This naturally occurring substance is produced and released by cells stimulated by sensory input, thus providing further evidence of the association between neuronal activity and neuronal viability and growth (Domenici *et al.* 1993).

Effects of sensory deprivation on development of brain functional organization follow from these effects on cell viability and growth. Neurons at each stage of processing compete for connections with neurons at each subsequent stage, with neurons that fire more often gaining territory. These effects were investigated systematically in Hubel and Wiesel's Nobel Prize winning studies of kittens and monkeys (Hubel 1988). Recording electrical activity from hundreds of cells in the area of the brain that receives visual information, they determined that in animals raised under normal conditions most cells respond to inputs from both eyes (approximately 85% in the kitten, 65% in the monkey). Many of these responded somewhat more frequently to input from one eye, with such eye preferences divided evenly between the eyes. Similarly, of the monocularly responsive cells, half responded exclusively to the right eye and half to the left. However, when an eye was sutured closed shortly after birth and then reopened 10 weeks later, 85% or more of cells responded preferentially to the previously non-deprived eye, and few if any cells responded exclusively to the previously deprived eye. Responses to stimulation of the previously deprived eye were slow to start, decreased in amplitude, and easily fatigued when present at all.

Hubel and Wiesel also demonstrated two additional features of the effects of sensory-induced neuronal activity on the development of brain structure and function that are of particular relevance to cultural evolution. When visual input to the deprived eye is restored, the altered pattern of cortical cell sensitivities persists despite the fact that both eyes are now receiving unobstructed visual input. As long as neurons from the previously non-deprived eye remain active, they are able to maintain their abnormally acquired hegemony. If, however, the previously non-deprived eye is occluded while the animal is still young enough, the abnormal response pattern can be normalized or reversed in favor of the previously deprived eye (Hubel 1988). The first conclusion of particular interest in relation to cultural evolution is that socially generated activity can create unusual structures that alter the interaction with the environment so as to maintain themselves. In this case, when the eye was occluded, cortical structure changed so as to be unusually responsive to input from only one eye. When the occlusion was removed and input was available to both eyes, the brain still registered input almost exclusively from only one eye. The neural resources necessary to process input now available from the previously occluded eye were absent. They had been appropriated by the active eye during the period of unilateral occlusion, and the active eye maintained the extra resources because it kept those resources actively engaged in processing input within the systems that had appropriated them. This situation could be reversed by occluding the previously open eye, demonstrating that the plastic potential remained, that the brain could be shaped or normalized by corrective intervention, and that without such active intervention the normal pattern could not reassert itself even in a normal situation. The second conclusion of particular interest is that active intervention to normalize or reverse the effects of the initial unilateral occlusion was only effective in young animals. After a certain stage in development, often referred to as the critical period, there is a higher degree of stability in established neural structures, in part because neurochemical mechanisms that support neuroplasticity are less powerful in older individuals.

In further work, Hubel and Wiesel demonstrated that altering the nature or content of the visual stimuli changes the functional organization of the visual cortex even when the stimuli are viewed normally by both eyes. For example, some cells in the visual cortex respond selectively to moving objects, with each cell having maximum sensitivity to movement in a particular direction. Other cells respond selectively to lines (i.e. object edges), with each of these cells having maximum sensitivity to lines of a particular orientation. Kittens raised in strobe light that prevents appreciation of movement have decreased numbers of motion sensitive cells (Cynader *et al.* 1973; Cynader and Chernenko 1976). Presumably cells that would have been specialized for movement detection became selectively responsive to some other aspect of visual information instead. Kittens raised in dark except for exposure to stripes moving from left to right have a marked increase in the proportion of cells selectively responsive to left/right rather than right/left movement (Tretter *et al.* 1975). Similarly, kittens exposed to vertical black and white stripes for a few hours each day, but otherwise reared in darkness, have cortical cells with vertical line orientation preferences, but none with preferences for other orientations (Blakemore and Cooper 1970). Kittens raised wearing goggles that allowed them to see only vertical lines in one eye and horizontal lines in the other, have fewer than the normal number of cells that respond to oblique lines. Moreover, cells responsive to vertical lines are active only with stimulation of the eye that had been exposed to vertical lines, and cells responsive to horizontal lines are active only with stimulation of the eye that had been exposed to horizontal lines (Hirsch and Spinelli 1970).

The extent of neuroplastic potential in the developing mammalian brain is remarkable. In adult rats that had an eye removed at birth, stimulation of their whiskers led to electrophysiological and metabolic activity within the visual cortex (Toldi *et al.* 1994). Apparently neurons in what is normally a visual processing area came instead to respond to input from the whiskers when deprived of input from the eye. In perhaps the most dramatic demonstration of plasticity, the optic nerve in 1-day-old ferrets was rerouted to provide visual rather than auditory input to what is normally the auditory cortex. The auditory cortex developed a functional organization of ocular dominance columns highly similar to the normal visual cortex rather than its usual tonotopic structure, and the ferrets saw with what would normally have been the auditory regions of the brain (Sharma *et al.* 2000).

The studies summarized in this section provide evidence that mammalian brains (and minds) develop concrete perceptual structures, capabilities, and sensitivities based on prominent features of the rearing environment, and then are more able and more likely to see those features in the sensory mix of new environments encountered subsequently. Or to turn it around, mammals have limited ability to see even prominent features of a new environment if those features were absent from their rearing environment.

SOCIAL INTERACTIONS AS THE SOURCE OF EARLY ENVIRONMENTAL STIMULATION

The class Mammalia is named on the basis of the presence of mammary glands. It is defined on the basis of nourishing young with milk and a series of physical features including a chain of small ear bones, four optic lobes in the brain, a particular mandibular structure, a muscular diaphragm separating the lungs and heart from the abdomen, only a left aortic arch, warm blood with red blood cells lacking nuclei, and viviparous reproduction. In studies of infant monkeys and wire mesh surrogate mothers, Harlow and Mears provided a radical correction to this definition, adding another central feature that in many ways is more important than all the others. Infant monkeys were separated from their mothers and raised in cages with access to both a wire mesh and a cloth surrogate mother. Both surrogate mothers were kept at the same temperature as normal monkey mothers. One-half of the monkeys received milk from the wire mesh mother and one-half from the cloth mother. Both groups spent much more time on the cloth than the wire mesh mother. The differential was greater by only a small amount when the cloth mother was the source of milk. The preference for the cloth mother became greater over time in both groups, the opposite of what would be expected from a food/hunger reduction conditioning model which would predict increasing preference over time for the food-providing surrogate mother. Harlow and Mears (1979, p. 108) concluded that "the disparity [in favor of selecting the cloth mother independent of which mother provides milk] is so great as to suggest that the primary function of nursing as an affectional variable is that of ensuring frequent and intimate body contact of the infant with the mother." In other words, instead of the provision of milk being the end goal of mother infant interaction in and of itself, it is a means of ensuring contact between the mother and the infant because this contact is essential for provision of sensory stimulation necessary for brain development, and for production of population variability through variability in that stimulation.

Real living mothers and other parenting figures vary in the ways they stimulate their infants and children. Naturally occurring differences in these parenting behaviors have life-long and specific effects on the brains and behavior of their offspring, and changes in DNA structure that mediate these effects have been identified in studies of rats (Weaver *et al.* 2004a,b). Mother rats differ in the amount of time they spend licking and grooming their pups, and the in the ways they position themselves for nursing. Michael Meaney and colleagues found that adult rats that had been licked more as pups had decreased behavioral and hormonal responses to stress, and greater spatial learning abilities—a capacity in which areas of the hippocampus play an important role (Weaver *et al.* 2004b). Examining brain chemistry and structure, they found greater levels of specific types of messenger RNA that carry the information from the DNA to parts of the cells that synthesize the glucocorticoid receptors important in regulating stress responses and the NMDA (N-methyl-D-aspartic acid) receptors important in promoting neuroplasticity. Direct examination of the hippocampus revealed that offspring of high licking mothers had longer neurons with more branches and interconnections (Figure 44.1) (Champagne *et al.* 2008). Direct examination of the DNA identified actual changes in the genes associated with stress response as a result of the degree of maternal licking. Shortly after birth, the surface of DNA is largely covered by small chemical complexes called methyl groups. These methyl groups limit access to the DNA and thereby limit activation or expression of genes. Experiences during the first weeks of life can lead to selective removal of these methyl groups, making some genes more active. The effects of experience on methylation are much greater during the first 3 weeks of a rat's life than thereafter, and changes induced by experience during this critical period usually remain relatively unchanged throughout the rat's adult life. Maternal licking initiates a series of neurochemical processes that selectively demethylate genes that produce the glucocorticoid receptors in the hippocampus and frontal lobes that turn off the stress response.

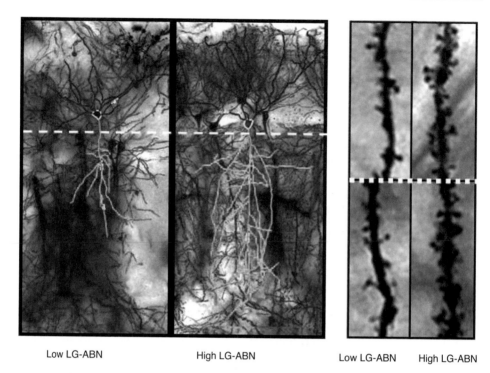

Low LG-ABN   High LG-ABN   Low LG-ABN   High LG-ABN

FIG. 44.1 (Also see Plate 11). Apical (blue) and basal (green) dendritic branching in adult rats who received lower (left) or higher (right) amounts of licking and grooming as infants. Stained neurons are pyramidal cells from the hippocampus. The study found significantly more branching in the rats who had received more licking and grooming. This is also visible in the photographs of branching points along the axonal spine shown on the right. (From Champagne *et al.* 2008).

To ensure that these observations were due to the differences in maternal behavior, and not to genes that high-licking mothers passed on to their offspring, Meaney and colleagues had pups born to low-licking mothers raised from birth by high-licking mothers, and vice versa (Weaver *et al.* 2004a,b). When these rats became adults, their stress responses and the methylation of their DNA (see Figure 44.2) (Weaver *et al.* 2004a) were both consistent with the type of mother that reared them and not with the type of their biological mother.

Two other aspects of this work are also of relevance to cultural evolution. First, when given learning tests in high stress environments, adult rats raised by low-licking mothers out performed rats raised by high-licking mothers. This demonstrates the adaptive value of the population variability induced by cultural evolution. Second, some of the persistent neuro-chemical and behavioral effects of maternal care of female infants affect the way the infant functions as a mother herself when she becomes an adult. Females that had been separated from their mothers when they were infants showed lower than normal gene expression in areas of the brain associated with maternal behaviors when they themselves became mothers (Fleming *et al.* 2002). They also licked and crouched over their pups less often than other mothers (Gonzalez *et al.* 2001), and their generally decreased ability to maintain attention

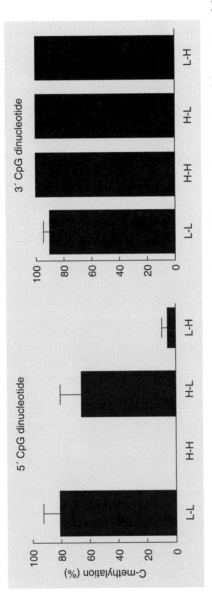

FIG. 44.2 Cross-fostering studies that maternal care and not maternal genes alter methylation and expression of the section of the genome that promotes expression of genes that code for the proteins that constitute neuroreceptors that regulate the stress response. The left side of the figure show low methylation (greater activity) in rats raised by high-licking grooming mothers if their biological mothers where high (H-H) of low-licking grooming (L-H) mothers, and high methylation (lower activity) in rats raised by low-licking grooming mothers with either high- (H-L) or low-licking grooming (L-L) biological mothers. The absence of such effects in another region of the DNA (right side of the figure) demonstrates specificity of the link between this aspect of maternal behavior and methylation of the part of the DNA associated with production of neuroreceptors regulating stress responsivity. Reprinted by permission from Macmillan Publishers Ltd: Nature Neuroscience, Weaver et al., Epigenetic programming by maternal behaviour copyright (2004).

and increased response to stress have been hypothesized to further compromise their maternal competence (Fleming *et al.* 2002). Such intergenerational effects are potentially self-propagating and even self-amplifying. Moreover, since litter size (Fleming *et al.* 2002; Jans and Woodside 1987) and food availability (Lyons *et al.* 2002) can influence the amount of licking and other behavioral interactions between mother and infant, a variety of environmental factors can influence maternal behaviors and their impact, across generations, on a range of individual and group behaviors. All this depends on the postnatal sensitivity of the mammalian brain to sensory stimulation, and the proximity of mammalian infants and mothers ensured by nursing.

THE HUMAN REARING ENVIRONMENT

Human rearing behaviors are more complex and more varied than those of other mammals, and include massive social components and influences from extended families, communities, and nation states. The extra-familial influences include schools, mass media, arts, laws, and customs. The human social and economic environments also affect the states of mind, time, and energy of the parents, thus affecting their interactions with their offspring in a manner analogous to the effects of food supply on rat maternal behavior. And although beyond the scope of this chapter to discuss, the huge role of language—spoken and written— in facilitating the influence of the human-made environment on the development of children must be noted, along with the fact that the latter is itself clearly a product of cultural evolution and it seems increasingly probable that the former is in large part as well.

At birth, human infants can distinguish their mother's language from other languages based on stimulation received in utero (Mehler *et al.* 1988). Within hours of birth they show a selective interest in looking at the human face, with the interest greatest for the full face as experienced in social interactions rather than for the face in profile. Within days they prefer their mother's face and voice to those of others (Carpenter 1974; Fifer and Moon 1994; Goren *et al.* 1975; MacFarlane 1978; Mehler *et al.* 1988; Mills and Melhursh 1974; Spitz and Wolf 1946). Within this context, parents provide objects of play and structure interactions and activities. As Kenneth Kaye (1982a, p. 193) has remarked, "social interference in the object-directed activities of babies is such a commonplace occurrence that few authors have remarked on its absolute uniqueness to our own species." The brains and minds of human infants and children develop while closely linked to the minds and brains of their biobehaviorally mature caregivers. The characteristics of the adults shape the stimulation that shapes the growing brains of the children through the small details and general rhythms of the child's experiences. The child integrates input from progressively larger circles of direct interaction, beginning with primary care givers and growing to include extended family members and then members of the community and society more broadly.

While some of the social input is actively shaped and provided by others, much is just absorbed through essentially constant imitation. Within 2 days of birth, infants will stick out their tongues and move their heads in imitation of an adult doing so (Meltzoff and Moore 1977, 1989). From infancy on, children learn how to do things simply by watching them done. They imitate the goals of action even by different means and imitate a parent's affective response to new stimuli (Kaye 1982b; Klinnet *et al.* 1986). Mirror neurons fire when people (and monkeys) watch an act being done, and many times these same neurons are then active when the individual performs the action previously observed (Iacoboni *et al.* 1999; Rizzolatti *et al.* 1996; Umilta *et al.* 2001). Similarly, looking at someone else in pain activates the same regions of the brain as are active when the observer experiences pain him or herself (Gu and Han 2007; Jackson *et al.* 2005; Singer *et al.* 2004). The earlier cited work of Hubel and Wiesel demonstrated that environmentally induced neuronal activity shaped the development of cerebral functional structures, following the principle that neurons that fire together wire together. In human development, active parental and community interventions and nearly constant imitation of what is seen and heard produce intensive and repetitive firing of neuronal ensembles and circuits. This environment-induced neural activation shapes brain development to be consistent with the largely human-made rearing environment.

Well before the relevant neuroscience research, psychologists were aware of the role of the social environment in shaping mental development, describing the processes in language remarkably similar to what would be suggested by the subsequent work of Hubel, Wiesel, Meaney and others. Writing in 1926, Fenichel (p. 57) states that "changes in the ego, in which characteristics which were previously perceived in an object [usually an important person] are acquired by the perceiver of them, have long since been familiar to psychoanalysis." Freud (1933, p. 47) described identification as "the assimilation of one ego to another one, as a result of which the first ego behaves like the second in certain respects, imitates it and in a sense takes it up into itself." Greenson (1954, pp. 160–1) stated that "identification with an object means that…a transformation of the self has occurred whereby the self has become similar to the external object…one can observe behavior, attitudes, feelings, posture, etc. which are now identical to those characteristics belonging to the external object," and that at early stages of development "perception implies transformation of the self." Reich (1954, p. 180) explained that "the child simply imitates whatever attracts his attention momentarily in the object…normally these passing identifications develop slowly into permanent ones, into real assimilation of the object's qualities." Writing from a different cultural and intellectual context, the Russian psychologist Lev Vygotsky described the process:

> "In the early stages of development the complex psychological function *was shared between two persons*: the adult *triggered* the psychological process by naming the object or by pointing to it; the child *responded* to this signal and picked out the named object either by fixing it with his eye or by holding it with his hand. In the subsequent stages of development…The function which hitherto was shared between two people now becomes a method of *internal organization of the psychological process*. From an external, socially organized attention develops the *child's voluntary attention*, which in this stage is an internal, self-regulating process."
> (Luria 1973, pp. 265–8)

BRAIN IMAGING DEMONSTRATIONS OF ENVIRONMENT INDUCED BRAIN ORGANIZATION IN HUMAN BEINGS

Brain imaging studies have now demonstrated changes in brain structure and function that result from unusual motor activity or sensory input during childhood and persist

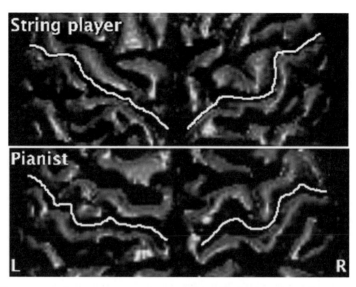

FIG. 44.3 Expansion of sensorimotor cortex unilaterally (right side) in long time players of string instruments and bilaterally in long-time piano players. These changes in brain structure result from many hours of music practice during childhood and are evident to the naked eye. Only the left sensorimotor cortex in string players is not affected by the practice since it controls the bowing (right) hand which makes many fewer and simpler movements than does the left hand. Thus, the left sensorimotor cortex in the string players serves as a reference that demonstrates the increase in size of the other sensorimotor cortexes. (From Bangert and Schlaug 2006.)

into adulthood. One set of studies has examined differences in brain structure and function as a result of practicing a musical instrument during childhood. A socially and culturally created and induced activity on multiple levels, intensive practice of string instruments leads to selective increase in volume of the right somatosensory and motor areas associated with the rapid, fine motor movements of the fingers of the left hand that provide intricate and fast moving sequences of pressure to the strings. The changes in the brain are greater in adults who practiced more hours and began practicing at younger ages (Schlaug 2001). Figure 44.3 shows this bulked up motor cortex in the right hemisphere of string players (the increase in volume is actually visible to the naked eye!) and bilaterally in piano players who practice with both hands (Bangert and Schlaug 2006).

The second set of studies looked at brain activations in the normal visual areas of the brain in adults who were blind at birth or shortly thereafter, or the normal auditory areas of the brain in adults who were deaf at or shortly after birth. Directly analogous to the selective sensory deprivation experiments of Hubel and Wiesel, the findings were also analogous. In early blind subjects, the area of the brain that is normally the site of early visual processing is activated instead by auditory and tactile stimulation (Figure 44.4) (Weaver and Stevens 2007), and is also more active during language processing tasks than is the case in sighted people (Amedi *et al.* 2003). Apparently, when the normal sensory input to the area was

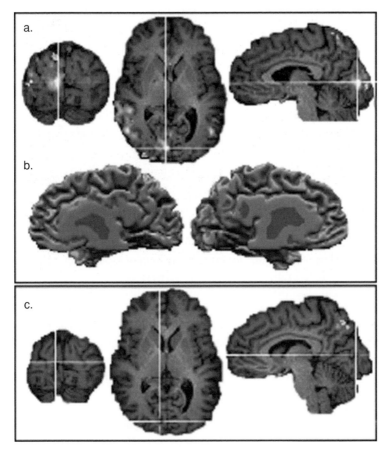

FIG. 44.4 Areas of the cortex that usually respond to visual sensory input are shown here to respond to auditory stimulation (white) and tactile stimulation (black) in individuals who were blind at birth or became so shortly after. (From Weaver and Stevens 2007)

absent, other sensory input and cognitive operations moved into the territory. Moreover, among the blind individuals, memory performance was higher in the individuals who made more use of the "visual" areas during the memory task.

The results of these new imaging studies in humans are what is expected based on the studies in animals, the increased plasticity of the human brain and the very active structuring by human adults of the rearing environment and developmental experiences of their offspring. As mentioned earlier, a 1994 study showed that if one eye of a rat is removed at birth, stimulation of their whisker when they are adults activates cells in what is usually visual cortex (Toldi *et al.* 1994). The demonstration of similar activation in the humans who are blind from early life, then, is no surprise. The demonstration of changes in brain morphology as a result of practicing a musical instrument extends things a bit beyond the animal studies in that practicing music is clearly a socially constructed human activity, and it is impressive that the environmentally induced changes can be seen with the naked eye when data from multiple individuals is averaged together. But the demonstration of changes is at a gross anatomic level and does not reveal more fine grained changes in structure and function. These studies, however, are important in the workman-like effort of science to test assumptions and build bridges that link different sets of data. We do not yet have methods and data in people to enable us to demonstrate effects of parental actions on axonal branching in the hippocampus, as Meaney and colleagues have done in rats, but by linking the data and theory from animal studies to human beings with the above cited imaging studies, scientists complete an evidentiary loop and increase confidence in the application to human beings of principles based on the data from animals.

Summary and conclusions

Functional properties of individual neurons in the human brain differ little from those of individual neurons in the brains of other primates. The large differences in function between the human brain and other primate brains result instead from the increased number of cells and interconnections among them, the extended period after birth during which the brain is highly susceptible to shaping by environmentally induced neuronal activity, and the fact that humans alone alter the environment that produces the neuronal activity that shapes the brains of their offspring. Together these factors constitute neuroplasticity and cultural evolution. Cultural evolution produces changes in human capabilities, desires, and expectations much more rapidly and through very different mechanisms than does Darwinian biological evolution. It is a cross-generational and social process that shapes individual actions, and these actions then in turn contribute to the social and cross-generational influences that shape other individuals.

We humans are not handed a set of fixed capabilities, developed desires and inclinations, and standards for ethical conduct. All three of these critical aspects of human being are in dynamic interplay through human history; such is our neurobiological relationship with our natural and human-made environments. Our ability to shape our environments, and through that to shape our minds, brains, and behavior, begets complex responsibility and promising opportunity. Both can only be met through new and thoughtful commentary. One challenge is to find solid ground amidst such plasticity.

References

Aghajanian, G.K. and Bloom, F.E. (1967). The formation of synaptic junctions in developing rat brain: a quantitative electron microscopic study. *Brain Research*, **6**, 716–27.

Amedi, A., Raz, N., Pianka, P., Malach, R., and Zohary, E. (2003). Early 'visual' cortex activation correlates with superior verbal memory performance in the blind. *Nature Neuroscience*, **6**, 758–66.

Bangert, M. and Schlaug, G. (2006). Specialization of the specialized in features of external human brain morphology. *European Journal of Neuroscience*, **24**, 1832–4.

Benson, T.E., Ryugo, D.K., and Hinds, J.W. (1984). Effects of sensory deprivation on the developing mouse olfactory system: a light and electron microscopic, morphometric analysis. *Journal of Neuroscience*, **4**, 638–53.

Berardi, N., Cattaneo, A., Cellerino, A., *et al.* (1992). Monoclonal antibodies to nerve growth factor (NGF) affects the postnatal development of the rat geniculocortical system. *Journal of Physiology-London*, **452**, 293P.

Berardi, N., Domenici, L., Parisi, V., Pizzorusso, T., Cellerino, A., and Maffei, L. (1993). Monocular deprivation effects in the rat visual cortex and lateral geniculate nucleus are prevented by nerve growth factor (NGF). I. Visual cortex. *Proceedings of the Royal Society of London*, B251, 17–23.

Blakemore, C. and Cooper, G.F. (1970). Development of the brain depends on visual experience. *Nature*, **228**, 477–8.

Carmignoto, G., Canella, R., Candeo, P., Comelli, M.C., and Maffei, L. (1993). Effects of nerve growth factor on neuronal plasticity of the kitten visual cortex. *Journal of Physiology-London*, **464**, 343–60.

Carpenter, G. (1974). Mother's face and the newborn. *New Scientist*, **21**, 742–4.

Champagne, D.L., Bagot, R.C., van Hasselt, F., *et al.* (2008). Maternal care and hippocampal plasticity: evidence for experience-dependent structural plasticity, altered synaptic functioning, and differential responsiveness to glucocorticoids and stress. *Journal of Neuroscience*, **28**, 6037–45.

Cragg, B.G. (1970). What is the signal for chromatolysis? *Brain Research*, **23**, 1–21.

Cynader, M. and Chernenko, G. (1976). Abolition of direction selectivity in the visual cortex of the cat. *Science*, **193**, 504–5.

Cynader, M., Berman, N., and Hein, A. (1973). Cats reared in stroboscopic illumination: effects on receptive fields in visual cortex. *Proceedings of the National Academy of Sciences of the United States of America*, **70**, 1353–4.

D'Esposito, M. (2007). From cognitive to neural models of working memory. *Philosophical Transactions of the Royal Society of London - Series B: Biological Sciences*, **362**, 761–72.

Domenici, L., Cellerino, A., and Maffei, L. (1993). Monocular deprivation effects in the rat visual cortex and lateral geniculate nucleus are prevented by nerve growth factor (NGF). II. Lateral geniculate nucleus. *Proceedings of the Royal Society of London*, B251, 25–31.

Fenichel, O. (1926). Identification, in G. Pollock (ed., 1993) *Pivotal Papers on Identification*, pp. 57–74. Madison, CT: International Universities Press.

Fifer, W.P. and Moon, C.M. (1994). The role of mother's voice in the organization of brain function in the newborn. *Acta Paediatrica*, **397**, 86–93.

Fifková, E. (1970). Changes of axosomatic synapses in the visual cortex of monocularly deprived rats. *Journal of Neurobiology*, **2**, 61–71.

Fleming, A.S., Kraemer, G.W., Gonzalez, A., Loveca, V., Reesa, S., and Meloc, A. (2002). Mothering begets mothering: the transmission of behavior and its neurobiology across generations. *Pharmacology Biochemistry and Behavior*, **73**, 61–75.

Freud, S. (1933). Excerpt from Lecture XXXI: The dissection of the psychical personality. In G. Pollock (ed., 1993) *Pivotal Papers on Identification*, pp. 47–52. Madison, CT: International Universities Press.

Friston, K.J., Price, C.J., Fletcher, P., Moore, C., Frackowiak, R.S.J., and Dolan, R.J. (1996). The trouble with cognitive subtraction. *NeuroImage*, **4**, 97–104.

Gaillard, W.D., Hertz-Pannier, L., Mott, S.H., Barnett, A.S., LeBihan, D., and Theodore, W.H. (2000). Functional anatomy of cognitive development: fMRI of verbal fluency in children and adults. *Neurology*, **54**, 180.

Goren, C.C., Sarty, M. and Wu, P.Y.K. (1975). Visual following and pattern discrimination of face-like stimuli by newborn infants. *Pediatrics*, **56**, 544–9.

Gonzalez, A., Lovic, V., Ward, G.R., Wainwright, P.E., and Fleming, A.S. (2001). Intergenerational effects of complete maternal deprivation and replacement stimulation on maternal behavior and emotionality in female rats. *Developmental Psychobiology*, **38**, 11–32.

Greenson, R.R. (1954). The struggle against identification. In G. Pollock (ed., 1993) *Pivotal Papers on Identification*, pp. 159–75. Madison, CT: International Universities Press.

Gu, X. and Han, S. (2007). Attention and reality constraints on the neural processes of empathy for pain. *NeuroImage*, **36**, 256–67.

Harlow, H.F. and Mears, C. (1979). *The Human Model: Primate Perspectives*. Washington, DC: V.H. Winston & Sons.

Hirsch, H.B. and Spinelli, D. (1970). Visual experience modifies distribution of horizontally and vertically oriented receptive fields in cats. *Science*, **168**, 869–71.

Hubel, D.H. (1988). *Eye, Brain and Vision*. Deprivation and development, pp. 191–217. New York: Scientific American Library.

Hubel, D.H. and Wiesel, T.N. (1970). The period of susceptibility to the physiological effects of unilateral eye closure in kittens. *Journal of Physiology*, **206**, 419–36.

Iacoboni, M., Woods, R.P., Brass, M., Bekkering, H., Mazziota, J.C., and Rizzolatti, G. (1999). Cortical mechanisms of human imitation. *Science*, **286**, 2526–8.

Jackson, P.L., Meltzoff, A.N., and Decety, J. (2005). How do we perceive the pain of others? A window into the neural processes involved in empathy. *NeuroImage*, **24**, 771–9.

Jans, J.E. and Woodside, B. (1987). Effects of litter age, litter size, and ambient temperature on the milk ejection reflex in lactating rats. *Developmental Psychobiology*, **20**, 333–44.

John, E.R., Tang, Y., Brill, A.B., Young, R., and Ono, K. (1986). Double-labeled metabolic maps of memory. *Science*, **233**, 1167–75.

Kaye, K. (1982a). Organism, apprentice, and person. In E. Tronick (ed.) *Social Interchange in Infancy: Affect, Cognition, and Communication*, pp. 183–96. Baltimore, MD: University Park Press.

Kaye, K. (1982b). *The Mental and Social Life of Babies: How Parents Create Persons*. Chicago, IL: University of Chicago Press.

Kelly, C., Foxe, J.J. and Garavan, H. (2006). Patterns of normal human brain plasticity after practice and their implications for neurorehabilitation. *Archives of Physical Medicine and Rehabilitation*, **87**, S20–9.

Klinnet, M., Emde, R.N., Butterfield, P., and Campos, J.J. (1986). Social referencing: the infant's use of emotional signals from a friendly adult with mother present. *Developmental Psychology*, **22**, 427–32.

Kumar, A. and Schliebs, R. (1992). Postnatal laminar development of cholinergic receptors, protein kinase C and dihydropyridine-sensitive calcium antagonist binding in rat visual cortex. Effect of visual deprivation. *International Journal of Developmental Neuroscience*, **10**, 491–504.

Kumar, A. and Schliebs, R. (1993). Postnatal ontogeny of $GABA_A$ and benzodiazepine receptors in individual layers of rat visual cortex and the effect of visual deprivation. *Neurochemistry International*, **23**, 99–106.

Kupfer, C. and Palmer, P. (1964). Lateral geniculate nucleus: histological and cytochemical changes following afferent denervation and visual deprivation. *Experimental Neurology*, **9**, 400–9.

Liang, H., Crewther, D.P., Crewther, S.G., and Barila, A.M. (1995). A role for photoreceptor outer segments in the induction of deprivation myopia. *Vision Research*, **35**, 1217–25.

Loubinoux, I., Carel, C., Alary, F., *et al.* (2001). Within-session and between-session reproducibility of cerebral sensorimotor activation: a test-retest effect evidenced with functional magnetic resonance imaging. *Journal of Cerebral Blood Flow and Metabolism*, **21**, 595–607.

Luria, A.R. (1973). *The Working Brain*. B. Haugh (trans.) New York: Basic Books.

Lyons, D.M., Afariana, H., Schatzberg, A.F., Sawyer-Glover, A., and Moseley, M.E. (2002). Experience-dependent asymmetric variation in primate prefrontal morphology. *Behavioural Brain Research*, **136**, 51–9.

MacFarlane, A. (1978). What a baby knows. *Human Nature*, **1**.

Mehler, J., Jusczyk, P., Lambertz, G., Halsted, N., Bertoncini, J., and Amiel-Tison, C. (1988). A precursor of language acquisition in young infants. *Cognition*, 29, 143–78.

Meltzoff, A.N. and Moore, M.K. (1977). Imitation of facial and manual gestures by human neonates. *Science*, **198**, 74–8.

Meltzoff, A.N. and Moore, M.K. (1989). Imitation in newborn infants: exploring the range of gestures imitated and the underlying mechanisms. *Developmental Psychology*, **25**, 954–62.

Mills, M. and Melhursh, E. (1974). Recognition of mother's voice in early infancy. *Nature*, **252**, 123–4.

Najbauer, J. and Leon, M. (1995). Olfactory experience modulated apoptosis in the developing olfactory bulb. *Brain Research*, **674**, 245–51.

Ogden, J.A. (1996). Phonological dyslexia and phonological dysgraphia following left and right hemispherectomy. *Neuropsychologia*, **34**, 905–18.

Pizzorusso, T., Fagiolini, M., Fabris, M., Ferrari, G., and Maffei, L. (1994). Schwann cells transplanted in the lateral ventricles prevent the functional and anatomical effects of monocular deprivation in the rat. *Proceedings of the National Academy of Sciences of the United States of America*, **91**, 2572–6.

Poldrack, R.A., Prabhakaran, V., Seger, C.A., and Gabrielli, J.D.E. (1999). Striatal activation during acquisition of a cognitive skill. *Neuropsychology*, **13**, 564–74.

Rakic, P., Suner, I., and Williams, R.W. (1991). A novel cytoarchitectonic area induced experimentally within the primate visual cortex. *Proceedings of the National Academy of Sciences of the United States of America*, **88**, 2083–7.

Rasch, E., Swift, H., Riesen, A.H., and Chow, K.L. (1961). Altered structure and composition of retinal cells in dark eared animals. *Experimental Cell Research*, **25**, 348–63.

Reich, A. (1954). Early identifications as archaic elements in the superego. In G. Pollock (ed., 1993) *Pivotal Papers on Identification*, pp. 177–95. Madison, CT: International Universities Press.

Rizzolatti, G., Fadiga, L., Gallese, V., and Fogassi, L. (1996). Premotor cortex and the recognition of motor actions. *Cognitive Brain Research*, **3**, 131–41.

Robner, S., Kumar, A., Kues, W., Witzemann, V., and Schliebs, R. (1993). Differential laminar expression of AMPA receptor genes in the developing rat visual cortex using *in situ* hybridization histochemistry. Effect of visual deprivation. *International Journal of Developmental Neuroscience*, **11**, 411–24.

Schlaug, G. (2001). The brain of musicians: a model for structural and functional adaptation. *Annals of the New York Academy of Sciences*, **930**, 281–99.

Sharma, J., Angelucci, A., and Sur, M. (2000). Induction of visual orientation modules in auditory cortex. *Nature*, **404**, 841–7.

Sherman, S.M. and Sanderson, K.J. (1972). Binocular interaction on cells of the dorsal lateral geniculate nucleus of visually deprived cats. *Brain Research*, **37**, 126–31.

Sherman, S.M., Hoffman, K.P., and Stone, J. (1972). Loss of a specific cell type from dorsal lateral geniculate nucleus in visually deprived cats. *Journal of Neurophysiology*, **35**, 532–41.

Singer, T., Seymour, B., O'Doherty, J., Kaube, H., Dolan, R.J., and Frith, C.D. (2004). Empathy for pain involves the affective but not sensory components of pain. *Science*, **303**, 1157–62.

Skeen, L.C., Due, B.R., and Douglas, F.E. (1986). Neonatal sensory deprivation reduces tufted cell number in mouse olfactory bulbs. *Neuroscience Letters*, **63**, 5–10.

Spitz, R. and Wolf, K. (1946). The smiling response: a contribution to the ontogenesis of social relations. *Genetic Psychology Monographs*, **34**, 57–125.

Stebbins, G.T., Carrillo, M.C., Dorfman, J., *et al.* (2002). Aging effects on memory encoding in the frontal lobes. *Psychology and Aging*, **17**, 44–55.

Tigges, M. and Tigges, J. (1993). Parvalbumin immunoreactivity in the lateral geniculate nucleus of rhesus monkeys raised under monocular and binocular deprivation conditions. *Visual Neuroscience*, **10**, 1043–53.

Toldi, J., Rojik, I., and Feher, O. (1994). Neonatal monocular enucleation-induced cross-modal effects observed in the cortex of adult rat. *Neuroscience*, **62**, 105–14.

Tretter, F., Cynader, M., and Singer, W. (1975). Modification of direction selectivity of neurons in the visual cortex of kittens. *Brain Research*, **84**, 143–9.

Umilta, M.A., Kohler, E., Gallese, V., *et al.* (2001). I know what you are doing: a neurophysiological study. *Neuron*, **31**, 155–65.

Vygotsky, L.S. (1978). *Mind in Society: The Development of Higher Psychological Processes.* Cambridge, MA: Harvard University Press.

Weaver, I.C.G., Cervoni, N., Champagne, F.A., *et al.* (2004a). Epigenetic programming by maternal behavior. *Nature Neuroscience*, **7**, 847–54.

Weaver, I.C.G., Diorio, J., Seckl, J.R., Szyf, M., and Meaney, M.J. (2004b). Early environmental regulation of hippocampal glucocorticiod receptor gene expression: characterization of intracellular mediators and potential genomic sites. *Annals of the New York Academy of Sciences*, **1024**, 182–212.

Weaver, K.E. and Stevens, A.A. (2007). Attention and sensory interactions within the occipital cortex in the early blind: an fMRI study. *Journal of Cognitive Neuroscience*, **19**, 315–30.

Werth, R. (2006). Visual functions without the occipital lobe or after cerebral hemispherectomy in infancy. *European Journal of Neuroscience*, **24**, 2932–44.

Wexler, B.E. (2004). Using fMRI to study the mind and brain. In R. Shulman and D. Rothman (eds.) *Brain Energetics and Neuronal Activity*, pp. 279–94. West Sussex: John Wiley and Sons.

Wexler, B.E. (2006). *Brain and Culture: Neurobiology, Ideology and Social Change.* Cambridge: MIT Press.

Wiesel, T.N. and Hubel, D.H. (1963). Effects of visual deprivation on morphology and physiology of cells in the cat's lateral geniculate body. *Journal of Neurophysiology*, **26**, 978–93.

....

CHAPTER 45

NEUROSCIENCE AND NEUROETHICS IN THE 21ST CENTURY

....

MARTHA J. FARAH

NEUROETHICS: FROM FUTURISTIC TO HERE-AND-NOW

....

ONE might not know it to see the numerous chapters of this Handbook summarizing progress on a wide array of topics, but the field of neuroethics is very young. Most would date its inception to the year 2002, when conferences were held on the ethical implications of neuroscience at Penn and at Stanford-UCF and a few early papers appeared (Farah 2002; Illes and Raffin 2002; Moreno 2002; Roskies 2002). Initially neuroethics was a predominantly anticipatory field, focused on future developments in neuroscience and neurotechnology. In his introduction to the Stanford conference, "Neuroethics: Mapping the Field," William Safire explained the distinctiveness of neuroethics, compared to bioethics more generally, by explaining that neuroscience "deals with our consciousness, our sense of self...our personalities and behavior. And these are the characteristics that brain science *will soon be able* to change in significant ways" (quoted in Marcus 2002, p. 7, emphasis added).

Neuroethics has developed rapidly since then, driven in large part by developments in neuroscience. The anticipation and extrapolation that characterized its earliest years, which some skeptics dismissed as science fiction, has receded. In its place has grown a body of neuroethics research and analysis focusing on actual neuroscience and neurotechnology. What accounts for this change? Part of the shift reflects the deepening neuroscience expertise of many neuroethicists and the migration of neuroscientists to the field of neuroethics. This important trend has enabled neuroethicists to identify real developments to analyze, as opposed to in-principle possible developments. However, a more fundamental cause can be found in the rapidly evolving state of neuroscience itself.

An example of the new immediacy of formerly hypothetical neuroethical discussions concerns the ability of brain imaging to deliver useful psychological information about individuals. In an early paper I concluded that "mind reading is the stuff of science fiction, and the current capabilities of neuroscience fall far short of such a feat. Even a major leap in the signal-to-noise ratio of functional brain imaging would simply leave us with gigabytes of more accurate physiological data, whose psychological meaning would be obscure" (Farah 2002, p. 1126).

Although this statement is true, noise in the acquired images was not the next technical barrier to fall. Rather, breakthroughs in the statistical analyses of brain images, including aspects of images previously treated as noise, have taken us a major step closer to deriving useful information about mental content from functional brain images. Starting around 2003, statistical methods from the field of machine learning were applied to the analysis of brain images, revealing the unexpectedly rich information that could be derived from the fine-grained patterns of activation in unsmoothed functional brain images (e.g. Cox and Savoy 2003; Haynes and Reese 2006).

In addition, not all consequential applications of brain imaging require decoding activity on the scale of small ensembles of neurons. Thanks to our growing knowledge of the psychological roles of large-scale brain systems, many applications require only the measurement of brain activity within macroscopic regions. For example, activation of the brain's reward system can be used to estimate product desirability in marketing, and activation of executive control circuits can be used as an indicator of deception. As a result, brain imaging for marketing and lie detection are now commercially available services. Let us leave aside for the moment the question of whether these companies' systems actually perform as claimed. The mere fact that the technology exists, and is being used, illustrates the shift from hypothetical to real problems for neuroethics.

In this chapter I will review neuroethics from the standpoint of its growing real-world relevance. I will begin with an analysis of the history of neuroscience that suggests the reason for the emergence of neuroethics now, in the early 21st century. I will proceed to survey current applications of neuroscience to diverse real-world problems. Finally, I will conclude with a discussion of the ethical issues raised by these developments, and outline three general challenges for society in the age of neuroscience.

THE HISTORY OF NEUROSCIENCE FROM 4000 BCE TO 2000 CE

If we define neuroscience as the systematic study of nervous system structure and function, then its history stretches back at least as far as the 4th millennium BCE, when Ancient Sumerians documented the effects of the poppy plant on mood. Neuroscientist Eric Chudler has constructed a timeline of neuroscience history with over 500 milestones representing important discoveries about the nervous system (http://faculty.washington.edu/chudler/hist.html). Although it might seem absurd to propose any generalization about 6000 years of history, or 500 scientific discoveries, I believe that the following is true, almost without exception: For the first 6000 years of neuroscience, each advance has been of one of just two types.

The first type of advance in neuroscience encompasses advances in basic science. These are the advances in our ability to describe and explain the workings of the nervous system, including brain-based explanations of human behavior. The second type of advance in neuroscience encompasses medical applications. These are the advances in pathophysiology, diagnosis, and treatment in the clinical neurosciences, chiefly neurology and psychiatry. Like other medical advances, many of these arose by accident, and were only understood after further research. The initial discovery and development of neuropsychiatric drugs are a prime example of this: Drugs used as antihistamines or antihypertensives had unanticipated psychiatric effects, which were then studied, refined, and used to treat psychiatric illnesses (Barondes 2003). Other advances in applied neuroscience were not accidental, but resulted from the deliberate application of basic neuroscience to medical problems. An example of this type of advance is structural and functional neuroimaging, based on developments in neurophysiology, radiochemistry and magnetic resonance physics, and used widely in the clinic (Savoy 2001).

THE AGE OF *NON-MEDICAL*
APPLIED NEUROSCIENCE

However the past 6000 years' advances in applied neuroscience came about, by accident or by scientific design, they were almost invariably directed toward the understanding and treatment of medical conditions. Since the turn of the century, however, a third category of neuroscience advance has joined the first two categories of basic neuroscience and medical applications. We are suddenly seeing many advances in non-medical applications of neuroscience. No longer is neuroscience confined to the research laboratory or the medical clinic. It is now finding applications in the home, office, school, courtroom, marketplace, and battlefield.

The explosion of non-medical neuroscience applications at this point in history is a straightforward result of developments in basic neuroscience, specifically cognitive and affective neuroscience. These are the branches of neuroscience with the most obvious and direct relevance to human behavior, and which form the scientific basis of most of the non-medical applications to be discussed here. Around the turn of the century they finally came of age. We now have a theoretical framework, derived from the cognitive and computational psychology of the late 20th century, within which we can formulate working hypotheses about the neural systems underlying human cognition and affect. We also have a variety of empirical methods suited to testing those hypotheses, including the powerful new techniques of functional neuroimaging, which became widely available for this purpose in the last decade of the 20th century. Of course we do not now have a complete understanding of the neural bases of human thought and feeling—far from it. But we do have a body of knowledge, some agreed-upon next questions, and an armamentarium of methods to address those questions with.

As a result of the maturation of cognitive and affective neuroscience, we can now bring neuroscience to bear on solving problems in all those spheres of human life that depend on being able to understand, assess, predict, control, or improve human behavior. This includes the spheres of education, business, politics, law, entertainment, and warfare—none of which are medical applications. Indeed, neuroscience is already been applied in these spheres.

In the remainder of this chapter I will review examples of these applications, by individuals and by the state, and discuss some of the ethical issues raised by these applications.

LIFESTYLE NEUROSCIENCE IN THE 21ˢᵀ CENTURY

Many of the new uses of neuroscience for non-medical purposes have found a place in the lives of private citizens, improving their lives at home, in school, and at the office. These applications of neuroscience, discussed in greater depth in other chapters within this volume, include the enhancement of individual psychological functioning, education, business, and a variety of other aspects of individual and community life.

Enhancement of mental function

The most familiar example of psychological enhancement by direct manipulation of brain function is the use of prescription stimulants by healthy individuals. Thanks to extensive media coverage, from "Desperate Housewives" to network news shows, the public has become aware that stimulants such as methylphenidate and amphetamine can be used to enhance concentration and productivity. Although the use of "speed" for non-medical purposes has a long history, almost as old as the synthetic stimulants themselves (Rasmussen 2008), its current use as a cognitive enhancement appears to be on the rise relative to recent years (Kroutil *et al.* 2006).

The segment of the population for which we have the best estimates of non-medical use of stimulants is the undergraduate student population on American college and university campuses. The results of a 2001 survey of over 10,000 such individuals showed that 7% had used a prescription stimulant non-medically, and this figure ranged as high as 20% on some campuses. This study was not designed to tell us why students were using the drugs. Studies of smaller and less representative samples of American college students have broached this subject and indicate that, for students who use methylphenidate and amphetamine non-medically, cognitive enhancement was the most common reason, although other "lifestyle" uses such as weight control were occasionally reported.

Anecdotal evidence, along with a variety of informal journalists' surveys, suggests that many students and professionals have added an array of different psychopharmaceuticals beyond the conventional stimulants to their work routines (Arrington 2008; Madrigal 2008; Maher 2008; Sahakian and Morein-Zamir 2007; Talbot 2009). These include newer compounds, originally intended for the treatment of neuropsychiatric disorders but already finding a role in the lives of normal healthy users.

Among the newer compounds that informal surveys suggest have already been taken up by healthy individuals for lifestyle reasons is modafinil. This drug was initially developed to reduce sleepiness in narcoleptic patients, but it also counteracts many of the cognitive symptoms of sleep deprivation in healthy normal users, allowing for more comfortable and productive "all-nighters" (Arrington 2008; Hart-Davis 2005; Madrigal 2008; Plotz 2003). Some research suggests that modafinil may also enhance aspects of cognition in healthy people who are not sleep-deprived (Turner *et al.* 2003). The ability to control when one gets sleepy, and perhaps even "work smarter" as well as work longer, has obvious lifestyle allure. Although healthy people comprise some of the market for this drug, how much of the market is not known. It is presumably limited by the expense of the drug, the need for a prescription and, last but not least, the unknown long-term effects of cheating one's body of sleep in this way.

In general, we know little about the lifestyle uses of cognitive enhancers outside the American college population. Do students generally leave their Adderall® behind on campus when they graduate and enter the world of work? Or do they carry this work habit over into their life at the office? We also know little about the prevalence and patterns of usage of other pharmaceuticals for cognitive enhancement, such as modafinil. Considering the likely public health implications of this phenomenon, as well as the potential impact on workplace hours, workforce competition and productivity, and the economy as a whole, the dearth of information is problematic.

Looking a bit farther out on the horizon, into the coming decades of the early 21st century, there are likely to be a number of new cognitive enhancers available. Several companies are developing drugs to manipulate learning and memory. Based on the research of Eric Kandel, Mark Bear, Gary Lynch, Tim Tully, and other molecular neurobiologists, molecules are being designed that will treat cognitive disorders and also enhance the memory abilities of normal people (Marshall 2004). If one projects the market for normal memory-enhancing drugs from sales of nutritional supplements sold for this purpose, it is clear that the economic motivation is huge to develop memory enhancing drugs to help normal people deal with their complex lives. Drugs to suppress unwanted memories are also the object of research and development (Singer 2009).

The enhancement of non-cognitive psychological processes is also a goal of corporations and the individuals who buy from them. Basic research has shown that trust and generosity can be manipulated neurochemically in humans through nasal administration of oxytocin (Fehr *et al.* 2005; Zak *et al.* 2007), an achievement with obvious potential for enhancing social and business interactions, not to mention forensic uses. A quick search online will turn up numerous companies selling oxytocin, although without evidence that the formulation being offered is effective.

Drugs with central nervous system targets can also be used to enhance sexuality. Testosterone patches and gels have been used to enhance libido in postmenopausal women (Fitzhenry and Sandberg 2005). A number of new drugs, including the serotonin agonist flibanserin, show promise for improving sexual function in otherwise healthy young women suffering from low libido, and are under review for this purpose with the US Food and Drug Administration (Fitzhenry and Sandberg 2005).

Pharmaceutical approaches to cognitive and affective enhancement have recently been joined by other technologies, including transcranial brain stimulation by magnetic fields (transcranial magnetic stimulation, TMS; e.g. Fecteau *et al.* 2007) or electric currents (transcranial direct current stimulation, tDCS), deep brain stimulation by implanted electrodes (Schiff and Fins 2007), stem cell grafts (Li *et al.* 2008), and gene knock-ins (Lehrer 2009). Most of these are too invasive or experimental to be considered for use by healthy humans, although the rapid pace of technological development makes this generalization a fragile one. In the past few years deep brain stimulation, for example, has been achieved non-invasively in animals using ultrasound (Tyler *et al.* 2008).

At present TMS and tDCS are the focus of active research programs on the manipulation of normal and abnormal brain function. In particular tDCS has earned the attention of researchers in recent years for its ability to enhance a variety of cognitive processes in healthy research subjects. Learning, working memory, decision making, and language have been enhanced under laboratory conditions using tDCS (e.g. Dockery *et al.* 2009; Floel *et al.* 2008; Fregni *et al.* 2006; Sparing *et al.* 2008). Unlike TMS, tDCS does not require expensive equipment, and online chatter indicates that people are experimenting with the method at home.

At present much brain enhancement in underground, with students illegally buying and selling stimulants in the college library and home hobbyists trying battery-powered tDCS. This may soon change, given the recent guidelines issued by the American Academy of Neurology's Ethics, Law and Humanities Committee (Larriviere *et al.* 2009). In a report entitled "Responding to requests from adult patients for neuroenhancements," they conclude that it is morally and legally permissible for physicians to prescribe brain enhancing medications to healthy individuals.

Neuroscience-based education

Education is an aspect of life that engages each of us growing up and, for most of us, again in adulthood as parents. For many years, stretching back well into the 20th century, educators sought guidance from neuroscience, especially the parts of neuroscience that address learning and development. Their hope was that neuroscience would inform the design of instructional systems based on knowledge of human brain function in general and would allow customization of instruction based on knowledge of individuals' brain function. Unfortunately, they were generally disappointed by a lack of relevant information in these areas of neuroscience. In 1997 John Bruer surveyed attempts to apply neuroscience to pedagogy and concluded that the relationship between neuroscience and educational practice was, in his words, "a bridge too far." It seemed a fair point. The understanding of long-term potentiation has little to say about the challenges of classroom learning, and critical periods for the development of stereopsis are no more than a metaphor for concepts of readiness to learn in school children.

Although it would be an exaggeration to say that Bruer's bridge now exists and supports heavy traffic, it is clearly under construction and has already enabled some transit between the two sides. Not surprisingly, the most common applications of neuroscience are found within education research—the kinds of research programs conducted in university departments of education—rather than in the instructional practices of classroom teachers. One would expect this to be the case, as new teaching methods ought to be subject to research before being implemented in the schools. Much of the progress in this area concerns reading, which is a difficult skill to teach, and which cognitive neuroscientists have learned a considerable amount about. An example of a research program with relevance to educational practice comes from the work of Fumiko Hoeft, John Gabrieli, and collaborators. They addressed the problem of evaluating when a child is ready to learn to read.

It has long been known that children become ready to learn to read at different ages, and assessing reading readiness is therefore an important task for kindergarten and first grade teachers. Traditionally, they have relied on tests of phonological processing, such as making rhymes and predicting what word you get by adding a hard "c" sound to the beginning of the word "at." Hoeft *et al.* (2007) scanned a sample of children and then looked to see which areas of functional activation, gray matter density, and white matter density are predictive of reading ability 1 year later. What they found is that the brain data is predictive and the traditional behavioral data is also predictive. More importantly, they found that if you take the traditional data into account, the brain imaging data can still further improve prediction of reading 1 year later, above and beyond what is possible with the traditional methods.

Children with reading difficulties are already being given computerized interventions produced by companies such as Scientific Learning (http://www.scilearn.com), which base their methods on general neuroscience principles such as the effects of timing and practice on neural plasticity.

The ratio of hope to proven benefits remains high in the area of education and the brain, but unlike the situation Bruer critiqued in the late 20th century, there is a growing body of research linking the study of brain function to educationally relevant aspects of human psychology. Reviews of recent neuroscience research on learning to read (e.g. Dehaene 2009), mathematical competence (e.g. De Smedt *et al.* 2010), and the socioeconomic achievement gap (e.g. Farah 2010) show that neuroscience can be fruitfully applied to education (see also Ansari and Coch 2006; Battro *et al.* 2008; Goswami 2006; Turner and Sahakian 2008).

Neuromarketing

Corporate strategies for advertising, positioning and pricing products are often informed by research on consumer psychology. The emotions and motivations of consumers are a particularly important focus for marketers, yet people are often unable to report accurately these aspects of their psychology. The prospect of directly "reading" the brain states of consumers is therefore of great interest to marketers. Compared to some psychological states, states of liking and wanting have a relatively straightforward relation to patterns of brain activity. Electroencephalography (EEG) and functional magnetic resonance imaging (fMRI) have therefore become widely used tools in market research, and in 2002 the term "neuromarketing" was coined to refer to this research (Lewis and Bridger 2005).

Published research in the field of neuromarketing is more focused on academic issues, such as the nature of the brain activity underlying consumer behavior and the accuracy of brain-behavior predictions, than it is on the real-world utility of neuromarketing for improving business. From the published research we have learned the ways in which packaging design, price, brand identity, spokesman celebrity and other marketing factors separate from the product itself affect neural responses to the product, and how accurately those neural responses predict purchasing decisions (for reviews see Hubert and Kenning 2008; Lee *et al.* 2006).

The success of neuromarketing as a business tool is harder to assess, but the list of companies paying for neuromarketing services suggests that many corporate decision-makers have faith in it. Forbes Magazine reported that this list includes Chevron, Disney, Ebay, Google, Hyundai, Microsoft, Pepsico, and Yahoo (Burkitt 2009).

The techniques of neuromarketing can also be used to study preferences for health behaviors (Langleben *et al.* 2009) and political candidates (Westen *et al.* 2006). The firm FKF Applied Research published advice to American presidential candidates for the 2008 election in

The New York Times Op Ed pages, based on their fMRI studies (Iacoboni *et al.* 2007). Their advice received widespread attention in the media and online (Aron *et al.* 2007; Farah 2007; see also Iacoboni 2008, Poldrack 2008). Less public attempts to understand voters' reactions to candidates based on measures of brain function have reportedly been carried out at the request of specific political campaigns (Linstrom 2008).

Other applications

Additional examples of new, non-medical applications of neuroscience that date from the turn of the century include entertainment, romance, and employment screening. To be sure, some of these examples involve products that have yet to demonstrate their effectiveness by objective criteria. But 15 years ago these applications did not exist whereas today they are beyond the prototype stage; they are products based on real neuroscience or neurotechnology, which have found at least a small initial market.

To start with the most light-hearted example, several companies offer EEG-based game controllers that allow video gamers to play with their brains instead of their hands (e.g. Emotiv, Mindball, Neurosky, OCZ). For example, the Neurosky "MindSet" headset uses a single electrode to detect EEG and enables owners to play specially designed games such as "The Adventures of NeuroBoy" by thought alone, as well as visualize their brain activity while they listen to music and measure their degree of attention or relaxation.

Several companies have developed ways to aid us in the search for love, focusing on the brain rather than the heart. Chemistry.com, which went live in 2006, characterizes potential mates according to various behavioral and morphological surrogates for neurotransmitter and neuroendocrine activity. For example, the degree of prenatal exposure to testosterone, which masculinizes brains, is estimated by the ratio of the lengths of the first and fourth fingers (pointer and ring fingers). This ratio has been found, empirically, to be related to prenatal testosterone exposure and later life behaviors.

The Amen Clinics, which offer SPECT scans for a variety of controversial diagnostic purposes (APACCAF 2005) have also begun to offer what they call "pre-screening of couples" (http://www.amenclinics.com). And for those who have found a date but want to confirm that this prospective partner is all that he or she claims to be, the company No Lie MRI offers fMRI-based lie detection for "dating risk reduction" and "trust issues in interpersonal relationships" (http://noliemri.com).

The same fMRI lie detection company offers brain-based employment screening. Their website states that brain imaging can "potentially substitute for drug screening, resume validation and security background checks" (http://noliemri.com). The Amen Clinics owner has proposed that presidential candidates be screened for psychological fitness to serve using brain imaging (Amen 2007).

In sum, the early 21st century has seen a proliferation of neuroscience products applied to everyday life. They vary in their maturity and effectiveness, and some will ultimately fail to deliver on their promises and succumb to market forces. However, this state of affairs represents a sea change from the preceding century. Before, applications of neuroscience were found almost exclusively in the biomedical realm. Now, a wide range of everyday human activities, from work to shopping, education to dating, and sleeping to voting, are being touched by neuroscience.

STATE USES OF NEUROSCIENCE IN THE 21ST CENTURY

The novel *Brave New World* painted a frightening picture of life under a totalitarian regime that used a variety of biotechnologies to maintain its control (Huxley 1932). Among these biotechnologies, neurotechnology figured prominently. Children's brain development was chemically manipulated to create biologically distinct social castes, including those who would not object to their lives of servitude. Citizens of all castes were encouraged to dose themselves with the imaginary drug, Soma, to replace their doubts and worries with feelings of contentment and bliss. In this way psychopharmacology was used for social control, to short-circuit the motivation of the citizenry to take back control of their lives.

Of course, state use of neuroscience is not intrinsically negative. Whether it is dystopian or utopian in nature depends on the state and its goals. The recently completed UK Foresight project surveyed the neuroscience of human capital development and preservation with the goal of increasing the cognitive capacity and mental health of the population (Cooper *et al.* 2010). Such a program would arguably increase, rather than decrease, individual autonomy. However, interventions that affect our brain can affect our attitudes, decisions and behavior in ways that we may not be aware of or be able to resist. For this reason state uses of neuroscience merit special attention. They differ from the "lifestyle" applications of neuroscience just reviewed, which tend to be used by individuals voluntarily.

Criminal justice and the law

Neuroscience is potentially applicable to all of the same areas of criminal justice and the law to which psychology has already been applied. Within the criminal justice system, this includes a variety of sentencing options referred to as "therapeutic justice," where offenders are sent for anger management classes, parenting classes, treatment for drug dependence, and a variety of other forms of behaviorally-based psychotherapy.

In many states within the US, one particular form of brain-based therapeutic justice is already being practiced: sex offenders may be given long-acting forms of anti-androgen medications. This so-called "chemical castration" is effective through its effects on the brain. Other psychopharmacologic treatments with potential for therapeutic justice include serotonergic drugs such as selective serotonin reuptake inhibitors (SSRIs), which have been found effective for reducing repeat offending in sex offenders, as well as reducing impulsive violence (Briken and Kafka 2007; Walsh and Dinan 2001).

Defendants' personal, medical, and psychological history and diagnoses have long been introduced in court as mitigating factors at the sentencing phase of criminal trials. Increasingly information about defendants' brain function has also been introduced (Miller 2009; Morse 2006). In principle, neuroscience can also play a role in assessing dangerousness and risk of recidivism. Such information, to date based on behavioral history and psychological examination, is used in sentencing and parole decisions. Brain imaging studies of murderers have distinguished between groups who committed their crime impulsively and groups who proceeded in a more planful way, the latter being more likely to murder again (Raine *et al.* 1998).

Other possible legal applications of neuroscience extend beyond the criminal law, to such general considerations as jury selection and the evaluation of testimony. In connection with jury selection, lawyers and the courts seek to eliminate jurors with biases that could impair their ability to deliberate in an open-minded way. This task is challenging because jurors may not report, or even be aware of, their biases. FMRI has been shown to assess certain types of unconscious bias in cooperative subjects (e.g. Stanley *et al.* 2008, Fiske and Borgida 2008).

As mentioned in the introduction, and discussed in other parts of this volume (see Chapters 21, 38, and 40), fMRI has also been used to measure the likely truthfulness of testimony, although to date such methods have not been admitted as evidence in a court of law. A different type of brain-based lie detection, based on event-related potentials (ERPs) has been admitted as evidence in the US (Harrington v. State of Iowa), and in India. Indeed, in India the method has helped convict at least two defendants of murder (Aggarwal 2009).

Security applications: intelligence and military

As Canli and coauthors (2007) have pointed out, national security concerns have driven the development of many technologies, including neurotechnologies. Much of the success of both intelligence and military operations depends on personnel, and specifically on the psychological strength and dependability of personnel, which are functions of the brain.

Of course, information about security applications of neuroscience is often not accessible to the public. On the basis of available information, it has been surmised that brain imaging is likely to be among the methods being studied or used for interrogation (Marks 2007). Recent research in cognitive and social neuroscience on mechanisms of deception, inhibitory control and trust has obvious relevance to the development of methods to weaken an interrogee's ability to withhold information (Luber *et al.* 2009).

Personnel selection is critical for both intelligence and military operations, where loyalty and psychological resilience may be challenged under extreme conditions. Despite its many shortcomings, the polygraph has a long history of use in security screening (Committee to Review the Scientific Evidence on the Polygraph 2003). Might ERP or fMRI systems for lie detection, as imperfect as they are, be used instead of, or in addition to, the polygraph to provide a degree of evidence on truthfulness? Might brain imaging markers of vulnerability to anxiety or other disorders have a place in screening personnel for the stress of combat?

In addition to assessing or predicting the psychological traits of personnel, there is a strong military interest in enhancing personnel (Kautz *et al.* 2007). It is well established that war-fighting personnel use a variety of psychopharmacologic agents to increase concentration, decrease fatigue and counteract anxiety. Amphetamine has a long history in the military (Rasmussen 2008), joined more recently by modafinil (Caldwell and Caldwell 2005), and SSRI use is reported to be common among American troops in Iraq and Afghanistan (Thompson 2008). Other enhancements under development by the military are quite different from those shared with the civilian world. One example is the US Defense Advanced Research Projects Agency project known as "Luke's binoculars" (Northrum Grumman 2008). The device uses EEG signals to alert the wearer to his or her own unconscious perception of a relevant stimulus or event. This enhancement of visual attention is projected to be in use within a few years. Another example is a portable TMS device for delivering brain stimulation in the field (MUSC press release 2002; Nelson 2007). A final area of military applications of neuroscience consists of the development of non-lethal weapons (Gross 2010; Moreno 2006). Methods that render the enemy temporarily sleepy, confused, in pain, or terrified would all have their effects by selectively influencing brain function.

In sum, the early 21st century has seen a proliferation of individual and state uses of neuroscience. Pharmacologic manipulation of brain function for lifestyle reasons is already commonplace on campuses and in some workplaces. A number of new drugs and non-drug methods for enhancing everything from cognition to libido are on the market or in development. Brain imaging has been commercialized for applications ranging from lie detection to the assessment of romantic compatibility, and all of these methods for monitoring and manipulating the brain have found their way into government uses, from criminal justice to warfare.

Neuroethical challenges
for the 21st century

How ought society to respond to the many new applications of neuroscience, which are beginning to influence human life at so many levels simultaneously? Simply avoiding or discouraging the application of neuroscience to non-medical problems would be neither feasible nor wise.

An across-the-board moratorium on non-medical applications of neuroscience would be unfeasible given that the genie is already out of the bottle; many of the relevant products exist and will continue to exist because of their medical applications (e.g. drugs, brain imaging). In addition, it would be unwise in that it would deprive us of the many benefits that these technologies offer. There is nothing inherently wrong with the application of neuroscience to any specific aspect of human life, and in many cases it is a means to indisputably good ends. Even state-imposed applications of neuroscience, which may conjure up the dystopian society of *Brave New World*, are not necessarily any more problematic than other ways in which the state exerts an influence on our lives. What matters, ethically, are the specifics of each case: How does it affect human health and well-being? Does it enhance or restrict freedom, enrich or diminish life's meaning, protect or undermine human dignity?

These questions are no different from the questions one would ask about any technology. In this regard neuroethics does not differ fundamentally from other branches of applied ethics. Some authors have accordingly questioned whether we need a new field, with a new name and its own journals and meetings and professional groups. They point out that most of the subject matter of neuroethics has precedents or analogous cases in bioethics more generally. This is true, and such precedents should of course be studied for the guidance they can offer.

Notwithstanding the progress we can make by piecemeal analogizing with earlier dilemmas in genetics, reproductive technologies, and other biomedical sciences, there is no precedent for the sudden and increasingly ubiquitous nature of neuroscience's influence on human life. Reproductive medicine and the molecular revolution in biology did not impact life outside the medical realm as neuroscience does, in business, education, law, warfare, and all the other areas of life discussed here. Among scientific and technological advances more generally—from the theory of natural selection to atomic physics—it is difficult to find any which intersect human life at so many points. The potential ubiquity of neurotechnology seems comparable only to that of information technology. Consider that in just a few decades IT has transformed work, education, individuals' social lives, and the global economy. For this reason, 21st century neuroscience warrants attention as a whole, and the emergence of neuroethics is a natural and useful response to the many inter-related changes being wrought by neuroscience.

In the sections that follow I will review some of the familiar and specific neuroethical issues, which have already been discussed in greater depth elsewhere (e.g. Farah 2005). I will then turn to three more general issues concerning the influence of neuroscience on society that emerge now with the proliferation of non-medical applications of neuroscience.

FAMILIAR NEUROETHICAL ISSUES: PRIVACY, SAFETY, FAIRNESS, FREEDOM

Brain imaging is already able to deliver a degree of personal information about people without an individual even knowing what traits or states are being assessed (Farah *et al.* 2009). We therefore need to think about how and when to protect "brain privacy" (Committee on Science and Law 2005; Hyman 2004; Illes and Racine 2005; Kennedy 2004). The same privacy-related issues have arisen in connection with genotyping. Although the brain is a causal step closer to the behavioral endpoints of interest than are genes and may therefore ultimately be more psychologically revealing (Canli and Amin 2002; Farah *et al.* 2009; Hamer 2002), brain imaging and genotyping are similar in that both involve measures that can be taken for one stated purpose and used for a different one, either contemporaneously or later. We can therefore turn to the past two decades of bioethical work on privacy and genetics for helpful guidance (Illes and Racine 2005).

Safety is a concern that is crucial to the assessment of the ethical, legal, and social implications of any neurotechnology, be it psychopharmacology, brain stimulation or high-field MRI. As with privacy concerns, there are precedents that provide a framework for addressing safety-related concerns. Methodologies for assessing risk and for relating risk to benefit have already been developed and used for a wide variety of drugs and procedures within the clinical neurosciences and in other fields of medicine. This includes drugs and procedures intended purely for enhancement purposes. While there are important gaps in our knowledge of both the risks and benefits of many neurotechnologies, this is not from any special difficulty with obtaining this knowledge, but simply because the knowledge has yet to be sought.

The issue of fairness arises in neuroethics mainly in connection with brain enhancement. In competitive situations, from college admissions testing to chess championships, brain enhancements could confer unfair advantage. One might be willing to accept the fairness of an enhanced admission test score for an individual who intends to continue using brain enhancement, as that score truly reflects the level of ability the individual is likely to bring to his or her studies. However, if someone were to use a temporary enhancer to improve a test score and then stop enhancing, this would be undeniably unfair. Another way that neuro-technology can lead to unfairness is related to socioeconomic disparities. Brain enhance-ments have so far been more available to wealthier and better connected members of society. In a world where basic healthcare, education and personal safety cannot be guaranteed to all, it seems unlikely that brain enhancements will be equitably distributed.

Finally, while neurotechnology can be enabling (Lynch 2009), it can also limit individual freedom. State uses of neurotechnology feature the most blatant opportunities for coercion, but even individually chosen lifestyle applications of neuroscience can exert indirect pressure on people. Take, for the example, the situation that would occur when one worker in an office uses modafinil to extend his work hours on a regular basis and his colleague then feels pressure from the boss to be as productive (see Appel 2008, for a discussion of worker protections).

The problems of fairness and freedom raised by neurotechnologies have many precedents. For example, access to the latest information technology confers a competitive advantage on students and employees. With a personal computer, high-speed Internet access and a color printer, the quality, speed, and polish of a student's homework is improved, yet many students do not have access to this technology from their homes, a situation which is not fair. The diffusion of IT and its benefits can also reduce freedom. For example, once it became commonplace for workers to check email throughout the day and on weekends, we all became less free to work offline for long periods.

In the next three sections I will outline three new neuroethical challenges of a general nature. These are not associated with any particular application of neuroscience, but rather with the growing role of neuroscience in society as a whole.

NEW CHALLENGE #1: NEUROLITERACY FOR THE NEUROCENTURY

Given its increasing influence on everyday life, the citizens of the 21st century will need at least a rudimentary grasp of neuroscience. Parents receiving educational recommendations based on their child's neuropsychological profile, workers looking to enhance work-related brain functions, judges presiding over trials involving brain imaging evidence on the truth-fulness of testimony or the mental state of a defendant, and businesspersons considering an investment in neuromarketing are just some of the people whose personal or professional decisions should be informed by a basic understanding of neuroscience. Common misun-derstandings about neuroscience, such as that brain differences are genetic and immutable, that neurotransmitter systems and psychological functions have a 1-to-1 relationship (enabling selective targeting of functions) or that brain images are more "objective" than behavioral measures, could contribute to poor decisions in the examples just mentioned.

Some professions have already taken steps to educate their practitioners about neurosci-ence. For example, educators can choose from a wide array of continuing education confer-ences, books, and journals, and even a graduate degree program on neuroscience and education (see, e.g. http://www.imbes.org/ and http://www.edupr.com/). Judges and attorneys also have access to workshops on neuroscience (see, e.g. http://www.gruterinstitute.org and http://www.aaas.org/spp/sfrl/projects/neuroscience/judicial.shtml). However, these professions are the exception.

If the trends discussed earlier in this chapter continue, neuroliteracy will be important for citizens in all walks of life, not just the professions. Yet neuroscience is barely represented in many school science curricula (see, e.g.http://www.collegeboard.com/prod_downloads/ap/students/biology/ap-cd-bio-0708.pdf). Much as environmental science and computer technology have entered the curriculum of most secondary schools over the past few decades, so neuroscience will need to be added in order to prepare students for life in the 21st century.

NEW CHALLENGE #2: OWNERSHIP AND CONTROL OF NEUROTECHNOLOGY

Who will control the applications to which neuroscience is put in the coming years? Who will determine which neurotechnologies are developed and which remain mere potential applications of neuroscience? For those neurotechnologies that are developed, who will determine who has access? And who will determine what users know about the technologies' effectiveness and safety? The answers depend in large part on who owns the technology. In turn, ownership of a technology depends in large part on who invested the money required to develop it.

Herein lays an important difference between medical applications of neuroscience and the non-medical applications that have been the focus of this chapter. Health-related research is supported by a diversity of funding sources from both the public and private sectors. The development of new neuropsychiatric drugs, for example, is supported by national funding agencies such as the National Institutes of Health (NIH) in the US, by private foundations with health-related missions, and by the pharmaceutical industry. The same mix of tax-payer, philanthropic and corporate investment has enabled the development of medical devices, from neural implants to new imaging modalities.

In contrast, once the pathway of developing a non-medical application of neuroscience diverges from clinical or basic neuroscience pathways of discovery and innovation, the cost is generally born by for-profit corporations. In the US, for example, NIH does not support research to develop methods for mainstream classroom education, the detection of deception or the enhancement of mental function in healthy normal individuals. Similarly, private foundations that support neuroscience generally focus on a disease entity. The National Science Foundation supports basic rather than applied neuroscience research. Therefore the task of shepherding non-clinical applications of neuroscience through the development process and into use falls mainly to business. The company Scientific Learning, rather than the US Office of Education Research and Improvement, is responsible for the development of Fast ForWord® and other computerized education programs. The company Cephos, rather than the National Institute of Justice, supported the largest study to date of fMRI-based lie detection (http://www.cephoscorp.com/about-us/index.php#about). This fact about the ownership of neurotechnology has important implications for which potential applications are and are not eventually developed, and for the availability of information about the products.

Concerning which non-medical applications of neuroscience are developed, the trend toward virtually exclusive private corporate funding implies that only the most profitable applications will be developed. While this is legitimate business practice, it will not necessarily give us the products that are the most beneficial to humanity. By analogy with morning television programming for young children, market forces give us the Mutant Ninja Turtle shows that children enjoy and advertisers pay for. In contrast, it is the Public Broadcasting System that gives us "Sesame Street," which the Education Resources Information Center finds beneficial to cognitive development and school readiness (1990) (http://www.eric.ed.gov).

Private ownership of neurotechnology also lessens incentive to evaluate the efficacy of popular products and communicate the evaluation results to users. Consider the case of Scientific Learning's flagship product, Fast ForWord®. This system has been in classrooms and clinics since the mid-1990s and has been used by an estimated 700,000 students worldwide. According to the company, "Based on more than 30 years of neuroscience and cognitive research, the Fast ForWord® family of products provides struggling readers with computer-delivered exercises that build the cognitive skills required to read and learn effectively." (http://www.scilearn.com/company/news/press-releases/20091009.php). In 2009 the Johns Hopkins University School of Education's Center for Data-Driven Reform in Education reviewed the evidence on the benefits of this product for struggling readers. They found little evidence available from appropriately designed studies. Furthermore, what evidence there was indicated that Fast ForWord® was of no value in improving the reading ability of struggling readers. Nevertheless, according to a recent press release, the company's third quarter revenue 2009 was $19-20 million (http://www.scilearn.com/company/news/press-releases/20091009.php), from sales to schools around the world. Lack of transparency and probable overclaim are also evident in the field of fMRI-based lie detection. For example, Cephos asserts that their method is 97% accurate (http://www.cephos.com), but the evidence for this claim in neither peer-reviewed nor published (S. Laken 2010, personal communication).

As the role of neurotechnology in society expands, we need a balance of public and private ownership to encourage the development of products whose social value is higher than their profit value, and to promote transparency concerning efficacy and, where relevant, safety. Public support, national and international, should be developed for non-medical applications of neuroscience.

New challenge #3: avoiding nihilism

A final neuroethical challenge for the 21st century will be to assimilate neuroscience's increasingly complete physical explanation of human behavior without lapsing into nihilism. If we are really no more than physical objects, albeit very complex objects containing powerful computational networks, then does it matter what becomes of any of us? Why should the fate of these objects containing human brains matter more than the fate of other natural or manmade objects? Why should we hold certain objects morally responsible for their actions and thus blame them rather than simply declaring them to be malfunctioning?

By showing how human behavior arises from mechanistic physical processes, neuroscience is eroding a fundamental distinction that underlies many of our moral intuitions: the distinction between persons and objects. Advances in basic science are revealing the necessary and sufficient neural processing underlying people's thoughts, feelings and personalities, the aspects of persons that seem to distinguish them from objects. Even the applications of neuroscience discussed earlier reinforce the view that we are physical objects. That is, to the extent that we increasingly manipulate our own and each others' brain functions in order to change abilities, moods and personality traits, we will be living with frequent reminders of the ultimately physical nature of our being.

The person–object distinction plays an important role in morality. First, we view persons as having agency and therefore generally hold them responsible for their actions. Although many people believe that, in principle, human behavior is the physical result of a causally determined chain of biophysical events, we tend to put that aside when making moral judgments. We do not say, "But he had no choice—the laws of physics made him do it!" However, as the neuroscience of decision making and impulse control begins to offer a more detailed and specific account of the physical processes leading to irresponsible or criminal behavior, the amoral deterministic viewpoint will probably gain a stronger hold on our intuitions. Whereas the laws of physics are a little too abstract to displace the concept of personal responsibility in our minds, our moral judgments might well be moved by a demonstration of subtle damage to prefrontal inhibitory mechanisms wrought by, for example, past drug abuse or childhood neglect. This has already happened to an extent with the disease model of drug abuse (Leshner 1997). As a result largely of neuroscience research showing how addictive behavior arises from drug-induced changes in brain function (Rogers and Robbins 2001; Verdejo-García *et al.* 2004), addiction is now viewed as more of a medical problem than a failure of personal responsibility.

We also view persons as having a special moral value, as distinct from all other objects in the universe. Persons deserve protection from harm just because they are persons. Whereas we value objects for what they can do—a car because it transports us, a book because it contains information, a painting because it looks beautiful—the value of persons transcends their abilities, knowledge, or attractiveness. Persons have what Kant called "dignity," meaning a special kind of intrinsic value that trumps the value of any use to which they could be put (Kant 1996). This categorical distinction would be difficult to maintain if everything about persons arises from physical mechanisms. Similarly, progress in neuroscience challenges the belief in immaterial souls, common to many religions (Farah and Murphy 2009).

In sum, neuroscience is calling into question our age-old understanding of the human person, and with it much of the psychological basis for morality. Much as the natural sciences became the dominant way of understanding the world around us in the 18th century, so neuroscience may be responsible for changing our understanding of ourselves in the 21st. Such a transformation could reduce us to machines in each other's eyes, mere clockwork devoid of moral agency and moral value. Alternatively, it could help bring about a more understanding and humane society, as people's behavior is seen as part of the larger picture of causal forces surrounding them and acting through them.

REFERENCES

Aggarwal, N.K. (2009). Neuroimaging, culture, and forensic psychiatry. *Journal of American Academic Psychiatry and Law*, 37, 239–44.

Amen, A.R. (2007). Getting inside their heads… really inside. *Los Angeles Times*, 5 December, 2007.

Ansari, D. and Coch, D. (2006). Bridges over troubled waters: education and cognitive neuroscience. *Trends in Cognitive Sciences*, 10, 146–51.

Appel, J.M. (2008). When the boss turns pusher: a proposal for employee protections in the age of cosmetic neurology. *Journal of Medical Ethics*, 34, 57–60.

Aron, A., Badre, D., Bratt, M., *et al.* (2007). Politics and the Brain. *New York Times*, 14 November, 2007.

Arrington, M. (2008). How Many Silicon Valley Startup Executives Are Hopped Up On Provigil? Los Angeles, *TechCrunch Online*, 15 July, 2008.

Barondes, S.H. (2003). *Better than Prozac: Creating the Next Generation of Psychiatric Drugs.* New York: Oxford University Press.

Battro, A.M., Fischer, K.W., and Léna, P. (eds.) (2008). *The Educated Brain: Essays in Neuroeducation.* Cambridge: Cambridge University Press.

Bert De Smedta, D.A., Grabnerc, R.H., Hannulad, M.M., Schneiderc, M., and Verschaffela, L. (2010). Cognitive neuroscience meets mathematics education. *Educational Research Review*, 5, 97–105.

Briken, P. and Kafka, M.P. (2007). Pharmacological treatments for paraphilic patients and sexual offenders. *Current Opinion in Psychiatry*, 20, 609–13.

Burkitt, L. (2009). Neuromarketing: Companies Use Neuroscience for Consumer Insights. *Forbes*, 29 October, 2009.

Caldwell, J.A. and Caldwell, J.L. (2005). Fatigue in military aviation: an overview of US military-approved pharmacological countermeasures. *Aviation Space Environmental Medical*, 76, C39–51.

Canli, T., Brandon, S., Casebeer, W., *et al.* (2007). Neuroethics and national security. *American Journal of Bioethics*, 7, 3–13.

Canli, T. and Amin, Z. (2002). Neuroimaging of emotion and personality: scientific evidence and ethical considerations. *Brain Cognition*, 50, 414–31.

Committee to Review the Scientific Evidence on the Polygraph (National Research Council (U.S.), National Research Council (U.S.). Board on Behavioral Cognitive and Sensory Sciences *et al.* (2003). *The polygraph and lie detection.* Washington, D.C., National Academies Press.

Committee on Science and Law. National Bar Association. (2005). *Are your thoughts your own? Neuroprivacy and the legal implications of brain imaging.* New York: Committee on Science and Law.

Cooper, C.L. (2009). *Mental Capital and Wellbeing.* Oxford: Wiley-Blackwell.

Cox, D.D. and Savoy, R.L. (2003). Functional magnetic resonance imaging (fMRI) "brain reading": detecting and classifying distributed patterns of fMRI activity in human visual cortex. *Neuroimage*, 19, 261–70.

Dehaene, S. (2009). *Reading in the Brain : the Science and Evolution of a Human Invention.* New York: Viking.

Dockery, C.A., Hueckel-Weng, R., Birbaumer, N., *et al.* (2009). Enhancement of planning ability by transcranial direct current stimulation. *Journal of Neuroscience*, 29, 7271–7.

Farah, M. (2007). This is Your Brain on Politics? *Neuroethics and Law Blog*. A. Kolber. 2009.

Farah, M.J. (2002). Emerging ethical issues in neuroscience. *Nature Neuroscience*, **5**, 1123–9.

Farah, M.J. (2005). Neuroethics: the practical and the philosophical. *Trends in Cognitive Sciences*, **9**, 34–40.

Farah, M.J. (2009). A picture is worth a thousand dollars. *Journal of Cognitive Neuroscience*, **21**, 623–4.

Farah, M.J. (2010). Mind, brain and education in socioeconomic context. In M. Ferrari and L. Vuletic (eds.) *The Developmental Interplay of Mind, Brian, and Education*. New York: Springer.

Farah, M.J. and Murphy, N. (2009). Neuroscience and the Soul. *Science*, **323**, 1168.

Fecteau, S., Knoch, D., Fregni, F., *et al.* (2007). Diminishing risk-taking behavior by modulating activity in the prefrontal cortex: a direct current stimulation study. *Journal of Neuroscience*, **27**, 12500–5.

Fiske, S.T. and Borgida, E. (2008). Providing expert knowledge in an adversarial context: Social cognitive science in employment discrimination. *Annual Review of Law and Social Science*, 123–48.

Fitzhenry, D. and Sandberg, L. (2005). Female sexual dysfunction. *Nature Reviews Drug Discovery*, 4, 99–100.

Flaherty, L.T., Arroyo, W., Chatoor, I., *et al.* (2005). *Brain imaging and child and adolescent psychiatry with special emphasis on SPECT*. New York: American Psychiatric Association, Council on Children, Adolescents and Their Families.

Floel, A., Garraux, G., Ben, B., *et al.* (2008). Levodopa increases memory encoding and dopamine release in the striatum in the elderly. *Neurobiology of Aging*, **29**, 267–79.

Goswami, U. (2006). Neuroscience and education: from research to practice? *Nature Reviews Neuroscience*, **7**, 406–11.

Gross, M. (2010). Medicalized Weapons and Modern War. *The Hastings Center Report*, **40**, 34–43.

Hamer, D. (2002). Rethinking behavior genetics. *Science*, **298**, 71–2.

Hart-Davis, A. (2005). The genius pill: would you be an idiot to take it? *The Evening Standard*, 22 November, 2005.

Haynes, J.D. and Reese, G. (2006). Decoding mental states from brain activity in humans. *Nature Reviews Neuroscience*, **7**, 523–34.

Hoeft, F., Ueno, T., Reiss, A.L., *et al.* (2007). Prediction of children's reading skills using behavioral, functional, and structural neuroimaging measures. *Behavioral Neuroscience*, **121**, 602–13.

Hubert, M. and Kenning, P. (2008). A current overview of consumer neuroscience. *Journal of Consumer Behaviour*, 7, 272–92.

Huxley, A. (1936). *Brave New World*. Garden City, NY: The Sun Dial Press.

Hyman, S.E. (2004). Introduction: the brain's special status. *Cerebrum*, **6**, 9–12.

Iacoboni, M. (2007). This is your brain on politics. *New York Times*, 11 November, 2007.

Iacoboni, M. (2008). Iacoboni Responds to Neuropolitics Criticism. *Neuroethics and Law Blog*. A. Kolber.

Illes, J. and Racine, E. (2005). Imaging or imagining? A neuroethics challenge informed by genetics. *American Journal of Bioethics*, **5**, 5–18.

Illes, J. and Raffin, T.A. (2002). Neuroethics: an emerging new discipline in the study of brain and cognition. *Brain Cognition*, **50**, 341–4.

Kant, I. (1996). *Critique of Pure Reason*. Indianapolis: Hackett Publishing Company.

Kautz, M.A., Thomas, M.L., and Caldwell, J.L. (2007). Considerations of pharmacology on fitness for duty in the operational environment. *Aviation Space Environment Medical*, **78**, B107–12.

Kennedy, D. (2004). Neuroscience and neuroethics. *Science*, **306**, 373.

Kosfeld, M., Heinrichs, M., Zak, P.J., Fischbacher, U., and Fehr, E. (2005). Oxytocin increases trust in humans. *Nature*, **435**, 673–6.

Kroutil, L.A., Van Brunt, D.L., Herman-Stahl, M.A., Heller, D.C., Bray, R.M., and Penne, M.A. (2006). Nonmedical use of prescription stimulants in the United States. *Drug Alcohol Depend*, **84**, 135–43.

Langleben, D.D., Loughead, J.W., Ruparel, K., *et al.* (2009). Reduced prefrontal and temporal processing and recall of high "sensation value" ads. *Neuroimage*, **46**, 219–25.

Larriviere, D., Williams, M.A., Rizzo, M., and Bonnie, R.J. (2009). Responding to requests from adult patients for neuroenhancements: guidance of the Ethics, Law and Humanities Committee. *Neurology*, **73**, 1406–12.

Lee, N., Broderick, A.J., and Chamberlain, L. (2007). What is 'neuromarketing'? A discussion and agenda for future research. *International Journal of Psychophysiology*, **63**, 199–204.

Lehrer, J. (2009). Neuroscience: Small, furry…and smart. *Nature*, **461**, 862–4.

Lewis, D. and Bridger, D. (July/August 2005). Market Researchers make Increasing use of Brain Imaging. *Advances in Clinical Neuroscience and Rehabilitation*, **5**, 35.

Li, J.Y., Christophersen, N.S., Hall, V., Soulet, D., and Brundin, P. (2008). Critical issues of clinical human embryonic stem cell therapy for brain repair. *Trends in Neurosciences*, **31**, 146–53.

Lindström, M. (2008). *Buy ology: Truth and Lies About Why We Buy*. New York: Doubleday.

Luber, B., Fisher, C., Appelbaum, P.S., Ploesser, M., and Lisanby, S.H. (2009). Non-invasive brain stimulation in the detection of deception: scientific challenges and ethical consequences. *Behavioral Science Law*, **27**, 191–208.

Lynch, Z. and Laursen, B. (2009). *The Neuro Revolution: How Brain Science is Changing Our World*. New York: St. Martin's Press.

Maher, B. (2008). Poll results: look who's doping. *Nature*, **452**, 674–5.

Madrigal, A. (2008). Readers' brain-enhancing drug regimens. *Wired Magazine*.

Marcus, S.J. (2004). *Neuroethics: Mapping the Field*. Chicago, IL: University of Chicago Press.

Marks, J.H. (2007). Interrogational neuroimaging in counterterrorism: a 'no-brainer' or a human rights hazard? *American Journal Law Medical*, **33**, 483–500.

Marshall, E. (2004). A star-studded search for memory-enhancing drugs. *Science*, **304**, 36–8.

McCabe, D.L. (2005). Academic dishonesty & educational opportunity. *Liberal Education*, **91**, 26–31.

Medical University of South Carolina. (2002). Press Release. Charleston, SC: Medical University of South Carolina.

Miller, G. (2009). fMRI Evidence Used in Murder Sentencing. ScienceDirect Online.

Moreno, J.D. (2003). Neuroethics: an agenda for neuroscience and society. *Nature Reviews Neuroscience*, **4**, 149–53.

Moreno, J.D. (2006). *Mind Wars: Brain Research and National Defense*. New York: Dana Press.

Morse, S.J. (2006). Addiction, genetics, and criminal responsibility. *Law & Contemporary Problems*, **69**, 166–207.

Nelson, J.T. (2007). Enhancing Warfighter Cognitive Abilities with Transcranial Magnetic Stimulation: a Feasibility Analysis. Air Force Research Laboratory (Technical Report AFRL-HE-WP-TR-2007-0095).

Northrup Grumann Corporation. (2008). Northrop Grumman-led team awarded contract to develop electronic binoculars that use brain activity to detect threats. Linthicum, MD: Northrop Grumann Corporation.

Phan, K.L., Wager, T., Taylor, S.F., and Liberzon, I. (2002). Functional neuroanatomy of emotion: a meta-analysis of emotion activation studies in PET and fMRI. *Neuroimage*, 16, 331–48.

Plotz, D. (2003). Wake Up Little Susie: Can we sleep less? *Slate Magazine Online*. Washington, DC: Newsweek.

Poldrack, R. (2008). Poldrack Replies to Iacoboni Neuropolitics Discussion. *Neuroethics and Law Blog*. A. Kolber.

Raine, A., Meloy, J.R., Bihrle, S., *et al.* (1998). Reduced prefrontal and increased subcortical brain functioning assessed using positron emission tomography in predatory and affective murderers. *Behavioral Sciences & the Law*, 16, 319–32.

Rasmussen, N. (2008). *On Speed: The Many Lives of Amphetamine*. New York: New York University Press.

Rogers, R.D. and Robbins, T.W. (2001). Investigating the neurocognitive deficits associated with chronic drug misuse. *Current Opinion Neurobiology*, 11, 250–7.

Roskies, A. (2002). Neuroethics for the new millenium. *Neuron*, 35, 21–3.

Sahakian, B. and Morein-Zamir, S. (2007). Professor's little helper. *Nature*, 450, 1157–9.

Savoy, R.L. (2001). History and future directions of human brain mapping and functional neuroimaging. *Acta Psychology*, 107, 9–42.

Schiff, N.D., Giacino, J.T., and Fins, J.J. (2009). Deep brain stimulation, neuroethics, and the minimally conscious state: moving beyond proof of principle. *Archives of Neurology*, 66, 697–702.

Singer, E. (2007). Erasing memories. *Technology Review Online*, 13 July, 2007.

Sparing, R., Dafotakis, M., Meister, I.G., Thirugnanasambandam, N., and Fink, G.R. (2008). Enhancing language performance with non-invasive brain stimulation – a transcranial direct current stimulation study in healthy humans. *Neuropsychologia*, 46, 8.

Stanley, D., Phelps, E., and Banaji, M. (2008). The neural basis of implicit attitudes. *Current Directions in Psychological Science*, 17, 164–70.

Talbot, M. (2009). Brain gain: The underground world of 'neuroenhancing' drugs. *The New Yorker*, 27 April, 32–43.

Thompson, M. (2008). America's Medicated Army. *Time*, 171, 138–42.

Turner, D.C., Robbins, T.W., Clark L, Aron, A.R., Dowson, J., and Sahakian, B.J. (2003). Cognitive enhancing effects of modafinil in healthy volunteers. *Psychopharmacology*, 165, 260–9.

Turner, D.C. and Sahakian, B.J. (2008). The cognition-enhanced classroom. In: L. Zonneveld, H. Dijstelbloem, and D. Ringoir (eds.) *Reshaping the Human Condition: Exploring Human Enhancment*, pp. 107–13. The Hague: Rathenau Institute.

Tyler, W.J. (2010) Noninvasive neuromodulation with ultrasound? A continuum mechanics hypothesis. *The Neuroscientist* [Epub before print 25 January].

Verdejo-Garcia, A., Lopez-Torrecillas, F., Gimenez, C. O., and Perez-Garcia, M. (2004). Clinical implications and methodological challenges in the study of the neuropsychological correlates of cannabis, stimulant, and opioid abuse. *Neuropsychology Review*, 14, 1–41.

Walsh, M.T. and Dinan, T.G. (2001). Selective serotonin reuptake inhibitors and violence: a review of the available evidence. *Acta Psychiatry Scandanavia*, 104, 84–91.

Westen, D., Blagov, P.S., Harenski, K., Kilts, C., and Hamann, S. (2006). Neural bases of motivated reasoning: an FMRI study of emotional constraints on partisan political judgment in the 2004 U.S. Presidential election. *Journal of Cognitive Neuroscience*, 18, 1947–58.

Zak, P.J., Stanton, A.A., and Ahmadi, S. (2007). Oxytocin increases generosity in humans. *PLoS One*, 2, e1128.

CHAPTER 46

NEUROSCIENCE AND THE MEDIA: ETHICAL CHALLENGES AND OPPORTUNITIES

ERIC RACINE

INTRODUCTION

THIS chapter provides a review and a perspective on the interaction between neuroscience and the media from an ethics standpoint. In the first part of the chapter, I situate public discourse and communication of neuroscience in an intricate web of social expectations and ethical responsibilities that converge and diverge between different stakeholders such as academic researchers, public sponsors of research, and the interested public. Second, based on previous research, I highlight some of the key ethical and social challenges that emerge when neuroscientists interact with the media. This review shows that the media manifests important shortcomings in matters of neuroscience explanations and fosters some unrealistic expectations for the outcomes of neuroscience. However, I argue that, in a democratic society, communication of science is not only a strategic and unidirectional process but also a social and multidirectional process with substantial ethical implications. The chapter concludes with attention to some of the research and practical questions that need further attention in matters of ethics and communication in neuroscience.

This chapter relies on a number of assumptions that need to be acknowledged from the onset. They explain the view that communication of neuroscience (and media coverage of neuroscience) is of crucial importance for neuroethics:

1) Ethics is multidimensional (Racine 2008a) and, for the sake of this chapter, inspired by pragmatic neuroethics that draws attention to social aspects of ethics and ethical contexts. Ethics seeks reasonable solutions for pluralistic and democratic societies but these solutions need to be tested in the real world and evaluated and revised if necessary (Racine 2008b, 2010).

2) Public communication is important, has important consequences and can influence behavior. From an ethical standpoint, it represents an act, reflects intents and, therefore, intersects with ethical responsibilities, duties, and obligations like other types of actions.

3) Communication and public discourse on neuroscience have meaning and implications beyond the interest of efficient communication of scientific content. The more fundamental recognition of the interest that multiple stakeholders have in voicing concerns, expressing interests, and discussing the social and ethical consequences of neuroscience is a recognition of common belonging to humankind. Acknowledging these implications signals a shared interest for the future of human welfare and the public good and is consistent with the fact that communication and open discourse are one of the pillars of democratic institutions as enshrined in democratic constitutions.

4) Public communication of science by neuroscientists, because of the values and principles underlying scientific knowledge, has a unique contribution to make to enlighten public discourse. It has the ability (in the case of neuroscience) to challenge and re-examine critically opinions and convictions about important social and medical subject matters (e.g. nature of mental health and behavior; personal responsibility for individual acts). This input could bring about more humanistic and comprehensive ways of dealing with healthcare and social problems as well as contributing to the renewal of thinking on social and mental health issues.

5) Empirical research is useful to understand ethical and social challenges and provide evidence on how ethical challenges are handled (or not) and how ethical issues are discussed in the media and other public fora.

ETHICS AND STAKEHOLDERS IN THE PUBLIC COMMUNICATION OF NEUROSCIENCE RESEARCH

The human nervous system is the most complicated biological system known to humankind and without surprise the organ that is least understood. The ethical landscape of healthcare and biomedical research on neurological and psychiatric disorders (as well as communication of this research) is shaped by this paradox. The availability of effective treatments for devastating neurodegenerative conditions such as Alzheimer's disease (AD); public comprehension of the complexity of mental health problems; and a good general scientific understanding of brain function and dysfunction would perhaps alleviate some (but certainly not all) of the current ethical and social challenges societies face. However, the current context is one where only limited treatments are available for many common and severe mental health and neurological disorders; one where there is much stigma related to mental illness and cognitive and motor disability; and where available tools to understand the nervous system are imperfect (Racine 2010). Multiple ethical–medical gray zones are created by this lack of effective treatment and ethical approaches.

The flip side of our limited understanding is that the evolution of neuroscience has now reached an exciting level of maturity. Work examining the biological underpinnings of neurological and psychiatric disorders is flourishing with unprecedented broad support and interest. Thousands of neuroscience researchers worldwide are engaged in research aimed at understanding the normal and pathological functions of the brain. Some of the basic knowledge generated by neuroscience is now translating into opportunities to apply discoveries and test novel insights in stroke, AD, and Parkinson's disease (PD) to name a few ethically salient examples (Ravina *et al.* 2003; Illes *et al.* 2007; Savitz and Fisher 2007; Bell *et al.* 2009; Weaver *et al.* 2009). In addition, national programs and initiatives to tackle mental health and to make it a priority are surfacing (Hickie 2004; Kirby 2008; Patel and Wells 2009).

The communication of neuroscience research is also shaped by underlying features of brain health and neuroscience research as well as the complexity of the interactions between neuroscience, on the one hand, and ethical, religious, and philosophical issues, on the other hand. The diverse roles and responsibilities of stakeholders (e.g. academic institutions, patients, academic researchers, and the media) involved in news construction, news dissemination, and news understanding reflect these features. Accordingly, and unsurprisingly, public communication of neuroscience is the meeting place of multiple and sometimes competing and even conflicting expectations and values. It is crucial to capture the ethical salience of communication of neuroscience and the pervasive pluralism that exists in this area. What follows are illustrations of multiple expectations and commitments at work between and within different stakeholders.

1) From an academic standpoint, the broader communication and discussion of neuroscience research and its implications for medicine, law, ethics, and society represent a growing area of scholarly interest, which is reflected in the dynamic growth of neuroscience and related specialties in academic programs. At the same time, academic institutions are under increasing pressure to augment their public visibility and their transparency to enhance their accountability for precious research dollars. They also have vested interests in attracting attention to their research activities. While intersecting with interest for strategic media visibility, modern academic institutions are rooted in the long tradition of Enlightenment thought that underscores the unique contribution of academic institutions to public education and informed democratic debates beyond the instrumental value of the media and of science communication.

2) In several research-intensive nations, neuroscience (including mental health, addiction, and neurological research) now represents one of the most active and dynamic areas of basic and applied biomedical investigation. Research sponsors are increasingly under pressure from their own funders, typically governments, to show the beneficial scientific, social, and economic outcomes of research. While the burden of neurological and mental health disorders justifies the eagerness to translate research, the complexity of the brain means that translation faces scientific, ethical, and social challenges. Like academic institutions, public funding bodies seek media exposure and encourage their researchers to participate responsibly in the effort of knowledge transfer.

3) The private research sector now views neuroscience as a promising area to invest in, where therapeutics can be developed to attract a huge consumer base (National Neurotechnology Initiative Act 2009). Neurological and psychiatric conditions represent a huge and growing health burden for many nations (World Health

Organization 2001, 2006; Kuehn 2009). For the private sector, chronic health conditions represent a stable consumer base and therefore a market to target with aggressive approaches (Hollon 2004; Racine *et al.* 2007b). For the private sector, interactions between the media and the public can come in service of creating interest for research activities, attract investment, and generate excitement for the treatments that may be yielded downstream (Eaton and Illes 2007).

4) Academics and research units are caught in a complex web of expectations. The commitment of academics to research and academic freedom is consistent with the goal of sharing knowledge with the public through teaching and training programs as well as broader public education through the media. At the same time, because of the stringency and rigor imposed by the nature of academic work, public discussion of research and interaction with the media are sometimes viewed as suspect by academic researchers. This is due to a number of factors including the sometimes sensational coverage of research and news in general (Caulfield 2004) and consequently the cultural distance between the ethos of the media and the academic culture. Therefore, many forces push and pull academics to and away from engaging with the media. As a consequence, academics face wide-ranging expectations of peers, private or public sponsors of research as well as those of the general public.

5) Media stakeholders have their own reasons for being interested in cutting edge research like neuroscience and its medical, ethical, philosophical, and social implications. The general public is fascinated by the brain (Frazzetto and Anker 2009). In the media, the brain has been depicted metaphorically as "the mystery we still can't penetrate" (Hall 2001), an "enigma" (Connor 1995), and the "terra incognita that lies between our ears" where one can find "the keys to the kingdoms of memory, of thought, of desire, of fear, of the habits and skills that add up to who we each are" (Hall 1999). Leading science journalists are themselves curious about neuroscience research. The media industry builds on this interest and needs to effectively reach its consumer base in a ferociously competitive media market where the status of traditional media like newspapers, radio, and television is constantly questioned with the emergence of more interactive forms of electronic media (Alessi and Alessi 2008).

6) Patients, caregivers, and patient groups look to neuroscience and neuroscientists in hope of potential cures and treatments for their health conditions. Headlines can become sources of hope and an impetus to participate to a clinical trial. But the reality of the slow and incremental nature of scientific progress means that disappointment can occur as neuroscientists slowly decipher the complexity of the biology of the brain.

Given the role and interest of different stakeholders in the public communication of neuroscience research, different logics are at play within and between different stakeholders meaning that pluralism is unavoidable and therefore dialogue necessary within a democratic framework. Table 46.1 provides examples of situations that involve ethical values and principles for some of the key stakeholders involved in the communication of scientific research based on the preceding explanations.

In response to the unavoidable conflicts created by the diverse roles and responsibilities of different stakeholders engaged at the intersection of neuroscience and the media, two distinct general responses have been put forward and are discussed in the following section.

Table 46.1 Examples of ethical tensions in the communication of neuroscience research based on the diverse role and responsibilities of different stakeholders

Academic institutions

The need to respect the slow and incremental nature of scientific knowledge and values of humility and integrity constitutive of the scientific research process *and* the need for immediate public exposure to increase visibility and augment institutional research activities

Public sponsors of research

The inherent unpredictability of funded scientific research *and* pressures to communicate tangible results and applications to decision-makers and public stakeholders to ensure ongoing public support for science

Private sponsors of research

The commitment to using the media as part of the development and marketing of economically viable scientific products and technologies that will be beneficial to individuals and society *and* pressures to yield return on investments rapidly while respecting standards of scientific integrity and academic freedom

Academic researchers

The careful reporting and discussion of research results to inform the public and be accountable (for receiving public funds for research) *and* the constraints of media reporting of research in contexts where simplified interpretations and hasty interpretations may cause harm to individuals, stakeholder groups, and science itself

Media stakeholders

The role of journalism for public interests, including commitment to balanced reporting of scientific news and facts *and* the commercial constraint of economic viability and sustainability in media most often rooted in the private sector

Public stakeholders

The interest in science and sometimes hope for better treatments yielded with insights into diseases *and* the need for individual efforts to understand how science and medicine relate to oneself (e.g. for one's healthcare) and to one's society (e.g. to take into consideration the scientific program of political parties)

Two sets of approaches to challenges and opportunities in the public communication of neuroscience in the media

The context I presented earlier makes it clear that different stakeholders come to the topic of public communication of neuroscience research with different logics and frameworks. On the one hand, differences in perspectives have been interpreted as creating obstacles for "efficient" or strategic communication of neuroscience research for stakeholders like academic institutions and academic researchers. This need for enhanced unidirectional channels of communication has been captured in the public understanding of science movement in the UK (Blakemore 2002; Rose 2003) as well as the so-called "deficit model" of science communication that stresses the need to bridge the gap between expert and lay citizens and minimize "distortions" of messages voiced by scientific experts. From an ethical standpoint, the underlying rationale of unidirectional approaches can be articulated as the search for enhanced information that supports the decision-making ability of citizens and also that protects citizens from uncritically accepting misleading and even harmful interpretations of neuroscience. However, this emphasis on the unidirectional aspects of communication processes can transform communication into a form of paternalism or a mere "selling of science" (Nelkin 1995) that presupposes that all of neuroscience is in the public's best interest without consultation of public stakeholders.

On the other hand, the conflicting rationales and goals of stakeholders can lead to a more open-ended examination of the underlying assumptions of efficient transfer of knowledge embedded in unidirectional approaches. Accordingly, unidirectional approaches need further consideration; not meaning that they are intrinsically shallow from an ethics standpoint but rather that it must be acknowledged that they reflect the perspective of some stakeholders but not of all (Racine *et al.* 2005a; Bubela *et al.* 2009). The broader critical perspective of ethics calls for open-ended perspectives and multidirectional approaches. Such approaches can welcome different discourses where competing goods and views on the public good can be put into question and re-examined, in the search for a common good beyond the interests of some specific stakeholders (Callahan 1994; Racine 2010). In this perspective, the broadly scoped neuroethical challenges contemporary societies are facing in dealing with the burden of brain health and the technological promises of neuroscience become occasions to acknowledge different values and ethical approaches. The following section explores challenges and opportunities for unidirectional and multidirectional approaches based on previous empirical research.

Table 46.2 illustrates the contrast between unidirectional and multidirectional approaches to public understanding of neuroscience and the role of science and its relationship to the media. Unidirectional and multidirectional approaches of communication also bring forward different scientific, social, and ethical concerns. Unidirectional approaches may be particularly interested and challenged by problems plaguing the quality and accuracy of neuroscientific content in media coverage of neuroscience. Multidirectional approaches stress that the scope of neuroscience and of its philosophical, social, and religious implications call for broader dialogue. Readers should keep in mind that I believe that both unidirectional and multidirectional approaches should serve complementary roles because they can not simply replace each other. Both pursue valuable goals from a scientific, ethics, and social perspective.

Unidirectional approaches and challenges of accuracy and reasonably balanced scientific content in the media

Traditionally, science communication has been viewed as a one-way process where scientists are considered content experts on the topic they are researching (Racine *et al.* 2005a).

Within unidirectional approaches, science communication is therefore viewed as the process of using an appropriate medium to transmit clearly, accurately, and without distortion the objective knowledge yielded by expert neuroscientists. Accordingly, unidirectional approaches stress the need for accurate messages and reliable transmission of neuroscience knowledge through "channels" like the media (Peters *et al.* 2008). This general approach assumes that researchers are in control of media content and are the primary gatekeepers of scientific knowledge. Additional assumptions inherent in this approach include the belief that science is primarily driven by value-free and rational knowledge that emerges from an intersubjective scientific community that validates the value, i.e. the scientificity of knowledge (Rose 2003; Racine *et al.* 2007a).

Within the framework of unidirectional approaches, some of the key challenges identified include problems related to over-interpretation of neuroscience research and poor explanation of neuroscience concepts and technologies, i.e. neuroscience literacy. In previous research, I have identified several over-interpretations of neuroscience research, especially of neuroimaging tools (Illes and Racine 2005; Racine *et al.* 2005a, 2006a, 2010). For example, results acquired by functional magnetic resonance imaging (fMRI) and positron emission tomography (PET) are portrayed as revealing direct images of the brain at work. The concept of neurorealism designates such beliefs that neuroimaging research yields direct data

Table 46.2 Unidirectional and multidirectional approaches of public science communication. Adapted from Racine *et al.* (2007)

Assumptions of unidirectional approaches of science communication	Assumptions of multidirectional approaches of science communication
Science is a discourse of experts	Science is a social discourse
Science is driven by knowledge	Applications lead interest in science
Science is a community	Media tends to emphasize scientific controversies and debates between researchers
Science is rational and free of value	Science includes applications and values sustaining them
Communication is initiated by individual researchers	Communication leads to involvement of multiple actors
Researchers are experts	Researchers voice non-expert comments
Distortion of message should be avoided	Some distortion is unavoidable and invites to broadening perspectives on science
Scientists control content	Scientists are one source of information
Science communication is a unidirectional process initiated by the expert community that targets non-experts	Science communication is a multidirectional process involving interactions between different stakeholders. It involves sharing of knowledge as well as debate and critical examination of different discourses.

on brain function (Racine 2010). Because of the visual simplicity of neuroimages, neuroimaging results can be hastily interpreted as the ultimate proof that a phenomenon is real, objective, and effective (e.g. in the case of health interventions such as hypnosis and acupuncture), often in spite of the complexities of the data acquisition and image processing involved. Another over-interpretation associated with neuroimaging, and more broadly with neuroscience research, is neuro-essentialism (Roskies 2002; Racine *et al.* 2005a), i.e. the interpretation of the brain as the self-defining essence of a person; a secular equivalent to the soul. Accordingly, the brain becomes short hand for concepts (e.g. the self, the person) that may serve to express other features of the individual not captured in the concept of the brain. Together the concepts of neuro-essentialism and neurorealism lay the theoretical groundwork for the hasty transfer of neuroscience research and attempts to apply this knowledge to a wide range of problems, or what is known as neuro-policy. Neuroscience may be made especially appealing when results seem to reflect the essence (neuro-essentialism) and the true nature of various phenomena (neurorealism). Examples of neuro-policy include education and childhood development programs, use of functional neuroimaging in the courtrooms, and direct sales of neuroimaging services to consumers (Illes *et al.* 2003; Illes 2004; Greely and Illes 2007; Gabrieli 2009; Meltzoff *et al.* 2009).

Another set of challenges related to the previously mentioned hype and over-interpretation, is the relative lack of explanations of neuroscience innovation and neurological concepts. Several studies have established that different forms of neuroscience innovations like fMRI (Racine *et al.* 2005a, 2006a), brain–machine interfaces (Racine *et al.* 2007a), neurostimulation techniques like deep brain stimulation (DBS) (Racine *et al.* 2007a) as well as PET and electroencephalography (EEG) (Racine *et al.* 2010) are infrequently and typically poorly explained in the media. Interestingly, a study of neuroscience literacy conducted in Brazil has identified amongst one hundred items of brain trivia knowledge that the principles of neuroimaging techniques figure amongst the most misunderstood items (Herculano-Houzel 2002). Studies that have examined media depiction of "cognitive enhancers" like methylphenidate and modafinil have also revealed broad frameworks that sometimes presuppose efficiency in spite of scant scientific evidence about non-medical uses of pharmaceuticals for performance enhancement (Williams *et al.* 2008; Coveney *et al.* 2009; Forlini and Racine 2009b; Racine and Forlini 2010). The depiction of psychiatric and neurological conditions can also suffer from partial media portrayals. Neurological conditions like coma and the persistent vegetative state (PVS) appear to be conveyed with confusing and at best ambiguous language. For example, studies have shown that the fundamentally different states of brain death, vegetative state, and coma are not well distinguished by the general public (Shanteau and Linin 1990; Siminoff *et al.* 2004). Many causes for this confusion are possible but Wijdicks and collaborators have shown in an innovative study how coma was generally ill-described and misinterpreted in 30 movies (1970–2004). Most (18/30) motion pictures represented patients who woke up, even from prolonged coma, with intact cognition; only two motion pictures provided a reasonably accurate depiction of coma (Wijdicks and Wijdicks 2006a). Definitional difficulties in distinguishing different neurological disorders have also been found in an examination of the depiction of coma in American newspapers (Wijdicks and Wijdicks 2006b). Similarly, an examination of media coverage of PVS in the Terri Schiavo case found important mischaracterizations of her prognosis and behavioral repertoire that are clearly inconsistent with the PVS diagnosis. For example, one-fifth of the 1141 articles examined contained unrealistic statements that she might recover after years in PVS. Additionally, it was not infrequent to encounter erroneous claims that she was responsive and reactive (Racine *et al.* 2008). This coverage could have direct consequences on healthcare delivery and legislative actions on sensitive end-of-life issues for this patient population (Bacon *et al.* 2007; Sudore *et al.* 2008). It is important to note that such observations are not restricted or unique to neuroscience research and neurotechnologies and have also been identified in media coverage of genetics and genomics research and technologies (Conrad 1996; Geller *et al.* 2002; Tambor *et al.* 2002; Smart 2003; Racine *et al.* 2006b).

Issues of neuroscience literacy and the need for reasonably balanced coverage of neuroscience research and technologies have been identified based on studies on the dissemination of neuroscience research in the media. These are issues at the core of unidirectional approaches. Even though these issues are typically associated with unidirectional approaches and an out-of-fashion "deficit model" of science communication and public understanding of science, they remain important from a scientific, medical, ethical, and social perspective (Bubela *et al.* 2009). The over-interpretation of data can have detrimental consequences for patients that place much hope in the promises of neuroscience which are still just that, only promises (Seale 2003). Poor explanations or reporting practices can also warp understandings of neurological and neuropsychiatric conditions or even exacerbate some aspects of mental disorders and behaviors like post-traumatic stress disorder and suicide (Collimore *et al.* 2008; Tor *et al.* 2008). At the same time, researchers and academic institutions risk a backlash from unfulfilled promises if policy makers and the public expect to be able to cash-in all of the hopes associated with neuroscience. Consequently, unidirectional approaches—stressing the need for accurate and balanced news coverage—bring to the forefront important and valuable concerns for enhanced neuroscience literacy and enlightened decision making. Nonetheless, unidirectional approaches focus on the needs of scientists and sponsors of research in matters of communication and do not fully capture the multidirectional nature of communication processes.

Multidirectional approaches and challenges for the broader implications of neuroscience

Traditional unidirectional approaches of science communication have been criticized in communication studies and bioethics. Major criticisms include the removal of science from its context of political, economical, and ideological pressures (Habermas 1968) as well as the lack of attention to the complexity of emitter–transceiver interactions in a multicultural context (van Djick 2003). These critiques have highlighted that traditional approaches can not fully support ethical approaches to science communication and public involvement (Goggin and Blanpied 1986; Joss and Durant 1995) since they foster an expert-non-expert divide within biomedical policy (Reiser 1991). Such approaches do not explicitly recognize the value of non-expert input in science policy and suggest an overly rational understanding of science and policy that dismisses non-scientific perspectives (Jennings 1990; Gutmann and Thompson 1997).

There is a clear need to adopt broad perspectives on communication in neuroscience given that at stake are concepts like human nature, responsibility, morality, and free will. Indeed, part of the interest in neuroscience stems from the hope for and pursuit of a deeper understanding of fundamental human phenomena such as emotion and cognition (Morein-Zamir and Sahakian 2010). A visionary 1998 *Nature Neuroscience* editorial about the relationship between neuroscientists and emerging public concerns that neuroscience could threaten human values, concluded that neuroscientists "should recognize that their work may be construed as having deep and possibly disturbing implications" (Editorial 1998). Indeed, neuroscience brings into play lay perspectives and scientific perspectives on a wide range of phenomena. It may be beneficial to interpret this interplay between scientific and non-scientific dimensions of these issues and their wider social depiction following philosopher Wilfred Sellars' distinction between the "manifest" and the "scientific" views of the world (Sellars 1963). The manifest image of the world is the common view of humans; it is the way humans are viewed in ordinary life based on free will and other cultural (folk-psychological) assumptions. Exploring the structure of the manifest image is largely the concern of the humanities even though this is changing with the advent of social neuroscience (Cacioppo and Bernston 2005) and the development of neuroscientific investigations, for example, in spirituality (Snyder 2008) and moral decision making (Greene *et al.* 2001). The scientific image of the world is the scientific view of ourselves and it can undermine or put in question the manifest image and beliefs underlying it, such as free will and moral responsibility. While the study of moral emotions and cooperation in the brain, for example, are in many ways enriching our scientific view of the world, some may interpret this trend as an impoverishment or a threat to our manifest image of the world, i.e. our common view of human phenomena based on existing human cultures (Frazzetto and Anker 2009).

The revisionary role of neuroscience for the manifest image is also captured in journalist and popular science accounts and interpretation of the broader implications of neuroscience (Johnson 2004). In the print media, neuroimaging technologies, for example, are depicted as allowing the exploration of "the secret, uncharted areas of the brain," and the identification of "the individual sources of all our thoughts, actions and behaviour" (Dobson 1997). Neuroscience is depicted therefore as revealing "life's ultimate mystery: our conscious inner selves" (Connor 1995) and is presented as science "gone in search of the soul" (Hellmore 1998). For example, several years ago, a contributor to *The New York Times*, Stephen Hall, self-reported his neuroprofiling experiences exploring his own personality based on functional imaging. In a stark example of the cultural impact of neuroscience, he compared his personal narratives (manifest image) to aspects of his brain's physiology as revealed by fMRI (scientific image). He concluded that:

> In our age-old struggle to understand the mind, we have always been empowered – yet oddly constrained – by the vocabulary of the moment, be it the voices of the gods in ancient myth, buried conflicts in the idiom of Freudian analysis or associative memories in Proustian terms. But as psychology and neuroscience begin to converge, brain imaging may provide a new, visual vocabulary with which to rethink, and perhaps reconcile, some of these older ideas on mind (Hall 1999).

The promises of the scientific image of ourselves has therefore cumulated in a lay neurophilosophy that promises to bring new views on important aspects of human existence and folk psychology (Racine and Illes 2009).

Neuroscience certainly does not warrant all the interpretations put forward in the media. But these interpretations illustrate how neuroscience interacts with wider cultural presuppositions and concerns. Such accounts also suggest that cultural assumptions such as free will or individual responsibility could be challenged fundamentally by neuroscience (Churchland 1986, 1995, 2002). However, according to some scholars, cultural beliefs could be dismissed prematurely if the persuasive power of neuroscience triumphs over other knowledge and belief systems (Stent 1990).

Multidirectional approaches to science communication try to reflect how neuroscience provokes fundamental debates on personhood and mental health. By recognizing the importance of human discourse based on broader interactions, multidirectional approaches resist the reduction of knowledge and science to mere acts of instrumental and strategic rationality (Habermas 1968). While not replacing the need for unidirectional science communication, they call for the inclusion of richer sources of ethics dialogue in public science policy. However, multidirectional approaches are—like unidirectional approaches— challenged by data on media coverage of neuroscience in at least two respects, notably (1) sporadic media coverage of ethical discourse and (2) the public's understanding of the coverage of neuroscience in the media.

An ethically-relevant aspect of the multidirectional approaches to the media coverage of neuroscience is the limited coverage of ethical and social challenges. This is important for multidirectional approaches because these approaches stress the need to engage in discussion about the multiple facets of the consequences of neuroscience, including social and ethical challenges. A few studies have found that the coverage of ethical challenges with techniques like fMRI and DBS is much lower than the discussion of such issues in news coverage of genomics and genetics research (Racine et al. 2006b). For example, a study of fMRI in the media indicates that news coverage had a mostly optimistic tone (79%), compared to 16% that were considered balanced or critical (5%) (Racine et al. 2005a). News coverage of fMRI featured scientific issues such as validity (18% of cases) more frequently than ethical issues such as confidentiality (7% of cases) (Racine et al. 2005a). An examination of DBS in a sample of US and UK media, found that the tone of the articles was mostly optimistic (51%), i.e. featuring benefits of research on neurostimulation and its applications. The tone for 31% of articles in this sample was balanced (featuring both benefits and risks or issues). The remaining articles were either neutral (14%; no benefits and no risks or issues) or critical (4%; emphasizing risks and issues) (Racine et al. 2007c). However, another examination of cognitive enhancement in the media found more extensive discussion of ethical and social issues associated with the use of methylphenidate for non-medical performance enhancement (Forlini and Racine 2009b). Another examination of ethical issues associated with media coverage of a brain–machine interface (Talwar et al. 2002) found that ethical issues (e.g. animal rights, "mind control") were featured prominently (Racine et al. 2007a). Similarly, media coverage of neurogenetics per se is associated with much more ethical discussion than fMRI or PET news coverage (Racine et al. 2005b). These data suggest that depending on the area of neuroscience involved, and what is at stake in a specific story, media coverage of neuroscience can attract substantial discussion of related ethical and social challenges. However, this means that the discussion of ethical issues is not necessarily systematic but rather contingent on the stakes involved. Moreover, in the media, ethics can be focused on controversial issues in contrast to substantial but less sensational or controversial ethical challenges. How public debate and knowledge is served or disserved by episodic discussion of ethics in the media remains open to debate. Some may feel like an ethics discussion is already in place where needed; while others might consider this discussion to be too sporadic and heavily dependent on specific public controversies (Simonson 2002).

A second aspect of media coverage relevant to multidirectional approaches concerns the understanding of media coverage by different stakeholders. This area is of fundamental importance for multidirectional approaches because these approaches stress the need to capture in depth the perspectives and values of stakeholders. As such, the study of the "reception" of news about science and technology is an established research area (Seale 2003) but little is known about how different groups understand neuroscience specifically. There are even more unknowns regarding the actual influence of media portrayals of neuroscience innovation on the actual decisions and behaviors of patients, caregivers, public stakeholders or healthcare providers and neuroscientists themselves (Condit *et al.* 2001; Conrad 2001; Geller *et al.* 2002; Seale 2003). Multiple factors complicate research in this area given the possible variables interfering with an individuals' understanding of media content. This complexity is increased when trying to determine what the impact of news coverage is on an individual's beliefs, attitudes, decisions, and behaviors. Although rather scarce, existing research into stakeholder views on media coverage of neuroscience highlights important challenges.

A few studies provide interesting insights. For example, one study (McCabe and Castel 2008), based on discussion of neurorealism's impact on the previous evaluation of the value of scientific validity and convictions (Racine *et al.* 2005a), examined the influence of adding brain images in articles that summarize neuroscience research. The investigators found that the presence of brain images—irrelevant of its connection and relevance to the actual explanation—increased the rated scientific value of these explanations in participants (McCabe and Castel 2008). Another similar study (although outside of the media context per se) considered if irrelevant neuroscience information in a psychological explanation increased the perceived value of good and bad psychological explanations (Weisberg *et al.* 2008). These investigators found that, generally speaking, explanations with neuroscience content were rated higher than those without neuroscience content. Interestingly, this study found an interaction between ratings of scientific value and explanation value (good or bad explanations). The positive evaluation of bad explanations by "naive individuals" (undergraduate students) increased significantly when accompanied by a neuroscience explanation. There was no such effect for experts in neuroscience.

A recently published focus group-based study has examined the perspectives of stakeholders (university students, parents, healthcare providers) on ethical issues related to non-medical cognitive performance enhancement using a common stimulant (methylphenidate) used for the treatment of attention deficit and hyperactivity disorder. This study found evidence that the optimistic and sometimes sensational coverage of this phenomenon in the print media (Racine and Forlini 2010) can actually incite the use of cognitive enhancers in students and other groups based on erroneous perceptions of safety and of supporting scientific evidence (Forlini and Racine 2009a,b,c). Representative of this view, one student said, in reaction to the media sample used as a prompt in the focus groups "I don't know why but it made me want to try Ritalin" (Forlini and Racine 2009c).

The media's impact on stakeholders like patients and research participants has been reported in other empirical neuroethics studies conducted by my group in the Canadian context. I have found that public understanding of neuroimaging ranked high amongst issues needing to be addressed in areas like neuroimaging research and DBS. First, Canadian neuroimagers reported concerns that fMRI was considered a mindreading device ready for real-world applications and that media coverage was fuelling misleading expectations

(Deslauriers *et al.* 2010). One-fourth of neuroimagers (27%) thought that actual research ethics governance dealt poorly or very poorly with this issue. Second, healthcare providers involved in Canadian DBS programs identified problematic media portrayals of DBS (Bell *et al.* 2010). DBS was judged to be reported as an effective treatment for all PD patients and a treatment without major side effects (e.g. "I think that what is shown in the media are the cases that really work fantastically well"; "They [the patients] have already decided that they want the surgery; they have seen it on TV and it is great. It is going to help them, it is going to solve their problems"). These providers reported that the build-up of patient expectations, notably by the media, creates substantial challenges for informed consent and post-surgical care for patients: "We (…) try to emphasize on a number of occasions what to expect, because very often (…) especially at the beginning of the procedure being introduced, people were seeing this as a (…) kind of a miracle" (Bell *et al.* 2010). The high expectations fuelled by enthusiastic media portrayals of neuroimaging and DBS therefore appear to have immediate consequences for researchers and clinicians.

In sum, there is limited data on the public's understanding of media coverage of neuroscience innovation and neurotechnologies but available data does suggests that the possible influence of neuroscience explanations on understanding of psychological and social phenomena merits close scrutiny and much further investigation. In addition, the possible consequences of media depictions of neuroscience innovation on cognitive enhancers and other neurotechnologies like neuroimaging and DBS also merits specific attention from ethics, communication sciences, and public health perspectives. While the public longs for research to better understand the impact of neuroscience innovation, and industry builds on the attractiveness of neuroscience explanations to increase support and consumer attention (Eaton and Illes 2007; Racine *et al.* 2007b). This has led neuroscientists and ethicists to call for greater discipline and self-regulation of the media and neuroscience (Racine and Illes 2006; Farah 2009).

These data on ethics discussion in the media and the public's understanding of neuroscience—although in need of further confirmation and international comparison—support the need for broadened multidirectional approaches to the understanding and practice of science communication (Secko *et al.* 2008). When neuroscience is conveyed in the media and touches upon the public domain, the meanings ascribed to the study and the fundamental goals of science communication change partly, because the possible real-world applications of neuroscience become drivers of interest instead of basic neuroscience knowledge. Other assumptions of unidirectional approaches of science communication (please consult Table 46.2) are challenged. The communication process is only partially controlled by researchers and engages expectations held by stakeholders. Independent researchers, non-researchers and other stakeholders provide divergent appreciations of neuroscience, thus showing the multifaceted aspects of science communication and dispelling the simplified image of a monolithic scientific community. In addition, the *act* of communicating is better captured as an *interaction* where researchers are brought to comment on the concerns of other stakeholders. These observations dissipate ideals of scientist control over media content and suggest that some distortion of messages is unavoidable.

The lacunae of unidirectional approaches have brought the recognition that alternate methods of science communication other than the media need to be explored. These range from citizens' juries to science workshops (Miller *et al.* 2009), theatre plays, and interactive forms of digital media (Racine 2010). Neuroscience exposition fairs have been used to introduce children to neuroscience principles (Zardetto-Smith *et al.* 2002). Citizens' conference and other deliberative public involvement mechanisms were used first in Denmark, and are now used in many other countries to promote multidirectional communication on controversial topics in healthcare policy (Abelson *et al.* 2003). Plays on science have also led to successful international initiatives (Frazzetto 2002).

Given the lack of strong evidence-based practices in matters of both innovative multidirectional approaches and even standard unidirectional approaches, many questions remain open at the intersection of neuroscience, the media, and ethics. Table 46.3 captures some of the questions that future research could tackle in matters of news construction, news dissemination, and news understanding. These include the possibility that official research ethics guidelines better reflect the salience of public understanding in neuroscience innovation as well as the ethical duties, obligations, and responsibilities of neuroscientists when

Table 46.3 Sample research questions at the crossroads of ethics and the public communication of neuroscience

Neuroscience news construction

Is there an ethical duty for neuroscientists to engage in the public communication of their results? Should researchers be held to higher standards of transparency and accountability in reporting their research activities, especially if their research is supported by public funds? What are the resources (e.g. training of neuroscientists, curricula design) needed to fulfill such responsibilities?

When, i.e. how early, should researchers initiate a process of public communication of their research results? Are there criteria that should be taken into consideration before doing so (e.g. maturity of the research area, potential for risks and misinterpretation; risks of dual or nefarious uses)? How is the responsibility shared between institutions, researchers, and funders of research?

Is there a social responsibility to provide additional support to experts in neuroscience news construction? Is this only a private sector responsibility or should public funds be involved?

Neuroscience news dissemination

Given some of the limitations of unidirectional approaches, what is the value of innovative and interactive forms of science communication such as cafés scientifiques, blogging, and citizen's forum? How and in what form should sensitive areas of neuroscience research be discussed publicly?

What is the current coverage of neuroscience internationally and what is the status of ethical debates on the social, legal, and policy consequences and implications of neuroscience in the media?

Neuroscience news understanding

Do controversial interpretations of neuroscience research in the forms of neuro-essentialism, neurorealism, and neuro-policy have a real negative impact on the understanding of neuroscience research? Do these interpretations shape the public's expectation regarding neuroscience and uptake of different forms of marketing claims?

How are technical neuroscience concepts and principles (e.g. neuronal plasticity, brain death) as well as neuroscience tools (e.g. fMRI, DBS) understood by the public? How do lay understandings interact with misunderstandings about brain function and "neuro-myths"? Can these misunderstandings be clarified and dealt with efficiently and proactively?

they communicate research results. The time has come for a broader culture shift in the academic realm to foster the development of expertise in public communication in neuroscience grounded in evidence-based practices to tackle public understanding challenges as well as neuroethical policy issues (Illes *et al.* 2010).

CONCLUSION

The interest and actions of different stakeholders in science communication can reflect different values and be guided by different ethical principles, duties, responsibilities, and obligations. Within the field of neuroethics, contemporary perspectives on the interaction of neuroscience and the media reflect a combination of unidirectional and multidirectional approaches. Unidirectional approaches stress the importance of accuracy and reasonably balanced portrayals of the benefits of neuroscience to avoid creating harm, to empower individuals and to avoid backlashes against undelivered promises of neuroscience. However, as reviewed, research has found that: reporting practices for neuroscience research are suboptimal; a balanced tone (that includes both the potential benefits and risks of neuroscience) is not predominant in media coverage; there are several shortcomings in scientific and medical explanations with regards to brain health and the portrayal of neuroscience technologies; there is content leading to misunderstanding, hype, and false expectations (e.g. neurorealism, neuroessentialism); there are multiples sources of ethics debates and controversies; and public understanding is identified by different stakeholders as a key socioethical issues. In spite of these findings, guidance in this area is scant for neuroscientists. In many respects neuroscience professional societies have initiated actions in this domain but formal ethics bodies and research ethics governance have been slow to consider the obligations and duties surrounding public communication of science and ethical challenges created by science communication. This led us to identify a number of questions for future research that should be investigated. A future paradigm shift at the intersection of neuroethics, and the communication sciences may be in order to instill substantial changes in academic institutions, the training of neuroscientists, and the further development of research at the intersection of neuroscience, neuroethics, and communication sciences (Illes *et al.* 2010; Morein-Zamir and Sahakian 2010). Much action and research is therefore needed to ensure that the full benefits of neuroscience be harvested in the interest of the common good.

ACKNOWLEDGMENTS

The author would like to acknowledge support from the Canadian Institutes of Health Research (New Investigator Award and States of Mind Network), the Fonds de la recherche en santé du Québec, the Institut de recherches cliniques de Montréal, and the Social Sciences and Humanities Research Council. Thanks to Mrs. Emma Zimmerman for feedback on this manuscript. I am indebted to colleagues with whom I have conducted research reviewed in this chapter.

REFERENCES

Abelson, J., Forest, P.G., Eyles, J., *et al.* (2003). Deliberations about deliberative methods: issues in the design and evaluation of public participation processes. *Social Science and Medicine,* **57**, 239–51.

Alessi, N.E. and Alessi, V.A. (2008). New media and an ethics analysis model for child and adolescent psychiatry. *Child Adolescent Psychiatric Clinics of North America,* **17**, 67–92.

Bacon, D., Williams, M.A., and Gordon, J. (2007). Position statement on laws and regulations concerning life-sustaining treatment, including artificial nutrition and hydration, for patients lacking decision-making capacity. *Neurology,* **68**, 1097–100.

Bell, E., Mathieu, G., and Racine, E. (2009). Preparing the ethical future of deep brain stimulation. *Surgical Neurology,* **72**, 577–86.

Bell, E., Maxwell, B., MacAndrews, M.P., Sadikot, A., and Racine, E. (2010). Hope and patient expectation in deep brain stimulation: healthcare provider perspectives and approaches. *Journal of Clinical Ethics,* **21**, 113–25.

Blakemore, C. (2002). From the "public understanding of science" to scientists' understanding of the public. In S.J. Marcus (ed.) *Neuroethics: Mapping the Field,* pp. 211–23. New York: The Dana Press.

Bubela, T., Nisbet, M.C., Borchelt, R., *et al.* (2009). Science communication reconsidered. *Nature Biotechnology,* **27**, 514–18.

Cacioppo, J.T. and Bernston, G. (2005). *Social Neuroscience: Key Readings in Social Psychology.* New York: NY Psychology Press.

Callahan, D. (1994). Bioethics: private choice and common good. *Hastings Center Report,* **24**, 28–31.

Caulfield, T. (2004). Biotechnology and the popular press: hype and the selling of science. *Trends in Biotechnology,* **22**, 337–9.

Churchland, P.M. (1995). *The Engine of Reason, the Seat of the Soul: A Philosophical Journey into the Brain.* Cambridge, MA: Bradford Books/MIT Press.

Churchland, P.S. (1986). *Neurophilosophy: Toward a Unified Science of the Mind-Brain.* Cambridge, MA: Bradford Book/MIT Press.

Churchland, P.S. (2002). *Brain-Wise: Studies in Neurophilosophy.* Cambridge, MA: MIT Press.

Collimore, K.C., McCabe, R.E., Carleton, R.N., and Asmundson, G.J.G. (2008). Media exposure and dimensions of anxiety sensitivity: differential associations with PTSD symptom clusters. *Journal of Anxiety Disorders,* **22**, 1021–8.

Condit, C.M., Ferguson, A., Thadhani, C., and Parrott, R. (2001). An exploratory study on the impact of news headlines on genetic determinism. *Science Communication,* **22**, 379–95.

Connor, S. (1995). Science; The last great frontier. *The Independent,* 21 May 1995.

Conrad, P. (2001). Genetic optimism: framing genes and mental illness in the news. *Culture, Medicine, and Psychiatry,* **25**, 225–47.

Conrad, P., Weinberg, D. (1996). Has the gene for alcoholism been discovered three times since 1980? A news media analysis. *Perspectives on Social Problems,* **8**, 3–24.

Coveney, C.M., Nerlich, B., and Martin, P. (2009). Modafinil in the media: metaphors, medicalisation and the body. *Social Science of Medicine,* **68**, 487–95.

Deslauriers, C., Bell, E., Palmour, N., *et al.* (2010). Perspectives of Canadian researchers on ethics review of neuroimaging research. *Journal of Empirical Research on Human Research Ethics,* **5**, 49–66.

Dobson, R. (1997). Navigating the maps of the mind. *The Independent*, March 1997.

Eaton, M.L. and Illes, J. (2007). Commercializing cognitive neurotechnology – the ethical terrain. *Nature Biotechnology*, 25, 393–7.

Editorial (1998). Does neuroscience threaten human values? *Nature Neuroscience*, 1, 535–6.

Farah, M.J. (2009). A picture is worth a thousand dollars. *Journal of Cognitive Neuroscience*, 21, 623–4.

Forlini, C. and Racine, E. (2009a). Autonomy and coercion in academic "cognitive enhancement" using methylphenidate: perspectives of key stakeholders. *Neuroethics*, 2, 163–77.

Forlini, C. and Racine, E. (2009b). Disagreements with implications: diverging discourses on the ethics of non-medical use of methylphenidate for performance enhancement. *BMC Medical Ethics*, 10, 9.

Forlini, C. and Racine, E. (2009c). "Pharmacology's delving into the matters of the brain: Ambiguities, uncertainties, and expectations for treatment and enhancement." At: Brain Matters: New Directions in Neuroethics [conference]. 24–26 September, 2009, Halifax, Nova Scotia, Canada

Frazzetto, G. (2002). Science on stage. *EMBO Reports*, 3, 818–20.

Frazzetto, G. and Anker, S. (2009). Neuroculture. *Nature Reviews Neuroscience*, 10, 815–21.

Gabrieli, J.D. (2009). Dyslexia: a new synergy between education and cognitive neuroscience. *Science*, 325, 280–3.

Geller, G., Bernhardt, B.A., and Holtzman, N.A. (2002). The media and the public reaction to genetic research. *Journal of the American Medical Association*, 287, 773.

Goggin, M.L. and Blanpied, W.A. (1986). *Governing Science and Technology in a Democracy*. Knoxville, TN: University of Tennessee Press.

Greely, H.T. and Illes, J. (2007). Neuroscience-based lie detection: the urgent need for regulation. *American Journal of Law and Medicine*, 33, 377–431.

Greene, J.D., Sommerville, R.B., Nystrom, L.E., Darley, J.M., and Cohen, J.D. (2001). An fMRI investigation of emotional engagement in moral judgment. *Science*, 293, 2105–8.

Gutmann, A. and Thompson, D. (1997). Deliberating about bioethics. *Hastings Center Report*, 27, 38–41.

Habermas, J. (1968). *Technik und Wissenschaft als "Ideologie"*. Frankfurt am Main: Suhrkamp.

Hall, C.T. (2001). Fib detector; Study shows brain scan detects patterns of neural activity when someone lies. *The San Francisco Chronicle*, 26 November, 2001.

Hall, S.S. (1999). Journey to the center of my mind. *The New York Times*, 6 June, 1999.

Hellmore, E. (1998). She thinks she believes in God. *The Observer*, 3 May, 1998.

Herculano-Houzel, S. (2002). Do you know your brain? A survey on public neuroscience literacy at the closing of the decade of the brain. *The Neuroscientist*, 8, 98–110.

Hickie, I. (2004). Can we reduce the burden of depression? The Australian experience with beyondblue: the national depression initiative. *Australasian Psychiatry*, 12, S38–46.

Hollon, M.F. (2004). Direct-to-consumer marketing of prescription drugs: a current perspective for neurologists and psychiatrists. *CNS Drugs*, 18, 69–77.

Illes, J. and Racine, E. (2005). Imaging or imagining? A neuroethics challenge informed by genetics. *American Journal of Bioethics*, 5, 5–18.

Illes, J., Fan, E., Koenig, B., *et al.* (2003). Self-referred whole-body CT imaging: current implications for health care consumers. *Radiology*, 228, 346–51.

Illes, J., Kann, D., Karetsky, K., *et al.* (2004). Advertising, patient decision making, and self-referral for computed tomographic and magnetic resonance imaging. *Archives of Internal Medicine*, 164, 2415–19.

Illes, J., Rosen, A., Greicius, M., and Racine, E. (2007). Prospects for prediction: ethics analysis of neuroimaging in Alzheimer's disease. *Annals of the New York Academy of Sciences,* **1097**, 278–95.

Illes, J., Moser, M.A., McCormick, J.B., and Racine, E., *et al.* (2010). Neurotalk: improving neuroscience communication. *Nature Reviews Neuroscience,* **11**, 61–9.

Jennings, B. (1990). Bioethics and democracy. *Centennial Review,* **34**, 207–25.

Johnson, S. (2004). *Mind Wide Open: Your Brain and the Neuroscience of Everyday Life.* New York: Scribner.

Joss, S. and Durant, J. (1995). *Public Participation in Science: The Role of Consensus Conference in Europe.* London: Science Museum with the support of the European Commission Directorate General XII.

Kirby, M. (2008). Mental health in Canada: out of the shadows forever. *Canadian Medical Association Journal,* **178**, 1320–2.

Kuehn, B.M. (2009). Mental health costs. *Journal of the American Medical Association,* **302**, 1162.

Marcus, S.J. (2002). *Neuroethics: Mapping The Field, Conference Proceedings.* New York: The Dana Foundation.

McCabe, D.P. and Castel, A.D. (2008). Seeing is believing: the effect of brain images on judgments of scientific reasoning. *Cognition,* **107**, 343–52.

Meltzoff, A.N., Kuhl, P.K., Movellan, J., and Sejnowski, T.J. (2009). Foundations for a new science of learning. *Science,* **325**, 284–8.

Miller, S., Fahy, D., and The Esconet Team (2009). Can science communication workshops train scientists for reflexive public engagement? *Science Communication,* **31**, 116–26.

Morein-Zamir, S. and Sahakian, B.J. (2010). Neuroethics and public engagement training needed for neuroscientists. *Trends in Cognitive Sciences,* **14**, 49–51.

National Neurotechnology Initiative Act, H. R. 1483. 111th cong. (2009).

Nelkin, D. (1995). *Selling Science: How the Press Covers Science and Technology.* New York: W.H. Freeman and Company.

Patel, K. and Wells, K. (2009). Applying health care reform principles to mental health and substance abuse services. *Journal of the American Medical Association,* **302**, 1463–4.

Peters, H.P., Brossard, D., De Cheveigne, S., *et al.* (2008). Science communication: interactions with the mass media. *Science,* **321**, 204–5.

Racine, E. (2008a). Enriching our views on clinical ethics: results of a qualitative study of the moral psychology of healthcare ethics committee members. *Journal of Bioethical Inquiry,* **5**, 57–67.

Racine, E. (2008b). Interdisciplinary approaches for a pragmatic neuroethics. *American Journal of Bioethics,* **8**, 52–3.

Racine, E. (2010). *Pragmatic Neuroethics: Improving Understanding and Treatment of the Mind-Brain.* Cambridge, MA: MIT Press.

Racine, E. and Forlini, C. (2010). Cognitive enhancement, lifestyle choice or misuse of prescription drugs? Ethics blind spots in current debates. *Neuroethics,* **3**, 1–4.

Racine, E. and Illes, J. (2006). Neuroethical responsibilities. *Canadian Journal of Neurological Sciences,* **33**, 269–77.

Racine, E. and Illes, J. (2009). "Emergentism" at the crossroads of philosophy, neurotechnology, and the enhancement debate. In J. Bickle (ed.) *Handbook of Philosophy and Neuroscience,* pp. 431–53. Oxford: Oxford University Press.

Racine, E., Bar-Ilan, O., and Illes, J. (2005a). fMRI in the public eye. *Nature Reviews Neuroscience,* **6,** 159–64.

Racine, E., Waldman, S., and Illes, J. (2005b). Ethics and scientific accuracy in print media coverage of modern neurotechnology. Society for Neuroscience Annual Meeting, November 12–16, Washington, D.C.

Racine, E., Bar-Ilan, O., and Illes, J. (2006a). Brain imaging: a decade of coverage in the print media. *Science Communication,* **28,** 122–42.

Racine, E., Gareau, I., Doucet, H., *et al.* (2006b). Hyped biomedical science or uncritical reporting? Press coverage of genomics (1992–2001) in Québec. *Social Science and Medicine,* **62,** 1278–90.

Racine, E., DuRousseau, D., and Illes, J. (2007a). From the bench to headlines: ethical issues in performance-enhancing technologies. *Technology,* **11,** 37–54.

Racine, E., Van Der Loos, H.A., and Illes, J. (2007b). Internet marketing of neuroproducts: new practices and healthcare policy challenges. *Cambridge Quarterly of Healthcare Ethics,* **16,** 181–94.

Racine, E., Waldman, S., Palmour, N., Risse, D., and Illes, J. (2007c). Currents of hope: neurostimulation techniques in US and UK print media. *Cambridge Quarterly of Healthcare Ethics,* **16,** 314–18.

Racine, E., Amaram, R., Seidler, M., Karczewska, M., and Illes, J. (2008). Media coverage of the persistent vegetative state and end-of-life decision-making. *Neurology,* **71,** 1027–32.

Racine, E., Bell, E., and Illes, J. (2010). Can we read minds? Ethical challenges and responsibilities in the use of neuroimaging research. In J. Girodano and B. Gordijn (eds.) *Neuroethics: Scientific, Philosophical, and Ethical Perspectives,* pp. 240–66, Cambridge: Cambridge University Press.

Racine, E., Waldman, S., Rosenberg, J., and Illes, J. (2010). Brain sciences and brain technology meet the media: media coverage of contemporary neuroscience innovation. *Social Science and Medicine,* **71,** 725–3

Ravina, B.M., Fagan, S.C., Hart, R.G., *et al.* (2003). Neuroprotective agents for clinical trials in Parkinson's disease: a systematic assessment. *Neurology,* **60,** 1234–40.

Reiser, S.J. (1991). The public and the expert in biomedical policy controversies. In K.E. Hanna (ed.) *Biomedical Politics.* pp. 325–31. Washington, DC: National Academy Press.

Rose, S.P.R. (2003). How to (or not to) communicate science. *Biochemical Society Transactions,* **31,** 307–12.

Roskies, A. (2002). Neuroethics for the new millennium. *Neuron,* **35,** 21–3.

Savitz, S.I. and Fisher, M. (2007). Future of neuroprotection for acute stroke: in the aftermath of the SAINT trials. *Annals of Neurology,* **61,** 396–402.

Seale, C. (2003). Health and media: an overview. *Sociology of Health and Illness,* **25,** 513–31.

Secko, D.M., Burgess, M., and O'Doherty, K. (2008). Perspectives on engaging the public in the ethics of emerging biotechnologies: from salmon to biobanks to neuroethics. *Accountability in Research,* **15,** 283–302.

Sellars, W. (1963). *Science, Perception, and Reality.* New York: Humanities Press.

Shanteau, J. and Linin, K. (1990). Subjective meaning of terms used in organ donation: analysis of word associations. In J. Shanteau and R. Harris (eds.) *Organ Donation and Transplantation: Psychological and Behavioral Factors,* pp.37–49. Washington, DC: American Psychological Association.

Siminoff, L.A., Burant, C., and Youngner, S.J. (2004). Death and organ procurement: public beliefs and attitudes. *Kennedy Institute of Ethics Journal,* **14,** 217–34.

Simonson, P. (2002). Bioethics and the rituals of media. *Hastings Center Report*, **32**, 32–39.

Smart, A. (2003). Reporting the dawn of the post-genomic era: Who wants to live forever? *Sociology of Health and Illness*, **25**, 24–49.

Snyder, S.H. (2008). Seeking god in the brain – efforts to localize higher brain functions. *NEJM*, **358**, 6–7.

Stent, G.S. (1990). The poverty of neurophilosophy. *Journal of Medicine and Philosophy*, **15**, 539–57.

Sudore, R.L., Landefeld, C.S., Pantilat, S.Z., Noyes, K.M., and Schillinger, D. (2008). Reach and impact of a mass media event among vulnerable patients: the Terri Schiavo story. *Journal of General Internal Medicine*, **23**, 1854–7.

Talwar, S.K., Xu, S., Hawley, E.S., *et al.* (2002). Rat navigation guided by remote control. *Nature*, **417**, 37–8.

Tambor, E.S., Bernhardt, B.A., Rodgers, J., Holtzman, N.A., and Geller, G. (2002). Mapping the human genome: an assessment of media coverage and public reaction. *Genetics in Medicine*, **4**, 31–6.

Tor, P.C., Ng, B.Y., and Ang, Y.G. (2008). The media and suicide. *Annals of the Academy of Medicine Singapore*, **37**, 797–9.

Van Djick, J. (2003). After the "Two Cultures": toward a "(multi)cultural" practice of science communication. *Science Communication*, **25**, 177–90.

Weaver, F.M., Follett, K., Stern, M., *et al.* (2009). Bilateral deep brain stimulation vs best medical therapy for patients with advanced Parkinson disease: a randomized controlled trial. *Journal of the American Medical Association*, **301**, 63–73.

Weisberg, D.S., Keil, F.C., Goodstein, J., Rawson, E., and Gray, J.R. (2008). The seductive allure of neuroscience explanations. *Journal of Cognitive Neuroscience*, **20**, 470–7.

Wijdicks, E.F. and Wijdicks, C.A. (2006a). The portrayal of coma in contemporary motion pictures. *Neurology*, **66**, 1300–3.

Wijdicks, E.F. and Wijdicks, M.F. (2006b). Coverage of coma in headlines of US newspapers from 2001 through 2005. *Mayo Clinic Proceedings*, **81**, 1332–6.

Williams, S.J., Seale, C., Boden, S., Lowe, P., and Steinberg, D.L. (2008). Waking up to sleepiness: Modafinil, the media and the pharmaceuticalisation of everyday/night life. *Sociology of Health and Illness*, **30**, 839–55.

World Health Organization (2001). *The World Health Report 2001. Mental Health: New Understanding, New Hope*. Geneva: World Health Organization.

World Health Organization (2006). *Neurological Disorders: Public Health Challenges*. Geneva, World Health Organization.

Zardetto-Smith, A., Mu, K., Phelps, C., Houtz, L., and Royeen, C. (2002). Brains rule! fun = learning = neuroscience literacy. *The Neuroscientist*, **8**, 396–404.

CHAPTER 47

ETHICAL ISSUES IN EDUCATIONAL NEUROSCIENCE: RAISING CHILDREN IN A BRAVE NEW WORLD

ZACHARY STEIN, BRUNO DELLA CHIESA, CHRISTINA HINTON, AND KURT W. FISCHER

A growing international movement, called educational neuroscience (or mind, brain, and education), aims to inform educational research, policy, and practice with neuroscience and cognitive science research. Usable knowledge from this field is already making important contributions to the field of education. However, this new field is also likely to radically alter our understanding of learning and schools. The research brings a powerful capability to directly intervene in children's biological makeup, stirring ethical questions about the very nature of child rearing, and the role of education in this process.

We argue that there is a key distinction between *raising children* and *designing children*, and that the ethical application of neuroscience research to education critically depends upon ensuring that we are *raising* children (Stein 2010). Designing children involves altering dispositions and behaviors by use of mainly physical means while adopting 3rd person perspectives and instrumental attitudes. Some current practices surrounding psychopharmacology in schools fit this description. Raising children, on the other hand, is a process in which dispositions and behaviors are altered mainly through the use of shared languages and values while adopting 1st and 2nd person perspectives and cooperative attitudes. We argue that designing children is ethically unacceptable, invoking Kant's categorical imperative and human rights issues, and we present a few case studies to highlight important ethical issues. We hope to provoke others to consider emerging ethical issues in mind, brain, and education, and to take preemptive action to protect children's right to participate in their own development.

FACING NEW EDUCATIONAL FRONTIERS

From Adderall® to zip drives, scientific and technological advances are transforming every aspect of schooling. People increasingly discuss learning and behavioral problems in biological terms, and psychopharmacology is a ubiquitous presence in North American schools. Computer technologies are transforming the nature of teaching and learning, and many adolescents are performing multiple tasks across multiple platforms at the same time for a large part of the school day. While there are major differences in these trends depending on national and cultural contexts, the nature of education is undergoing profound change everywhere on the planet, bringing new challenges for human beings and their brains. The future of education and the future of neuroscience are linked (OECD 2007a). This chapter addresses some of the ethical issues likely to be encountered as our societies move into new educational frontiers where neuroscience and education intertwine.

Educational neuroscience (or the broader field of mind, brain, and education) is an emerging polycentric transdisciplinary movement (Fischer *et al.* 2007, 2010; Koizumi 1999) aimed at helping to reform educational research, practice, and policy in light of brain research and cognitive science. The first section briefly looks at this field and two of its important organizations. Generally, the field is shaped by concerns about the nature of usable knowledge, especially concerns about what constitutes a valid application of neuroscience in an educational context. The limits of neuroscience methods and the complexity of relations between research and practice take center stage in debates about how the field can move forward responsibly.

However, as the second section makes clear, a host of ethical issues pervade the field. These ethical issues range from the equitable distribution of benefits to the privacy rights of people studied in research and the sensitivity of conducting research in schools. We focus on a central issue in the third section—the distinction between two general types of educational interventions informed by neuroscience, *designing children* versus *raising children*.

We explicate the meaning of this distinction and ground it in several case-study scenarios in the fourth section. These scenarios envision educational reforms that might follow in the wake of advances in understanding the biological bases of ethical behaviors. Some approaches aim to physiologically alter a child's brain with the goal of correcting an organic dysfunction or creating a desirable ability or characteristic—that is *designing children* so that they behave the way the designer wants. Other approaches provide children with a variety of educational and social contexts, informed by probabilistic neuropsychological profiles—that is *raising children* to be ethical. Critical differences between these two types of approaches hinge on issues of basic justice and fairness—the manner with which a child's right to autonomy is respected and fostered or overridden and denied.

The future of education and its relation to neuroscience revolve around the way knowledge is put to use with those most affected by it. The central issue is how education systems and families intervene in children's lives. Educational applications of neuroscience that favor designing children over raising them are unacceptable in so far as they change behavior through *coercion* as opposed to *persuasion*. Such educational interventions run the risk of creating individuals who are incapable of assuming authorship for their own life. We share Habermas' (2003) worry that the careless use of biomedical advances may undermine the organismic conditions that allow for ethical self-understanding and responsible agency. When mature individuals do a retrospective review of their lives, they ought to be capable of taking responsibility for their own lives. This possibility is denied to someone who has been made into who they are by irrevocable instrumental interventions into their biological makeup. All children have a right to participate in their own development, as stated in the Convention on the Rights of the Child: "Parties shall assure to the child who is capable of forming his or her own views the right to express those views freely in all matters affecting the child, the view of the child being given due weight in accordance with the age and maturity of the child" (United Nations 1989, article 12). Educational institutions and societies more generally need to take preemptive action to ensure that children exercise this right in the wake of biotechnologies that allow adults to directly intervene in children's neurobiology.

Educational neuroscience—a growing global movement

Education is emerging as one of the central concerns for humanity in the 21st century. The most pressing global challenges—from climate change to terrorism to economic globalization—all hinge upon quality education. Mounting evidence points toward the efficacy of education in international development, economic growth, and social equity (OECD 2009). Access to education is a central civil rights issue, along with access to basic life-sustaining necessities such as food and shelter (OECD 2009; Obama 2008). International communities of political and business elites are beginning to see what devoted educators have always known—that the future of civilization hinges upon the ability to educate coming generations (Coulombe *et al.* 2004; OECD 2007b; OECD 2009).[1]

Although education is now recognized as important for the present and future, it still lacks an essential foundation for quality that is pervasive in other industries: Education has little research and development (Fischer 2009; Hinton and Fischer 2008). As a result, *there is not a clear science of education*. As demands for high quality education proliferate around the globe the need for a science of education looms large—and many are beginning to look to brain research and cognitive and affective science for help in establishing this science of education.

The emerging field of *educational neuroscience* is as much a response to pervasive social need as it is an outgrowth of progress in the relevant sciences. As a result, the field is dynamic, heterogeneous, and contested, as a wide variety of stakeholders maneuver for influence. Responsible brain and cognitive scientists and open-minded educational leaders stand in

---

[1] While this attitude is universally adopted on paper, the degree to which governments and business communities are truly committed to having a highly educated population is debatable (Bourdieu and Passerson 1964/1990). Some argue that there may be some resistance to education systems that are too successful because they might breed social changes considered dangerous by dominant elites who are keen to reproduce the current social structures (della Chiesa 2008; della Chiesa and Christoph 2009; OECD 2007c).

stark contrast to entrepreneurs spinning off biomedical technologies and snake-oil sales-men selling so-called "brain-based pedagogy." Several international organizations and initiatives have emerged to give shape to these burgeoning and widespread efforts to build a science of education. Of particular note are the International Mind, Brain, and Education Society (IMBES) and the Brain Research and Learning Sciences project at the Organization for Economic Cooperation and Development's (OECD) Center for Education Research and Innovation (CERI) (OECD 2007a).

These initiatives serve an important dual role. On the one hand, they function to facilitate the growth of educational neuroscience. IMBES launched the journal *Mind, Brain, and Education* in 2007 to encourage and disseminate research and best practices. IMBES also coordinates a set of research school collaborations (Hinton and Fischer 2008) as part of growing efforts to bridge theory and practice in a rigorous, sustainable manner. Leading educators, neuroscientists, and cognitive scientists attend biennial IMBES conferences to build the field and to draw positive public attention to the field's important aspects and prospects. Moreover, in conjunction with these efforts, a group of major universities—including Harvard University, the University of Texas, and Cambridge University—now offer degrees in mind, brain, and education or educational neuroscience, as well as workshops for educators and scientists who want to learn about and contribute to connecting mind, brain, and education.

At the same time, a pressing need to combat market forces and misinformation has these organizations issuing warnings concerning misapplications, neuromyths, and overzealous bridge-building from basic research to classroom practice. In this capacity they serve to focus the attention of researchers, practitioners, and the public on the limits of brain and cognitive science methods and knowledge. They issue a call for humility and caution, and a call for the kind of concerted transdisciplinary efforts needed to build usable knowledge in the field (della Chiesa *et al.* 2009; Fischer 2009; Koizumi 1999).

Valid usable knowledge stands in contrast to prevalent neuromyths (OECD 2002, 2007a). For example, several popular educational products claim that neuroscientific evidence demonstrates that infants' development and intelligence is enhanced by exposure to stimuli such as paintings, classical music, or flash cards. Others claim that certain types of physical exercise and movement (such as specific regimens of finger maneuvers) stimulate brain health and increase memory and academic performance. Still others make claims that individuals can be classified in terms of their hemispheric dominance ("left brain" people and "right brain" people), for which they sell diagnostics and related educational interventions. The research claims for these products are totally fallacious. The products are merely *marketed* using the language of neuroscience because using brain images and neuroscience terms makes people more likely to believe the ideas (McCabe and Castel 2008; Weisberg *et al.* 2008). There are many plausible explanations for the effects of neuroscience claims on marketing, including that the Western world is dominated by a positivistic/scientistic mindset that preferentially accepts material explanations and that the media promotes neuroscience as innovative and fashionable. Regardless of the underlying cause, as Dewey (1929) saw decades ago, people will flock to anything claiming a "scientific seal of approval" as long as a true science of education is absent.

One more subtle example of brain science being misapplied to education concerns the issue of "critical periods"—phases of brain development that are seen as narrow windows of opportunity for the acquisition of key skills, such as learning a second language.

Inappropriate claims are made about the *narrowness* and *criticalness* of the periods (Neville and Bruer 2001), with some suggesting that if a person misses a small window of opportunity his or her chance to acquire the skill is gone forever. The issue exemplifies the kind of oversimplified moves from research to practice that need to be avoided. In order to avoid misunderstandings, careful scientists ban the phrase "critical period" when it comes to teachable/learnable knowledge and skills in formal education contexts, and replace it with the phrase "sensitive period," which suggests a much broader time-line flexibility (OECD 2002, 2007a). Unfortunately, the media is not always this careful, leading to a quick proliferation of misconceptions (Bourdieu 1998; della Chiesa 1993, 2008).

A common problem is that these kinds of claims do not recognize the limits of cognitive neuroscience methods. Most studies to date neglect or ignore individual differences, treat the pervasive variability and diversity of human behavior as error or noise, and use samples that do not represent the full range of human beings. When research focuses on variability and diversity, learning and development display individual differences and variability everywhere (Fischer and Bidell 2006; Mascolo and Fischer 2010; Rose and Dalton 2009)—even more so when researchers consider groups that are not highly educated in industrialized Western societies (Henrich *et al.*, 2010). Researchers making claims about the *narrowness* and *criticalness* of phases of brain development and how these are related to optimal educational environments need to stop assuming that all people are the same. When research conclusions are to be connected to educational practice and policy, researchers need to consider the relation of their samples to the whole population. They need to analyze variability when they attempt to move from description to prescription. The lack of research and development about educational practice creates major difficulties in connecting research on learning and development with practice and policy (della Chiesa *et al.* 2009; Fischer 2009; Hinton and Fischer 2008).

These calls for caution are calls for *epistemic responsibility*. What do we really know? What does research demonstrate that is clearly relevant for educational practice? Is a given practice truly based on valid research? To make valuable advances in the coming decades, the field of educational neuroscience will require principles for quality control that are widely agreed upon and forged at the interface of research and practice. IMBES and OECD/CERI have made this problem explicit and called for innovative collaboration between researchers, teachers, and others in fostering the co-construction of valid usable knowledge for education.

In addition to ethical issues concerning the limits of scientific methods and the need to more directly connect research with practice, major ethical issues are emerging that reach into the very fabric of human society and culture (Spitzer 2004; Koizumi 2007). IMBES and OECD/CERI have called for *ethical responsibility* in research and practice, and in the remainder of this paper we propose a key ethical distinction for grounding discourse about responsibility in educational neuroscience.

CONTEXTUALIZING ETHICS IN EDUCATIONAL NEUROSCIENCE

Right now all across the planet, researchers and educators are working to bring advances from neuroscience and cognitive science into educational research, policy, and practice.

Educational neuroscience (or mind, brain, and education) has a wide range of applications, from psychopharmacology to brain-based pedagogy; from the search for biomarkers of risk and disability (Goswami 2009; Singh and Rose 2009) to programs focusing on the importance of health, stress reduction, and sleep (Golombek and Cardinali 2008). Of course, some of the issues facing educational neuroscience are not new. There is a long history of discourse about the ethical issues involved with educational research (Lagemann 2000, 2008).

Here are a few important examples of classic ethical issues that carry over to educational neuroscience:

1) In a study using quasi-experimental designs in classrooms or schools, a neuroscientific intervention is hypothesized to benefit those exposed to it. If it is effective, it will leave the control group potentially educationally disadvantaged, an unjust situation for the students involved.

2) Researchers conspire with publishing houses and school leaders to roll out new practices based on neuroscientific educational research, thus *unilaterally* affecting the lives of students and teachers, precluding their involvement in deciding how they will be educated.

3) The benefits of new research-based practices are inequitably and unfairly distributed among those who stand to benefit.[2]

4) Diagnostic categories developed by neuroscience researchers come to function as labels used to stereotype individuals, typically damaging the school culture in which they are used and the emotional lives of those labeled.

This list could be extended. Educational neuroscience inherits these kinds of classic ethical issues from educational research, but the power of brain research and cognitive science intensifies many of them—such as (3) and (4)—while also creating radically new ones.

The radically new ethical issues raised by educational neuroscience, such as changing a child's brain through surgery or pharmacology, or changing genes to create a "better" child, have important overlaps with issues in related fields. Bioethics (Glannon 2007; Singer and Kuhse 2000) and neuroethics (Illes 2005; Marcus 2002) offer insights into some of the issues raised by educational neuroscience. There are also important connections to medical ethics (Beauchamp and Childress 2008) and the ethics of human enhancement (Savulescu and Bostrom 2009).

However, education is distinct from medicine and related biomedical practices in both its ends and its means. Education is concerned with, among other things, the transmission of cultural values and skills (Dewey 1916). The philosophy of education addresses normative questions that do not arise in the same way in the context of medical practice and public health. Questions about which skills and cultural practices are worth instilling in the next generation have implications for the kinds of societies people want to live in and the general

---

[2] This is a long-standing issue in education. Some countries continue to maintain policies that are explicitly inequitable despite OECD's PISA studies clearly showing since 2001 that inequity in education, on top of being ethically questionable, is also inefficient in terms of overall education outcomes (OECD 2007b, 2007c). Moreover, these policies could create a social time bomb that could eventually explode in conflict and disrupt political stability (della Chiesa and Christoph 2009).

shape of a life worth living. These questions transcend but include those about how to ensure that individuals are physically healthy or how to extend life or improve human well-being and achievement.

Clearly relevant are issues about psychopharmacology and the violations of privacy that are likely to accompany emerging brain imaging technologies. Issues surrounding the ethics of human enhancement are just beginning to take shape, but already concerns about the proliferation and side effects of cognitive-enhancement technologies have significant implications for educational neuroscience.

Importantly, there are central issues for which ethicists already have relevant concepts and frameworks, for example, those concerning social justice and reform. Concerns about the fair distribution of benefits loom large and are relevant for sanitation or vaccination as well as educational neuroscience. Educational applications of the brain and cognitive sciences serve a wide range of social functions and create a unique problem-space for questions of distributive justice, responsible reform, and social transformation (Cremin 1976; Dewey 1916; Rawls 1968). Education is a basic social good that sustains group life. Broad changes to education are everyone's concern. We will argue that they play a central role in an important distinction about how parents and scientists shape their children.

Sheridan *et al.* (2005) and Fischer *et al.* (2010) point out the unique problems that arise at the interface of neuroethics and education. The complexity of knowledge production in the field and the possibilities for misuse demand attention from experts devoted and trained to think through new issues. They suggest that the new role of "neuroeducator" is needed—a person explicitly devoted to bridging the gaps between neuroscience and education responsibly. This is an example of the kinds of institutional innovations and policy recommendations on the horizon.

In impending policy debates, concerns about the distribution of benefits and the shape of future institutions are necessarily preceded by concerns about what is really beneficial for growing, learning human beings. What can be drawn from new neuroscientific knowledge that is *good* for children and society? Generally, these kinds of everyday moral judgments should play an important role in legislation and the formation of democratic will (Habermas 1996). When neuroscience creates radically new possibilities, people do not even know how to think about what is at stake. Can a line be drawn between *treatment* and *enhancement* for possible uses of brain science that look like human engineering or "cosmetic psychopharmacology" (Marcus 2002; Wolpe 2002)? Will wielding the power of the neurosciences lead down dubious paths, away from humanity and towards something else? These kinds of dystopian visions[3] are valuable in drawing attention to important moral issues that are still difficult to define.

---

[3] Aldous Huxley's *Brave New World* (1932/2010) is obviously relevant. Huxley wrote to George Orwell on October 21, 1949: "...the world's leaders will discover that infant conditioning and narco-hypnosis are more efficient, as instruments of government, than clubs and prisons, and that the lust for power can be just as completely satisfied by suggesting people into loving their servitude as by flogging them and kicking them into obedience". Beyond Huxley's well-known warnings, the dystopian tradition (up to the "cyberpunk" movement in the 1980's and 90's) has dealt often with ethical issues which revolve around the fundamental question "What does it mean to be human?" This direction culminated with the visionary work of Philip K. Dick (1963/2002, 1968/2007).

We propose a fundamental ethical distinction that is crucial for addressing the ethical implications of advances in educational neuroscience (or mind, brain, and education). In contrast to most prior arguments, this distinction concerns different ways of intervening in children's lives. It is less about what humanity is becoming as neuroscience begins to change people and more about the kinds of interpersonal interactions that people are willing or unwilling to condone. Framing the problems this way brings much needed clarity and insight to the ethical problems facing educational neuroscience.

THE DIFFERENCE BETWEEN DESIGNING CHILDREN AND RAISING CHILDREN

Aristotle (2002), the first ethologist to study the human species, outlined the various basic practices and attitudes that constitute our everyday lives. He showed that there is a difference between the *theoretical* and the *practical*, between the *ethical* and the *political*, and between *healing*, *breeding*, and *building*. To this day, in everyday life, people routinely mark off these kinds of differences between, for example, attitudes toward the organic nature of plants and animals versus attitudes toward the inorganic, social, and political products made by human beings. Most would agree that people *cultivate* living things, a process involving a respect for the inherent dynamics of their auto-regulated nature, while we *build* artifacts, a process involving the strategic planning of fitting means to an end. Sellars (2006) and Habermas (1987) argue for the importance of these kinds of basic common-sense distinctions, and suggest that the background knowledge forming people's shared life-world grounds mutual understanding and shared orientations.

Drawing a line between the practices of *building/designing* and *cultivating/raising* has high face validity as well. It marks a deep-seated distinction between two modes of production, invoking two distinct semantic networks of meanings (Habermas 2007). Recent debates over genetically engineered agricultural products often revolve around this basic distinction.

Of course, when the "products" are people, as opposed to plants, the distinction is much weightier. Institutions and relationships have always shaped lives, thus "producing" certain types of people as opposed to others. The question of *how* a life is shaped, by what actions and methods, and in light of which attitudes, is an essential question for education and child-rearing. Typically, educational methods are characterized as akin to cultivation; the fostering or growing—in short, the *raising* of children—is the standard conception of the process of education (broadly construed, including not only schools but a wide range of learning environments). This definition contains a sense of respect for the internal regulative processes of individuals. Cultivation entails *working with* the unfolding of an already self-directed life. Raising a child is a process of co-constructing goals and shared values alongside the inculcation of skills and practices. Communication, compromise, and relationships of mutual expectation are essential, as are the mutual understanding of social norms and the dynamics of authority. Educational processes—the raising and cultivating of the next generation—depend upon actions, methods, situations, and attitudes that rely heavily on 1st- and 2nd-person perspectives and on the use of language and (at least some) cooperation. We offer reasons to those we educate, seeking to convince and persuade them of what is in their interest—ideally, raising a child involves shaping behavior through the garnering of consent.

For most of history the main alternative to this view was a conception of education as coercive *training* (Cremin 1976; Lagemann 2000, 2008). But even training, if it is to be effective, still requires a respect for the limits and internal dynamics of the life being shaped, involving issues such as motivation and differential individual capacities. However, the birth of psychological science, and especially the rise of behaviorism, brought with it the idea that education is akin to building or engineering—in short, over a century ago some social scientists began to favor the prospect of *designing* children (Pavlov 1927; Skinner 1938). As the metaphor implies, the internal dynamics and growth processes themselves are taken as an object of manipulation. This is *working on* the life being shaped, as opposed to *working with* it. The life is made to fit ends specified by the designer, as opposed to being shaped toward ends that fit it.

Designing children is a process in which an instrumental intervention changes behaviors, dispositions, and capabilities, affecting processes and mechanisms that change who the children will become. These are actions that rely mainly on 3rd-person perspectives, which (in principle) need to make no use of relationships built on communication, compromise, or mutual expectation. The unilateral *construction* of future generations has long been the dream of social engineers. One example is the crude wedding of IQ testing with overly simple notions of genetic heritability, which led to eugenics, including the sterilization of thousands of people in post-bellum America (Gould 1981). Thankfully, such flagrant violations of human rights have been widely condemned—state sanctioned eugenics programs are nearly universally opposed. But what has not changed is the basic idea that future generations might be shaped strategically by means of instrumentally targeted interventions that change their biological nature.

Critically, this distinction between raising children and designing them is not simply a distinction between physical and non-physical intervention. All educational processes have an effect on student's brains. Instead, the distinction concerns the structure of the educational relationship in question—how the elders intervene in children's lives. The line is drawn between relationships that respect the child's (limited and burgeoning) autonomy and those that override the child's nascent autonomy in the interest of goals to be imposed upon the child.

In the raising of a child the relationship has a dialogical structure of relative reciprocity, established in light of the child's input and an awareness of how the child's goals, capabilities, and dispositions do or do not fit with the surrounding norms and expectations of the educational environment. The child *participates* in the shaping of her life, and knows she is doing so.

In the design of a child the relationship has a monological structure of non-reciprocal imposition, established in light of the designer's goals for the child without input from the child or consideration/awareness of the child's goals. The child does *not* participate in shaping her life, but is acted on from the outside. The child experiences behavioral and dispositional changes imposed by processes beyond her control, with results she is not involved in producing.

The distinction focuses on the way people intervene in children's lives. The distinction actually establishes a continuum applicable in the analysis of any educational relationship. As it happens, many biologically focused interventions tend toward design. They make it possible to get results—to change behavior as desired—without establishing the kinds of relationships typically associated with the raising of children.

For example, psychopharmacology allows people, in principle, to change the behaviors of children without the establishment of shared goals or a situation of mutual understanding. As biochemical knowledge increases, the effectiveness of pharmacological interventions is also increasing. In some current situations brain imagining technology can similarly be used to target special populations for invasive sub-cranial interventions, such as neural implants for mediating behavior or emotions in people. As biomedical advances begin to address cognitive functions such as memory, situations will emerge where parents choose to bestow a "competitive advantage" on their child by purchasing biomedical enhancement packages.

The feasibility of these various scenarios is not the point. Regardless of the specific advances, brain and cognitive sciences will increasingly give schools and parents choices in shaping their children's lives. As opportunities to design children become increasingly available, defending the value of raising them becomes a necessity—if human beings decide that design is to be avoided.

WHAT IS THE TROUBLE WITH DESIGN?

Most people seem to have an intuitive moral aversion to the idea of designing children (Glover 2006). Still, we need to clarify and explicate what is troublesome about treating children this way. Explicating the ethical issues will provide the beginnings of a moral framework for facing the future of educational neuroscience.

The difference between designing children and raising them retrofits loosely Kant's (1785/2008, 1788/1996) famous articulation of the categorical imperative—that one should treat others always as an end in themselves and never as a mere means to an end. This basic insight at the heart of Kant's deontology has been enriched by recent theorists (Habermas 1990; Rawls 1968; Scanlon 1998; Sellars 2006) and rearticulated in terms of communicative rationality. Acceptable interactions are those in which all people who are possibly affected agree to—or could be reasonably expected to agree to—the norms being followed. In the ideal interaction the norms that govern it are co-constructed. We should agree on how we want to interact with one another.

But of course we often cannot ask a child how she or he wants to be treated—perhaps because s/he is too young to understand what is at stake. Then we must act on the child's behalf, which means we must act in light of a reasonable belief that our action would be justified in the child's eyes (were she or he granted full knowledge of the situation). This principle does not rule out disagreement and conflict; it merely suggests that disagreements over actions and norms should be *reasonable* and *considered* ones. That is, we are obliged *not* to act towards a child in a way that disregards her considered acceptance of our actions. We are also obliged *not* to act towards a child such that our actions would be, by our own estimation, inevitably unjustifiable to the child. Perhaps no rational person would agree to being treated that way.

These are some of the kinds of considerations that bear on the ethical dimensions of educational neuroscience, and the related prospect of designing children. Thinking in these terms, it is unacceptable to instrumentally intervene in the life of another—to work *on* them as opposed to *with* them. Actions carried out by engaging mainly 3rd-person perspectives are not performed with a concern for the potential agreement of those affected. Only taking the role of others or talking to them—engaging 1st- and 2nd-person perspectives—allows for the assumption that we are acting with shared interests in mind. Some of the ethical concerns facing educational neuroscience arise from the fact that biomedical technologies make it possible for authorities to change behavior without dealing with mutually understood norms and goals. The ideal, of course, would be to work jointly to co-construct norms and goals.

In the US, some schools require the administration of psychopharmacological agents such as Ritalin[4] to students with certain behavioral profiles. One danger of these policies is that little is known about the effects of long-term usage or of drug administration early in childhood. More is at stake, however, than the potential physical risk (although this is not a trivial issue). Mandated prescriptions establish an educational process in which the failure to meet specific behavioral expectations is thought to warrant a physical intervention aimed at changing the brain chemistry of the child—the strategic alteration of the child's dispositions, regardless of the child's (or her parent's) dissent. Most educationally relevant "disabilities," such as ADHD (attention deficit hyperactivity disorder) and dyslexia, arise at the interface of individual differences and the normative expectations from the school environment. In fact, the status of ADHD and dyslexia as diseases caused by localized organic dysfunction has been questioned by some writers (Diller 1996; Rose and Dalton 2009) who have also suggested that prescription of Ritalin® may sometimes be a response to a child's failure to comply with norms and expectations rather than an attempt to heal brain and body.

It is worth noting that mandating prescriptions is different from issuing punishments, even physical punishments. Punishments, as inappropriate and ineffective as they may be in some cases, are typically issued with a communicative intent: They are meant to teach a lesson. Even if a child changes her behavior simply so as not to get punished again, she has made a *choice* in light of an understanding of the norms in play (whether she agrees with them or not). The forced administration of psychotropic substances, on the other hand, changes behavior in a different way. It goes *around* the judgment and choice of the child, changing her behavioral dispositions by acting on mechanisms "behind the scenes," as it were. So the child can be designed to behave, regardless of her consent—regardless even of her understanding of the expectations and norms in question. The outcome of this design process is a system of norms that is insensitive to dissent and that literally relies on its ability to design children who will conform.

Also, the mandated prescription of psychotropic agents to children in educational contexts significantly differs from situations in which adults freely choose to undertake comparable treatments in order to relieve symptoms such as depression or PTSD (post-traumatic stress disorder). In the first case, an individual's brain-chemistry is strategically changed by authorities in order to alter behaviors deemed undesirable by those authorities. In the other,

---

[4] It is important to note that, internationally, the use of drugs such as Ritalin varies greatly. The Italian government, for example, first banned Ritalin. That move was again authorized in Italy April 8, 2007, as a consequence of a law ("legge n. 49/2006", known as "legge Fini-Giovanardi"), applied from December 30, 2005.

an individual chooses to change her own brain chemistry with help from authorities (doctors) in order to relieve symptoms that she deems undesirable. The structure of the relations and actions here are strikingly dissimilar. Surprisingly, the implications of this difference are often overlooked in neuroethical discussions of psychopharmacology (Levy 2007). The risks, harms, and benefits that may accompany psychopharmacological treatments administered to consenting adults raise important ethical issues (and they become even more complex with issues of strategic self-enhancement or "cosmetic psychopharmacology"). But in a way, these debates about the future of the mental health care system deflect attention from the key point—a simple focus on the way people act toward their children.

The objection against mandating the prescription of psychotropic agents stems not from issues of physical risk or changing the brains of future generations. These issues require empirical evidence, with consequent ethical implications; but the jury is out. The objection is that prescribing such drugs is unfair, that it is unjust to treat children this way. There is no need to engage in quasi-metaphysical debate about what is natural or unnatural or to stir up fears of a post-human future in which the overuse of psychopharmacology has radically altered our species-specific behaviors. Prior to those issues, examining the dynamics of the relationships in question is enough to clarify that certain uses of biomedical technologies for educational purposes are unacceptable. It is unethical to design children.

Issues of identity formation

Another way to frame these issues of justice and fairness is to consider the impact on the formation of identity in people who have been designed by an authority. Again, this shifts the argument away from unproductive debates towards a hard look at the *relationships* being built around neuroscience-based biomedical interventions. Habermas (2003) and others (Fukuyama 2002; Glover 2006) have raised concerns about the unprecedented intergenerational dynamics that could result from certain kinds of biotechnologies in educational contexts. Parents have always affected their children, and teachers affect their students. People establish their identities in close relationships within cultural contexts. The preferences and values embodied in the relationships and cultures thus shape the lives of future generations. In this dynamic process of individuation through socialization, an individual *negotiate*s her identity in relation to the desires of significant elders and broad cultural patterns. However, when authorities use biomedical technologies to affect the outcome of identity formation, a child's ability to negotiate her own identity can be lost, as the preferences of parents or prevalent cultural norms are literally *built* into her biology. Will science provide the capacity for one generation to strategically and irreversibly alter the biological substrate of another?

Having the sense that one's identity has been *imposed* rather than negotiated can lead to an inability to claim authorship for one's own life. The result is loss of autonomy and undercutting of responsibility and agency. This loss would have dramatic consequences for societies as well as individuals. Consider, for example, how we could structure a criminal justice system in a society where citizens did not feel a sense of personal responsibility. Before neuroscientific interventions, many contexts in which children form their identities have been dysfunctional or unjust—for example, situations in which children are forced into certain roles (such as child soldiers) or denied a reasonable range of opportunities. Parents or cultures that severely constrain the choices during their children's identity formation are seen as repressive. All children have "the right to an open future," in which they can act autonomously and responsibly (Feinberg 1992) and a right to participate in their own development (United Nations 1989). Some types of biomedical advances make possible more radical methods for *imposing* parental or cultural preferences onto children. As the technology advances, the impacts will become increasingly predictable and effective. For example, parents and schools may soon choose to use biomedical technologies to enhance working memory, mathematical/ spatial intelligence, emotional self-regulation, or talent at sports.

Imagine a high-school culture in which key characteristics of the nascent identities of the young adults have been chosen for them—built into them, as it were— and they have full awareness of this fact. They've been designed and they know it. What would it be like for them to work through the problems that typically face adolescents? What would it mean to "find a voice of one's own" or even to "consider career options" when one's basic capabilities and dispositions were chosen by others? How would close friendships and first romances be understood in light of knowledge that the qualities of one's emotional life are the result of technical biomedical interventions made by authority figures? These are disturbing questions, arising from the unjust use of newly wrought powers stemming from neuroscience.

Injustice is the pejorative of choice here because these children have been denied their *right* to an open future, denied the right to negotiate their identities. Designing children denies them the possibility of autonomous identity formation. Yes, there are other issues, such as empirical questions about unpredictable side effects of interventions, but the fundamental starting point is the social relationships established by designing children instead of raising them. In the next section two brief case studies clarify and elaborate this way of thinking about ethical issues in educational neuroscience.

Case studies on neuroscience and the future of moral education

In recent years there have been major advances in our understanding of the biological underpinnings of key aspects of moral judgment and ethical behavior (Gazzaniga 2006; Zelazo *et al.* 2010). Neuroscientists are beginning to understand the biological basis of ethical judgment, and have discovered a candidate mechanism for the neurological substrate of empathy, which involves mirror neurons that mimic the experience of others (Gallese 2003; Ganoczy 2008; Roth 2003, 2009; Spitzer 2004). These kinds of advances are likely to continue, and they are already leading some to suggest possible educational implications and applications.

The goal of this section is to look at two case studies (Boxes 47.1 and 47.2) concerning the future of moral education, a future radically affected by advances in the brain and cognitive sciences. After presentation of the two cases we will discuss them in light of the distinctions and terms introduced earlier. This exercise will elaborate how the difference between designing children and raising them involves treating them unjustly versus justly; it is not merely about whether biological interventions are used or not. There is not space to tackle all the issues raised by each scenario. Instead, this final section serves to open up possibilities and raise awareness. It is a conclusion that serves to raise more questions.

These case studies are models of possible futures, models that distort features of interest and frame critical properties for discussion. The focus on morality and moral education is

Box 47.1 David and Maggie

Maggie got pregnant at a young age and found it hard to change her lifestyle in a responsible way. David was born premature after spending 7 months in a womb that was often saturated with drugs and other toxins. At the age of 4 David is kicked out of preschool, and becomes almost impossible for Maggie to control. By the age of 8 David has already acted violently toward other children on many occasions and expresses ideas and beliefs about himself and others that his teachers describe as "frightening." In order to avoid expulsion from yet another school Maggie enrolls David in a new treatment program advertised (and mandated in some school districts) for children with problematic histories of antisocial behavior. The program joins advances in brain-imaging technology with psychopharmacology to "improve basic moral functions" such as empathy, positive emotion, and docility. After 2 months of treatment David's behavior begins to change. For the first time he tells his mother he is sorry for how he acted, explains that he used to always feel "out of control," and expresses thankfulness for the treatment he is receiving. After 2 years David, now 10 years old, is succeeding in school and no longer gets negative attention from teachers. However, for a class assignment in social studies, David writes a paper that prompts a teacher–parent conference. In this paper he suggests that everybody should get treatment like he does to "make them behave," that the world would be better if "kids with broken brains had them fixed" and argues further that "criminals probably just have broken brains." Maggie is concerned and talks to David about these beliefs. He says he is confused about why some kids can "be good without pills," and wonders if she would "still love him if he stopped taking his."

Box 47.2 Paula and Rick

Rick is the principal of Westbrook Prep, one the premier private college preparatory schools in the Northeastern US, boasting competitive admissions and a challenging curriculum. Paula is 16 years old, described as bright, sociable, and promising. But after 2 years at Westbrook Paula begins to falter. She explains to her guidance counselor that she feels her friends are "fake" and that her parents only care about whether or not she gets into the right college. She says she thinks there is "more to life than where you go to college," and says she thinks about dropping out to "start trying to help people, like at a soup kitchen or something." That week, a cheating scandal erupts at Westbrook. Six high-profile seniors are implicated, one a star football player. Rick's attempts to control the situation involve a community assembly, including parents, teachers, and students, where he reiterates the code of ethics at Westbrook, but expresses leniency and forgiveness toward the students caught cheating. At this point Paula erupts indignantly in front of the whole community, yelling about the "hypocrisy" of the school and "how fake everyone is." The outburst puts Paula at odds with her parents, her friends, and Principal Rick. Her behavior changes as a result. She is increasingly isolated from her peers. Her teachers begin to describe her as defiant. Twice more she openly speaks out against the school's culture. Her grades plummet. Rick meets with Paula's parents, explains that she is becoming a major distraction, and hands them a pamphlet for a company that uses advances in brain-imaging technology and psychopharmacology to "improve basic moral functions" such as empathy, positive emotion, and docility. One week later Paula is taken in for treatment, despite her complaints and wishes to transfer schools. Her parents explain that they have "invested in her education at Westbrook" and want her to "succeed at fitting in." Paula's lack of compliance changes the treatment modality and a series of high doses are administered during her first several visits. Over the next 6 weeks, Paula's attitudes change drastically. She meets with Rick and expresses remorse for her prior transgressions, thanks him for intervening, explaining that her "life's true purpose should have always been to succeed at Westbrook and get into Yale."

purposeful and non-trivial. Other possible futures that deserve consideration include brain-science-informed strategies for altering memory and attention. Moral education is, and probably should be, controversial, with or without brain-based approaches in the mix, because it aims to foster the growth of personal character, not just academic skills. Thus, these scenarios may give even the staunchest proponent of psychopharmacology in schools cause for pause. Usable knowledge about the biological substrates associated with moral dispositions, judgments, and action is immanent (it is fast becoming a major focus of research (Greene and Haidt 2002; Immordino-Yang *et al.* 2009)). This knowledge, like all knowledge, will bring power in its wake. Specifically, it will bring the power to intervene in the biology of individuals with the goal of changing basic aspects of their moral lives.

These two cases have many similarities. They both involve young people who are struggling to fit in and succeed in school, and who have, as a result, been placed in a treatment program that utilizes biomedical interventions aimed at altering their moral dispositions. Both David and Paula embrace their new dispositions and express some gratitude for undergoing the treatment. In both cases the intervention is a "success." However, many people are left feeling uneasy about the stories. The case of David and Maggie (Box 47.1) exemplifies in many respects how advances in biomedical technologies can contribute to the careful *raising* of a child. And yet, there are lingering and complex concerns about the identity-formation of a child whose brain has been so radically and instrumentally changed by his caregivers. The case of Paula and Rick (Box 47.2) is more openly problematic and exemplifies our deepest concerns about the possibilities of *designing* children. In this case, both the reasons for the intervention and its supposed "success" must be questioned.

As noted earlier, the distinction between raising children and designing them does not mark the difference between biomedical and non-biomedical interventions. Before his treatment, David is, arguably, incapable of being raised because he is not consistently able to share in the experience and goals of others and is insensitive to linguistic-emotional persuasion. Maggie cannot control him and his teachers find his ideas frightening. Moreover, these behavioral dispositions continue over the long term, making it clear that the difficulties are not a transient phase. The circumstances surrounding his birth suggest that his central nervous system may not provide the conditions for communicative relationships that form the groundwork for early childhood socialization. The treatment is an attempt to get him "up to" normal, and to make certain basic capabilities—such as self-control—available to him. Despite the need for proxy consent, the biomedical intervention is in line with goals valued by reasonable people: David would want this for himself if he could decide such things—the intervention provides a boon to his autonomy and facilitates the formation of relationships where he can build his identity. One can argue that it is a fair thing to do to David, in his best interests. Children like David are one reason that our fears about designing children should not be used to radically constrain research and development efforts.

But of course there are trade-offs. For the purpose of our argument, risks and long-term physical side effects are not at issue (although they would be very real concerns in cases like this). The issue is that David will come to understand himself differently from other children. He knows that who he is, how he acts, and what he thinks are all, somehow, the result of the treatment his Mom and teachers have arranged for him to receive. Thankfully, in this case, he is surrounded by caregivers who are concerned about his welfare and identity as well as the reasonableness of his views about himself and others. His worldview has been affected; he has positioned himself and partitioned the world in terms of unique ideas that are at the core of his identity. His concerns about his love-worthiness are important and poignant. As David matures these concerns may deepen. As his awareness of the treatment-dependency of his accomplishments increases, he may question the authenticity of his relations and identity. In this case, if the sensitivity and communicativeness of his caregivers remains intact, David may navigate this complex mode of identity formation with success, but there are real, potentially difficult issues for him and his family and teachers to navigate.

There is less reason for optimism regarding the case of Paula and Rick. The episodes and behaviors that prompt treatment for Paula are not suggestive of long-term dispositions or deep-seated biological dysfunctions. She is open, communicative, capable of relationships (she is actually longing for them), and reflective about who she is and what she values. Her outbursts are, in fact, an expression of certain *reasonable* grievances with her surrounding culture. The problem resides at the *interface* of her emerging identity and the values of her parents and school. The problem is not merely between Paula's ears, but it is co-located in the culture. Moreover, the situation should be handled as a reasonable disagreement and an opportunity for communicative exchange, not as evidence of a brain abnormality best treated with drugs. The deepest dangers of design reside in this kind of possibility, that disagreements can become cast as biological dysfunctions and that coercive biomedical interventions can be used to insulate cultural norms from criticism.

Thus, the big issue here is that it is *unjust* for Rick and Paula's parents to exercise their authority in this way and oversee her forced compliance to a biomedical treatment. They choose to design her instead of working to raise her. This is an unacceptable response to Paula's dissent because it does not adequately engage her perspective. Instead of embracing dialogue and a willingness to more flexibly co-construct educational goals, the specific values of the school are literally built into her. The biomedical intervention is not guided by uncontroversial goals because it is, in fact, *reasonable* to disagree about educational values and the shape of the good life. Rick and her parents, in effect, override Paula's right to negotiate her identity by denying her right to *choose* the values she wants to live by. Her post-treatment espousal of new values is disturbing because she appears to be merely a mouthpiece; she has lost her unique voice.

There is more to say about these case studies. In these stories, an industry has been built around advances in usable knowledge about the brain's moral circuitry. Both Maggie and Rick utilize the services of a company specializing in biomedical technologies that "improve basic moral functions." There are many issues that need to be discussed, with this chapter providing only a starting point for dialogue, focusing on a likely future educationally oriented medical-industrial complex. Other central worries include inaccurate and questionable mass-media dissemination (Bourdieu and Passeron 1990) and simplistic popularization of educational neuroscience (Hinton and Fischer 2008; OECD 2007a). The goal of this discussion has simply been to discuss possible futures in terms of the ways we should intervene in children's lives. The distinction between designing children and raising them discloses central features of the new and complex intergenerational relationships that will become possible in the coming decades.

CONCLUSION: ENTHUSIASM AND ETHICS

Educational neuroscience (or mind, brain, and education) is gaining in momentum and is beginning to produce usable knowledge with profound implications. Enthusiasm is growing that a true science of learning is on the horizon. But there are concerns, and perhaps even liabilities surrounding the use in educational and family contexts of approaches inspired by brain science and biomedical technologies. *Epistemological responsibility* is needed, as the complexities of bridging research and practice are confronted. What can brain scans really tell us? What do we really know? These are legitimate questions, but at the core of neuroethics is the question of *ethical responsibilities*—specifically, how we ought to intervene in children's lives. The key issue is: What are acceptable or unacceptable relationships for adults to have with the children who depend on them? Our distinction—between designing children and raising them—helps draw attention to what really matters: the lives of children and the kinds of relationships they have with adults. Some relationships made possible by educational neuroscience may not ultimately be viewed as acceptable. In relationships of design, 3rd-person perspectives dominate, and the voice and autonomy of the child are neglected. Fortunately educational neuroscience can also enable relationships with powerful positive possibilities, better ways of raising children instead of designing them. In these relationships people use the best knowledge about mind and brain in the service of children's welfare, sensitive to individual differences, values, and goals.

References

Aristotle (2002). *Nicomachean ethics* (R. Crisp, Trans.). Cambridge: Cambridge University Press.

Beauchamp, T. and Childress, J. (2008). *Principles of Biomedical Ethics*. Oxford: Oxford University Press.

Bourdieu, P. (1998). *On Television*. New York: New Press.

Bourdieu, P. and Passeron, J.-C. (1990). *Reproduction in Education, Society and Culture* (Theory, Culture, and Society series). Newbury Park: Sage.

Coulombe, S., Tremblay, J.-F., and Marchand, S. (2004). *International adult literacy survey: literacy scores, human capital, and growth across fourteen OECD countries*. Ottawa: Statistics Canada.

Cremin, L. (1976). *Public Education*. New York: Basic Books.

della Chiesa, B. (1993). Ein knappes Ja: die Franzosen und die Verträge von Maastricht. In H. Rust (ed.) *Europa-Kampagnen: Dynamik öffentlicher Meinungsbildung in Dänemark, Frankreich und der Schweiz*, pp.101–46. Vienna: Facultas wuv Universitätsverlag.

della Chiesa, B. (2008). Introduction. In P. Léna and B. Ajchenbaum-Boffety (eds.) *Education, sciences cognitives et neurosciences*. Sous l' égide de l' Académie des Sciences, pp.7–20. Paris: Presses Universitaires de France.

della Chiesa, B. and Christoph, V. (2009). Neurociencia y docentes: Crónica de un encuentro. *Cuadernos de pedagogía*, Madrid, **386**, 92–6.

della Chiesa, B., Christoph, V., and Hinton, C. (2009). How many brains does it take to build a new light: knowledge management challenges of a transdisciplinary project. *Mind, Brain, and Education*, 3, 17–26.

Dewey, J. (1916). *Democracy and Education*. New York: The Macmillan Company.

Dewey, J. (1929). *The Sources of a Science of Education*. New York: Liveright.

Dick, P.K. (1963/2002). *The Simulacra*. New York: Vintage.

Dick, P.K. (1968/2007). *Do Androids Dream of Electric Sheep?* (reprinted as *Blade Runner*). New York: Del Rey.

Diller, L.H. (1996). The run on Ritalin: Attention deficit disorder and stimulant treatment in the 1990s. *Hastings Center Report*, **26**, 12–18.

Feinberg, J. (1992). *Freedom and Fulfillment. Philosophical Essays.* Princeton, NJ: Princeton University Press.

Fischer, K.W. (2009). Mind, brain, and education: Building a scientific groundwork for learning and teaching. *Mind, Brain, and Education,* 3, 3–16.

Fischer, K.W. and Bidell, T. (2006). Dynamic development of psychological structures in action and thought, in W. Damon and R.M. Lerner (ed.) *Handbook of Child Psychology: Theoretical Models of Human Development,* 6th edn., pp. 313–99. New York: John Wiley & Sons.

Fischer, K.W., Daniel, D.B., Immordino-Yang, M.H., Stern, E., Battro, A., and Koizumi, H. (2007). Why mind, brain, and education? Why now? *Mind, Brain, and Education,* 1, 1–2.

Fischer, K.W., Goswami, U., and Geake, J. (2010). The future of educational neuroscience. *Mind, Brain, and Education,* 4, 68–80.

Fukuyama, F. (2002). *Our Posthuman Future.* New York: Farrar, Straus, and Giroux.

Gallese, V. (2003). The roots of empathy: The shared manifold hypothesis and the neural basis of intersubjectivity. *Psychopathology,* 36, 171–80.

Ganoczy, A. (2008). *Christianisme et Neurosciences.* Paris: Odile Jacob.

Gazzaniga, M. (2006). *The Ethical Brain: The Science of our Moral Dilemmas.* New York: HarperCollins.

Glannon, W. (2007). *Bioethics and the Brain.* New York: Oxford University Press.

Glover, J. (2006). *Choosing Children: The Ethical Dilemmas of Genetic Intervention.* New York: Oxford University Press.

Golombek D. and Cardinali, D. (2008). Mind, brain, education, and biological timing. *Mind, Brain, and Education,* 2, 1–6.

Goswami, U. (2009). Mind, brain, and literacy: Biomarkers as usable knowledge for education. *Mind, Brain, and Education,* 3, 176–84.

Gould, S. J. (1981). *The Mismeasure of Man.* New York: Norton.

Greene, J. and Haidt, J. (2002). How (and where) does moral judgment work? *Trends in Cognitive Sciences,* 6, 517–23.

Habermas, J. (1987). *The Theory of Communicative Action: Lifeworld and System, A Critique of Functionalist Reason* (T. McCarthy, Trans. Vol. 2). Boston, MA: Beacon Press.

Habermas, J. (1990). *Moral Consciousness and Communicative Action* (C. Lenhardt and S. Nicholsen, Trans.). Cambridge, MA: MIT Press.

Habermas, J. (1996). *Between Facts and Norms: Contributions to a Discourse Theory of Law and Democracy* (W. Rehg, Trans.). Cambridge, MA: MIT Press.

Habermas, J. (2003). *The Future of Human Nature.* Cambridge, UK: Polity Press.

Habermas, J. (2007). The language game of responsible agency and the problem of free will: How can epistemic dualism be reconciled with ontological monism? *Philosophical Explorations,* 10, 13–50.

Henrich, J., Heine, S.J., and Norenzayan, A. (2010). The weirdest people in the world? *Behavioral and Brain Sciences,* 33, 61–135.

Hinton, C. and Fischer, K.W. (2008). Research schools: Grounding research in educational practice. *Mind, Brain, and Education,* 2, 157–60.

Huxley, A. (1932/2010). *Brave New World.* New York: Harper Perennial Modern Classics.

Illes, J. (ed.) (2005). *Neuroethics: Defining the issues in theory, practice, and policy.* New York: Oxford University Press.

Immordino-Yang, M.H., McColl, A., Damasio, H., and Damasio, A. (2009). Neural correlates of admiration and compassion. *Proceedings of the National Academy of Sciences, USA,* 106, 8021–26.

Kant, I. (1788/1996). *Kritik der praktischen Vernunft* (*Critique of practical reason*) (Gregor & Wood, Trans.). Cambridge, UK: Cambridge University Press.

Kant, I. (1785/2008). *Grundlegung zur Metaphysik der Sitten* (*Groundwork for the Metaphysics of Morals*). Berlin: L. Heimann & Radford: Wilder.

Koizumi, H. (1999). A practical approach to transdisciplinary studies for the 21st century – The centennial of the discovery of radium by the Curies. *Journal of Seizon and Life Sciences,* **9**, 19–20.

Koizumi, H. (2007). The concept of 'brain-science and ethics'. *Journal of Seizon and Life Sciences,* **17B**, 13–32.

Lagemann, E.C. (2000). *An Elusive Science: The Troubling History of Educational Research.* Chicago: University of Chicago Press.

Lagemann, E.C. (2008). Education research as a distributed activity across universities. *Educational Researcher,* **37**, 424–9.

Levy, N. (2007). *Neuroethics: Challenges for the 21st Century.* Cambridge, UK: Cambridge University Press.

Marcus, S.J. (ed.) (2002). *Neuroethics: Mapping the Field.* New York: Dana Press.

Mascolo, M.F. and Fischer, K.W. (2010). The dynamic development of thinking, feeling, and acting over the lifespan. In R. M. Lerner and W. F. Overton (eds.) *Handbook of Life-Span Development. Vol. 1: Biology, Cognition, and Methods Across the Lifespan.* Hoboken: Wiley.

McCabe, D.P. and Castel, A.D. (2008). Seeing is believing: The effect of brain images on judgments of scientific reasoning. *Cognition,* **107**, 343–52.

Neville, H.J. and Bruer, J.T. (2001). Language processing: how experience affects brain organization. In D.B. Bailey, Jr., J.T. Bruer, F.J. Symons and J.W. Lichtman (eds.) *Critical Thinking about Critical Periods,* pp. 151–72. Baltimore: Paul H. Brookes Pub. Co.

Obama, B. (2008). Speech to the 146th Annual Meeting and 87th Representative Assembly of the National Educational Association. Delivered July 5th, 2008.

OECD (2002). *Understanding the Brain: Towards a New Learning Science.* Paris: OECD.

OECD (2007a). *Understanding the Brain: The Birth of a Learning Science.* Paris: OECD.

OECD (2007b). *Understanding the Social Outcomes of Learning.* Paris: OECD.

OECD (2007c). *No More Failures: Ten Steps to Equity in Education.* Paris: OECD.

OECD (2009). *Education at a Glance 2009: OECD Indicators.* Paris: OECD.

Pavlov, I.P. (1927). *Conditional Reflexes.* New York: Dover Publications.

Rawls, J. (1968). Distributive justice: Some addenda. *Natural Law Forum,* **13**, 51–71.

Rose, D. and Dalton, B. (2009). Learning to read in the digital age. *Mind, Brain and Education,* **3**, 74–83.

Roth, G. (2003, 2009). *Aus Sicht des Gehirns.* Frankfurt: Suhrkamp.

Savulescu, J. and Bostrom, N. (ed.) (2009). *Human enhancement.* New York: Oxford University Press.

Scanlon, T.M. (1998). *What We Owe to Each Other.* Cambridge, MA: Harvard University Press.

Sellars, W. (2006). *In the Space of Reasons.* Cambridge, MA: Harvard University Press.

Sheridan, K., Zinchenko, E., and Gardner, H. (2005). Neuroethics in education. In J. Illes (ed.) *Neuroethics: Defining the Issues in Theory, Practice, and Policy.* New York: Oxford University Press.

Singer, P. and Kuhse, H. (ed.) (2000). *Bioethics: An Anthology.* Malden, MA: Blackwell.

Singh, I. and Rose, N. (2009). Biomarkers in psychiatry. *Nature,* **460**, 202–7.

Skinner, B.F. (1938). *The Behavior of Organisms: An Experimental Analysis*. New York: Appleton-Century-Crofts.

Spitzer, M. (2004). *Selbstbestimmen. Gehirnforschung und die Frage: Was sollen wir tun?* München: Spektrum.

Stein, Z. (2010). On the difference between designing children and raising them: Ethics and the use of educationally oriented biotechnology. *Mind, Brain, and Education*, 4, 53–67.

United Nations (1989). Convention on the Rights of the Child. New York. Available at: http://www2.ohchr.org/english/law/crc.htm (accessed 15 November 2009).

Weisberg, D.S., Keil, F.C., Goodstein, J., Rawson, E., and Gray, J.R. (2008). The seductive allure of neuroscience explanations. *Journal of Cognitive Neuroscience*, 20, 470–7.

Wolpe, P.R. (2002). Treatment, enhancement, and the ethics of neurotherapeutics. *Brain and Cognition*, 50, 387–95.

Zelazo, P.D., Chandler, M., and Crone, E. (eds.) (2010). *Developmental Social Cognitive Neuroscience*. New York: Psychology Press.

CHAPTER 48

....

FROM THE INTERNATIONALIZATION TO THE GLOBALIZATION OF NEUROETHICS: SOME PERSPECTIVES AND CHALLENGES

....

DAOFEN CHEN AND REMI QUIRION

INTRODUCTION

....

MAJOR challenges have marked the field of bioethics over the past two decades. The revolutionary genome project and the promising development of personalized medicine have led to the creation of multiple international bodies aimed at reflecting and eventually adopting international guidelines and even regulations on various aspects of ethics, law, and society (ELSI) related to biomedical research and health practice. The United Nations Educational, Scientific and Cultural Organization (UNESCO) has been particularly active in that regard with the creation in 1993 of the International Bioethics Committee (IBC). Significant progress has been made on various fronts, especially in the field of genomics (Carson and Rothstein 1999; Launis and Raikka 2008).

Parallel to rapid expansion of knowledge in genomics and molecular biology, the field of neuroscience has markedly expanded to become one of the leading topics in biomedical science and health research worldwide, generating an endless stream of exciting new discoveries and development. This is partly due to major investments in initiatives such as the Decade of the Brain in the 1990s in the US, and to investments by many other countries, from Japan and Singapore to Germany and the UK. Professional societies such as the Society for Neuroscience (SfN) and the International Brain Research Organization (IBRO) have seen their memberships increase sharply and now range in tens of thousands of scientists from all over the world (Carew 2009).

In that context, it is not surprising that the rather novel field of neuroethics (Marcus 2002) has recently experienced significant expansion in breadth and depth, much of this being reflected in the topics and areas covered in the various chapters of this volume. As the number and the scope of neuroscience studies on cognitive and social behavior are still rapidly expanding, issues related to either the ethics of neuroscience or the neuroscience of ethics continue to emerge, challenging academicians, governments and the civil society as a whole (Roskies 2002). This is particularly true in the field of cognitive enhancers (Farah 2004), brain imaging (Illes *et al.* 2003), mindreading (Haynes *et al.* 2007), and direct-to-consumer advertising (Frazzetto and Anker 2009). The reader is invited to consult various chapters of this book for detailed information on the state of affairs in each of these subfields.

THE INTERNATIONALIZATION OF NEUROETHICS

As for other subject areas of bioethics, the internationalization of various aspects of neuroethics was rapidly considered as a means to increase knowledge in the field by sharing expertise and the cross-fertilization of ideas. The Dana Foundation (US) played a seminal leadership role in that regard with the organization of the first meeting ever devoted solely to neuroethics (Marcus 2002) as well as multiple follow-up initiatives aimed at increasing awareness about this emerging field of bioethics having a unique set of challenges locally, nationally, and internationally. Various other organizations have followed in the footsteps of the Dana Foundation including UNESCO, as well as the creation in the US of the Neuroethics Society in 2005.

Canada also played a key role in the internationalization of perspectives in neuroethics. Under the early leadership of Quirion, Eberhart, and Illes at the Institute of Neurosciences, Mental Health and Addiction (INMHA) of the Canadian Institutes of Health Research (CIHR), the International Neuroethics Network (INN) was launched in 2005 with annual gatherings at the SfN meetings ever since. One of the main objectives of the INN is to foster communication and support among neuroethicists around the world. Also key is the development of international training and funding opportunities in neuroethics, as well as increased awareness about neuroethics by neuroscientists and the general public (Illes 2005). The INN currently includes representatives from the US, Canada, Great Britain, Germany, Italy, Japan, Switzerland, and Venezuela.

While the far-reaching impact of brain science on our lives and its ethical, legal, and social implications are relevant to all societies and should be recognized by all of them, intense and in depth discussions on neuroethical issues are still mostly concentrated in North America, and in Europe with British neuroscientists being particularly active (Lombera and Illes 2009). The field was created by leading neuroscientists and ethicists from these countries. These individuals or groups of individuals are still today the main architects shaping the scope and directions of neuroethics, providing the great majority of the most influential perspectives as found in a few published volumes on this topic (Illes 2006; Glannon 2007).

The increasingly global nature of scientific inquiries and healthcare research requires international participation to address all key issues related to biomedical ethics in general.

This is also true for neuroethics. Its internationalization is at least partly driven by the rapidly increasing global and economic needs related to the treatment of brain disorders, mental illnesses, and addiction; by the worldwide interests in research and innovation in neurosciences and neurotechnologies; by the increasing international presence and commercial interests of the pharmaceutical and biotechnology industries; and above all by the strong common desire to pursue one of humankind's last frontiers, namely unlocking the mysteries of the brain and the mind. In addition, ideas, concepts, and images derived from neuroscience research have spread beyond the scientific and educational domains to become widely portrayed in literature, movies, and works of art, with related mass media and commercial products shaping social values and consumer practices around the world (Frazzetto and Anker 2009). While these are all genuinely international aspects of neurosciences and neuroethics, they have yet to become truly global, taking into account different cultural and societal backgrounds and beliefs. In the remaining sections of this chapter, we will thus focus on challenges related to the true globalization of neuroethics or perspectives in neuroethics.

THE GLOBALIZATION OF NEUROETHICS

In which ways can neuroethics be considered to be truly global? Answers to this question can be multifaceted. But major goals for a more global perspective in neuroethics should at least include identifying and seeking sets of rules and norms that reflect a common core of values that ideally can be shared by societies from all over the world. In spite of increasing globalization resulting from major economic development, fast travel, and instant communication, moral differences between societies, regions, or populations remain and even thrive. As our world is socially getting much smaller, we are often physically and ideologically interacting with people who have different core values, reflecting diversities partly in religions, partly in cultures. Ethics is considered as a branch of philosophy, concerned with uncovering the truth about a transcendent aspect of reality, often referred to as 'Good' or morality. As an area of interdisciplinary study of problems created by medical values and neuroscience progress, or a "field of philosophy that discusses the rights and wrongs of the treatment of, or enhancement of, the human brain" (Safire 2002), neuroethics, especially in its global perspective, inevitably will have to deal with the cultural dimensions of ethical reasoning. Much of the discussions of mainstream neuroethics, or for that matter bioethics in general, have so far focused on issues from the perspective of Anglo-European and North American rooted philosophical tradition and reasoning. These rights and wrongs are more or less based on values in societies that have a long tradition of emphasis on free will or autonomy from the perspective of the individuals living in those regions. They reflect ethos that are perceived by a significant proportion of populations living in other world region as representing very different values; e.g. by continental Europeans as values based on liberal principles, or by Asians as values centered around Judeo-Christian culture. In contrast, the ethical principles and values held in many societies in continental Europe and Asia have an emphasis on striving for a balance between the rights of the individual versus the good of the community or society (Engelhardt and Rasmussen 2002).

Multicultural perspectives in global neuroethics

Issues and challenges related to multicultural perspectives in global neuroethics are not new. They have been faced and continuously been taken on by efforts of the globalization of bioethics over the past decades. Both lessons and wisdom should be drawn from those experiences. While a global focus on bioethics was not institutionalized until 1993 with the establishment of the IBC with a work program and budget for international activities under the UNESCO, there had been significant international outreach efforts made by American bioethicists to other countries and regions. In almost all these efforts, the notion that a universal set of rules and norms for a global bioethics can be found has often been challenged (Baker 1998; Takala 2001; Nie 2005).

Indeed, the moral pluralism and clashes between cultures are not unique even when comparing cultures that shared common traditions or philosophical roots. While both have Judeo-Christian values at their roots, continental Europeans see their bioethical principles to be very different from those of North Americans. They consider the principles of dignity, precaution, and solidarity to reflect the European ethos better than the North American liberal concepts of autonomy, nonmaleficence, beneficence and justice. They tend to value prudence over hedonism, communality over individualism, and moral sense over pragmatism (Hayry 2003). Somewhat similar sets of values are said to be shared by many countries in Eastern Europe, Africa, and South America even if changes are certainly occurring, especially in the context of modern instant communications (Prodanov 2001; Toscani and Maestroni 2006; Kara 2007; Fox and Swazey 2008).

The outreach effort of bioethicists has faced even more challenges in Eastern Asia, where such efforts began in earnest in the late 1970s. In his essay "Bioethics in the plural: an introduction to taking global moral diversity seriously," H. Tristram Engelhardt Jr. vividly described his first visit to Japan in 1979 with a group of American bioethicists to engage scientists, physicians, and philosophers there on topics concerning the philosophy of medicine. At that time, Japanese hosts and audience were "politely puzzled" by the claims made by the Americans on bioethics, and saw issues of bioethics "from radically different perspectives." The visiting Americans, on the other hand, were "of the view that the critical reflective character of Western philosophy had brought them to understand the conceptual assumptions at the root of proper moral deportment"; and they were sincerely "convinced that, with analysis and reflection, the considered judgments of Japanese philosophers and physicians would come to accord with that of American bioethics" (Engelhardt and Rasmussen 2002). It took many years of numerous encounters and exchanges between American and Japanese groups, and the significant participation of Western-trained Japanese scholars of bioethics, such as Kazumasa Hoshino, for the difference between American and Japanese approaches to become apparent to the Americans. Both Japanese and American scholars came to the recognition that "Japanese bioethics distinguishes itself from American bioethics by the former's focusing on deeply developed senses of moral virtue and character, which were understood to guide the harmonious interaction between physicians, patients, and their families, and by the latter's focusing on individuals, their autonomy, and their good" (Hoshino 1997; Takahashi 2005).

That same year, Engelhardt has also visited for the first time the People's Republic of China (PRC) with a group of American bioethicists, which he had documented in the Hastings Center Report (Engelhardt 1980). Similar to what they had experienced in Japan, Engelhardt and his fellow American bioethicists encountered puzzled responses from their Chinese audience when American bioethics was discussed. Engelhardt concluded in his report that "there is no bioethics in the PRC as a scholarly subdiscipline," and he attributed the moral viewpoint of the Chinese with whom they discussed ethical matters to be solely related to Marxism-Leninism-Maoism upraising, instead of any possible link to Confucian, Taoist, or Buddhist influences. Interestingly, in the following year after Engelhardt's China report was published, two other American bioethicists, Renee Fox and Judith Swazey, went to China for a 6-week sociological field research project at a major hospital in northern China. Although having read Engelhardt's China report prior to their trip, Fox and Swazey came away with a very different impression after their own China experience. Unlike Engelhardt, Fox and Swazey saw a "Chinese-ness" of the Taoist, Confucian, Buddhist, and Maoist-Marxist ideas that had been "blended into" Chinese medical morality, a system they viewed as distinctively different from American bioethics (Fox and Swazey 2008). Obviously, what the two American groups had learned from their experiences in the respective China trips was quite different, and so were the perspectives they have taken from their observations.

GEOGRAPHY OF THOUGHT, AND PHILOSOPHICAL OR ETHICAL REASONING

The effect of cultural difference on our ability of perspective taking, or "mindreading," has been well documented in studies using different multidisciplinary experimental measures (psychology or neurophysiology; e.g. see Wu and Keysar 2007). While we all share the same organ or biological structures used for cognitive and executive functions, our different cultural backgrounds tend to make us think about the world differently. This particular topic of cultural psychology has been comprehensively explored and studied by many cognitive and behavioral psychologists, notably in the recent work by the psychologist Richard Nisbett and his students, many of whom are of Asian background. In his influential 2002 book *The Geography of Thought – How Asians and Westerners Think Differently… and Why*, Nisbett described how he was intellectually challenged by questions asked by one of his first students from China, Kaiping Peng, and how he came to realize that "indoctrination into distinctive habits of thought from birth could result in very large cultural differences in habits of thought" and that there is "a gulf that separates the children of Aristotle from the descendants of Confucius" in the ways they view the world" (Nisbett 2003). He and his group collected a significant amount of experimental evidence suggesting that cultural difference could affect or even dictate the way people view causality and exercise their logic (Peng and Nisbett 1999). Many similar studies also support the notion that there are culturally and geographically based basic but contrasting patterns of thought between Westerners and Easterners (Sabbagh *et al.* 2006).

Cultural perspectives can be manifested in multiple dimensions—and a dichotomy between East and West is somewhat simplistic (Chan and Yan 2007), but a good place to start. In fact, many argue that we all think both ways, and just some of us tend to lean more toward one perspective than the other. The ways we think have been shaped as much by our cultural and philosophical background as by contributing back to that culture. Those influential philosophers such as Aristotle and Confucius would not have had the enormous impact on intellectual, social, and political aspects of our societies, had they not reflected the way people thought in the societies they lived in. It is still interesting for us today to try to figure out why it is Aristotle (but not the "Eastern-like" Heraclitus) and Confucius (not the "Western-like" Mo-Tzu), whom eventually succeeded in setting the long-lasting tradition in the West and East, respectively. It is therefore important that the examination of ethical issues within a contextual framework that assumes dominant cultural values that are very different from the traditional cultural and spiritual perspectives or values in other regions of the world should be highly sensitive to these differences. Accordingly, it is to be expected that in addition to the perspective of a given dominant culture or philosophy, debate or discussion on neuroethical issues could have distinct social or political implications or solutions in societies with a unique set of cultural values or different political and demographical structures, such as between societies that are relatively homogeneous culturally and demographically (Japan, Korea, Finland, or others) versus "diverse-but-isolated" type such as Switzerland or "diverse melting-pots" type like the US, Canada, or Singapore.

NEUROSCIENCE OF THINKING HABITS AND PERSPECTIVE TAKING IN NEUROETHICS

Multicultural perspective will not only be highly relevant and important for a truly global neuroethics' perspective to develop and mature (Chen 2007), but it should also become a neurobiology research topic for neuroscientists to explore. Indeed, one could investigate what role our brain machinery and cognitive ability play in forming our cultural perspective, and how cultural backgrounds and beliefs would in turn shape functional brain systems and behavioral abilities, i.e., the neuroscience of our thinking habits or the nature of human morality (Haidt 2007; Hsu *et al.* 2008; Lahat *et al.* 2010). Given the innate capacities we humans have, it would be interesting to see if there is a continued divergent spectrum in habits of thought, or whether some of the cognitive differences identified turn out to be of historical interest and undergoing transformation as social systems and values are converging. Neurotechnology will continue to provide tools that give us insight into the relationship and integration of the mind and body in sensing and interacting with the world. It is important that we develop a framework and a strategy for examining cognitive and behavioral concepts such as self, consciousness, or fairness not only within the context of research in neurosciences, psychology, and mental health, but also from a multicultural perspective including relevant societal and spiritual values or beliefs. In view of the current effort in studying the psychobiology of the "self" by exploring how the brain manages to form and maintain a sense of self with a goal of better understanding dementia and other mental disorders (Feinberg and Keenan 2005; Gillihan and Farah 2005; Zimmer 2005), attempts at finding a scientific definition of "self" with a culturally relevant perspective will likely generate interesting discussions and debates particularly in Asian and African societies (Nakayama 2005; Cho 2006).

As debates on neuroethical issues are moving onto the global stage, it is imperative to engage participation at the societal level. It is also both exciting and encouraging to appreciate the distinct advantage that different societies have in addressing these issues in the context of their cultural identity and strength. As discussion is just getting underway in eastern Asian societies and their respective scientific communities (Chen 2007; Fukushi *et al.* 2007), it is also important to realize that Asia's post-war economic success has presented a variety of political and cultural landscapes, most still rapidly evolving or changing. Each of these societies and regions could play different roles in the process of the globalization of neuroethics, and takes its own pace in developing its own culturally appropriate "indigenous" neuroethics as well as contributing to a more global perspective (Nie 2000). Japan, for instance, has for centuries taken a leading role among the Far Eastern societies in approaching European and North American civilizations, coping at the same time with the influences of these civilizations, especially in the area of science and technology, and trying to maintain a Buddhist and Confucian philosophies based on cultural values. With a current political system, a constitution, and an economy very much Westernized, discussions on neuroethics in Japan should provide much insight regarding contemporary Asian social and cultural issues and challenges (Akabayashi *et al.* 2008). Let us hope that such discussion and debate on various aspects of neuroethics will lead to solutions that are truly relevant to issues in these societies, and not just as another "Western import." Indeed, in order for this to happen, we must engage in genuine two-ways exchanges and discussions that go well beyond the more traditional import model (Campbell 2008). The key here will not just be to understand the neuroethics issues at hand but to strike on deeper cords of respective values and beliefs. It may also be important to invite experts in other disciplines (Asian studies, Transcultural studies, Religious studies, Indigenous studies, African studies, others) to our discussions and exchanges on neuroethics if we are genuinely interested in ensuring their globalization and relevance to all.

Besides Asia, significant differences toward the very concept of neuroethics can be expected to be seen in other parts of the world such as various countries in Africa and South America. Again, open, frank and frequent genuine dialogs will be critically important to ensure that different aspects of neuroethics take into consideration the societal and cultural fabrics of these nations. This will certainly be challenging but at the same time rewarding and exciting, ensuring that the discipline of neuroethics is in constant evolution thanks to the open mindedness and critical thinking of its disciples.

A ROLE FOR THE PUBLIC TOWARD THE GLOBALIZATION OF NEUROETHICS

Any healthy societal debate or discussion on neuroethical issues will require a reasonably solid public understanding of neuroscience as well as neuroscientists' understanding of public concerns (Blackmore 2002; Friedman 2008). To that end, a scientifically well-informed public that can objectively digest research findings and appreciate their potentials, in a fair-minded way, is essential for integrating neuroscientific knowledge with ethical and social thought (Roskies 2002; Illes 2005). Such an educated public can only be cultivated from a combination of the public's general level of educational preparation in biomedical science and the media's objective and adequate reporting of a scientific result with its potential applications. The process of the public understanding of neurosciences in general, neuroethical issues in particular, and their implications to society can only be realized by a two-way interaction between scientists and the public through open dialogue.

Among all the biomedical subjects, brain science is relatively more complex and difficult to understand. Perhaps the biggest challenge for the globalization of neuroethics for most part of the world is the public understanding of our brain. Even for well-informed and well-educated developed countries, there will still be a gap between the lay public's understanding of neuroscience and the level of understanding necessary to comprehend neuroethical issues or arguments about neurotechnology. In comparison, public engagement activities in underdeveloped countries are rather limited. In addition to the disparity in national/regional resources, the current "regional disparities" reflected in the lack of neuroscientific knowledge in underdeveloped regions may further complicate any effort of global initiative in neuroethics. Unlike the creation of a new antibiotic or a cancer treatment, the successful use of an equally regarded effective new psychopharmacological agent for ameliorating a psychiatric disorder would have to take into consideration of potential social issues as a result of the public's lack of adequate knowledge on related science and ethical implications (Jamison *et al.* 2006). For eastern Asian countries, the language barrier poses even more challenges toward efforts at narrowing the knowledge gap—without a good comprehension of historical and cultural context, subtle meaning could get lost in translation and major points could be misinterpreted simply due to a lack of adequate grasp of the language or accurate translation of biomedical definitions and terminologies (Pusey 1983).

New opportunities for a globalized neuroethics

The revolutionary development in life sciences in recent decades has been made practically side by side with that in the information and communication technologies. In fact, the 40-year history of our Society for Neuroscience has been almost exactly in parallel with the 40-year history of the development of the Internet. Mobile phones, at the same time, became the most popular and widespread personal communication device on the planet, winning the status of probably being the most rapidly adopted technology in history. According to recent figures provided by the International Telecommunications Union (http://www.itu.int/ict), there were an estimated 4.6 billion mobile phone subscriptions globally by the end of 2009, equivalent to a penetration rate of 70%, and more than a quarter of the world's population are using the Internet. While a significant digital (or broadband) divide still remains for internet use and particularly for the availability of broadband connection, the majority of underdeveloped nations/regions are only a few years behind, should the current trend continues.

These new information and communication technologies have significantly transformed every aspect of our society in ways that were unthinkable in the past. Our lives are constantly being shaped by the new tools of the 21st century: Facebook, Twitter, LinkedIn, and YouTube. These new social media, coupled with "older" traditional technologies, are transforming the way we interact with each other, creating completely new forms of communities and cultures (Rheingold 2002). While it remains to be seen whether and to which extent these social media will affect the way by which our habits of thinking (or geography of thought) are developed and shaped (Begley 2010), the new ways of social networking are highly significant to the mission of global bioethics or neuroethics. They are changing the way we engage the public, not just in the forms of news and social media, but also in the ways of delivering education or knowledge and conducting public discourse, creating unprecedented opportunities for cross-cultural knowledge translation and exchange capacity building. It is exciting to observe that new tools are being used in overcoming the barriers stated above, with the hope that the internet may eventually help flatten out the information and knowledge gap (Yang 2009). For instance, the International Neuroethics Education Online (http://www.hso.info), a web-based curriculum developed by the Canadian National Core for Neuroethics at the University of British Columbia, and the Neuroscience Wikipedia Initiative by the Society for Neurosience (SfN 2009), both took the advantage of the cyber-infrastructure to either engage a broader community in discussion of international neuroethics, or make new neuroscientific knowledge available to the wired general public (Illes *et al.* 2010).

With the goal of seeking multicultural perspectives in mind, it is important to realize that "education" in global neuroethics, or bioethics, is not value-neutral, and cannot be value-neutral: what information was to be conveyed, who was its audience, whose moral views should be included, how different perspectives can be represented, and which social values should be incorporated. For global neuroethics, our goal should be to promote healthy debate and dialogue, and try to help each other to understand and internalize different perspectives, but not to universalize any particular ethical claims. It is also important not to underestimate the risk of online public engagement. Efforts should be made to make sure that the online dialogue will be appropriately moderated, and that the cyberspace is for constructive discussions on controversial issues and for acculturating the world netizens to the common values identified, but not for polarized views and extreme positions.

In summary, the continued development of new neurotechnology and our ever-increasing understanding of how the brain works present us with new treatment opportunities, as well as challenging ethical issues. The globalization of perspectives in neuroethics is essential for increasing knowledge of neuroscience and cross-fertilizing ideas for global health in neurological and psychiatric domains. These perspectives will be multicultural in nature, and should be respected and incorporated in our effort of seeking common values for different communities to adapt and not just to adopt. In that effort, it is also important to recognize that knowledge occupies the center stage of global health and international bioethics. Continued outreach efforts will also be essential in capacity building in neuroscientific knowledge expansion, translation, and exchange. New tools from information and communication technologies provide unprecedented opportunity for the globalization of neuroethics, making it possible for both a significant debate and public dialogue on neuroethical issues and a global public outreach about neuroscience knowledge.

DC and RQ have served as the country representative for the USA and Canada respectively in the International Neuroethics Network (INN). The views expressed herein are solely of the authors and do not represent the viewpoint of any entity, including the US Government.

REFERENCES

Akabayashi, A., Kodama, S., and Slingsby, B.T. (2008). Is Asian bioethics really the solution? *Cambridge Quarterly of Healthcare Ethics*, 17, 270–2.

Baker, R. (1998). Negotiating international bioethics: A response to Tom Beauchamp and Ruth Macklin. *Kennedy Institute of Ethics Journal*, 4, 423–53.

Begley, S. (2010). Your Brain Online: Does the Web change how we think? *Newsweek*, 8 January, 2010 (also see http://Edge.org, accessed 15 January 2010).

Blackmore, C. (2002). From the "public understanding of science" to "scientists' understanding of the public". In S.J. Marcus (ed.) *Neuroethics: Mapping the Field*, pp. 211–23. New York: The Dana Press.

Campbell, C. (2008). *The Easternization of the West: A Thematic Account of Cultural Change in the Modern Era*. Boulder, CO: Paradigm Publishers.

Chan, H.M. and Yan, H.K.T. (2007). Is there a geography of thought for East-West differences? Why or why not? *Educational Philosophy and Theory*, 39, 383–403.

Chen, D. (2007). Toward a clearer understanding of the multi-cultural perspectives concerning pressing neuroethical issues. *Eubios Journal of Asian and International Bioethics*, 17, 78.

Cho, F. (2006). Buddhist perspectives on brain function and personhood. Presentation at the symposium on "Ethics of Neuroscience: Lack of Consciousness and Assessment of Personhood", AAAS annual meeting, St. Louis. 16–20 February, 2006.

Carew, T.J. (2009). A Message from the President. Society for Neuroscience. Available at: http://www.sfn.org/skins/main/pdf/annual_report/fy2009/message.pdf (accessed 31 December 2009).

Carson, R.A. and Rothstein, M.A. (1999). *Behavioral Genetics, the Clash of Culture and Biology*. Baltimore, MD: The Johns Hopkins University Press.

Engelhardt, H.T. Jr. (1980). Bioethics in the People's Republic of China. *The Hastings Center Report*, 10, 7–10.

Engelhardt, H.T. Jr. and Rasmussen, L.M. (2002). *Bioethics and Moral Content: National Traditions of Health Care and Morality*. Boston, MA: Kluwer Academic Publishers.

Farah, M.J., Illes, J., Cook-Deegan, R., *et al.* (2004). Science and society: Neurocognitive enhancement: what can we do and what should we do? *Nature Reviews Neuroscience*, 5, 421–5.

Feinberg, T.E. and Keenan, J.P. (2005). *The Lost Self: Pathologies of the Brain and Identity*. London: Oxford University Press.

Fox, R.C. and Swazey, J.P. (2008). *Observing Bioethics*. New York: Oxford University Press.

Frazzetto, G. and Anker, S. (2009). Neuroculture. *Nature Review Neuroscience*, 10, 815–21.

Friedman, D.P. (2008). Public outreach: A scientific imperative. *Journal of Neuroscience*, 28, 11743–5.

Fukushi, T., Sakura, O., and Koizumi, H. (2007). Ethical considerations of neurosicnece research: the perspectives on neuroethics in Japan. *Neuroscience Research*, 57, 10–16.

Gillihan, S.J. and Farah, M.J. (2005). Is self special? A critical review of evidence from experimental psychology and cognitive neuroscience. *Psychological Bulletin*, **131**, 76–97.

Glannon, W. (2007). *Defining Right and Wrong in Brain Science: Essential Readings in Neuroethics*. Washington DC: The Dana Press.

Haidt, J. (2007). The new synthesis in moral psychology. *Science*, **316**, 998–1002.

Haynes JD, Sakai K, Rees G, Gilbert S, Frith C., and Passingham RE. (2007). Reading hidden intentions in the human brain. *Current Biology*, **17**, 323–8.

Hayry, M. (2003). European values in bioethics: Why, what, and how to be used? *Theoretical Medicine*, **24**, 199–214.

Hoshino K. (1997). *Japanese and Western Bioethics*. Boston, MA: Kluwer Academic Publisher.

Hsu, M., Anen, C., and Quartz, S.R. (2008). The right and the good: distributive justice and neural encoding of equity and efficiency. *Science*, **320**, 1092–5.

Illes, J. (2006). *Neuroethics: Defining the Issues in Theory, Practice, and Policy*. New York: Oxford University Press.

Illes, J., Kirschen, M.P., and Gabrieli, J.D.E. (2003). From neuroimaging to neuroethics. *Nature Neuroscience*, **6**, 205.

Illes, J., Blakemore, C., Hansson, M.G., *et al.* (2005). Science and society: International perspectives on engaging the public in neuroethics. *Nature Reviews Neuroscience*, **6**, 977–82.

Illes, J., Moser, M.A., McCormick, J.B., *et al.* (2010). Neurotalk: improving the communication of neuroscience research. *Nature Reviews Neuroscience*, **11**, 1–9.

International Telecommunication Union. http://www.itu.int/ict and http://www.itu.int/ITU-D/ict/material/Telecom09_flyer.pdf; see also: http://www.internetworldstats.com/stats.htm (both accessed 31 December 2009)

Kara, M.A. (2007). Applicability of the principle of respect for autonomy: the perspective of Turkey. *Journal of Medical Ethics*, **33**, 627–30.

Jamison, D.T., Breman, J.G., Measham, A.R., *et al.* (2006). *Disease Control Priorities in Developing Countries, Second Edition*. New York: Oxford University Press and the World Bank.

Lahat, A., Todd, R.M., Mahy, C.E., Lau, K., and Zelazo, P.D. (2010). Neurophysiological correlates of executive function: a comparison of European-Canadian and Chinese-Canadian 5-year-olds. *Frontiers in Human Neuroscience*, **3**, 72.

Launis, V. and Raikka, J. (2008). *Genetic Democracy, Philosophical Perspectives*. New York: Springer.

Lombera, S. and Illes, J. (2009). The international dimensions of neuroethics. *Developing World Bioethics*, **9**, 57–64.

Marcus, S.J. (2002). *Neuroethics: Mapping the Field*. New York: The Dana Press.

Nakayama, S. (2005). On human dignity: Japan and the West, In "Taking Life and Death Seriously – Bioethics from Japan". *Advances in Bioethics*, **8**, 47–64.

Nie, J.B. (2000). The plurality of Chinese and American medical moralities: toward an interpretive cross-cultural bioethics. *Kennedy Institute of Ethics Journal*, **10**, 239–60.

Nie J.B. (2005). Cultural values embodying universal norms: a critique of a popular assumption about cultures and human rights. *Developing World Bioethics*, **5**, 251–7.

Nisbett, R.E. (2003). *The Geography of Thought: How Asians and Westerners Think Differently... and Why*. New York: The Free Press.

Peng, K. and Nisbett, R.E. (1999). Culture, dialectics, and reasoning about contradiction. *American Psychologist*, **54**, 741–5.

Prodanov, V. (2001). Bioethics in Eastern Europe: a difficult birth. *Cambridge Quarterly of Healthcare Ethics*, **10**, 53–61.

Pusey, J. (1983). *China and Charles Darwin*. Boston, MA: Harvard University Asia Center.

Rheingold, H. (2002). *Smart Mobs: The Next Social Revolution*. Cambridge, MA: Perseus Publishing.

Roskies, A. (2002). Neuroethics for the new millennium. *Neuron*, **25**, 21–3.

Sabbagh, M.A., Xu, F., Carlson, S.M., *et al.* (2006). The development of executive functioning and theory of mind. *Psychological Science*, **17**, 74–81.

Safire, W. (2002). Introduction. Visions for a new field of "neuroethics". In: S.J. Marcus (ed.) *Neuroethics: Mapping the Field*, pp. 3–9. New York: Dana Press, New York.

SfN (2009). Neuroscience Wikipedia Initiative by the Society of Neuroscience, http://www.sfn.org/index.aspx?pagename=neuroscienceQuarterly_09spring_wikipedia (accessed 31 December, 2009).

Takahashi, T. (2005). Introduction: A Short History of Bioethics in Japan, in "Taking Life and Death Seriously – Bioethics from Japan". *Advances in Bioethics*, **8**, 1–18.

Takala, T. (2001). What is wrong with global bioethics? On the limitations of the four principles approach. *Cambridge Quarterly of Healthcare Ethics*, **20**, 72–7.

Toscani, T. and Maestroni, F.L. (2006). Deception, Catholicism, and hope: understanding problems in the communication of unfavorable prognoses in traditionally-Catholic countries. *The American Journal of Bioethics*, **6**, W6–18.

Wu, S. and Keysar, B. (2007). The effect of culture on perspective taking. *Psychological Science*, **18**, 600–6.

Yang, G. (2009). *The Power of the Internet in China: Citizen Activism Online*. New York: Columbia University Press.

Zimmer, C. (2005). The Neurobiology of the Self. *Scientific American*, November, 92–101.

CHAPTER 49

GLOBAL HEALTH ETHICS

JESSICA EVERT, ROBERT HUISH, GARY HEIT,
EVALEEN JONES, SCOTT LOELIGER,
AND STEVE SCHMIDBAUER

GLOBAL health ethics is a burgeoning field of thought and application. This expansive topic spans biomedical, clinical, and public health ethics (Velji 2007). As evidenced by the organizations discussed in this chapter, it also encompasses institutional ethics. Global health ethics has roots in the four traditional pillars of biomedical ethics—autonomy, non-maleficence, justice, and beneficence. However, the ethical charge of the globally active healthcare provider goes beyond these principles (Velji 2007). Dr. Carl E Taylor, founder of Johns Hopkins Department of International Medicine, espoused ethical principles for the international physician. Taylor's "Free version of the Hippocratic Oath" embodies these principles, as follows:

> I will share the science and art by precept, by demonstration, and by every mode of teaching with other physicians regardless of their national origin.
>
> I will try to help secure for the physicians in each country the esteem of their own people, and through collaborative work see that they get full credit.
>
> I will strive to eliminate sources of disease everywhere in the world and not merely set up barriers to the spread of disease to my own people.
>
> I will work for understanding of the diverse causes of diseases, including social, economic, and environmental.
>
> I will promote the well-being of mankind in all its aspects, not merely the bodily, with sympathy and consideration for a people's culture and beliefs.
>
> I will strive to prevent painful and untimely death, and also help parents to achieve a family size conforming to their desires and to their ability to care for their children.
>
> In my concern with whole communities I will never forget the needs of its individual members. (Taylor 1966)

The ethical underpinnings of four global health organizations/institutions, Americare Neurosurgery International, Child Family Health International, Mark Stinson Fellowship in Underserved and Global Health, and the Latin American School of Medicine, are described in this chapter. Importantly, these organizations are not merely touting ethical ideals; they are putting these concepts into practice. The ethical challenges and mandates of each organization can guide health care providers and institutions engaged in global health work. In addition, the variation of these organizations depicts the multiple facets and approaches to global health work. Although their missions and focus differ, common ethical threads, as well as unique ethical priorities, create an illustrious overview of global health ethics. While they apply broadly to medicine, we will draw upon examples from the domain of neurology and neurosurgery wherever possible to illustrate salient principles.

Practical ethical considerations in international subspecialty care: Americare Neurosurgery International

Americare Neurosurgery International (AMCANI; see http://www.amcani.org) was founded in 2001 with the objective of developing sustainable local medical practices while also improving resource distribution by the recycling of so-called capital medical items. Much of modern neurosurgery is embodied in complex and expensive technologies. Core to neurosurgical practice is the operating microscope, capable of being moved in multiple axes of space with two fingers; high-speed pneumatic drills; and bipolar coagulators. These instruments have substantially curtailed the morbidity and mortality of surgery, while significantly expanding the anatomical locations and types of pathology that can be addressed. Unfortunately, most neurosurgeons trained in the developing world do not have access to critical instruments secondary to their high cost. For example, an operating microscope can cost up to US $250,000 and a cranial air drill system can cost up to US $40,000. A belief of AMCANI is that training practitioners within the context of the person's practice environment will lead to more efficient healthcare delivery than training that person in a developed country, on advanced technological instruments that are ultimately unavailable in the home country.

AMCANI missions start with simultaneous outreach to local neurosurgeons within potential target countries. Once a suitable group has been found, a site visit is done to assess the needs and capabilities of the local community and to explore practical means to effectively address them. Preference is given to teaching hospitals or large clinics serving indigent people to maximize the benefit of donated materials. Subsequent visits then involve the installation of the infrastructure and donated equipment, and training in the maintenance and use of the items. Optimally, this leads to the local practitioner performing more complex and difficult cases over time as the local neurosurgeon now has the capacity to perform procedures that they did not posses the technology to do. A consequence of this is that there is an increase in morbidity and mortality due to the advanced pathologies and more difficult locations within the neuroaxis than the neurosurgeon can approach surgically. Therefore, subsequent trips also include training of ancillary medical personal (e.g. speech therapy, neurorehabilitation) to assist in the maximization of clinical outcomes following an intervention. A Memorandum of Understanding is drafted and signed by both parties after the site visit to ensure that all parties are in concordance over what will transpire and respective responsibilities. Typically it covers importation cost, customs, tariffs, duties and clearance, temporary clinical licenses, and indemnification from malpractice if appropriate.

The ethical principles governing AMCANI operations can be grouped under two categories: core guiding elements and operating principles. The latter is more fluid and dynamic as dictated by varying situations.

Core ethical principles

Benevolence

A strong guiding principle for AMCANI is that the individuals or collectives have an ethical duty to alleviate suffering for no overt personal gain. To that end, the principle mission of AMCANI is to improve the local medical care in communities where there is no, or limited access, to neurosurgery. All participants are volunteers and donate their time and often cover the expense for travel. One example is the recently completed work cycle in the Department of Neurosurgery, Hue Medical College, Hue, Vietnam. The Medical College is the only teaching hospital in Central Vietnam. Since completion of the 4-year mission, few if any patients are now transferred to Hanoi or Ho Chi Minh City (Saigon) for care (1200km away) which was formerly the only option for them. In Vietnam, families provide the bulk of floor nursing care, feeding, and attendance to the activity of daily living. As most families in the Hue catchments are from rural areas or are impoverished, travel to these cities is financially prohibitive. Prior to the work of AMCANI, patients transferred due to the lack of local technical capabilities created a stressful financial or social burden on their families and often the patients' postoperative care was compromised. The activity of AMCANI in Hue has improved the overall delivery of neurosurgical care in central Vietnam at minimal cost to the recipients; the bulk of the expenditures were from donors and the mission volunteers.

Social justice and distributed good

Rationing in the developing world is primarily due to lack of finances to procure the modern tools of medicine as well as to support the practitioners, whereas rationing in the developed world is explicitly enforced by governments or implicitly through market forces. AMCANI addresses the disparate distribution of global resources and the inherit waste of developed societies by recycling abandoned but still highly functional capital equipment to environments that would never have access to them. Furthermore, AMCANI believes that much of the equipment has multispecialization use, and therefore the resource is distributed to a larger target population then neurosurgical disease. For example, pneumatic air drills used by neurosurgeons to open the skull can also be used by orthopedic surgeons for their work on joint transplants and repairs. Ophthalmology and vascular surgery can use the microscope for their microsurgery procedures and portable monitors, X-ray, and hand instruments can be used by the entire operating room complex.

A secondary fulfillment of social justice is that this used equipment is not re-sold to developing countries. Often used medical equipment is sold as scrap or a third-party company will remove it for a fee. These corporations in turn, will resell the items to medical systems in the developing world, diverting resources from the delivery of healthcare. This then limits access to the served population and strains the financial resources of the caregivers in developing countries. In order to optimize the social justice of equipment re-use, there needs to be a supply chain directly from providers and institutions in the developed world to our resource-strapped colleagues in low-income countries. This supply chain circumvents unethical fees charged by for-profit entities for used equipment. These fees further detract resources from already strained systems and do more to exacerbate global health inequalities.

Paternalism

Paternalism has been the most difficult and dynamic ethical principle to work with. As opposed to a core ethical principle that drives an organization's agenda, paternalism has direct effects on operational execution. While trying to increase the capacity and competency of local practitioners, one must recognize the established priorities and local wishes that are often dictated by cultural and resource allocations, and not assume that the non-government organizations (NGOs) imperatives are the correct ones to apply. This was evident early on in the work in Hue where there appeared to be low rates of brain tumors in the elderly (over age 60) compared to similar populations in the US. On investigation, we learned that this was not due to an epidemiological phenomenon, but because of pragmatic resource rationing. Many patients were not treated optimally from a Western medical, evidence-based standard as the infrastructure to support optimal treatment was lacking. To accommodate the local resource limitations and approach to delivery of care, AMCANI physicians (acting from a paternalistic role) were required to change their perspective on the definition of a substandard care level. The rationale to continue to use a treatment algorithm that was substandard by Western practices, even after delivery of the modern technology, became rooted in the local sense of "primum non nocere." Notably over time, the neurosurgeons are now more aggressively treating tumors as their technical competence increases, and the treatment algorithms are now approaching Western medical standards.

We have found that the sudden introduction of advanced technologies into a medical practice can lead to a wave of excessive morbidity in the absence of appropriate counseling regarding that possibility. A delicate interplay of paternalism, cultural appreciation, respect for a practitioner's autonomy and clinical skills and acumen, as well as benevolence to the local population comes into play in these conversations about what case types should be attempted after AMCANI has departed and the local neurosurgeons are working with the new technologies on their own. These interactions modulate the paternalistic drive to introduce and rapidly accelerate the neurosurgical care locally and profoundly affect how AMCANI operates in its missions.

AN ETHICAL FRAMEWORK FOR GLOBAL HEALTH IMMERSION PROGRAMS: CHILD FAMILY HEALTH INTERNATIONAL

Child Family Health International (CFHI) is a non-profit organization dedicated to improving the delivery of healthcare in underserved communities in some of the poorest parts of the world. The primary means toward this end is working with local health professionals to create global health immersion experiences for Western health sciences trainees, predominantly medical students, within a framework that is socially responsible and financially just. These immersion experiences lay the groundwork for global citizenship and dedication to underserved populations domestically and globally. This primary charge is augmented by secondary mandates to promote professional development opportunities for international partners, to invest in community-based projects, and to provide needed medical supplies or equipment when possible. The ethical pillars of CFHI include justice, equity, sustainability, professionalism, consciousness and authenticity. These ethical principles are not merely the philosophical footing of CFHI programs; they pervade the operational components of the organization.

CFHI's ethical underpinnings stem from its origins. CFHI was established two decades ago by one of the authors—Evaleen Jones MD, a family physician—who desired to create a mechanism for health science students to rotate abroad in a fashion that prioritized just compensation of partners in-country for the time and energy devoted to absorbing and educating such students. Jones was bothered by the dilemma that Western students rotating at low resource sites often serve to further extract resources from that environment, as clinicians and staff spend time and energy educating and hosting the visitor. In the immediate sense this serves to further global health inequities and subvert the priorities of the in-country hosts to those of the Western students. Jones decided it was imperative that physicians, clinical officers, midwives, and other health professionals who host Western colleagues and students are appropriately compensated, both financially and intangibly.

Currently, CFHI offers 21 rotations in five countries. Participants include medical students, public health students, resident physicians, nurses, and other health science trainees and practitioners. In addition to providing rotations, CFHI invests in community projects that originate in the minds and hearts of their international partners. These include, for example, disability awareness and training for community health workers in rural Mexico for care of neurologically impaired wheelchair bound patients, prevention of secondary complications, such as decubitus ulcers, and physical therapy rehabilitation. Other examples include lay health promoter training in rural India, establishment of a clinic for children living in Bolivian jails with their incarcerated parents, and supporting a clinic (salaried physician, equipment, and medications) in the Himalayan foothills.

Core ethical principles

Equity

World health organization (WHO) Director-General Margaret Chan recently reframed the global health equity charge as follows, "Greater equity in the health status of populations, within and between countries, should be regarded as key measure of how we, as a civilized society, are making progress" (World Health Organization 2009). Many global health education programs proclaim they address inequities. However, far too many programs fail to reflect on their actual impact and motivations. CFHI prioritizes self-reflection and transparency of its impact and limitations therein.

CFHI furthers the ideal of global health equity by exposing health science trainees and professionals to the vast differences in healthcare that exist between the developed and developing countries. CFHI conceptualizes itself as a stepping stone program for introductory exposure to these inequities. Thirty-seven per cent of CFHI participants report that their immersion experience affected their career choice, presumably in the direction of lessening the healthcare divide (Unpublished survey, CFHI 2009). Once this exposure has occurred, CFHI challenges its alumni to partake in global citizenship. The roots of global citizenship can be traced to Thomas Paine who wrote in the Rights of Man, "My country is the world, my religion is to do good" (Paine 1791). CFHI's alumni network serves as a vehicle for participants to take the mutually supported next step toward global citizenship.

Currently, there are more than 5000 CFHI program alumni. The immediacy and intensity of the observational experience they receive through CFHI makes each of its alumni potential change agents who are uniquely qualified to advocate for underserved communities and to educate others on the realities of resource-poor clinical settings and overburdened health systems. They are eyewitnesses to the sheer dedication and determination of local health professionals committed to providing the highest level of care possible in some of the least optimal environments.

CFHI makes direct investments in local communities and the healthcare workforce to combat global health inequities. For example, CFHI funds the clinic infrastructure in the remote Himalayan foothills of northern India where there had previously been no access to formal healthcare. CFHI provides professional development grants for their health partners who have utilized these grants to conduct and present research, provide training in childhood development, cardiovascular resuscitation, and train support staff, including nurses and community health workers. Other direct investments have included a variety of efforts such as: (1) the creation of a clean drinking water system for a village, (2) establishment of a domestic violence program, (3) completion of health and developmental assessments for high-risk pre-school children, and (4) provision of medical and social services to young children living in jails with their incarcerated parents. Through the alumni network, investment in local health systems and sponsorship of professional development, CFHI actively pursues equity, both for patients and healthcare professionals.

Justice

The unique justice of CFHI's model cannot be over emphasized. Two important and unique aspects of the CFHI model include recognizing local community members to serve as experts, and providing compensation. These two features most exemplify the organization's attempt to live out its values. From the beginning of relationship building in an underserved community, CFHI intentionally identifies the local community members and healthcare providers as the experts of their local situation. Too often the knowledge and skills of students arriving from the global north may be over-estimated simply by the level of their education. In some cases, students have even been treated as the expert *over and above local health professionals* who have spent their entire career serving the local community. CFHI values the role and the experience of local preceptors and works to help students understand that there is much that can be learned at the grassroots level—lessons that will never be found in a text book.

As part of recognizing the expertise of the local preceptors, CFHI also offers a compensation model for international partners. There are hundreds of organizations that send students, professionals, and other interested persons abroad to rotate at healthcare facilities. Participants are charged a fee that supports the Western-based organization sending them abroad. Usually there is compensation paid to home-stay sponsors and logistical persons on the ground in-country. It is very rare for the healthcare personnel that precept participants to receive any financial compensation for the time and energy devoted to rotating Westerners. As CFHI Founder Evaleen Jones MD articulates, CFHI is based on the premise that the world is a classroom, and we must pay for our instruction, wherever and to whomever, that happens to be (unpublished 2009). CFHI proposes a universal standard that compensates healthcare professionals who absorb Westerners rotating in their clinics, hospitals, and medical facilities by providing a stipend for their role as mentors. It must be pointed out that in some countries, health professionals are government employees and are not allowed to accept compensation. In these settings, CFHI works with the local clinic and hospital administration to utilize or create a special fund. CFHI contributes the equivalent of the preceptor compensation to that fund and, over time, these proceeds can be used to acquire much needed supplies/equipment, or further professional training. In addition to being a just model of compensation, this rectification exemplifies the non-paternalistic underpinnings of CFHI, unlike Americare Neurosurgery International described in the previous section.

When in-country preceptors are not compensated, it sends a message that Western visitors are due gratis time and energy. This premise is based on the assumption that the Western visitor is a "have" who is bringing something to the "have-nots," even if that Westerner fails to inject more resources than extract. For years clinical sites have accepted rotating Westerners, often with the hope that such Westerners will become benefactors. These hopes often fail to materialize. Consequently, the entire dynamic operates on an inequitable, unjust assumption.

CFHI recognizes the reality of a default power differential between a school or an organization based in a more developed country partnering with clinical sites based in a developing country. CFHI believes that this creates an ethical mandate to strive for equity between collaborators and justice for low-resource partners. The organization naturally assumed to have a greater advantage must consistently look for ways to level the playing field. This leveling occurs by focusing on the strengths and inherent wisdom of hosting partners. It takes hold by establishing a flexible relationship that maintains transparency in its organizational process. Recognizing local experts, offering a fair compensation model, and creating a communication structure that invites local collaborative participation are ways that create a culture of respect and trust throughout the organization, which in turn, is recognized and felt by participants.

Social justice involves not only creating new paradigms but rejecting old ones (Stuart 2008). One common historical educational convention has been for academic institutions to require students rotating abroad to participate in some form of research. This may be realistic for students going for longer periods of time (6–12 months), but it is not practical, nor beneficial, to the host community for 1-month rotations. Short-term immersion programs are highly valuable experiences that can be academically rigorous without the exercise of a research project. For example, CFHI has piloted a 20 hour/week Emotional Intelligence curriculum for participants. This is one mechanism to satisfy US Institutional Partnerships and medical faculty who often worry that students going abroad are simply going on an academic vacation (Editorial 1993). This curriculum has also proven extremely valuable to our partners in creating dialogue on professionalism, cross cultural differences, and self-care.

When research is conducted, ethics approval from the student's home institution is required. Usually the institutional review process does not involve participation from the host community, as only occasionally will the process include input from a professor native to the host country. With the increase in numbers of students going abroad and the likelihood that more research will be conducted over time, the ethics of such research projects and relationships is undergoing greater scrutiny (Pinto 2009). Toward this end, the Community-Campus Partnerships for Health (CCPH), with input from CFHI, has created ethical paradigms for such activities urging institutions to examine the motivations, outcomes and approval process for such research, especially with grassroots organizations in the global setting.

The motto of CFHI speaks volumes, "Let the world change you." It is important to remember that international colleagues and their clinical sites provide education, fulfillment, and enlightenment to rotating Westerners. It is often the Westerners who gain the most in this equation. On many levels the Westerners who undertake these trips are operating in self-interest, a desire to see the world and gain the fulfillment by positively affecting others. This is the paradox of selfishness and altruism debated in many philosophical circles (see "Authenticity," later in this chapter). Westerners, and the organizations that facilitate global health educational opportunities, should compensate international partners for the benefits of global experiences. This is the just approach to global health education program structures.

Sustainability

Sustainability is paramount to CFHI's programming, as evidenced by its approach to working relationships and longevity within communities. Instead of conducting a needs assessment to find what a community is lacking, CFHI takes an asset mapping approach, beginning with a community's strengths rather than its weaknesses. This approach strengthens sustainability for several reasons. As the programs and projects are driven at a pace that is consistent with local capacity, the community takes ownership much more quickly, and an inherent check is placed on the donor organization from imposing its agenda, consciously or unconsciously. Moreover, consistently addressing issues from the perspective of what the community lacks can create a mindset that unconsciously promotes a neediness and dependence on help from outside the community. Approaching the same issues by intentionally seeking, celebrating, and building on the strengths of the community can engage people in a process that implements successful development, while at the same time builds self-esteem, local pride, and ownership. This asset mapping approach is the cornerstone of sustainability for CFHI community projects and engagement.

This cornerstone is augmented by the longevity of CFHI relationships with its partner sites. CFHI constantly reviews the internal motivations and external pressures to expand programs and scale up projects to ensure that such stressors do not compromise the capacity to maintain and nurture existing relationships and sites. CFHI has been operating at its existing sites for 15–20 years, it is confidence built with international partners over time that allows CFHI to execute continuing quality improvements and other program expansions with buy-in and cooperation from partners.

Professionalism

Professionalism and professionalization are emphasized in multiple facets of CFHI programming. *A Physician Charter. Medical Professionalism in the New Millenium* (2002) defines the fundamental principles of professionalism in terms of: (1) the primacy of patient welfare; (2) patient autonomy; (3) social justice. Two important demonstrations of these concepts are explicit. First, the role of CFHI participants is qualified as that of observer within the clinical setting. This role acknowledges that Western medical training does not necessarily prepare a person for work in a foreign context. It prioritizes patient welfare by appropriately acknowledging the skill sets of native practitioners which is both biomedically and culturally rooted. The explicit designation of observer status for rotating students and trainees also implies that clinical experimentation, such as doing procedures for the first time, is not an appropriate exploit of global health rotations.

CFHI has also created a professional structure for its program administration. This institutionalization and professionalization establishes clarity for both CFHI and its partners. An administrative structure is often taken for granted or is merely implicit. However, in the realm of global health medical education and related immersion programs, a purposeful, longstanding administrative structure at each rotation site is essential but often lacking. It is this attention to detail of the administrative structure, and the standardization of professional roles, which distinguishes CFHI's ethical matrix. Each CFHI site has a site coordinator who is usually non-medical and is skilled at program administration, trouble shooting, liaising between the US-based home office, and programmatic technicalities. In addition, there is a medical director for each site, a physician or nurse practitioner who usually holds a position of authority within the local medical community. The role of this individual is to be the main contact point for CFHI, to oversee clinical preceptors, to provide didactic sessions with CFHI participants, and to function as liaisons between the healthcare system and CFHI programs.

The third layer of structure is the clinical preceptors. Each CFHI participant is assigned a preceptor who is shadowed in a clinical setting. These individuals are usually medical officers or physicians. They are accountable to medical directors.

This structure allows for program implementation and improvements to occur through official communication vehicles and within a seniority structure that is appropriate to the local environment. It also provides a structure for accountability and delineates responsibility. CFHI's respect for this administrative structure is conscientious and longstanding so that partners have a clear understanding of their individual roles and interactions with other members of the administrative structure.

Consciousness and authenticity

CFHI proactively fosters consciousness and authenticity among its participants. In *The Ethics of Authenticity*, Charles Taylor asserts that the path to understanding ourselves and our intentions is through dialogue (Taylor 1992). Rousseau elucidated the following about consciousness: "conscience, indestructible in us but easily defeated, is the feeling that urges us, in spite of contrary passions, towards the two harmonies: the one within our minds and between our passions, and the other within society and between its members" (Plamenatz 1963, p. xxii). Since its inception CFHI has required participants to complete pre-departure online training that includes factual and hypothetical case scenarios. This preparation has set the tone for participants to invoke consciousness and authenticity while abroad and in their post-immersion lives.

As we described earlier, the Emotional Intelligence curriculum was implemented recently to formalize the cultivation of consciousness and authenticity. In the words of its founder, Daniel Goleman, Emotional Intelligence provides for "the added value of an empathetic physician or nurse, attuned to patients, able to listen and be heard. This means fostering "relationship-centered care...self-awareness and the arts of empathy and listening" (Goleman 1995, p. 183). Two tenets emphasized by CFHI's curriculum are cultural humility and humanism. Cultural humility has several components. It requires that healthcare personnel be reflective practitioners, be aware of inner assumption and biases, and utilize patient-focused interviewing to correct power imbalances between providers and patients.

The implementation of the Emotional Intelligence curriculum has been a collaborative venture with medical directors at partner sites. Buy-in from these partners was obtained through collaborative discussions and bilateral adjustments to the curriculum. The feedback from partners has been very positive and indicates that emphasis on consciousness and authenticity has been internalized by the entire organizational structure and is not limited to program participants.

Authenticity within the framework of CFHI's work involves challenging traditional notions of altruism. A common reaction of homebound participants is that their international experience helped them exponentially more than they contributed to the underserved environment. "Let the world change you" reflects the notion of changing the world that differentiates CFHI from many other organizations. In essence, the immersion experience, done in a just, sustainable fashion, exudes an authenticity that challenges the core altruistic notions of global health work. It is the exposure and process of "[letting] the world change you" that plants the seeds necessary to develop authenticity around the self-serving, self-fulfilling outcomes of global health activities. Viewed through the lens of the altruism debate, this approach is aligned with what Arne Naess (1989) characterizes as the ecological self, and Mendonca (2001) calls mutual altruism. The ecological self fosters a self-actualization that service for the good of others is, in actuality, an enlightened form of self-interest (Seed *et al.* 1988). In Mendonca's estimation, certain acts exhibit mutual altruism in which they are bilaterally beneficial and represent enlightened self-interest. Contrary to Comte's (1875) original definition of altruism, that such actions are undertaken purely in service to the goods of others, CFHI disseminates a model that acknowledges the inestimable benefits to self by serving the global health cause.

Conclusions for CFHI

Global health medical education is brimming with idealism and ethical mandates. Far too often the pursuit of these good intentions is fraught with hypocritical paradoxes. In consideration of the growing burden of neurologic and psychiatric disease in the developing world (Johnston 2009; Kessler *et al.* 2009), there is a great need for considerate global health immersion programs. CFHI aims to avoid common pitfalls by allowing basic ethical principles to pervade not only its mission, but also its operational framework. The process of self-examination is not merely a lesson taught to participants, it is an ongoing conscientious process undertaken by the organization. As Arne Naess espouses, "there must be identification in order for there to be compassion, and among humans, solidarity" (Seed *et al.* 1988, p. 22). Through this consciousness, the pursuit of equity, justice, sustainability, and authenticity is realized.

Born of a socially responsible county healthcare system and integrated family medicine residency: The Mark Stinson Fellowship in Underserved and Global Health

Contra Costa Regional Medical Center is a county-based facility that exists primarily to serve the population of Contra Costa County, east of San Francisco, California, USA. As with many county-sponsored or county-operated facilities, its primary clients are the underserved, the uninsured, and those covered by the public healthcare systems known as Medicaid and Medicare in the US. It has been in existence since the early 1880s when the County of Contra Costa purchased land and built a hospital to care for the area's indigent patients. Thus, this healthcare system has provided both inpatient and outpatient care to residents of this county who are unable to obtain care from the private healthcare system for over 125 years.

The mission statement reads as follows:

> Contra Costa Health Services (CCHS) cares for and improves the health of all people in Contra Costa County with special attention to those who are most vulnerable to health problems.
>
> We provide high quality health services with respect and responsiveness to all.
>
> We are an integrated system of health care services, community health improvement and environmental protection.
>
> We anticipate community health needs and change to meet those needs.
>
> We work in partnership with our patients, cities and diverse communities, as well as the health, education and human service agents.
>
> We encourage creative, ethical and tenacious leadership to implement effective health care policies and programs.
>
> We have a department-wide goal to reduce health disparities by addressing issues of diversity and linguistic and cultural competence. (http://www.cchs.org/aboutus/missionstatement/20090927/en.html)

Characteristics of a socially responsible institution

Operating ethics principles

Historically in the US, county health services were primarily managed by general practitioners. In the pre-specialist era, before the 1960s, generalists took care of the mentally ill, delivered babies, treated infectious, acute and chronic disease, and performed many general surgeries.

In the late 1970s, soon after family medicine was established as a specialty in the US, a 3-year family medicine residency was instituted at central county hospital and several clinics in Contra Costa. The character of the residency program was to produce physicians that practiced a broad-spectrum version of family medicine—inpatient and outpatient care, chronic and neurological disorders, surgery and obstetrics, intensive care and pediatrics. The general goal was to produce young, broadly trained physicians who would serve those without access to more specialized care in almost any underserved locale, mainly concentrating in the more urban, suburban areas of the US. The family medicine residency in Contra Costa County became well known for its training program, clearly embedded in a culture of caring for the underserved and reaching out to the most vulnerable in the county. Over the years community clinics in both rural and urban centers were added to improve access to services and were later included as training sites for residents.

The residency program attracted individuals driven by visions of old-fashioned practice; many of the graduates went on to work on reservations, in inner-city clinics and for other county healthcare systems. Many had already worked with underserved populations before, during and after medical school: as Peace Corps volunteers, community activists, and employees in public health departments. Many already had advanced degrees, such as a Masters in Public Health (MPH), that had solidified their experience with communities and broader health policy and social justice issues that impact health and healthcare.

An excellent example of the residents' commitment to the underserved occurred in 2009. As a result of the government financial crisis at federal, state and local levels, county financial experts decided that the healthcare system could save millions of dollars by ending care for undocumented persons. Upon learning that many of their clinic patients would lose access to basic healthcare the residents organized protests and media events that clearly highlighted how well they understood the nature of their training and their role as family physicians in the larger social and healthcare system. Their clear commitment to social justice and healthcare access forced other, older physicians to examine their roles with the county healthcare system and caused a larger participation among a community of physicians that is often silent about such matters.

Many graduated residents have stayed to work in the Contra Costa healthcare system, continuing to see the primarily Medicaid-funded population and to continue to teach both residents and new registrars who would carry on the tradition of full-spectrum service. Others have left to work in rural California, China, Indonesia, and Western Native-American reservations. The fellowship director works abroad with several organizations that focus on training family physicians for primary healthcare systems and for promoting the vision of social justice and accountability. Each graduate serves as a role model for others and encourages the sustained participation of equally focused staff and residents. Over the years this tradition of work and study in and out of the US continues to infuse the home institution with vitality, curiosity and dedication of purpose in serving the most vulnerable of the population. It is definitely a part of why medical students interested in some lifetime work with the underserved, both in the US and a global setting, continue to seek training there.

Finding the right candidates

A recent review of the applications of residents graduated and admitted during the last 5 years reveals the following goals and beliefs in the statement of purpose.

- Commitment to the underserved and reducing barriers to healthcare.
- Commitment to family and community.
- Prior work in the Third World and the inner city.
- Dedicated to the underserved.
- Rural upbringing.

Onto this fertile environment of practice and training—outside of the traditional academic framework of professorships, multispecialty training programs, and publish or perish mentality—was grafted a new, integrated post-residency fellowship focusing on both underserved and global health. It likely would never have come into existence without the elements of community service, social justice, reducing disparities and barriers to care and family- centered medical practice already in place. However, it might be argued that research aimed at Third World and underdeveloped countries could potentially have larger effects in terms of impact than the limited number of patients that any one doctor could see in those places.

In 2004, a small group of family medicine residents and faculty/staff met and started a process towards a fellowship offered after completion of a family medicine residency. This group included one resident who, as an undergraduate, worked in an Indonesian rainforest studying threatened orangutans and who now runs an isolated family medicine clinic in West Kalamatan. Another member of the early group, Dr. Mark Stinson, was a graduate of the Contra Costa residency program but worked full-time in the emergency department while doing significant and frequent work in conflict zones overseas, including Bosnia, and disaster scenes such as the Indonesian tsunami and the site of the 9/11/01 disaster in New York City.

The initial proposed goal of the new fellowship was to create an educational/service oriented training program coordinated with an international relief organization and the existing family medicine residency program. A handwritten note from that developmental period promoted a vision to "create a new super-specialty of global family physicians that are driven by social justice and humanitarianism to provide medical services in areas where medical resources are limited, whether due to geography, poverty, disaster, war, barriers to care or lack of medical insurance."

Along the way the initial 1-year program, started formally in 2006, transformed into a full-fledged, 2-year fellowship that combines a basic grounding in public health ideals and principles—through an MPH at the University of California School of Public Health (SPH)—with ongoing training and immersion in family medicine residency training. Fellows are given opportunities to increase skills and competency in obstetrics, gynecology, and outpatient care with an underserved population in the county clinic system. They are also encouraged to join the ranks of faculty that promote the culture of the county/residency mission. This environment of commitment, ongoing participation in equity and social justice issues and the current ethical crisis in providing care to the under-insured and the uninsured should influence and shape the fellow. There is ongoing development of curriculum that covers ethics and professionalism that is purposely part of the fellowship's self-study and development of a required project based in an underserved community.

Exposure to, and treating, the poor and the underserved during residency training does not by itself create a cadre of committed, socially responsible family doctors. Physicians in the US are paid an admirable amount of money whether they work for a county, an academic institution, or a private system; there are clearly providers in the county system without a commitment greater than coming to work in a clinic every day. A moral commitment is instilled in all the residents, fellows and faculty to look far beyond the clinic visit or daily hospital rounds to the factors that made these patients ill, often why they presented so late in the course of their illness, and what prevents them from following recommendations of care, treatment and follow-up visits.

Such institutional characteristics have been discussed in some international literature about ethics. At the Latin America School of Medicine (ELAM) thousands of young medical students from around the world, including the US, are entering their studies with a moral commitment to provide care in underserved and vulnerable communities (Huish 2009). For years, Charles Bolen and others have challenged medical schools to integrate social accountability into their mission and curriculum. The social accountability of these institutions is defined by World Health Organization as "the obligation to direct their education, research and service activities towards addressing the priority health concerns of the community, the region and/or the nation they have a mandate to serve. The priority health concerns as to be identified jointly by governments, health care organizations, health professionals and the public" (Bolen 1995). Such directed social focus in education and mission would seem to have equal importance in family medicine training programs such as that in Contra Costa County and will be further refined by the post-graduate fellowship in existence.

The fellowship itself continues to survive in an environment of funding scarcity that is adversely impacting on all social programs in the US. Only at the last minute did funding get approved. Programs that promote social change and dedication to community must clearly struggle to emerge in an environment that values physicians only as skillful technicians and not committed agents of change. As a component of the training mission in Contra Costa County, great commitment will be required from the faculty and administration to grow and adapt. Its most recent stepchild is a nascent underserved and global health track within the residency program developed by residents themselves. One Contra Costa resident recently returned from Uganda after a month of training under a local family physician in a rural hospital. Of interest, at about the same time in late 2009, the Institute of Medicine's Forum on Neuroscience and Nervous System Disorders convened a workshop that addressed the quality of care, sustainability and ethical issues of mental health and neurological issues in Sub-Saharan Africa (http://www.iom.edu/en/Activities/Research/NeuroForum/2009-AUG-04.aspx). With the proper preparation and under direct supervision of host faculty, these experiences and workshops will continue to prepare family physicians for socially responsible and ethical work in a new medical home model, one without political and geographical boundaries.

PLACING HUMAN RIGHTS AT THE HEART OF MEDICAL EDUCATION: THE NORMATIVE ETHICS OF CUBA'S LATIN AMERICAN SCHOOL OF MEDICINE

ELAM (Cuba's Latin American School of Medicine) was born out of a desperate scenario. With close to 40,000 dead and over a million persons displaced after Hurricane Mitch (1998) immediate medical relief, including Cuban medical brigades was too limited to overcome the massive structural inequities that made Central America so vulnerable to this natural disaster. Cuba had an impressive track record of international relief assistance throughout the Americas and Africa, but with Mitch the medical brigades witnessed hopelessness for many vulnerable communities because of a lack of resources and a lack of trained medical personnel.

Cuban medical internationalism took a bold and innovative approach: train medical personnel from vulnerable communities for those communities on a massive scale (Huish and Kirk 2007). In 1999, Cuba's Ministry of Health (MINSAP) established ELAM; a medical school offering a free 6-year education for those willing to serve in underserved regions. The scholarship was initially offered to victims of Mitch (Guatemala, Honduras, El Salvador, and Nicaragua) but quickly expanded to involve 30 countries around the world, including the US. Since 1999, over 14,000 students have come to ELAM, and over 5000 have graduated. Not all students have been able to secure work in their home countries, but the overwhelming majority of graduates have applied their skills to some of the world's most vulnerable communities, which demonstrates a strong institutional ethic of medical service as social justice.

ELAM is grounded in a simple premise: medical professionals desire to serve underserved communities. Students and graduates are under no fixed contract while attending the school. If a student drops out of the program, or if they choose to serve in a more affluent setting, Cuba does not demand any sort of tuition repayment or retraction of degree. Instead, the commitment to serve the vulnerable is enforced only through a moral obligation that values medicine as a method of social justice and service to the poor as the top priority.

How is it possible then for a program like ELAM to see the majority of its graduates serve the underserved without a mandatory contract or generous remuneration? It contradicts the majority of human resource for health literature that argues that one, if not both, of these elements are necessary in order to bolster service to the underserved (Brown and Connell 2004; Dovlo 2003; Labonte et al. 2006; Schrecker and Labonté 2007).

The answer lies in understanding the school's institutional ethics and normative values (Huish 2009). Based on extensive review of medical curriculum and interviews with faculty, administrators and students, ELAM's institutional ethics stem from four key elements: ethical recruitment, catered curriculum, clinical confidence, and practical moral instruction (Huish 2008a). Combined, they create a powerful service ethic where the vast majority of individuals willingly choose to provide care for the destitute rather than to pursue self-interest for financial gain.

Operating ethics principles

Discontent with the acquiescence of healthcare inequity

Cuba's commitment to global health is a rejection of what Thomas Pogge has referred to as an acquiescence of world poverty (Pogge 2008). Building capacity for healthcare systems is typically deemed to be a national pursuit rather than a product of international cooperation. While prosperous nations could do more to assist the needs of the poor, they often do not, because as Pogge (2008) suggests, "failing to save lives is not morally on par with killing...if we do less or even nothing, we are not therefore responsible for any poverty deaths we might have prevented" (p. 14). Furthermore, it is tacitly accepted that nations will look out for the interests of their own before the needs of others.

Cuba's approach is a radical departure from this paradigm. With 36,000 of its own health-care workers practicing in vulnerable communities in 72 countries, Cuba has demonstrated a discontent to accept the healthcare inequity that stems from global poverty. Likewise, it has challenged the idea that training healthcare workers need only be a nationalist pursuit. These normative ethics are not rooted in a devotion to philanthropy; rather they are rooted in a commitment to cooperation with other countries that, like Cuba, are struggling to over-come underdevelopment. In some cases, Cuba receives remuneration from other countries, such as South Africa, or subsidized imports from countries like Venezuela (Muntaner *et al.* 2006; Schuyler 2002). Other countries such as The Gambia, Honduras, and Haiti offer little in return other than their support for Cuba to be included in regional trade discussions, and solidarity against the nearly 50-year embargo of the country by the US.

While the number of international cooperation projects is impressive, the international support for Cuban medical internationalism, including ELAM, is grounded in institutional ethics that see Cuban-trained healthcare workers practice in some of the poorest and vul-nerable populations, from the slums of Caracas to rural Ghana. Cuban healthcare workers have earned international accreditation because they are well prepared to work in challeng-ing conditions throughout the developing world. Looking specifically at ELAM, this readi-ness is the product of a medical education with the central tenet that healthcare is a human right. This value is taken to the heart of the program and is strengthened by four pillars of recruitment, catered curriculum, clinical confidence, and mentorship.

Ethical recruitment of students to ELAM

The school recruits students mostly from vulnerable communities and humble economic backgrounds. Cuban solidarity organizations, labor movements and leftist political parties in the students' countries, informally help out in the application process by spreading word of the program and providing assistance with applications prior to submission to the Cuban embassy who sends the final applications to ELAM. Candidates from more humble back-grounds, indigenous communities, and rural areas will likely have better access to such soli-darity groups, rather than those who see the Cuban education as a stepping stone to the North. In countries such as Guatemala, Honduras, and Nicaragua, Cuban healthcare work-ers help to coordinate applications directly to the embassy. This again has a filtering effect, as the Cuban medical brigades are already in contact with some of the most needy communities in the country.

Catered curriculum

The Cuban medical education curriculum focuses heavily on social and environmental determinants of health. It focuses on the two-volume set by Alvarez Sintes (2001), *Temas de Medicina General Integral* (MGI; Themes in Integral General Medicine). MGI is considered the foundation for students during their studies and afterwards for their practice. While basic science, clinical practice, and various pre-specialties, including neurology are integral to the program, the emphasis is on incorporating medical science into social and environ-mental determinants of health. The goal is to train physicians to have a role in recognizing and treating the patient in order to maintain health rather than repair its loss. The curriculum deals with health risks that impact low-resource communities, such as basic sanitation, proper nutrition, vector diseases, and workplace health and safety. For MGI, the physician works in the community to deeply understand the particular localized risks that impact health. MGI encourages intersectoral collaboration with other health professionals, but in their absence, the physician has the skills to identify potential health risks. The text approaches diagnosis and treatment through investigations into patients' general health history and how it could relate to current conditions. This sort of methodology bodes well for students who would continue on in neurology, which demands careful inquiry into a patient's history in order to help isolate and identify pathologies. Chapters such as community health, epidemiology in primary care, demographics, communication, and research methods have a dedicated focus on how to recognize and measure health determinants at the community level (Álvarez Sintes and et al. 2001).

Clinical confidence

Students develop their clinical skills by working with doctors in groups of four or fewer in *polyclinicos* and in hospitals by their second year of studies. Bedside instruction is kept purposefully small to foster attentive mentorship and to afford students the time to interact with both patients and instructors. Through hands-on experience in the clinic, students also gain clinical confidence from the early stages of their medical education. The expectation is that by the end of their tenure they will be confident leaders in the clinic in their home communities.

The students have repeatedly expressed readiness to work in underserviced conditions even if it means facing a lacking infrastructure or poor access to tertiary care. In a 2009 first-person interview, one student from California noted that:

> In Cuba you are not just tested on the standard routines. They want you to be innovative in your diagnostic and prognostic analysis. For example, if you were to order an X-ray, the professor might come back and say, "well, the machine is not working, or there is no power" so then what do you do? You learn to find alternative means to diagnose and treat the patient until that service is ready.

Many students have pursued advanced training after their 6-year program. Specializations in neurology or neurosurgery are available to students at no additional cost. MINSAP requires that postgraduate specialization include a specialization in public health in addition to any other area of study, including neurology. The idea is that even highly skilled neurosurgeons would still have robust understanding of popular health needs and risks.

Lead by example

Cuban medical education involves the many faculty members who have participated in the over 100 international health cooperation missions since 1960 (Feinsilver 1993; Kirk and Erisman 2009). ELAM's faculty has experienced working in challenging conditions, but they also bring a sense of pride and valor for service to the poor. The faculty is comprised of 466 doctors who have had extensive teaching experience; most have practiced overseas on medical brigades and through cooperation efforts. Teaching at ELAM is considered a prestigious posting for Cuban faculty. Rector Juan Carrizo Estévez claimed that elite faculty come to ELAM: "The best professor of anatomy will teach to a thousand students" (Huish 2008b, p .146). The school boasts some of the most highly-decorated researchers in medicine and science throughout Cuba. Several faculty members are associated with Cuba's Centro Internacional Restauracion Neurologica (CIREN), founded in 1989 which is Cuba's premiere neurological teaching and research centre. The centre pursues advanced research in an interdisciplinary spirit on a wide range of neurological procedures, but it is especially focused on advancing procedures for structural and functional recuperation. As part of Cuba's broad program of medical internationalism CIREN has received 40,000 patients from 85 countries for advanced neurosurgery and therapeutic treatment. Faculty from CIREN lecture at ELAM, and students have the chance to do rounds there with specialists.

ELAM's institutional ethics

Ethical recruitment, tailored curricula, clinical confidence, and appropriate mentorship produce an institutional culture that not only values service to the vulnerable, but equips students with the necessary knowledge, confidence, and mentorship to realize that their skills and compassion are desperately needed. Furthermore, ELAM instills a confidence in its students that their efforts can make a difference in the lives of the poor.

ELAM's mission has proved to be partially fulfilled. 5500 trainees have graduated since 2005, but many national and private physicians' associations have refused to recognize the Cuban medical degree. Peru, Argentina, Uruguay, Belize, and Antigua, have all advised ELAM graduates to retrain. In Ecuador the graduates are permitted to practice for 1 year, but are left with few options for residency. Many have returned to Cuba to continue training, and some have joined the Barrio Adentro program in Venezuela. Others offered their time in rural outposts in Honduras and Nicaragua, working alongside other Cuban-trained doctors. Private practices in Spain and the US have extended numerous offers for employment and migration to ELAM graduates, along with other Cuban healthcare professionals, to work in wealthier settings. According to both Cuba and US sources only about 3% of Cuban healthcare workers (ELAM graduates included) have taken up such offers.

At one level, ELAM's institutional ethics offer a unique aperture for medical education to be about accessibility to the vulnerable as much as it is an understanding of curative practice. On a larger scale, programs like ELAM demonstrate Cuba's commitment to global health and the normative values of treating those who need it the most. At both the individual level and the structural level this program demonstrates that acquiescence to global health inequity does not have to dominate as a normative approach to ensuring health as a human right.

CONCLUSION

Globally, it is estimated that one in every nine individuals dies of a disorder of the nervous system (Murray 1996). The lack of access to care for neurological disorders in low-income and developing countries has been documented through collaboration between the World Federation of Neurology (WFN) and WHO (Janca *et al.* 2006). The gross inequalities that exist in the realm of neurological care create an ethical imperative for physicians and institutions from resource-rich countries to establish mechanisms to expose such inequalities and contribute to their rectification. Concurrently, there is an increasing globalization within Western societies and focus on global health among medical trainees and practitioners (Drain 2009). Meanwhile there are potential ethical pitfalls of global health activities, including paternalism, power imbalances, and cultural incompetency (Pinto 2009; Velji 2007). Cost effectiveness and sustainability are among others.

Critics might argue that a number of factors, including quality of life, the reality of large student loans, and safety jeopardize the feasibility of some global health initiatives. However, opportunities with competitive salaries for physicians who have a unique skills set or level of experience are available. Some practitioners combine research and global health clinical work, utilizing research dollars to support related clinical practices. Depending on the specific program, funding for salaries may also be subsidized by private funding, domestic governments, medical schools, and scholarships. Practitioners with loans have the option to claim economic hardship or other deferments to postpone repayment, or to seek loan forgiveness for domestic underserved work. There are current proposals in the US legislature to provide loan forgiveness for global underserved clinical practice, as well. Safety issues are a concern, some of which are unique to women working abroad. Regardless of gender, however, the most common causes of morbidity and mortality include traffic accidents, diseases of poor sanitation, infectious diseases, and mental health challenges. It is critical to have a primer in culture, language, history, environmental challenges, and disease profiles before one descends on an international site.

The organizations described in this chapter operate unique programs in global health. AMCANI distributes subspecialized neurosurgical instruments with attention to sustainable training and ongoing evaluation of morbidity outcomes. CFHI provides global health immersion programs for trainees and individuals wanting an initial exposure to healthcare provision in developing countries. The Mark Stinson Fellowship in Underserved and Global Health creates a postgraduate training opportunity that draws parallels between domestic and globally underserved populations. ELAM brings to fruition a country's commitment to addressing the global health workforce crisis and to harnessing healthcare as a means to diplomacy. Although each organization has a unique means to addressing common global health needs, they are based on common ethical foundations. In addition, each organization demonstrates how global health ethics are not merely intangible principles, but rather directives for operational functions of each institution.

REFERENCES

Álvarez Sintes, R., Díaz Alonso, G., Salas Mainegra, I., *et al.* (2001). *Temas de Medicina General Integral.* (vol. 1 Salud y Medicina). La Habana: Editorial Ciencias Médicas.

Boelen, C. and Heck, J.E. (1995). *Defining and measuring the social accountability of medical schools,* WHO document WHO/HRH/957. Geneva: World Health Organization.

Brown, R.P.C. and Connell, J. (2004). The migration of doctors and nurses from south pacific island nations. *Social Science & Medicine,* **58**, 2193–210.

Comte, I.A. (1875). *System of positive polity* (vol. 1). London: Longmans, Green.

Contra Costa Health Service. Website, Martinez, CA. http://cchs.org/aboutus/missionstatement/20090927.en.html (accessed 27 September 2009).

Dovlo, D. (2003). *The Brain Drain and Retention of Health Professionals in Africa. Report to Regional Training Conference on Improving Tertiary Education in Sub-Saharan Africa: Things that work!* [Electronic version], Available at: http://medact.org/content/health/documents/brain_drain/Dovlo%20-%20brain%20drain%20and%20retention.pdf

Drain, P.K., Holmes, K.K., Skeff, K.M., Hall, T., and Gardner, P. (2009). Global health training and international rotations during residency: current status, needs, and opportunities. *Academic Medicine*, **84**, 320–5.

Editorial (1993). The overseas elective: purpose or picnic? *Lancet*, **342**, 753.

Feinsilver, J. (1993). *Healing the masses: Cuban health politics at home and abroad*. Berkeley, CA: University of California Press.

Goleman, D. (1995). *Emotional Intelligence*. New York: Bantam.

Huish, R. (2008a). Going where no doctor has gone before: The role of Cuba's Latin American School of Medicine in meeting the needs of some of the world's most vulnerable populations. *Public Health*, **122**, 552–7.

Huish, R. (2008b). "Going Where No Doctor Has Gone Before: The Place of Cuba's Latin American School of Medicine in Building Health Care Capacity for Ecuador" (Ph.D. Dissertation). Department of Geography, Simon Fraser University, Burnaby British Columbia, Canada.

Huish, R. (2009). How Cuba's Latin American School of Medicine challenges the ethics of physician migration. *Social Science and Medicine*, **69**, 301–4.

Huish, R. and Kirk, J.M. (2007). Cuban Medical Internationalism and the Development of the Latin American School of Medicine. *Latin American Perspectives*, **34**, 77–92.

Janca, A., Aarli, J.A., Prilipko, L., Dua, T., Saxena, S., and Saraceno, B. (2006). WHO/WFN Survey of neurological services: A worldwide perspective. *Journal of Neurological Sciences*, **247**, 29–34.

Johnston, S.C., Mendis, S., and Mathers, C.D. (2009). Global variation in stroke burden and mortality: estimates from modeling, surveillance, and modelling. *Lancet Neurology*, **8**, 345–54.

Kessler, R.C., Aguilar-Gaxiola, S., Alonso, J., *et al.* (2009). The global burden of mental disorders: an update from the WHO World Mental Health (WMH) surveys. *Epidemiologia e psichiatria sociale*, **18**, 23–33.

Kirk, J.M. and Erisman, M.H. (2009). *Cuban Medical Internationalism: Origins, Evolution and Goals*. New York: Palgrave Macmillan.

Labonte, R., Packer, C., Klassen, N., *et al.* (2006). *The Brain Drain of Health Professionals from Sub-Saharan Africa to Canada* (Vol. 2). Cape Town and Kingston: Idasa & Queen's University.

Mendonca, M. (2001). Preparing for ethical leadership in organizations. *Canadian Journal of Administrative Sciences*, **18**, 266–76.

Muntaner, C., Salazar, R.M.G., Rueda, S., and Armada, F. (2006). Challenging the neoliberal trend – The Venezuelan health care reform alternative. *Canadian Journal of Public Health-Revue Canadienne De Sante Publique*, **97**, I19–24.

Murray, C.J.L. and Lopez, A.D. (1996). *The Global Burden of Disease*. Boston, MA: Harvard School of Public Health.

Næss, A. (1989). *Ecology, Community and Lifestyle*. Cambridge: Cambridge University Press.

Paine, T. (1791). *Rights of Man*. London. Available at: http://www.ushistory.org/Paine/rights/singlehtml.htm

Pinto, A. and Upshur, R. (2009). Global Health Ethics for Students. *Developing World Bioethics*, **9**, 1–10.

Plamenatz, J. (1963). *Man and Society (vol. 1).* London: Longmans.

Pogge, T. (2008). *World Poverty and Human rights,* 2nd edn. Cambridge: Polity Press.

Project of the ABIM Foundation, ACP–ASIM Foundation, and European Federation of Internal Medicine (2002). Medical Professionalism in the New Millennium: A Physician Charter, *Annals of Internal Medicine,* **136,** 243–6.

Schrecker, T. and Labonté, R. (2007). "Globalization and Health Equity: Globalization and Health Equity: Investigating the Connections." Paper presented at the Basic Science Departments presentation to the Dean of Medicine, University of Ottawa.

Schuyler, G.W. (2002). Globalization and health: Venezuela and Cuba. *Canadian Journal of Development Studies-Revue Canadienne D Etudes Du Developpement,* **23,** 687–716.

Seed, J., Macy, J., Naess, A., and Fleming, P. (1988). *Thinking Like a Mountain: Towards a Council of All Beings.* Canada: New Society Press.

Rennie, S. and Mupenda, B. (2008). Living Apart Together: reflections on bioethics, global inequity and social justice. *Philosophy, Ethics, and Humanities in Medicine,* **3,** 25.

Taylor, C. (1992). *The Ethics of Authenticity.* Cambridge, MA: Harvard University Press.

Taylor, C.E. (1967). Ethics for an international health profession. *Science,* **153,** 716–20.

World Health Organization (2009). *Greater equity in health should be a progress indicator.* Availableat:http://www.who.int/mediacentre/news/releases/2009/health_policies_20090615/en/index.html (accessed 28 September, 2009).

Velji, A. and Bryant, J.H. (2007). Global health ethics. In W.H. Markle, M.A. Fisher, and R.A. Smego (eds.) *Understanding Global Health,* pp. 295–317. New York: McGraw Hill.

....

CHAPTER 50

ETHICAL PERSPECTIVES: CLINICAL DRUG TRIALS IN DEVELOPING COUNTRIES

....

CRAIG VAN DYKE

GLOBALIZATION

....

GLOBALIZATION, driven by the rapid spread of the Internet and mobile devices, has transformed the world's landscape. New technologies have allowed information to be transmitted across vast distances quickly, easily, and inexpensively and have facilitated capital flow, the spread of technology, and the transfer of goods and services across national boundaries. Globalization has increased economic growth in high-, middle-, and low-income countries and facilitated the emergence of powerful economic development, perhaps most noticeably in China and India, where a third of the world's population resides (Osland 2003). The expansion of the middle class population in low- and middle-income countries (LMICs) (i.e. developing countries) holds the potential for an increase in the marketing of consumer goods, especially products from high-income countries (HICs).

Concomitantly, globalization has led to ever widening social inequalities and has increased the disparity between the "haves" and "have-nots" and between those who are technologically enabled and those who are not (Frank and Cook 1995; Pritchett 1997). There are now substantial differences between the wealthiest individuals and the over one billion people living on less than a dollar per day (United Nations Development Programme 2001). In addition, the advent of rapid mass communication has raised concerns amongst social conservatives everywhere about the breakdown of local cultures and the creation of a worldwide monoculture. This may be counterbalanced, however, by the development of local or regional cultural media with indigenized program content. Accompanying this is a growing movement in many countries to maintain and promote ethnic identity (Osland 2003; Karliner 2008).

Moreover, the global economy and multinational corporations have become so powerful that they have altered the autonomy of countries by pushing for fewer barriers to trade and by altering many of the social structures that were traditionally supported by national governments (Cox 1996; Lee 1996, 1997; Champlin and Olsen 1999; Yergin and Stanislaw 2000). This inexorable spread of power from sovereign nationals and organized labor to global markets, international organizations, and multinational corporations has been accompanied by concerns about environmental contamination, global warming, and human rights abuses (Lechner and Boli 2000). In 1999 then UN Secretary General, Kofi Annan, expressed it this way:

> The spread of markets outpaces the ability of societies and their political systems to adjust to them, let alone to guide the course they take. History teaches us that such an imbalance between economic, social and political worlds can never be sustained for very long. (Annan 1999)

Two of the processes that have pushed the spread of multinational enterprises are "outsourcing" and "offshoring." In *The World is Flat*, Thomas Friedman writes:

> Outsourcing means taking some specific, but limited, function that your company was doing in-house – such as research, call centers, or accounts receivable – and having another company perform that exact same function for you and then reintegrating their work back into your overall operation. Offshoring, by contrast, is when a company takes one of its factories that it is operating in Canton, Ohio, and moves the whole factory offshore to Canton, China. There, it produces the very same product in the very same way, only with cheaper labor, lower taxes, subsidized energy, and lower health-care costs. (Friedman 2005)

This chapter addresses the expansion of clinical trials to the developing world as part of the globalization process. The opportunity to reduce costs with less expensive labor and to access patient populations in developing countries was the initial motivation for offshoring clinical trials. As the enterprise has grown the complexity of the ethical issues has become more apparent. Clinical trials of medications and procedures for neuropsychiatric conditions raise particular ethical concerns, especially protecting vulnerable subjects in developing countries during the consent process. However, the most critical ethical issue is ensuring that clinical trials in these countries are relevant to the population being studied. Focusing on this issue provides an opportunity for improving health care in LMICs.

THE GLOBALIZATION OF THE PHARMACEUTICAL INDUSTRY

There are several reasons behind the pharmaceutical industry's expansion to the developing world. First is the size of the potential marketplace. At present, the industry has annual revenues of $770 billion (approximately 8% of the total represents central nervous system medications), which have largely been generated in HICs. However, this pattern may be changing, since several pharmaceutical companies now view LMICs as a potential cure for diminishing sales. For the first time in over 50 years, sales of prescription medications are forecast to decline in the US. While the US remains the most profitable market, the expiration of patents (70% of prescriptions in the US are for generics) and healthcare reform are threatening profits and there is a push for examining LMICs as a source to supplement profits for the pharmaceutical industry. The sales of prescription drugs in emerging markets rose to US $153 billion in 2008 which represents a marked increase from the US $67 billion in 2003. It is anticipated that by 2013 this figure will be US $265 billion (Di Masi *et al.* 2003; Adams and Brantner 2006; Garnier 2008; Boguski *et al.* 2009; Johnson 2009; Okie 2009).

Previously in LMICs, sales efforts focused on the wealthy and middle class, but now there is an increasing emphasis on marketing medications to the "bottom of the pyramid." Because patented medications are perceived as safer and more effective than generics, they are often thought to be worth the extra premium. In many developing countries generic drugs do not face stringent requirements to be the equivalent of brand name versions. In fact, the World Health Organization (WHO) estimates that up to 25% of all medications sold in low-income countries are counterfeit and may be quite ineffective. This is now a growing concern in HICs where the quality of generic drugs is coming under increased scrutiny, since they may include chemicals originating in places with uncertain quality control procedures and safeguards (Okie 2009).

The second reason for global expansion is the financial advantage of outsourcing and off-shoring clinical trials to LMICs (U.S. Food and Drug Administration 2007). For each drug that is successfully developed many more are eliminated at different stages of development because of toxicity or ineffectiveness. Including the research and developmental expenses of failed drugs, the pharmaceutical industry expends approximately US $1 billion for each drug that makes it to market. These costs are increasing at about 7% per year above inflation (Di Masi *et al.* 2003; Adams and Brantner 2006; Garnier 2008; Boguski *et al.* 2009). Approximately two-thirds of this expense is the cost of clinical trials and by moving these studies offshore, expenses can be reduced by 30–50% (Sinha 2004; Rai 2005; Duley *et al.* 2008; Bailey *et al.* 2009).

As one measure of this shift to developing countries, the number of clinical investigators in the US decreased by 5.5% annually since 2006. In contrast, the number of US Food and Drug Administration (FDA) registered principal investigators not located in the US or Western Europe increased from 5% of all registered investigators in 1997 to 29% in 2007. India, China, Russia, and Argentina had the most rapid growth (Schmidt 2001; Getz 2007; Jack 2008; Theirs *et al.* 2008).

In addition to financial considerations, other factors have driven the migration of clinical trials to developing countries. One is access to millions of potential patients/subjects, many of whom are treatment naïve. By residing in LMICs, these individuals frequently have not had ready access to diagnosis and treatment. As a consequence, each trial site may have access to a large number of potential subjects allowing more rapid recruitment. Phase 3 trials can be completed sooner and drugs can be brought to market more rapidly (Jack 2008; Bailey *et al.* 2009).

This is in contrast to the US and Europe where there may be competition for subjects, many of whom have already received treatment and may include a disproportionate number of individuals who are refractory to treatment. Furthermore, patients in HICs may be reluctant to participate in clinical trials, preferring to access standardized care. Conducting clinical trials in HICs frequently requires enrolling a small number of subjects at multiple sites to achieve the required number. The lack of economy of scale along with high labor costs increases expenses significantly (Schmidt 2001; Getz 2007; Jack 2008; Theirs *et al.* 2008).

There are also advantages for pharmaceutical companies to conduct trials in multiple countries simultaneously. By doing so data may be forwarded to regulating agencies simultaneously rather than sequentially. Conducting trials in multiple countries may facilitate the creation of new commercial markets, since it is not uncommon for regulating agencies in developing countries to require testing on their population. Seasonal patterns of certain infectious diseases can allow drugs to be tested year round on a global scale and expedite the time to market for a new medication (Schmidt 2001; U.S. Department of Health and Human Services 2001).

There are also unique scientific opportunities for conducting clinical trials in LMICs. Longitudinal data sets may be available in certain LMICs that do not exist in HICs. The genetic makeup of certain populations in LMICs may provide valuable information about the efficacy or toxicity of drugs that would be difficult or impossible to evaluate in populations residing in HICs (Seitz *et al.* 2001; Goldstein *et al.* 2003; Larson *et al.* 2007; Jack 2008). For example, gefitinib, a drug used for the treatment of lung cancer, failed to win approval in the West but was found to be more effective in Asian populations and is marketed in China and Japan (Jack 2008; Mok *et al.* 2009). Conversely, one emerging factor that may slow the expansion of trials to offshore sites is concern about the generalizability of information on the efficacy and safety of a particular medication that is evaluated in a LMIC population and used in a HIC. This is likely to be more of an issue in the future as emphasis shifts to personalized medicine and the use of genetic markers to stratify smaller groups of patients (Goldstein *et al.* 2003; Jack 2008; Boguski *et al.* 2009; Garbar and Tunis 2009).

Contract research organizations

Over the past 50–60 years, there has been an increasing necessity to employ randomized clinical trials (RCTs) with a large number of subjects to demonstrate effectiveness. As trials moved from infectious diseases with large effect size (significant decrease in death rate) to chronic illnesses with more modest treatment effects, an increased number of subjects was required to provide adequate statistical power. While controversial, the latest trend pushing the need for large study populations is the pressure for comparative-effectiveness research to demonstrate that an experimental treatment is better, safer, or more cost effective than a standard treatment (Garber and Tunis 2009; Naik and Petersen 2009; Zhang 2009). Being better than a placebo is less compelling where an effective treatment already exists, and it is often considered to be unethical as well (Angell 1997; Lurie and Wolfe 1997; Varmus and Satcher 1997; Annas and Grodin 1998; Shapiro and Meslin 2001; Council for International Organizations of Medical Sciences 2002; Steiner 2007, 2008; Glass 2008, 2008). It should be noted, however, that not all standard treatments have been tested for safety and effectiveness (Califf 2005; Nissen and Wolski 2007; Garber 2009; Zhang 2009).

To cope with the complexities of clinical trials, the pharmaceutical and medical device companies have progressively outsourced these functions. Originally trials were conducted largely by academic institutions, but over time, contract research organizations (CROs) have risen to prominence because of greater efficiency and now dominate the clinical trials field. CROs offer many advantages for the pharmaceutical industry. They specialize in clinical trials and have the potential for standardizing practices across countries. They often have expertise in conducting trials in a particular country with staff that speak the language, are familiar with the culture, and know the local rules and regulations. There were more than 1000 CROs with gross revenues of US $17.8 billion in 2007. Each of the four largest had greater than US $1 billion in annual revenues. The next two largest, had greater than US $0.5 billion in annual revenue. In 2004 the 10 largest CROs had enrolled 640,000 subjects in clinical trials (Schmidt 2001; Di Masi *et al.* 2003; Rowland 2004; Shuchman 2007).

MORAL IMPERATIVE FOR CONDUCTING CLINICAL TRIALS IN DEVELOPING COUNTRIES

Separate from financial and business considerations, clinical trials offer the prospect of improving the health status of the population in developing countries. For this to occur the intervention being evaluated must have relevance to the population being studied and be available after the trial is completed. Failure to meet these criteria represents exploitation of the LMIC population in the service of HICs (Angell 1997; Lurie and Wolfe 1997; Varmus and Satcher 1997; Annas and Grodin 1998; Council for International Organizations of Medical Sciences 2002; Killen *et al.* 2002; Jack 2008).

There are several challenges in meeting these goals. First is that the diseases and medications under study are frequently not chosen by the developing country and often do not represent local priorities (Duley *et al.* 2008). For example, it is estimated that of all the drugs developed in the past quarter century only 1% were for tropical diseases (Nundy *et al.* 2005). However, many endemic diseases in developing countries may not present a sufficient market to attract the attention of pharmaceutical industry based in HICs. Nevertheless, there is a moral imperative to address the imbalance when 90% of research expenditures are for medications for the richest 10% of the world's population (Nuffield Council on Bioethics 1999; Global Forum for Health Research 2000; Shapiro and Meslin 2001). Other barriers to making medications available to the broader population are the meager and insufficient healthcare budget in many LMICs and the limited healthcare delivery system. While it might be reasonable to expect the pharmaceutical industry to fund treatment for the study population after completion of the study, it is often times unrealistic to expect them to fund this care indefinitely for the entire population of the LMIC. To ensure handoff to the health sector, governments and foundations must intervene (Council for International Organizations of Medical Sciences 2002; Jack 2008).

CHALLENGES FOR CONDUCTING CLINICAL TRIALS IN DEVELOPING COUNTRIES

Many challenges relate to the implementation of clinical research in LMICs. These include: lack of trained or licensed clinical research personnel, inadequate clinic or hospital infrastructure, absent or poorly staffed and trained institutional review boards (IRBs), absent monitoring, restrictive laws, administrative and bureaucratic delays, conflicts of interest, and both language and cultural barriers (Nuffield Council on Bioethics 1999; Srinivasan and Loff 2006; Abbas 2007; U.S. Department of Health and Human Services 2007; Duley *et al.* 2008; Zhang *et al.* 2008). Of particular concern to the pharmaceutical industry is that in many LMICs there may not be exclusive rights to the clinical data that is generated. Rather trial reports may be part of the public domain and can serve as a basis for generic drug manufacturers to bring their version of the drug to market (Nundy *et al.* 2005).

Furthermore, certain countries have made it difficult for pharmaceutical companies to patent medications unless they are truly new or for new indications (Whalen and Greil, 2009). This has been incorporated into national law in some cases so that companies cannot patent new versions of older drugs unless they offer significantly better efficacy. Such laws have limited "me too" drugs (the FDA estimates only 20% of drugs are breakthrough agents) that either extend the patent life or allow a company to enter a proven market. It permits less expensive generic medication to compete in the marketplace with lower costs and greater accessibility (Nundy *et al.* 2005; Psaty and Charo 2007).

INFORMED CONSENT

Beginning with the doctors' component of the Nuremberg War Trials one of the core principles of human experiments is that subjects must provide informed consent. This has been both refined and reinforced with the Declaration of Helsinki, the Belmont Report, and more recently by the International Conference on Harmonization (ICH), which emerged from European countries wanting to standardize regulations for the pharmaceutical industry (Trials of War Criminals before the Nuremberg Military Tribunals under Control Council Law No. Ten 1949; The National Commission for the Protection of Human Subjects of Biomedical and Behavioral Research 1979; Schmidt 2001; U.S. Department of Health and Human Services 2001; Council for International Organizations of Medical Sciences 2002; Jack 2008; World Medical Association 2008; Annas 2009). The Belmont Report emphasized three ethical principles, namely respect for the research subject, beneficence for society, and justice towards subjects (i.e. equal access to participation and equal treatment). Key elements include informed consent, impartial selection of subjects, and risk/benefit analysis. (The history of human research regulation is nicely summarized by Howland in 2008.)

Inherent in informed consent is the assumption that subjects have sufficient decisional capacity. There are several elements in decisional capacity, namely understanding the provided information, appreciating its significance, using the information in reasoning, and having the ability to express a choice (Dunn *et al.* 2006). This capacity may be limited in subjects with dementia or psychiatric illnesses (Fisk 2007; Palmer *et al.* 2007). There are many factors that need to be weighed during the assessment of capacity and there is no simple method for determining it (Dunn *et al.* 2007; Jacob and Chowdhury 2009). Where there are serious concerns about a subject's ability to understand and appreciate the risks and benefits of a particular study, participation by a family member or caregiver in the consent process is often required. It should be noted, however, that the legal status of proxy or surrogate consent is poorly defined in both HICs and LMICs (Kim *et al.* 2004).

In addition, subjects must be free of undue or coercive influences and provide a voluntary consent (Dunn *et al.* 2007). The latter issue can be quite subtle and complex in LMICs where individuals may be placed in a vulnerable position by dint of the economic power of multinational pharmaceutical enterprises and by the educational and economic differential with the clinical investigators (Angell 1997; Nuffield Council on Bioethics 1999). In this context, vulnerability represents a threat to self-determination and equality that exists independent of research. In such situations individuals may think they will receive special consideration if they participate or will be subject to discrimination if they do not. Decisions are often deferred to more powerful authorities (Eckenweiler 2001; Council for International Organizations of Medical Sciences 2002; London 2002; Rowland 2004; Hill *et al.* 2006; Malhotra and Subodh 2009). Whenever vulnerability exists, it is incumbent on investigators to take the necessary steps to protect potential subjects during the consent process.

As one example of vulnerability, can informed consent validly exist in a country with little if any healthcare services? In these situations, individuals may feel compelled to participate in a study regardless of its risks as a preferable alternative to being without healthcare altogether. It is extremely difficult for a clinical trial to be conducted in this setting in a way that allows individuals not to feel overly enticed into participating (Annas and Grodin 1998; Hutton 2000; London 2002; Hill *et al.* 2008).

Certain segments of the population may be particularly vulnerable. Children are always vulnerable, but in certain countries the authority of the parent is absolute, and it may be impossible for children to develop and assert their own opinion about participation. Likewise, women are often socially conditioned to submit to authority, accept pain, and not ask questions. Being impoverished makes one extremely vulnerable. What might appear to investigators as a small sum of money for participating in a study can represent a substantial sum and be extraordinarily persuasive. Therefore, there may be direct and indirect coercion due to financial payments for conducting studies with the money being paid either to subjects and patients directly or to governments, institutes, and hospitals. Individuals who are illiterate or have little education are also extremely vulnerable during the consent process. Where education is lacking there may be great disparities between local concepts of health and disease and scientific understanding and practices. Issues such as the randomization process and use of placebo may be very difficult to communicate and have understood. In the developing world, seriously mentally ill individuals are often placed in asylums, chained or caged, socially isolated and subject to other abuses (Council for International Organizations of Medical Sciences 2002; Nundy *et al.* 2005; Smith-Tyler 2007; Hill *et al.* 2008; Kleinman, 2009; Malhotra and Subodh 2009). Because of these extreme circumstances, alternative psychiatric populations should be sought for study.

One of the critical precepts on which informed consent rests is the assumption of patient autonomy. These issues and rights have been well developed in Western countries. This does not hold true for much of the world where the values of families, communities, and the larger society may take precedent over that of individual rights and autonomy. For example, China's long tradition of medical ethics, based in Confucianism, often leads to considerable differences between Western and Chinese clinical ethical practice. In China, individuals are considered to be embedded in the greater context of family and society. It is quite common that when an individual contracts an illness that has serious prognostic implications the family is informed, and it is left to them to make a determination about informing the patient. This practice may further isolate the patient.

One very controversial area of neuropsychiatric research is deep brain stimulation (DBS) for disorders of mood, behavior, and thought (MBT). It is controversial because of the problematic history of psychosurgery, the perception that neuropsychiatric patients are vulnerable, the concerns that DBS may alter an individual's personality or identity, and the risk of an invasive surgical procedure. A recent consensus conference on this issue made a number of recommendations about future research (Rabins *et al.* 2009). The conference supported future research and emphasized that DBS was at an early-proof-of-principle stage and had to be considered investigational. Of relevance to our discussion, it was recommended that DBS for MBT required a multidisciplinary team (i.e. neurologists, neurosurgeons, psychiatrists, neuropsychologists, bioethicists, and case managers), an independently reviewed research protocol, subjects to be adults and thoroughly evaluated, and subjects be followed for 5–15 years. Given the sensitivity surrounding the procedure, the conference recommended that an IRB approved assessment of the subject's capacity be utilized as part of the consent process. An additional recommendation was that the patient's caregiver or partner ("a close third") participate and witness the provision of information and the consent process.

Given its controversial nature and the extensive resources required to evaluate and treat patients with DBS, conducting such trials in LMICs will be extremely challenging. Moreover, the relevance of this procedure for populations in the developing world is highly questionable. Can DBS be a priority in countries struggling to provide basic neurologic and mental health care?

Genomic studies in LMICs raise particular concerns. One key issue is how genetic material will be handled downstream from the specific trial, particularly the possibility of performing studies on human tissue beyond the scope of the original consent. It is also of concern that political or tribal leaders might consent for an entire population without gaining individual consent (Council for International Organizations of Medical Sciences 2002; Smith-Tyler 2007). This has raised questions about the rights to profits and the commercial development of products. Should individuals or governments be entitled to share in future product revenues? It may be particularly difficult for vulnerable individuals and populations to pursue their rights, because of insufficient economic, legal, and political resources. When should the issue of potential commercial rights be raised? At the beginning of the study, such information might be coercive, especially for the impoverished, and lead individuals or populations to agree to studies that they might otherwise not agree to. However, failing to raise it may lead to mistrust at a later date (Ellerin *et al.* 2005).

What are possible solutions to the problems of informed consent outlined earlier? Brody (2001) argues that informed consent procedures have failed because it is seen as a basic right and not as a value. More emphasis has been placed on conveying information and making sure the subject understands what is being conveyed than on working with the individual to help them form an autonomous decision. To do this requires an ongoing dialogue where interactive questioning between investigators and potential subjects can improve understanding (Palmer *et al.* 2008). It is a process and not an event. How else can this capacity be developed and built? How can vulnerable individuals become empowered as agents of their own welfare to be able to take the initiative and organize their own health ethical review? Even the best IRBs in LMICs are placed in very difficult positions in terms of balancing both the legislative and ethical issues in the context of cultural, educational, and language differences (London 2002; Nundy *et al.* 2005).

It is no wonder that IRBs frequently revert to focusing on issues of informed consent documentation and legal issues since documentation is easier and addresses accountability and concerns about financial or legal penalties (London 2002). In addition, the sponsors of clinical trials and the investigators may be caught between meeting the provisions and standards of HICs and addressing ethical issues and local cultural traditions. At its worst, a strict constructionist approach to meeting the letter of the law from HICs, complete with multi-page consent forms, may confuse and overwhelm potential subjects and be entirely inappropriate given local practices and cultural values (Duley *et al.* 2008). This approach is often more concerned with protecting the investigator and sponsor than the subject (London 2002).

In these circumstances, it is often the best that IRBs can do, to make the values, pressures, and requirements of the different stakeholders explicit and transparent. Ways of doing this include making IRB deliberations public and transparent, expanding the IRB membership to include members of the population being studied, and to work vigorously to educate the community, local government and national government about the issues involved in the study (Hutton 2000; Council for International Organizations of Medical Sciences 2002; London 2002; Stough *et al.* 2007; Hill *et al.* 2008; Jaspan *et al.* 2008; Sumathipala *et al.* 2008). As one example of the barriers that must be overcome to increase transparency and cultural sensitivity there is often reluctance to include members of the study population at the same table as scientists and policy makers, particularly if subjects are from stigmatized or devalued groups (e.g. mentally ill individuals, intravenous drug users, or commercial sex workers).

Given these considerations, it is easy to understand the challenges and the time and effort required for both investigator and subject in a vulnerable population to achieve informed consent. It is not surprising that when tested at later dates, subjects have significant gaps in their knowledge and understanding of key elements of the study in which they are participating (Hill *et al.* 2008).

Conflict of interest

Conflict of interest policies are intended to prevent bias and should be forward looking (Steinbrook 2009a). There have been many instances where profit motive, desire for professional advancement, or favors to family and friends have created undue influence and bias in investigators and educators. This has undermined public trust and distorted the practice of medicine and medical education (Armstrong 2009; Kaiser 2009). One of the fundamental approaches to conflict of interest policy has been the disclosure of financial interests (Okike *et al.* 2009; Steinbrook 2009b, c). However, this does not necessarily address the question of bias or eliminate undue influence.

Under external pressure from governments and NGOs, a number of pharmaceutical companies now either voluntarily disclose payments to physicians and medical investigators or do so as the result of legal settlements. In addition, certain states (e.g. Massachusetts) now require this disclosure. There is a nascent movement to standardize the format for reporting activities for which medical investigators are being reimbursed (Steinbrook 2009b, c). For example, the International Committee of Medical Journal Editors has recently adopted a uniform disclosure form (Drazen *et al.* 2009). Four types of information are required: (1) support by commercial entities for the work reported, (2) associations with commercial organizations that might have an interest in the area reported in the manuscript, (3) spouse or children less than 18 years old who have similar financial associations, and (4) non-financial interests that have relevance to the manuscript.

Several analyses indicate that industry sponsored studies are much more likely to have a positive outcome than trials supported by other organizations (Bekelman *et al.* 2003; Lexchin *et al.* 2003; Tungaraza and Poole 2007). This is in part because pharmaceutical companies are unlikely to bear the expense of clinical trials they judge as unlikely to succeed. In addition, selective publication, that favors positive results, can produce unrealistic estimates of the effectiveness of drugs and can distort judgments about their cost/benefit ratio (Turner *et al.* 2009; Vedula *et al.* 2009). There is evidence that not all clinical trials are published (Schmidt 2001; Whittington *et al.* 2004; Kyzas *et al.* 2005; Adams and Brantner 2006; Turner *et al.* 2008). Reasons for this are many, including methodological flaws, manuscripts that were not submitted because authors and sponsors failed to do so, and journal editors, who decided not to publish them. However, it is unfair and potentially a breach of contract to expose subjects to risk during clinical trials that do not lead to publication. Failure to publish (especially negative studies) may lead to studies being repeated and placing subjects at risk unnecessarily (Schulman *et al.* 2002).

While all of these issues apply equally well to developing countries, they are likely to have fewer safeguards to prevent potential conflicts of interest. Government regulation, laws, and monitoring may be weak or absent, professional organizations less well developed, medical schools may have fewer resources to devote to the teaching of ethics, and often there is the absence of whistle-blowing laws or a free press. What are the requirements for financial disclosure in developing countries? What are the reporting requirements for physicians and clinical investigators in developing countries? If an adverse event occurs, is it reported to the sponsor or to regulating agencies? This last issue has been quite controversial in HICs and is likely to be equally problematic in developing countries (Schafer 2004).

Whistle-blowing protection laws in certain HICs represent another safeguard and non-systematic monitoring system. In the US, federal whistle-blowing laws not only protect the individual bringing the complaint against retaliation and retribution, but they also financially incentivize individuals to file complaints by allowing them to share in funds that are recovered by the government. Quite often the whistleblower is a member of an organization, who possesses privileged information. For instance, a recent civil complaint unsealed by the US Department of Justice alleged that one drug was illegally marketed in pediatric patients when it was approved only for adults. Of relevance to our discussion, the company is accused by one of its former employees of promoting positive results of a US study while not disclosing a negative study in Europe (Kaplan 2009).

The potential for misconduct in clinical trials in LMICs exists just as it does in HICs, but the absence of whistle-blowing laws in most developing countries is one less defense against such abuses. In countries that lack such legal protections, it is practically impossible and potentially dangerous for an individual citizen to mount a complaint about exploitation, abuse, or misrepresentation of information by CROs, academic institutions, government agencies, foundations, or pharmaceutical or medical device companies.

Another safeguard, again seldom discussed in this context, is the power of a free press. Shining the media spotlight on abusive practices can be an effective deterrent. For instance, in Ireland and the Netherlands adverse publicity either prevented the opening of commercial stem cell clinics or resulted in closing them. This has not occurred in certain LMICs (e.g. India and Thailand) where "stem cell tourism" is flourishing (Jayaraman 2005; Boseley 2006; The Netherlands Health Care Inspectorate 2006; Ebbin 2007; Price 2007; Royal Gazette 2008; Kiatpongsan and Sipp 2009). Another concern is countries with government censorship of the press. In these settings it is likely that many aspects of the clinical trials process will lack transparency and as a result protections and safeguards for human subjects will be compromised.

MONITORING AND TRANSPARENCY OF RESULTS

From the sheer size of the industry, number of trials, locations, countries, and IRBs it is obvious that monitoring and regulating it is a challenge (U.S. Department of Health and Human Services 2007). Most countries do not have the equivalent of the FDA. If they do, it is often understaffed and lacks the expertise to evaluate protocols and the resources to monitor and enforce regulations (Nundy *et al.* 2005). Because of this, the FDA serves as the *de facto* drug regulating agency for much of the developing world since most drugs are marketed in the US. The FDA is concerned with the integrity of the data and protection of human subjects. As such, foreign investigators are required by the FDA to sign attestations of intent to comply with ethical guidelines if their studies are to serve as a basis for FDA review (U.S. Department of Health and Human Services 2001).

However, the FDA, with limited resources, faces an enormous task in regulating products that represent 25% of US GDP. As just one example of the magnitude of the problem, there are currently 6,350 IRBs registered with the Department of Health and Human Services (Mundy 2009). While the FDA is able to inspect approximately 1% of clinical trial sites each year, its ability to inspect sites in non-US jurisdictions is severely constrained by legal issues, logistics, budgetary restrictions, language barriers, and a host of other problems (Psaty and Charo 2007; U.S. Food and Drug Administration 2007). The FDA is taking steps to increase inspections of non-U.S. sites, but the challenges in doing so are significant (Shuchman 2007; Okie 2009). As a result FDA oversight occurs primarily before a study starts by reviewing the qualifications of the investigators and the quality and safety of the protocol. There is much less monitoring and surveillance once a study is underway (U.S. Department of Health and Human Services 2007).

The FDA is particularly challenged in post-approval powers to maintain surveillance of medications that expand to the care of the general public. The main component of this is the Adverse Event Reporting System (AERS) which collects information on suspected cases but represents a relatively weak and non-systematic surveillance system. This should improve dramatically with the Sentinel Initiative that will provide electronic post-marketing surveillance on 100 million people starting in 2012 (Platt *et al.* 2009). Post-marketing commitments made by sponsors (i.e. phase 4 studies) are another form of post-approval surveillance; however, the completion rate for these studies has decreased dramatically. All of these issues are particularly critical for LMIC populations where post-approval surveillance is even weaker or entirely absent (Nuffield Council on Bioethics 1999; Psaty and Charo 2007; Avron and Schneeweiss 2009; Boguski *et al.* 2009; Okie 2009).

There are also increasing requirements for clinical trials to be included in one or more registries that are part of the public domain and electronically searchable (Laine *et al.* 2007; Theirs *et al.* 2008). The largest registry, http://www.ClinicalTrials.gov, had 67,000 registered trials by early 2009. Often these registries contain information about the trial methods but much less information about results. Outcome results are considered confidential in order to protect intellectual property rights (Kesselheim and Mello 2007; Wood 2009). However, arguments in support of keeping safety information confidential are less compelling and in the US there are challenges to this through the Freedom of Information Act (Turner 2004; Kesselheim and Mello 2007). The FDA requires trials to be registered, including results, and the International Committee of Journal Editors requires this for manuscripts submitted for publication (Schulman *et al.* 2002; International Committee of Medical Journal Editors 2007, 2008; Laine *et al.* 2007). Even with more transparency, populations in developing countries may be disadvantaged in accessing this information because of low literacy rates, language barriers, and limited access to the Internet (Nundy *et al.* 2005). In such settings it is critical that sponsors and investigators bring all available information to the attention of potential subjects (Lenzer 2005; Avron and Schneeweiss 2009; Schwartz and Woloshin 2009).

Future considerations

The overriding challenge for the ethics of clinical trials in developing countries is to link them directly to improving the health status of the population being studied. Responding to the moral imperative requires that a greater proportion of research expenditures be devoted to addressing the specific health needs of LMICs. It is not morally justifiable that 90% of research expenditures are targeted to the medical problems of the wealthiest 10% of the world's population. Clinical drug trials in developing countries must evaluate the effectiveness and safety of products that are relevant to the population being studied. Realistic plans to provide these treatments to the entire population if the study is successful need to be in place before the study is implemented (Council for International Organizations of Medical Sciences 2002).

If such a commitment were to be made by governments, academic institutions, the pharmaceutical industry, international health organizations, and foundations, it would change the entire ethical dynamic. The focus of discussion would no longer include concerns about protecting vulnerable populations from being exploited by HICs. Rather, discussions could concentrate on the potential risks and benefits of the study in the population being studied. To accomplish this requires an active effort of engaging the population being considered for study in a process to define their health needs and empowering them to participate in the process to find solutions (Rudan *et al.* 2007; Tomlinson *et al.* 2009). This requires relationship building and the development of mutual respect and trust. It is best achieved in the context of a long-term relationship.

Furthermore, it seems reasonable to develop pathways for sponsors of externally driven clinical trials to contribute to LMIC infrastructure. This would reflect a true partnership in developing sound priority setting, procedures, and capacity. Examples of such efforts include training personnel in clinical research methods and research administration. Modest training efforts are underway, but much more needs to be done. Training IRB leadership through courses of instruction and scholarships to visit model IRBs in other settings needs to be a priority. Working with IRB leadership to identify and address specific issues relevant to the vulnerabilities of their populations in the consent process is another priority. A neglected area is training personnel in LMIC academic institutions to administer clinical research grants and contracts and to understand the organizational structures required to ensure the integrity of the process. Working to standardize rules and regulations across countries would simplify training, regularize ethical practices and lower costs (Schulman *et al.* 2002; Yusuf 2004; Dilts and Sandler 2006; Duley *et al.* 2008; Eisenstein *et al.* 2008).

Glickman and others (2009) recommend increasing use of centralized IRBs. There is much to recommend with this approach since centralized IRBs are in a better position to evaluate scientific merit, research methods, and the qualifications of investigators. They can also provide uniform practices and standards. However, they may not necessarily be in a good position to offer an understanding of local culture and what adjustments are required for a trial to be ethical in a particular setting. One way to address this is to pair centralized IRBs with local IRBs that have membership of the populations being studied (Council for International Organizations of Medical Sciences 2002).

Another complexity requiring attention is that authorities responsible for the delivery of health services, the education and training of health professionals, the development of science and technology, and the safeguarding of human rights in LMICs are often in separate governmental structures. For example, there may be separate ministries of health, education, and science and technology. Clinical trials will benefit from efforts to establish close collaboration through joint sponsorship of programs and activities across these structures.

One encouraging factor is the growth and development of a broadly based pharmaceutical effort in middle income countries such as India and China. This represents a combination of multinational pharmaceutical enterprises and the development of national enterprises that are investing in both basic and applied research (Johnson and Whalen 2009). It is reasonable to anticipate that this trend will expand to other LMICs over the next few decades. To be successful, these efforts will need to develop treatments for endemic diseases and to be responsive to the health requirements of the local population.

A recent IOM report recommends that ethics should be taught in US professional schools and that the medical profession address this as a fundamental form of self-regulation (Institute of Medicine 2009; Steinbrook 2009a). This is consistent with a recent meeting between the Chinese Association of Science and Technology and American Association for the Advancement of Science on research ethics. Although not focused on clinical trials, it identified certain potential projects to address misconduct in research. These included: (1) misconduct surveys, (2) exchange programs on training ethics educators, (3) compiling case studies of ethical misconduct, and (4) developing a guidebook on ethics in science. It was in response to a relatively high percentage of scientists in both countries, who engage in either misconduct or have little if any education in research ethics (Lempinen 2009).

One extremely important issue relates to the governance of the entire enterprise. Issues of concern include the transparency of the process and trial results, the rights and jurisdictions of the many different stakeholders, and the basis for regulation and enforcement. Electronic registries of trials are a major step forward, but more can be done to ensure all trials are included and to standardize reporting requirements. Who will fund the maintenance of these databases? What are the rights of investigators to access the data of a clinical trial and to publish the results, including adverse events and negative outcomes (Drazen 2002; Schulman *et al.* 2002; International Committee of Medical Journal Editors 2007)? How are the intellectual property rights of commercial enterprises balanced against the needs of developing country health care needs? What are the financial and legal rights of individuals in developing countries, who suffer adverse outcomes as a result of trial participation (Nuffield Council on Bioethics 1999)?

Much of the responsibility for these issues rests with the pharmaceutical industry, CROs, academic institutions, local and national governments, IRBs, journal editors, and many others. But to the extent clinical trials occur in multiple countries and there are power differentials between HICs (and their multinational enterprises) and LMICs, it calls for international organizations to increase their involvement. Possibilities include the WHO, United Nations, World Bank or the World Trade Organization.

CONCLUSION

Driven initially by the need to reduce costs and the potential to access subject populations, the pharmaceutical enterprise has greatly expanded the number of clinical trials in LMICs. At the same time, this expansion has facilitated the development of new commercial markets and presented unique scientific opportunities.

However, as the number and complexity of clinical trials has grown, the challenges have become more apparent. Challenges include: poorly trained personnel, insufficient medical infrastructure, inadequate institutional review boards, lack of monitoring, conflicts of interest, and many ethical issues, especially protecting the rights of vulnerable populations during the informed consent process. Just as in HICs, special precautions are required when obtaining informed consent from those with dementia or serious mental illness. However, there is the added burden in LMICs of protecting those who are vulnerable as the result of minimal education, limited literacy, extreme poverty, inadequate health care, and marked social inequalities for women, children, and ethnic minorities.

Of particular ethical concern is that many of the trials being conducted do not reflect the health priorities of the population being studied. This practice often represents exploitation of LMIC populations by HICs and is not morally justified. It is one obvious manifestation of the 90/10 gap, namely 90% of health research expenditures are targeted to the problems of the wealthiest 10% of the world's population. Correcting this inequity is the overriding ethical priority. To effect this requires an active engagement of the LMIC population in defining their health needs and finding potential solutions. HICs can also play a critical role in helping the developing world build their clinical research capacity. Such efforts offer the very real prospect of improving healthcare in the developing world.

REFERENCES

Abbas, E.E. (2007). Industry-sponsored research in developing countries. *Contemporary Clinical Trials*, **28**, 677–83.

Adams, C.P. and Brantner, V.V. (2006). Estimating the cost of new drug development: is it really $802 million? *Health Affairs*, **25**, 420–8.

Angell, M. (1997). The ethics of clinical research in the Third World. *New England Journal of Medicine*, **337**, 847–9.

Annan, K. (1999). *Address to Davos World Economic Forum, Davos, Switzerland* (31 January 1999) Available at: http://www.un.org/News/ossg/sg/stories/statments_search_full.asp?statID=22 (accessed 6 March 2009).

Annas, G.J. (2009). Globalized clinical trials and informed consent. *New England Journal of Medicine*, 360, 2050–3.

Annas, G.J. and Grodin, M.A. (1998). Human rights and maternal-fetal HIV transmission prevention trials in Africa. *American Journal of Public Health*, 88, 560–3.

Armstrong, D. (2009). New conflict rules at medical journals. *The Wall Street Journal*, 14 October, 2009.

Avorn, J. and Schneeweiss, S. (2009). Managing drug-risk information – what to do with all those new numbers. *New England Journal of Medicine*, 361, 647–9.

Bailey W., Cruickshank, C., and Sharma, N. *Make your move: taking clinical trials to the best location.* Available at: http://www.atkearney.com/main.taf?p=5,1,1,116,3,1/ (accessed 30 October 2009).

Bekelman, J.E., Li, Y., and Gross, P.C. (2003). Scope and impact of financial conflict of interest in biomedical research. A systematic review. *Journal of the American Medical Association*, 289, 454–65.

Boguski, M.S., Mandl, K.D. and Sukhatme, V.P. (2009). Repurposing with a difference. *Science*, 324, 1394–5.

Boseley, S. (2006). Stem cell firm uses Swansea ferry to evade Irish block on controversial treatment. *The Guardian*, 1 May. Available at: http://www.guardian.co.uk/society/2006/may/01/health.medicineandhealth (accessed 6 March 2009).

Brody, B.A. (2001). Making informed consent meaningful. *IRB*, 23, 1–5.

Califf, R.M. (2005). Simple principles of clinical trials remain powerful. *Journal of the American Medical Association*, 293, 489–91.

Champlin, D. and Olson, P. (1999). The impact of globalization on U.S. labor markets: redefining the debate. *Journal of Economic Issues*, 33, 443–51.

Cox, R.W. (1996). A perspective on globalization. In J.H. Mittelman (ed.) *Globalization: Critical reflections*, pp. 21–30. Boulder, CO: Lynne Rienner.

Council for International Organizations of Medical Sciences. (2002). *International ethical guidelines for biomedical research involving human subjects.* Available at: http://www.cioms.ch/frame_guidelines_nov_2002.htm (accessed 6 March 2009).

Dilts, D.M. and Sandler, A.B. (2006). Invisible barriers to clinical trials: the impact of structural, infrastructural, and procedural barriers to opening oncology clinical trials. *Journal of Clinical Oncology*, 24, 4545–51.

DiMasi, J.A., Hansen, R.W., and Grabowski, H.G. (2003). The price of innovation: new estimates of drug development costs. *Journal of Health Economics*, 22, 151–85.

Drazen, J.M. (2002). Institutions, contracts, and academic freedom. *New England Journal of Medicine*, 347, 1362–3.

Drazen, J.M., Van Der Weyden, M.B., Sahni, P., *et al.* (2009). Uniform format for disclosure of competing interests in ICMJE journals. *New England Journal of Medicine*, 361, 1896–7.

Duley, L., Antman, K., Arena, J., *et al.* (2008). Specific barriers to the conduct of randomized trials. *Clinical Trials*, 5, 40–8.

Dunn, L.B., Nowrangi, M.A., Palmer, B.W., Jeste, D.V., and Saks, E.R. (2006). Assessing decisional capacity for clinical research or treatment: a review of instruments. *American Journal of Psychiatry*, 163, 1323–34.

Dunn, L.B., Palmer, B.W., Appelbaum, P.S., Saks, E.R., Aarons, G.A., and Jeste, D.V. (2007). Prevalence and correlates of adequate performance on a measure of abilities related to decisional capacity: differences among three standards for the MacCAT-CR in patients with schizophrenia. *Schizophrenia Research*, 89, 110–18.

Ebbin, M. (2007). A Sun investigation: Are we ready for a stem cell clinic? The Premier and his wife believe so, but are any checks and balances in place? *Bermuda Sun*, 14 September. Available at: http://www.bermudasun.bm/main.asp?SectionID=24&SubSectionID=270&ArticleID=34993 (accessed 6 March 2009).

Eckenweiler, L. (2001). Moral reasoning and the review of research involving human subjects. *Kennedy Institute of Ethics Journal*, 11, 37–69.

Eisenstein, E.L., Collins, R., Cracknell, B.S., *et al.* (2008). Sensible approaches for reducing clinical trial costs. *Clinical Trials*, 5, 75–84.

Ellerin, B.E., Schneider, R.J., Stern, A., Toniolo, P.G., and Formenti, S.C. (2005). Ethical, legal, and social issues related to genomics and cancer research: the impending crisis. *American College of Radiology*, 2, 919–26.

Fisk, J.D. (2007). Ethical considerations for the conduct of antidemetia trials in Canada. *Canadian Journal of Neurological Sciences*, 34(Supplement 1), S32–36.

Frank, R.H. and Cook, P.J. (1995). *The winner-takes-all society*. New York: Free Press.

Friedman, T.L. (2005). *The World Is Flat*. New York: Farrar, Straus and Giroux.

Garber, A.M. (2009). An uncertain future for cardiovascular drug development? *New England Journal of Medicine*, 360, 1169–71.

Garber, A.M.and Tunis, S.R. (2009). Does comparative-effectiveness research threaten personalized medicine? *New England Journal of Medicine*, 360, 1925–31.

Garnier, J.P. (2008). Rebuilding the R&D engine in big pharma. *Harvard Business Review*, 86, 68–76.

Getz, K.A. (2007). Global clinical trials activity in the details. *Applied Clinical Trials*, 16, 42–4.

Glass, K.C. (2008). Ethical obligations and the use of placebo controls. *Canadian Journal of Psychiatry*, 53, 4328–9.

Glass, K.C. (2008). Rebuttal to Dr. Streiner: can the "evil" in the "lesser of 2 evils" be justified in placebo-controlled trials? *Canadian Journal of Psychiatry*, 53, 433.

Glickman, S.W., McHutchinson, J.G., Peterson, E.D., *et al.* (2009). Ethical and scientific implications of the globalization of clinical research. *New England Journal of Medicine*, 360, 816–23.

Global Forum for Health Research (2001). *The 10/90 report on health research 2000*. Geneva: World Health Organization.

Goldstein, D.B., Tate, S.K., and Sisodiya, S.M. (2003). Pharmacogenetics goes genomic. *Nature Reviews Genetics*, 4, 937–47.

Hill, Z., Tawiah-Agyemang, C., Odei-Danso, S., and Kirkwood, B. (2008). Informed consent in Ghana: What do participants really understand? *Journal of Medical Ethics*, 34, 48–53.

Howland, R.H. (2008). How are drugs approved? Part 2: ethical foundations of clinical research. *Journal of Psychosocial Nursing*, 46, 15–20.

Hutton, J.L. (2000). Ethics of medical research in developing countries: the role of international codes of conduct. *Statistical Methods in Medical Research*, 9, 185–206.

Institute of Medicine. (2009). Conflict of interest in medical research, education, and practice. Washington, DC: National Academies Press. Available at: http://www.iom.edu/CMS/3740/47464/65721.aspx.

International Committee of Medical Journal Editors. (2007). Sponsorship, authorship, and accountability. Available at: http://www.icmje.org/update_sponsor.html (accessed 6 March 2009).

International Committee of Medical Journal Editors. (2008). Uniform requirements for manuscripts submitted to biomedical journals: writing and editing for biomedical publication. Available at: http://www.icmje.org/2007_urm.pdf (accessed 30 October 2009).

Jack, A. (2008). New lease on life? The ethics of offshoring clinical trials. *Financial Times*, 28 January, 2008, p .58.

Jacob, R. and Chowdhury, A.N. (2009). Assessment of mental capacity in patients recruited in clinical trials in psychiatry and its relationship to informed consent. *Indian Journal of Medical Ethics*, 1, 43–4.

Jaspan, H., Nosiphiwo, F.S., Strode, *et al.* (2008). Community perspectives on the ethical issues surrounding adolescent HIV vaccine trials in South Africa. *Vaccine*, 26, 5679–83.

Jayaraman, K.S. (2005). Indian regulations fail to monitor growing stem-cell use in clinics. *Nature*, 434, 259.

Johnson, A. (2009). Drug firms see poorer nations as sales cure. *The Wall Street Journal*, 7 July, 2009.

Johnson, I. and Whalen, J. (2009). Novartis mounts ambitious push into China: pharmaceutical giant commits $1 billion, citing rapidly growing market driven by health-care reform. *The Wall Street Journal*, 4 November, 2009.

Kaiser, J. (2009). Private money, public disclosure. *Science*, 325, 28–30.

Kaplan, A. (2009). Forest under fire. *Psychiatric Times*, 26, 1–7.

Karliner, J. (2008). Grassroots globalization: reclaiming the blue planet. In F.J. Lechner and J. Boli (eds.) *The Globalization Reader*, pp. 34–8. Oxford: Blackwell.

Kesselheim, A.S. and Mello, M.M. (2007). Confidentiality laws and secrecy in medical research: improving public access to data on drug safety. *Health Affairs*, 26, 483–91.

Kiatpongsan, S. and Sipp, D. (2009). Monitoring and regulating offshore stem cell clinics. *Science*, 323, 1564–5.

Killen, J., Grady, C., Folkers, G.K., and Fauci, A.S. (2002). Ethics of clinical research in the developing world. *Nature*, 2, 210–15.

Kim, S.Y., Appelbaum, P.S., Jeste, D.V., and Olin, J.T. (2004). Proxy and surrogate consent in geriatric neuropsychiatric research: update and recommendations. *American Journal of Psychiatry*, 161, 797–806.

Kleinman, A. (2009). Global mental health: a failure of humanity. *Lancet*, 374, 603–4.

Kyzas, P.A., Loizou, K.T., and Ioannidis, J.P.A. (2005). Selective reporting biases in cancer prognostic factor studies. *Journal of the National Cancer Institute*, 97, 1043–55.

Laine, C., De Angelis, C., Delamothe, T., *et al.* (2007). Clinical trial registration—looking back and moving ahead. *New England Journal of Medicine*, 356, 2734–6.

Larson, H.N., Zhou, J., Chen, Z., Stamler, J.S., Weiner, H., and Hurley, T.D. (2007). Structural and functional consequences of coenzyme binding to the inactive Asian variant of mitochondrial aldehyde dehydrogenase: roles of residues 475 and 487. *Journal of Biological Chemistry*, 282, 12940–50.

Lechner, F.J. and Boli, J. (eds.) (2000). *The Global Reader*. Oxford: Blackwell.

Lee, E. (1996). Globalization and employment: Is anxiety justified? *International Labour Review*, 135, 486–97.

Lee, E. (1997). Globalization and labour standards: A review of issues. *International Labour Review*, 136, 173–89.

Lempinen, E.W. (2009). China, U.S. plan projects in S&T ethics education. *Science*, 324, 1159.

Lenzer, J. (2005). FDA warns about using antipsychotic drugs for dementia. *British Medical Journal*, 330, 922–3.

Lexchin, J., Bero, L.A., Djulbegovic, B. and Clark, O. (2003). Pharmaceutical industry sponsorship and research outcome and quality: systematic review. *British Medical Journal*, 236, 1167–70.

London, L. (2002). Ethical oversight of public health research: can rules and IRBs make a difference in developing countries? *American Journal of Public Health*, **92**, 1079–84.

Lurie, P. and Wolfe, S.M. (1997). Unethical trials of interventions to reduce perinatal transmission of human immunodeficiency virus in developing countries. *New England Journal of Medicine*, **337**, 853–6.

Malhotra, S. and Subodh, B.N. (2009). Informed consent & ethical issues in paediatric psychopharmacology. *Indian Journal of Medical Research*, **129**, 12–32.

Mok, T.S., Wu, Y.L., Thongprasert, S., *et al.* (2009). Gefitinib or carboplatin-paclitaxel in pulmonary adenocarcinoma. *New England Journal of Medicine*, **361**, 947–57.

Mundy, A. (2009). Drug-study reviewer halted n safety issue. *The Wall Street Journal*, 15 April, 2009.

Naik, A.D. and Petersen, L.A. (2009). The neglected purpose of comparative-effectiveness research. *New England Journal of Medicine*, **360**, 1029–31.

Nissen, S.E. and Wolski, K. (2007). Effect of Rosiglitazone on the risk of myocardial infarction and death from cardiovascular causes. *New England Journal of Medicine*, **356**, 2457–71.

Nuffield Council on Bioethics. (1999). *The ethics of clinical research in developing countries*. London: Nuffield Council on Bioethics.

Nundy, S. Chir, M., and Gulhati, C.M. (2005). A new colonialism?—Conducting clinical trials in India. *New England Journal of Medicine*, **352**, 1633–6.

Okie, S. (2009). Multinational medicines – ensuring drug quality in an era of global manufacturing. *New England Journal of Medicine*, **361**, 737–43.

Okike, K., Kocher, M.S., Wei, E.X., Mehlman, C.T., and Bhandari, M. (2009). Accuracy of conflict-of-interest disclosures reported by physicians. *New England Journal of Medicine*, **361**, 1466–74.

Osland, J.S. (2003). Broadening the debate: the pros and cons of globalization. *Journal of Management Inquiry*, **12**, 137–54.

Palmer, B.W., Cassidy, E.L., Dunn, L.B., Spira, A.P., and Sheikh, J.I. (2008). Effective use of consent forms and interactive questions in the consent process. *IRB*, **30**, 8–12.

Palmer, B.W., Dunn, L.B., Depp, C.A., Eyler, L.T., and Jeste, D.V. (2007). Decisional capacity to consent to research among patients with bipolar disorder: comparison with schizophrenia patients and healthy subjects. *Journal of Clinical Psychiatry*, **68**, 689–96.

Platt, R., Wilson, M., Chan, K.A., Benner, J.S., Marchibroda, J., and McClellan, M. (2009). The new Sentinel Network – improving the evidence of medical-product safety. *New England Journal of Medicine*, **361**, 645–7.

Price, S. (2007). Stem cell clinic closed. *Nation News*, 26 November. Available at: http://web.archive.org/web/20080128173958/http://www.nationnews.com/story/315095110731643.php (accessed 6 March 2009).

Pritchett, L. (1997). La distribution passee et future du revenue mondial. [The once (and future) distribution of world income]. *Economie Internationale*, **0**, 19–42.

Psaty, B.M. and Charo, R.A. (2007). FDA responds to Institute of Medicine drug safety recommendations—in part. *Journal of the American Medical Association*, **297**, 1917–20.

Rabins, P., Appleby, B.S., Brandt, J., *et al.* (2009). Scientific and ethical issues related to deep brain stimulation for disorders of mood, behavior, and thought. *Archives of General Psychiatry*, **66**, 931–7.

Rai, S. (2005). Drug companies cut costs with foreign clinical trials. *New York Times*, 24 February, 2005.

Rowland, C. (2004). Clinical trials seen shifting overseas. *International Journal of Health Services*, 34, 555–6.

Royal Gazette (2008). *Stem cell firm drops Bermuda from website*. Available at: http://www.royalgazette.com/rg/Article/article.jsp?sectionId=60&articleId=7d8893730030001 (accessed 6 March 2009).

Rudan, I., Gibson, J., Kaipirini, L., *et al.* (2007). Setting priorities in global child health research investments: Assessment of principles and practice. *Croatian Medical Journal*, 48, 595–604.

Schafer, A. (2004). Biomedical conflicts of interest: a defence of the sequestration thesis – learning from the cases of Nancy Olivieri and David Healy. *Journal of Medical Ethics*, 30, 8–24.

Schmidt, C.W. (2001). Monitoring research overseas. Clinical trial conduct reaches global harmonization. *Modern Drug Discovery*, 4, 25–6.

Schulman, K.A., Seils, D.M., Timbie, J.W., *et al.* (2002). A national survey of provisions in clinical-trial agreements between medical schools and industry sponsors. *New England Journal of Medicine*, 347, 1335–41.

Schwartz, L.M. and Woloshin. (2009). Lost in transmission – FDA drug information that never reaches clinicians. *New England Journal of Medicine*, 361, 1717–20.

Seitz, H.K., Matsuzaki, S., Yokoyama, A., Homann, N., Väkeväinen, S. and Wang, X.D. (2001). Alcohol and cancer. *Alcoholism: Clinical and Experimental Research*, 25, 137S–43S.

Shapiro, H.T. and Meslin, E.M. (2001). Ethical issues in the design and conduct of clinical trials in developing countries. *New England Journal of Medicine*, 345, 139–42.

Shuchman, M. (2007). Commercializing clinical trials – risks and benefits of the CRO boom. *New England Journal of Medicine*, 357, 1365–8.

Sinha, G. (2004). Outsourcing drug work: pharmaceuticals ship R & D and clinical trials to India. *Scientific American*, 291, 24–5.

Smith-Tyler, J. (2007). Informed consent, confidentiality, and subject rights in clinical trials. *Proceedings of the American Thoracic Society*, 4, 189–93.

Srinivasan, S. and Loff, B. (2006). Medical research in India. *Lancet*, 367, 1962–4.

Steinbrook, R. (2009). Controlling conflict of interest – proposals from the Institute of Medicine. *New England Journal of Medicine*, 21, 2160–3.

Steinbrook, R. (2009). Online disclosure of physician-industry relationships. *New England Journal of Medicine*, 360, 325–7.

Steinbrook, R. (2009). Physician-industry relations – will fewer gifts make a difference? *New England Journal of Medicine*, 360, 557–8.

Stough, W.G., Zannad, F., Pitt, B., and Goldstein, S. (2007). Globalization of cardiovascular clinical research: the balance between meeting medical needs and maintaining scientific standards. *American Heart Journal*, 154, 232–8.

Streiner, D.L. (2007). Alternatives to placebo-controlled trials. *Canadian Journal of Neurological Sciences*, 34, S37–41.

Streiner, D.L. (2008). The lesser of 2 evils: the ethics of placebo-controlled trials. *Canadian Journal of Psychiatry*, 53, 430–2.

Sumathipala, A., Siribaddana, S., Hewage, *et al.* (2008). Informed consent in Sri Lanka: a survey among ethics committee members. *BMC Medical Ethics*, 9, 10.

Theirs, F.A., Sinskey, A.J., and Berndt, E.R. (2008). Trends in the globalization of clinical trials. *Nature Reviews Drug Discovery*, 7, 13–14.

The National Commission for the Protection of Human Subjects of Biomedical and Behavioral Research. (1979). *The Belmont report: Ethical principles and guidelines for the protection of human subjects of research.* Available at: http://ohsr.od.nih.gov/guidelines/belmont.html (accessed 6 March 2009).

The Netherlands Health Care Inspectorate. (2006). *Inspectorate orders PMC of Rotterdam to stop stem cell treatment.* Available at: http://www.igz.nl/uk/files/379598 (accessed 6 March 2009).

Tomlinson, M., Rudan, I., Saxena, S., Swartz, L., Tsai, A.C., and Patel, V. (2009). Setting priorities for global mental health research. *Bulletin of the World Health Organization*, 87, 438–46.

Trials of War Criminals before the Nuremberg Military Tribunals under Control Council Law No. 10. (1949). *Nuremberg Code.* Washington, DC: U.S. Government Printing Office.

Tungaraza, T. and Poole, R. (2007). Influence of drug company authorship and sponsorship on drug trial outcomes. *British Journal of Psychiatry*, 191, 82–3.

Turner, E.H. (2004). A taxpayer-funded clinical trials registry and results database. *PLos Medicine*, 1, 180–2.

Turner, E.H., Matthews, A.M., Linardatos, E., Tell, R.A. and Rosenthal, R. (2009). Selective publication of antidepressant trials and its influence on apparent efficacy. *New England Journal of Medicine*, 358, 252–9.

United Nations Development Programme (UNDP). (2001). *Human development report 2001.* New York: Oxford University Press.

U.S. Department of Health and Human Services. (2001). *The globalization of clinical trials.* Available at: http://oig.hhs.gov/oei/reports/oei-01-00-00190.pdf (accessed 4 March 2009).

U.S. Department of Health and Human Services. (2007). *The Food and Drug Administration's oversight of clinical trials.* Available at: http://oig.hhs.gov/oei/reports/oei-01-06-00160.pdf (accessed 4 March 2009).

U.S. Food and Drug Administration. (1997). *Food and Drug Administration Modernization Act of 1997. Congressional Record, Public Law No. 105-115.* Available at: http://www.fda.gov/CDER/guidance/105-115.htm (accessed 11 March 2009).

U.S. Food and Drug Administration. (2007). *Food and Drug Administration Amendments Act of 2007. Congressional Record, Public Law No. 110-85.* Available at: http://www.fda.gov/RegulatoryInformation/Legislation/FederalFoodDrugandCosmeticActFDCAct/SignificantAmendmentstotheFDCAct/FoodandDrugAdministrationAmendmentsActof2007/default.htm (accessed 11 March 2009).

Varmus, H. and Satcher, D. (1997). Ethical complexities of conducting research in developing countries. *New England Journal of Medicine*, 337, 1003–5.

Vedula, S.S., Bero, L., Scherer, R.W., and Dickersin, K. (2009). Outcome reporting in industry-sponsored trials of gabapentin for off-label use. *New England Journal of Medicine*, 361, 1963–71.

Whalen, J. and Greil, A. (2009). Novartis patent rejected in India. *Wall Street Journal*, 7 July, 2009.

Whittington, C.J., Kendall, T., Fonagy, P., Cottrell, D., Cotgrove, A., and Boddington, E. (2004). Selective serotonin reuptake inhibitors in childhood depression: systematic review of published versus unpublished data. *Lancet*, 363, 1341–45.

Wood, A.J.J. (2009). Progress and deficiencies in the registration of clinical trials. *New England Journal of Medicine*, 360, 824–30.

World Medical Association. (2008). *World Medical Association Declaration of Helsinki, Ethical Principles for Medical Research involving human subjects.* Available from: http://www.wma.net/en/30publications/10policies/b3/index.html (accessed on 11 March 2009).

Yergin, D. and Stanislaw, J. (2000). The commanding heights: The battle between government and the marketplace that is remaking the modern world. In F.J. Lechner and J. Boli (eds.) *The Globalization Reader*, pp. 212–20. Oxford: Blackwell.

Yusuf, S. (2004). Randomized clinical trials: slow death by a thousand unnecessary policies? *Canadian Medical Association Journal*, **8**, 889–92.

Zhang, D., Yin, P., Freemantle, N., Jordan, R., Zhong, N., and Cheng, K.K. (2008). An assessment of the quality of randomised controlled trials conducted in China. *Trials*, **9**, 22.

Zhang, J. (2009). Push to compare treatments worries drug, device makers. *The Wall Street Journal*, 14 April, 2009.

CHAPTER 51

LEARNING ABOUT NEUROETHICS THROUGH HEALTH SCIENCES ONLINE: A MODEL FOR GLOBAL DISSEMINATION

KATE TAIRYAN AND ERICA FRANK

There is no prescription more valuable than knowledge.
C. Everett Koop, MD, Former US Surgeon General

INTRODUCTION

DESPITE the importance of information for both health and development, the world's vast store of knowledge and high-quality education remains largely out of reach for health professionals in many countries. Health personnel regularly confront new and sometimes critical situations that add to the already heavy burden of providing healthcare with inadequate resources. At the same time, health sciences students may complete their training insufficiently prepared to cope with the health problems they will encounter in practice with their local communities (World Health Organization 2006a).

Here we describe Health Sciences Online (HSO; http://www.hso.info), an initiative to improve professional educational resources for those in the global health community interested in neuroethics and other health sciences disciplines. We place HSO in the context of online health professional education and the technological advances that make such education possible, present the strategic components of HSO project development and implementation in neuroethics and overall, and address some issues of future developments in distance learning.

BACKGROUND

The World Health Organization (WHO) has identified a need for 4 million additional healthcare workers, recognizing the lack of a trained health workforce as a threat for global public health: "Pressing health needs across the globe cannot be met without a well-trained, adequate and available health workforce" (WHO 2006b). Many national education systems are unable to provide basic or continuing education, and many countries lack sufficient resources to ensure that current knowledge, methods and materials are used in teaching. As an urgent step toward solving the emerging public health problem, the WHO calls for more direct investment in the training and support of health workers (WHO 2006b).

Aging and growing populations, and a dramatic increase in chronic diseases worldwide including a high burden of neurological and psychiatric disorders, are placing new demands on a health workforce that is already inadequate. Not only are there insufficient numbers of health workers, they are also unequally distributed, as shown in Table 51.1.

In industrialized societies where neurotechnology rapidly advances the field of neuroscience and the understanding of brain functions, health providers and researchers in clinical and academic settings are facing new challenges. The need for proactively identifying and addressing those challenges and recognizing the ethical, legal, and social implications of neuroscience research has been emphasized repeatedly by many pioneers in neuroethics (Roskies 2002; Illes, et al. 2006; Illes and Atlas 2007). Academic centers and universities in Canada, US, Europe, and Japan have responded to the urgent need to align advances in neurosciences and societal values. The newly established neuroethics centers and programs are becoming hubs for mobilizing resources and addressing neuroethical dilemmas through empirical research and knowledge translation. The federal governments and private funds support many of those centers, and many of them have vital information to share.

Additionally, the media and public show ever-increasing interest around neuroethics issues. As predicted by Sahakian and Morein-Zamir (2009) in *Science*, "neuroethical issues are surely going to become ever more pertinent" with new developments in imaging analysis techniques, imaging modalities, and means to link genetics with functional brain maps (Tairyan and Illes 2009). In the new era of neuroscience development and neuroethical dilemmas, there is a growing need for applied neuroethics training to be integrated into neuroscience education (Sahakian and Morein-Zamir 2009; Lombera *et al.* 2010). This is

Table 51.1 The health workforce in the Americas versus sub-Saharan Africa

The Americas	Sub-Saharan Africa
14% of the world's population	11% of the world's population
10% of the global burden of disease	25% of the global burden of disease
42% of the world's health workers	3% of the world's health workers
>50% of global health expenditure	<1% of global health expenditure

Reproduced from the World Health Organization. The global shortage of health workers and its impact. Fact sheet N° 302, April 2006. Available at: http://webcache.googleusercontent.com/search?q=cache:MWQ24Udr1l8J:www.who.int/mediacentre/factsheets/fs302/en/index.html+%22Americas+versus+sub-Saharan+Africa%22&cd=1&hl=en&ct=clnk&gl=ca&source=www.google.ca (accessed 14 December 2009) © 2009 WHO with permission.

critical for the responsible and appropriate use of emerging brain-related technologies and methods; neuromarketing and cognitive enhancement; management of incidental findings among healthy volunteers and other research participants; public perception; and the management of hyperbole around potential implications of neuroscience research results, especially for patients with persistent vegetative states (Greely *et al.* 2008; Murphy *et al.* 2008; Racine *et al.* 2008; Wolf *et al.* 2008). Although the importance and the timeliness of neuroethics content in existing neuroscience programs has been emphasized by many neuroscience researchers around the world, two independent reports from the UK (Sahakian and Morein-Zamir 2009) and Canada (Lombera *et al.* 2010) have shown that neuroethics training is not commonly a formal part of neuroscience programs in those countries, and the majority of neuroscience students do not receive formal education about ethics in neuroscience. However, the Canadian study revealed that there is a strong interest in including more ethics content in programs among both faculty and students. The vast majority—more than 90%—of participating faculty program directors endorsed the importance of including formal ethics training in neuroscience programs. Despite the interest in and perceived need for more formal ethics content in the neuroscience curricula, lack of time and expertise, as well as lack of relevant resources were identified as the main barriers to incorporating ethics into the neuroscience education. This led the authors to recommend the development of more tailored educational tools to promote neuroethics expertise, and to offer more appropriate educational media to reduce time constraints. Similarly, the UK-based investigators suggested that academic programs should also have mechanisms in place for offering neuroethics teaching, although they were less specific with ideas of how this can be achieved. Investigators in both groups also commented on the already heavily loaded neuroscience training agenda, posing challenges for effective scheduling and inclusion of any new topics. Therefore, new models of training and innovative ways of delivering such training should be further explored and tested in order to make neuroethics content widely available, not only in countries with relatively high volume of neuroethics content development, but also to their eager colleagues globally.

TECHNOLOGICAL DEVELOPMENT AND E-LEARNING

The Internet offers a well-developed and cost-effective option for delivering and enhancing professional education in high-income countries. Increasingly, as both Internet access and user-capability improve, the same option is becoming available in developing countries. Computers are also becoming increasingly prevalent in medical practices, regardless of location or relative wealth of the local healthcare community (Richwine and McGowan 2001). Computer-assisted training programs delivered through the Internet now make education and training increasingly available at a relatively low per-unit cost. As a result, health sciences education provided through cost-effective, largely available and acceptable, innovative initiatives such as Web-based virtual educational centers are expanding globally (Harden and Hart 2002).

The emergence of the Internet has introduced new ways for users to access information resources and has shaped user behavior and expectations. Users now expect instant and constant access to information, often from distant locations (MacCall 2006). However, rapid change in information technologies also means that users need to adapt to the changing environment faster than ever before. Then, as users' perspectives change, online resource providers also have to keep up by anticipating the needs of users and updating, organizing, and managing resources effectively and seamlessly (Blansit and Connor 1999).

The rapid development of digital technologies combined with the growth of the Internet in the past decade has revolutionized traditional methods of research and teaching and has led to a proliferation of digital material. The amount of health-related material generated in digital format has also increased tremendously over a short period of time (Blansit and Connor 1999). Digital materials come in the form of online courseware, lab image files, statistical files and databases, clinical and research publications, reports, electronic books, and many other formats.

Today, world-class universities are developing and promoting online courses and degree offerings, extending their programs to meet the needs of local students as well as working professionals (Smith 2002). Faculty and staff in the health sciences arena now use and create digital material for their research and teaching on a daily basis. While campus-based education may continue to be the first choice of many students and institutions, the benefits of distance learning have increased international demand for access to virtual universities and other electronic educational resources (Phipps and Merisotis 1999; McKimm *et al.* 2003).

Online access to open-source education portals is growing every year; the increase is documented not only in industrialized countries, but also outside of the developed world. For instance, the OpenCourseWare of the Massachusetts Institute of Technology (MIT) recorded a 56% increase in visits in 2005; 61% of visits were from non-US users (MIT 2006).

In order to make the educational experience relevant, information must be accessible from anywhere and anytime, directly delivered to the end-user. Changes in information technology have allowed the world's biomedical information to be available on a physician's computer desktop. Changes in the practice of medicine, and technological developments are creating unprecedented opportunities to select and organize electronic resources, using the Web to deliver content throughout the world, and enhance knowledge. Ronald Phipps and Jamie Merisotis, of the USA Institute for Higher Education Policy, noted in their 1999 report on distance education:

> Technology is having, and will continue to have, a profound impact on colleges and universities in America and around the globe. Distance learning, which was once a poor and often unwelcome stepchild within the academic community is becoming increasingly more visible as a part of the higher education family. (Phipps and Merisotis 1999, p. 29)

Educators even warned that universities that failed to transform courses and degree programs for Internet delivery would not survive long into the next century (Harden and Hart 2002; Endler 2005).

E-LEARNING AND CONTINUING MEDICAL EDUCATION

Health professionals increasingly rely on the Internet not only to obtain information on clinical issues and research, but also to fulfill continuing medical education (CME) requirements. A 2001 study on physician preferences for CME reported that only 2.7% of North American physicians used the Internet for CME (Brown *et al.* 2001), whereas more recent figures show use of the Internet by physicians to be closer to 31% (Rossett and McDonald 2006). Access to CME is one of the most commonly reported Internet uses by physicians. These data are consistent with reports by the US Accreditation Council for Continuing Medical Education (ACCME) of an upward trend in online CME offerings, with Internet CME activities increasing by 121% from 2003 to 2004. In 2003, De Groote and Dorsch found that, at the University of Illinois at Chicago, 95% of the users of health sciences library (medical students, faculty, and residents) reported having access to a computer with Internet access outside of the library, and 53% of these users reported that they searched MEDLINE at least once a week. This study also found that only 16% of users depended entirely on the library to access its online resources, while 39% of users never entered the library to access online resources. In an especially remarkable attitudinal change, 71% of users indicated a preference for online over print resources when possible (De Groote and Dorsch 2003).

POTENTIAL BENEFITS AND SOME CHALLENGES OF E-LEARNING

The reusable learning object

E-learning, or technology-enhanced learning has grown in popularity because of ever-improving quality, convenience, and flexibility, increasing availability of computers, and students' familiarity with them. Many researchers have predicted that future students will be educated in a context where considerable time is spent online, regardless of their educational institutions' locations. Some researchers suggest that e-learning will fundamentally alter traditional modes of higher education. Rather than being affiliated with a single institution, learners will be associated concurrently with multiple content providers throughout the world. The "reusable learning object" approach is the most powerful feature of e-learning. For example, the same learning object created in one educational institution can be used by different teachers and learners in different ways and may be reused a number of times in different learning contexts. This scenario assumes unbundled education, with students having greater control over their educational experiences and programs that fit their own special needs for content, length, delivery mode, time, and location.

Harden and Hart (2002) summarize the benefits of e-learning for students, partner institutions, and society (Figure 51.1). The benefits involve important aspects of e-learning such as quality, flexibility and cost-effectiveness, innovation, responsiveness to social needs, and collaboration nationally and internationally.

Global perspectives and universal delivery

Benefits of remote access for students include a high-quality unique education program, with expert-designed learning systems. Such online programs can offer a global perspective,

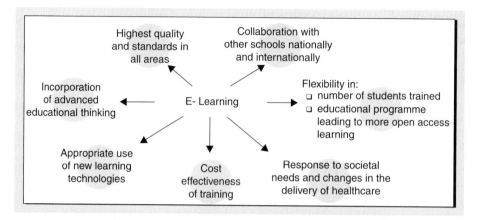

FIG. 51.1 Benefits of e-learning. Adopted from Harden and Hart (2002).

with students becoming part of an international community offering cultural diversity, a flexible and adaptive curriculum to fulfill individual needs, a wide range of learning opportunities and approaches, home-based learning (with the benefit of saving on relocation costs), experience gained with new technologies, preparedness for lifelong learning, and continuous professional development (Harden and Hart 2002).

Other obvious advantages of electronic formats include essentially universal delivery of high-quality information and learning materials at nominal costs, with the benefits of desktop access, searchable text, and flexible editing options, and without the inconvenience and costs of accessing information at traditional libraries. These costs can be both individual (both time and opportunity costs, often quite steep for trained health providers), and institutional, as libraries can decrease their commitments to subscribing, shelving, reshelving, binding, and housing a given journal title (Blansit and Connor 1999).

Computer-assisted instruction (CAI) is an efficient means of conveying knowledge to large numbers of health professionals given the small marginal costs of providing access to already-developed computer-based materials. This is especially the case if connectivity, hardware, and software are already present (an increasingly common situation). While the cost of educating a physician in developing countries is far less than in industrialized countries, the relative expenditure for educating a physician, adjusted for per capita GNP, can be very high. For example, relatively speaking, Vietnam spends 2.8 times the US average (Bicknell *et al.* 2001). Further, while educating the 100th student in a bricks-and-mortar institution costs nearly as much as educating the 10th student, the cost of educating an additional health provider using computer-assisted instruction is zero for material development and can be negligible for material distribution and usage. While the current cost of computers and Internet access still limits their use by many health professionals in less-developed countries, these limits will shrink as the costs of handheld devices with Internet access, PCs, and CDs continue to plummet and Web access grows.

Effectiveness and quality

New learning technologies and e-learning will clearly have an increasingly important role to play in neuroethics and other aspects of medical education. However, the extent and the nature of developments in the area of e-learning are difficult to predict. The scientific world is only beginning to investigate the possibilities offered by the Internet for education, and is coming to recognize its strengths and limitations (Freeman *et al.* 2000). The need to foster the development of truly international learning experiences and make that learning universally available has been described previously (Harden and Hart 2002). A recent US Department of Education publication entitled *Evaluation of Evidence-Based Practices in Online Learning: A Meta-Analysis and Review of Online Learning Studies* revealed many interesting findings over 1000 empirical studies conducted between 1996 and 2008. In particular, it reports that students in online learning conditions perform better on average than those receiving face-to-face instruction (U.S. Department of Education 2009)

Extensive research has shown that online learning is at least as effective as traditional classroom formats (Lewis *et al.* 1999; Levine 2002), and that CAI may be superior to traditional didactic techniques (Chan *et al.* 1999; Phipps and Merisotis 1999; Greenhalgh 2001; Mazmanian and Davis 2002). But what of integrating and applying knowledge to practice (Giani and Martone 1998) in the context of CAI? This may be accomplished by blending CAI with face-to-face and community/skills-based learning. E-learning need not replace traditional forms of learning, but it clearly can complement and enhance training, and improve continuing education (Harden and Hart 2002). Online education or supplementary online courses can enhance learning particularly in such fundamental medical sciences as human anatomy. Experiences in the dissection laboratory allow researchers to conclude that such comprehensive online programs could also be effective in other disciplines where human resources for teaching are a limiting factor (Granger *et al.* 2006).

There is an enormous volume of readily accessible Web-based health information resources, allowing health professionals to retrieve current information with unprecedented ease and speed. These attributes can be of particular assistance to clinicians and scientists working in areas in which scientific and clinical developments move quickly (Peters and Sikorski 1998) or are new and fast-developing (such as neuroethics). However, an immediate limitation is that the quality of these resources is variable. Given the evolving state of the Internet, it may be difficult or even inappropriate to develop a static tool or system for assessing health-related websites (Kim *et al.* 1999). Users may feel overwhelmed by the range and variety of information and uncertain about which resources are most useful in their specialty areas.

A second limit is that providers who are more familiar with older print media may not have the skills to use new databases and information formats efficiently and correctly. In fact, one study shows that while many clinicians have adapted quickly to the new digital environment, at least 59% experience difficulty navigating or searching for biomedical information (Richwine and McGowan 2001). The situation is even more difficult in developing countries, where limited Web-use skills are often exacerbated by technical access and cost issues, reducing the quality and quantity of accessed materials even further.

Third, there are issues around the extent to which CAI can produce active learning. A review of medical teaching web sites for evidence of active learning showed that although most sites met criteria for a "general informational website," only 17% had all components of the "learning paradigm" that involves the critical thinking, independent learning, evidence-based learning, and feedback that are so important for health sciences education (Cook and Dupras 2004).

Access

Digital libraries represent the most common form of online access to current medical information. Many biomedical libraries and publishers have set up remote access to their collections, allowing physicians to use online resources from their campus office, hospital workstation, and off-campus office computers, whether the physical library is open or closed (Beam *et al.* 2006). Medical information is also increasingly portable—physicians can quickly download, email, and save content to computers or personal digital assistants. Access to online health-sciences libraries can offer comprehensive collections of credible, up-to-date resources, and create opportunities for quality research, education, and patient care for healthcare professionals and students (Sheffield 2006). One study demonstrated that information services provided by hospital librarians in support of clinical decision-making had a significant positive impact on healthcare outcomes, as measured by the physicians' self-reported evaluation of impact of the library's information on diagnosis, choice of tests and drugs, reduced length of hospital stay, and advice given to the patient (Marshall 1992). It has become ever more important to explore new and more effective ways of information delivery to ensure that all healthcare providers have good access to necessary information to support their decision making, regardless of their geographic location.

The importance of online access to health sciences information cannot be overstated, especially in the context of rural, sparsely populated, medically underserved areas. Clinicians in remote and rural areas (even in developed countries) face geographic isolation. Health professionals in those settings often lack training and proper academic support due to distance from large, central hospitals and academic centers of excellence (Richwine and McGowan 2001). Professionally isolated health practitioners may fall behind in their continuous professional development. Distance education courses can reverse this sense of isolation and, in this context, learner support is vital, and social interaction and virtual collaboration become highly desirable features of the learning product (Boulos *et al.* 2006). A virtual library implemented in rural areas in southern Indiana confirmed that the impact of the project for healthcare outcomes was comparable to that found in the Marshall study (Richwine and McGowan 2001). The authors reported that two elements of the virtual library project contributed to its success: (1) well-organized and appropriate electronic resources that support clinical decision making; and, (2) training offered to facilitate use of the resources (Richwine and McGowan 2001).

In past few years, the medical community also has witnessed a rapid increase in the use of Web-based "collaborationware," so-called Web 2.0 tools: wikis, blogs, and podcasts. These applications have been increasingly adopted by many online health-related professional and educational services. They offer the opportunity for powerful information sharing and ease of collaboration. Wikis are Web sites that can be edited by anyone who has access to them. The word "blog" is an online Web journal that can offer a resource-rich multimedia environment. Podcasts are repositories of audio and video materials. These audio and video files can be downloaded to portable media players that can create "anytime, anywhere" learning experiences (i.e. mobile learning) (Boulos *et al.* 2006).

HEALTH SCIENCES ONLINE: A MODEL FOR MAXIMIZING BENEFITS AND OVERCOMING CHALLENGES OF E-LEARNING

Attributes

Maximizing the use of online education for healthcare professionals will save time, money, and other critical resources. In the past, the majority of online educational website course offerings have been devoted to a single area of expertise. Other sites are affiliated with associations or publishers and have educational content reflecting the specific focus of the association or periodical. As a result, before the advent of HSO (http://www.hso.info), healthcare practitioners needed to spend a considerable amount of time searching the Web for sites offering courses on their specific area of expertise, rather than going to a single site that serves as a clearinghouse for courses and offers one-stop services for information across many health-related disciplines. Systematically designed filtering mechanisms have allowed HSO to accumulate only high-quality, current and credible learning resources, using clearly-defined content criteria for relevance/independence, objectivity, credibility/currency, and design (Frank 2004). As pointed out by Garcia, a comprehensive online education portal site minimizes the amount of resources that clinicians and healthcare systems need to devote to education-seeking, thus improving patient care (Garcia 2000).

Martinez has suggested:

> The dream to deliver personalized learning using learning objects that fit the real-time, anywhere, anytime, just-enough needs of the learner is about to become a reality.... The most obvious benefit of these innovations is the creation of a learning ecology that shares resources from large reservoirs of content where learning objects are shared individually, widely and more economically. (Martinez 2002, p. 24)

With founding collaborators and funders including the US Centers for Disease Control and Prevention, Emory University, the University of British Columbia, the Ulrich and Ruth Frank Foundation for International Health, the World Bank, WHO, and the American College of Preventive Medicine, HSO meets the emerging need for increased access to health sciences education with innovative thinking new learning technologies such as virtual reality, and an international perspective on health sciences education for the benefit of communities on a global scale. To this end, HSO's audience is health professionals, researchers, and policy makers both in training and practice in developing countries. Its content covers topics in medicine, public health, nursing, dentistry, and other healthcare and health sciences disciplines, with learning objects including textbooks, journals, databases, and interactive media tools and is constantly being updated. In Table 51.2 we present sample online resources on neuroethics.

Table 51.2 Sample online resources in neuroethics

Title	Description	Content provider and URL
Neuroethics: Implications of Advances in Neuroscience	Online course with 4 modules	Columbia University, NY http://ccnmtl.columbia.edu/projects/neuroethics/index.html
Neuroethics – A literature review prepared for Toi te Taiao: the Bioethics Council	Review of the current literature on neuroethics	Toi te Taiao: The Bioethics Council, New Zealand http://ndhadeliver.natlib.govt.nz/ArcAggregator/arcView/IE1074184/http://www.bioethics.org.nz/publications/neuroethics-review-jul06/index.html
Health Sciences Online: Neuroethics Resources And References	Introduction to current topics and the landmark papers in neuroethics	National Core for Neuroethics, University of British Columbia http://neuroethics.ubc.ca/National_Core_for_Neuroethics/Initiatives_files/NeuroethicsReferences&Resources.pdf
Filmed Course Lectures	Lecture Series on various neuroscience topics with neuroethics content	The Science Network http://thesciencenetwork.org/search?q=neuroethics&tx=0&ty=0
Ethics in Medicine (Ethics and Law; Termination of Life-Sustaining Treatment; Confidentiality, etc.)	Online modules with case studies	University of Washington, School of Medicine http://depts.washington.edu/bioethx/topics/index.html
Decision Making in a Case of Personality Change	Clinical Cases	American Medical Association, Virtual Mentor http://virtualmentor.ama-assn.org/2008/03/ccas1-0803.html
Ethics Videos on The Web	Lectures, presentations, course and conference talks	University of San Diego http://ethics.sandiego.edu/video/APA/Pacific/2002/index.html
Penn Media Seminar on Neuroscience and Society	Series of expert talks	University of Pennsylvania http://www.neuroethics.upenn.edu/index.php/resource-center/videos-and-podcasts
Facts, Ethics, and Policy Guiding Neuroscience Today (Michael Gazzaniga, Hank Greely, William Safire)	Science and the City Podcasts	The New York Academy of Sciences http://www.nyas.org/Publications/Media/PodcastDetail.aspx?cid=9a4d84cb-3bb9-47f9-9f24-47789e884a21
Gray Matters	Podcasts	The Dana Foundation http://www.dana.org/danaalliances/programs/graymatters/

Limitations

Easy, reliable and affordable access to the Internet is crucial for incorporating online learning initiatives into basic and continuous education for healthcare professionals and successful implementation of HSO. Although the Internet is available in most countries and continues to expand rapidly, access to Web-based learning opportunities is limited in many countries—especially in remote and rural areas, where healthcare providers are most in need of current information and education. Thus, infrastructure shortcomings and the cost of telecommunications are key obstacles to using the Internet and Web-based learning.

Happily, intellectual property and copyright issues have not been impediments, and this is true for at least three reasons. First, because essentially all the learning objects HSO uses are from links already publicly posted on the Web (and our other learning objects were given directly to us), links that were posted expressly with the hope of being shared and used among the health sciences and health education communities. Second, because our efforts are legally and ethically considered "fair use": it is our intention for http://www.hso.info to always be completely free and open to anyone with web access to learn about the health sciences, and this is also fair use. In Phase II, where we will begin to charge people small amounts for training and certification, we will also be considered fair use, as our activities will constitute the non-profit use of freely posted materials (and we will also email all authors whose materials we use for our charged-for trainings, to give them an opportunity to withdraw access. We have been advised that this meets or exceeds terms of fair use by Steve Carson (HSO Advisory Committee member who also is Senior Strategist at MIT's Open Courseware initiative), and by our pro bono counsel, the international intellectual property lawyers at Latham and Watkins (a 2000-attorney firm with 29 legal offices around the world).

Accomplishments to date and future steps

In December 2008 we officially launched HSO, the first website to deliver authoritative, comprehensive, free, and ad-free health sciences knowledge (with over 50,000 hand-selected resources, and 1000+ visits/day). HSO has been well-received by reviewers, including the WHO stating as early as 2006 that "HSO is expected to make a considerable contribution to the advancement of e-learning worldwide" (WHO 2006a), and AltSearchEngines calling HSO in 2008:

> The Internet at its finest... an incredibly worthwhile enterprise... a boon... a model of what Health 2.0 and Science 2.0 can be... a pioneering project in health sciences education and medical information dissemination. Let us hope that every major medical school in the world jumps onto the bandwagon... **Projects like this give me hope for the future.** (emphasis theirs, AltSearchEngines.com 2008)

For HSO's next phase, we are beginning work with colleagues around the world to create what we hope will be one of the largest, most accessible, and best health sciences universities— all done with distance HSO-based didactics, local hands-on mentoring, and peer-to-peer distance feedback. In beta-testing until mid-2011, we have launched the world's first free university. We plan to train many thousands of trainees at a time, particularly in developing countries, with the students remaining in their home environments to build capacity. Among our offerings in 2011 will be:

- Residencies in Ob-Gyn, Women's Health, Pediatrics, and Adolescent Health, in partnership with WHO, the international Federation of Gynecologists and Obstetricians, Medical Women's International Association, the American College of Preventive Medicine, and others
- A Master's degree in Public Health offered with Jilin University (the 9th ranked Chinese University, with 1800 public health students), the Public Health Foundation of India (we'll be using the same tests as their conventionally-trained MPH students for our students), and the American Association of Public Health Physicians
- Hospital and Clinic-based Infection Control, in collaboration with WHO
- Introduction to General Surgery, with Global Surgery at the Center for Surgery and Public Health at Brigham and Women's Hospital, the University of Zambia, and the Education Committee of the College of Surgeons in East, Central and Sourthern Africa (who will authorize these graduates to take surgical boards in 9 sub-Saharan countries)
- Exercise and Health, in partnership with the U.S. CDC, the American College of Sports Medicine, and the Fundacion Santa Fe Bogota
- A Pre-Medical Curriculum and a training on the Prevention and Cessation of Tobacco Use, both with the International Federation of Medical Student Associations
- Prevention and Treatment of Alcohol Abuse, in collaboration with the Betty Ford Institute, and the Annenberg Physician Training Program in Addiction Medicine
- A comprehensive, competency-based training program in neuroethics in collaboration with the Canadian National Core for Neuroethics at the University of British Columbia

CONCLUSIONS

The demand for equal access to high-quality, health sciences education is enormous, especially in the developing world. HSO is designed to help meet this overwhelming educational need regardless of geographical location and field of study, specialization, or practice, by providing a critical means to improve the health of the developing and industrialized world through free online access to high-quality, up-to-date courses and references for health professionals in training and practice. HSO's collection is vast spanning diagnostic and therapeutic advances in medicine, as well as over 400 resources in biomedical ethics to neuroethics. It is a model for far-reaching innovative learning throughout the world in neuroethics, and beyond.

REFERENCES

AltSearchEngines.com. *Hope for the future – Health Sciences Online.* Available at: http://www.altsearchengines.com/2008/12/26/hope-for-the-future-health-sciences-online/ (accessed 18 February 2010).

Beam, P.S., Schimming, L.M., Krissoff, A.B., and Morgan, L.K. (2006). The changing library: what clinicians need to know. *Mount Sinai Journal of Medicine,* 73, 857–63.

Bicknell, W.J., Beggs, A.C., and Tham, P.V. (2001). Determining the full costs of medical education in Thai Binh, Vietnam: a generalizable model. *Health Policy & Planning,* 16, 412–20.

Blansit, B.D. and Connor, E. (1999). Making sense of the electronic resource marketplace: trends in health-related electronic resources. *Bulletin of the Medical Library Association,* 87, 243–50.

Brown, T.T., Proctor, S.E., Sinkowitz-Cochran, R.L., Smith, T.L., and Jarvisia, W.R. (2001). Physician preferences for continuing medical education with a focus on the topic of antimicrobial resistance: Society for Healthcare Epidemiology of America. *Infection Control and Hospital Epidemiology*, **22**, 656–60.

Boulos, M.N.K., Maramba, I., and Wheeler, S. (2006). Wikis, blogs and podcasts: a new generation of Web-based tools for virtual collaborative clinical practice and education. *BMC Medical Education*, **6**, 41.

Chan, D.H., Leclair, K., and Kaczorowski, J. (1999). Problem-based small-group learning via the Internet among community family physicians: a randomized controlled trial. *MD Computing*, **16**, 54–8.

Cook, D.A. and Dupras, D.M. (2004). A practical guide to developing effective web-based learning. *Journal of General Internal Medicine*, **19**, 698–707.

De Groote, S.L. and Dorsch, J.L. (2003). Measuring use patterns of online journals and databases. *Journal of Medical Library Association*, **91**, 231–40.

Endler, P.C. (2005). New initiative–Interuniversity European Union project: distance learning program in integrated health sciences. *Journal of Alternative & Complementary Medicine*, **11**, 203–4.

Frank, E. (2004). HSO Content Criteria. Available at: https://docs.google.com/viewer?url=http://hso.info/about/hso-guidelines.pdf (accessed 20 March 2010).

Freeman, H., Routen, T., Patel, D., Ryan, S., and Scott, B. (2000). *The Virtual University: The Internet and Resource-Based Learning*. London: Kogan Page Limited.

Garcia, L. (2000). Maximizing the online education experience. *Health Management Technology*, **21**, 68.

Giani, U. and Martone, P. (1998). Distance learning, problem based learning and dynamic knowledge networks. *International Journal of Medical Informatics*, **50**, 273–8.

Granger, N.A., Calleson, D.C., Henson, O.W., Juliano, E., Wineski, L., and McDaniel, M.D. (2006). Use of Web-based materials to enhance anatomy instruction in the health sciences. *Anatomical Record, New Anatomist*. **289**, 121–7.

Greely H., Sahakian, B., Harris, J., Kessler, R.C., Gazzaniga, M., Campbell, P., and Farah, M.J. (2008). Towards responsible use of cognitive-enhancing drugs by the healthy. *Nature*, **456**, 702–5.

Greenhalgh, T. (2001). Computer assisted learning in undergraduate medical education. *British Medical Journal*, **322**, 40–4.

Harden, R.M. and Hart, I.R. (2002). An international virtual medical school (IVIMEDS): the future for medical education? *Medical Teacher*, **24**, 261–7.

Illes, J., DeVries, R., Cho, M.K., and Schraedley-Desmond, P. (2006). ELSI priorities for brain imaging. *American Journal of Bioethics*, **6**, W24–31.

Illes, J. and Atlas, S. (2007). Risks and benefits of the new medical imaging enterprise. *American Medical Association Journal of Ethics: Virtual Mentor*, **9**, 99.

Kim, P., Eng, T.R., Deering, M.J., and Maxfield, A. (1999). Published criteria for evaluating health related web sites: review. *British Medical Journal*, **318**, 647–9.

Levine, A.E. (2002). Evaluation of World Wide Web-based Lessons for a First Year Dental Biochemistry Course. *Medical Education Online*, **7**, 13.

Lewis, L., Snow, K., and Farris, E. (1999). *Distance Education at Postsecondary Education Institutions*: National Center for Education Statistics, US Department of Education, Office of Educational Research and Improvement.

Lombera, S., Fine, A., Grunau, R.E., and Illes, J. (2010). Ethics in Neuroscience Graduate Training Programs: Views and Models from Canada. *Mind, Brain and Education*, **4**, 20–7.

MacCall, S.L. (2006). Online medical books: their availability and an assessment of how health sciences libraries provide access on their public Websites. *Journal of the Medical Library Association,* **94,** 75–80.

Marshall, J.G. (1992). The impact of the hospital library on clinical decision making: the Rochester study. *Bulletin of the Medical Library Association,* **80,** 169–78.

Martinez, M. (2002). Designing learning objects to personalise learning, in **D.A. Wiley** (ed.), *The Instructional Use of Learning Objects.* Bloomington, IN: Agency for Instructional Technology, Association for Educational Communications and Technology.

Massachusetts Institute of Technology OpenCourseWare Group. *2005 Program Evaluation Findings Report* (2006), MIT OpenCourseWare.

Mazmanian, P.E. and Davis, D.A. (2002). Continuing medical education and the physician as a learner: guide to the evidence. *Journal of the American Medical Association,* **288,** 1057–60.

McKimm, J., Jollie, C., and Cantillon, P. (2003). ABC of learning and teaching: Web based learning. *British Medical Journal,* **326,** 870–3.

Murphy, E., Illes, J., and Reiner, P.B. (2008). Neuroethics of neuromarketing. *Journal of Consumer Behavior,* **7,** 293–302.

Peters, R. and Sikorski, R. (1998). The AIDS Net: HIV/AIDS resources on the World Wide Web. *Journal of the American Medical Association,* **280,** 2037–8.

Phipps, R. and Merisotis, J. (1999). *What's the Difference? A Review of Contemporary Research on the Effectiveness of Distance Learning in Higher Education* (Policy report): Washington, DC: The Institute for Higher Education Policy.

Racine, E., Amaram, R., Seidler, M., Karczewska, M., and Illes, J. (2008). Media coverage of the persistent vegetative state and end-of-life decision-making. *Neurology,* **71,** 1027–32.

Richwine, M.P. and McGowan, J.J. (2001). A rural virtual health sciences library project: research findings with implications for next generation library services. *Bulletin of the Medical Library Association,* **89,** 37–44.

Rossett, A. and McDonald, J.A. (2006). Evaluating technology-enhanced continuing medical education. *Medical Education Online,* **11.**

Roskies, A. (2002). Neuroethics for the New Millennium. *Neuron,* **35,** 21–3.

Sahakian B.J. and Morein-Zamir, S. (2009). Neuroscientists need neuroethics teaching. *Science,* **325,** 147.

Sheffield, C. (2006). e-Learning Object Portals: a new resource that offers new opportunities for librarians. *Medical Reference Services Quarterly,* **25,** 65–74.

Smith, R. (2002). Online Degrees Multiply. *International Herald Tribune*

Tairyan, K. and Illes, J. (2009). Imaging genetics and the power of combined technologies: a perspective from neuroethics. *Neuroscience,* **164,** 7–15.

U.S. Department Of Education (2009). *Evaluation of Evidence-Based Practices in Online Learning: A Meta-Analysis and Review of Online Learning Studies.* Washington, DC: U.S. Department Of Education.

Wolf, S.M., Lawrenz, F.P., Nelson, C.A., *et al.* (2008). Managing incidental findings in human subjects research: analysis and recommendations. *Journal of Law, Medicine and Ethics,* **36,** 219–24.

World Health Organization. *Building Foundations for E-Health* (2006a). Available at: http://www.who.int/kms/initiatives/ehealth/en/ (accessed 19 February 2010).

World Health Organization. *The global shortage of health workers and its impact. Fact sheet.* №.302, (2006b). Available at: http://webcache.googleusercontent.com/search?q=cache:MWQ24 Udr1l8J:www.who.int/mediacentre/factsheets/fs302/en/index.html+%22Americas+versus+sub-Saharan+Africa%22&cd=1&hl=en&ct=clnk&gl=ca&source=www.google.ca (accessed 14 December 2009).

EPILOGUE

CHAPTER 52

··

NEUROETHICS AND THE LURE OF TECHNOLOGY

··

JOSEPH J. FINS

NEUROETHICS AS AN ETHICS OF TECHNOLOGY

If there is a unifying theme to neuroethics, and this anthology, it is the predominance of technology. Neuroethics is both made necessary by technology and utterly dependent upon it. Without resort to hyperbole, it could be asserted that *neuroethics is essentially an ethics of technology*.

Indeed, if a derivative neuroethics can be distinguished from "conventional" medical ethics (Fins 2008), that differentiation would hinge upon neuroethics' overwhelming preoccupation with, and reliance upon, technology. Simply stated, without the dramatic confluence of progress in the related realms of computer science, nuclear physics, electrical engineering, and pharmacology, neuroethics would never have emerged as a discipline. Neuroethics, as a domain of inquiry, was made necessary by this interdisciplinary march of technology and the resulting synergism which resulted in the development of neuroimaging, deep brain stimulation, and advanced neuropharmaceutics. Each of these developments have been borne of technological advance and become the subject of neuroethical critique.

In just a couple of decades technology has yielded tools that have altered how the mind interfaces with the brain. Through visual proxies, electrical connections, and pharmacologic manipulation, technology has enabled a connection with the brain and central nervous system, heretofore unimagined, much less imaged. What had once been the realm of science fiction, an impenetrable black box, has now come into focus through techniques which provide both structural and functional knowledge of the living brain. These insights have, in turn, led to new ways to manipulate cognitive processes, develop mind–brain interfaces and prompted deeper reflection on questions like personhood and the self.

The pace of technological advance only adds to its significance. In the 25 years since I graduated from medical school the resolution of brain images have gone from clunky black and white box-like grainy pixels to a degree of resolution on diffusion tensor imaging tractography—a type of advanced functional magnetic resonance imaging (fMRI)—that permits the visualization of single axons (Filler 2009). This is an unprecedented advance when placed into an historical context. It is not even 100 years ago that the Hopkins neurosurgeon Walter Dandy developed the ventriculogram, a way to see inside the brain by injecting air into the spinal column and identifying air–fluid–tissue interfaces on a conventional x-ray (Fox 1984). As recently as 1921, Wilder Penfield, then a novice neurosurgeon, traveled urgently to Baltimore to learn this *new technique in neuroimaging* to determine whether to operate on a young child with a deep brain tumor (Penfield 1977; Fins 2008).

It is a long way from those shadowy images to modern tractography, although the motivations of investigators over the decades have remained the same: to discern the workings of the brain. The only difference now is the power, and complexity, of the tools at the disposal of modern investigators, which—as Susan Wolf suggests—erodes the simple dichotomy between research and clinical practice upon which so much of our normative and regulatory standards are founded (Wolf 2011). The pace is now so quickened that it is increasingly difficult to draw a neat line between investigational work and therapeutics.

If we consider modern neuroradiology, we will note that it has already enabled hypotheses into the mechanisms of major depression through the work of neurologist Helen Mayberg (Mayberg *et al.* 2005). Mayberg has created a synthetic mechanistic model based on an array of neuroimaging techniques that have begun to localize the disorder to circuits converging in the subcallosal cingulate gyrus (SCG), including Brodmann area 25 (Mayberg 2003). Her structure and function correlations have been facilitated by translational neuroimaging (Mayberg 2009). More recently her hypotheses have been tested—some might say validated—by clinical trials with deep brain stimulation with targets further refined through tractography, a newer fMRI technique which can identify isolated fiber tracts (Gutman *et al.* 2009).

FROM FRANKLIN TO FUNCTIONAL ELECTRICAL STIMULATION

Closing the loop from discovery of basic mechanisms of illness to knowledge of structure and function en route to restorative therapeutics is a long way from earlier efforts to use electrical stimulation to address human maladies. All we have to do is recall Ben Franklin's very plausible musings that paralysis might be treated with an electrical current (Goodman 1931). It was a good idea that wanted for an effective technology. In a letter dated 1757 to John Pringle he writes encouragingly of the "immediate greater sensible warmth in the lame limbs" and the "prickling sensation" felt by some the night after their treatments. He laments that he never saw a permanent change and that his temporary success might have been an 18th-century placebo effect. He wondered:

> ...And how far the apparent temporary advantage might arise from the exercise of the patients' journey, and coming daily to my house, or from the spirits given by the hopes of success, enabling them to exert more strength in moving their limbs, I will not pretend to know. (Goodman 1931)

Franklin concludes by critiquing his methodology and wondering:

> Perhaps some permanent advantage might have been obtained, if the electric shocks had been accompanied with proper medicine and regimen, under the direction of a skillful

physician. It may be, too, that a few great strokes, as given in my method, may not be so proper as many small ones.... (Goodman 1931)

Franklin pursued a good hypothesis, an idea which was limited by available technology rather than by scientific creativity. Today, two and a half centuries later, we are on the cusp of realizing Franklin's therapeutic vision for paralysis. Neuroprosthetic experts, engineers Joseph Pancrazio and P. Hunter Peckham, report that the experimental use of electrical stimulation in paralysis recently has been achieved in an animal model and predict that proof of concept for functional electrical stimulation (FES) will be achieved within the next 5 years (Pancrazio and Peckham 2009).

As these remarkable examples of depression and paralysis illustrate, technology has given form to hypotheses and accomplishments which have long eluded humankind. It has made the impossible possible. It has deepened knowledge of complex biological systems and expanded diagnostic and therapeutic horizons. But as Helen Mayberg reminded me in a recent conversation, in quoting the physicist David Goldstein in his review of *Einstein's Unfinished Symphony, Listening to the Sounds of Space-Time* (Bartusiak 2000):

> The cutting edge of science is not about the completely unknown. It is found where we understand just enough to ask the right question or build the right the instrument. (Goldstein 2000)

Our progress has been through the pursuit of good questions using the right instruments. But if that progress has been made possible by new tools, it is, in an equally dramatic fashion, vulnerable to technology. Misunderstood, technology can become an object of desire to which we aspire, forgetting the pragmatic dictum of true instrumentality in which *usefulness* is the marker of a worthy tool or intervention. If we hope to realize the promise that technology might offer we also have to be cognizant of its own seductions, lest we miss opportunities that predict progress or ignore occasions which portend problems.

The promise and peril of technology

Perhaps the most challenging aspect about neuroethics is that the technology used by neuroscientists needs to be understood in order to offer responsible neuroethical critique. Regrettably, many who comment on the normative implications of the field know too little about the capabilities and limits of tools used by investigators and their relationship to the current state of scientific knowledge. Although this is not unique to neuroethics—similar challenges were commented upon by the late bioethicist, Marc Lappe, with the advent of recombinant DNA in the 1970s and the advent of molecular biology (Martin 2005)—I would maintain that the challenges posed to neuroethics by technology are on a grander scale because so many modalities have converged to give birth to this investigative and clinical endeavor. The challenge is deepened by public ignorance of, or distrust in, science and its methods (Kitchner 2010). As Alan I. Leshner observes trenchantly in his essay on neuroscience and public engagement:

> On the one hand, the purpose of science is to tell us about the nature of the natural world, whether we like the answer or not. On the other hand, only scientists are obliged to accept

scientific explanations, again whether they like them or not. The rest of the public is free to disregard or, worse, to distort scientific findings at will, and with rather limited immediate consequences. Scientific understanding is only binding on scientists. (Leshner 2011)

This relative ignorance of technology can lead to normative distortions, even errors. The first sort of error imbues technology with more capability than it actually possesses or is likely to possess in the near future. Instead of describing the crudeness of initial prototypes, laden with margins of error, the forward-looking ethicist imagines all the possibilities that *might* result from the invention. This leads to hyperbolic, almost science fiction scenarios which, in turn, are either bright and optimistic or dark and glum (Fins 2005).

Over its short academic life neuroethics has been the tale of two disciplines. One iteration sees promise while the other envisions peril. It is an overly dichotomous view of the field which persists into this handbook and which, I must admit, threatens its longevity as a mature academic field.

Neuroimaging work—as Federico, Lombera, and Illes claim as a scholarly pillar for neuroethics (Federico *et al.* 2011)—has been particularly prone to such extreme characterizations, especially those publications which depict how neuroimaging is exploring the hither lands of consciousness and disorders like the vegetative and minimally conscious states. The response to Owen *et al.*'s 2006 *Science* paper (Owen *et al.* 2006) and Monti *et al.*'s more recent *New England Journal of Medicine* paper (2010) demonstrating command-following in some minimally conscious and vegetative patients and the ability of one vegetative patient to respond to simple yes/no questions using fMRI is an example of worrisome hyperbole exemplifying a pattern of journalism noted by Racine (2011), as well as Zarzeczny and Caulfield in this volume (2011), building upon earlier work by Racine, Bar-Ilan, and Illes, and others (Racine *et al.* 2005). Although the technology is in its infancy the immediate question posed by media invested the method with far greater capabilities than it possessed: namely, whether patients could use this crude communication channel as a way to express their wishes regarding life-sustaining therapies, whether they would want to live or die (Carey 2010).

To this commentator, it seemed a bit premature to generalize the findings (Fins and Schiff 2010a). After all, of the 54 subjects studied, only five demonstrated command-following and all of these patients had traumatic and not anoxic brain injury. This phenomenological study took no account of the variance seen in which patients were responding, a seemingly key part of the puzzle before this technique is applied more broadly. The science tells us that a response is only dispositive of consciousness absent a mechanistic explication of responsiveness. Absent that deeper scientific knowledge, a failure to respond to a query could stem from a methodological error and not indicate that the patient is unconscious. A non-response could also be the result of: a failure to ask the question in a proper fashion; the patient's inattention; or even failing to wait long enough for a response. Normatively, even if the patient were to respond, would his binary answers satisfy a "sliding scale of competence" where the gravity of a patient's choice is matched by proportionate evidence of understanding and explication (Drane 1984)? Doubtful, at best, at least for now (Fins and Schiff 2010).

And yet despite these highly significant scientific and normative limitations some view neuroimaging as a powerful threat to our human nature. In these speculative scenarios the functional magnetic imager has the power to decode mental states and read minds, alter relationships, detect criminality, or pose a threat to national security (Haynes 2011; Leshner 2011).

While such speculations, *generally about non-medical applications,* are intellectually inter-esting and often elegantly Talmudic in their reasoning, the hyperbole often does not take account of the technical limits of neuroscience to read minds, as Emily Murphy and Hank Greely wisely warn us. They advise a healthy dose of humility when predicting the future, especially when it comes to decoding "the most complicated thing in the universe" (Murphy and Greely 2011).

Untempered by prudence and caution, hyperbolic predictions can create fears that under-mine legitimate uses of still nascent technology for populations in need, and as Eric Racine importantly observes, impedes credible knowledge dissemination inimical to an open and democratic society (Racine 2011). So while we should imagine future uses of still primitive devices and their possible implications, it is especially critical to distinguish the probable from the implausible, and—as Hildt and Metzinger rightly suggest—distinguish the needs of individuals from public policy and draw a line between the medical and non-medical uses of emerging technologies even if a distinction can not easily be discerned between the therapeutic and enhancement at the level of the individual (Hildt and Metzinger 2011).

Truth be told, one needs to be something of a scientific polyglot to make sense of the many developments which are taking place. This need for specialized knowledge to under-take ethical analysis suggests that we will see areas of subspecialization within neuroethics much earlier than might have been the case for other areas of ethical reflection and this vol-ume's many focused essays suggest that this process is already occurring so that responsible and informed critiques can take place.

Although this is a necessary trend, it is also regrettable because of the further fragmenta-tion that will occur as commentators focus on new developments in self-imposed silos of splendid isolation. Many insights will be lost through this process of sequestration and we must be careful to avoid too narrow a focus as we seek to balance the need to be informed about relevant scientific details while contextualizing this knowledge against a larger back-drop. From personal experience, I can attest that my own work considering the use of deep brain stimulation in disorders of consciousness was enriched by considering the history of psychosurgery and its relevance to modern neuromodulation and the application of deep brain stimulation to psychiatric disorders (Fins 2003b).

Hans Jonas and technoprudence

If we place our current tendency to hyperbole into that earlier historical context, we see that we are not alone in being vulnerable to the lure of technology. Even Hans Jonas, a philoso-pher I admire, expresses a technophobia—or better yet a *technoprudence*—written during the psychosurgery era. In "Technology and Responsibility", an essay published in 1974, he worries about longer-term consequences of "novel" technology and questions whether our traditional framework of an age-old proximate ethics can accommodate technological forces which make man—and the species—vulnerable in an unparalleled manner:

> To be sure, the old prescriptions of the "neighbor" ethics—of justice, charity, honesty, and so on—still hold in their intimate immediacy of the nearest, day by day sphere of human inter-action. But this sphere is overshadowed by a growing realm of collective action where doer,

deed, and effect are no longer the same as they were in the proximate sphere, and which by the enormity of its powers forces a new dimension of responsibility never dreamt of before. (Jonas 1980)

Although psychosurgery is not his exclusive concern, he does worry about behavior control and the rather imminent morphing of laudable medical goals into worrisome societal ones:

It is similar with all the other, quasi-utopian powers about to be made available by the advances of biomedical science as they are translated into technology. Of these, behavior control is much nearer to practical readiness that the still hypothetical prospect I have been discussing, (the prospect of prolonged, even immortal life) and the ethical question it raises are less profound but have a more direct moral bearing on the moral conception. Here again, the new kind of intervention exceeds the old ethical categories. They have not equipped us to rule, for example, on mental control by chemical means of by direct electrical action of the brain via implanted electrodes –undertaken lest us assume, for defensible even laudable ends. The mixture of beneficial and dangerous potentials is obvious, but the lines are not easy to draw. Relief of mental patients from distressing and disabling symptoms seems unequivocally beneficial. But from the relief of the patient, a goal entirely in the tradition of the medical art, there is an easy passage to the relief of society…this opens up an indefinite field with grave potentials. (Jonas 1980)

From there Jonas worries about the effect mind control for "social management" would have on "human rights and dignity." He shared the modern neuroethicist's concerns about the loss of *free will* through "circumventing the appeal of autonomous motivation," *enhancement* by inducing "learning attitudes in school children by mass administration of drugs" and "performance increase" at work, and the generation of "sensations of happiness or pleasure or at least contentment…independent, that is, of the objects of happiness, pleasure or content and their attainment in personal living and achieving." (Jonas 1980).

It is a remarkable passage for its resonance with the preceding pages of this volume. But was Jonas a sage or a hysteric? Despite Harris's claim for the social utility of pharmaceutical enhancements (Harris 2011), I am with Jonas and share his concern about children receiving pharmaceutical enhancement with drugs like Ritalin® (methylphenidate). Along with others, I endorse advocacy for non-pharmacological efforts at "enhancement" such as proper education and exercise (Morein-Zamir and Sahakian 2011).

Having said that, I also worry about the therapeutic index that might exist between the treatment of some neuropsychiatric disorders with deep brain stimulation and the induction of addiction—in some but not all putative targets (Synofzik *et al.* under review). While the use of deep brain stimulation in depression remains investigational, the concerns raised by Kringelbach and Berridge in their essay about happiness (2011), reminds us that we need a systems approach to neurobiology to understand affect and reward, as Suhler and Churchland indicate (2011), as well as addiction, as Reske and Paulus suggest (2011), and that functional networks are interrelated, sometimes presenting a fine line between benefit and burden (Morein-Zamir and Sahakian 2011).

Yet, despite Jonas' prescience on the aforementioned points, it must be said that most of his ruminations, written with such urgency, *have yet to come to pass*. In fact, contemporaneous allegations of mind control applied to vulnerable members of our citizenry via psychosurgery during that time was debunked by scholarly reports from The Hastings Center and the National Commission just a few years after Jonas published his essay (Blatte 1974; The National Commission 1977; Fins 2003b).

Perhaps more to the point, in contrast to Jonas' concerns about the circumvention of autonomy with manipulation of the brain, psychosurgery's modern successor—deep brain stimulation—has actually helped to restore a degree of personal agency in minimally conscious subject. My colleagues and I have recounted how a severely injured individual whose highest level of interaction was inconsistent command-following via eye movements prior to stimulation regained the ability to voice preferences at the level of assent (Schiff *et al.* 2007, 2009).

Similarly, in this volume, legal scholar Stacey Tovino has argued that additional knowledge of neurobiological differences between the sexes constitutes not a threat to women's rights but rather might afford additional protections in criminal law and civil procedure although she cautions that there might be correlative implications that warrant concern and dictates prudence against precipitous application in law and society (Tovino 2011). Joshua Greene and Jonathan Cohen also indicate that while neuroscience will change the law, it will not do so by altering current legal assumptions (Greene and Cohen 2011).

These examples, taken together, suggest that Jonas' pessimism may not have been warranted and that while we should heed Jonas' precautionary principle, a point made by Steve Hyman in his essay on the neurobiology of addiction and its implications for voluntary control of behavior. Hyman tempers the tendency towards viewing addiction as beyond individual control. He urges that we neither revamp our legal nor normative structures about responsibility and culpability based on interim data and adds that a proportionate dose of moral outrage and punishment for drug-related activity is warranted, if it is a deterrent (Hyman 2011).

Prudence is further warranted because the outcome that we should fear may be the exact *opposite* of the one Jonas predicted. Jonas was concerned about the loss of free will and the circumvention of autonomy through enhancement efforts. The more likely scenario, as elegantly argued by Chneiweiss is a hyperautonomous enhanced brain bound up in itself and disconnected from the constraints imposed by society (Chneiweiss 2011). Such an outcome, a sort of *Civilization and its Malcontents*—to remind us of Freud's counter example of the repressions imposed by society upon the individual (Freud 1961)—is something to be heeded and far better understood, lest we create a class of sociopaths who know only their own self-imposed limits on normative behavior (Stout 2005).

Chneiweiss's argument is reinforced, in my view, by Wexler who correctly observes that humans are social and historical creatures and that our capabilities, desires, and proclivities develop through a complex interaction between our neurobiology and the natural and built environment (Wexler 2011). To limit these interactions through enhancement of the self at the expense of one contextualized within community, would as Chneiweiss warns us lead to:

> The risk is creating isolated super-brains lost within a self-centered, self-organized, virtual world wherein the absence of the eyes of the other blurs the fundamental meaning of "telling the truth" on oneself. (Chneiweiss 2011)

This is a critical point echoed as well by Haggard in his essay on the societal constraints placed on free will (Haggard 2011) and by Reiner in his essay on the limits of "neuroessentialism" (Reiner 2011). Taken together, these essays suggest that whatever our intrinsic neurobiology, our brains—if not our very selves—are social entities that must and need to take account of societal and normative externalities. They also demonstrate that the landscape of speculative ethical commentary since Jonas has shifted from fears about mind control and the loss of autonomy or free will through manipulation of the brain to worries about an overly atomistic self disconnected from societal correctives, clues and constraints through technological or pharmacological intervention in the brain.

While it is too early to know what will come to pass, the shifting debate over agency and free will in the decades since Jonas point out that wise commentators may in fact be wrong and that ill-informed prudence or excessive hype comes at a cost.

NEUROETHICS AND POLITICAL ECONOMY

The cost of these normative errors is amplified by the economics of the technologies which have led to neuroethical critique. If we misconstrue these technologies we might find that they are perceived as neither affordable nor worth the investment.

The technocentricity of neuroscience makes it especially vulnerable to broader market forces and the sway of political economy, all of which might be exacerbated by the recent fiscal melt down and recent trends in healthcare reform. Because of endowment losses amongst universities and philanthropies (of over 20% for leading research universities) (Lewis 2010) and dollar cost averaging in payouts, there is less philanthropic money in the system to support—or even sustain—research programs. Government support in developing countries is essentially flat. The passage of healthcare reform in the United States, which laudably enfranchises millions who have been uninsured, consciously does so through parsimonious entitlements, which for patients with historically marginalized and high-cost neuropsychiatric disorders, raise the question, "access to what?"

My concern is that the high costs of such interventions will become a new excuse to neglect another generation of patients with neuropsychiatric disorders (Fins 2003a) whose hope and vulnerability lie in the promise and expense of technologies upon which they may vitally depend.

These challenges are illustrated by our investigational work exploring the use of deep brain stimulation in the minimally conscious state (Schiff et al. 2007). Despite the preliminary nature of this study, (Schiff et al. 2009) whenever I discuss it in public, I am invariably asked about its cost as if this emergent response to disorders of consciousness were somehow responsible for creating a market for new expenditures. Closer reflection on the putative cost–benefit analysis of this intervention, again should it be deemed therapeutic, might reveal that neuromodulation might actually cut into fixed costs associated with the chronic sequelae of severe head injury and associated chronic care costs (Fins 2010a).

The problem here, it seems to me, might be one of unrealized expectations. Although the response to our work was laudatory, the hype with which it was greeted—despite our effort to be understated with our claims (Schiff et al. 2007)—led invariably to a critique which asked if whatever good was achieved was good enough to warrant ongoing support. Like most innovations, our efforts were a step forward, not a leap across the finish line, notwithstanding how it might have been portrayed. Instead, it was, what the late physician-scientist Lewis Thomas called a "half-way technology" (Thomas 1974; Schiff et al. 2009). Dr. Thomas' description is apt because it is a preventive against hyperbole which mischaracterizes incremental progress as a final product, a distinction which needs to be carefully delineated when considering distributive justice questions.

This question of access is perhaps most compelling when we consider the emergent use of neuroimaging methods as communication tools. This work's potential is epitomized by Monti's recent proof of principle using fMRI as a communication paradigm in patients with disorders of consciousness. Suppose this ability to query those with disorders of consciousness evolves beyond the binary capabilities of yes/no responses and becomes a link for those who have heretofore been beyond our shared community of communication? Imagine a tool that can pierce the isolation of those who are conscious but can not speak, *but whose voices can now be heard through a prosthetic intermediary* (Fins and Schiff 2010a)? What price can be placed upon this capability, which might be viewed more as a basic civil right than as an entitlement (Fins 2011)?

And even as we worry about a lack of access to innovation and care, we need to be concerned about the influence of corporate interests and intellectual property law on the use of these technologies (Fins 2010b; Fins and Schiff 2010b). Such market forces can lead to the premature or inappropriate dissemination of new technologies as vetted diagnostic or therapeutic tools when they have yet to be fully evaluated for efficacy. An example of the former would be the use of investigational neuroimaging techniques in clinical practice at this juncture outside of a clinical research context prepared to interpret and generalize results (Fins *et al.* 2008).

An example of the latter is the corporate branding of investigational applications of devices as therapeutic when they have not been fully vetted in a clinical trial. An example of such behavior is the marketing of deep brain stimulation for the "treatment" of obsessive-compulsive disorder by one manufacturer when the actual FDA approval under which that advertising campaign is occurring is a Humanitarian Device Exemption (HDE) (US FDA 2009). This is in lieu of the more costly and extensive vetting that would occur through an Investigational Device Exemption under which a proper clinical trial would have been conducted to demonstrate safety and efficacy (Fins *et al.* under review).

Conclusion

The fundamental mind–brain question, raised here by Beauregard (2011) and Levy (2011)—and by Wilder Penfield (Fins 2008) posthumously in *The Mystery of The Mind* (Penfield 1978; Lipsman and Bernstein 2011)—remind us to be cautious with claims about our current state of knowledge. Despite all our stunning progress in the past decade, we remain relatively ignorant. Although we have progressed, we need to avoid hubris and remain humble about our mastery of neuroscience and the ability to predict the interplay of technology and society.

Future generations will view our prized technologies as crude and our hypotheses as naïve. They will likely view our neuroimaging efforts as reductionistic post-phrenological—or better yet *phenomenological* flares—which distracted us from important questions in systems neurobiology. They will supply an explication of how deep brain stimulation actually works, a question that Lipsman and Bernstein reminds us remains unknown (2011). And in answering these questions, they generate many others of more complexity and challenge.

Each generation will have its own questions to answer and be tempted by the lure of its technology. The key for us and our successors is to be wary of technology's sway and recall

C.P. Snow's admonition decades ago: "Technology, remember, is a queer thing; it brings you great gifts with one hand, and it stabs you in the back with the other." (Lewis 1971). What was prescient then remains timely now.

ACKNOWLEDGEMENTS

Dr. Fins gratefully acknowledges funding from an Investigator Award in Health Policy Research from the Robert Wood Johnson Foundation, The Buster Foundation, and additional support from the NIH Clinical & Translational Science Center UL1-RR024966 Weill Cornell Medical College Research Ethics Core.

DISCLOSURES

IntElect Medical, Inc. provided partial support for the deep brain stimulation in the minimally conscious state clinical trial described and considered in this paper and the author was an unfunded coinvestigator.

REFERENCES

Bartusiak, M. (2000). *Einstein's Unfinished Symphony, Listening to the Sounds of Space-Time.* Washington, DC: Joseph Henry Press.

Beauregard, M. (2011). Neural foundations to conscious and volitional control of emotional behavior: a mentalistic perspective. In J. Illes and B.J. Sahakian (eds.) *Oxford Handbook of Neuroethics*, pp.83–100. Oxford: Oxford University Press.

Blatte, H. (1974). State prisons and the use of behavior control. *The Hastings Center Report*, **4**, 11.

Carey, B. (2010). *Trace of thought is found in "vegetative" patient.* Available at: http://www.nytimes.com/2010/02/04/health/04brain.html (accessed 4 February 2010).

Chneiweiss, H. (2011). Does cognitive enhancement fit with the physiology of our cognition? In J. Illes and B.J. Sahakian (eds.) *Oxford Handbook of Neuroethics*, pp.295–308. Oxford: Oxford University Press.

Drane, J. (1984). Competency to give an informed consent. A model for making clinical assessments. *Journal of the American Medical Association*, **252**, 925–7.

Federico, C.A., Lombera, S., and Illes, J. (2011). Intersecting complexities in neuroimaging and neuroethics. In J. Illes and B.J. Sahakian (eds.) *Oxford Handbook of Neuroethics*, pp.377–388. Oxford: Oxford University Press.

Fins, J.J. (2003a). Constructing an ethical stereotaxy for severe brain injury: balancing risks, benefits and access. *Nature Reviews Neuroscience*, **4**, 323–7.

Fins, J.J. (2003b). From psychosurgery to neuromodulation and palliation: history's lessons for the ethical conduct and regulation of neuropsychiatric research. *Neurosurgery Clinics of North America*, **14**, 303–19.

Fins, J.J. (2005). The Orwellian threat to emerging neurodiagnostic technologies. *American Journal of Bioethics*, **5**, 56–8.

Fins, J.J. (2008). A leg to stand on: Sir William Osler and Wilder Penfield's "neuroethics." *American Journal of Bioethics*, **8**, 37–46.

Fins, J.J. (2010a) Deep brain stimulation: Calculating the true costs of surgical innovation. *Virtual Mentor*, **12**, 114–18. Available at: http://virtualmentor.ama-assn.org/2010/02/msoc1-1002.html

Fins, J.J. (2010b). Deep brain stimulation, free markets and the scientific commons: is it time to revisit the Bayh-Dole Act of 1980? *Neuromodulation: Technology at the Neural Interface*, **13**, 153–9.

Fins, J.J. (2011). Minds apart: severe brain injury, citizenship, and civil rights. In M. Freeman (ed.) (Volume 13), *University College of London Faculty of Laws' Law and Neuroscience – Current Legal Issues*. Oxford: Oxford University Press.

Fins, J.J. and Schiff, N.D. (2010a). In the blink of the mind's eye. *The Hastings Center Report*, **3**, 21–3.

Fins, J.J. and Schiff, N.D. (2010b). Conflicts of interest in deep brain stimulation research and the ethics of transparency. *Journal of Clinical Ethics*, **2**, 125–32.

Fins, J.J., Illes, J., Bernat, J.L., Hirsch, J., Laureys, S., Murphy, E., and Participants of the Working Meeting on Ethics. (2008). Neuroimaging and limited states of consciousness. Neuroimaging and disorders of consciousness: envisioning an ethical research agenda. *American Journal of Bioethics*, **8**, 3–12.

Fins, J.J., Mayberg, H.S., Nuttin, B., *et al.* (Under review). Neuropsychiatric Deep Brain Stimulation Research and the Misuse of the Humanitarian Device Exemption.

Filler, A. (2009). Magnetic resonance neurography and diffusion tensor imaging: origins, history, and clinical impact of the first 50,000 cases with an assessment of efficacy and utility in a prospective 5000-patient study group. *Neurosurgery*, **65**, A29–43.

Fox, W.L. (1984). *Dandy of Johns Hopkins*. Philadelphia: Williams & Wilkins.

Freud, S. (1961). *Civilization and its Discontents*. New York: W.W. Norton.

Goldstein, D. (October 29, 2000). Sounds of gravity, an account of the project to detect and measure gravitational waves. *The New York Times*.

Goodman N.G. (ed.) (1931). *The Ingenious Dr. Franklin: Selected Scientific Letters of Benjamin Franklin*. Philadelphia: University of Pennsylvania Press.

Greene, J. and Cohen, J. (2011). For the law, neuroscience changes nothing and everything. In J. Illes and B.J. Sahakian (eds.) *Oxford Handbook of Neuroethics*, pp.655–674. Oxford: Oxford University Press.

Gutman, D.A., Holzheimer, P.E., Behrens, T.S., Johansen-Berg, H., and Mayberg, H.S. (2009). A tractography analysis of two deep brain stimulation white matter targets for depression. *Biological Psychiatry*, **65**, 276–82.

Haggard, P. (2011). Neuroethics of free will. In J. Illes and B.J. Sahakian (eds.) *Oxford Handbook of Neuroethics*, pp.219–226. Oxford: Oxford University Press.

Harris, J. (2011). Chemical cognitive enhancement: is it unfair, unjust, discriminatory or cheating for healthy adults to use smart drugs? In J. Illes and B.J. Sahakian (eds.) *Oxford Handbook of Neuroethics*, pp.265–284. Oxford: Oxford University Press.

Haynes, J.D. (2011). Brain reading: decoding mental states from brain activity in humans. In J. Illes and B.J. Sahakian (eds.) *Oxford Handbook of Neuroethics*, pp.3–14. Oxford: Oxford University Press.

Hildt, E. and Metzinger, T. (2011). Cognitive enhancement. In J. Illes and B.J. Sahakian (eds.) *Oxford Handbook of Neuroethics*, pp.245–264. Oxford: Oxford University Press.

Hyman, S.E. (2011). The neurobiology of addiction: implications for voluntary control of behaviour. In J. Illes and B.J. Sahakian (eds.) *Oxford Handbook of Neuroethics*, pp.203–218. Oxford: Oxford University Press.

Jonas, H. (1974, 1980). Technology and responsibility. In *Philosophical essays: from ancient creed to technological man*, pp. 3–20. Chicago, IL: The University of Chicago Press.

Kitchner, P. (2010). Two forms of blindness: on the need for both cultures. *Technology in Science*, **32**, 40–8.

Kringelbach, M.L. and Berridge, K.C. (2011). The neurobiology of pleasure and happiness. In J. Illes and B.J. Sahakian (eds.) *Oxford Handbook of Neuroethics*, pp.15–32. Oxford: Oxford University Press.

Leshner, A.I. (2011). Bridging neuroscience and society: Research, education and broad public engagement. In J. Illes and B.J. Sahakian (eds.) *Oxford Handbook of Neuroethics*, pp.v–xii. Oxford: Oxford University Press.

Lewis, A. (1971). Dear Scoop Jackson. *The New York Times*. Available at: http://select.nytimes.com/mem/archive/pdf?res=F30A11F73454127B93C7A81788D85F458785F9 (accessed 15 March 2010).

Lewis, T. (2010). Investment losses cause steep dip in university endowments, study finds. *The New York Times*. Available at: http://www.nytimes.com/2010/01/28/education/28endow.html (accessed 28 January 2010).

Levy, N. (2011). Neuroethics and the extended mind. In J. Illes and B.J. Sahakian (eds.) *Oxford Handbook of Neuroethics*, pp.285–294. Oxford: Oxford University Press.

Lipsman, N. and Bernstein, M. (2011). Ethical issues in functional neurosurgery: Emerging applications and controversies. In J. Illes and B.J. Sahakian (eds.) *Oxford Handbook of Neuroethics*, pp.405–416. Oxford: Oxford University Press.

Martin, D. (2005). Marc Lappé, 62, dies; fought against chemical perils. *The New York Times*. Available at: http://www.nytimes.com/2005/05/21/national/21lappe.html (accessed 21 May 2010).

Mayberg, H.S. (2003). Positron emission tomography imaging in depression: a neural systems perspective. *Neuroimaging Clinics of North America*, **13**, 805–15.

Mayberg H.S. (2009). Targeted electrode-based modulation of neural circuits for depression. *Journal of Clinical Investigation*, **119**, 717–25.

Mayberg, H.S., Lozano, A.M., Voon, V., *et al.* (2005). Deep brain stimulation for treatment-resistant depression. *Neuron*, **45**, 651–60.

Monti, M.M., Vanhaudenhuyse, A., Coleman, M.R., *et al.* (2010). Willful modulation of brain activity in disorders of consciousness. *New England Journal of Medicine*, **362**, 579–89.

Morein-Zamir, S. and Sahakian, B.J. (2011). Pharmaceutical cognitive enhancement. In J. Illes and B.J. Sahakian (eds.) *Oxford Handbook of Neuroethics*, pp.229–244. Oxford: Oxford University Press.

Murphy, E.R. and Greely, H.T. (2011). What will be the limits of neuroscience-based mind-reading in the law? In J. Illes and B.J. Sahakian (eds.) *Oxford Handbook of Neuroethics*, pp.635–654. Oxford: Oxford University Press.

Owen, A.M., Coleman, M.R., Boly, M., Davis, M.H., Laureys, S., and Pickard, J.D. (2006). Detecting awareness in the vegetative state. *Science*, **313**, 1402.

Pancrazio, J.J. and Peckham, P.H. (2009). Neuroprosthetic devices: how far are we from recovering movement in paralyzed patients? *Expert Reviews in Neurotherapeutics*, **4**, 427–30.

Penfield, W. (1977). *No Man Alone: A Neurosurgeon's Life*. Boston, MA: Little, Brown and Company.

Penfield W. (1978). *Mystery of the Mind*. Princeton, NJ: Princeton University Press.

Racine, E. (2011). Neuroscience and the media: ethical challenges and opportunities. In J. Illes and B.J. Sahakian (eds.) *Oxford Handbook of Neuroethics*, pp.783–802. Oxford: Oxford University Press.

Racine, E., Bar-Ilan, O., and Illes, J. (2005). fMRI in the public eye. *Nature Reviews Neuroscience*, 6, 159-64.

Reiner, P.B. (2011). The rise of neuroessentialism. In J. Illes and B.J. Sahakian (eds.) *Oxford Handbook of Neuroethics*, pp.161–176. Oxford: Oxford University Press.

Reske, M. and Paulus, M.P. (2011). A neuroscientific approach to addiction: ethical concerns. In J. Illes and B.J. Sahakian (eds.) *Oxford Handbook of Neuroethics*, pp.177–202. Oxford: Oxford University Press.

Schiff, N.D., Giacino, J.T., Kalmar, K., *et al.* (2007). Behavioral improvements with thalamic stimulation after severe traumatic brain injury. *Nature*, 448, 600–3.

Schiff, N.D., Giacino, J.T., and Fins, J.J. (2009). Deep brain stimulation, neuroethics and the minimally conscious state: moving beyond proof of principle. *Archives of Neurology*, 66, 697–702.

Stout, M. (2005). *The Sociopath Next Door*. New York: Broadway Books.

Suhler, C. and Churchland, P. (2011). The neurobiological basis of morality. In J. Illes and B.J. Sahakian (eds.) *Oxford Handbook of Neuroethics*, pp.33–58. Oxford: Oxford University Press.

Synofzik, M., Sclaepfer, T.E., and Fins, J.J. (Under Review). How happy is happy enough? Euphoria, neuroethics and deep brain stimulation of the Nucleus Accumbens.

The National Commission for the Protection of Human Subjects of Biomedical and Behavioral Research (May 23, 1977). Use of psychosurgery in practice and research: report and recommendations of national commission for the protection of human subjects of biomedical and behavioral research. *Federal Register*, 23, 26318–32.

Thomas, L. (1974). *The Lives of a Cell: Notes of a Biology Watcher*. New York: The Viking Press.

Tovino, S.A. (2011). Women's neuroethics. In J. Illes and B.J. Sahakian (eds.) *Oxford Handbook of Neuroethics*, pp.701–714. Oxford: Oxford University Press.

US FDA (2009). Approval Order H05003. Letter to Patrick L. Johnson, Medtronic Neuromodulation from Donna-Bea Tillman, Ph.D, M.P.A., Director, Office of Device Evaluation, Center for Devices and Radiologic Health, FDA.

Wexler, B.E. (2011). Neuroplasticity, culture and society. In J. Illes and B.J. Sahakian (eds.) *Oxford Handbook of Neuroethics*, pp.743–760. Oxford: Oxford University Press.

Wolf, S.M. (2011). Incidental findings in neuroscience research: A fundamental challenge to the structure of bioethics and health law. In J. Illes and B.J. Sahakian (eds.) *Oxford Handbook of Neuroethics*, pp.623–634. Oxford: Oxford University Press.

Zarzeczny, A. and Caulfield, T. (2011). Public representations of neurogenetics. In J. Illes and B.J. Sahakian (eds.) *Oxford Handbook of Neuroethics*, pp.715–728. Oxford: Oxford University Press.

Subject Index

AUTHOR INDEX